Urologic Pathology

Robert O. Petersen, M.D., Ph.D.

Department of Pathology
Fox Chase Medical Center
Jeanes Hospital
American Oncologic Hospital
Philadelphia, Pennsylvania

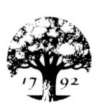

J. B. Lippincott Company
Philadelphia
London   Mexico City   New York   St. Louis   São Paulo   Sydney

Urologic Pathology

Acquisitions Editor: Lisa A. Biello
Sponsoring Editor: Sanford Robinson
Manuscript Editor: Virginia M. Barishek
Indexer: Julia Schwager
Design Director: Tracy Baldwin
Production Supervisor: Kathleen Dunn
Production Coordinator: George V. Gordon
Compositor: Progressive Typographers
Printer/Binder: Halliday Lithograph

6 5 4 3 2 1

Library of Congress Cataloging-in-Publication Data

Petersen, Robert O.
    Urologic pathology

    Includes bibliographies and index.
    1. Genito-urinary organs—Diseases. I. Title.
[DNLM: 1. Genitalia, Male—pathology. 2. Urinary
Tract—pathology. 3. Urologic Diseases—pathology.
WJ 100 P484u]
RC873.9.P47   1986   616.6   85-23247
ISBN 0-397-50626-0

The author and publisher have exerted every effort to ensure that drug selection and
dosage set forth in this text are in accord with current recommendations and practice
at the time of publication. However, in view of ongoing research, changes in govern-
ment regulations, and the constant flow of information relating to drug therapy and
drug reactions, the reader is urged to check the package insert for each drug for any
change in indications and dosage and for added warnings and precautions. This is
particularly important when the recommended agent is a new or infrequently employed
drug.

This book is dedicated to:

my wife, Olga, whose encouragement and unfailing support transformed a dream into a book

my children, Kim and Chris, for their patience

my parents, who made my medical education possible

my teachers, from whom I continue to learn

> *A. M. Jensen, M.D.*
> *Aaron Learner, M.D.*
> *Renato Baserga, M.D.*
> *Benjamin Castleman, M.D.*
> *Robert E. Scully, M.D.*
> *Wallace H. Clark, Jr. M.D.*
> *Paul B. Putong, M.D.*
> *Yung H. Kim, M.D.*

Contributors

Arnold C. Friedman, M.D.

*Department of Diagnostic Imaging
Temple University Medical Center
Philadelphia, Pennsylvania*

Paul D. Radecki, M.D.

*Department of Diagnostic Imaging
Temple University Medical Center
Philadelphia, Pennsylvania*

Francis J. Shea, M.D.

*Department of Diagnostic Imaging
Temple University Medical Center
Philadelphia, Pennsylvania*

Barry S. Stein, M.D.

*Department of Urology
Brown University Medical Center
Rhode Island Hospital
Providence, Rhode Island*

Preface

The advances in urologic pathology occurring in recent years have no equal in any comparable period of time. Significant advances in our understanding of the etiology, pathogenesis, pathology, and natural history of many diseases of the urinary tract and male genital system have been recorded. The introduction and application of technical advances including histochemical staining, immunoperoxidase staining with tumor markers, and diagnostic electron microscopy have greatly increased the diagnostic armamentarium of the surgical pathologist interested in disorders of the urogenital system. These advances are of such a fundamental nature that the classification of urogenital disorders has undergone significant revision in recent years. The very language used in discussing many of these disorders has changed. Not only have numerous new diseases been described, but previously described disorders are identified with new terminology.

The scope of these advances has created a major challenge for both the urologist and the surgical pathologist. Although monographs dealing with the pathology of disorders of individual organs of the urinary tract and the male genital system are currently available, I am unaware of any standard textbook published since 1952 that deals with the entire field of urologic pathology.* The major advances noted above have been the product of studies during the subsequent years and in particular during the 1970s. Currently, awareness of these advances, by necessity, requires referral to available monographs, chapters in textbooks of surgical pathology, and the increasing volume of journal articles.

This book is written in an attempt to synthesize these new advances and thereby update the established body of knowledge in urologic pathology. Although it reflects the viewpoint of a surgical pathologist, this book is intended for use by all those interested in the pathologic basis of urogenital disorders, including surgical pathologists, urologists, oncologists, and all those in the training

---

* Herbut, PA: In *Urologic Pathology*. Philadelphia, Lea & Febiger, 1952

programs of these medical specialties. The practical significance of these recent advances can be realized only through a close working relationship of the surgical pathologist and his clinical colleagues. With the application of these advances, the potential contribution of the surgical pathologist to quality patient care is unprecedented.

The book is presented in 11 chapters. The first five chapters are devoted to the organs of the urinary tract including kidney, renal pelvis, ureter, urinary bladder, and urethra. Chapters 6 through 10 discuss the pathology of the male genital organs including testis, testicular adnexa, prostate, penis, and scrotum. Disorders of the adrenal gland are presented in Chapter 11. Each chapter is introduced with a review of embryologic development, normal structure, and age-related changes, with particular emphasis on their histogenetic and topographical relationship to diseases of the respective organ. The diseases of each organ are organized in the traditional manner with non-neoplastic disorders (congenital, inflammatory, vascular, and proliferative diseases) followed by presentations of primary and metastatic neoplastic lesions.

Each section devoted to a disease process (*i.e.,* congenital, inflammatory, neoplastic) is introduced by a classification of the specific disease entities accompanied by a discussion of the histogenetic and pathologic basis for the classification. The current terminology of disease classification is emphasized.

With the exclusion of those renal diseases treated by nephrologists (*i.e.,* glomerulopathies and systemic vascular diseases with renal involvement), I have attempted to include all diseases traditionally within the spectrum of disorders treated by urologists. Within the scope of urologic pathology, I intended for the book to be comprehensive in both the total number of diseases discussed and the depth of the discussion of each disorder. The epidemiology, etiology, and histogenesis of each disorder is reviewed. The gross and microscopic features of the typical lesion and variants are discussed and illustrated in over 300 photographs. Where appropriate, I have contrasted the most important diagnostic features with those characteristics of other lesions in consideration of the differential diagnosis. When of diagnostic value, photomicrographs of special staining techniques, including histochemical and immunoperoxidase stains, as well as electron micrographs are included. Finally, discussions of the clinical–pathologic aspects of the natural history of each disease, including results and complications of therapy, unusual clinical presentations, local and distant dissemination, and where applicable, the findings reported in autopsy studies are included.

Special emphasis has been given to recent developments dealing with the embryology of the kidney, testis, and prostate, with reference to disorders of these organs ranging from cysts to neoplasms; the early morphologic changes in cryptorchidism; the etiology, pathogenesis, and natural history of urinary tract infections including xanthogranulomatous pyelonephritis and malakoplakia; the biologic significance of metaplastic and dysplastic changes of the urothelium and their relationship to urothelial neoplasia; and the current staging and grading protocols of all urogenital malignancies.

The illustrations derive primarily from cases studied in the Departments of Pathology of Temple University Hospital, Fox Chase Medical Center, and St. Christopher's Hospital for Children in Philadelphia. The text reflects a synthesis of 4300 references from the appropriate urology and pathology literature of the last eight decades, and my studies and personal experience of the last decade. During this time I have been the beneficiary of a close and productive working relationship with the Departments of Urology and Radiology at Temple University Hospital, Jeanes Hospital, and American Oncologic Hospital in Philadelphia. The book fundamentally reflects the perspective of a surgical pathologist, but the influence of my clinical colleagues is present throughout.

The preparation of this book is the result of the cumulative contributions of many, to whom I express my gratitude. The entire manuscript was typed with critical review and comments by my wife, Olga, to whom I am also indebted for countless hours of assistance in the many medical libraries in Philadelphia and with the task of translating hundreds of articles from foreign journals. We shared the journey to completion of this book.

To the four contributors of this textbook, Drs. Stein, Shea, Radecki, and Friedman, I express my gratitude for their added perspective afforded this textbook. Their additional dimension will be of future benefit to all pathologists approaching diagnostic problems in urologic pathology.

I express my gratitude to Otto Lehman and Ski Scarano whose expert photographic developing assistance is demonstrated throughout the book.

Contribution of pathologic material was graciously provided by many to whom I express my gratitude and acknowledgment including: A. Bernard Ackerman, M.D., New York; Arthur Aufderheide, M.D., Duluth; J. Bruce Beckwith, M.D., Denver; Norman Coopersmith, M.D., Trenton; Ian D. Craig, M.D., London, Ontario; Richard Estensen, M.D., St.Paul; Dale Huff, M.D., Philadelphia; Frank B. Johnson, M.D., Washington, D.C.; Yung Kim, M.D., Trenton; Anand Lattanand, M.D., Philadelphia; Michael T. Mazur, M.D., Birmingham; John W. Roberts, M.D., Berkeley; Livia Ross, M.D., Oakland; Robert E. Scully, M.D., Boston; Joseph Sherrick, M.D., Chicago; Harvey Slater, M.D., Pittsburgh; John K. Wyatt, M.D., London, Ontario; Charles Yang, FRACP, Melbourne; Nayere Zaeri, M.D., Philadelphia.

To Ivan Damjanov, M.D., Donald F. Gleason, M.D., Wayne Johnson, M.D., and Edith Potter, M.D., I express my gratitude for major contributions of photographic material utilized in this book.

Finally, I wish to express my gratitude for the support and patience provided by the publishers, J. B. Lippincott Company. The greatest tribulations of publishers wrought by first time authors were graciously endured by Lisa Biello, Sanford Robinson, and Virginia Barishek. I will be forever in their debt for their guidance and patience.

Robert O. Petersen, M.D., Ph.D.

Contents

Urologic Pathology

Kidney

1

Normal Kidney

Embryologic Development

The kidney in the newborn is embryologically the final kidney in a series of three that develop during gestation, its two predecessors having sequentially regressed in the events leading to the development of the final kidney.[5,8,12]

The first excretory system is the pronephros, which develops from dorsal specialized mesenchyme at about 3 weeks' gestation. The paired solid cord forms caudally, gradually develops a lumen, and enters the cloaca. The pronephric kidney consists of tubules (pronephric tubules) that develop laterally from the pronephric duct. The pronephric kidney never attains functional capacity, but rather evidences regression at the cephalad end even as the most caudal pronephric tubules are forming.

The second excretory system, the mesonephric (or wolffian) system, begins development during the fourth gestational week. Solid cords, which soon demonstrate a lumen, develop from the specialized mesenchyme (nephrostome). The mesonephric duct courses dorsolaterally and connects with the pronephric duct, the most cephalad portion of which has regressed. The pronephric duct is now called the mesonephric or wolffian duct. Branches of the abdominal aorta grow laterally to connect with the most proximal ends of the mesonephric tubules, forming a glomerulus structure. It is unsettled whether the mesonephric kidney functions, albeit transiently, in the human embryo.

The subsequent function of the mesonephric duct, exclusive of its role in the urinary tract, occurs only in the male. In the female the duct regresses, but it can be found as vestigial rudimentary tubules in the ovarian hilum, walls of the fallopian tubes, and uterus as paroophoron, hydatids of Morgagni, and Gartner's ducts. This association with the female gonadal structures is the result of the close proximity of the mesonephric duct to the precursors of the genital organs. In the male the mesonephric duct, in the proximity of the gonad (future testis), develops as the efferent ductules of the epididymis. Vestigial terminal ends of the mesonephric duct are also observed as appendices of epididymis (see Chap. 7).

The final kidney, the metanephric kidney, takes origin at the caudal end of the mesonephric duct, just proximal to the duct's ostium in the cloaca. In the fifth gestational week the metanephric diverticulum, or ureteric bud, develops and grows in a dorsocephalad direction into a specialized mesenchyme, the metanephric mesoderm, which forms a cap on the advancing ureteric bud. Both migrate in a cephalad direction to arrive ultimately at the position of the normal kidneys. These events occur bilaterally to result in the paired metanephric or final kidneys.

The advancing end (the ampulla) of the ureteric bud undergoes dichotomous branching within the metanephric blastema with corresponding segmentation of the latter around the clusters of metanephric duct branches. By sequential generations of branches, the renal pelvis, major and minor calyces, and terminal collecting ducts are formed (Fig. 1-1).[5,8,12] Nephrons begin to form within the metanephric blastema; these are initially observed as oval condensations of blastemal cells in the vicinity of the terminal collecting duct ampulla. This mass of blastemal cells forms cords that develop a lumen, and these nephrons subsequently make connections with the collecting duct. Osathanondh and Potter describe four stages of growth of the collecting ducts (Figs 1-2 to 1-4).[6,8] During stage 1, there is active branching of the collecting ducts. In stage 2, there is reduction of tubule branching and attachment of the nephrons to the collecting tubules in arcades. In stage 3, branching stops, but nephrons continue

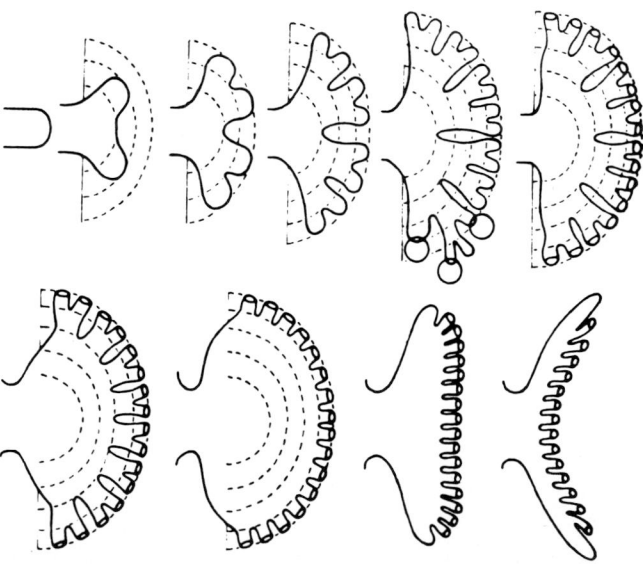

Figure 1-1   *Embryologic development of minor calyx of kidney.*
Sequential branching and intrapyramid growth of the terminal collecting tubules results in the configuration of the minor calyx. (Potter EL: Normal and Abnormal Development of the Kidney. Copyright © 1972 by Year Book Medical Publishers, Inc, Chicago. Used by permission.)

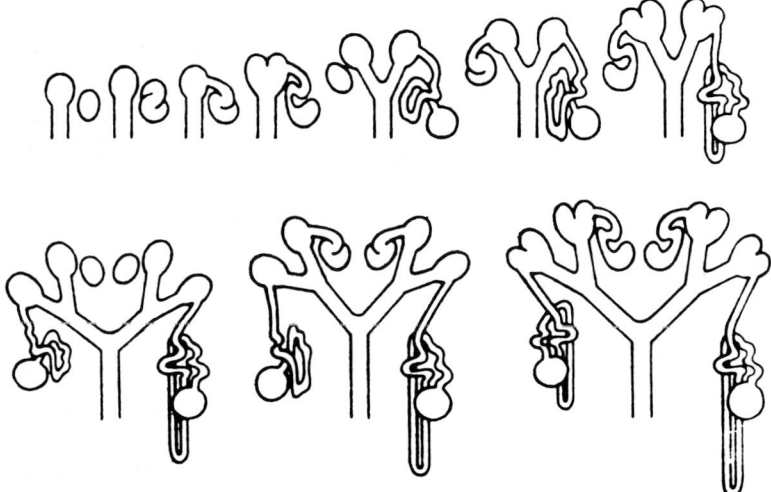

Figure 1-2 *Embryologic development of nephron and terminal collecting tubules, period 1. During period 1 there is active growth of the terminal collecting tubule and ampullary branching. Developing nephrons attach to the ampullae. (Potter EL: Normal and Abnormal Development of the Kidney. Copyright © 1972 by Year Book Medical Publishers, Inc, Chicago. Used by permission.)*

to form and attach to the terminal ends of the collecting ducts. The final stage, stage 4, is characterized by collecting tube elongation (interstitial growth) and cessation of all branching and nephron formation. Ultimately, the nephron, derived from the metanephric blastema, gives origin to the glomerulus, proximal convoluted tubule, loop of Henle, and distal convoluted tubule. The metanephric duct gives origin to the collecting tubules (attached to the distal convoluted tubules of the nephron), the minor and major calyces, the renal pelvis, and the ureter.

Renal disorders, including congenital anomalies, renal dysplasias, and renal cystic diseases, are significant manifestations of disordered embryogenesis. Understanding these disorders requires an understanding of the sequential events in the normal embryologic development of the final or metanephric kidney.

Anatomy and Histology

The metanephric (or final) kidneys, located on each side of the great vessels within the abdomen, increase in length from 6 cm at birth to a maximum of 13 cm at 25 years to 30 years of age. Thereafter a gradual decrease in size and weight continues. At birth the kidneys weigh 26 g, increasing progressively to an average of 150 g to 160 g attained in the third decade.[3,4] In the kidneys' normal position, between T-12 and L-3, the anterior surface of the left kidney lies adjacent to the tail of the pancreas, the ipsilateral adrenal, the fundus of the stomach, the posterior-inferior surface of the spleen, the splenic flexure of the colon, and the proximal jejunum. The anterior surface of the right kidney is adjacent to the ipsilateral adrenal, the posterior surface of the liver, and the hepatic flexure of the

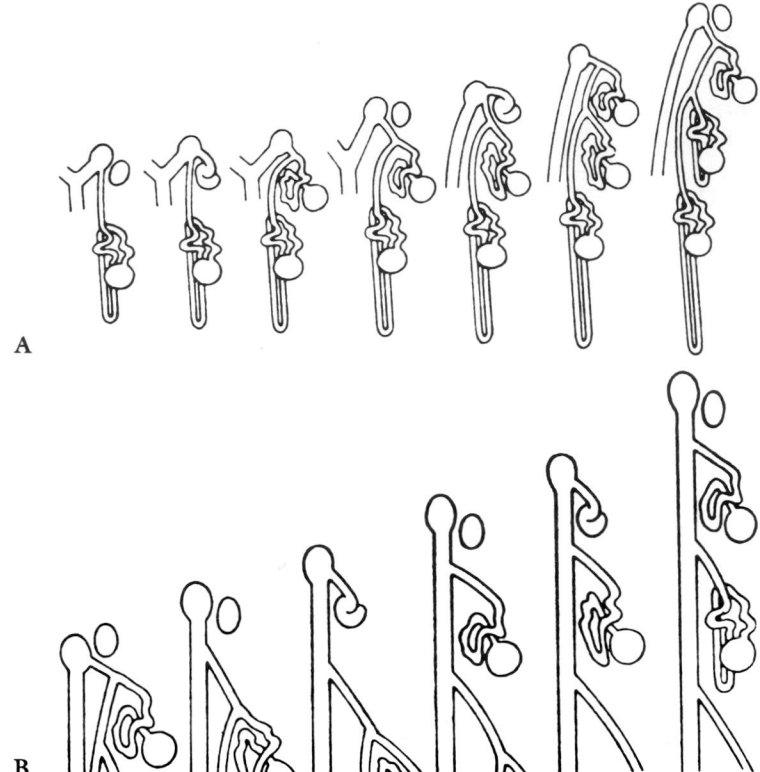

Figure 1-3   **Embryologic development of nephron and terminal collecting tubules, periods 2 and 3.** *(A) Decreased ampullary branching and development of nephron arcades characterize period 2. (B) Cessation of ampullary branching with continued direct attachment of nephrons to advancing ampullae occurs in period 3. (Potter EL: Normal and Abnormal Development of the Kidney. Copyright © 1972 by Year Book Medical Publishers, Inc, Chicago. Used by permission.)*

colon. Enveloping the kidney immediately outside the capsule is the perirenal adipose tissue within Gerota's fascia.[9]

The renal arterial supply is highly variable. The most common pattern includes a single renal artery that takes origin from the aorta and traverses laterally to divide into anterior and posterior arterial branches. These segments, still within the extrarenal hilum, divide as follows: the anterior branch gives origin to the apical segmental artery supplying the entire superior pole, a lower pole artery, and the upper and middle segmental arteries; the posterior branch supplies only the middle posterior segment of the kidney. All segmental arteries enter the renal parenchyma at the renal columns of Bertin, which protrude into the renal sinus of the hilar region.[2,11]

Upon entering the kidneys, the segmental arteries are called the interlobar arteries. These give rise to numerous arcuate arteries traversing the renal parenchyma near the corticomedullary junction. These arterial segments in turn give rise to the interlobular arteries, from which originate numerous afferent arterioles that course into the glomerular capillary tufts. The vascular supply to the renal medulla is through the vasa recta, which take origin from the efferent arterioles and alternatively directly from the interlobular arteries.[7] The renal

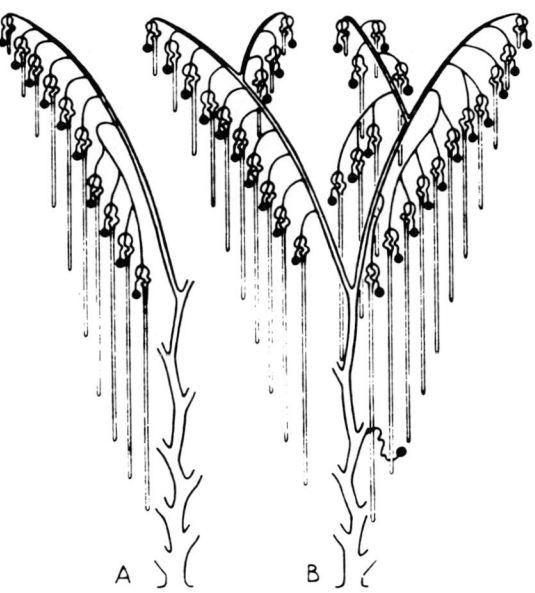

Figure 1-4   *Embryologic development of nephron and terminal collecting tubules, final period. The ampullae disappear, nephron formation ceases, and further elongation of the terminal collecting tubules is the result of growth of the more distal segments. The final arborizing patterns of terminal collecting ducts and nephrons are depicted in their usual (A) and variant (B) patterns. (Potter EL: Normal and Abnormal Development of the Kidney. Copyright © 1972 by Year Book Medical Publishers, Inc, Chicago. Used by permission.)*

capsule has a dual arterial supply from anastomosing intrarenal and the extra-renal arteries. Capsular arteries, taking origin from the segmental arteries, anastomose with capsular perforating arteries arising from interlobular arteries. The venous system follows the arterial tributary pattern in reverse.

The lymphatic vessels are located in the cortex adjacent to the interlobular vessels. Lymphatic drainage exits the kidney at the hilum where the vessels join the left and right lumbar lymphatic chains, either directly into para-aortic nodes or through lymph nodes within the renal hilum.[1,10] No direct connections from one kidney to the contralateral kidney were identified by Parker (1935).[1]

The structural unit of the kidney is the lobe, of which there are about 14 in the organ. The individual lobes can be identified from the cortical surface in the newborn, but thereafter the surface depressions defining the adjacent lobes gradually disappear in most people, resulting in a smooth cortical surface. The lobe is composed of a cortical zone that is draped over the medulla and tapers to form the renal pyramid indenting a calyx. The cortex of a lobe, in three dimensions, overlies the medullary component in a configuration resembling the cap of a mushroom. The convergence of the cortical areas of adjacent lobes forms the column of Bertin, into which the arterial supply enters the kidney as noted above. The lobe is composed of multiple repeating functional units, lobules, composed of glomeruli and their contiguous tubules coursing internally into the medulla and ultimately opening at the tip of the pyramid as converging collecting tubules. The lobule is bordered by the interlobular arteries, which radiate toward the capsule from the arcuate arteries. The clustered tubules running parallel to each other and subserving the glomeruli of a lobule are called medullary rays. They are adjacent to and intermingled with the vasa recta and the parallel medullary rays, and vasa recta can be observed in the outer medulla on close gross inspection of the kidney cut surface. The contents of the cortex include the glomeruli, segments of the proximal and distal convoluted tubules, straight segments of the loop of Henle, and collecting tubules (Fig. 1-5). The outer medulla, immediately within the cortex at the corticomedullary junction, contains the collecting tubules and straight segments of the loops of Henle with admixed blood vessels (the vasa recta) (Fig. 1-6). The inner medulla contains the converging collecting tubules, sparse capillaries surrounding the tubules, and minimal interstitium, which for practical purposes is not apparent in the normal cortex and outer medulla because of tight packing of the nephron components. Interstitial cells, although they are sparse in numbers, can be identified most readily in the inner medulla. By electron microscopy these cells have ultrastructural features differing from those of fibroblasts (refer to the discussion of renomedullary interstitial cell tumors, later in this chapter).

The ostium of the collecting tubules at the papillary tip is the location where the tubular epithelium makes a transition to the urothelium of the calyx and

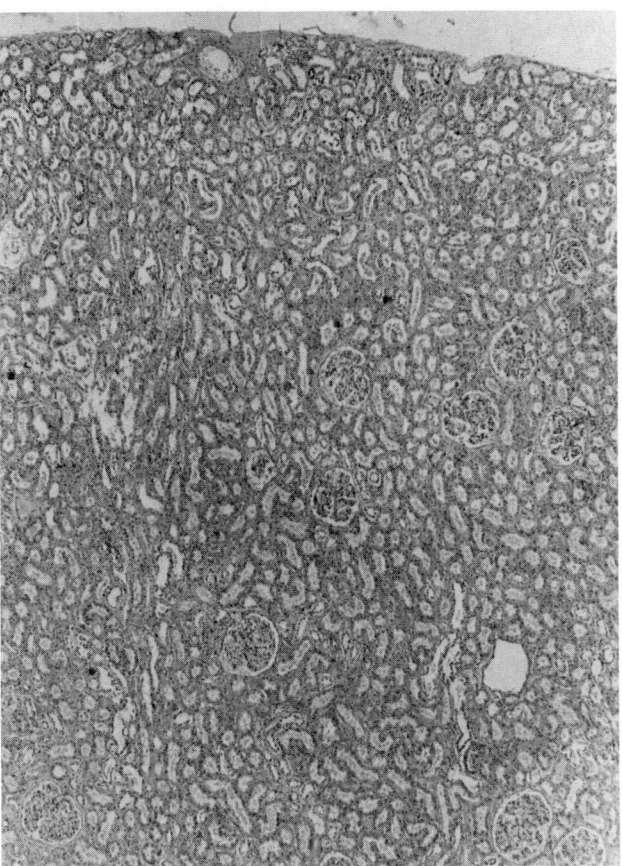

Figure 1-5   **Normal kidney.** *The renal cortex is composed predominantly of segments of the proximal and distal convoluted tubules with their respective glomeruli.*

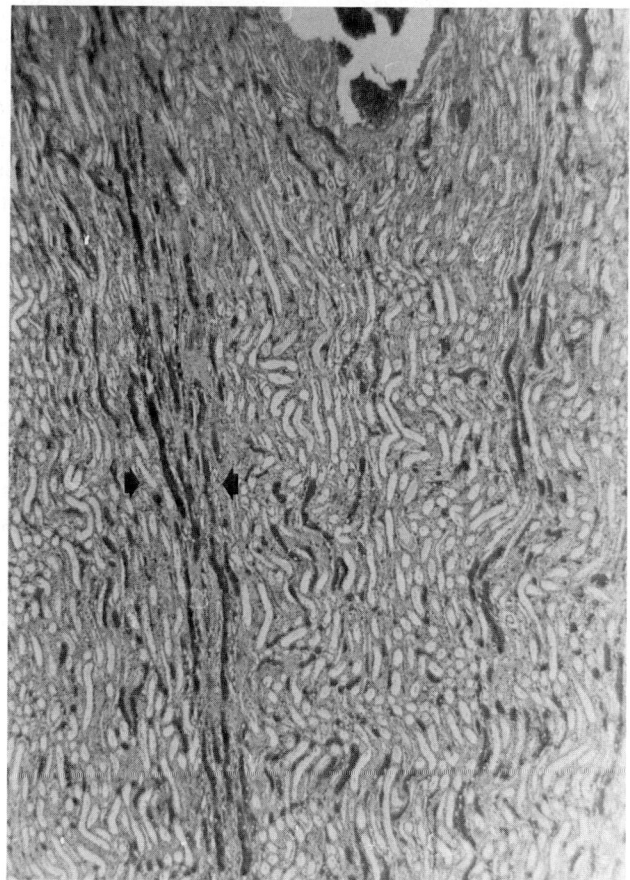

Figure 1-6   *Normal kidney. The outer zone of the renal medulla is composed of clusters of collecting tubules and straight segments of the proximal convoluted tubules together comprising the components of the medullary rays of the cortex. The vasa recta of the medulla (arrows) is found between the tubular components of the medullary rays.*

becomes continuous with the epithelium of the renal pelvis and the remainder of the lower urinary tract.

Congenital Anomalies

Agenesis

Unilateral renal agenesis may occur as an isolated congenital anomaly or in association with a wide variety of urinary, genital, and nongenitourinary anomalies.[13,15,16] It occurs with a frequency of approximately 1 in 1000 adults but, based on pediatric autopsy studies, has been reported to be more common in children. This difference in frequency can be partly attributed to the significant mortality resulting from renal disease affecting the extant kidney or from associated congenital disorders found with unilateral renal agenesis.[16-22]

Early literature reviews by Campbell (1928), Collins (1932), and Doroshow and Abeshouse (1961) indicate that this congenital anomaly is more common in males (64%) and slightly more frequent on the left side (56%).[16,17,19] The majority of reported cases occur in adults, but unilateral renal agenesis has been observed in persons ranging in age from the newborn to 92 years. The early literature is dominated by the cumulative experience obtained from autopsy studies. Unilateral renal agenesis is no longer regarded as a relatively innocuous anomaly adequately compensated for by enlargement of the contralateral kidney. Significantly higher frequencies of renal infection and lithiasis with resulting renal failure have been observed in these patients.[21] Associated congenital anomalies, especially among female patients, are reported in approximately 20% of cases.[20] In females, unicornuate uterus and absence of fallopian tubes, ovaries, or all Müllerian organs have been observed.[19,20] Cryptorchidism, absence of the ipsilateral seminal vesicle, seminal vesicle cyst, and absence of epididymis or testis are most common in the male.[20,22] The ipsilateral ureter is absent or rudimentary in most cases, and a complete and patent ureter is distinctly rare.[19] Nongenitourinary anomalies associated with unilateral renal agenesis include cardiovascular (septal defects, pulmonary artery stenosis, tricuspid atresia, and others with lesser frequency), gastrointestinal (imperforate anus, anal atresia, and duodenal atresia), and musculoskeletal defects (spinal deformities, absence of thumb, and multiple others).[20,21]

The frequent absence of the ureter underlies one pathogenetic explanation of this anomaly. The failure of the ureteric bud to contact and stimulate the metanephric blastema to differentiate into kidney results in the renal agenesis.[8,16] Alternatively, Ashley and Mostofi (1960) believe the metanephric blastema is capable of differentiation without the ureteral bud stimulus, an explanation based on the observations of 11 kidneys without ipsilateral ureters.[18] This interaction of ureteral bud and metanephric blastema remains unresolved.

Bilateral renal agenesis is incompatible with life, and the majority of afflicted newborns die within days of birth.[13-15] A significant number of affected infants are stillborn. Associated oligohydramnios is characteristic of such pregnancies. There are also associated findings of pulmonary hypoplasia and characteristic abnormalities of the head and face (Potter facies), including large, low-set ears, wide-set eyes, flattening of the nose, receding chin, and a prominent skin fold below the eyes and extending downward and lateral from the inner canthus.[13,14]

Bilateral renal agenesis is more frequent in males.[13,14] Associated anomalies include absence or abnormal development of the Müllerian organs, imperforate anus, and musculosketetal abnormalities.[15]

Hypoplasia

Renal hypoplasia is a rare congenital defect of unknown cause. It is most commonly unilateral, but it may be bilateral. True hypoplasia is characterized by a reduction in the number of renal papillae and minor calyces (fewer than six). For unknown reasons, renal hypoplasia is more common in males and the left kidney.[23,24] Boissonnat described three patterns of renal hypoplasia based on extent of involvement (partial or complete) of the kidney.[23]

Renal hypoplasia, when unilateral, is commonly associated with adequate compensatory enlargement of the contralateral kidney. The diagnosis is best achieved by combining the observations of specimen x-ray examinations with contrast material in the pelvicalyceal system with gross and microscopic observations of size of the kidney. True hypoplasia must be differentiated from renal dysplasia, "end-stage" kidney of vascular origin, and pyelonephritis. This latter distinction may be difficult or impossible in some cases.[23,24]

Segmental Hypoplasia (Ask-Upmark Kidney)

In 1929 Ask-Upmark described a unique form of hypoplasia characterized by renal hypoplasia (unilateral or bilateral), a circumferential cortical groove overlying an enlarged calyx, and intervening renal tissue devoid of the normal parenchymal architecture but rather occupied by dilated tubules, interstitial fibrosis, and thick-walled vessels (Figs. 1-7 and 1-8).[25] This lesion was most common in adolescent girls who frequently demonstrated systemic hypertension. Since the original description by Ask-Upmark, approximately 200 similar cases have been reported.[26-32] The emerging clinical picture features a female preponderance (2 : 1), unilateral involvement (2 : 1), and a wide age range, including children and older adults, 75% of whom have hypertension.[25,29]

Morphologic studies including microangiographic investigations have shown that rudimentary glomeruli, frequently sclerotic to the point of virtual obliteration, are present with the tubules that were originally noted by Ask-Upmark.[25,26,29] The vascular pattern has been found to recapitulate that in the uninvolved renal segments.[26]

The pathogenesis is unsettled. Ask-Upmark regarded the lesion as a congenital segmental hypoplasia.[25] More recent studies have suggested that the lesion

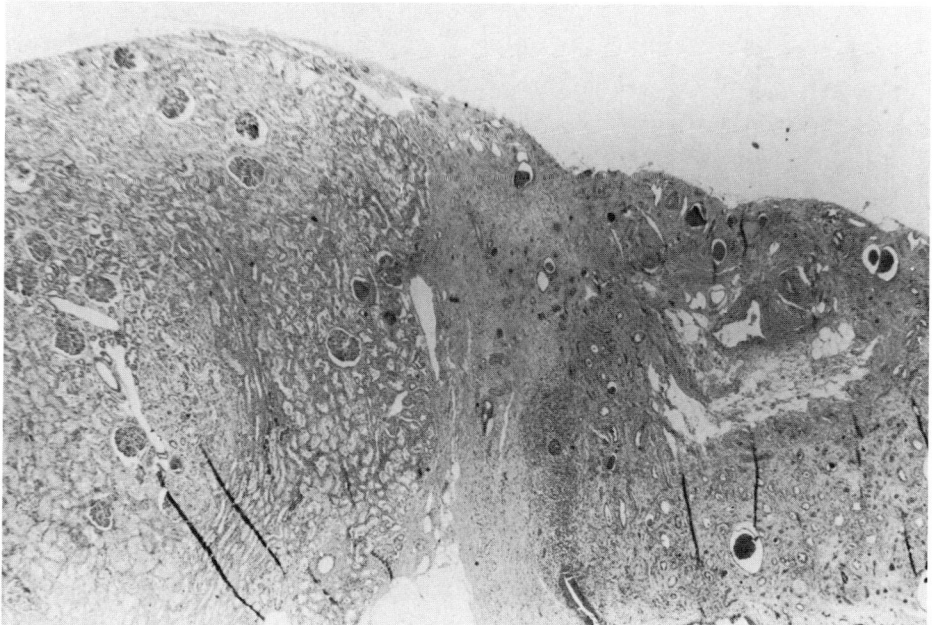

Figure 1-7 *Segmental hypoplasia (Ask-Upmark kidney). The circumferential cortical groove characteristic of Ask-Upmark kidney occupies the right half of the figure. Stromal fibrosis with disorganized renal tubules overlie a dilated calyx* (lower right).

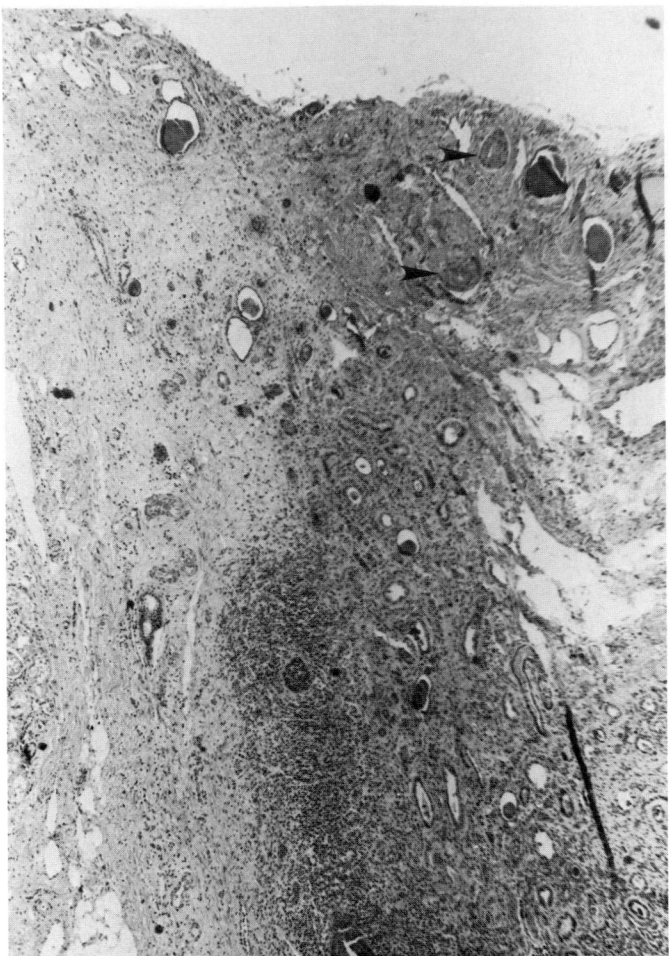

Figure 1-8   *Segmental hypoplasia (Ask-Upmark kidney). Sclerotic vessels*
(arrows) *and dilated renal tubules are present within abundant*
stromal fibrosis of hypoplastic segment.

may be acquired and may be the result of segmental vascular compromise or of
vesicoureteral reflux and associated urinary tract infection.[32] In 1979, Valderrama and Beckman reported a case in a premature infant documenting the
prenatal development of this lesion.[30]

Renal Hypoplasia With Oligomeganephronia

Renal hypoplasia with oligomeganephronia is a rare form of renal hypoplasia,
first described by Royers and colleagues and Habib and colleagues in 1962.[33,34]
This congenital disorder usually presents in infancy and childhood and is clinically characterized by slowly progressive renal failure occurring during the second decade. Nausea, vomiting, episodic dehydration, polyuria, proteinuria, systemic acidosis, and growth retardation are characteristic of the clinical progression.[33–41] No inheritance pattern is associated with this disorder, but congenital
renal lesions have been reported in family members of some patients.[41] It is

bilateral in all reported cases with the exception of two patients who were noted to have agenesis of the contralateral kidney.[36]

Morphologically the kidneys show marked reduction in size with a simplified calyceal system characteristic of hypoplasia. The corticomedullary junction is poorly delimited. The histologic features vary with the stage of disease progression, but a reduction of the number of glomeruli (nephrons) and marked enlargement of the extant glomeruli are characteristic of all stages.[33-41] Initially the proximal tubules are markedly dilated, a feature that gradually changes to tubular atrophy and accompanying interstitial fibrosis.[35] The late stages of the disease are characterized by enlarged and sclerotic glomeruli, tubular atrophy, and interstitial fibrosis, all nonspecific features of end stage renal disease with the exception of the enlarged glomeruli. There is no histologic evidence of renal dysplasia.[36] Ultrastructurally, the glomeruli show nonspecific increase in mesangial matrix and increased pericapsular stromal collagen.[37,39]

The pathogenesis of this disorder is unknown. The combined clinical and histologic features differentiate this renal hypoplasia with oligomeganephronia from other hypoplastic and dysplastic disorders of the kidney.

Malposition

Ectopia

Congenital renal ectopia is characterized by an abnormally located kidney (or kidneys) supplied by the vasculature in its immediate vicinity. This congenital disorder is to be differentiated from excessively mobile kidneys and from ptotic kidneys, which have a vascular supply from a renal artery originating from the aorta at the normal lumbar level. The ectopic kidney may be located ipsilateral to its normal location (simple ectopia) or contralateral (crossed ectopia). In addition, examples of ectopia with contralateral renal agenesis (congenital unilateral renal ectopia), and crossed ectopia with contralateral renal agenesis (solitary crossed ectopia) have been reported.[45,46] The most frequent of the renal ectopia variants is simple ectopia (1 per 800 autopsies).[44] All other variants are distinctly rare.[42,43,45-48]

The vast majority of all ectopic kidneys, whether simple or crossed, are located caudal to the normal anatomic site of the kidneys. The cephalad migration of the kidney occurring during the second month of gestation may become arrested at any site above its point of origination in the pelvis. Vessels within the vicinity of the migrating kidney, normally only temporary vessels during embryologic development of the organ, become the permanent vasculature of the kidney when the migration is arrested. The cause of the migratory inhibition is unknown. Conversely, in rare instances, the ascending kidney apparently "overshoots" and migrates to a location cephalad of normal, resulting in a thoracic kidney.[46,47] In such rare instances, the renal vascular supply may have a normally located origin from the abdominal aorta. The renal artery is, however, stretched cephalad to the ectopic kidney in the thorax.[47] Such kidneys most commonly come to medical attention as incidental opacities on chest x-ray films.[47]

Among the recent and most complex forms of ectopia are the crossed ectopic kidneys. In approximately 85% of such cases, the crossed kidney is fused with the contralateral kidney. There are multiple types of crossed renal ectopia based on the configuration of the fused kidney.[42,45,48] A wide spectrum of associated anomalous vascular and ureteral configurations are associated with the various crossed ectopic variants.

Ectopic kidneys, especially simple ectopia, may be without clinical significance and may be detected only at the time of autopsy as an incidental finding. Clinical significance of ectopia has been reported most commonly with pelvic kidneys and the various forms of crossed ectopia, which are associated with a significant frequency of associated congenital anomalies of the genitourinary, skeletal, and cardiovascular systems.[46] In addition, crossed renal ectopia is commonly associated with recurrent urinary tract infections, pyelonephritis, and renal lithiasis.[46]

For unknown reasons, renal ectopia is more common in males and affects the left kidney more than the right.[42]

Supernumerary Kidney

The term *supernumerary kidney* describes a ". . . free accessory organ, which is a distinct, encapsulated, large or small parenchymatous mass, topographically related to the usual kidney by a loose, cellular attachment at most, and often by no attachment whatsoever," as originally suggested by Geisinger (1937).[52] Fused kidneys (duplex kidneys) with duplication of the renal pelvis and ureter are thus differentiated.[52] Fewer than 70 authenticated cases have been reported in the literature.[49-59] The majority of supernumerary kidneys are smaller and lower than the ipsilateral "normal" kidney, located on the left side, and diagnosed in adults (average age in the fourth decade).[55,58,59] Males and females are equally affected. Approximately one third of the reported cases have a completely duplicated ureter. More commonly the ureter of the supernumerary kidney joins the ipsilateral ureter, forming a bifid ureter.[59] Rarely, junction with the ipsilateral renal pelvis is observed.[59] Seventy-five percent of the cases with a double ureteral system show vesicle insertions that conform to the Weigert-Meyer principle (see Chap. 3).[59]

Supernumerary kidneys may either be incidental findings at autopsy or underlie clinical symptoms due to secondary development of hydronephrosis, pyelonephritis, or (in extremely rare instances) renal cell carcinoma.[53,55]

The diagnosis of supernumerary kidney is based on the finding of an extra kidney fulfilling Geisinger's criteria (see above) that microscopically may show evidence of distal obstruction with or without superimposed pyelonephritis. Preoperative radiologic diagnosis has been reported in rare instances.[57,58] When supernumerary kidney has been diagnosed in children, multiple nongenitourinary and genitourinary malformations have been observed.[57,59]

The embryogenesis of this rare malformation is thought to involve ureteral buds that independently interact with separate metanephric blastemal masses, ultimately producing two separate kidneys on the ipsilateral side.[59]

Horseshoe Kidney

Horseshoe kidney is a common congenital anomaly of kidneys that results from the fusion of the independent metanephric blastema during the second gestational month, prior to their cephalad migration. The fusion, which in 90% of cases involves the lower poles, prevents normal rotation of the kidneys, which in turn requires the ureter to arise anterior to, and pass over, the fused lower renal poles.[62,66] The ultimate position of the fused kidneys tends to be lower than normal. Multiple variations of the renal vasculature are encountered in such kidneys.[62,71] Partial ureteral obstruction results, with an associated increased risk of renal infection and lithiasis.[63,64] The frequency of horseshoe kidneys has been variously estimated to be from 1 in 350 to 1 in 1800.[62,66] There is a male preponderance.[62,64,66]

The discovery of horseshoe kidney most commonly occurs accidentally, as an incidental finding in radiologic or postmortem examinations (Figs. 1-9 and 1-10). Less frequently, horseshoe kidney is diagnosed in the course of examinations prompted by symptomatology referable to the anomaly itself.[66,68] Radiologic diagnosis can frequently be made on flatplate of the abdomen showing the midline soft tissue mass of the isthmus. Intravenous pyelography (IVP) or retrograde studies disclose the ectopic location and abnormal orientation of the renal pelvis. Arteriography frequently reveals anomalous vascular supply to the fused kidneys.[62,71]

The literature has increasingly concerned itself with the clinical complications of horseshoe kidney and the results of surgical correction.[60,62,63] This has tended to give an exaggerated impression of the complication rate associated

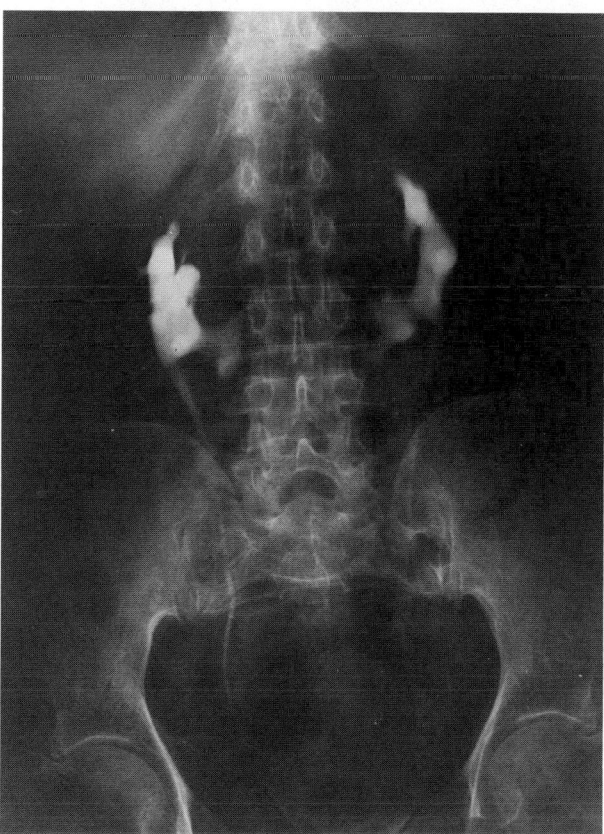

Figure 1-9   *Horseshoe kidney. An intravenous urogram shows the lateral rotation of the renal pelvis and ureters that is characteristic of horseshoe kidneys.*

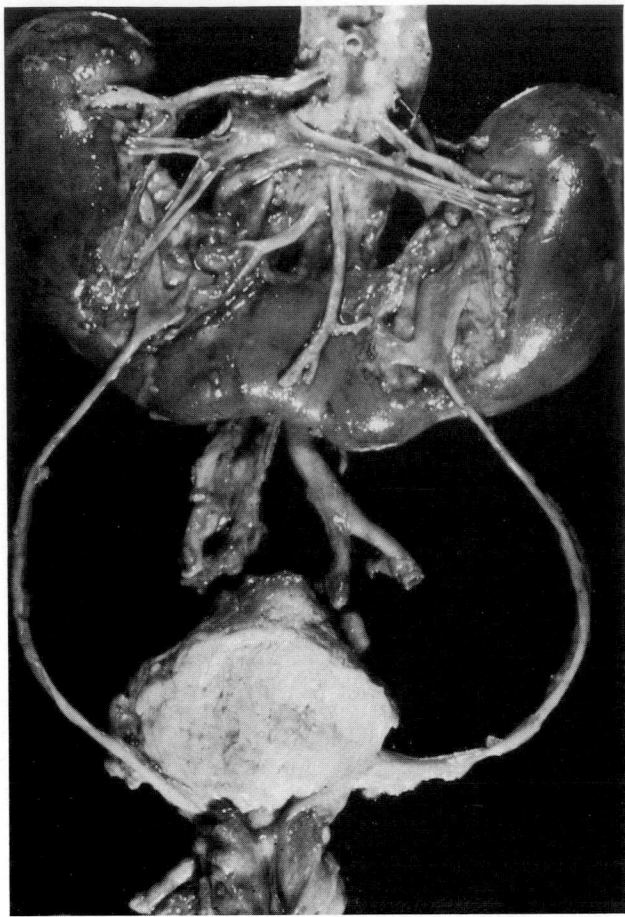

Figure 1-10   *Horseshoe kidney. The posterior view of the horseshoe kidney reveals the associated anomalous renal arterial supply in abnormal locations of the renal pelvis.*

with this common renal anomaly.[60-66] Urinary tract infection and renal calculus disease account for the majority of clinically treated complications of horseshoe kidney.[63,64] Less frequently, neoplasms originating in either the kidney or the renal pelvis are discovered.[67,69,70,72,73] Buntley recorded 55 cases of renal cell carcinoma, 22 renal pelvic transitional cell carcinomas, 25 Wilms' tumors, and 9 additional neoplasms of various histologic types arising in horseshoe kidneys reported up to 1975.[70] One additional example of renal cell carcinoma and one of transitional cell carcinoma were recently reported.[72,73] Patients with symptomatology referable to the anomaly per se are the least frequent encountered clinically.[66,68] Pain related to compression of the isthmus of the fused kidneys on the vena cava and aorta, accentuated by hypertension and associated with a sensation of fullness and nausea, forms the symptom complex referred to as Rovsing syndrome.[64,65] Various surgical procedures, including pyeloplasty, resection of isthmus, heminephrectomy, and nephrectomy, have been required for surgical correction of the clinical complications of this common anomaly.[60-66]

Renal Dysplasia

Renal dysplasia is characterized by disorganized organogenesis with primitive tubules surrounded by concentric fibromuscular stromal sheaths; focal areas of cartilaginous metaplasia; and primitive glomerular structures, frequently showing sclerosis.[74] Cystic changes commonly accompany renal dysplasia. The disorder is congenital and sporadic, with no documented mode of inheritance.[74-76] The cause is unknown. Renal dysplasia may be unilateral or bilateral and may involve the entire kidney or only segments of the organ. The dysplastic kidney may be smaller than normal or markedly enlarged, the latter occurring when cystic change is prominent. Associated congenital anomalies of the lower urinary tract are present in a high percentage of cases.[74-76] Multicystic dysplastic kidney is the most completely defined entity in the spectrum of dysplastic renal disorders.

Multicystic Dysplastic Kidney

History

Multicystic dysplastic kidney has been reported under multiple names including unilateral polycystic disease, aplasia with cystic degeneration, cystic hypoplasia, metanephric cystic remnants, congenital cystic hydrocalicosis, unilateral multilocular cyst, multiple simple cysts, congenital cystic disease with hydronephrosis, metanephric cystic tumor, cystic hamartoma, tuber kidney, congenital unilateral multicystic disease, unilateral multicystic disease, cystic dysplastic kidney, multicystic dysplasia, and multicystic dysplastic kidney.[97,108] The most frequently employed term is *unilateral multicystic disease,* introduced by Schwartz in 1936,[93] and more recently, *multicystic dysplastic kidney* (MDK).[74-76, 101,103,105,106] The latter term reflects the dysplastic nature of the disorder and the more recently appreciated fact that some cases are not unilateral.

The first description of this cystic lesion was recorded by Cruveilhier in 1836.[113] The illustrated example was observed in a 3-year-old boy at autopsy. Normal renal parenchyma was not found in the multicystic kidney. Schwartz (1936) is attributed with the first description of this entity in the U.S. literature.[93] A possible example was reported by Wakeley (1931) 5 years before, but insufficient details were given to allow distinction from a multilocular cyst.[92] Spence (1955) presented four cases and reviewed fifteen previously reported cases, including the questionable case of Wakeley (1931).[95] In subsequent years many reported individual cases and series of cases appeared in the literature, clarifying both the clinical and pathologic features of MDK.[96-117]

Clinical Features

Most cases of MDK are diagnosed in the neonatal period and manifest as either unilateral or (less frequently) bilateral masses.[102,106,111,117] MDK is the most common lesion producing an abdominal mass in the newborn, congenital hydronephrosis being more common in older infants during the first year.[102,104,116] Because the affected kidney has no functioning renal tissue, all patients with bilateral MDK exhibit Potter facies at birth and die within a few days. The majority of unilateral cases also manifest at or shortly after birth but may escape detection until adolescence or even adulthood.[107,109,110,116,117] Approximately 25 cases of MDK have been reported in adults.[107,109,110,116,117] A predilection for males and for the left kidney is observed.

The majority of recorded cases have not been correctly diagnosed preoperatively. Recent reports describe successful preoperative radiologic diagnosis by percutaneous injection of contrast material and by ultrasound.[106,112] Excretory urography (IVP) discloses apparent absence of a kidney on the affected side, and retrograde pyelography discloses absence or obstruction of the ipsilateral ureter.[105–107] Calcification of the cyst walls has been reported in adult cases.[106,107,110] Occasional cases with associated hypertension have been reported.[117] Malignancy in association with MDK has been reported in two patients.[96,115]

Pathologic Features

The affected kidney appears as a multilobulated mass composed of multiple thin-walled cysts containing clear fluid surrounding a more or less centrally located solid core of fibrous tissue (Fig. 1-11). No cortical or medullary landmarks are observed in this central fibrous core. The affected organ has totally lost an overall reniform configuration and resembles a cluster of grapes. The ipsilateral calyceal system, renal pelvis, and ureter are commonly atretic.[105,106,111] When atresia is limited to the calyceal system and the renal pelvis, it is associated with a lower frequency of congenital anomalies in the contralateral kidney than when it extends to the entire length of the ipsilateral ureter as in cases of MDK.[111] The vessels of the renal pedicle show no consistent changes. Vascular hypoplasia is observed in some cases.

Microscopically, the cysts are lined by a single layer of cuboidal cells. The cyst walls are composed of fibrous tissue without evidence of renal structures (Fig.

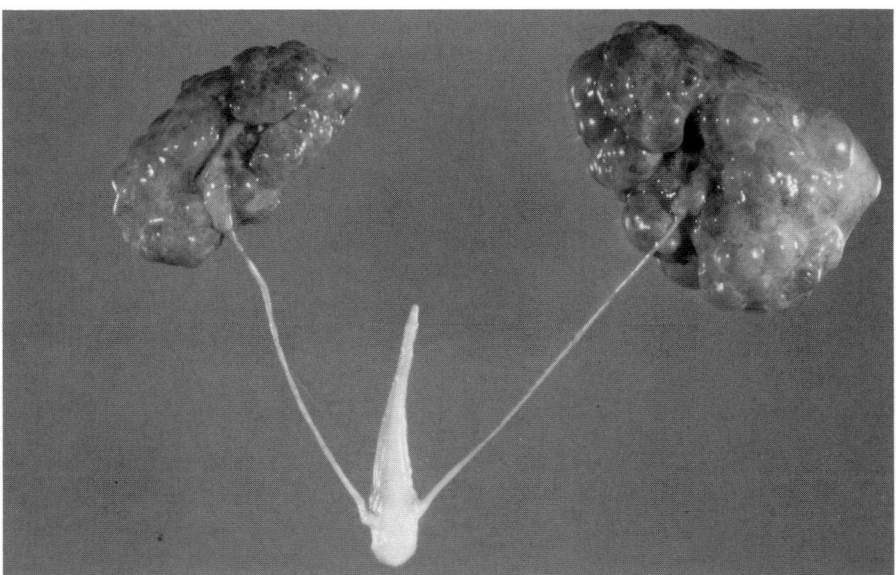

Figure 1-11   *Multicystic disease of the kidney. The affected kidney is composed of clustered cysts of varying size with total loss of the normal renal configuration.*

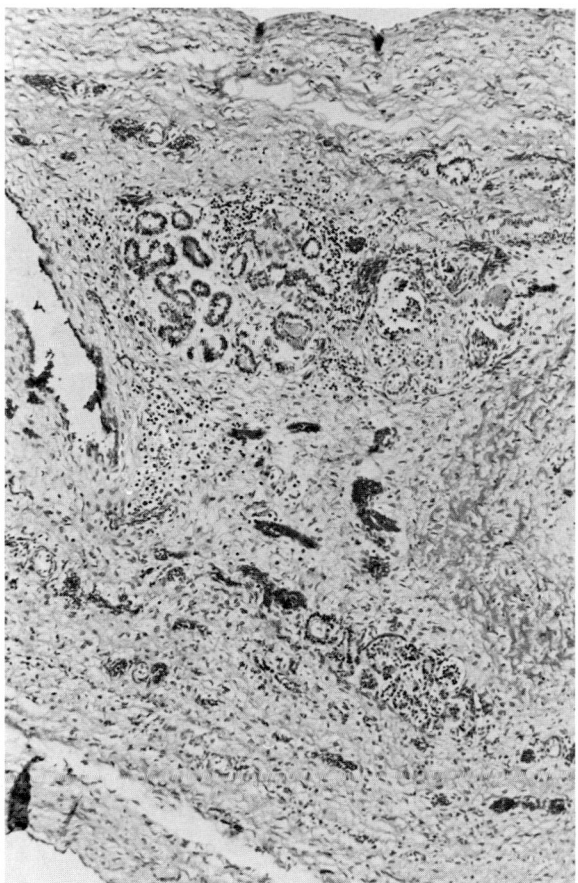

Figure 1-12 *Multicystic disease. The walls of the cyst are composed primarily of collagenous fibrous tissue with a few scattered primitive tubules.*

1-12). Primitive tubules with surrounding concentric fibromuscular tissue and islands of cartilaginous metaplasia are dispersed in a loose stroma. Occasionally, primitive glomeruli are present, frequently showing sclerotic changes. Neither normal renal parenchyma nor evidence of cytologic atypia of the primitive tubules or stroma is observed.

The diagnosis of MDK requires distinction of this lesion from polycystic renal disease, both infantile and adult types; multilocular cystic kidney; and simple cyst. In polycystic renal disease, the renal contour and normal calyceal pattern are retained. Normal renal parenchyma is present between the cysts. Also, the associated liver cysts and the established genetic transmission characteristic of polycystic renal disease further aid in differentiating these cystic renal diseases from MDK. The segmental involvement of the kidney and the cyst structure (multiloculated) characteristic of multilocular cyst allow differentiation of this disorder from MDK. Multiple simple cysts are distinguished by the presence of intervening mature renal parenchyma not present in MDK. As fully discussed by Bernstein (1968), a diagnostic challenge is presented in trying to distinguish

MDK from chronic pyelonephritis, with the spectrum of secondary changes including cystic dilatation and atrophy of renal tubules, and from glomerular sclerosis.[74]

Pathogenesis

The microdissection studies of Osathanondh and Potter disclosed failure of branching of the ampullary portion of the collecting ducts in MDK.[76,86] In Osathanondh and Potter's suggested classification of cystic diseases of the kidney, MDK is an example of Type II.[76,86] It is proposed that branching failure results in a failure to induce nephron formation. The theory that there is a primary defect in the ureteral bud is supported by the high frequency of abnormalities observed in the ipsilateral ureter.

Segmental Renal Dysplasia

Relatively little recorded experience with subtotal or segmental renal dysplasia is available in the literature.[74,75,109] Segmental dysplasia may be unilateral or bilateral, and it frequently is associated with lower urinary tract obstruction.[75,109] Affected patients are frequently hypertensive.[109] The possible role of reflux from congenital lower urinary tract obstruction in the cause of dysplasia is unsettled, but it is most likely an associated but independent lesion.[74,75]

Distinction of true renal dysplasia in these cases rests on the finding of primitive tubules and chondroid metaplasia in a focal region of a kidney. These features allow accurate identification of renal dysplasia and differentiation from severe chronic pyelonephritis and unilateral renal hypoplasia. In fact, pyelonephritis frequently accompanies the segmental form of renal dysplasia.[74,109]

Cystic Diseases of the Kidneys

Although several classifications of cystic renal diseases have been formulated, none is completely satisfactory because they are based on a mixture of descriptive clinical or pathologic features that reflect our limited understanding of the etiology and pathogenesis of these disorders.[77-91] Variants of cystic renal diseases with differences in clinical presentation, mode of inheritance, associated abnormalities, and age of onset continue to be reported, making all working classifications tentative. Substantial progress has been made in recent decades in understanding both clinical and pathologic aspects of these disorders.

From the latter half of the 19th century through the first half of the 20th century, the origin and nature of the renal cysts were regarded as being due to (1) obstruction of normal tubules (Virchow, 1869), (2) embryologic nonunion of the nephron and ureteral bud (Hildebrand, 1896), (3) failure of regression of "first generation nephrons" or failure of attachment of "later generations of nephrons" to the collecting tubules (Kampmeier, 1923), or (4) secondary focal degeneration of renal tubules with segmental isolation (Norris and Herman, 1941).[77,78,81,82] In addition, others thought the lesions to be fundamentally proliferative lesions of hamartomatous (Herxheimer, 1906) or neoplastic nature (Staemmler, 1921).[79,80] At present, although the ultimate answers to questions of cause are unknown, we can relegate to history and dismiss for lack of supportive evidence theories of hamartomatous and neoplastic origin, tubular obstruction, nonunion, nephron regression and failure of attachment, and secondary segmental isolation. All of these theories have been disproven.

As a result of microdissection studies, most notably those of Osathanondh and Potter (1964), the location of the cysts in various clinical forms of cystic renal disease has been identified, and the absence of nonunion of ureteral bud–derived tubular renal nephron was demonstrated.[83-89] Four types of renal cystic disease were described on the basis of location of the cystic abnormality of the renal tubular system. Type I, exemplified by the heritable disorder infantile polycystic disease, showed cystic enlargement of the ampullary collecting ducts.[85] Type II, characteristic of dysgenetic cystic disease and multilocular cystic disease, showed cystic enlargement of the terminal ends of the ampullary collecting ducts with reduced numbers of both collecting tubule branches and nephrons.[86] Type III, characteristic of adult polycystic disease, showed variable cystic dilatation of the ampullary collecting branches and segments of tubular system of nephron origin (*i.e.,* Bowman's capsule and the proximal convoluted tubule).[87] Type IV, originally described in association with urethral obstruction of the lower urinary tract, results in back pressure that affects the embryologic development of the ampullary collecting ducts with dilatation accompanying dilatation of Bowman's capsule.[88] Similar changes observed in glomerulocystic disease occur without evidence of urethral obstruction. These studies, identifying the tubular segment undergoing cystic enlargement in renal cystic disease, do not answer the question of underlying cause. More recently, ultrastructural studies of young persons genetically at risk to develop adult polycystic disease disclosed splitting of the tubular lamina densa with possible implications of structural weakness contributing to cystic enlargement of the tubule.[143]

The cumulative clinical and pathologic observations reported in recent decades form the basis for the current working classifications of cystic diseases of the kidney. Features of diagnostic importance include (1) evidence of possible genetic transmission, (2) age predilection, (3) associated congenital anomalies, and (4) gross and microscopic features of the renal cysts, including uninvolved renal parenchyma. In the absence of more definitive understanding of the pathogenesis of these disorders, these features currently serve as the basis for diagnosis of the recognized forms of cystic diseases of the kidney.

Polycystic Renal Disease

Infantile Type

There is evidence that infantile polycystic renal disease, an inherited form of cystic renal disease, is actually a disease spectrum with variable severity of renal and liver involvement.[120,121,124,126] It is inherited as an autosomal recessive disorder that in its most severe or typical form manifests in the newborn or young infants with renal failure.[118,122,123] In the majority of patients, the disorder becomes clinically manifest before the age of 3 months.[119,124,125] Evidence of respiratory distress associated with a protuberant abdomen leads ultimately to the radiologic diagnosis of bilateral renal enlargement. A prolonged nephrogram, resulting from the cystically dilated renal tubules transiently entrapping the excreted contrast material, is characteristic.[124] Some patients are hypertensive. Microdissection studies by Osathanondh and Potter (1964) revealed the consistent finding of dilatation of the terminal portions of the ampullary collecting tubules producing the renal cysts.[85,89]

Invariably associated with the renal cysts are liver changes, including bile duct proliferation with portal fibrosis. In cases demonstrating less severe cystic change of the renal tubules, survival is prolonged with a concomitant development of more severe portal fibrosis.[125,127] It is unsettled whether all cases of "congenital hepatic fibrosis" represent extrarenal manifestations of infantile polycystic renal disease or whether they may represent a unique clinicopathologic entity.[120,121,124–127]

Pathologic Features

The kidneys are bilaterally enlarged but retain their reniform configuration (Fig. 1-13). Innumerable cortical and medullary cysts, lined by flattened epithelium, are present throughout the kidney as observed on the cut surface (Fig. 1-14). The cysts tend to be linear and to radiate in the orientations typical of renal collecting tubules (Fig. 1-15). Uninvolved nephrons are present in the intervening renal tissue. The relative severity of the cystic change varies, with the most extensive

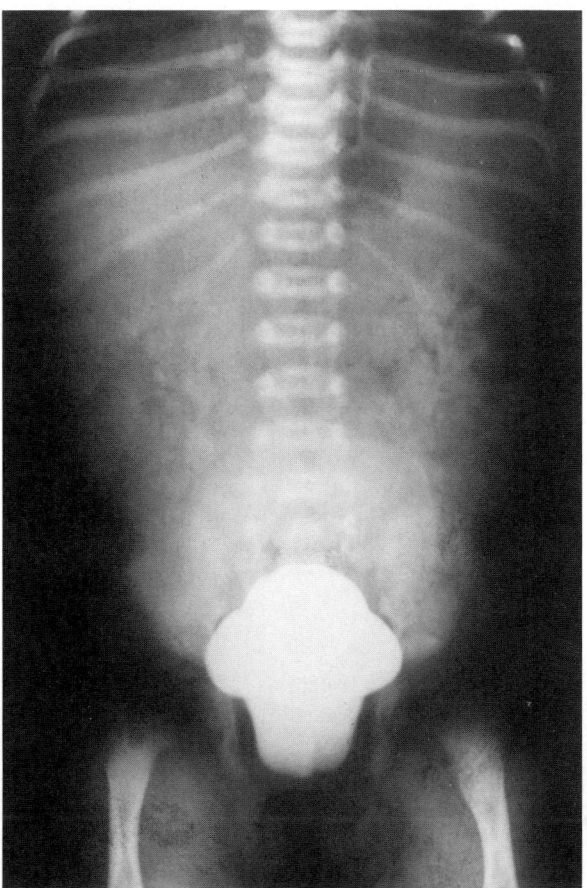

Figure 1-13   *Infantile polycystic disease. An intravenous urogram demonstrates diffusely enlarged kidneys in a 6-day-old infant. Multiple avascular (cystic) structures are present in both kidneys.*

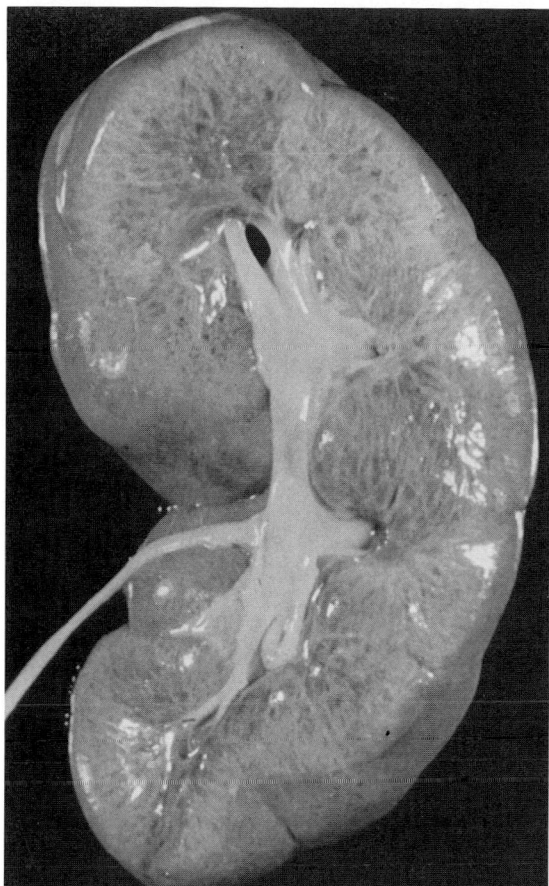

Figure 1-14 *Infantile polycystic disease.* The characteristic widespread small cysts with retention of the overall configuration of the kidney is seen in this example of infantile polycystic disease.

cyst formation observed in those patients dying of renal failure in the neonatal period.[124,125,128]

Infantile polycystic disease must be differentiated from other cystic disorders commonly manifesting in infants, including multicystic dysplasia, medullary cystic disease, and glomerulocystic disease (see separate discussions). The accurate diagnosis of infantile polycystic disease, an inherited disease capable of manifesting in siblings of the identified patient, is required for the appropriate genetic counseling of parents.

Adult Type

Polycystic disease of the adult type is an inherited autosomal dominant disorder with variable penetrance.[76,118,122] This disorder typically manifests in the fourth to fifth decades with a gradual onset of renal failure.[118,122,131] Occasionally flank pain attributed to associated lithiasis, hemorrhage into a cyst, or ureteral obstruction by blood clot is reported as the initial clinical presentation.[144] Asso-

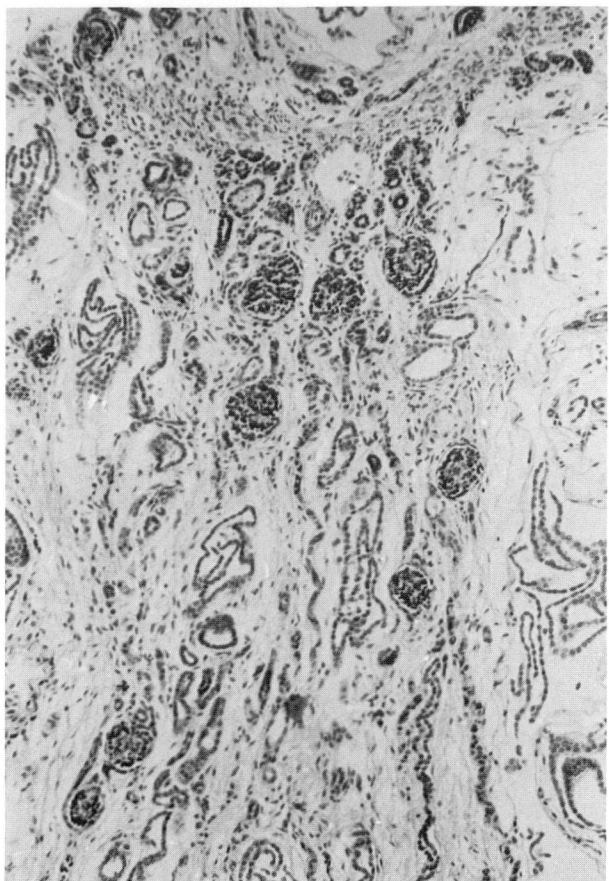

Figure 1-15   *Infantile polycystic disease. Normal glomeruli are present between the numerous linear cysts lined by low cuboidal tubular epithelium.*

ciated hypertension is common. Rare examples have recently been reported in children and young adults.[134,137,140]

Adult polycystic disease is always bilateral, but significant asynchrony of involvement of the kidneys may be observed in occasional cases.[151] Such cases may present as radiologically unilateral. Typical radiologic findings include hypovascular enlargement of the kidneys with distortion of the calyceal system (Figs. 1-16 and 1-17). Angiography demonstrates stretching and thinning of the vessels around the cysts. The nephrogram shows multiple radiolucent areas with an irregular renal outline.[150] Calcification of the cyst wall is uncommon, but calculi are present in 20% of cases.[144] Rarely, kidneys of normal size are observed radiographically.[145]

Liver cysts are present in approximately one third of patients with adult polycystic disease.[144,149] The frequency of associated liver cysts increases with age.[148] Milutinovic and co-workers reported observing no cysts in the livers of patients at risk younger than 19 years.[148] The frequency increased to 40% at 50 years to 59 years and to 77% in all patients older than 60 years.[148] Liver cysts were not observed in patients at risk but without demonstrated renal cysts. The hepatic cysts rarely, if ever, cause functional impairment or portal hypertension. Manes

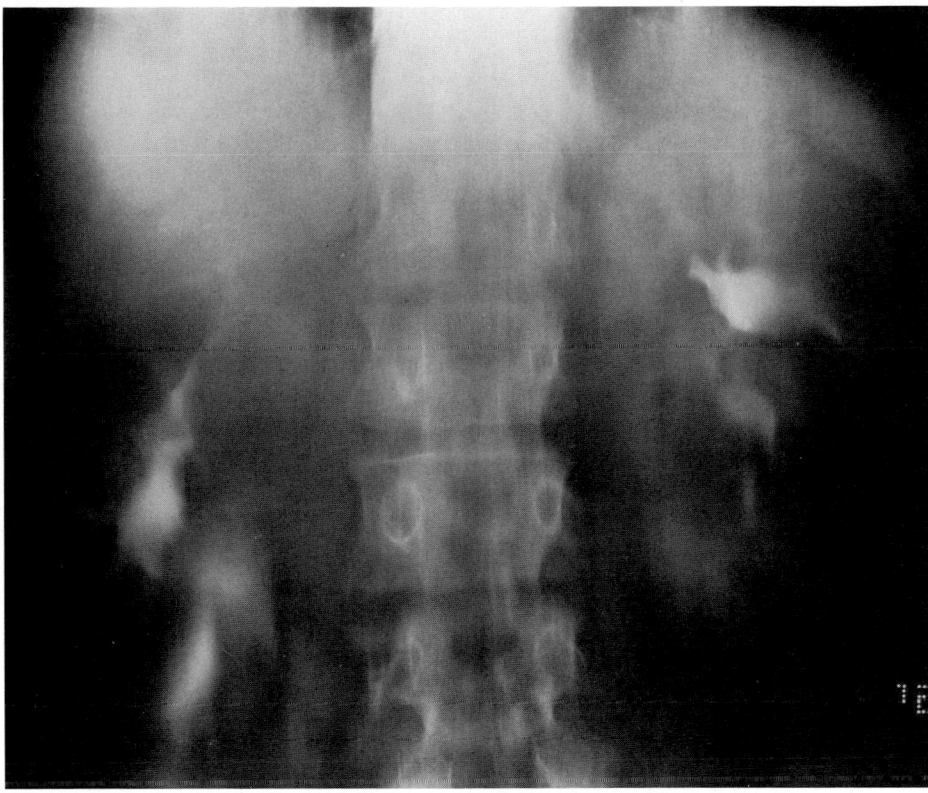

Figure 1-16 *Adult polycystic disease. Intravenous urogram shows bilateral renal enlargement with stretched and distorted calyces. Multiple avascular masses within the kidney project beyond the renal contour consistent with polycystic disease in this 68-year-old woman.*

and colleagues (1977) reported a 69-year-old man with polycystic disease and associated hepatoma superimposed on congenital hepatic fibrosis, the latter a disorder that is generally associated with infantile polycystic disease.[142]

Approximately 20 cases of adult polycystic renal disease with associated renal cell carcinoma have been reported.[129,130,136,138,139,141,147] Barbour and Casali (1978) reported a unique case of a renal cell carcinoma and an angiomyolipoma taking origin in a polycystic kidney.[147] Association of adult polycystic disease with congenital cerebral arterial aneurysms has also been observed.[132]

Pathologic Features

The typical case of polycystic renal disease is characterized by enlargement of both kidneys, which show a bosselated outer cortical surface produced by the innumerable cysts (Figs. 1-18 and 1-19). The cysts may be so numerous that normal renal parenchyma is apparent only microscopically in the intervening renal tissue. The cysts, ranging in size from millimeters to several centimeters, are thin-walled, unilocular, and filled with clear fluid. Hemorrhage into a cyst is occasionally apparent. The calyceal system may be so distorted as to be outlined with difficulty. The renal pelvis and ureter show no abnormalities, with the possible exceptions of lithiasis and secondary inflammatory changes of pyelonephritis.

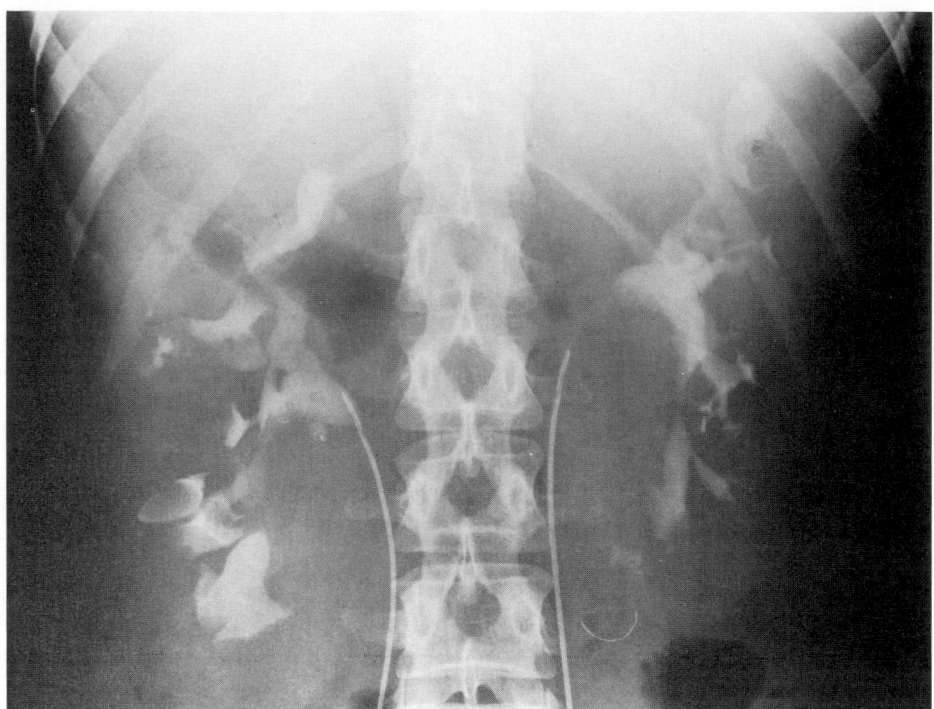

Figure 1-17   *Adult polycystic disease. Retrograde pyelogram shows bilateral renal enlargement and distortion of the calyceal system due to multiple cysts.*

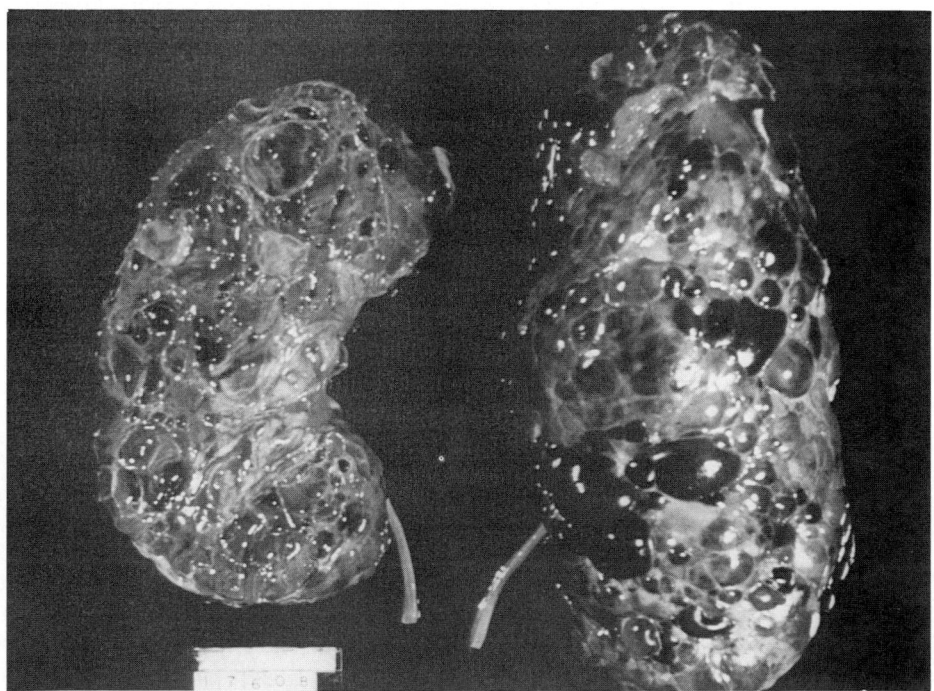

Figure 1-18   *Adult polycystic disease. The cortical and cut surfaces reveal the number and widespread distribution of the thin-walled cysts in this enlarged polycystic kidney.*

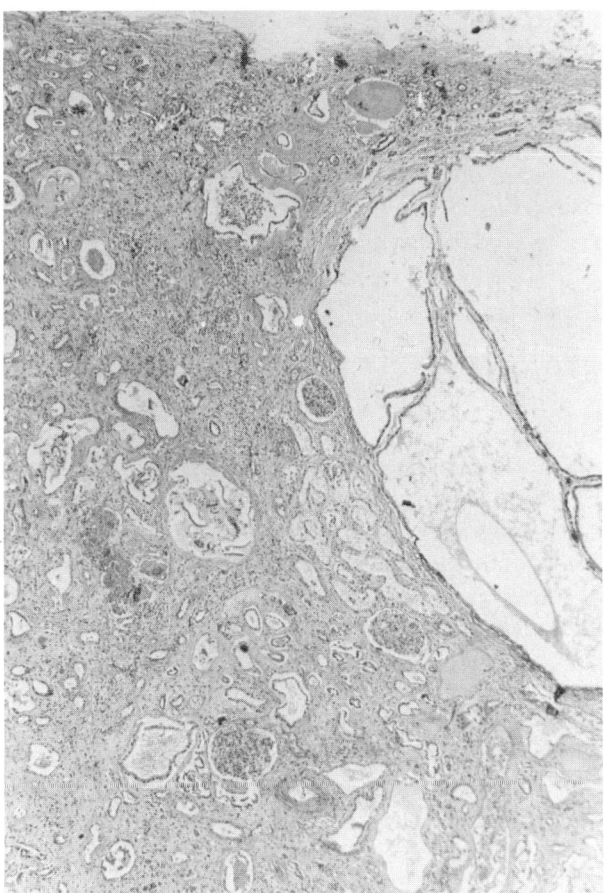

Figure 1-19 **Adult polycystic disease.** *The cysts are adjacent to areas of the renal cortex with interstitial fibrosis, tubular atrophy, and scattered histologically normal glomeruli.*

Microscopically, the cysts are lined by flattened epithelial cells with occasional hyperplastic foci of these lining cells.[87] The intervening renal parenchyma contain normal nephrons, commonly evidencing atrophic changes with or without associated changes of pyelonephritis.

Pathogenesis

The pathogenesis of this inherited renal disorder remains unknown. Osathanondh and Potter (1964) demonstrated cystic dilatation of the collecting tubules and of segments of the nephron including Bowman's space, the proximal convoluted tubule, and the loop of Henle.[87] Baert (1978) reported similar findings but did not observe the abnormal branching of collecting ducts previously reported by Osathanondh and Potter.[146] The retained functional capacity of cystically dilated tubules in adult polycystic disease has been documented.[133,135,143] Gardner (1969), measuring the amino acids of the cyst fluid, raised the possibility that these substances could act as osmotically active agents contributing to tubular dilatation.[135] In 1980, Milutinovic and co-workers examined renal biopsies from 16 asymptomatic patients aged 11 to 26 years who were at risk, as determined by family history, for the development of adult polycystic renal disease.[149] Some of these individuals showed focal tubular dilatation and, ultrastructurally, delamination or splitting of the tubular lamina densa.[149] Such changes are the earliest reported in patients at risk for the development of clinically significant adult polycystic disease, typically two decades later.

The correct diagnosis of this inherited form of cystic renal disease in the typical case is rarely difficult, but it may prove a challenge when encountered in older children or adolescents. A detailed family history is required.

Medullary Cystic Disease and Juvenile Nephronophthisis

History

In 1945, Smith and Graham reported a case of an 8-year-old girl with anemia and previously undiagnosed azotemia.[152] Within 1 year the patient died with refractory anemia and progression of the azotemia. At autopsy the medullary regions of the kidneys contained numerous cysts 1 mm to 5 mm in diameter. Neither cortical cysts nor cysts within other organs were present. Extensive glomerular fibrosis was also recorded. No similar previously reported cases were found in the literature.

In 1951, Fanconi and co-workers reported a small group of young patients with salt wasting, anemia, and azotemia, all of whom showed medullary cysts, prompting the authors to introduce the name *familial juvenile nephronophthisis* for what they regarded as a newly described renal disease.[153] This disorder was subsequently reported in the European literature but did not appear in the American literature until the publication in 1964 of the study by Mangos and colleagues, who confirmed the documented familial nature of the disorder.[156] Furthermore, the clinical and pathologic features reported in this study resembled those observed in the previous European reports. Multiple reports of juvenile nephronophthisis have subsequently appeared in the American literature.[157-167] The association of juvenile nephronophthisis complex with retinal disorders has been observed.[165,166]

In 1962, 2 years prior to the first report of juvenile nephronophthisis by Mangos and co-workers (1964) in the American literature, Strauss reported three patients and reviewed fifteen previously reported cases of medullary renal cysts associated with salt wasting, anemia, and azotemia occurring in patients 8 to 56 years of age.[154] Strauss (1962) introduced the term *medullary cystic disease* for this clinicopathologic disorder.[154]

Publications subsequent to these initial descriptions have dealt principally with resolving whether medullary cystic disease and familial juvenile nephronophthisis are different disorders with overlapping features or whether they represent the same disease, as originally suggested by Winberg (1964).[155] Gardner (1971), reflecting on previously reported cases and a personal series, concluded that the clinical and pathologic similarities did not offset the differences of recorded modes of inheritance and age of onset.[161] He regarded it more appropriate to consider them separately, regarding juvenile nephronophthisis as a recessively transmitted disorder with onset in infancy and childhood and medullary cystic disease as a disorder with dominant mode of transmission and onset in adult years.

Pathologic Features

The affected kidneys are smaller than normal, with variable numbers of medullary cysts apparent on the cut surface. The cysts vary in size from microscopic to 1 cm and show a distinct predilection for the outer medulla near the corticomedullary junction.[157-159,165,166] The cortex of the kidney is commonly diminished, with an underlying reduction in both number and size of extant glomeruli with interstitial fibrosis. The medullary collecting ducts are cystically dilated or alternatively atrophic. The cysts are lined by flattened epithelium. Interstitial fibrosis and chronic inflammatory cells reflect a superimposed chronic pyelonephritis, which may obscure the underlying cystic disorder.[157-159]

Diagnosis requires differentiation of this medullary cystic disorder, with its characteristic clinical picture and familial history, from other renal cystic disorders, especially medullary sponge kidney and polycystic diseases.

Medullary Sponge Kidney

The original report of the cystic renal disorder ultimately known as medullary sponge kidney was presented as a description of the characteristic radiologic features by Lenarduzzi in 1939.[168] Ten years later, Cacchi and Ricci reported the pathologic and corresponding radiologic features of this disorder, coining the term *sponge kidney*.[169] The disorder is uncommon, and virtually all initial reports of this entity were found in the European literature. In 1960, Abeshouse and Abeshouse collected 131 previously reported cases and added 5 new cases.[172] Since this review, several reports have appeared in the literature.[173-189]

Medullary sponge kidney is of unknown cause and without evidence of genetic transmission.[172,183] It is most commonly observed in adults in the fourth to sixth decades, but it has been reported in young children.[172] There is a male preponderance.[172] Approximately 80% of cases are bilateral.[172] Most cases are discovered as incidental radiographic findings on IVP performed for unrelated reasons. Less frequently, patients have symptomatic urinary tract infections and lithiasis, both conditions that are apparently more frequent in patients with underlying medullary sponge kidney.[179,186] Associated disorders including renal tubular acidosis, hemihypertrophy, Ehlers-Danlos syndrome, and Sjögren's syndrome have been reported in some patients.[168,177,178,180-182,185,187,188] Radiologic findings characteristically include multiple minute renal calculi within the renal papillae observed on scout film and blush of the renal papillae with linear streaks identifying the dilated collecting tubules within the renal medulla (Fig. 1-20). However, these findings are not regarded as diagnostic.[168,173,175,189] The radiologic differential diagnosis includes medullary cystic disease and polycystic renal disease.[173,175,189]

This disorder is regarded as a developmental defect of the collecting tubules, which exhibit dilatation throughout their course in the renal papilla. The ostium of each tubule at the renal calyx is of normal diameter.[187] Osathanondh and Potter's initial microdissection studies prompted their classifying this disorder as type III with the prototype of this category, adult polycystic renal disease, an inherited form of cystic disease that is invariably bilateral.[87] The microdissection studies of Baert (1978), however, disclosed no cystic changes in the nephrons as previously reported in type III cystic lesions by Osathanondh and Potter.[87,187]

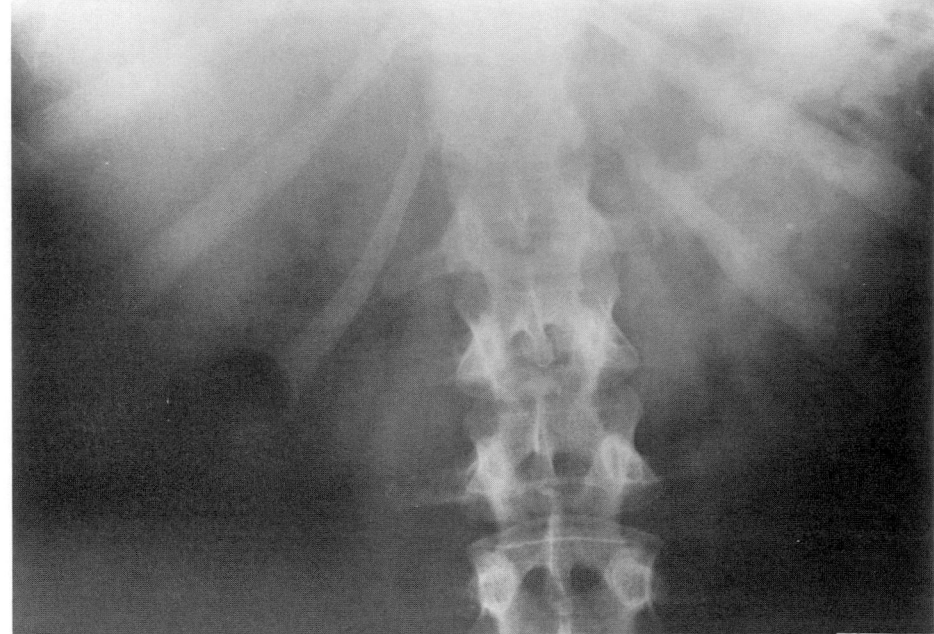

A

B

Figure 1-20   ***Medullary sponge kidney.*** *(A) Abdominal scout film shows multiple small calcifications in kidneys. (B) Intravenous urogram shows intracalyceal and intratubular calcification. Dilated (ectatic) collecting tubules are apparent in the renal papillae.*

Although no subsequent support has appeared in the literature, Vermooten (1951) has suggested that the cystic change in medullary sponge kidney may be due to uric acid crystal obstruction of the tubules.[170]

Pathologic Features

The cysts are multiple, small (1–5 mm), and limited to the renal medulla, to which they impart a spongy appearance.[169,171,183,184] The cysts are prevalent at the papillary tip. One or multiple papillae may be involved. Twenty percent of cases are unilateral.[172] The dilated tubules frequently contain microcalculi with associated changes of superimposed infection. Lithiasis may be evident within the calyceal system.

Microscopically typical are medullary cysts lined by flattened epithelium, commonly showing concretions within the lumen and inflammatory changes in the interstitium.

Diagnosis requires the synthesis of all available clinical, radiologic, and pathologic information. The disorder must be differentiated from medullary cystic disease.

Glomerulocystic Disease

Glomerulocystic disease is a rare nonhereditary form of renal cystic disease that had been observed exclusively in neonates and children until the recent report of this disorder in a 25-year-old man.[194] The majority of reported examples were discovered as incidental autopsy findings; however, in some instances, clinical evidence of progressive renal failure is recorded.[190-193] The cysts are found exclusively in the renal cortex and represent cystic dilatation of Bowman's capsule as determined histologically and confirmed by microdissection studies.[190,191] The lesion bears superficial resemblance to a Potter type IV renal cystic change, but the reported cases of glomerulocystic disease do not show evidence of distal urinary tract obstruction, a requisite feature of true type IV cystic disease.[88,194] Taxy and Filmer (1976) introduced the term *glomerulocystic disease.*[192]

The cause of glomerulocystic disease is unknown. In microdissection studies, Roos was unable to find cystic glomeruli attached to proximal tubules.[190] Baxter found both unattached and attached glomeruli.[191] Dosa and co-workers suggested that as the disease progresses, the increasing periglomerular fibrosis may contribute to proximal tubular atrophy and ultimate dissociation of the cystic glomerular structure from its previously attached proximal tubule.[194]

Characteristically, the cortices of both kidneys show innumerable cystic glomerular spaces, commonly with atrophic glomerular tufts attached to the wall. Periglomular fibrosis and tubular atrophy are the histologic features allowing the diagnosis. As the cysts range in size from microscopic to 3 mm, the affected kidney retains its reniform shape. No congenital anomalies of the lower urinary tract are associated with this form of renal cystic disease.

Multilocular Cyst and Benign Multilocular Cystic Nephroma

The relevant history of the renal disorders known as multilocular cyst and multilocular cystic nephroma is relatively brief but controversial. Originally regarded as a developmental defect, these lesions' similarities to Wilms' tumors with cystic change prompted some to reinterpret them as neoplasm – cystic variants of Wilms' tumors showing variable degrees of differentiation. The matter remains unsettled as judged by the pertinent literature of the past decade. Reflecting my opinion that the two lesions are distinct, they will be discussed separately, with the final judgment to be rendered only after more recorded experience clarifies the dilemma. Multilocular cystic nephroma is discussed in detail later in the chapter, in the section on neoplastic disorders.

Multilocular Cyst

In 1951, Powell and associates reported two cases of multilocular renal cysts and proposed a set of eight criteria for the diagnosis of this cystic lesion:[197]

1. Lesions are unilateral.
2. Lesions are solitary.
3. Lesions are multilocular.
4. Cysts do not communicate with the renal pelvis.
5. Loculi do not communicate with one another.
6. Loculi are lined by epithelium.
7. The interlocular septae are devoid of renal parenchyma.
8. Residual renal tissue, if present, should be normal.

Applying these criteria, the authors accepted only 13 examples of the 22 reported cases of multilocular renal cysts commencing with the first recorded case by Edmunds in 1892.[195–197]

Five years later, Boggs and Kimmelstiel (1956) reported two cases noting that only their second case fulfilled the criteria of Powell and associates (1951).[197,199] The first case contained "solid cords and tubules" within the interlocular septal walls, prompting the authors to modify the seventh criterion of Powell and associates and substitute an exclusion of cases with mature renal tissue.[199] These authors further interpreted the cords and tubules as evidence of the neoplastic nature of their case and "the entire group of so-called multilocular cysts of the kidney."[199] They abandoned the term *multilocular cyst,* renaming the lesion *benign multilocular cystic nephroma* (Fig. 1-21).

In the years following the studies of Powell and associates (1951) and Boggs and Kimmelstiel (1956), numerous case reports were published, all of which reflected the features of the lesions described by these two studies and were correspondingly divisible into two histogenetic schools, the developmental defect and the neoplastic interpretations.

Cases fulfilling the criteria for multilocular cyst of the kidney as proposed by Powell and associates are presented in Table 1-1. In spite of the uniform features of all cases listed in the table, there is no uniformity of reported diagnoses. The majority are appropriately called multilocular cysts, but some authors reported identical cases as benign multilocular cystic nephroma, multilocular cystic nephroma, or just cystic nephroma.[199,219,224] This inconsistent application of established criteria has served to complicate further the task of unraveling real histogenetic differences among these lesions, if indeed these differences exist.

Clinical Features

The ages of the patients with multilocular cysts of the kidney range from 8 months to 71 years.[197,219] Approximately half of these patients are less than 2 years of age, with a second age peak from 40 to 69 years (approximately 40% of cases). Patients most commonly present with a flank mass with or without hematuria. Flank pain and hypertension have been reported but are uncommon. One case of bilateral multilocular renal cysts has been reported in a 57-year-old woman.[220]

Radiologically, an avascular mass with calyceal distortion showing curvilinear blushes and irregular central vessels are suggestive but not diagnostic of this disorder.[209,210,214,218,220,221]

With the exception of the one patient with bilateral multilocular renal cysts,

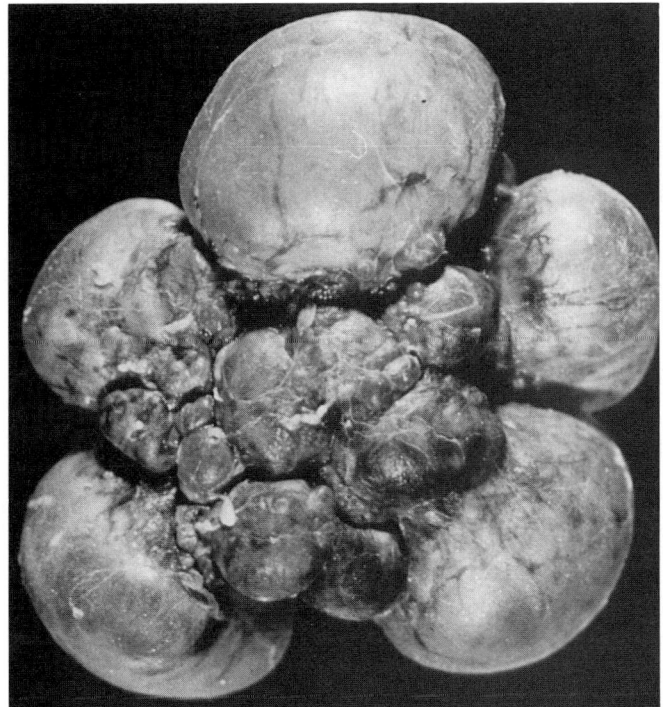

A

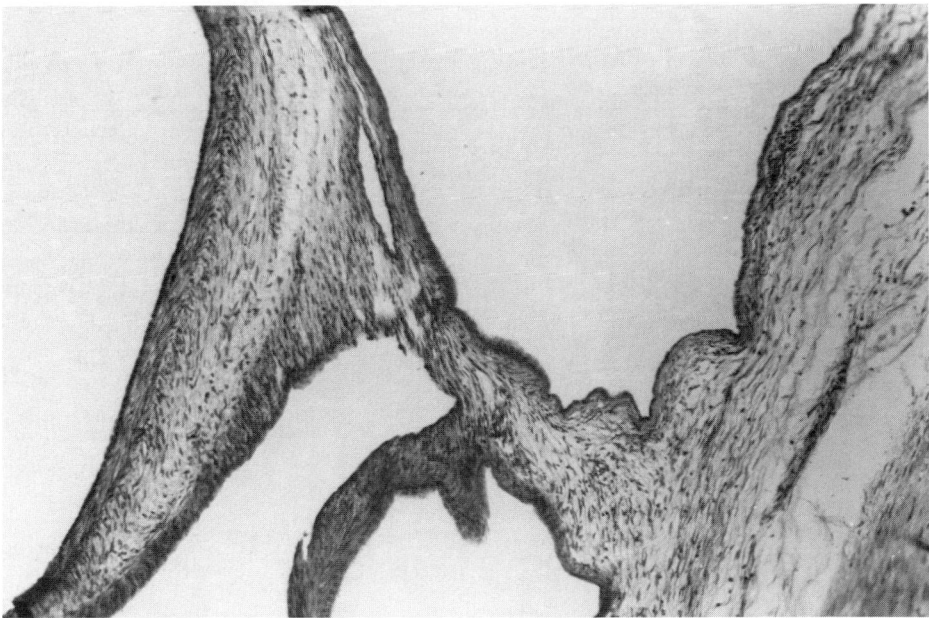

B

Figure 1-21   ***Benign multilocular cystic nephroma.*** *This rare example of bilateral multilocular cystic nephroma is associated with hypoplasia of the ureters and bladder. (A) Multilocular cyst. (B) The septae between the numerous cysts contain only fibrous tissue. There is no evidence of primitive glomerular or tubular structures. The stroma has no blastemal component.*

in whom renal functional impairment was observed, all other patients have been treated by nephrectomy, frequently with the preoperative diagnosis of renal malignancy.

Pathologic Features

The pathologic features of multilocular cystic kidneys conform to the diagnostic criteria set forth by Powell and associates (1951) as outlined above. The cyst loculi range in size from millimeters to multiple centimeters and are separated by thin septae. The multilocular cyst is separated from the remaining renal tissue by a fibrous capsule. The cysts contain clear yellow fluid. Calcification is occasionally reported in cyst walls. The remaining renal parenchyma is compressed around the outer capsule of the lesion.

Multilocular cystic disease of the kidney must be differentiated from multicystic dysplastic disease (refer to prior discussion in this chapter) and polycystic renal disease (bilateral, in contrast to the unilateral multilocular cystic kidney). Differentiation from multilocular cystic nephroma is discussed later in the chapter.

Pathogenesis

Multilocular cysts as defined by Powell and associates' criteria and exemplified by the clinical and pathologic features of the cases listed in Table 1-1 are regarded as developmental defects of unknown cause. There is no evidence of a genetic basis

Table 1-1   ***Cases of Multilocular Cyst of the Kidney Fulfilling the Criteria of Powell and Associates (1951)***

Author	Year	No. of Cases	Author's Diagnosis
Powell et al[197]	1951	2	Multilocular cyst of kidney
Frazier[198]	1951	1	Multilocular cyst of kidney
Boggs, Kimmelstiel[199]	1956	1	Benign multilocular cystic nephroma*
Attwood, Grieve[200]	1958	1	Multilocular cyst of kidney
Dainko et al[204]	1963	1	Multilocular cyst of kidney
Davides et al[214]	1976	1	Multilocular cyst of kidney
Baldauf, Shultz[215]	1976	3	Multilocular cyst of kidney
Epstein et al[218]	1978	2	Multilocular cyst of kidney
Fobi et al[219]	1979	2	Multilocular cyst of kidney†
Fobi et al[219]	1979	3	Multilocular cystic nephroma†
Geller et al[220]	1979	1 (bilateral)	Multilocular cyst of kidney (bilateral)
Hunt et al[221]	1979	1	Multilocular cyst of kidney
Abt et al[224]	1979	1	Cystic nephroma‡

* Boggs and Kimmelstiel (1956) postulated that all multilocular cysts, including those fulfilling Powell and associates' criteria as well as those showing primitive tubules in intracyst septae, were to be regarded as a neoplastic, benign cystic counterpart of nephroblastoma.

† Fobi et al (1979) provide no explanation as to why, among the five cases reported, all of which fulfilled Powell's criteria, three were designated as multilocular cystic nephroma and two were diagnosed as multilocular cyst of kidney.

‡ Abt et al (1979) presented a case fulfilling Powell's criteria without reference to these criteria. Instead, they referred to the proposed criteria of histogenesis and the name introduced by Boggs and Kimmelstiel (1956), which they adopted, naming their multilocular cyst *cystic nephroma.*

of this renal cystic disorder. Arey regards this lesion as a renal hamartoma.[201] The microdissection studies of Osathanondh and Potter were interpreted as showing a defect in the ampullary portion of the collecting duct with decreased branching and cystic terminal ends, prompting a classification of this lesion as type II cystic disease.[89]

Simple Cysts

Simple cysts are undoubtedly the most common cystic lesions occurring in the kidney. The vast majority are clinically insignificant and are detected as incidental findings at autopsy. Their frequency increases with age, with only rare examples reported in children. There is no sex predilection. Their occurrence in the majority of patients older than 50 years, as observed at autopsy, coupled with their infrequency in younger age groups, has been regarded as supportive of their acquired nature.[230,231,233] Hepler (1930), citing unsuccessful previous attempts to produce renal cysts by circumferential ligature of a renal papilla, produced experimental renal cysts by concurrent vascular compromise and tubular obstruction.[228] The application of these findings to the pathogenesis of simple cysts was based on the prevalence of these cysts in older patients who exhibit a significant frequency of tubulo-interstitial disease and intrarenal vascular disease. Since Hepler's report, little attention has been given to the question of pathogenesis of these cysts and the matter remains unsettled.

These cysts were previously called "serous cysts" or "solitary cysts."[228] In the more recent literature, they have been generally referred to as *simple cysts,* a term introduced by Braasch and Hendrick (1944), recognizing that most are not solitary.[230] Clarke and co-workers (1956) reported that the cyst fluid is a transudate with electrolyte concentration similar to serum levels.[234] Cyst fluid levels of albumin and globulins were below serum levels.

Clinical Features

Simple cysts most commonly come to clinical attention as incidental radiologic findings. Rarely, associated hypertension or polycythemia has been reported.[242] Approximately 25 cases of infected simple cysts have been reported.[229,235,242] This complication shows a significant predilection for young women (92%), with a mean age of 27 years.[242] For unknown reasons, 73% of cases involve the right kidney. Patients present with fever and flank pain; urinalysis shows pyuria in the majority of cases. Culture of cyst contents is positive in most cases, with *Escherichia coli* the most frequent organism detected.

Pathologic Features

Grossly, the cysts are commonly located in the subcapsular location, with a predilection for the lower pole, where they produce a focal distortion of the cortical surface (Fig. 1-22). Alternatively, those located in the medulla may distort the calyceal configuration by compression. They are commonly multiple and vary in size from a few millimeters to several centimeters. The precise site of origin of the largest examples is impossible to determine. These unilocular cysts compress the adjacent renal parenchyma.

Microscopically, they are lined by a flat epithelium overlying a thin fibrous wall. Atrophy of the adjacent glomeruli and tubules is variable and proportional

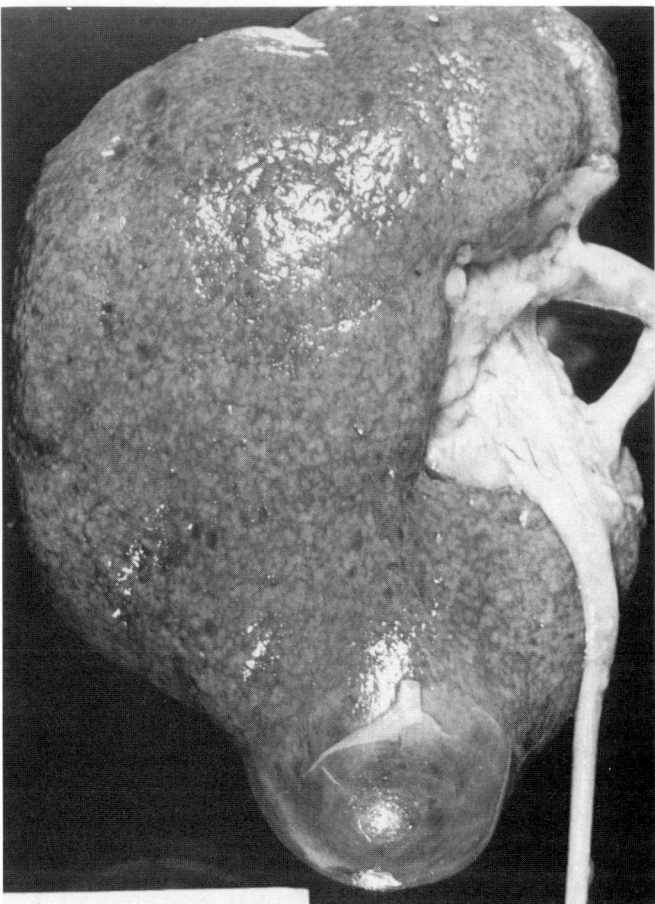

Figure 1-22   *Simple (retention) cyst. The single thin-walled cyst at the lower
pole contains clear serous fluid. The cortical surface elsewhere
shows a fine granularity characteristic of benign nephrosclerosis.*

to the size of the cyst. Calcification in the cyst wall occurs but is uncommon in the
absence of associated neoplasm.

The association of renal malignancies with cysts of the kidney has been the
subject of considerable attention, especially in the radiologic literature, reflecting the difficulty and potentially disastrous results of inaccurately differentiating
these two lesions. The relationship of these two renal disorders is best put into
perspective by reference to the classification suggested by Gibson (1954), who
proposed four possible interrelationships of a renal neoplasm and a cyst within
the same kidney:[232]

1. Widely separated and unrelated in origin
2. Origin of cyst within the tumor
3. Origin of tumor within the cyst
4. Occurrence of cyst distal to tumor

The most commonly observed relationship of cyst and tumor is origin of a cyst
within the tumor. More accurately, this reflects cystic degeneration due to necrosis of the tumor. Examples of number 1 above are uncommon, but the independent occurrence of cyst and tumor is not surprising considering the predilec-

tion of both diseases for the same age group (*i.e.,* 50 years and older). Occurrence of the cyst distal to the tumor, possibly recapitulating the combined vascular and ductal compromise created experimentally by Hepler, is rare in my personal experience and in the literature.[236] Neoplasms taking origin from the cyst wall are distinctly rare, with less than 20 cases recorded.[236-241]

Acquired Cysts in Renal Dialysis Patients

In 1977, Dunnill and co-workers described the development of bilateral renal cystic disease in 14 of 30 patients on long-term hemodialysis.[244] They further reported that six of the patients were observed to have papillary neoplasms associated with the cysts, one example giving origin to metastatic carcinoma and resulting in the death of the patient.[244] These two complications, acquired renal cysts and occasional associated epithelial neoplasms, have since been repeatedly confirmed by others.[243,245,247-249] Indeed, the interest in the histogenesis and clinical aspects of the associated neoplasms has partially eclipsed interest in the origin and histogenesis of these cysts (which remains unresolved).

These acquired cysts, which are most commonly but not invariably bilateral, have been observed in patients on renal dialysis for as short a period as 4 months, with a mean duration of 3.4 years as reported by Dunnill and colleagues.[244] More recently, Ishikawa and associates (1980) reported a frequency of renal cysts of 43.5% in patients on dialysis less than 3 years, rising to 79.3% in a group on dialysis longer than 3 years.[248] Patients present with hematuria, a complication of hemorrhage into the cysts.

The affected kidneys contain multiple cysts varying in size from microscopic to 2 cm. In some specimens the extent of cyst formation virtually replaces all renal parenchyma. Cortical cysts are more common than medullary cysts, but the reverse distribution has been observed.[244] Kidney size may be reduced or modestly enlarged, the latter being more common in patients on dialysis longer than 3 years.[248]

Microscopically, the cysts are most commonly lined by a flattened epithelium. However, in specimens harboring associated neoplasms as noted above, foci of hyperplasia, commonly in papillary configuration, are observed in scattered cysts. Cytologic atypia is observed in such proliferations.[247] The associated neoplasms are commonly multiple, and they range from cytologically benign "adenomas" to overtly malignant renal cell carcinomas with histologic evidence of invasion of the adjacent renal parenchyma and the ultimate capacity to metastasize.[244,247-249]

The etiology and pathogenesis of these acquired cysts are unknown. Dunnill and co-workers (1977) raised the possibility that the oxalate crystals commonly observed within the cysts were involved by causing tubule obstruction.[244] The reason why such kidneys with dialysis-related cysts are at significantly greater risk of neoplasia is also unknown.[244,247,249]

Endometriosis

Renal endometriosis is rare, with only eight recorded cases (Table 1-2).[250-257] The reported patients range in age from 20–48 years; however, six of the eight patients were in the fifth decade. Six of the recorded cases presented with flank

Table 1-2　　　*Reports of Renal Endometriosis by Characteristics and Patient's Age*

Author	Year	Age of Patient	Side	Clinical Presentation	Hematuria	Endometriosis Elsewhere
Marshall[250]	1943	40	L	Flank pain, mass	−†	None
Maslow, Learner[251]	1950	20	R	Hematuria	+	None
Fruhling, Blum[252]	1951	42	*	Flank pain	+	
Fruhling et al[253]	1952	22		Flank pain		
Kamaev, Vigorskii[254]	1963	46	R			
Miles, Falconer[255]	1969	43	R	Hematuria	+	Ovary
Hajdu, Koss[256]	1970	48	L	Asymptomatic, incidental findings at autopsy		
Bazaz-Malik et al[257]	1980	40	R	Flank pain, mass	−	None

* Blank spaces denote lack of information.
† + denotes presence of hematuria; − denotes absence.

pain, a palpable mass, or hematuria. The endometriotic lesions of the kidney were isolated lesions in all cases with the exception of the patient reported by Miles and Falconer (1969), who previously had ovarian endometriosis.[255] This is in contrast to the reported cases of ureteral and vesicle endometriosis, which are commonly accompanied by more widespread pelvic endometriosis (refer to discussions of endometriosis in Chaps. 3 and 4).

The pathogenesis of renal endometriosis remains unsettled. The contending theories include Müllerian metaplasia, migration of endometrium, and embryonic nests resulting from displaced Müllerian tissue within the urogenital ridge.[251,255,257] Implantation during prior surgery is a possibility, albeit remote, in only one of the reported cases of renal endometriosis.[255]

With the exception of one case found incidentally at autopsy, the diagnosis of renal endometriosis was made only after histologic examination of the hemorrhagic nodules and cysts within the nephrectomy specimens of the other cases. Endometrial glands within typical stroma accompanied by old and recent hemorrhage are the diagnostic features of endometriosis in all locations.

Inflammatory Disorders

Renal Tuberculosis

Virtually all of our knowledge about the pathology and natural history of tuberculous renal disease was recorded in the first half of the 20th century, prior to the introduction of effective chemotherapy.[252-262] Currently, the principal challenge of tuberculosis lies not in the therapy of this disease but in its clinical diagnosis. Previously undiagnosed cases of tuberculosis are still discovered at the time of autopsy. The prevalance of tuberculosis continues to be higher in urban areas than in rural sections of the United States.[267] The low frequency of renal tuberculosis currently experienced is in contrast to the 1930s, when 30% of renal lesions in surgical specimens were of a tuberculous etiology.[258]

Prior to the advent of effective nonsurgical therapy of tuberculous infections, renal tuberculosis was regarded as an inexorably progressive infection, ultimately leading to destruction of the entire organ. Renal infection accompanied clinically known pulmonary involvement, either concurrently or years after apparent resolution of the lung lesions. Approximately 75% of affected patients were young or middle-aged adults (20 – 49 years).[259,267] Most studies found both renal and pulmonary tuberculosis to be more frequent in males. A significant number of patients in whom acid-fast organisms were detected in the urine by smear or guinea pig inoculation were asymptomatic.[261] However, most had clinical evidence of frequency, dysuria, or hematuria. Hypertension attributable to the tuberculous renal involvement is common, and in the majority of cases it is cured by the nephrectomy procedure.

The majority of cases evidenced bilateral renal involvement, but frequently the extent of the renal infection in one kidney far exceeded that of the opposite, and surgical excision of enlarged nonfunctioning tuberculous kidneys became a standard form of therapy. This disparity of renal involvement raised the question of possible spontaneous resolution of some tuberculous infections, a finding not documented until 1926 by Medlar and later confirmed by Baggenstoss and Greene (1941).[258,262] These investigators studied small fibrotic nodules in the kidneys of autopsied patients with active tuberculosis and interpreted them as "burned-out" granulomas.[262] The distribution of these healed granulomas showed the same strong predilection for cortical locations (80%) as observed in early active tuberculous lesions of the kidney.[258,262]

Further studies of renal tuberculosis described two types of renal lesions, fundamentally reflecting the extremes of the spectrum of the lesions produced in the kidney. The earliest lesions were virtually limited to the cortex and took the form of miliary granulomas up to a few millimeters in size.[258,260,265] The hematogenous route of infection, most frequently from pulmonary lesions, was indicated by the prevalance of glomerular involvement in the apparent absence of medullary and tubular infection. Some of these lesions apparently underwent spontaneous arrest and produced fibrous scars as noted above.

Alternatively, others progressed and ultimately produced often multiple and confluent tuberculous abscess cavities that involved both cortex and medulla (Fig. 1-23). Not uncommonly, these lesions ruptured into the calyceal system. Tuberculous involvement of the lower urinary tract, especially the bladder, is common.

Microscopically, the typical caseating granulomas with Langhans' giant cells characteristic of tuberculosis are the diagnostic features. Ziehl-Neelsen stain detects the acid-fast bacilli within the granulomas. The larger cavitating lesions are accompanied by a correspondingly greater structural destruction of the renal parenchyma with marked calyceal distortion and ulceration of the renal pelvic urothelium.

Tuberculosis of the kidney can bear a striking resemblance to renal cell carcinoma, xanthogranulomatous pyelonephritis, and malakoplakia involving the kidney. These non-neoplastic and neoplastic disorders are distinguished histologically (refer to the discussions of these disorders, later in this chapter).

Clinical suspicion is of paramount importance in the diagnosis of renal tuberculosis. Historical evidence of current or past pulmonary tuberculosis associated with local renal symptoms and signs of dysuria, with or without flank plain and hematuria, is sufficiently suggestive to warrant radiologic evaluation. The

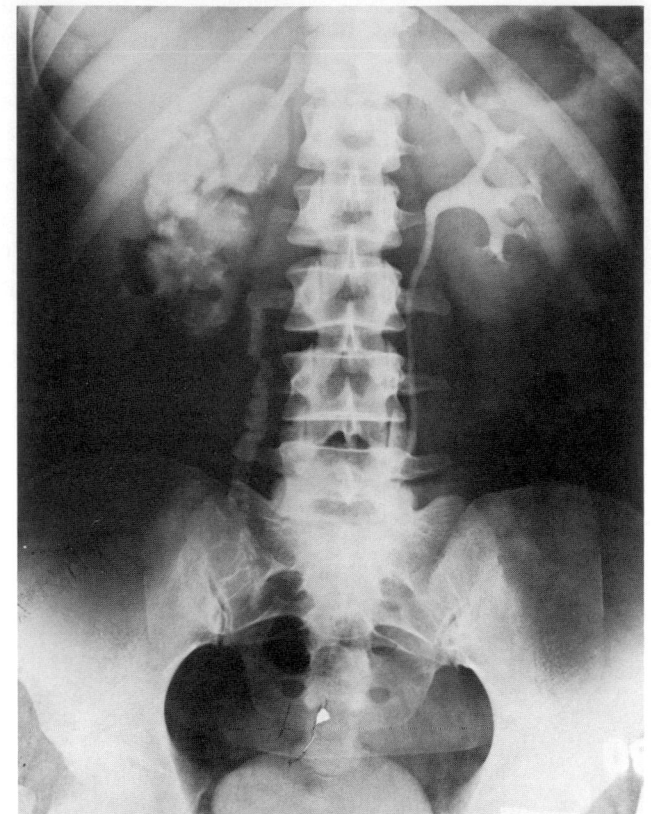

A

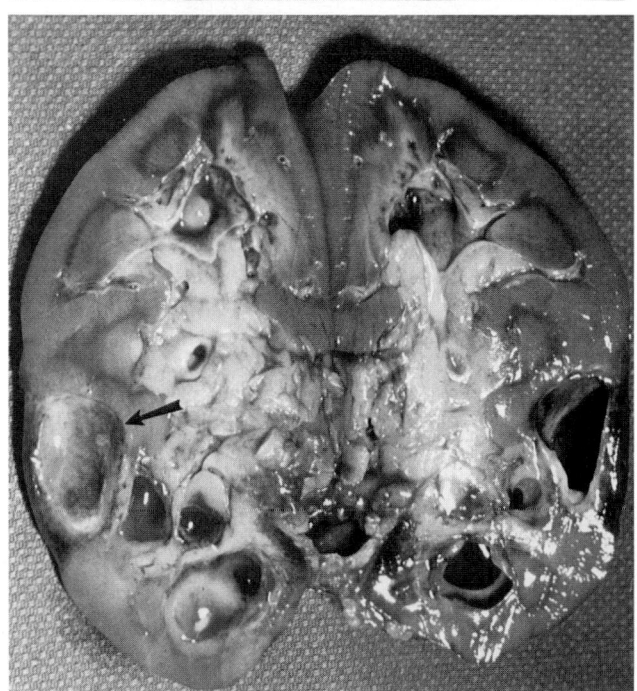

B

Figure 1-23 **Tuberculosis.** (A) *Abdominal scout film shows widespread calcification throughout right kidney and ureter. A diffuse lobular form of calcification is characteristic of the caseous form of renal tuberculosis. (B) The cut surface of the kidney reveals multiple tuberculous cavities (arrow) with necrosis and hemorrhage in the affected regions of the kidneys.*

most common findings on IVP reflect the morphologic lesions described above and include calyceal dilatation and distortion, parenchymal calcification, poor concentration on nephrogram phase, cavitation, and nonvisualization.[267]

Current therapy includes chemotherapy regimens of streptomycin, isoniazid, and para-aminosalicylate sodium (PAS) or rifampin, isoniazid, and ethambutol.[264,266] Surgical excision of an enlarged, nonfunctioning tuberculous kidney is still advocated by some because the frequency of delayed complications of flank sinuses and hypertension is greater in the group of patients who receive only chemotherapy.

Pyelonephritis

Few renal disorders have provided the diagnostic and therapeutic challenge of pyelonephritis. Furthermore, none rivals the complexity of the etiologic and pathogenetic problems posed by this disease. Readers are referred to more comprehensive available texts, monographs and reviews of this renal inflammatory disorder that supplement the presentation herein.[268,291-193]

Clinical Features

Clinically, pyelonephritis is encountered in the acute and chronic forms, the latter being further subclassified depending on whether there is associated lower urinary tract obstruction. Pyelonephritis is encountered in all age groups but with well-recognized peak ages including (1) infancy, especially in girls; (2) the childbearing years for women; and (3) the elderly, especially men with prostatism. The relatively short urethra in infant girls, the contribution of urinary tract obstruction produced on an intermittent basis by the enlarging uterus during pregnancy, and the chronic obstruction resulting from prostatic hyperplasia all directly contribute to the increased risk of the indicated groups.[292] These factors directly or indirectly contribute to the relative risk of bacterial infection of the urinary tract. Additional factors increasing the risk of urinary tract infection are instrumentation of the urinary tract and vesicoureteral reflux, each of which contributes to introduction of bacteria into the bladder and retrograde spread of bacteria to the ureters, renal pelvis, and ultimately the renal parenchyma.

Acute pyelonephritis presents characteristically with fever, chills, flank pain, and malaise.[272] Concurrent bladder infection is common as evidenced by dysuria and urgency. Examination of the urine discloses bacteriuria and pyuria. *E. coli* is the bacterial agent in the vast majority of initial infections, with relatively higher frequencies of *Proteus, Pseudomonas,* and *Klebsiella* encountered in recurrent and chronic pyelonephritic attacks.[269,273,276,281,292] Appropriate antibiotic treatment following culture and sensitivity testing is successful in sterilizing the urine in the majority of cases. Clinical studies continue to report less than uniform success in eradicating bacteria from the urine on follow-up examination.[282,287] Apparent perpetuation of the infection and compromise of renal function in a small percentage of patients is observed.[282,287] Clinically symptomatic recurrences are uncommon, but the frequency of clinically asymptomatic recurrences is unknown.

Chronic pyelonephritis most frequently presents insidiously with progressive renal failure, not uncommonly with associated hypertension. Less frequently, the symptomatology characteristic of acute pyelonephritis is observed.

A history of prior urinary tract infections may be recorded. Bacteriuria and pyuria are again encountered. Radiologic examination of the upper collecting system demonstrating calyceal contraction and deformity, most commonly unilateral, strongly support the diagnosis of chronic pyelonephritis.[271]

Pathogenesis

The pathogenesis of pyelonephritis has been the focus of enormous clinical and experimental research, only a brief outline of which is possible here.[270,274,276-279,281,283-290]

There is general agreement that the ascending route of infection underlies cases of acute pyelonephritis.[270,292] Conditions contributing to contamination of bladder urine include age and sex (*e.g.,* short urethra in young infant girls), instrumentation, poor personal hygiene, and undoubtedly other factors.[292] The most commonly involved *E. coli* serotypes reflect the bacterial population in the colon contents.[274,276] Contributing to the establishment of contaminated bladder urine are obstructive lesions of the urethra (*i.e.,* valve obstruction, strictures, and prostatic hyperplasia). Vesicoureteral reflux, observed in a significant number of young girls with urinary tract infection, further contributes to the retrograde spread of bacteria from the bladder to the kidney.[284,287] There has been a recent discovery that bacterial fimbriae in *E. coli* organisms assist the bacteria in adhering to the surface of urothelium, further contributing to establishment of infection and possibly retrograde ureteral spread.[288-291]

Chronic obstructive pyelonephritis, far exceeding the nonobstructive type in frequency, results from bacterial infection in a progressive manner, attributable to the persistent influence of the urinary tract obstruction.[268,293] The portal of entry and retrograde spread to the kidney are influenced by the same factors as noted under acute pyelonephritis. The pathogenesis of the less frequent examples of nonobstructive cases of chronic pyelonephritis is less well understood. The detection of asymptomatic bacteriuria in young girls, some of whom have radiologic evidence of established vesicoureteral reflux and established renal scars, suggests that in combination with persisting reflux, the renal damage may also continue.[277,283,284,287] The vesicoureteral reflux may contribute both to the retrograde access of bacteria to the calyceal system and also to increased intracalyceal pressure. The increased intracalyceal pressure in turn results in pyelotubular backflow, especially in areas of established medullary scars and in the compound papillae found in the kidney poles.[286,292,293] The capacity of sterile urine reflux to produce renal scars has not been demonstrated. The detection of bacterial antigens in the pyelonephritic scars of patients with sterile urine and without history of previous urinary tract infection was not confirmed in a similar subsequent study.[278,283] The perpetuation of renal scar formation appears not to be the result of possible immunologic injury resulting from persistence of bacterial antigenic substances. Continued scar structural injury of the kidney results most probably from recurrent subclinical urinary tract infections.

Pathologic Features

Acute Pyelonephritis

As observed at the time of autopsy, the typical gross features of acute pyelonephritis include punctate abscesses present on both the cortical and cut surfaces of the kidney, with an apparent predilection for the cortex (Fig. 1-24). These abscesses are well delineated and outlined by a thin red margin corresponding to

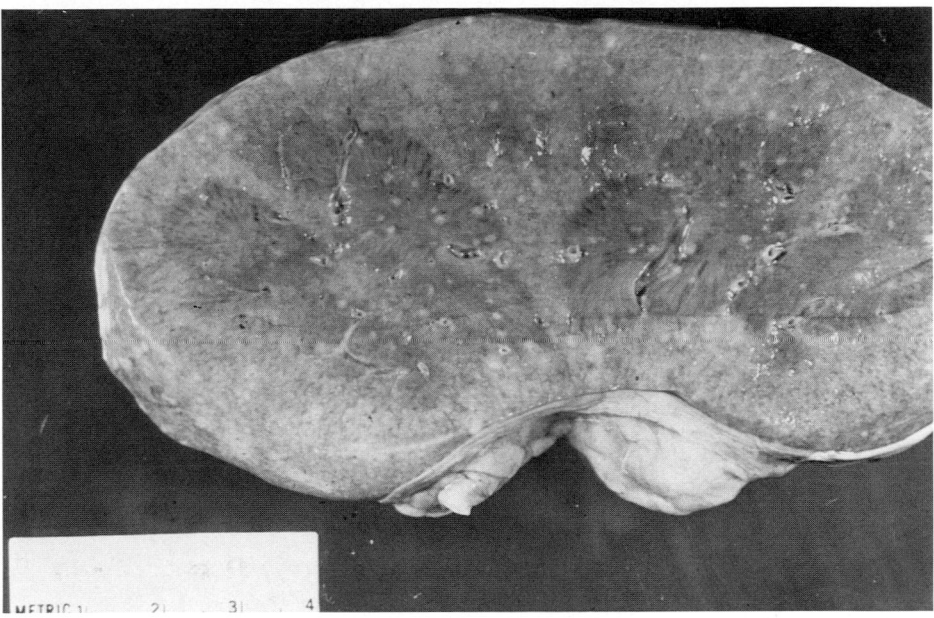

Figure 1-24 *Acute pyelonephritis. The cut surface of the kidney reveals numerous small abscesses in the cortex and medulla.*

marginal vascular dilatation. The number of such abscesses is highly variable and correlates roughly with the extent of swelling and corresponding renal enlargement. Yellow-white linear streaks reflecting medullary tubular segments filled with pus may be apparent. The urothelial mucosa of the calyceal system commonly shows patchy hyperemia. The urine in the collecting system is cloudy, reflecting the bacteriuria.

Microscopically, the abscesses are characterized by innumerable neutrophils with fewer lymphocytes in foci of parenchymal destruction, the completeness of which is variable and correlated with abscess size. The interstitium in areas adjacent to the abscesses is edematous and has scattered neutrophils (Fig. 1-25). The medulla contains tubules, frequently clustered, filled with innumerable neutrophils. Characteristic of acute pyelonephritis is the patchy distribution of the intense inflammatory foci with intervening areas of normal renal parenchyma. The calyceal and pelvic urothelium shows acute inflammation in a patchy distribution, occasionally with mucosal ulceration.

Chronic Pyelonephritis

The cardinal gross features of chronic pyelonephritis are the patchy cortical scars related to distorted and enlarged subjacent calyces. The parenchymal loss between the scar and the distorted calyx is evident and is accompanied by variably complete loss of an identified corticomedullary junction (Fig. 1-26). The reduction in kidney size is related to the extent and number of cortical scars and dilated calyces, which in turn reflect the severity of the inflammatory destruction of the kidney (Fig. 1-27). Unilateral involvement is typical and in this context can produce kidneys among the smallest encountered at the autopsy table. Focal hyperemia and mucosal ulcerations are common in the calyceal urothelium. These findings are the rule when chronic pyelonephritis is associated with calculi.

The patchy distribution of the gross scars correlates with the microscopic

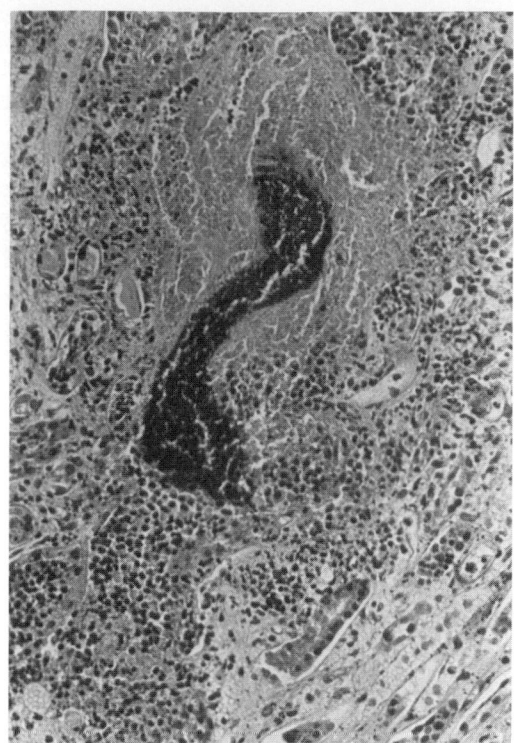

Figure 1-25   *Acute pyelonephritis. An abscess with local tubular destruction is surrounded by numerous acute inflammatory cells in the medullary interstitium and in adjacent renal tubular segments.*

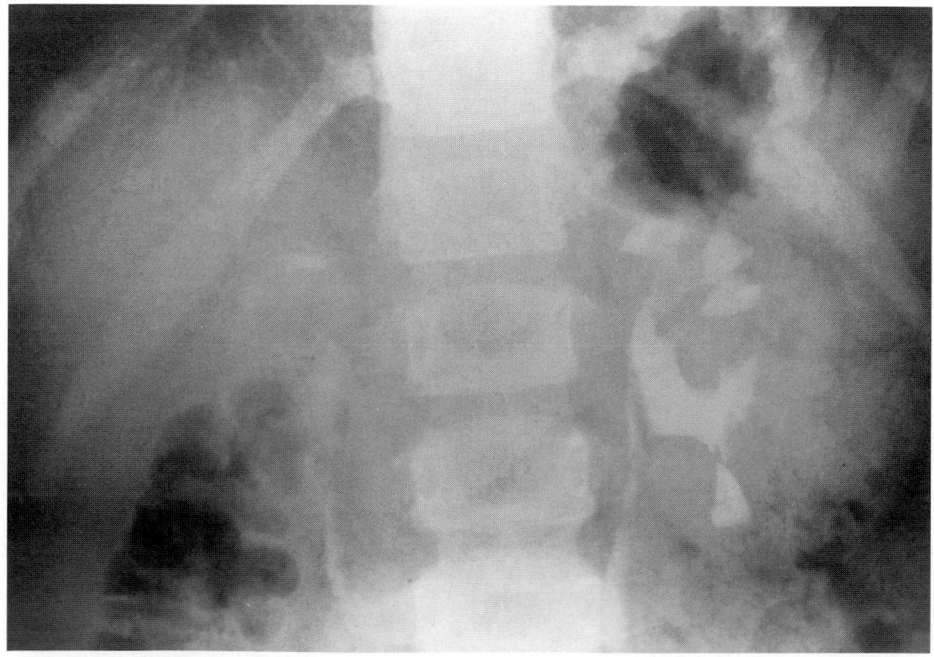

Figure 1-26   *Chronic pyelonephritis. Cortical loss and calyceal clubbing are characteristic.*

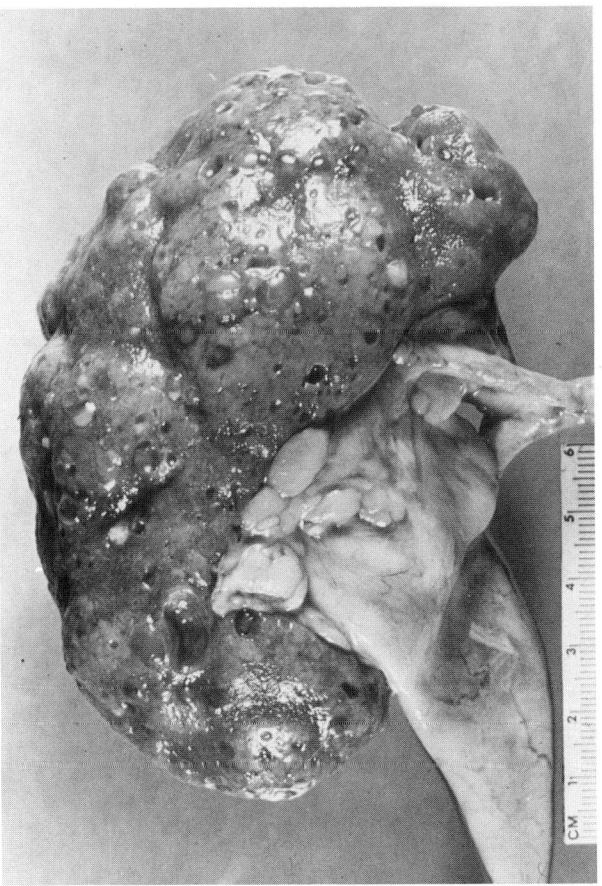

Figure 1-27   *Chronic pyelonephritis. The cortical surface of this small kidney contains numerous irregular linear and confluent depressions resulting from inflammatory destruction of underlying parenchyma.*

distribution of interstitial fibrosis, with nephron atrophy and destruction and periglomerular and perivascular fibrosis. A variably dense infiltrate of chronic inflammatory cells with scattered neutrophils and eosinophils is present (Fig. 1-28). The changes are most pronounced in the region judged to be the remnant of the inner cortex and outer medulla. In the areas of greatest destruction, landmarks identifying cortex and medulla are largely obliterated. In this background are dilated tubular segments with atrophic epithelium and eosinophilic casts, traditionally called "thryoidization" of the kidney. The calyceal mucosa characteristically contains an intense lymphocytic infiltrate, frequently with lymphoid aggregates showing germinal centers (Fig. 1-29). Urothelial atrophy, hyperplasia, prominence of Brunn's epithelial nests, and pyelitis cystica are typical changes within the affected calyces.

Differential Diagnosis

The gross and histologic picture of acute pyelonephritis, encountered most frequently at autopsy and described above, is characteristic and poses little diagnostic challenge. The frequency of these findings at autopsy in patients without

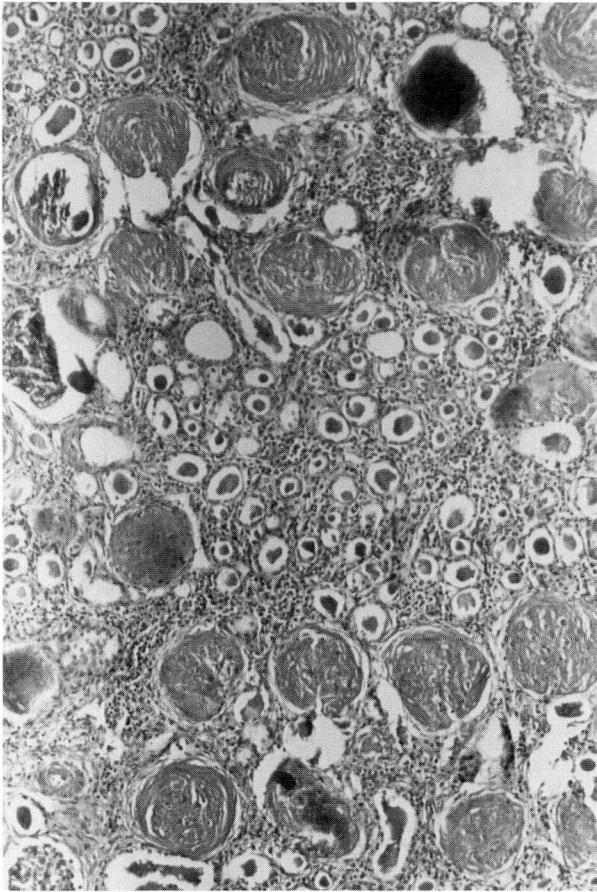

Figure 1-28   *Chronic pyelonephritis. Numerous lymphocytes infiltrate the renal parenchyma between atrophic tubules (containing proteinaceous secretions) and many fibrotic remnants of glomeruli.*

clinical evidence of acute pyelonephritis is not rare and raises the question of the true frequency of apparent clinically asymptomatic acute pyelonephritis. The answer to this is unknown, but most probably the majority of such cases encountered at autopsy reflect undetected terminal renal infection in the background of systemic disease, commonly neoplastic in my experience.

The morphologic features of chronic pyelonephritis as outlined above are far from specific and can be the result of numerous diverse etiologic factors including bacteria, ischemia, various drugs, radiation, urinary tract infection, and factors secondary to papillary necrosis of analgesic etiology.[268,275,280,285,292,293] All of these factors can produce essentially identical gross and especially histologic changes that are termed "chronic interstitial nephritis." The burden of responsibility of making an accurate diagnosis requires evaluation of the morphologic features and an investigation of all clinically relevant information to identify the specific etiologic agent(s).

Differentiating unilateral renal hypoplasia and chronic pyelonephritis can pose a diagnostic challenge on occasion (refer to the discussion of renal hypoplasia, earlier in this chapter).

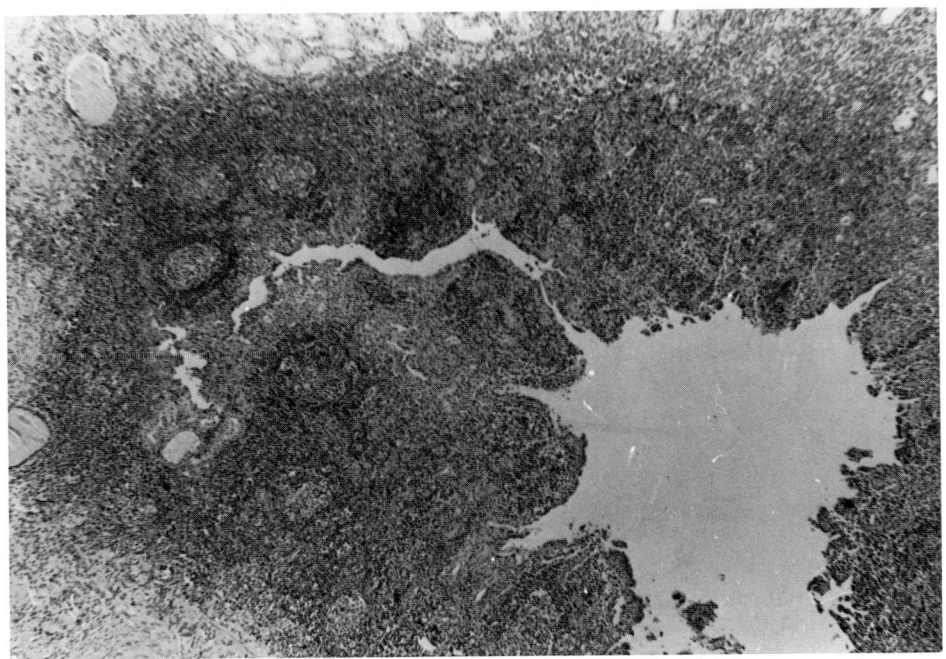

Figure 1-29 **Chronic pyelonephritis.** *A dense lymphocytic infiltrate, focally organized in lymphoid follicles, is present beneath the pelvic urothelium.*

Papillary Necrosis

Although recognized long before 1950, especially in diabetics developing pyelonephritis, papillary necrosis has dramatically increased in frequency in the past 3 decades.[294] This increased frequency was originally reported by Zollinger and Spuhler (1950), who recorded a high intake of the analgesic phenacetin among a group of patients with papillary necrosis.[295] This observation has been confirmed in numerous subsequent studies from many parts of the world.[292,300,302,304] Other analgesics including aspirin have been implicated in more recent studies.[292] In addition to an increased risk of papillary necrosis associated with pyelonephritis, especially among diabetics, recorded cases associated with systemic vasculitis, sickle-cell disease, and recently Wegener's granulomatosis have appeared in the literature.[297,299,303,305,307]

Papillary necrosis is most commonly observed in women of late middle-age but has been observed at all ages in both sexes.[292,307] Varying degrees of azotemia and hypertension are present at initial diagnosis. Uncommonly, colic may indicate the sloughing of the necrotic papillae with ureteral obstruction. The diagnosis has been made on histologic examination of the urinary sediment, which may contain fragments of the necrotic papillae.

Radiologic examination discloses calyceal irregularity, extravasation of contrast material from mid-calyx into a cleavage plane of completely or incompletely sloughed papillae, ring shadows around sloughed papillae within the calyx, and calyceal clubbing (Fig. 1-30 *A* and *B*).[296,306]

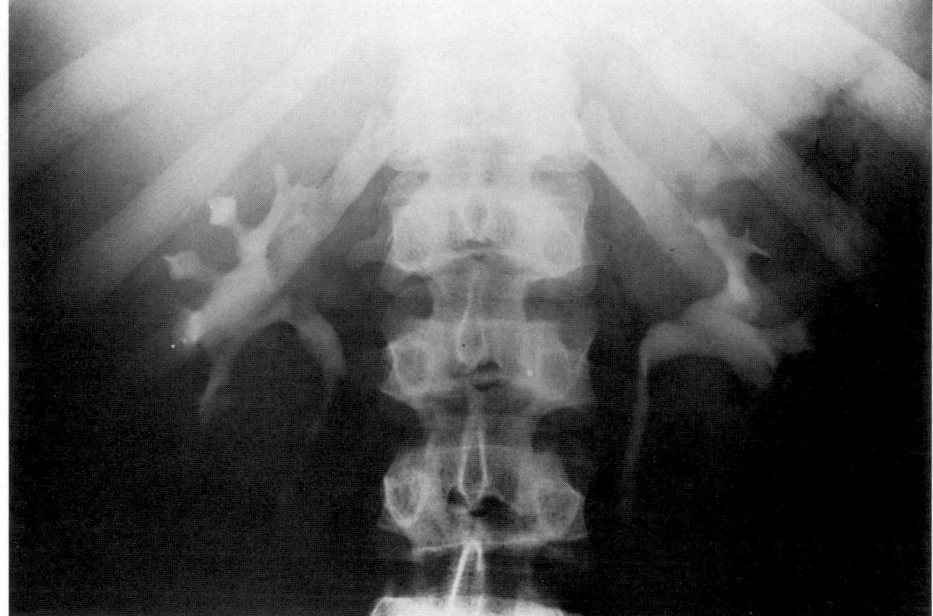

A

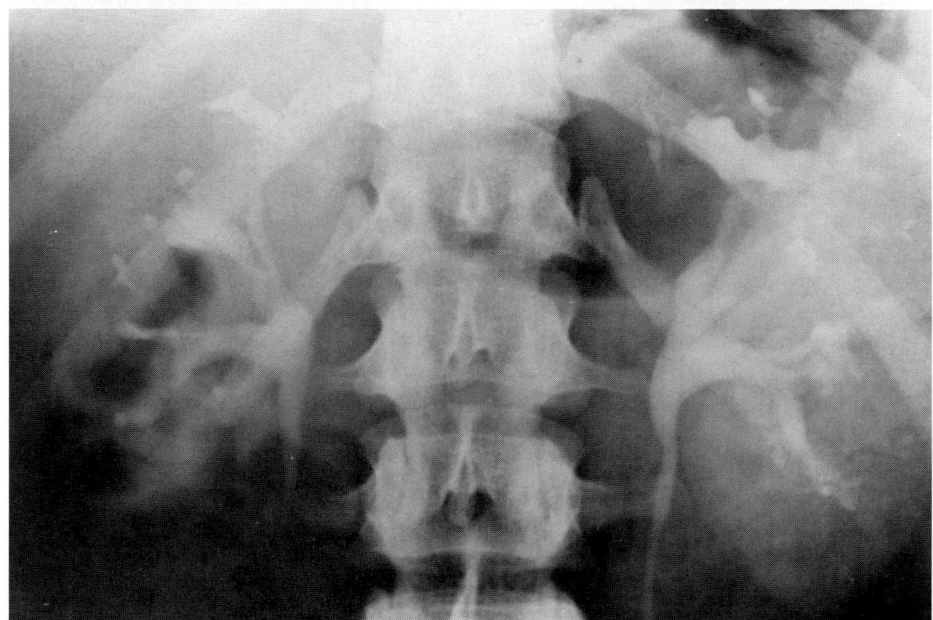

B

Figure 1-30   ***(A and B) Papillary necrosis.*** *Calyceal blunting with clefts of contrast material in mid-calyx cleavage plane of incompletely sloughed papillae.*

Pathologic Features

The pathologic features of papillary necrosis vary with the extent of renal involvement. Necrosis may be patchy, as when associated with pyelonephritis, or diffuse. Pathologic features also vary with the stage of development.[301] Burry has described three stages of papillary necrosis, each with characteristic gross and microscopic features.[301] In the early phase, the involved papillae are normal in size

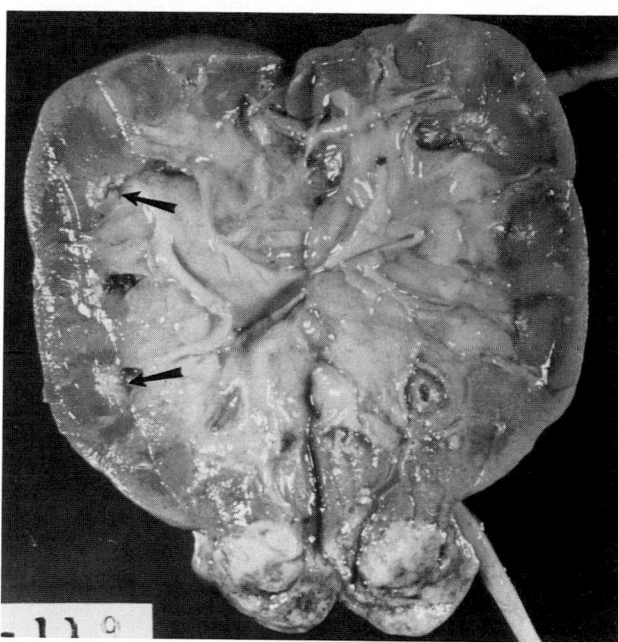

Figure 1-31 *Papillary necrosis. The cut surface of the kidney shows multiple papillae with granular, pale tips (arrows). An incidental renal cell carcinoma is present in the inferior pole of the kidney.*

and show minimal changes in color. As the duration increases, the renal papillae shrink and appear dark red – brown. Still later in phase of total papillary necrosis, the structure is pale, reduced in size, and may show focal calcification (Fig. 1-31). The medullary pyramid may slough and lie free in the calyx, with a rough cleavage plain apparent at the point of origin. The overlying cortex, frequently initially swollen, later shows loss of parenchyma, which microscopically corresponds to tubular atrophy and interstitial fibrosis.

Microscopically, the early stage shows interstitial edema and thickening of both tubular and vascular basement membranes. Foci of tubular necrosis with associated neutrophil infiltrate and calcific stippling is common. Later, the extent of coagulative necrosis of the tubular epithelium becomes more widespread, ultimately including all tubules within the affected renal pyramid. The infarcted pyramid is well outlined by a wide band of neutrophils at the outer limit of the infarcted area, with few neutrophils infiltrating the area of infarction, which now appears as a virtually acellular structure with ghostlike structures of necrotic tubules (Fig. 1-32). The overlying cortex, as previously noted, shows variable tubular atrophy and interstitial edema and fibrosis.

Pathogenesis

The pathogenesis of papillary necrosis involves the dual injury of direct toxic effects of the offending agent, as in the case of phenacetin abuse, and vascular compromise and resultant ischemia to the involved pyramid.[298,301] The vascular component is less well understood, but there is evidence of endothelial and basement membrane injury to the vasa recta.[292,293,301]

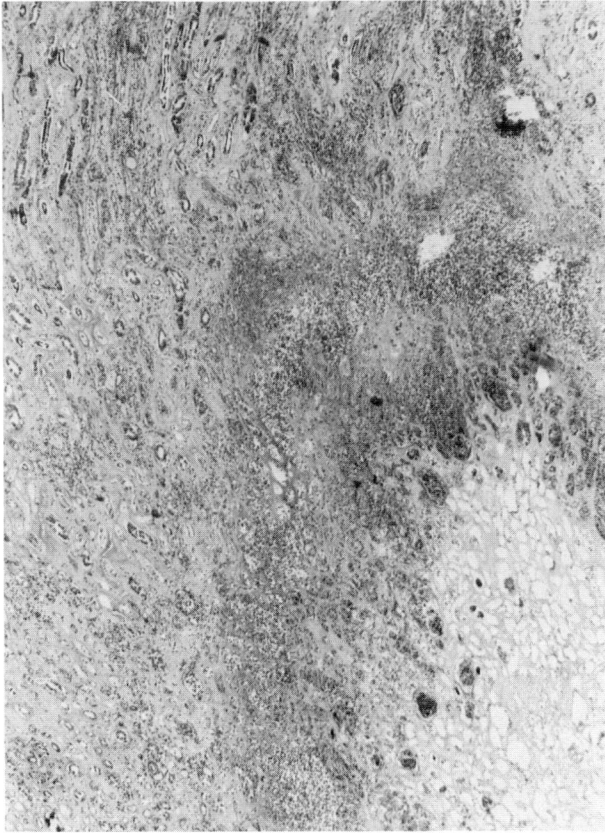

Figure 1-32   **Papillary necrosis.** *The necrotic papillary tip is virtually acellular, but the tubular outlines have been preserved. The upper margin of the necrotic area has a dense infiltrate of neutrophils located in the upper medulla.*

Xanthogranulomatous Pyelonephritis

History

The first descriptions of the distinctive gross and microscopic features of xanthogranulomatous pyelonephritis, an uncommon inflammatory disorder, were reported by Schlagenhaufer (1916) and Putschar (1934).[308,309] These authors noted the preponderance of foamy histiocytes in the inflammatory cell infiltrate, which Putschar observed to be of such magnitude as to give the lesion a yellow color resembling that of butter.[309] In 1944, Osterlind reported three similar cases, which he called "pyelonephritis xanthomatosa."[310] Barrie (1949) reported a case of "foam-cell granuloma in chronic pyonephrosis."[311] In the early 1950s the lesion was reported as "pyogenic (foam cell) granuloma" and "chronic pyelonephritis with xanthogranulomatous change."[312,313] In 1957, Selzer and associates collected 24 reported cases, described 7 additional examples, and introduced the term *xanthogranulomatous pyelonephritis.*[314] The number of reported cases gradually increased, with Anhalt (1971) collecting 90 published prior to 1970.[327] Numerous series, the largest reported by Tolia (1981), bring the total number to greater than 200.[344]

Xanthogranulomatous pyelonephritis is an uncommon disorder of unknown etiology, demonstrating extensive destruction of the organ by an inflammatory process, often in nodular configuration with abscess formation. The color of these lesions and the distinctive microscopic features are attributed to large numbers of "foamy macrophages" (histiocytes) predominating in the inflammatory cell infiltrate. Although the majority of patients have associated gram-negative urinary tract infection and renal lithiasis, the etiology and pathogenesis of this morphologically distinctive lesion remains unknown. Similarities among malakoplakia, megalocytic interstitial nephritis, and xanthogranulomatous pyelonephritis suggest that these disorders may represent variants of the same disease process.[323,340] There is currently no proof of this hypothesis. However, this remains within the realm of possibility, and any commonality will require future clarification of possible acquired metabolic defects of the histiocytes of each of these renal disorders. There is no evidence of a genetic influence operative in xanthogranulomatous pyelonephritis. Experimental production of morphologically similar renal lesions resulted from permanent ligature of the ureter followed by intravenous injections of *E. coli* 04:H5 as reported by Povysil and Konichova (1972).[329]

Clinical Features

Xanthogranulomatous pyelonephritis is observed more commonly in women (70%) than in men. It is most frequent during the fourth to seventh decades, but approximately 35 cases have been reported in patients less than 20 years old, the youngest a 6-month-old infant.[318,319,326,331-337,339,342,344-346] The mean ages in multiple series are in the fifth and sixth decades (Table 1-3). Patients present most frequently with flank pain, fever, a palpable mass, weakness, and anemia, as observed in the majority of cases. A history of urinary tract infection is common and urine culture at the time of presentation reveals *E. coli, Proteus mirabilis, Aerobacter,* or other gram-negative organisms in most cases. Sterile urine cultures are obtained in about 30% of reported cases. Abnormalities of liver function tests are not uncommon, and these tests are observed to return to normal following surgical excision of the involved kidney. Radiologic evidence of renal calculi is recorded in the majority of patients. Additional radiologic findings include evidence of (1) a hypovascular mass or masses, (2) calyceal distortion, (3) renal enlargement, or (4) nonfunction.[318,319,324,331-333,337,338] Differentiating xanthogranulomatous pyelonephritis from other non-neoplastic and neoplastic disorders on radiologic grounds has proved difficult in the recorded series. Bilateral renal involvement has been reported only once.[324] Single cases of xanthogranulomatous pyelonephritis with accompanying adult polycystic disease, renal cell carcinoma, and a transitional cell carcinoma have been reported.[332,344]

Pathologic Features

The majority of cases of xanthogranulomatous pyelonephritis are treated by nephrectomy. Less frequently there is treatment by partial nephrectomy when renal involvement is segmental. The extent of involvement by this inflammatory disorder has been described by Malak and associates in a formalized staging protocol.[330]

Stage I — nephric; involvement limited to the kidney

Stage II — nephric and perinephric; involvement of kidney and perirenal fat within Gerota's fascia

Stage III — nephric, perinephric, and paranephric; extension into adjacent organs or diffuse retroperitoneum

The involved kidney is invariably enlarged. Capsular and pericapsular fibrosis commonly accompanies lesions limited to the kidney. On occasion, the capsule is disrupted and the inflammatory process extends into the perirenal fat or beyond. This feature, combined with the appearance on cut surface, is reminiscent of tuberculosis and renal cell carcinoma.[317,321,338] Renal – enteric fistulas have been reported. On cut surface, the typical appearance is variable numbers of single or confluent yellow nodules with central necrosis and cavity formation (Fig. 1-33). The smaller nodules are solid without cavity formation. Abundant admixed and surrounding gray-white fibrous tissue is associated with these nodules. The lesions may be medullary or cortical, and commonly both locations are involved. The largest lesions extend from the distorted calyceal system to the cortical surface or beyond. Hydronephrosis with relatively uniform calyceal dilatation is common. Renal calculi, frequently staghorn calculi, are present in the majority of cases.

Microscopically, large numbers of large foamy histiocytes infiltrate fibrous tissue or form expansive sheets, with fewer numbers of plasma cells, lymphocytes, and neutrophils found within the yellow nodules. In the center of the lesions, no remaining renal parenchyma is apparent (Fig. 1-34). Cholesterol clefts with associated foreign body – type multinucleated giant cells are common

Table 1-3   ***Age – Sex Distribution and Presentation of Xanthogranulomatous Pyelonephritis***

Author	Year	No. of Patients	Sex	
			Males	*Females*
Selzer[314]	1957	7	4	3
Hooper et al[315]	1962	15	*	
Friedenberg et al[319]	1963	12	4	8
Saed, Fine[316]	1963	4		
Rios-Dalenz, Peacock[322]	1966	4	0	4
Noyes et al[325]	1969	5	4	1
Anhalt[327]	1971	4	0	4
Mering[332]	1973	5	2	3
Gammill[333]	1975	13	2	13
Malek et al[338]	1978	26	11	15
Goodman et al[341]	1979	23	7	16
Moller, Kristensen[342]	1980	19	8	11
Tolia et al[344]	1981	29	8	21
Total		166	50	99

* Blank space denotes unavailability of information.

within the infiltrate. Isolated nephrons are present at the periphery of the inflammatory infiltrate. The intervening parenchyma may be normal but more commonly shows nonspecific acute and chronic interstitial inflammation. Special stains fail to disclose organisms, but confirmation of the intracellular lipid of the histiocytes is achieved with oil red-O. In addition, faint periodic acid-Schiff (PAS)-positive granules are observed within the histiocyte cytoplasm.

The diagnosis of xanthogranulomatous pyelonephritis can be made when encountering a kidney with the above typical features. Misinterpretation of the histiocytes has led to the misdiagnosis of renal cell carcinoma, clear cell type.[320,328] Attention to the smaller nuclei of the histiocytes and the mixed cell infiltration will allow distinction from this renal malignancy. Ballesteros and associates report the diagnosis of xanthogranulomatous pyelonephritis by urinary cytology.[343] Distinguishing malakoplakia requires determining the absence of the diagnostic inclusions, Michaelis-Gutmann bodies, which are not observed in cases of xanthogranulomatous pyelonephritis (refer to the discussion of malakoplakia, below). Other specific infectious granulomas are distinguished by special stains for acid-fast organisms and fungi.

Malakoplakia

Malakoplakia is a chronic granulomatous inflammatory disorder originally described early in the 20th century and until 1958 regarded as unique to the urinary tract. This disease has now been observed in the gastrointestinal tract, genital tract, lungs, skin, adrenal gland, central nervous system, and other sites. (Refer to

Age (years)		Presentation			
Range	Mean	Lithiasis	Mass	Fever	Pain
30–70	53	2 (29%)	3 (43%)	3 (43%)	7 (100%)
29–79	46.5	12 (80%)	6 (40%)	9 (60%)	13 (87%)
13–82	51	8 (67%)	4 (33%)	7 (58%)	11 (97%)
30–54	42	3 (75%)	4 (100%)	3 (75%)	2 (50%)
42–73	60.6	4 (80%)	3 (60%)		3 (60%)
28–67	48.5	4 (100%)	0	2 (50%)	3 (75%)
11 mo–63 yr	45	2 (40%)	1 (20%)	1 (20%)	2 (40%)
14–72	43	8 (61%)			
15–82	50	10 (38%)	16 (62%)	18 (69%)	18 (69%)
16–70	44	7 (30%)	8 (35%)	14 (61%)	17 (74%)
8–81	56	14 (74%)		8 (42%)	8 (42%)
9.5–87	55.6	14 (48%)	2 (7%)	16 (55%)	12 (41%)
11 mo–87 yr	42–60.6				

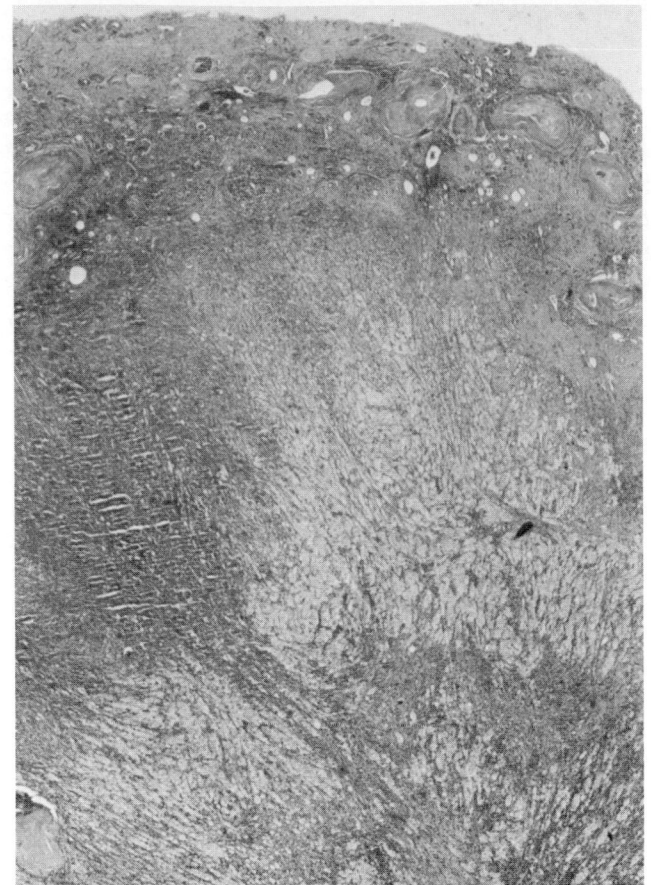

A

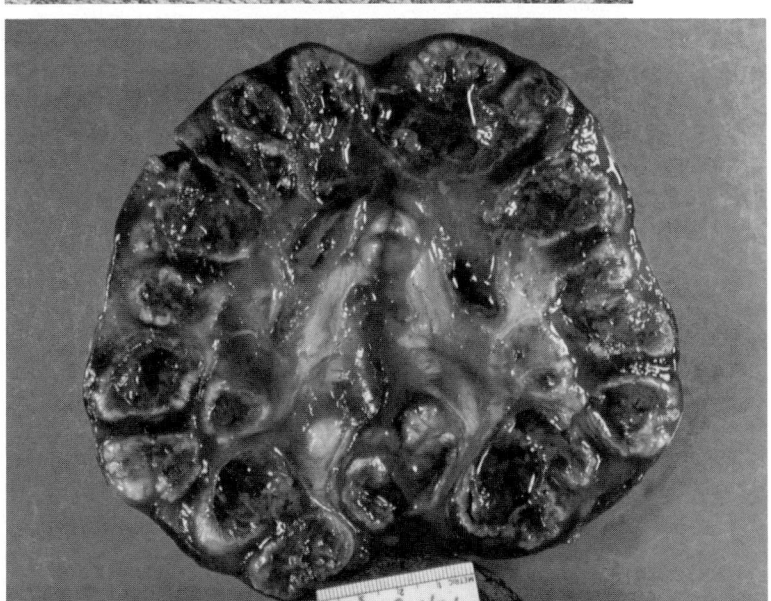

B

Figure 1-33   ***Xanthogranulomatous pyelonephritis.*** *(A) The lower cortex and medullary region contain an area composed exclusively of large foamy histiocytes. The renal parenchyma in this xanthogranulomatous lesion has been entirely destroyed. (B) The cut surface of the kidney shows distorted calyces rimmed by yellow-tan renal parenchyma containing a heavy infiltrate of histiocytes.*

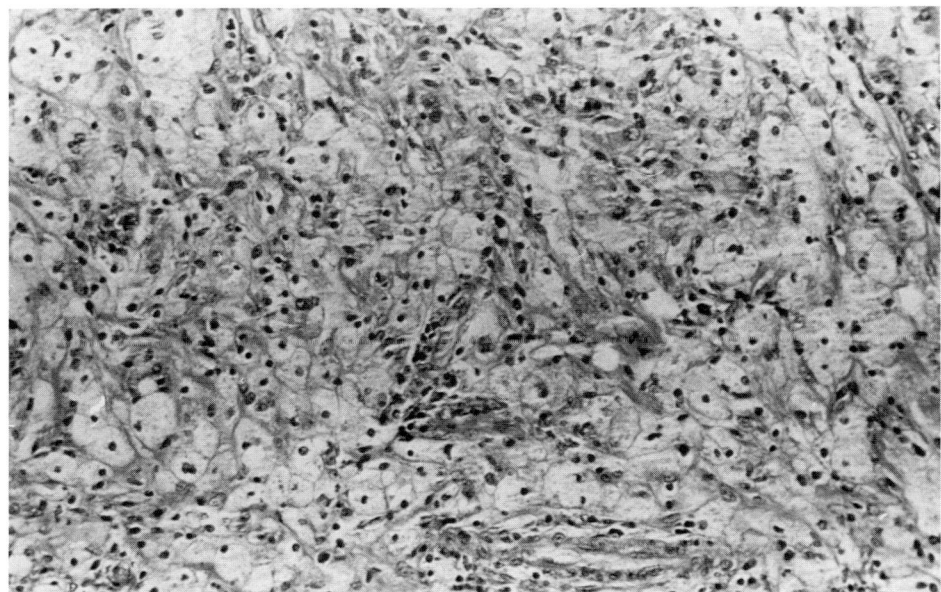

Figure 1-34   *Xanthogranulomatous pyelonephritis. The inflammatory-cell infiltrate is chiefly composed of large foamy histiocytes with admixed lymphocytes and occasional neutrophils. The renal parenchyma has been destroyed in the region of the lesion.*

Chap. 4 for further discussion.) Regardless of site of involvement, malakoplakia has characteristic gross and microscopic features, the most specific being abundant histiocytes (von Hansemann cells) associated with inclusions, the Michaelis-Gutmann bodies, representing calcified bacterial debris.

The first case of renal malakoplakia was reported in a 42-year-old woman by Michaelis and Gutmann in 1902.[347] Fifty-three additional cases were reported by 1982.[348-396] Renal involvement is exceeded in frequency only by reported cases in the urinary bladder, with fewer cases involving the renal pelvis, ureter, and organs of the male genital tract (refer to malakoplakia discussions in corresponding chapters). Approximately 55% of all recorded cases of renal malakoplakia have been reported in the past 10 years, suggesting an increased frequency of recognition of this disorder in the kidney (Table 1-4). Previously, malakoplakia was most likely interpreted as xanthogranulomatous pyelonephritis, with which it bears considerable resemblance.

Malakoplakia in the kidney (as in all other sites of the urinary tract) shows a striking female sex preponderance, with 80% (44 cases) reported in women. A wide age range (3–82 years) is observed, but 80% of the reported cases have been diagnosed in patients 30 to 69 years of age. The disease has not been reported in males younger than 50 years. The right and left kidneys are affected with equal frequency. Bilateral renal malakoplakia has been observed in 20 patients (37% of all reported cases). Approximately half of the cases of renal malakoplakia are associated with concurrent involvement of the renal pelvis, ureter, and bladder, and less frequently testis and adrenal. The majority of patients' past medical histories shows prior compromising systemic disorders including alcoholism, diabetes, renal transplantation with immunosuppressive therapy, and long-standing urinary tract infections.

Patients most commonly present with fever, flank pain, pyuria, and hematuria. Azotemia is present in most cases of recorded bilateral involvement. A flank mass is detected in some cases. With rare exceptions, urine culture is positive for *E. coli.* Purpon and Tamayo (1960) reported a positive culture with *Proteus vulgaris* and nonhemolytic streptococci.[358] IVP shows an irregularly enlarged kidney with filling defects that may distort the calyceal pattern. Angiography characteristically shows a hypovascular lesions, most commonly without neovascularization at periphery. The renal abnormalities may be single or multiple.

Table 1-4   **Renal Malakoplakia: Age–Sex Distribution, Location, and Associated Lesions**

Author	Year	Patient Age	Patient Sex	Location	Associated Lesions
Scheiner et al[370]	1975	74	M	No information	None
L'Hermite et al[371]	1975	64	F	Right	Bladder
Clarke et al[372]	1975	46	F	Left	Bladder
Deridder et al[376]	1977	3	F	Left	None
Osborn et al[373]	1977	46	F	Bilateral & transplant	Renal pelvis, ureter, bladder
Cavins, Goldstein[375]	1977	60	M	Right	None
McClure et al[378]	1977	61	M	Left	Testis
Lamb, Ayers[377]	1977	54	M	Bilateral	None
Arnesen[379]	1977	37	F	Transplant kidney	Bladder
Trillo et al[374]	1977	9.5	F	Left	None
Trojani et al[380]	1977	49	F	Bilateral	None
Raymond et al[383]	1978	50	F	Left	None
Cadnapaphornchai et al[384]	1978	35	F	Bilateral	None
Cadnapaphornchai et al[384]	1978	56	F	Bilateral	Bladder
Galla, Bhathena[381]	1978	31	F	Bilateral	None
Mullan, Hesse[382]	1978	42	F	Transplant kidney	Left
Ho et al[385]	1979	35	F	Bilateral	None
Charpin et al[387]	1980	74	M	Right	None
Griggs, Hemstreet[388]	1980	54	M	Left	None
Hartman et al[386]	1980	68	F	Right	Renal pelvis
Hartman et al[386]	1980	51	F	Left	None
Hartman et al[386]	1980	56	F	Right	None
Hartman et al[386]	1980	42	F	Right	Renal pelvis
Hartman et al[386]	1980	25	F	Right	None
Hillion et al[389]	1980	81	F	Bilateral	None
Benjamin, Fox[391]	1981	68	F	Left	Adrenal
Moller, Gerdes[392]	1981	56	F	Left	None
Carney et al[390]	1981	25	F	Left	Bladder
Katske et al[393]	1981	51	M	Bilateral	None
Moussu et al[396]	1982	73	F	Bilateral	Ureters, bladder

Pathology

Gross Features

Renal involvement by malakoplakia produces gross changes very suggestive of a number of disorders with similar features, including xanthogranulomatous pyelonephritis, renal tuberculosis, extensive pyelonephritis, and renal cell carcinoma. The kidney is generally enlarged and may have fibrous adhesions or extension of the lesion apparent on the cortical surface. The cut surface discloses streaks, nodules, or masses, which tend to bulge from the cut surface and in which all remnants of renal parenchymal landmarks are lost. The smaller nodules may be either exclusively cortical or medullary, localization that is lost when encountering larger lesions, which may distort the calyceal system and extend to and deform the outer cortical contour. Occasional cases are represented by one mass, the majority showing multiple nodules, frequently confluent, and replacing most of the renal parenchyma. The nodules may be soft to firm, depending on the extent of central necrosis. The color of the nodules varies from gray-tan to yellow-white, the latter being more characteristic. Most nodules are well demarcated with an irregular overall spherical configuration. There is no evidence of encapsulation. The remainder of the kidney may appear normal or show evidence of lesser degrees of involvement suggested by yellow streaks. The calyceal system may be either reduced in size or dilated, depending on the size of the renal parenchymal lesions and possible concurrent involvement of the ipsilateral renal pelvis and ureter.

Microscopic Features

The diagnosis of renal malakoplakia may be suggested by consideration of the clinical, radiologic, and gross morphologic features of the kidney specimen but may be established with certainty only by microscopic evaluation of the lesions in the resected kidney. Although regarded as pathognomonic of malakoplakia regardless of site of involvement, the Michaelis-Gutmann bodies may not be present in early lesions as originally reported by Smith (1965).[355] In the early phase of malakoplakia, the inflammatory lesion is composed of a dense infiltrate of von Hansemann cells, plasma cells, and lymphocytes with a background of tissue destruction and stromal edema. Michaelis-Gutmann bodies are typically not present in this early phase. In the next phase (the classic phase), histiocytes are the predominant inflammatory cells, with fewer lymphocytes and plasma cells. Hematoxylin-staining calcospheres, the Michaelis-Gutmann bodies, $5\,\mu$ to $10\,\mu$ in diameter, are found both within the von Hansemann cells and extracellularly in the stroma. Variably complete renal tubular destruction occurs within the focus of inflammation, with only a fragmented reticulin framework background for the inflammatory cell infiltrate. These calcospheres or Michaelis-Gutmann bodies stain positively with PAS, von Kossa's, and Prussian blue stains, assisting in their detection when present in sparse numbers (Fig. 1-35). The von Hansemann cells show PAS-positive intracytoplasmic granules. Later, in the fibrosing phase, the lesion shows fibroblast proliferation and collagen deposition throughout, with a corresponding reduction in the density of the inflammatory cells. Histiocytes and Michaelis-Gutmann bodies are still identified (Fig. 1-36).

This histologic picture characterized by predominance of histiocytes and featuring the diagnostic Michaelis-Gutmann bodies, all accompanied by the typical clinical and radiologic characteristics of malakoplakia, allows the diag-

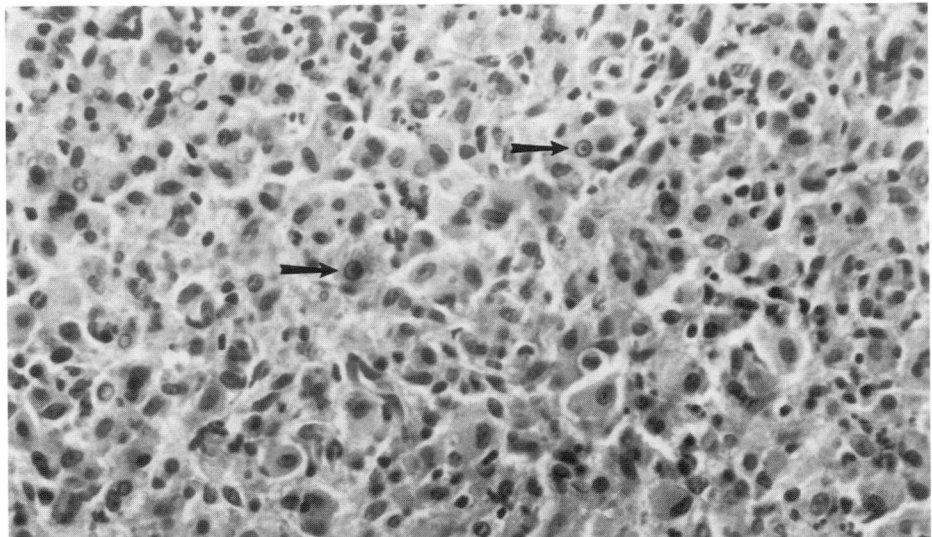

Figure 1-35   ***Malakoplakia.*** *The presence of Michaelis-Gutmann bodies* (arrows) *is demonstrated by use of the PAS stain. The predominant cells are histiocytes, with fewer numbers of neutrophils and lymphocytes.*

nosis of this rare disorder. The distinction of malakoplakia from tuberculosis is accomplished by the absence of detectable acid-fast organisms and paucity or absence of Langhans' giant cells. Xanthogranulomatous pyelonephritis does not show the Michaelis-Gutmann bodies, but it is similar in other respects. This similarity has prompted some investigators to suggest that malakoplakia, xanthogranulomatous pyelonephritis, and megalocytic interstitial nephritis all represent different phases or variants of the same disease (refer to the preceding discussion of xanthogranulomatous pyelonephritis).[394,395]

Natural History

Until the advent of dialysis and transplantation, bilateral involvement by malakoplakia has resulted in renal failure, progressive over weeks to months. The majority of reported examples of unilateral renal malakoplakia have been treated by nephrectomy, commonly with a preoperative diagnosis of renal neoplasm. Rarely the disorder has been successfully treated conservatively with antibiotics with apparent success.

Etiology and Pathogenesis

The cause of this disorder is unknown. The frequent association of *E. coli* infection of the urinary tract with malakoplakia in the kidney and other sites has implicated this organism. However, the disparity of the high frequency of *E. coli* urinary tract infections and the rarity of malakoplakia of all sites within the urinary system casts doubt on the possibility that the disorder represents a simple infection by this organism. Furthermore, there is no evidence that malakoplakia is associated with a unique, particularly virulent strain of the organism (refer to the discussion on malakoplakia in Chap. 4).

Attention has been focused on host factors, including immunologic status and macrophage function, as possible dominant contributions to the develop-

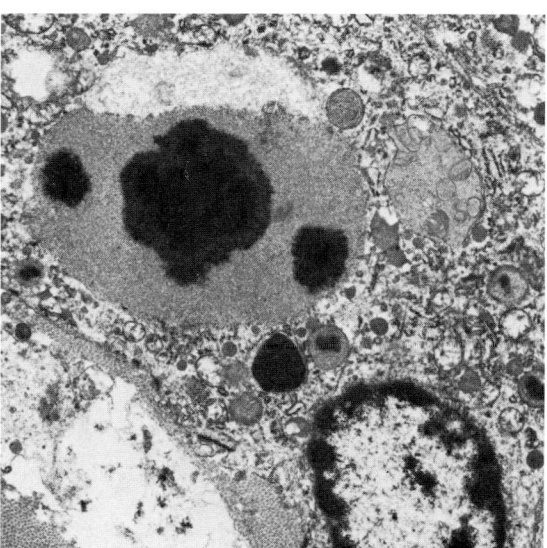

Figure 1-36   *Malakoplakia. Ultrastructural features of Michaelis-Gutmann body.*

ment of malakoplakia. There is no evidence of a genetic basis for this disorder (see also Chap. 4).

Neoplastic Disorders

Metanephric Blastemal Neoplasms

Nodular Renal Blastema and Nephroblastomatosis

The presence of nodular collections of undifferentiated renal blastema cells in the kidney following birth is termed *nodular renal blastema* (NRB), a term introduced by Bove and co-workers in 1969.[399] Such collections are observed at the periphery of renal lobules, most commonly in the superficial cortex immediately beneath the renal capsule. Less frequently they are found in the deeper cortex along the lobule septum. Bennington and Beckwith (1975) reported finding 12 examples in a consecutive pediatric autopsy series of 2452 patients for a frequency of 1 in 204 children.[401] The greatest frequency was found in children younger than 3 months. The lower frequency of NRB in older children suggested that most cases spontaneously regress with age. The true frequency of these nodules of renal blastema is yet to be determined by a systematic prospective study.

The majority of nodules of renal blastema are microscopic foci, most commonly multiple and bilateral. Associated nonurologic or urologic malformations are frequent.[399,401] Such nodules are not formed during normal nephrogenesis and are regarded as focal maturation arrests by Bove.[399,403] The predominant cells are primitive undifferentiated cells resembling those of the normal renal blastema. No epithelial differentiation is apparent in most cases, but dysplastic tubules at the periphery or in adjacent cortex have been reported.[403]

The significance of these discrete microscopic nodules of renal blastema is related to their association with Wilms' tumor.[399,402-406] The true frequency of NRB foci in kidneys harboring Wilms' tumor is currently unknown, but their association has prompted speculation that NRB may be a precursor stage of Wilms' tumor.[399,402-406]

Similarly, a more diffuse, characteristically bilateral form of NRB is called *nephroblastomatosis,* a term introduced by Hou and Holman (1961).[397] Typically involved kidneys are enlarged, and on cut surface they show confluent, subcapsular nodules clearly demarcated from the underlying compressed renal cortex. Patients range in age from birth to the oldest case of a 13-year-old girl reported by Pichler and associates (1982).[407] Systemic hypertension is common.[407] The microscopic features may be identical to those of NRB or may alternatively evidence varying tubular differentiation.[397,398,400,402,403] No mesenchymal differentiation is observed as in Wilms' tumors.[406]

Origin of nephroblastomatosis from NRB is suggested by the case reported by Rous and associates (1976) and generally accepted by others.[402,407] Further, a histogenetic relationship, linking NRB, nephroblastomatosis, and Wilms' tumor has been suggested.[401,402,407]

Wilms' Tumor (Nephroblastoma)

The original clinical and histologic descriptions of Wilms' tumor date back to the 19th century. Since then there has been sufficient time for innumerable descriptive studies and histogenetic hypotheses, and there have been equally numerous names suggested. Because the histogenesis remained controversial through most of the 20th century, the proposed names reflected either the German surgeon Max Wilms, who described this "mixed tumor of the kidney," or descriptive synonyms including adenosarcoma, embryonal adenocarcinoma, embryonal nephrosarcoma, myochondroadenocarcinoma, and carcinosarcoma to name but a few.[401,441] The histologic evidence of stromal and epithelial differentiation with blastemal tissue suggested a neoplasm of embryonal tissue origin. Views differed concerning the specific embryonal tissue source, either from undifferentiated mesenchyme prior or subsequent to nephrogenic differentiation. Currently, with evidence far short of what could be regarded as providing proof, Wilms' tumor (nephroblstoma) is thought to arise from metanephric blastema that undergoes malignant transformation either before or after birth.[408,411,413] Persistent blastema in the kidneys of newborn infants has been reported, documenting the presence of the proposed tissue of origin at an age consistent with the peak occurrence of the clinical development of malignant renal tumor (refer to the preceding discussion of nodular renal blastema and nephroblastomatosis). The mechanisms of neoplastic change of blastemal tissue with resultant Wilms' tumor have been discussed by Knudson and Strong (1972).[413]

Wilms' tumors are most common in the 2- to 5-year-old age group with no sex predilection. There is no geographical or race predilection of Wilms' tumor, which is reported with the above demographic features throughout the world. The typical case presents as a unilateral mass in an infant, but uncommonly this malignant neoplasm can be bilateral and can occur in adults (see Clinical Presentation, below). There is no genetic component in the vast majority of patients with Wilms' tumor, but genetic contribution to some cases with familial examples demonstrating autosomal dominant transmission are recorded.[401,413,460,485] Association of this malignancy with Beckwith-Wiedemann syndrome is reported.[401]

Clinical Features

Wilms' tumor is most frequently diagnosed between the ages of 1 and 5 years, with only 20% to 30% of cases observed in older children.[408,412,414,415,417,422,424,433] Approximately 3% of cases occur in children older than 10 years.[408,417,433] Wilms' tumor has been observed in adults, with about 150 cases reported in the literature.[441–449] There is no sex predilection.[412,414,415,417,419,423] The right and left kidneys are affected with approximately equal frequency, but two studies observed slight left-side predominance.[412,423] Bilateral Wilms' tumors are observed in 2% to 14% of large series.[450–462] Nineteen cases of extrarenal Wilms' tumors could be found in the literature (Table 1-5).[463–477]

Patients typically come to medical attention following detection of an abdominal mass by a family member. Ninety percent to one hundred percent of infants with this renal malignancy have an evident mass at the time of initial

Table 1-5   *Age–Sex Distribution and Location of Extrarenal Wilms' Tumors*

Author	Year	Age (years)*	Sex	Location	Comment
Fruhling et al[442]	1954	60	F	Posterior peritoneum, mesentery	No teratoma
Toudoire, Neveux[465]	1960	16	M	Posterior retroperitoneum	No teratoma
Toudoire, Neveux[465]	1960	23	M	Posterior retroperitoneum	No teratoma
Moyson et al[466]	1961	3	F	Posterior mediastinum	Origin from teratoma
Bhajekar et al[467]	1964	2	M	Posterior retroperitoneum	No teratomatous component
Nicod[468]	1965	35	F	Ovary	No teratoma
Edelstein et al[469]	1965	3	M	Retroperitoneum	No teratomatous component
Malik et al[470]	1967	6	F	Retroperitoneum	Origin in teratoma
Wu, Garcia[471]	1971	7	F	Posterior pelvic wall	Supernumerary kidney
Thompson et al[472]	1973	3	M	Inguinal canal	No teratomatous component
Thompson et al[472]	1973	4.5	F	Inguinal canal	No teratomatous component
Tebbi et al[473]	1974	3	F	Sacrococcygeal location	Origin from teratoma
Ward, Dehner[474]	1974	3	F	Sacrococcygeal location	Origin from teratoma
Carney[475]	1975	41	M	Retroperitoneum	Origin from teratoma; associated renal cell carcinoma
Akhtar et al[476]	1977	2 mo	M	Inguinal canal	No teratomatous component
Madanat et al[477]	1978	9	F	Lateral chest wall	No teratomatous component
Madanat et al[477]	1978	3 mo	M	Inguinal canal	No teratomatous component
McCauley et al[478]	1979	4.5	F	Retroperitoneum	No teratomatous component
Adam et al[479]	1983	10	M	Retroperitoneum	No teratomatous component

* Age given in years, except where otherwise noted.

examination.[409,415,417,423] Abdominal pain and (less frequently) hematuria may accompany the mass, with reported frequencies of 33% to 50% and 12% to 25%, respectively.[412,415,417,423] Other findings reported include hypertension, fever, and anemia, all observed in a minority of patients at presentation.[409,415–417,423] Uncommonly, clinical presentation is related to massive intratumor hemorrhage, a surgical emergency, or metastases.[427]

A variety of associated malformations including hemihypertrophy, aniridia, multiple urogenital tract anomalies, harelip, cleft palate, and mental retardation are reported in 10% to 15% of infants with nephroblastoma.[478–486]

Radiologic Features

The combined radiologic modalities of excretory urogram, renal angiography, and ultrasound provide the correct preoperative diagnosis of Wilms' tumor in the vast majority of cases.[415,432,437] The National Wilms' Tumor Study I encountered radiologic diagnostic errors in 5% of over 600 submitted cases.[432] The neoplasm is radiologically characterized by a well-defined margin, calyceal distortion, abnormal tumor vessels, and stretching of renal parenchymal vessels on angiography.[415,437] Calcification is present in occasional cases. The entities posing the greatest differential diagnostic challenge are neuroblastoma, mesoblastic nephroma, and polycystic renal disease. Ultrasound assists in distinguishing cysts from nephroblastoma and can give additional information relative to the presence and extent of tumor necrosis.[436] Included in the radiologic examination are chest x-ray examination and computed tomography (CT) scan evaluation of the lungs and abdomen for evidence of metastases. Bone metastases from Wilms' tumor are distinctly uncommon (refer to the discussion of clear cell sarcoma later in this chapter).

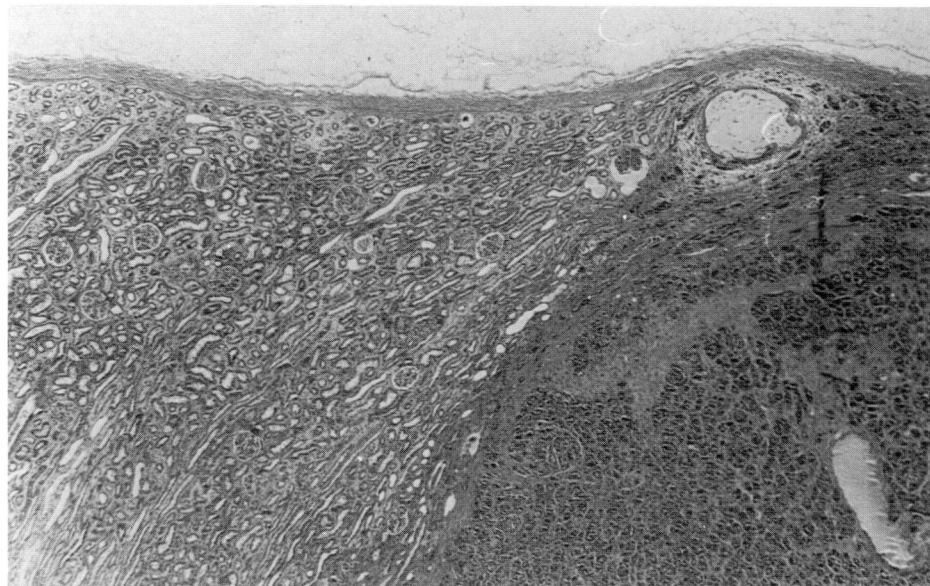

Figure 1-37   *Wilms' tumor. The expanding neoplasm on the right is well demarcated from the normal cortex on the left. The neoplasm is composed of poorly developed tubular structures with varying amounts of intervening stroma.*

Pathologic Features

Consistent with the high frequency of a clinically palpable mass, 80% to 90% of Wilms' tumors are more than 5 cm in diameter.[401,414,423] Approximately one third to one half of cases are larger than 10 cm.[414,423] Examples reported by Breslow and co-workers (1978) weighed up to 2500 g, with a mean of 572 g.[429] The cut surface of the tumor typically shows a prominent pseudocapsule enclosing a solid, soft to firm, gray-white to gray-tan mass. Focal areas of hemorrhage, necrosis, and cystic change are not uncommon but not prominent. Occasional cases will have extensive secondary changes. The most diagnostically atypical Wilms' tumors are those cases with prominent and diffuse cystic change as discussed in the section on multilocular cystic nephroma, which follows. Evidence of capsular, vascular, and renal hilar lymph nodes may be observed in the nephrectomy specimen; if present, these should be adequately documented in the final report.[418,435]

The microscopic evaluation of Wilms' tumor requires the synthesis of both the histologic and cytologic features present in a specimen thoroughly sampled to document the presence and extent of variability of the three components: epithelial, stromal, and blastemal.[414,420,421,424,428,430] In addition, the degree of differentiation of the epithelial and stromal components and the presence and extent of anaplastic cytologic features (abnormal mitoses, nuclear pleomorphism, and hyperchromaticity) are recorded. The typical case of Wilms' tumor shows varying proportions of epithelial components composed of tubules and glomerular structures in the background of spindle cell stromal components and undifferentiated, densely cellular blastemal tissue (Figs. 1-37 and 1-38). Tumors are classified as epithelial, stromal, or blastema predominant or as mixed if no one component is clearly dominant.[428,514]

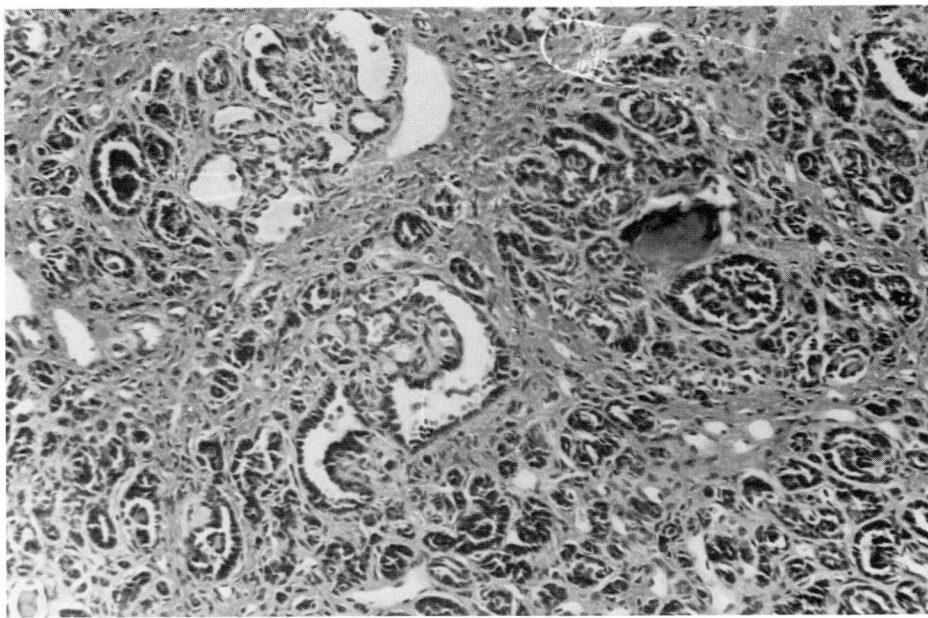

Figure 1-38 **Wilms' tumor.** *Primitive tubule and glomerulus-like structures are separated by collagenous stroma containing individual spindle and polygonal cells with hyperchromatic nuclei.*

The stromal component is myxoid or fibroblastic, commonly with evident admixtures of smooth muscle or skeletal muscle (Fig. 1-39). Rare cases of Wilms' tumor, called rhabdomyomatous nephroblastomas, are composed virtually exclusively of fetal striated muscle with only inconspicuous foci of the more typical histologic components of Wilms' tumor.[438,439] Additional forms of stromal differentiation include fat cells and chondroid differentiation.

The blastemal cells, which are small and with sparse cytoplasm, tend to be present in clusters, with dissimilar spindle cell stroma intervening. Beckwith describes uncommon variants showing blastemal cell collections separated by large thin-walled cysts resembling lymphatic channels (Fig. 1-40).[401,428]

The tubular differentiation of the epithelial component is variable, with some structures devoid of a lumen and with a limited degree of tubular epithelial differentiation. Uncommon variants of epithelial differentiation include squamous metaplastic foci and mucin-producing cells.[401,514,517]

The histogenesis of neural components reported in rare cases of Wilms' tumors, and recently within the pulmonary metastases of one case, remains controversial.[440]

The above histologic and cytologic features have been organized into multiple tumor grading protocols currently applied to identify prognostically important features (refer to the discussion of prognosis, below).[414,415,420,423,428,430]

Natural History

Tumor Staging

The clinical groups (tumor stages) of Wilms' tumor proposed by the National Wilms' Tumor Study are presented in Table 1-6. This protocol has received general acceptance, and it is one of the major contributions of this cooperative study group.

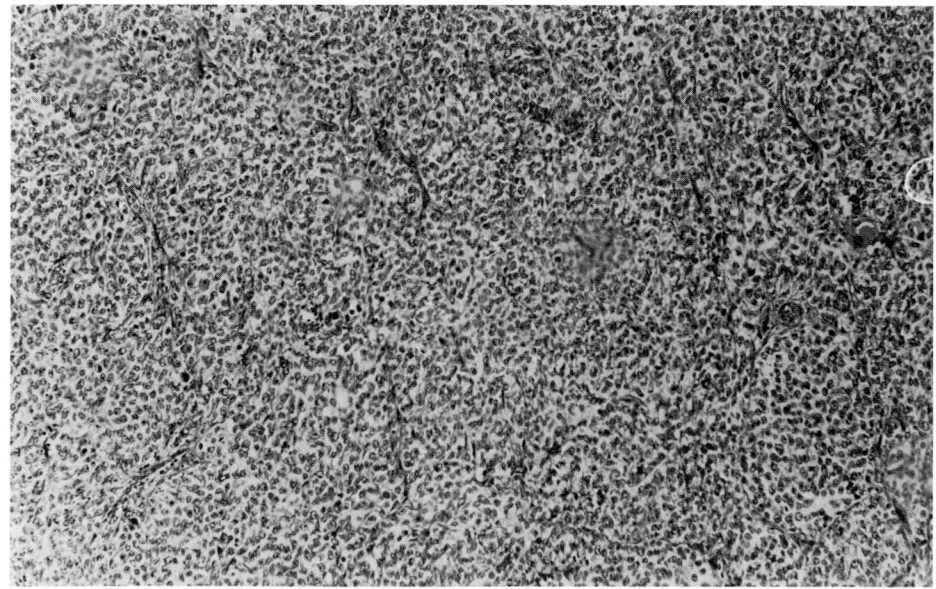

Figure 1-39   *Wilms' tumor. An example of monophasic Wilms' tumor composed of primitive mesenchymal cells without evidence of epithelial structures.*

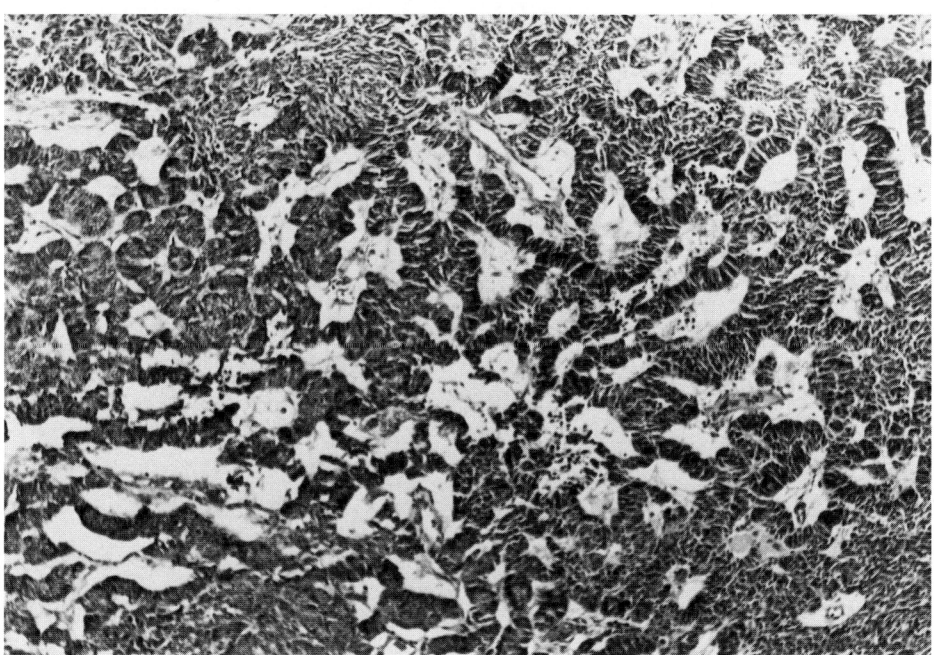

Figure 1-40 **Wilms' tumor.** Blastemal cells arranged in a trabecular pattern with intervening fibrovascular stroma.

The reported distribution of tumor stage (clinical groups) in recent studies of Wilms' tumor appear in Table 1-7. An average of 36% of Wilms' tumors are confined to the kidney and are completely excised at the time of nephrectomy. An additional 26% (mean of six studies) have invaded beyond the kidney but are still regarded as completely excised.

Metastases

As summarized in Table 1-7, 34% of patients have intra-abdominal or other distant metastases at the time of initial presentation. Among those patients with localized tumor regarded as completely resected, 29% will subsequently demonstrate recurrence in the form of distant metastases.[417] Ninety-one percent to one

Table 1-6 **Clinical Grouping of Wilms' Tumor by the National Wilms' Tumor Study Committee***

Group	Description
I	Tumor limited to kidney and completely resected
II	Tumor extends beyond the kidney but is completely resected
III	Residual nonhematogenous tumor confined to the abdomen
IV	Hematogenous metastases
V	Bilateral renal involvement either initially or subsequently

* For complete description, refer to D'Angio GJ, Evans AE, Breslow N et al: The treatment of Wilms' tumor: Results of the National Wilms' Tumor Study. Cancer 38:633, 1976.

Table 1-7   **Wilms' Tumor Clinical Group (Tumor Stage) Distribution**

Author	Year	No. of Patients	Tumor Stage				
			I	II	III	IV	V
Jereb, Sandstedt[414]	1973	112	42%	19%	29%	10%	0
Perez et al[415]	1973	49	31%	18%	18%	20%	12%
Aron[417]	1974	81	41%	23%	16%	10%	10%
Bond[419]	1975	78	44%	17%	15%	19%	5%
Lemerle et al[424]	1976	219	21%	45%	23%	11%	0
Kheir et al[430]	1978	26	35%	31%	27%	8%	0
Total		565					
Range			21%–44%	17%–45%	15%–29%	10%–20%	5%–12%
Mean			36%	26%	21%	13%	9%

hundred percent of these metastatic recurrences will appear within the first 2 years following nephrectomy.[415,417,423,429] The single most common metastatic site is pulmonary, comprising 80% to 90% of cases.[417,419,423,429] Other common sites, in order of decreasing frequency, are intra-abdominal and hepatic.[417,423,429] Bone metastases are uncommon. Multiple other reported sites are rare.[487–489] Breslow and co-workers (1978) reported that approximately 50% of patients die within 18 months of diagnosis of tumor recurrence.[429]

Prognosis

Multiple studies have demonstrated that the principal factors related to prognosis are tumor stage, patient age, and histologic differentiation of the tumor. The relationship of tumor stage (patient group) and survival with Wilms' tumor as reported in studies is presented in Table 1-8.

The survival data show reference points of variable duration (2–5 years) following diagnosis and initial treatment (Table 1-8). The justification for judging survival at intervals as short as 2 or 3 years rests on the observed chronology of recurrences and metastases. In summary, multiple studies have shown that tumor-related deaths occurring later than 2 years following diagnosis and initial therapy are uncommon to rare.[408,410,423,429] Aron (1974) observed no tumor-re-

Table 1-8   **Wilms' Tumor Clinical Group (Tumor Stage) vs. Survival Rates***

Author	Year	No. of Patients	Tumor Stage					Survival End Point
			I	II	III	IV	V	
Jereb, Sandstedt[414]	1973	112	55%	29%	6%	0%	—	2 yr
Perez et al[415]	1973	49	80%	55%	0%	30%	50%	3 yr
Aron[417]	1974	81	85%	73%	32%	37%	47%	5 yr
Bond[419]	1975	78	87%	36%	8%	33%	50%	2 yr
Lemarle et al[424]	1976	219	74%	59%	38%	21%	—	5 yr
Kheir et al[430]	1978	26	78%	75%	43%	0%	—	2 yr

* Survival rate variously defined as survival at 2–5 years. Refer to text.

lated deaths after 2 years among patients with localized disease; conversely, all tumor-related deaths among stage IV cases occurred within the first 2 years.[417] The definition of the period of risk was originally proposed by Collins and associates (1956).[408] Their proposal, known as Collins' rule, defined this period of risk as equal to the patient's age plus 9 months on the assumption that the origin of the neoplasm could be dated in early gestation. With the further assumption of constant growth rate, tumor metastases or recurrences would be detected within the same time frame. Subsequently, Platt and Linden (1964) demonstrated that the period at risk could be redefined as 2 years, independent of the age of the patient at the time of diagnosis, with the same low probability of later recurrence as observed applying Collins' rule.[408,410]

Survival rates among patients less than 2 years of age are observed to exceed those of older patients.[412,415,417,419,423,429] When studied by multivariant analysis, the effect of age on survival is indirect, reflecting the higher frequency of low-stage tumors in patients less than 2 years of age than in older patients.[412,415,417] Some, but not all, studies have demonstrated that the survival of patients both younger and older than 2 years with Wilms' tumors of equivalent stage is comparable.[415,417,419] However, Aron (1974) reported younger patients with stage I Wilms' tumor fared better than older children with Wilms' tumor of the same stage.[417]

Clinical factors including presenting symptoms, patient sex, and laterality of the tumor have no bearing on survival rate.[412,415,417,423,429]

Pathologic features (exclusive of tumor stage) bearing on prognosis include tumor size, hemorrhage, and capsular invasion.[414,415,418,423] Tumor size positively relates to survival only when tumors smaller and larger than 5 cm are compared.[414] Incremental increases in size of tumors larger than 5 cm do not show a corresponding progressive decrease in survival.[414] Finally, microscopic features constituting criteria for tumor grading associated with poor prognosis include predominant sarcomatoid pattern with sparse or absent differentiation toward tubules and glomeruli, cytologic atypia, and abnormal mitoses.[414,415,423,428,430] The histologic evaluation of Wilms' tumors with attention to the above criteria allows classification into favorable and unfavorable patterns predictive of ultimate outcome.[414,415,421,423,424,428,430] In the original investigation of Beckwith and Palmer (1978), the identified unfavorable patterns included those cases showing anaplasia and sarcomatoid features, comprising 11.6% of a series of 427 cases of Wilms' tumor.[428] In subsequent studies the sarcomatoid group was reclassified into the clear cell sarcomas and the malignant rhabdoid tumors. These neoplasms are currently regarded as entities nosologically separate from Wilms' tumors and not as aggressive variants of this neoplasm (refer to the discussions of clear cell sarcoma and malignant rhabdoid tumors later in this chapter).

With improvement in surgical technique, and most importantly with the introduction of combined radiation and chemotherapy for this malignancy, the survival rates currently achieved (85% compared with 15% in 1920) reflect one of the major medical achievements of the 20th century.[401,425,426] The development of cooperative study groups such as the National Wilms' Tumor Study has provided the opportunity to study large numbers of this uncommon neoplasm.[422,428,429,431,432,434,514] Major contributions to our understanding of clinical and pathologic features of prognostic significance, and to therapy protocols, can be directly attributed to the National Wilms' Tumor Study investigations.

Differential Diagnosis

The diagnosis of Wilms' tumor requires differentiation of this malignancy from (1) multilocular cystic nephroma, (2) mesoblastic nephroma, (3) malignant rhabdoid tumor, and (4) clear cell sarcoma, each of which has distinct biologic, clinical, and pathologic features (refer to the respective discussions elsewhere in this chapter).

Benign Multilocular Cystic Nephroma

The historical significance of Boggs and Kimmelstiel's report in 1956 rests not with their suggested change in the diagnostic criteria for multilocular cysts *per se,* but with their interpretation of these cysts as neoplasms related to Wilms' tumors.[199] Indeed the change in criteria is inconsequential because they postulated that all such cystic lesions with primitive tubules, glomeruli, and blastemal stroma (or their absence) were benign neoplastic lesions. Thus, the multilocular cyst as a developmental defect, as earlier described by Powell and associates (1951), was invalidated.[197]

Following the report of Boggs and Kimmelstiel (1956), others reported cases of multilocular cystic lesions that contained foci of renal blastema, tubular or glomerular structures, skeletal muscle, or combinations of these tissues (Table 1-9). As the number of such reported cases increased, so did both the suggested histogenetic explanations and the proposed names for these multilocular cystic lesions (Table 1-10).[211–213,217,223,225–227]

In 1967, Christ reported a case of diffuse organoid features including glomerular and tubular structures with associated foci of blastema within the septae of the cysts.[206] The lesion was interpreted as a cystic variant of a well-differentiated nephroblastoma (Wilms' tumor), and Christ coined the term *polycystic nephroblastoma.*

In 1971, Fowler presented a case containing only tubules within the septae, which he called "differentiated nephroblastoma."[208] The chosen term accurately conveyed the histogenesis favored by Fowler (*i.e.,* origin from a nephroblastoma [Wilms' tumor] that showed differentiation, contrasting with a benign neoplasm developing *de novo,* as postulated by Boggs and Kimmelstiel [1956]).[199]

In 1975, Brown presented a case showing focal glomerular and tubular structures, renal blastema, and skeletal muscle.[212] In contrast to Fowler's case, which was regarded as fully differentiated, this case was interpreted as a "cystic partially differentiated nephroblastoma."[208,212]

Thus, the full spectrum of histogenetic possibilities was presented in these four reports ranging from the proposed benign variant of Wilms' tumor favored by Boggs and Kimmelstiel (1956) to the partially and fully differentiated nephroblastoma, views held by Brown (1975), Christ (1967), and Fowler (1971).[199,208,212] Subsequent authors, although tampering with the previously suggested names, did not substantively alter the conceptual framework of this spectrum of neoplastic lesions.

However, the premises on which this conceptual framework is constructed warrant critical scrutiny. The question of whether Wilms' tumors can show extensive cystic change has been settled by examples published by Uson and associates (1960).[202] However, differentiation of Wilms' tumor as proposed by Christ (1967), Fowler (1971), and Brown (1975) among others has never been

Table 1-9   ***Reports of Kidneys With Multilocular Cysts***
                             as Related to Composition of Intracystic Septae

Author	Year	Cases	Author's Diagnosis
Blastema only			
Uson, Melicow[205]	1963	Case #3	Multilocular cyst
Gallo, Penchansky[216]	1977	Case #1	Cystic nephroma
Gonzalez-Crussi et al[226]	1982	Case #3	Cystic nephroma
Tubules only			
Frazier[198]	1951	Case #2	Multilocular cyst
Boggs, Kimmelstiel[199]	1956	Case #1	Benign multilocular nephroma
Gibson[203]	1961	1 case	Multilocular cyst
Kawamura, Miyakawa[207]	1969	1 case	Multilocular cyst
Fowler[208]	1971	1 case	Differentiated nephroblastoma
Datnow, Daniel[213]	1976	1 case	Polycystic nephroblastoma
Gallow, Penchansky[216]	1977	Case #2	Cystic nephroma
Coleman[225]	1980	1 case	Multilocular cyst
Gonzalez-Crussi et al[226]	1982	Cases #1,5	Cystic nephroma
Andrews, et al[227]	1983	Case #2	Cystic partially differentiated nephroblastoma
Tubules and blastema			
Andrews et al[227]	1983	Case #1	Polycystic Wilms' (polycystic nephroblastoma)
Tubules, blastema, glomerular structures			
Christ[206]	1967	1 case	Polycystic nephroblastoma
Behr, Duasi[211]	1975	1 case	Cystic nephroblastoma
Keegan et al[223]	1979	1 case	Cystic partially differentiated nephroblastoma
Tubules, blastema, skeletal muscle			
Gallo, Penchensky[216]	1977	Case #3	Cystic nephroma
Gonzalez-Crussi et al[226]	1982	Cases #2,4,6	Cystic nephroma
Tubules, blastema, glomerular structures, skeletal muscle			
Brown [212]	1975	1 case	Cystic partially differentiated nephroblastoma
Joshi et al[217]	1977	3 cases	Cystic partially differentiated nephroblastoma

proven. Further, primitive tubules and renal blastemal mesenchyme, the basis for regarding many cases as cystic variants of nephroblastoma, are not unique to Wilms' tumors, but can be observed in dysplastic kidneys (refer to the discussion of renal dysplasia, earlier in this chapter). The absence of such primitive tissues in the intercystic septae has been attributed to inadequate sampling and microscopic examination.[199] This most certainly is a possibility, but it is a totally inadequate basis for including cases lacking these structures among the neoplastic multilocular cysts. Finally, among those cases in which only rare or occasional foci of tubules are found in the septae, the theory has not been disproven that their presence results from sequestration into the cyst as opposed to representing an integral part of the alleged neoplastic process.

As attention has been focused primarily on clarifying the histogenesis of cystic "benign" or "differentiated" variants of nephroblastoma during the past 2 decades, the status of the multilocular cyst of Powell and associates (1951) has remained unsettled. The theory that multilocular cysts result from developmental error has been accepted by some (Christ, 1967; Joshi, 1977) but rejected by others (Boggs, Kimmelstiel, 1956; Fowler, 1971; Gallo and Penchansky, 1977).[199,206,208,216,218] This distinction is not academic but carries obvious potential practical significance related to biologic behavior and patient prognosis. The fundamental conceptual problems noted above must be solved before a clear understanding of all of these multilocular renal lesions can be achieved.

In the meantime, the classification of all multilocular cysts as benign or differentiated variants of Wilms' tumor appears unjustified. Clarification of histogenesis will in turn solve the secondary problem of the currently encountered plethora of suggested names, which frequently seem to be applied with random chance (Tables 1-1, 1-9, 1-10).

Congenital Mesoblastic Nephroma

History

The term *congenital mesoblastic nephroma* was coined by Bolande and associates in 1967 for a renal neoplasm most commonly observed in the newborn period and bearing gross and microscopic resemblance to leiomyomas.[491] This neoplasm is predominantly composed of interlacing spindle cells. However, it inconstantly shows foci of undifferentiated mesenchyme, primitive tubules, and foci of chondroid differentiation, suggesting a histogenetic relationship to Wilms' tumor.[504,505] In contrast to patients with Wilms' tumors, however, patients do

Table 1-10 **Proposed Names of Lesions in Kidneys With Multilocular Cysts Fulfilling Criteria of Boggs and Kimmelstiel[199]**

Proposed Name	Author and Year
Benign multilocular cystic nephroma	Boggs, Kimmelstiel (1956)[199]
Polycystic nephroblastoma	Christ (1968)[206]
Multilocular cyst	Kawamura, Miyakawa (1969)[207]
Differentiated nephroblastoma	Fowler (1971)[208]
Cystic partially differentiated nephroblastoma	Brown (1975)[212]
Cystic nephroma	Gallo, Penchansky (1977)[216]

uniformly well (with one exception noted below) following surgical excision during prolonged follow-up observation periods.

Prior to the report of Bolande and associates, similar, if not identical, congenital tumors were previously reported as leiomyomas and leiomyomatous-type renal hamartoma.[490] The histogenetic and neoplastic nature of congenital mesoblastic nephroma proposed by Bolande and associates was not generally accepted in the years following its publication. The same tumor was subsequently reported variously as fetal hamartoma of kidney,[493] fetal mesenchymal hamartoma,[499] fibromyomatous hamartoma,[492] and leiomyomatous hamartoma.[496]

Numerous ultrastructural studies attempting to clarify this tumor's histogenesis variously reported features of fibroblast, myofibroblast, and smooth muscle differentiation.[492,497,502,504–506] In addition, interpretation of the tubules and glomeruli found within the tumor has varied. Some authors regarded them as entrapped by the infiltrating tumor cells and not as an intrinsic part of the lesion.[492,494,496,500–502] The absence of tubules in recurrences and in metastases indirectly supported this view.[503,506] Others disagreed and regarded the epithelial component as an intrinsic part of the tumor.[498] Although most authors reported foci of cartilage, Favara (1968) and Shen and Yunis (1980) noted its absence.[492,502]

Potter (1972) and more recently Snyder and colleagues (1981) and Ganick and colleagues (1981) have suggested that the congenital nature of the neoplasm suggests a relatively early origin during embryologic development of the kidney.[76,504,505] This is consistent with the predominant mesenchymal nature of this tumor, because metanephric blastema is primarily stromagenic in the early phases of metanephrogenesis.[76]

With rare but important exceptions, all studies reported the uniform experience of cure by surgical excision. The first exceptions to this rule were reported by Fu and Kay (1973) and Walker and Richard (1973), who described local recurrences 4 months after diagnosis and surgical excision in a newborn and a 3-month-old infant, respectively.[495,497] The only other example was recently reported by Levin and co-workers (1982), who recorded the recurrence of a mesoblastic nephroma 21 years following surgical excision of the primary tumor.[506] The only case of mesoblastic nephroma demonstrating metastases was reported by Gonzalez-Crussi and associates in 1980.[503] This case not only put to rest prior suggestions of the hamartomatous nature of mesoblastic nephroma, but it also defined one end of the biologic spectrum of this neoplasm.

Through 1984, approximately 70 examples of congenital mesoblastic nephroma have been reported, virtually all diagnosed in infants less than 6 months old.[490–506] The first report of mesoblastic nephroma occurring in an adult (a 31-year-old woman) was reported by Block and co-workers.[498] The example reported by Levin and colleagues noted above, which was recurrent after 21 years, was originally diagnosed in a 19-year-old girl.[506]

Clinical Features

The diagnosis of mesoblastic nephroma is made following the detection of an abdominal mass in a newborn or young infant. The preoperative differential diagnosis includes Wilms' tumor, multicystic dysplastic kidney, and multilocular cyst and multilocular cystic nephroma. Wilms' tumor is more common in children older than 6 months of age, and multicystic dysplasia can frequently be differentiated from the solid mesoblastic nephroma by radiologic means.[500] An increased frequency of polyhydramnios has been reported among mothers giving birth to infants in whom mesoblastic nephroma is diagnosed.[492,501,504]

Pathologic Features

The affected kidneys are distorted and enlarged, up to 800 g as reported by Bogdan and associates.[496] On cut surface, most of the kidney is replaced by a solid pink-gray, firm mass. The surface of the tumors shows a whorled pattern without the lobulation more typical of Wilms' tumors. Most reports make reference to the gross features bearing a resemblance to uterine leiomyomas. Minute cysts may be present. Deviation from this typical appearance, including gross cystic change and focal hemorrhage and necrosis observed in the "cellular variants," has been reported (refer to the discussion of microscopic features, below).[502–505] The neoplasm is not encapsulated, and the local invasion characteristically observed microscopically is commonly evident on gross examination.

Histologically, the neoplasm is composed of interlacing broad bundles of spindle cells with the cytologic appearance of fibroblasts predominating (Fig. 1-41).[491] In some areas, cells more typical of smooth muscle may be present. At the periphery of the neoplasm, the neoplastic spindle cells infiltrate the adjacent renal parenchyma, isolating and entrapping renal glomeruli and tubules (Fig. 1-42).[491,492,494,496,497,502–504] Nuclear pleomorphism and mitoses are not prominent features in typical cases.[494,496] Foci of cartilage and primitive mesenchyme and tubules may be identified in the neoplasm.[491,495–498,500,505]

Recently, cellular variants of the typical mesoblastic nephroma have been described. Associated findings with the increased cellularity are greater numbers of mitoses and nuclear pleomorphism.[502–504] Hemorrhage and necrosis are more common.[502–504] This morphologic appearance has been associated with recur-

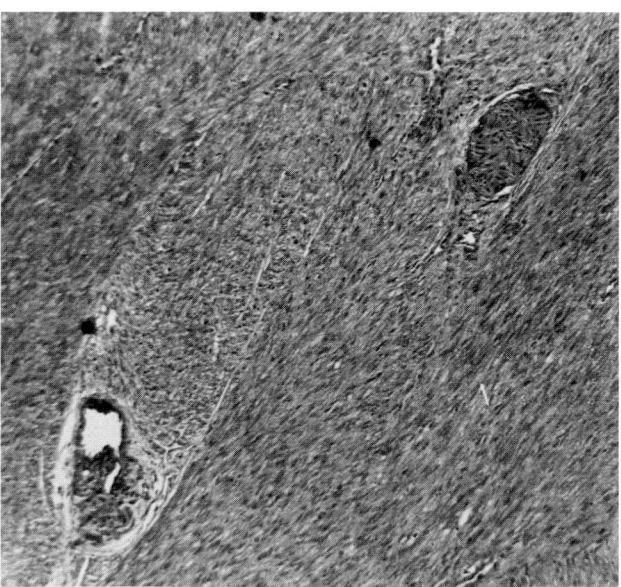

Figure 1-41   *Congenital mesoblastic nephroma. Bundles of spindle cells encircle a nerve within the kidney. No necrosis, nuclear atypia, or mitotic figures are present.*

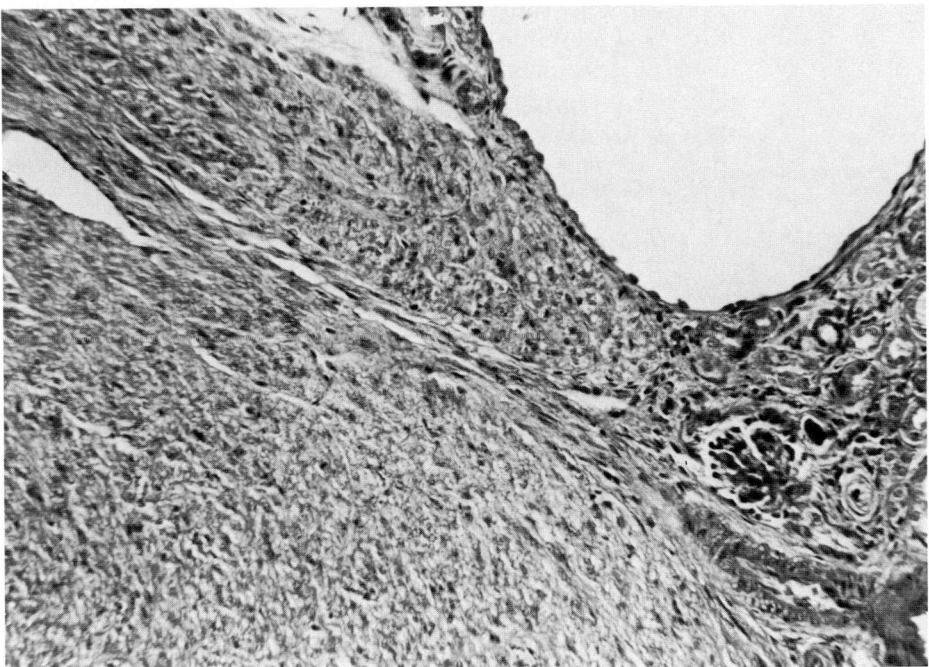

Figure 1-42   *Congenital mesoblastic nephroma. Spindle cells compress and infiltrate the adjacent renal parenchyma.*

rence and was observed in the only reported example demonstrating metastases.[503] The true frequency of atypical clinical behavior observed in examples with these ominous histologic features is currently unknown.

Differential Diagnosis

The diagnosis of congenital mesoblastic nephroma rests on the gross and histologic features outlined above. The major disorders to be differentiated are Wilms' tumors with or without cystic changes, multilocular cystic nephroma, and leiomyomas (refer to the corresponding sections of this chapter).

Clear Cell Sarcoma

Clear cell sarcoma (bone metastasizing renal tumor of childhood) is a rare renal neoplasm of children that was independently described in 1978 by three groups of pathologists.[507,508,509,517] In all of these reports, the recognition of this entity resulted from retrospective reviews of large numbers of neoplasms previously diagnosed as Wilms' tumors. Beckwith and Palmer reported 11 cases that they termed *clear cell sarcoma of the kidney.*[517] Morgan and Kidd reported nine renal tumors, which they called *undifferentiated sarcoma of kidney.*[509] Marsden and Lawler reported 15 cases that they termed *bone metastasizing renal tumor of childhood.*[507,508] A review of the clinical and pathologic features described in each of these publications reveals that the tumors were one and the same, the three different names notwithstanding. In the years following these initial reports, approximately 130 additional cases have been reported, virtually all initially diagnosed as Wilms' tumor, reflecting the lack of general recognition of this newly described childhood neoplasm.[510-515] Indeed, this neoplasm was initially tentatively regarded as a sarcomatous variant of Wilms' tumor.[517] However, there is now general agreement that clear cell sarcoma (bone metastasizing renal tumor of childhood) is a distinct nosologic entity unrelated to Wilms' tumor.[514-515]

Clinical Features

This renal neoplasm is most commonly diagnosed in children 1 to 5 years of age, with reported age means of 30 to 42 months.[507,510,513,515] It has been diagnosed in children as young as 3 months and as old as 14 years.[515] All studies indicate a male preponderance of 1.2 – 7.6 : 1.[507,511,513,515] Most patients present with a renal mass. Hematuria is recorded uncommonly. Prominent in the clinical course, and on occasion present at the time of diagnosis, is the unusual predilection of this tumor to metastasize to bone. Osseous metastases were observed in 40% to 100% of the earliest reported series.[507,509,511,517] More recently, Haas and associates (1984) reported bone metastases in only 17% of a series of 75 cases. Even this lowest reported frequency exceeds the frequency of bone metastases observed with Wilms' tumors.[515] The mortality rate of clear cell sarcoma is significantly higher than observed with Wilms' tumors, with the majority of patients dying with metastases to bone and other sites.[507,509,511,517] Haas and co-workers (1984) report 2-year survival rates of two groups of patients from the National Wilms' Tumor Study of 39% and 49%, respectively.[515]

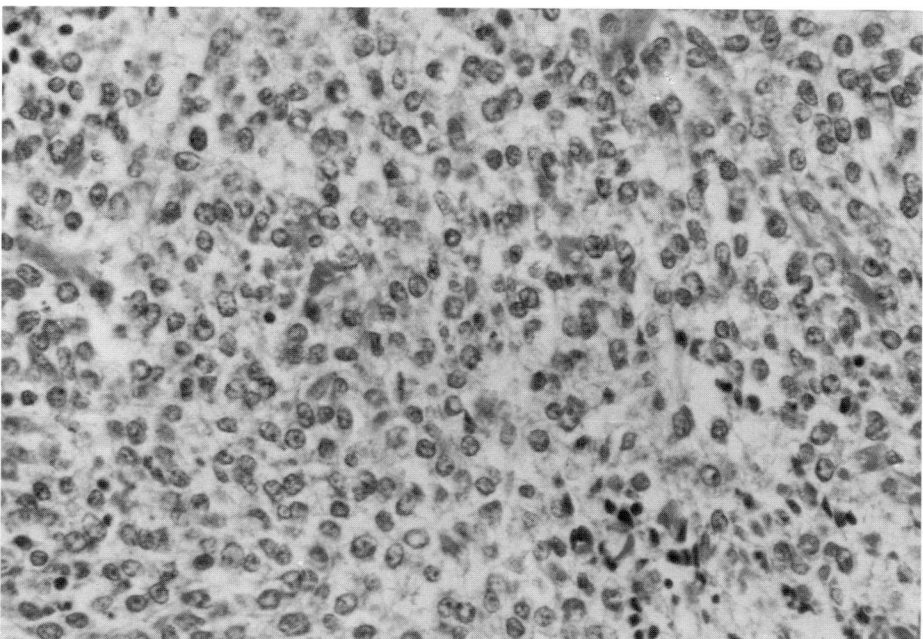

Figure 1-43   *Clear cell sarcoma. This neoplasm, devoid of histologic structural features, contains sheets of poorly defined cells with clear cytoplasm, and round or oval nuclei. The chromatin is finely dispersed. Nucleoli are present but are not prominent. (Microscopic slide courtesy of J. Bruce Beckwith, M.D., Denver, CO)*

Pathologic Features

Clear cell sarcomas are solid neoplasms, commonly with scattered small cysts. Uncommonly, cysts are prominent. The cut surface is described as buff, gray-white, or tan. Hemorrhage and necrosis may be present but are not prominent features. The neoplasm replaces much of the kidney, with an infiltrating border showing invasion of the adjacent renal parenchyma and renal capsule commonly reported. Metastatic tumor may be present in the hilar lymph nodes.

Microscopically, Beckwith (1983) describes a "classic pattern" and variants.[514] As suggested by the descriptive name *clear cell sarcoma,* the tumor cells have clear or very poorly staining cytoplasm (Fig. 1-43). Cytoplasmic vacuoles may be present in focal areas of the tumor. Cell boundaries are indistinct. The nuclei are oval or round, lack significant pleomorphism, and have a finely dispersed chromatin. Nucleoli are not prominent, and mitotic figures are uncommon. The histologic pattern characteristic of most examples is nests of tumor cells without apparent organization, separated by a prominent capillary network

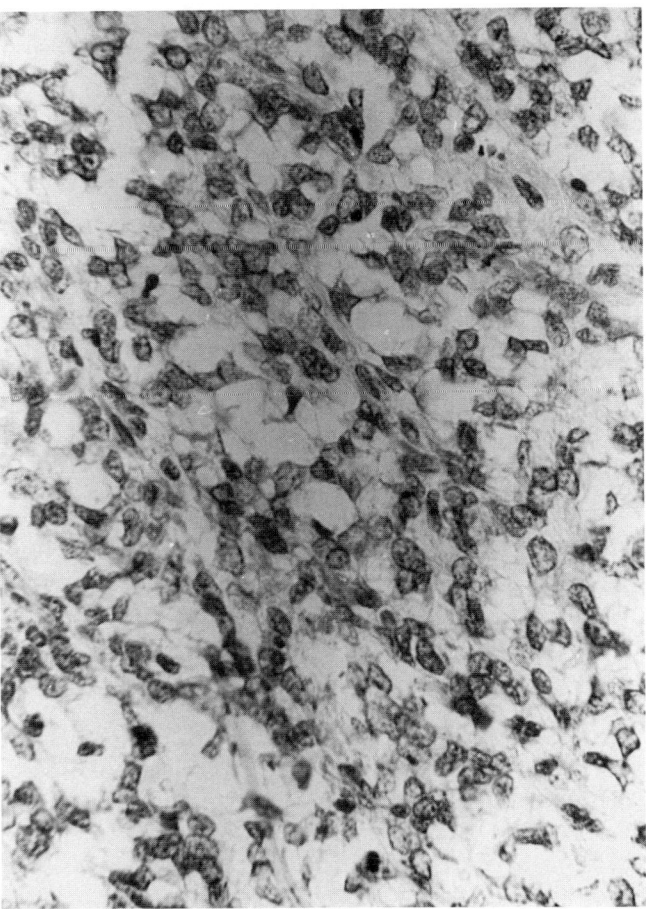

Figure 1-44   *Clear cell sarcoma. The tumor cells are dispersed in sheets without apparent structure. Individual tumor cells have a clear or lightly staining cytoplasm within distinct cell borders. Nucleoli are not prominent. (Microscopic slide courtesy of J. Bruce Beckwith, M.D., Denver, CO)*

with spindle stromal cells (Fig. 1-44). At the periphery, entrapped renal tubules confirm the infiltrative border observed grossly. A reticulin stain accentuates the vascular trabeculae separating the tumor cell nests.

Variant patterns include cases with increased prominence of the vascular septae, hyalinization of the stroma, accentuated stromal spindle cell proliferation, and cystic dilatation of entrapped renal tubules.[514] Additionally, nuclear palisading may mimic neurilemmoma. Finally, a trabecular pattern mimicking tubular differentiation of Wilms' may be prominent. Thorough microscopic examination of the tumor will disclose more characteristic areas of the tumor, allowing differentiation from Wilms' tumor.

Histogenesis

The histogenesis of clear cell sarcoma remains unsettled. Novak and associates (1980) proposed origin from blastemal cap cells on the basis of ultrastructural studies.[512] In a subsequent electron microscopic study, Haas and associates (1984) illustrated extracellular matrix entrapped in cytoplasmic extensions, imparting the clear cytoplasmic features observed with light microscopy.[515] On the basis of the observed ultrastructural features, Haas and colleagues (1984) regarded the neoplasm to be of primitive mesenchymal origin and not of blastemal cap cells, but more precise determination was not accomplished.[515] The exact histogenesis of clear cell sarcoma (bone metastasizing renal tumor of childhood) remains unknown, and the descriptive name must serve in the absence of such clarification.

Malignant Rhabdoid Tumor

The first description of the aggressive neoplasm malignant rhabdoid tumor was reported by Beckwith and Palmer (1978) in their review of cases submitted to the National Wilms' Tumor Study.[517] The unique pathologic features were accompanied by clinical characteristics that were unique and unlike those of typical Wilms' tumors. Beckwith and Palmer tentatively regarded this neoplasm as a "sarcomatoid variant" of Wilms' tumor, but they recognized the possibility that further study may indicate that this neoplasm was unique and distinct from Wilms' tumors. Their prediction proved accurate.

In their original report, Beckwith and Palmer (1978) indicated tht preliminary ultrastructural studies supported skeletal muscle origin of the tumor, prompting the name *malignant rhabdoid tumor.*[517] Subsequent studies by Beckwith and associates, as well as others, have not confirmed these preliminary findings.[518-520,523,524] The originally suggested name is descriptively accurate on the light-microscopic level, and it has been retained in the absence of a more appropriate term based on histogenesis, which at present remains unresolved.[518,523,524] Of interest is the finding that this neoplasm is not unique to the kidney, with recently published examples taking origin in the thymus, chest wall, liver, paravaginal and paravertebral soft tissue, and heart.[516,520,522,524,525] Approximately 30 cases have been reported, all taking origin in the kidney with the exception of the six cases of extrarenal malignant rhabdoid tumor noted above.[517-521,523]

Clinical Features

This neoplasm has been reported in children 3 months to 42 months of age, with a median age of approximately 1 year. The recent extrarenal example reported by Frierson and co-workers occurring in a 14-year-old girl is unique.[524] At the time

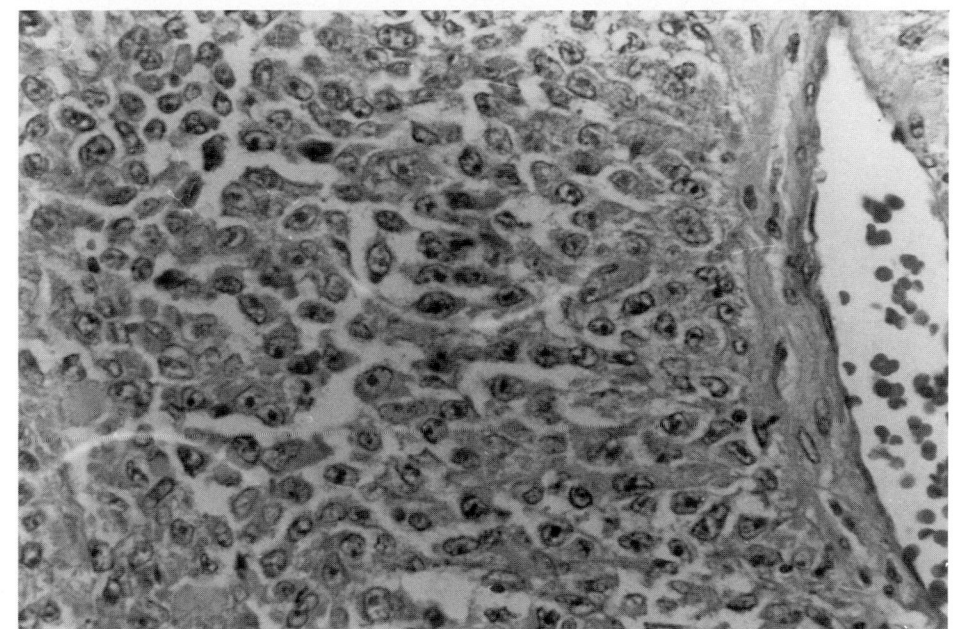

A

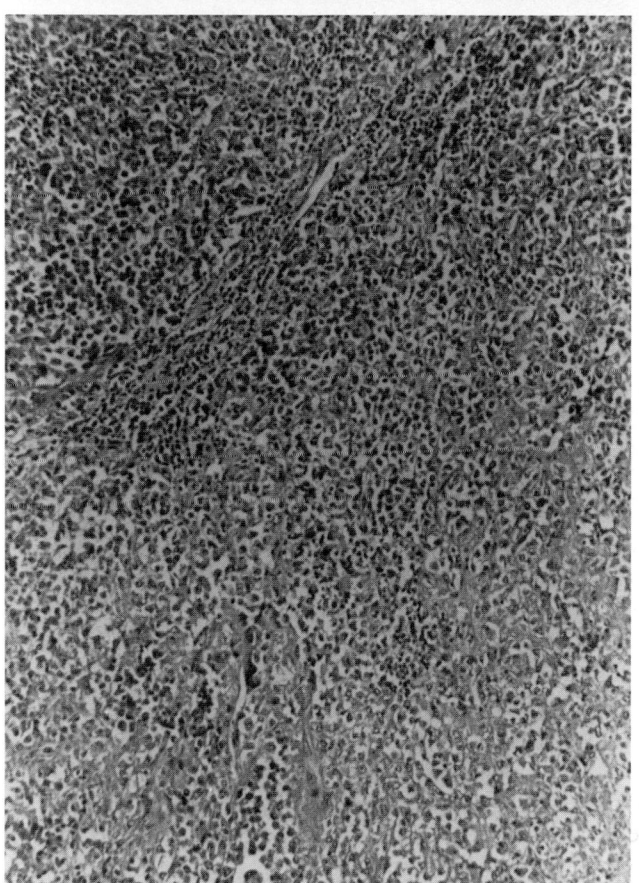

B

Figure 1-45   *Malignant rhabdoid tumor.* (A) *The pleomorphic tumor cells have abundant eosinophilic cytoplasm, occasionally with a hyaline droplet inclusion. The vesicular enlarged nuclei contain prominent nucleoli.* (B) *Sheets of cytologically malignant cells with abundant eosinophilic cytoplasm characterize the neoplasm. (Microscopic slide courtesy of J. Bruce Beckwith, M.D., Denver, CO)*

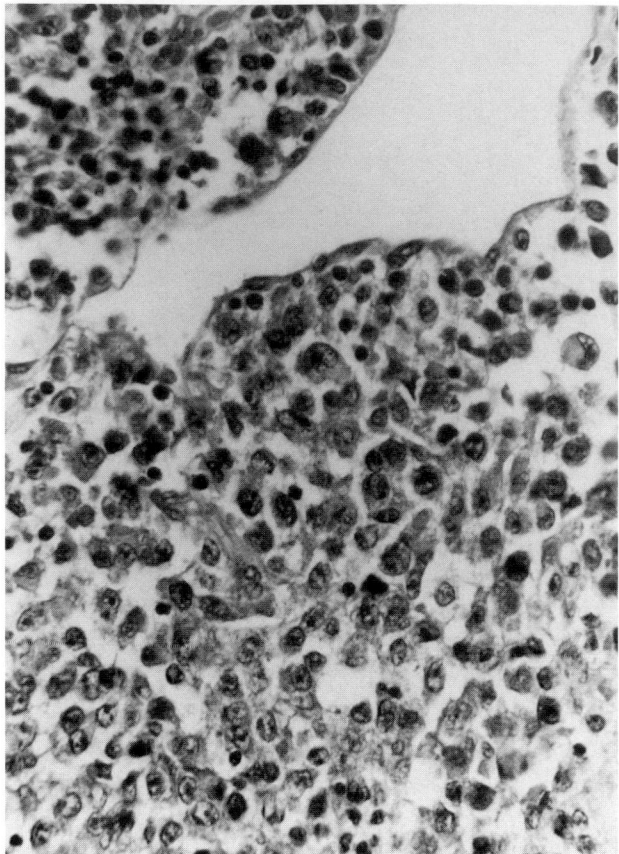

Figure 1-46   *Malignant rhabdoid tumor. The tumor cells demonstrate
prominent nucleoli, clumped chromatin, and irregularity of
the nuclear configuration. Occasional cells show eosinophilic
hyaline inclusions, and the majority show a granular
cytoplasm.*

of diagnosis, an abdominal mass is detected in the young patients. The tumor is
highly lethal, frequently with lung and brain metastases.[517-521,523] Nineteen of
twenty-one patients reported by the National Wilms' Tumor Study Group suc-
cumbed to their malignancy.[523]

Pathologic Features

Grossly, the solid tumor characteristically has infiltrating borders. The majority
of the cases reported by Beckwith and Palmer (1978) showed evidence of invasion and growth beyond the kidney at the time of initial diagnosis.[517] Microscopically, the polygonal tumor cells, growing in sheets and nests, have abundant
eosinophilic cytoplasm, commonly with prominent hyaline cytoplasmic inclusions (Fig. 1-45). Nuclei are vesicular, and they characteristically contain a prominent nucleolus (Fig. 1-46). Ultrastructural studies demonstrate masses of
whorled filaments corresponding to the cytoplasmic inclusions observed with
light microscopy.[518,519] In spite of the resemblance of the cells to myoblasts in
routine stains, as judged by light microscopy, no cross striations are detected

with phosphotungstic acid hematoxylin (PTAH). Furthermore, all electron microscopic studies have failed to demonstrate Z-bands.[518,519] Immunoperoxidase staining for myoglobin has similarly been uniformly negative.[519]

Differential Diagnosis

Occasional foci of spindle cells may resemble the histologic features of mesoblastic nephroma. The significantly different clinical behavior patterns of these two neoplasms underscores the importance of making this diagnostic distinction. Finally, there is no evidence of blastemal or epithelial components, which, when coupled with the features of malignant rhabdoid tumor, allows differentiation of this highly lethal tumor from Wilms' tumor.

Epithelial Neoplasms

Oncocytoma

History

The term *oncocytoma* was introduced by Jaffe (1932) as a synomym for adenolymphomas of the salivary gland.[526] The term made reference to large polygonal cells possessing abundant eosinophilic cytoplasm called oncocytes. In 1962, Hamperl suggested that the term *oncocytoma* be restricted to neoplasms composed exclusively of oncocytes.[578] Lesions fulfilling this criterion have been reported in several sites, including salivary glands, thyroid, parathyroid, and until recently, only rarely in the kidney.[534] Regardless of the organ of origin, ultrastructual studies of oncocytes characteristically show abundant mitochondria filling the cytoplasm of the cells.[534]

The recognition of renal oncocytomas in the American literature is a relatively recent event, dating back only to 1976 when Klein and Valensi reported 13 cases in a retrospective study at one institution.[534] Seven of the thirteen cases were encountered during the years 1964 to 1973, and an additional six cases occurred from 1973 to 1975. All cases were originally interpreted as renal cell carcinomas. In a review of the literature, these same authors found six previously reported cases, all in European journals.[527,529-532] The first case of renal oncocytoma was reported by Zippel in 1942.[527] Klein and Valensi (1976) summarized the features of these neoplasms including their tendency to (1) be incidental findings unaccompanied by symptoms, (2) be large in size, (3) have well-defined borders without evidence of typical microscopic appearance of the oncocytes, and (4) exhibit benign clinical behavior with long recurrence-free intervals recorded.[534] Subsequent to the study of Klein and Valensi (1976), renal oncocytomas have been reported with increasing frequency (Figure 1-47).[533,535-573] Approximately 230 cases were found in the literature, of which 80% have been reported since 1980.[547-573] Based on the cumulative reported experience, renal oncocytomas have developed a generally benign reputation and are regarded as variants of cortical adenomas. These "adenoma variants" are capable of attaining large size, with a paradoxical lack of the relationship between tumor size and risk of metastases that generally characterizes the behavior of typical so-called cortical adenomas and renal cell carcinomas.

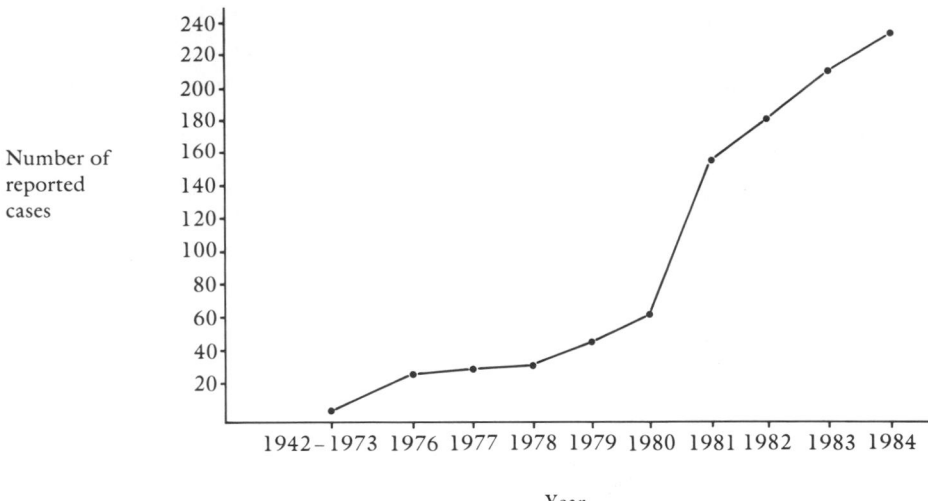

Figure 1-47   *Reported cases of renal oncocytoma.*

Frequency

The frequency of renal oncocytomas among renal neoplasms in adults averages about 5%, with reported percentages of 1% to 16%, the higher figures being reported in the most recent studies.[534,548,557,558,566] An apparent increase in frequency of this neoplasm was first suggested by Klein and Valensi (1976), who noted seven of their thirteen cases occurring between 1964 and 1973, with the remaining six cases diagnosed during the subsequent 3 years, 1973 to 1975, prior to publication.[534] Of the total cases reported to date, approximately 140 cases (60%) represent oncocytomas discovered only at the time of retrospective review of cases originally diagnosed as renal cell carcinoma. A real increase in the frequency of this neoplasm has not been demonstrated, and I find it doubtful.

Age and Sex Distribution

Renal oncocytomas are more frequent in males, who represent 161 cases (69%) of the total 232 cases reported to 1985. The patients range in age from 15 years (Pearse and Haughton, 1979) to 102 years (Milstoc, 1977) with a peak frequency in the sixth to eighth decades (75% in ages 50–79 years).[535,540]

Clinical Features

Approximately 65% of the reported cases were asymptomatic and were discovered as incidental findings on IVP performed for unrelated reasons or at autopsy (Table 1-11). Symptomatic patients (35% of reported cases) presented with pain (flank or abdominal), hematuria, or a mass, in order of decreasing frequency.

Radiologic Features

The consensus of numerous radiologic studies of renal oncocytomas is that although there are characteristic angiographic features, none individually or together are diagnostic of this neoplasm. Renal cell carcinoma cannot be differentiated with complete assurance by radiologic means. Ultrasound, IVP, and CT scan procedures are of less value in differentiating renal cell carcinoma. The angiographic features characteristic of renal oncocytomas were originally described by Sos and co-workers (1976), Weiner and Bernstein (1977) and Ambos and associates (1978) and include (1) uniform blush during nephrogram phase; (2) well-marginated lesion with smooth contour, frequently with vessels stretched around the tumor; (3) hypervascular neoplasm without evidence of puddling; and (4) "spoke-wheel" pattern of tumor vascularity, with vessels converging toward the center.[533,536,539] An IVP commonly demonstrates a mass lesion with distortion of the calyceal system. Ultrasound shows a solid mass, confirmed by CT scan, which further shows the characteristic sharp demarcation of this neoplasm.[547,551,557,568]

Pathology

Gross Features

The gross features of renal oncocytomas are sufficiently characteristic to suggest strongly the correct diagnosis and differentiate this neoplasm from renal cell carcinoma. The reported cases of oncocytoma average 6.9 cm in diameter, with a range of millimeters to the largest reported case, 26 cm in diameter.[555] Fifty-three percent of the reported cases measure 3 cm to 7 cm in diameter. The typical example is solid and well demarcated, with a surrounding capsule of variable thickness and a color of red-brown to mahogany on cut surface (Fig. 1-48). A central fibrous scar is typically but not invariably present.[566,571,572] Characteristically absent are extensive areas of hemorrhage and necrosis, although small focal areas showing these changes have been reported.[570] Only two examples of extensive hemorrhage within the tumor, one requiring an emergency nephrectomy, have been reported.[535,558] I have encountered a third example also requiring emergency nephrectomy because of the spontaneous hemorrhage and rupture of the tumor into the perirenal adipose tissue. Uncommon variations from the above typical features include focal cystic change, associated polycystic disease, and a renal cell carcinoma.[555,563,572]

Table 1-11 **Clinical Presentation of 232 Cases of Renal Oncocytoma Reported Between 1942 and 1984**

Clinical Presentation	No. of Cases
Asymptomatic; discovered during IVP for unrelated disorder	135 (58%)
Incidental finding at autopsy	13 (6%)
Incidental finding at surgery	1 (0.5%)
Pain	44 (19%)
Hematuria	27 (12%)
Mass	8 (3%)
No information	4 (2%)

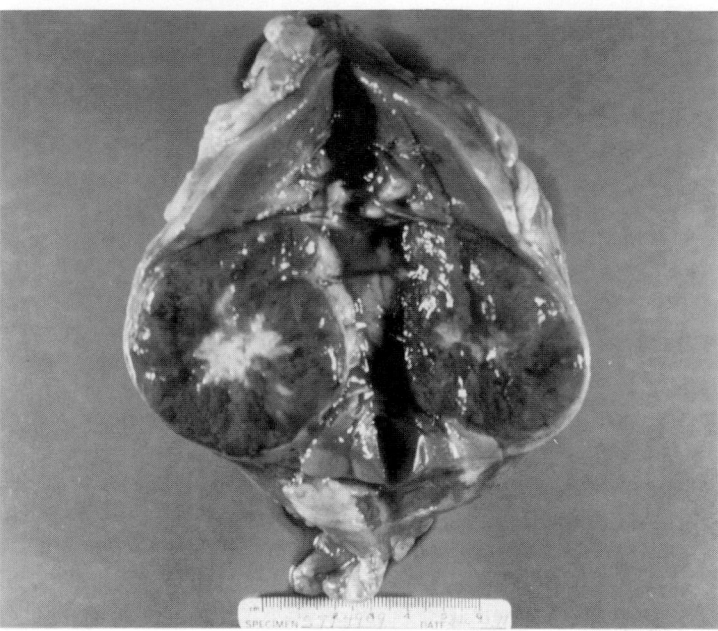

Figure 1-48   *Renal tubular oncocytoma. The well-circumscribed neoplasm has a central area of fibrosis surrounded by tumor similar in color to the normal renal parenchyma.*

Although renal oncocytomas are typically unilateral and single, examples of bilateral and multicentric oncocytomas have been reported.[559,560,562,564,565,567,570,572,573] Multicentricity in the ultimate sense is demonstrated by the case reported by Warfel and Eble (1982), which showed bilateral "oncocytomatosis" with 27 separate tumors in the right kidney and 26 in the left, each measuring 1 mm to 3 mm in diameter.[562]

Microscopic Features

The histologic organization of the oncocytes is variable but most commonly features nests, cords, or tubules of tumor cells in a loose, edematous stroma (Fig. 1-49*A*). Less commonly, sheets of tumor cells or microcysts lined by oncocytes are observed. The typical cells are polygonal with abundant eosinophilic stroma (Fig. 1-49*B*) and round to oval, hyperchromatic nuclei, generally with minimal pleomorphism (Figs. 1-50 and 1-51). Nucleoli may be inconspicuous or prominent. Mitoses are rarely present. Occasionally cells with enlarged, rarely bizarre nuclei are found in an otherwise typical oncocytoma. The spectrum of nuclear pleomorphism that is acceptable without anticipated change in clinical behavior is currently not defined with certainty and awaits greater cumulative experience. Among the cases reported to date are examples with readily identifiable nuclear pleomorphism without associated aggressive clinical behavior.[555,563,571]

In contrast to all other reported cases of renal oncocytomas are the six cases (among 90 cases of a retrospective series) reported by Lieber and associates (1981) that demonstrated metastases, two to regional lymph nodes and four to unstated distant sites, with ultimate death of the patients.[555] All six cases con-

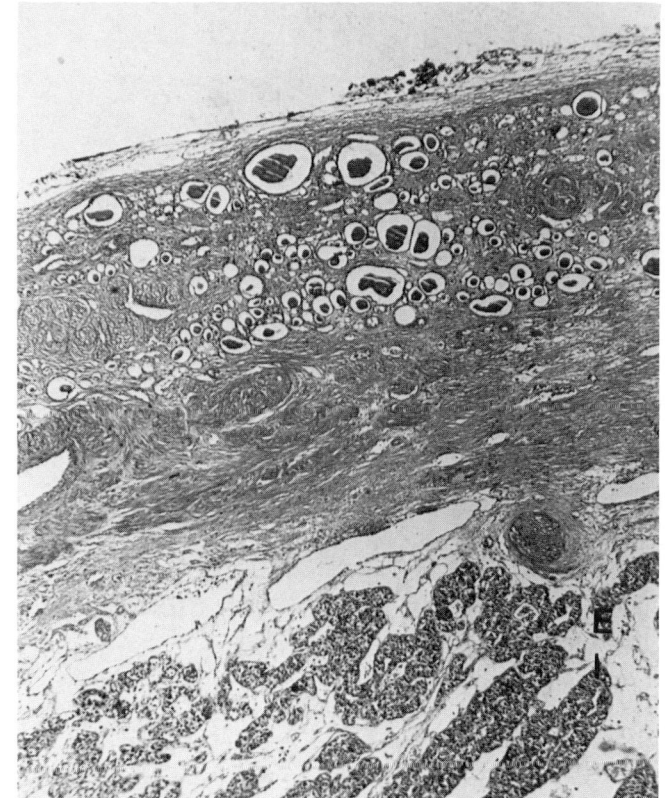

A

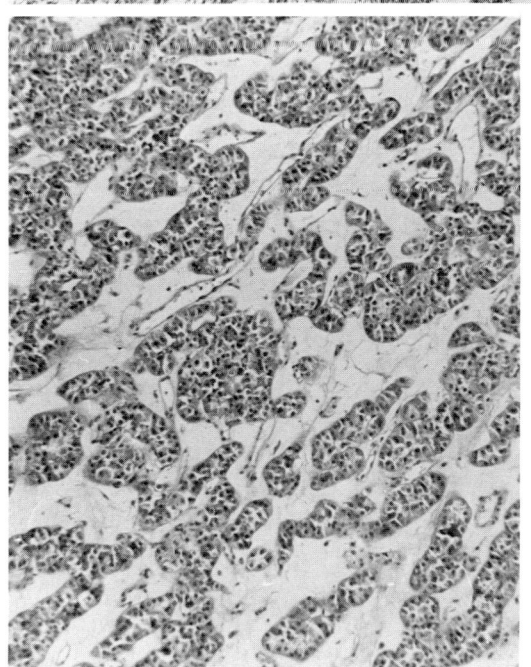

B

Figure 1-49   ***Oncocytoma.*** *(A) The renal cortical structures beneath the capsule include sclerotic glomeruli and dilated tubules, the result of chronic pyelonephritis found in association with the renal oncocytoma at the bottom of the photograph. The tumor is composed of cords of oncocytic cells separated by an edematous stroma. (B) The oncocytic cells with abundant eosinophilic cytoplasm are arranged in irregular cords with intervening edematous stroma containing thin-walled blood vessels.*

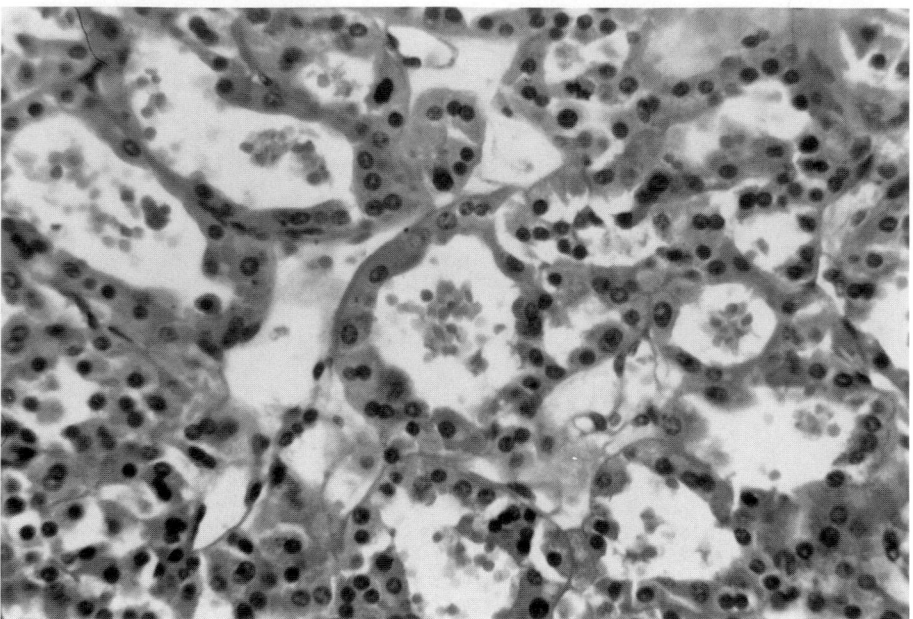

Figure 1-50   **Renal tubular oncocytoma.** *The oncocytic cells are arranged in tubules. There is an absence of tumor necrosis, mitoses, and significant pleomorphism.*

formed to grade 2 criteria in a tumor grading protocol proposed for renal oncocytomas as described below:

Grade 1 — Tumor composed of cells with uniform, round nuclei with abundant cytoplasm

Grade 2 — Tumor composed of cells showing greater pleomorphism with larger, more irregular nuclei

Grade 3 — Tumor composed of cells with greater variation than demonstrated by grade 2 tumors and possibly accompanied by bizarre cells and mitoses

Among the 90 oncocytomas reported by Lieber and associates (1981), 62 (69%) were grade 1 and 28 (31%) were grade 2.[555] No other cases of renal oncocytomas evidencing metastases have appeared in the literature in the few years since Lieber and associates' study (refer to further discussion of natural history, below).

Ultrastructural Features

The ultrastructural features of renal oncocytomas were first described by Blessing and Wienert in 1973, and the basic features have been confirmed in numerous subsequent studies.[532] The cytoplasm of the tumor cells is virtually filled with innumerable mitochondria with a paucity of other cell organelles including Golgi apparatus, rough endoplasmic reticulum, and lipid vacuoles, all features that tend to be prominent in clear cells of renal cell carcinoma.[534,544,545,548,561,571] The mitochondria are variously described as normal or swollen, frequently showing stacking of the cristae. Cytoplasmic filaments described by Yu and associates (1980) have been reported in subsequent studies.[548,561,571] One feature, microvilli, is observed inconstantly among different studies and among

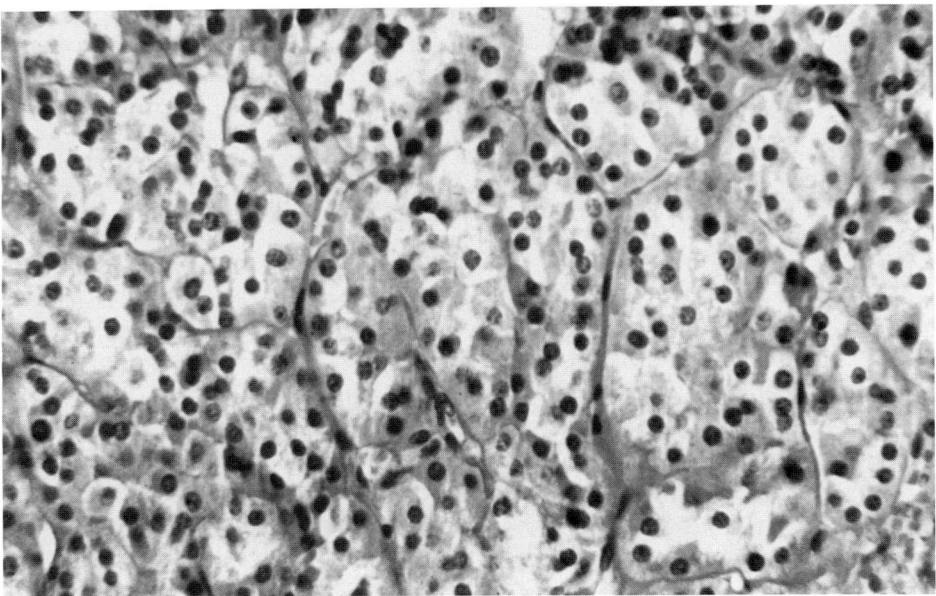

Figure 1-51   *Oncocytoma. The oncocytic cells, here showing the absence of significant nuclear pleomorphism, are arranged in nests separated by thin fibrous trabeculae.*

tumors within the same series.[534,548,561,571] Klein and Valensi (1976) proposed the proximal tubules as the origin of renal oncocytomas, based on their observations of microvilli in the tumor cells.[534] This conclusion has recently been challenged by Eble and Hull (1984), who described complex basal plasmalemma interdigitations, a feature of distal tubules.[571] However, Marino and Livolsi (1982) observed positive immunoperoxidase staining for lysozyme in tumor cells, which they proposed supported origin from proximal tubules.[561] This matter awaits further study.

Natural History

As previously discussed, renal oncocytomas, unknown in the United States prior to the report of Klein and Valensi in 1976, have been reported with increasing frequency in recent years.[534] The cumulative weight of these studies is best described in the introduction of a recent study: "Subsequent reports of these lesions further established their clinical validity as benign entities."[571] Two considerations underscore the need for caution in the acceptance of this view of the biologic potential of renal neoplasms meeting the criteria of oncocytomas.

The first consideration centers on the study reported by Lieber and associates (1981), which recorded six examples of oncocytomas demonstrating metastases.[555] The authors discussed the inherent limitation of the study imposed by its retrospective nature. The six cases showing metastases were not described in any detail beyond their assignment to a grade 2 category. Information referable to size of primary tumor, stage of primary tumor, and time interval between diagnosis and detection of metastases was not provided. Of greater importance was the limited number of slides available for review, which may have precluded identification of features of the tumors (*e.g.*, clear cells) allowing the alternative diagnosis of renal cell carcinoma. However, within the constraints of the available information, we have six possible renal oncocytomas among the 232 published cases that demonstrated metastases. With more experience the biologic continuum of these oncocytic neoplasms, from benign to clinically malignant, as suggested by Lieber and colleagues (1981) may prove to be the more accurate view of their natural history.

The second consideration relates to the soundness of the current data supporting the biologic benignity of renal oncocytomas, exclusive of the six disturbing cases reported by Lieber and associates. Specifically, a critical review of the recorded follow-up information of the 232 cases reported to 1985, outlined in Table 1-12, discloses a very meager data base on which conclusions can be made. Ninety-one of the reported cases are of limited or no value in evaluating clinical behavior because (1) either no follow-up or no tumor size data are provided; (2) neither tumor size nor follow-up data are provided; (3) follow-up information is provided but is of limited duration (less than 4 years); or (4) the neoplasm was diagnosed at autopsy. Furthermore, an additional 120 cases are reported without relating follow-up information to tumor size, thereby limiting the value of these reports. In sum, only 21 cases, 20 larger than 3 cm, were reported with both tumor size and follow-up information 5 years in duration or longer. Thus, the characterization of renal oncocytomas as clinically benign entities rests solidly on these 21 cases. In fact, we know little of the natural history of these interesting neoplasms.

Table 1-12   **Renal Oncocytoma, 1942 – 1984**

Follow-up Information	Number of Cases
No follow-up information	20 ⎫
No tumor size data	14 ⎪
Neither follow-up nor tumor size data	2 ⎬ 91
Diagnosis at autopsy	10 ⎪
Follow-up information ≤ 2 years	40 ⎪
Follow-up information > 2 years, ≤ 4 years	5 ⎭
Follow-up information not related to tumor size	120*
Tumors > 3 cm followed < 5 years with NED	20 ⎫ 21
Tumors < 3 cm followed ≥ 5 years with NED	1 ⎭
Total reported cases	232

* Ejeckam et al (1979) presented 7 cases, including 3 diagnosed at autopsy with size range of 2.5 cm – 10 cm. Of 4 cases diagnosed antemortem, only 2 had follow-up information > 1 year (5 years and 6 years).
   Lieber et al (1981) presented 90 cases with size distribution data but with follow-up information not related to tumor size. Sixty-six patients (73%) were alive, 20 (22%) had died of other causes, and importantly, 4 (4.4%) had died of metastatic disease during the 15 years of observation.
   Merino and Livolsi (1982) presented 14 cases ranging in size from 2.5 – 14 cm, and followed 1 – 14 years (average, 5 years). Thirteen patients had no evidence of disease at last follow-up. One patient had died of cardiovascular disease 6 years after diagnosis without evidence of tumor recurrence.
   Maatman et al (1984) presented 11 cases, including 1 diagnosed at autopsy and another patient, with a 3 cm tumor, who died 11 years after diagnosis of unrelated cause (CVA) and who had no evidence of disease at the time of death. The remaining 9 cases were followed 3 months to 7 years, without evidence of recurrence, but without details relating duration of follow-up to the tumor size. The 9 patients had tumors that ranged in size from 1.5 cm – 13 cm, including 1 case of bilateral oncocytomas.

Renal Cortical "Adenoma"

Recognition of small epithelial proliferations, frequently tubular or papillary in configuration, located under the renal capsule dates back to the late 19th century. The earliest focus of interest in these nodules was primarily in the context of the ongoing debate referable to histogenesis — renal tubule versus ectopic adrenal tissue. Decades later, with the histogenesis controversy unresolved, studies centered on the relatively high incidence of these tumors encountered as incidental findings at autopsy.[578,579,585,586,590,598] Overall frequencies of 7% to 23% were reported in adult autopsy studies.[578,579,586,590,598] The frequency increased with age, with few such cortical neoplasms observed in children and young adults. These proliferative lesions were frequently multiple.[584] The significance of these lesions was unsettled, with some regarding them as benign while others thought they were potentially malignant.[576,580,582,583,588,597]

In 1938, Bell studied a series of renal "adenoma–carcinomas" with reference to the relationship of tumor size to the frequency of metastases.[582] This series was expanded in the subsequent publication of his book.[588] Among 65 tumors less than 3 cm in diameter, metastases were observed in only three cases (4.6%). One of these three tumors measured only 1.5 cm in greatest diameter. In addition, Bell makes reference to another case demonstrating metastases in spite of the small size (5 mm) of the renal primary.[588] Bell showed that 35%, 72%, and 85% of tumors measuring 3 cm to 6 cm, 6 cm to 10 cm, and more than 10 cm demonstrated metastases, respectively.[588]

The data clearly showed an increased risk of metastases associated with an increase in tumor diameter, bearing in mind that 15% of the largest tumors in the series (>10 cm) showed no metastases. The author's interpretations will be quoted: "We may conclude that the small tumors (so-called adenomas) are early stages of the large growths and that no certain distinctions can be made between adenoma and carcinoma." Further, "The histologic structure of the tumors did not afford a reliable means for distinguishing adenoma from carcinoma."[588]

Unfortunately, Bell, admitting the criterion was arbitrary, disregarded the data and his interpretations as cited above, and curiously felt compelled nonetheless to classify those nodules less than 3 cm as adenomas and those larger as carcinomas.[588] This dissociation of conclusion from the data is most regrettable.

In subsequent years, textbooks and many studies focused on Bell's classification and joined the original author in disregarding the data in the final analysis. Bell's classification translated into working definitions of benign cortical adenomas (those tumors less than 3 cm), and renal adenocarcinomas (those tumors of larger dimensions). This succeeded in establishing cortical adenoma as a distinct nosologic entity (based on size criterion) which is completely contrary to Bell's and to all other available data.

Defying this working definition of adenoma and carcinoma, isolated case reports of large, symptomatic adenomas encountered clinically appeared in the literature.[574,575,577,581,587,589,592,594,602] Alternatively, sporadic reported cases of renal cortical neoplasms less than 3 cm in diameter demonstrate widespread metastases (Table 1-13). By definition, these cases are carcinomas, and they thereby require a "temporary suspension of the rules." A review of the included microscopic descriptions in these case reports does not provide a consistent set of histologic features allowing reliable identification. Indeed, there have been no reported histologic features of these metastasizing neoplasms that would allow

Table 1-13   **Small Renal Cell Carcinomas Demonstrating Metastases**

Author	Year	Tumor Size (cm)
Hale, Burkland[583]	1943	1.5
Bell[586]	1950	0.5
Bell[586]	1950	1.5
Bell[586]	1950	<3.0
Bell[586]	1950	<3.0
Hajdu, Thomas[851]	1967	<1.5
Hajdu, Thomas[851]	1967	<1.5
Hajdu, Thomas[853]	1970	<1.5
Evins, Varner[600]	1979	1.3
Talamo, Shonnard[651]	1980	0.9

reliable distinction from other cortical neoplasms of similar size not demonstrating metastases.

The current status of this dilemma can be summarized. It has been determined that both renal cell carcinoma and so-called cortical adenoma have a common origin in the proximal convoluted tubules of the kidney (Figs. 1-52 and 1-53) (refer to the discussion of renal cell carcinoma, below). Bell's data relating an increased probability of metastases associated with an increase in tumor size generally holds true. Exceptional cases behave in a manner markedly different

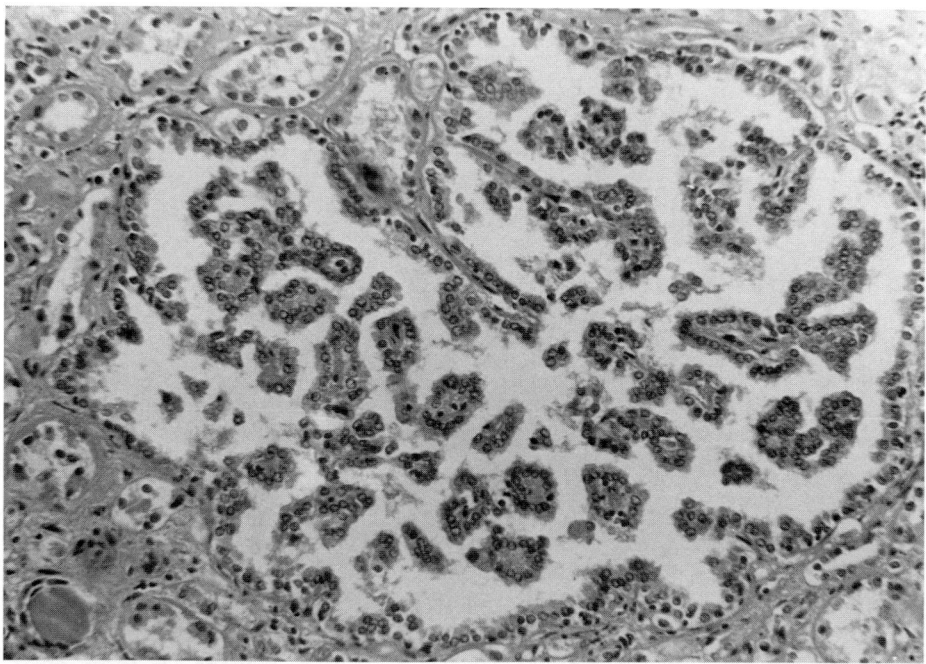

Figure 1-52   **Renal cortical adenoma.** *This cystic structure with numerous papillary projections into the lumen is lined by epithelial cells with features suggesting their renal tubular origin. No mitoses or significant pleomorphism is present.*

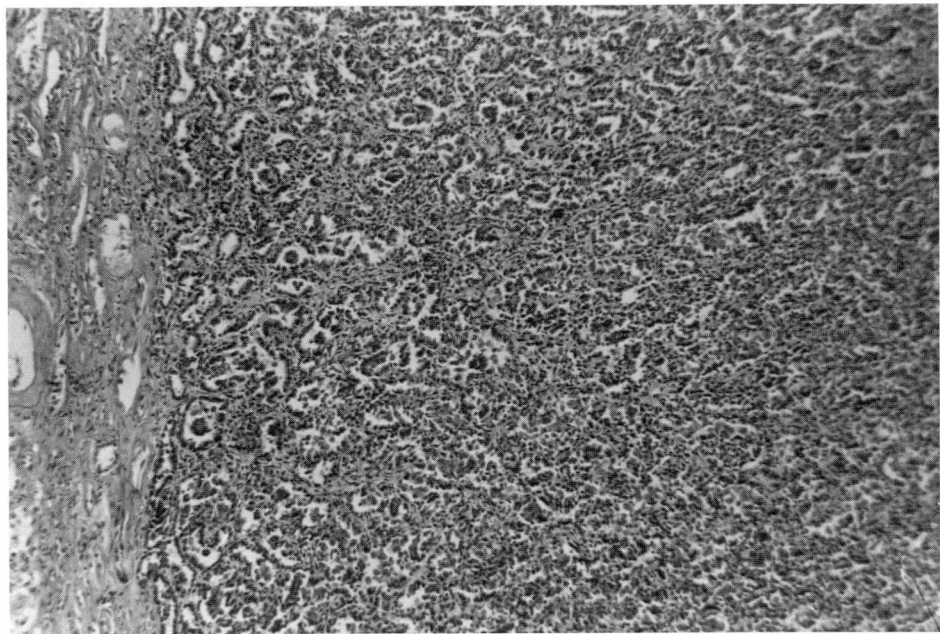

Figure 1-53   *Renal cortical adenoma. This cortical adenoma is composed of a complex pattern of small tubules with little intervening stroma. There is an absence of pleomorphism and necrosis, and no mitotic figures are present. The interface with the adjacent normal cortex is seen near the left margin of the photograph.*

from that expected from the work of Bell. There are rare examples of small tumors demonstrating malignant behavior and slightly more frequently examples of large tumors exhibiting benign behavior in spite of their very large size. Although Mostofi has reported identifying benign adenomatous areas giving origin to carcinomas based on histologic grounds, others, including Bennington and Beckwith, report that adenomas and carcinomas are not distinguishable.[600,601] Bennington summarizes the clearest position, which I share, that there are neither gross, microscopic, ultrastructural, nor histochemical features that reliably allow distinction between so-called cortical adenomas and renal adenocarcinomas.[600]

The adoption of this view requires a full understanding of the practical consequences of rendering a diagnosis of renal adenocarcinoma when encountering a small (< 3 cm) neoplastic nodule in a nephrectomy specimen. The probability of metastatic dissemination from such a lesion is low, as discussed above, and this information should be part of the rendered diagnosis. A suggested term for such neoplasms is *renal adenocarcinoma of low metastatic potential.*

It is hoped that future studies demonstrating the reliability of tumor grading will resolve this dilemma.[591,604]

Renal Cell Carcinoma

Renal malignancy in childhood is virtually synonymous with Wilms' tumor; in the adult, renal malignancy is virtually synonymous with renal cell carcinoma (renal adenocarcinoma). Renal cell carcinoma constitutes 80% to 90% of primary malignant renal neoplasms in the adult age group, with the remainder represented by urothelial malignancies of the renal pelvis, primarily transitional cell carcinoma, renal sarcomas, rare examples of adult Wilms' tumor, and mixed tumors (carcinosarcomas) in order of decreasing frequency.

The historical controversies related to the histogenesis of this neoplasm, renal versus "adrenal rests" within the kidney, reflected in previous names such as Grawitz tumor and hypernephroma, have been settled with the application of the electron microscope.[758,760] The challenges currently posed by renal cell carcinoma are manifold and are principally related to the undetermined etiology, infrequency of early clinical diagnosis, identification of morphologic features of predictive value, and most certainly, the development of effective adjuvant therapy. Directly related to these limitations, this fascinating neoplasm remains a very dangerous malignancy and a major challenge to surgical pathologist and oncologist alike.

Epidemiology and Etiology

Etiology will be dealt with briefly. The cause of renal cell carcinoma remains unknown. The experimental production of so-called cortical adenomas has been reported in rats by the injection of nitrosamines.[667,676] Carcinogens of this type are present in cigarette smoke, which has been reported in two studies to be associated with increased risk of development of renal cell carcinoma.[666,675] The report of Bennington and Laubsches (1968) implicated pipe and cigar smoke.[666] There is neither experimental nor epidemiologic evidence supporting viruses, radiation, or industrial carcinogen exposure to the development of renal cell carcinoma.[675,677,678] Genetic factors are evident in only rare, invariably reported cases.[670,671,679]

Table 1-14   *Demographic Characteristics of Renal Cell Carcinoma*

Author	Year	No. of Patients	Age		Sex Distribution		Side Distribution*	
			Range	Mean	Male	Female	Right	Left
Hand, Broders[605]	1932	193	29–93	6th decade	70%	30%	49.2%	50.8%
Priestly[606]	1939	482	—†	6th decade	70%	30%	—	—
Griffith, Thackray[607]	1949	103	24–83	6th decade	67%	33%	50%	50%
Claes[613]	1963	92	38–81	59	60%	40%	—	—
Arner et al[617]	1965	197	20–90	6th decade	60%	40%	—	—
Myers et al[622]	1968	533	8–83	6th decade	70%	30%	53%	47%
Robson[625]	1969	88	19–81	53	76%	24%	—	—
Rafla[628]	1970	244	10–>70	7th decade	76%	33%	44%	56%
Ochsner et al[636]	1973	103	35–77	56.8	78%	22%	38%	62%
Mancilla-Jimenez et al[639]	1976	224	10–82	51	65%	35%	—	—
Patel, Lavengood[642]	1978	166	24–85	6th decade	61%	39%	56%	44%
Selli et al[662]	1983	115	30–84	59	60%	40%	—	—

* Five percent of patients had bilateral neoplasms.

† Dash denotes lack of information.

Renal cell carcinoma is most common in males, with most studies showing a male to female ratio of approximately two to one (Table 1-14). This ratio tends to decrease with increasing age.[677] The peak age frequency is in the sixth decade, with 80% of cases reported between ages 40 and 69 years (Table 1-14). The neoplasm is uncommonly observed in young adults.[681] Although still rare, increasing numbers of reports of this neoplasm arising in children are found in the literature. Approximately 200 cases of renal cell carcinoma have been reported in children and adolescents below the age of 20 years.[665,668,669,672–674,680,682] Rare examples of this neoplasm occurring in siblings and in parent and child are reported.[670,671]

Referable to other epidemiologic factors, this neoplasm appears to be more frequent in urban environments, but there is no identifiable correlation with socioeconomic status, previous medical history, or coffee or alcohol consumption.[677–679]

Significant geographic variation in incidence of renal cell carcinoma is observed throughout the world.[677] The highest recorded frequencies are found in two Scandinavian countries, Denmark and Sweden, with death rates of approximately 4.5 to 5.0 per 100,000 persons.[677] Frequencies approximately half that rate are observed in England, France, the United States, and Israel. The lowest frequencies, less than 1 death per 100,000, are observed in widely dispersed countries including Yugoslavia, Venezuela, and Japan.[677] The relative frequencies in these countries are exhibited by both sexes of the respective nationalities.

Clinical Features

The single most frequent manifestation of renal cell carcinoma is hematuria (Table 1-15). The relative frequencies of gross hematuria and microscopic hematuria are not separately recorded in most studies. The importance of thorough determination of the origin of microscopic hematuria cannot be overemphasized; this determination has ultimately led to the discovery of renal malignancies in a significant number of cases as reflected in published studies and my experience. Associated flank pain is reported in 14% to 51% of cases (Table 1-15). A palpable mass is recorded in 21% to 47% of cases of renal cell carcinoma. The classic triad of hematuria, flank pain, and a flank mass is observed in very few

Table 1-15 **Clinical Presentation of Renal Cell Carcinoma: Frequency of Signs and Symptoms Referable to Primary Tumor**

Author	Year	Hematuria	Flank Pain	Mass	Asymptomatic
Griffiths, Thackray[607]	1949	48%	51%	37%	8%
Hajdu, Thomas[851]	1968	60%	40%	38%	—
Skinner[631]	1971	60%	—†	—	7%
Ochsner et al[636]	1973	40%	48%	39%	5%
Patel, Lavengood[642]	1978	35%	34%	30%	27%
Waters, Richie[650]	1979	52%	38%	21%	23%
Fuselier et al[660]	1983	35.6%	—	—	22%
Petersen*	1984	29%	36%	21%	21%

* Personal observations
† Dash denotes lack of information.

patients, with a recorded range of 4% to 17% (Table 1-16). On rare occasions, massive hemorrhage into an undetected renal cell carcinoma results in a surgical emergency at the time of presentation.[648]

In addition to signs and symptoms directly referable to the renal malignancy, there is increasing appreciation of the systemic manifestations observed in the context of renal cell carcinoma. The following list summarizes such systemic abnormalities in terms of their relative frequencies:

Commonly Observed

    Anemia[629,685,689,691,698]

    Fever[629,685,689,691,698]

    Elevated sedimentation rate[629,685,689,691]

Uncommon

    Hepatorenal dysfunction[684,686,688,690,694]

    Amyloidosis[685,699,703]

    Polycythemia[689,691,696,698]

    Hypercalcemia[683,687,689,693,698,702]

    Thrombophlebitis[685,697]

    Thromboembolism[641]

    Nephrotic syndrome[821]

Rare

    Insulin, glucagon secretion[700]

    Gonadotropin secretion[692,695]

    Renin secretion[696]

    Mineralocorticoid deficiency[701]

Unexplained anemia, fever, and elevated sedimentation rate, all entirely nonspecific, are observed with renal cell carcinoma. Uncommonly, tumor-related eryth-

Table 1-16   ***Clinical Presentation of Renal Cell Carcinoma: Frequency of Patients Presenting With Classic Triad****

Author	Year	No. of Patients	Frequency of Patients Presenting With Classic Triad
Griffith, Thackray[607]	1949	103	17%
Hajdu, Thomas[851]	1968	100	15%
Skinner[631]	1971	309	9%
Ochsner et al[636]	1973	103	11%
Patel, Langengood[642]	1978	166	5%
Waters, Richie[650]	1979	130	4%
Fuselier et al[660]	1983	161	5.7%
Petersen†	1984	80	11%

* Hematuria, flank pain, palpable mass
† Personal observations

rocytosis, hepatorenal dysfunction, amyloidosis, hypercalcemia, and thrombophlebitis are observed. Rare examples of tumor-related hyperinsulinism and increased glucagon and gonadotropin levels are reported.

Disquieting is the not uncommon experience of detecting a renal cell carcinoma in a routine physical examination or in radiologic examination of the urinary system for unrelated medical reasons, in the total absence of any other signs or symptoms referable to the renal primary.[637,638] The frequency of fortuitous detection varies among studies providing this information, but its occurrence is in the range of 10% to 25% of all cases.

Alternatively, a patient may present with complaints referable to a metastatic lesion of an undiagnosed renal primary (Table 1-17). The lungs are the most common anatomical site among such symptomatic metastases from an occult renal cell carcinoma. However, as is evident from the above table, the list of such recipient sites, each with unique attendant clinical symptomatology, is both long and diverse. Indeed, one patient in four has distant metastases at the time of initial presentation (see Table 1-22). These are most commonly detected in the lungs, bones, and brain, in order of decreasing frequency (refer to discussion of metastatic renal cell carcinoma).

Radiologic Features

Radiologic evaluation of a renal mass consistent with or suspicious of renal cell carcinoma on clinical grounds is indispensable and can achieve an accuracy in excess of 95% according to Ney and Friedenberg.[710] The scout film may show diffuse or regional irregular enlargement of the kidney. The majority of renal cell carcinomas show no calcification, but calcification is observed in a small percentage of cases with variable patterns.[709,710] An IVP demonstrates the irregular outline of a mass, commonly with calyceal distortion.[704] Renal arteriography characteristically shows a hypervascular mass with tortuous irregular vessels, diffuse hypervascularity, contrast pooling, and a diffuse tumor blush (Fig. 1-54).[704-708,710] On occasion, hypovascularity may be observed, a finding most commonly associated with a specific histologic type of renal carcinoma, the papillary-cystic variety (Mancilla-Jimenez, 1976) (Fig. 1-55).[639] Ultrasound distinguishes renal cysts from the solid renal cell carcinoma in most cases.[710]

Diagnostic challenge may be produced by specific circumstances including association of the neoplasm with renal cysts, small size, abundant tumor necrosis, occurrence of the papillary-cystic variety as noted above, and occasional examples of large so-called renal cortical adenomas and radiologically atypical oncocytomas of the kidney. A characteristic spoke-wheel angiographic pattern has been observed with oncocytomas, but its presence is inconstant (refer to the preceding discussion of oncocytoma).

Pathology

Gross Features

The gross features of renal cell carcinoma show variation to the extreme with reference to size, color, consistency, extent of hemorrhage and necrosis, and characteristics of the tumor margin (Figs. 1-56 and 1-57).

The majority of reported renal carcinomas measure 5 cm to 10 cm in diameter when size information is detailed.[655,663] Hand and Broders (1932), however, reported that 72% of their 193 cases were larger than 10 cm, suggesting that more current studies reflect earlier detection of these neoplasms than occurred

Table 1-17　　*Metastatic Renal Cell Carcinoma as Initial Manifestation by Site of Metastases*

Site	Author	Year	Age	Sex	Follow-up
Brain	Chute[610]	1958	54	M	D, 11 mo
	Taxy[841]	1981	60	M	D, "several months"
Spinal cord	Weigensberg[816]	1972	48	M	D, 2 mo
Orbit	Chute[610]	1958	64	M	D, 8 mo
Ear	Sellstrom[800]	1962	66	M	A, NI
	Weigensberg[816]	1972	65	M	NI
Nasal cavity	Burns et al[796]	1956	74	F	A, NI
	Eneroth et al[799]	1961	76	F	A, NI
	Bernstein et al[806]	1966	58	F	A, NED, 1 yr
	Bernstein et al[806]	1966	68	F	D, 1 mo
Palate	Susan et al[647]	1979	53	M	D, 9 mo
	Susan et al[647]	1979	62	M	A, NED, 3 yr
Uvula	Lansigan[634]	1973	74	F	NI
Lung	Maytum, Vinson[790]	1936	63	M	NI
	Greenberg, Young[611]	1958	34	M	D, 5 mo
	Gerle, Felson[801]	1963	81	M	D, 3 wk
	Gerle, Felson[801]	1963	51	M	D, 2 mo
	Gerle, Felson[801]	1963	59	M	D, 3 days
	Gerle, Felson[801]	1963	65	M	D, 3 wk
	Trinidad et al[803]	1963	74	M	D, 4 days
	Trinidad et al[803]	1963	56	M	D, 3 mo
	Trinidad et al[803]	1963	72	M	D, 3 mo
	Adolfsson[621]	1967	28	F	A, NED, 5 yr
	Silverberg et al[624]	1969	53	M	A, NED, 2 yr
	Weigensberg[816]	1972	68	M	D, 16 mo
	Katzenstein et al[831]	1978	*	M = 15	13 — D, 2–28 mo
				F = 4	3 — A, NED, 21–75 mo
					2 — NI
Hilar nodes	Lang[828]	1977	†	NI	Mean survival — 1.4 mo
Chest wall	Chute[610]	1958	42	M	A, NED, 8 yr
	Silverberg et al[624]	1969	55	M	A, with tumor, 15 mo
Breast	Silverman, Oberman[817]	1974	NI	F	D, NI
	Chica et al[652]	1980	47	F	D, with tumor, 4 yr
Testis	Creevy[789]	1935	NI	M	NI
	Bandler, Roen[792]	1946	47	M	A, NED, 2 yr
	Talerman, Kniestadt[819]	1974	68	M	A, NED, 4 mo
Penis	Begg[788]	1928	62	M	D, 6 wk
	Burrell[793]	1948	39	M	D, 1 wk
	Weisman et al[810]	1969	66	M	D, 3 mo
	Katz, Davis[823]	1976	55	M	D, 1 yr
	Narayana et al[826]	1977	75	M	D, post-op
	Ordonez et al[846]	1982	69	M	D, 2 wk
	Sarma et al[850]	1985	83	M	D, 2 mo

Table 1-17 (continued)

Site	Author	Year	Age	Sex	Follow-up
Prostate	Cihak et al[836]	1980	81	M	D, 6 mo
Vagina	Mulcahy, Furlow[814]	1970	56	F	NI
	Weigensberg[816]	1972	50	F	NI
	Yamasaki et al[820]	1975	51	F	A, NI
	Redman, Roman-Lopez[824]	1977	62	F	A, NED, 2 yr
	Knight[825]	1977	79	F	A, NED, NI
	Sogani et al[835]	1979	47	F	D, 11 mo
	Sogani et al[835]	1979	47	F	D, 1 yr
	Sogani et al[835]	1979	75	F	A, NED, 6 yr
	Sogani et al[835]	1979	62	F	A, NED, 7 yr
	Nocks[837]	1980	64	F	NI
Bone					
Frontal	Scudder[787]	1906	40	F	D, mo
Humerus	Freid[791]	1946	69	F	D, mo
Pelvis	Freid[791]	1946	71	M	NI
Humerus	McClanahan, Bonann[794]	1953	54	M	D, 13 mo
Humerus	McClanahan, Bonann[794]	1953	59	M	D, 8 mo
Humerus	McClanahan, Bonann[794]	1953	59	M	A, NED, 2 yr
Mandible	Castigliano, Rominger[795]	1954	‡		
Clavicle	Weigensberg[816]	1972	NI	F	A, with tumor, 18 yr
Humerus	Jackman et al[818]	1974	55	M	NI
Humerus	Kagan, Steckel[827]	1977	53	M	A, NED, NI
Temporal	Taxy[841]	1981	65	M	NI
Clavicle	Ritch[847]	1983	75	M	A, NI
Scapula	Ritch[847]	1983	69	F	A, NI
Humerus	Ritch[847]	1983	70	M	A, NI
Muscle	Alexios et al[849]	1984	74	M	NI

A, NED—alive, no evidence of disease; D—dead; NI—no information

* 19 cases

† 8 cases

‡ 19 cases—literature review

50 years ago.[605] Bell (1947) subsequently reported that 43% of a series measured greater than 10 cm.[586] Further supporting a tendency toward smaller tumors at the time of diagnosis are the data of Petkovic (1959) and Kay (1968), who recorded only 29% and 39% of their respective series measuring larger than 10 cm.[612,623] In a personal series spanning the years 1960 to 1980, I encountered only 11% of tumors in excess of 10 cm. Finally, Fuhrman and associates (1982) reported that only 9% of their series measured larger than 12 cm.[655] In my experience, the mean diameter of 7.5 cm compares favorably with previous published data. Rare examples of renal cell carcinomas demonstrating metastases and measuring less than 2 cm, and even less than 1 cm, have been reported (see Table 1-13). At the other extreme, tumors measuring in excess of 25 cm are observed.[614]

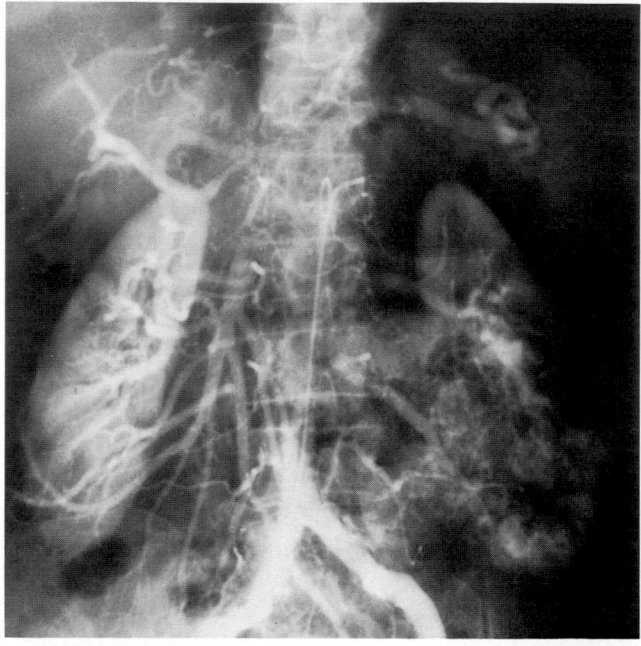

A

B

Figure 1-54   ***Renal cell carcinoma.*** *(A) Arteriogram demonstrates*
hypervascular renal cell carcinoma in lower pole of left kidney.
(Compare with Fig. 1-55.) (B) Retrograde pyelogram
demonstrates filling defects of renal pelvis and ureteropelvic
junction produced by the lower pole neoplasm.

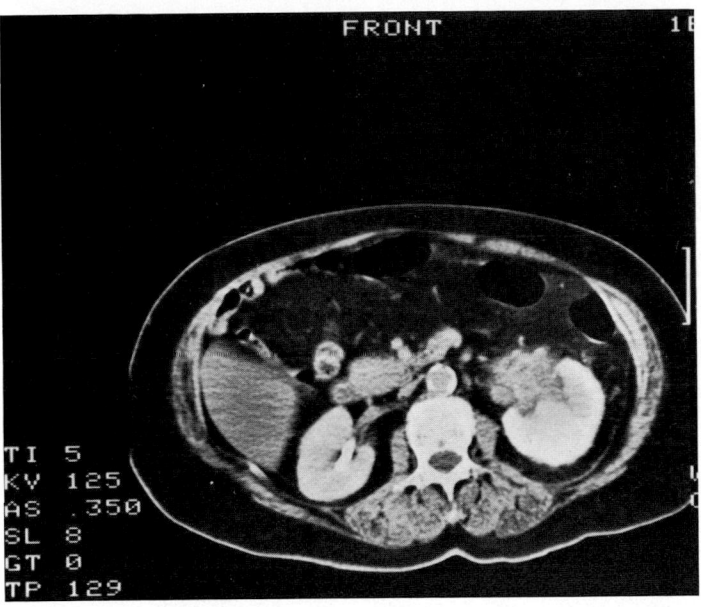

Figure 1-54 (Continued) (C) *The CT scan shows a solid lower pole neoplasm extending anteriorly and medially.*

The color of the cut surface of the kidney reflects the presence and extent of hemorrhage, necrosis, and lipid content of the neoplastic cells, the latter being more abundant in tumors of the clear cell variety. The predominant color is commonly white-yellow, rust, yellow-red, or yellow-brown. The tumor is lobulated, with a tendency to bulge from the cut surface. White-gray fibrous trabeculae separate the lobules and peripherally merge with the fibrous pseudocapsule. The hemorrhage and necrosis may be associated with cyst formation or central liquification of the tumor without the formation of a cyst. One histologic variety, the papillary-cystic type (refer to p. 109), deceptively suggests total necrosis of the tumor within a fibrous cyst wall (Fig. 1-58). Histologic examination of such a tumor commonly discloses that the central soft-granular contents are composed of viable neoplastic cells in papillary configuration, often with minimal necrosis present. Focal calcification may be apparent on the cut surface in occasional cases. In the absence of significant necrosis, and exclusive of examples of the papillary-cystic variety mentioned above, the typical renal cell carcinoma has a firm consistency.

The perimeter of the neoplasm is commonly well demarcated, with compression of the adjacent renal parenchyma. In some cases, the pseudocapsule is incomplete and an infiltrative border of the tumor appears at the irregular interface with the adjacent uninvolved kidney.

In most instances the tumor is a single mass. Less commonly, satellite nodules are present adjacent to the main mass. It is not rare to see scattered, small "cortical adenomas" with different histologic features or, alternatively, nodules with histologic features resembling the main neoplasm in the adjacent parenchyma. In the latter case, the question of multicentricity or intrarenal metastases is encountered.

The examination of a radical nephrectomy specimen in the clinical context of renal cell carcinoma requires further attention at both the gross and microscopic

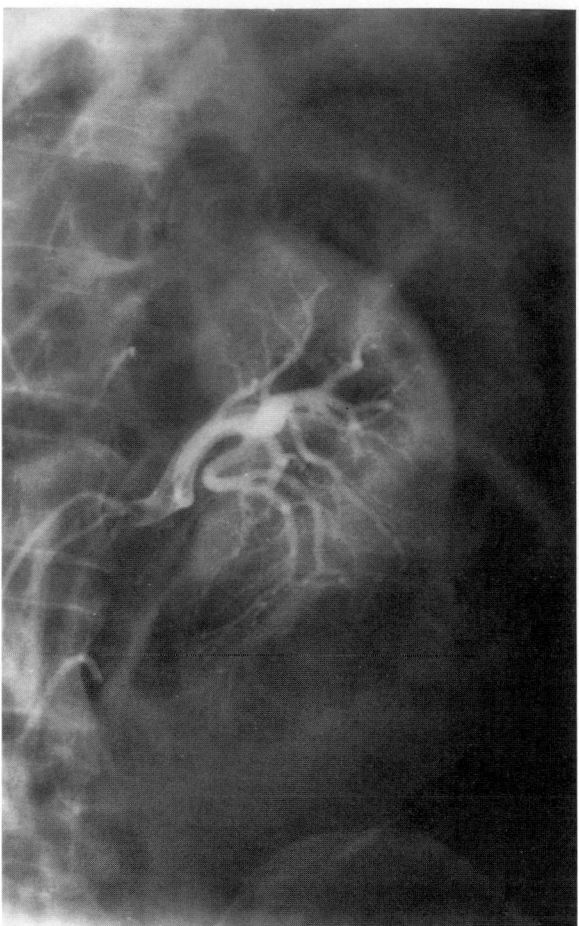

Figure 1-55   *Renal cell carcinoma. Arteriogram demonstrates hypovascular renal cell carcinoma in lower pole of kidney. (Compare with Fig. 1-54A.)*

levels of (1) the renal capsule, (2) the renal vein, (3) included hilar lymph nodes, and (4) the renal calyceal system, in order of their frequency of tumor involvement.[608,626] Tumor present in the perirenal tissue and not apparent at the time of gross examination can be accurately and reliably identified microscopically by painting the exterior of the specimen with india ink. The hilar adipose tissue should be dissected for purposes of identifying included lymph nodes to be submitted for microscopic examination. This is to be done after the vascular pedicle has been sectioned with the intent of detecting grossly apparent renal vein invasion. The renal calyceal system, invaded only infrequently by renal cell carcinoma, may on rare occasions be associated with apparent downstream implants in the ureter (see the discussion of metastatic tumors in Chap. 3).

Finally, rare examples of spontaneous hemorrhage with rupture of the renal carcinoma may be seen.[648] The massive retroperitoneal hematoma may be of such magnitude that the presence of the neoplasm may be obscured by the abundant blood clot included in or with the nephrectomy specimen. Adequate histologic sectioning will assist in detecting the tumor, frequently evidencing abundant

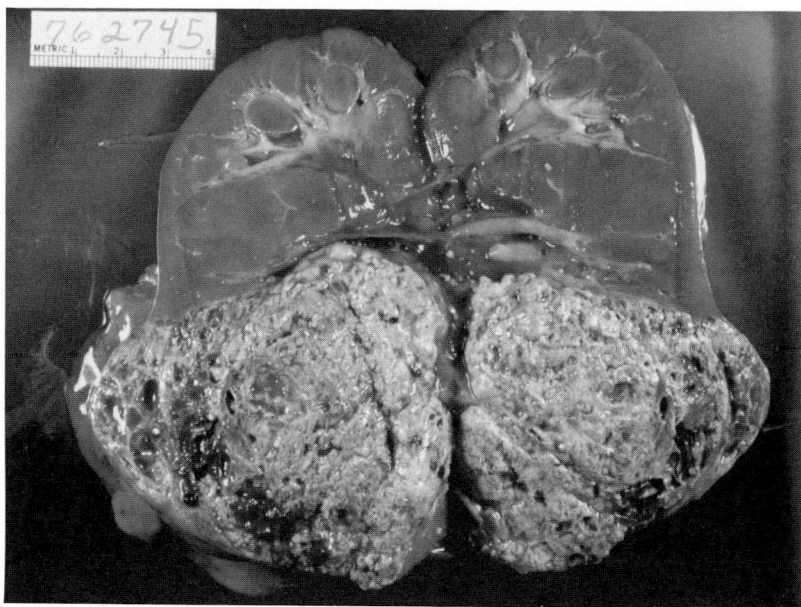

Figure 1-56　　**Renal cell carcinoma.** *The deceptively well-delineated renal cell carcinoma shows extensive necrosis and hemorrhage with penetration of the overlying capsule.*

necrosis and few viable diagnostic neoplastic cells. Alternatively, a wide spectrum of concurrent renal disorders has been uncommonly observed in association with renal cell carcinoma including cysts, inflammatory lesions, and other neoplasms on rare occasions, as listed below:

Congenital Disorders
    Supernumerary kidney[53]
    Horseshoe kidney[67,69,70,73]
    Multicystic dysplasia[115]
    Adult polycystic disease[130,136,141,147]

Acquired Cysts
    Simple cysts[237,239,240]
    Cysts in dialysis patients[247,248,249]
    Multilocular cyst[658]

Systemic amyloidosis[699]

Inflammatory Disorders
    Tuberculosis[263]
    Xanthogranulomatous pyelonephritis[332,653]

Neoplasms
    Cortical adenoma, so-called (common observation)
    Wilms' tumor[473]
    Angiomyolipoma[147]
    Transitional cell carcinoma, renal pelvis (refer to Chap. 2)
    Sarcomas (collision tumors)[1078,1080]
    Carcinosarcoma[1080,1085]

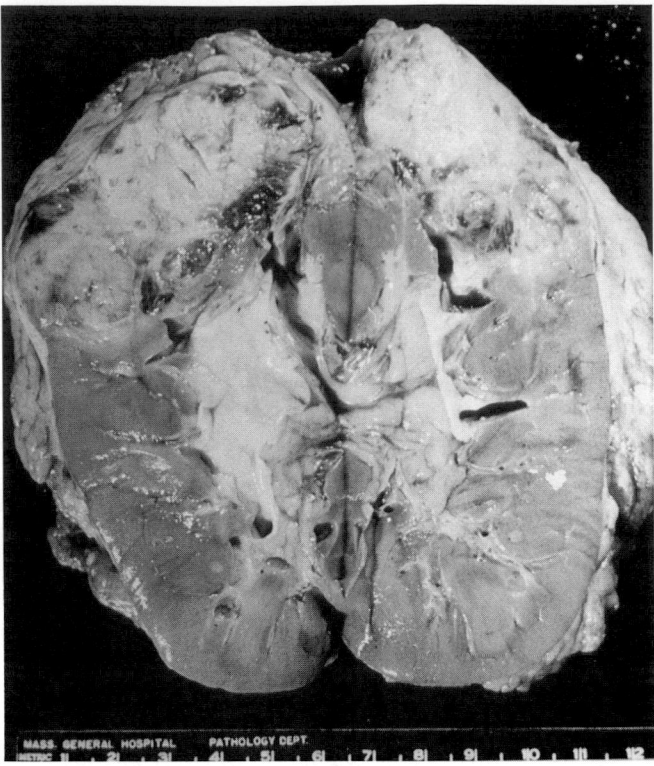

Figure 1-57   *Renal cell carcinoma. The tumor replaces the upper pole of the kidney, and the cut surface shows the characteristic features of focal hemorrhage and necrosis with expansion of the renal capsule and apparent compression without invasion of the adjacent renal parenchyma. Microscopic invasion of both capsule and adjacent kidney cortex was found.*

The apparent receptivity of renal cell carcinomas to metastatic neoplasms is well known.[664] The 32nd example of a renal cell carcinoma's serving as the recipient for a metastatic carcinoma (a malignant melanoma) was recently reported by Singh and associates.[664] All metastatic neoplasms may serve to obscure the presence of the renal cell carcinoma.

Rarely, renal cell carcinoma may occur bilaterally. These bilateral neoplasms may be either synchronous or asynchronous in their occurrence, with about equal frequency.[711-750] When they are asynchronous, the diagnosis of the second renal malignancy may occur as long as several years after the nephrectomy for the contralateral renal cell carcinoma. When the tumors occur synchronously, a diagnostic and therapeutic challenge presents itself. Under such circumstances, the initial surgical resection is commonly a nephron-saving partial nephrectomy. If the entire surgical resection margin is not carefully examined grossly and by frozen section for the presence of tumor, a major disservice will have been done. The possible successful subsequent contralateral radical nephrectomy will accomplish little if the kidney initially treated by partial nephrectomy contains residual tumor at the resection margin.

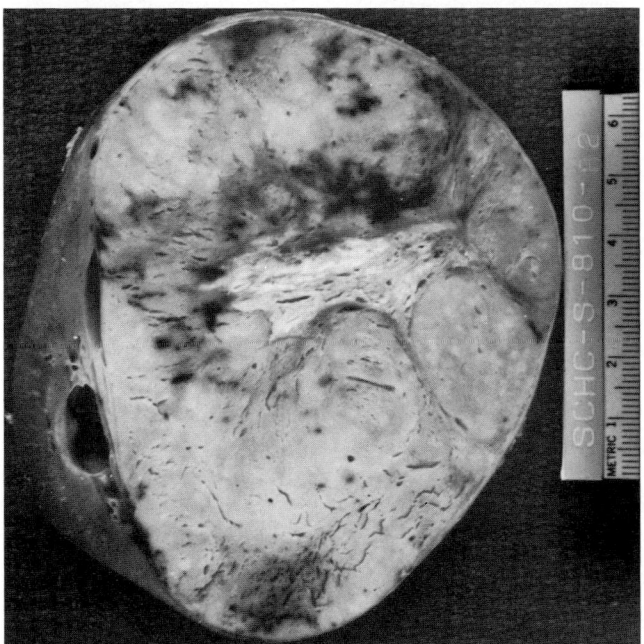

A

B

Figure 1-58   ***Renal cell carcinoma.*** *(A) Tumor virtually replaces kidney, which is present along the left rim of the tumor. (B) The tumor expands and distorts the lower pole of the kidney. Histologic examination of the overlying capsule revealed microscopic penetration by tumor cells.*

Microscopic Features

Two types of cells, the clear cell and the granular cell, comprise renal cell carcinomas, either exclusively or more commonly as mixtures of the two cell types (Figs. 1-59, 1-60, and 1-61). A rare variant of this neoplasm, the sarcomatoid type, is characterized by spindle cells in haphazard bundles or sheets, bearing no resemblance to cells of carcinomatous origin (Fig. 1-62).[751-757] The true nature of these cells can usually be determined by adequate sectioning with disclosure of more typical malignant epithelial cells showing sarcomatoid transition. Ultrastructural studies further document their epithelial nature.[754-756]

The typical renal carcinoma shows no such sarcomatoid areas but is unmistakably carcinomatous with tubular, acinar, alveolar, or papillary histologic patterns. Alternatively, the carcinoma cells grow in expansive sheets with only focal areas of the structural patterns noted above. With the exception of two patterns, the papillary-cystic variety and the sarcomatoid variety, with well-documented tendencies for nonaggressive and aggressive behavior, respectively, the other histologic patterns convey no unique prognostic information.

The gross features of hemorrhage, necrosis, fibrosis, and focal calcification have their histologic counterpart and form the admixed, non-neoplastic background of the tumor. Associated histologic hallmarks of these secondary changes include foamy histiocytic macrophages, some with phagocytized hemosiderin; cholesterol clefts; and focal collections of foreign body giant cells. Psammoma bodies are commonly observed in the papillary tumors. The prognostic significance of an associated lymphoplasma-cell infiltrate associated with the tumor cells is unsettled.[633]

Although no current staging system gives significance to invasion of intrarenal vascular tributaries, it is hoped that this current protocol shortcoming will

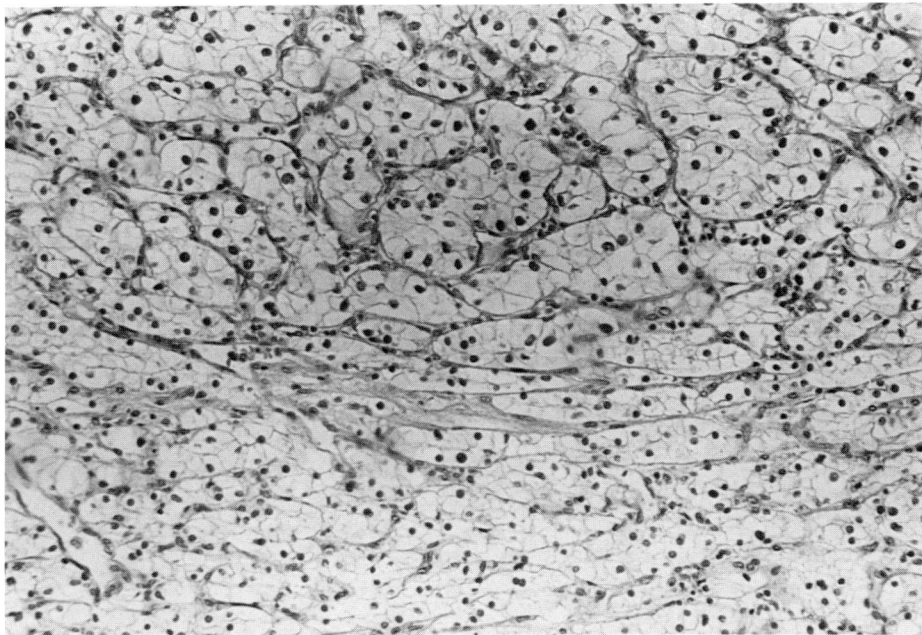

Figure 1-59   *Renal cell carcinoma. The tumor cells are arranged in an alveolar or nest pattern and are exclusively of the clear-cell type.*

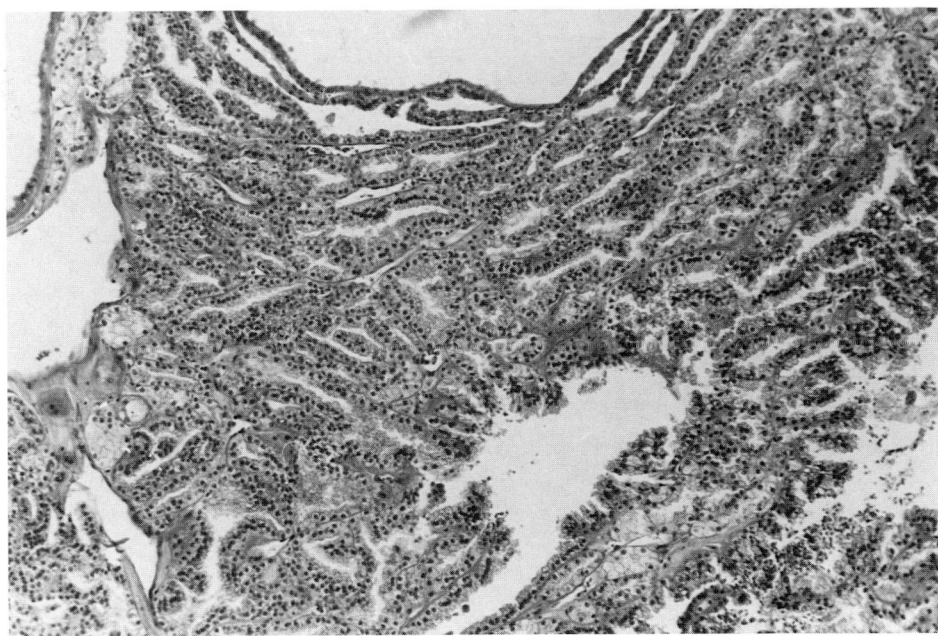

Figure 1-60 *Renal cell carcinoma. This renal cell carcinoma is composed predominantly of granular cells, with fewer clear cells in a tubular and microcystic pattern.*

be corrected in the future. Such vascular invasion and capsular invasion or penetration by tumor cells should be determined and recorded. Histologic evidence of renal vein (extrarenal) and renal pelvic invasion, as well as regional lymph node metastases, is recorded in the final diagnosis, serving as integral information on which the final pathologic stage is determined.

Histochemical and ultrastructural studies of the two common cell types of renal cell carcinoma disclose the resemblance of these cell types to the cells of the proximal convoluted tubules of the kidney, thus clarifying their histogenesis.[758-760] No ultrastructural features allow distinguishing the so-called adenoma from renal cell carcinoma.[759,760] The clear cells are characterized by abundant glycogen and lipid, demonstrated by the PAS stain with and without diastase pretreatment and the oil red-O stain, respectively. Ultrastructural studies confirm these staining results. In addition, the clear cells have few mitochondria and sparse endoplasmic reticulum. The granular cells tend to have less glycogen and lipid but numerous mitochondria and prominent Golgi apparatus and endoplasmic reticulum.[758-760] Both cell types share ultrastructural features identifying the proximal tubular origin, including pinocytotic vesicles at the cell membrane and numerous microvilli on cell luminal surface.[758-760] The mitochondria commonly have abnormal configurations.

The significant cytologic features of these neoplastic cells are outlined in the protocols for tumor grading.

Tumor Grading

Tumor grading protocols reported in the literature with varying claims of prognostic value have actually met with only limited success and correspondingly limited general acceptance. Three such protocols are oulined in Table 1-18. The

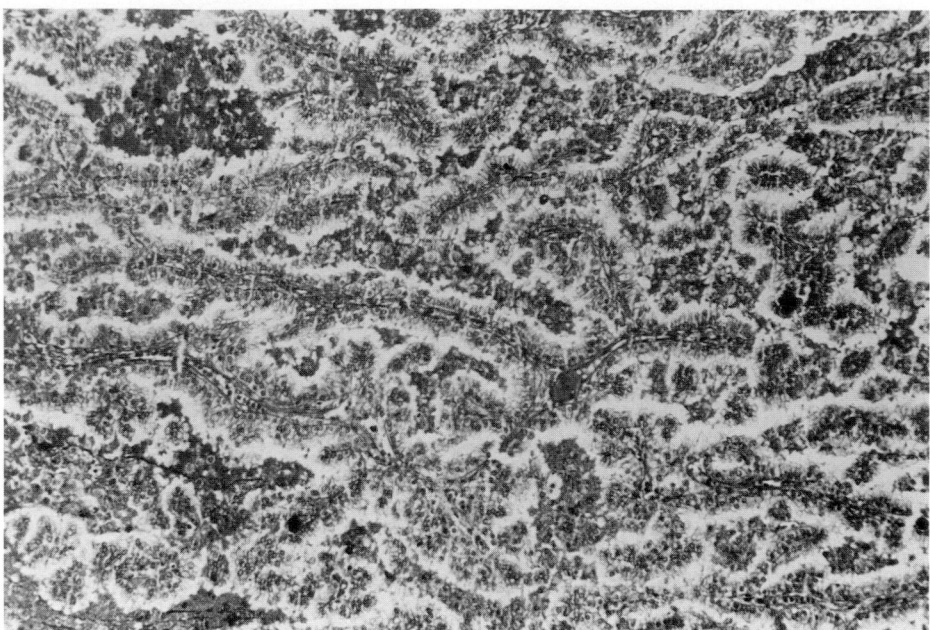

Figure 1-61   *Renal cell carcinoma. This neoplasm contains clear cells in a tubular-papillary pattern. Malignant cells line the thin fibrovascular septa.*

Table 1-18   **Renal Cell Carcinoma Tumor Grading Protocols**

Grade	Description
Arner et al (1965)[617]	
I	Highly differentiated tumors, sharply demarcated from surrounding tissue
IIA	Moderately differentiated tumors, locally well circumscribed, but not necessarily provided with capsule
IIB	Moderately differentiated tumors, poorly circumscribed but not diffusely infiltrating and/or markedly polymorphous
III	Poorly differentiated, markedly polymorphous tumor, which are diffusely infiltrating tumors with abundant growth in capillary vessels
Skinner et al (1971)[631]*	
I	Nuclei indistinguishable from normal tubular cells
II	Nuclei only slightly larger than normal tubular cells; nuclear outline slightly irregular
III	Nuclei moderately enlarged, pleomorphic, and with irregular outline
IV	Occasional common bizarre, giant nuclei present
Fuhrman et al (1982)[655]†	
1	Small, round, uniform nuclei with inconspicuous or absent nucleoli
2	Larger nuclei with irregular outline and small nucleoli present
3	Larger nuclei with irregular outline and prominent nucleoli
4	Grade 3 features with bizarre, multinucleated cells, with or without spindle cells

* No evaluation of histologic pattern
† Graded by most malignant features, even if only focal

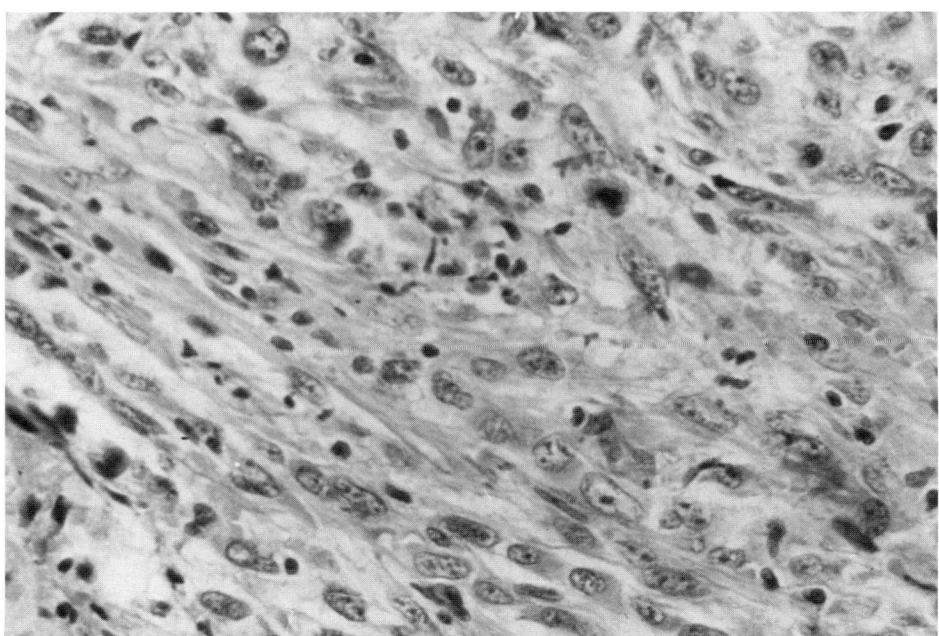

Figure 1-62   **Renal cell carcinoma.** *The sheets of elongated and spindle cells without tubular differentiation are characteristic of the sarcomatoid pattern of renal cell carcinoma.*

protocol of Arner and colleagues (1965) incorporates gross, histologic, and cytologic features into the final tumor grades (I–III).[617] Because differentiation of renal cell carcinomas has never been formally defined, the basis for regarding papillary, tubular, or acinar patterns on a scale of differentiation has not been clarified. Indeed, as noted above, only two histologic patterns, the papillary-cystic and sarcomatoid patterns, have demonstrated prognostic value. Importantly, I am unaware of any study relating prognostic value to any of the other patterns comprising the overwhelming majority of renal cell carcinoma cases. Thus, on both practical and conceptual grounds, the grading system incorporating evaluation of histologic and certainly gross features has little to recommend it.

Unfortunately, the alternative grading protocols devised by Skinner and colleagues (1971) and Fuhrman and co-workers (1982), although based solely on evaluation of nuclear features of the tumor cells and therefore relatively simple and reproducible, do not adequately stratify the vast majority of cases of renal cell carcinoma.[631,655] Each of these protocols has four tumor grade categories, and each grading protocol was capable of identifying the relatively few patients with the prognostically best and worst tumors, grades I and IV, respectively. However, the vast majority of patients have tumors with intermediate morphologic features and survival rates. Thus the stratification capabilities are limited to three groups: the best, the worst, and the large percentage of patients in between. When the relationship of tumor grade to frequency of subsequent tumor metastases was studied, only two groups were identified: grade 1 tumors and grades 2 to 4 tumors.[655] The frequency of metastases of grades 2, 3, and 4 tumors was not significantly different.

These limitations are not trivial. They are the results that can be achieved with a grading system that has the highest demonstrated level of objectivity, simplicity, and reproducibility of any system yet devised. The limited prognostic value of these nuclear grading systems can possibly be improved when combined with other recorded features of the primary tumor as discussed below.

Natural History

Tumor Stage

Stratification of cases of renal cell carcinoma based on extent of disease spread, or tumor staging, is a relatively recent advance in the study of this neoplasm. The first staging protocols by Flocks and Kadesky (1958) and Petkovic (1959) served as the basis for Robson's staging system, proposed in 1969 (Table 1-19).[609,612,625] Robson's staging protocol has received widespread acceptance and is currently the protocol most frequently applied to the study of this malignancy as reflected in the urologic literature. The newest staging system referable to renal parenchymal malignancies is the TNM system, the 1983 version of which is outlined in Table 1-20. The adoption of this more elaborate staging system is urged despite its apparent greater demand on memory than the relatively simple Robson staging protocol. The adoption of the TNM system is encouraged primarily because it allows clear stratification of cases with various combinations of regional tumor spread, which the Robson system does not recognize. With the Robson staging protocol, patients with tumors either limited to the kidney (stage I), infiltrating the perirenal adipose tissue (stage II), or showing distant metastases (stage IV B) all belong to clearly defined groups that have stage-related relative survival rates. The problem with this staging system is its inapplicability to patients with combined features of stages II and III (*i.e.,* perirenal invasion and either renal vein invasion or hilar node metastases). The current controversy over the prognostic significance of renal vein invasion would probably have never evolved had the opportunity to compare stratified cases based on the Robson system not taken place. In this context, the application of the Robson system has clarified its inherent shortcomings. Further, the higher survival rates reported among stage III patients compared with stage II patients, observed in several studies, suggest that the risk value assigned to stage II and III tumors by this staging protocol must be thoroughly re-evaluated (Table 1-21).

Stage Distribution

The inherent limitations of the Robson staging protocol notwithstanding, it has served as the stratification guideline in studies of renal malignancies published to

Table 1-19   **Renal Cell Carcinoma Staging Protocols: Protocol of Robson (1969)**

Stage	Description
I	Confined to kidney
II	Perirenal fat invasion, but confined to Gerota's fascia
IIIA	Gross renal vein or inferior vena cava involvement
IIIB	Lymphatic involvement
IIIC	Vascular and lymphatic involvement
IVA	Adjacent organs other than adrenal involved
IVB	Distant metastases

Robson CJ, Churchill BM, Anderson W: The results of radical nephrectomy for renal cell carcinoma. J Urol 101:297, 1969; ©1969, The Williams & Wilkins Co, Baltimore

this time. The distribution of tumor stage at the time of diagnosis observed in 14 studies of renal cell carcinoma is presented in Table 1-22. Tumors limited to the kidney (stage I) comprise an average of 40% of the total cases. In contrast, 3% to 36% (mean 25%) of patients have distant metastases at the time of initial clinical presentation. Regional spread of tumor, stages II and III, is observed in approximately one third of all patients at the time of initial diagnosis and surgical therapy.

Prognosis. The prognostic value of clinical and morphologic features of renal cell carcinoma is presented in the following list:

Significant
    Tumor stage[609,612,619,625,631,632,640,643,649,654,655,657,660–663,834]
    Tumor grade[616,631,649,654,655,660,662]
    Sarcomatoid histologic pattern[631,649,655,663,751,753]
    Papillary-cystic pattern[639]

Without Significance
    Patient age, sex

Table 1-20   **TNM Staging Protocol (American Joint Committee)**

Stage	Description
Primary Tumor (T)	
TX	Minimum requirements to assess the primary tumor cannot be met
T0	No evidence of primary tumor
T1	Small tumor; minimal renal and calyceal distortion or deformity; circumscribed neovasculature surrounded by parenchyma
T2	Large tumor with deformity or enlargement of kidney or collecting systems
T3a	Large tumor involving perinephric tissues
T3b	Tumor involving renal vein
T3c	Tumor involving renal vein and infradiaphragmatic vena cava
T4	Tumor extending into neighboring organs or abdominal wall
Nodal Involvement (N)*	
NX	Minimum requirements to assess the regional nodes cannot be met
N0	No evidence of involvement of regional nodes
N1	Single, homolateral regional nodal involvement
N2	Involvement of multiple regional or of contralateral or bilateral nodes
N3	Fixed regional nodes (assessable only at surgical exploration)
Distant Metastasis (M)	
MX	Minimum requirements to assess the presence of distant metastasis cannot be met
M0	No (known) distant metastasis
M1	Distant metastasis present
	Specify site†

* The regional lymph nodes are the para-aortic and paracaval nodes.

† Pulmonary = PUL; Pleura = PLE; Brain = BRA; Lymph nodes = LYM; Bone marrow = MAR; Hepatic = HEP; Eye = EYE; Osseous = OSS; Skin = SKI; Other = OTH

American Joint Committee for Cancer Staging and End-Results Reporting of the American College of Surgeons: Manual for Staging of Cancer, 2nd ed. p 177. Philadelphia, JB Lippincott, 1983

Presence and type of local symptoms[631,636,649,663]
Renal pelvis invasion[634,661]
Histologic pattern other than sarcomatoid[649] or papillary-cystic

Significance Controversial
Renal vein invasion[605,606,623,625,649,650,654,660–662]
Tumor size[623,640,655]
Cell type[613,618,623,631,649,654,655,660,662,663]

The evaluated parameters are classified into those with or without prognostic value and those with currently unsettled prognostic value. In sum, the only important prognostic guidelines of renal cell carcinoma of consistent value are (1) tumor stage, (2) tumor grade, and (3) histologic patterns, namely the sarcomatoid pattern and the papillary-cystic pattern (Figs. 1-62 and 1-63). The clinical behavior of renal cell carcinoma bears no direct relationship to the multitude of clinical parameters exhibited by patients with this malignancy. Older studies suggesting prognostic importance of specific signs and symptoms and laboratory values are flawed by the inadequate number of patients studied or the absence of appropriate controls with stratification on the basis of tumor stage.

The responsibility of prognosticating renal cell carcinoma rests principally

Table 1-21   *Renal Cell Carcinoma: Tumor Stage vs. Prognosis*

Author	Year	5-Year Survival		
		I	*II*	*III*
Riches[615]	1963	58%	26%	
Kaufman, Mims[620]	1966	61%	24%	31%
Kay[623]	1968	63%	25%	39.5%
Grumstadt, Wahlquist[705]	1969	86%	33%	47%
Robson[625]	1969	66%	64%	42%
Bottinger[630]	1970	76%	65%	35%
Rafla[628]	1970	51%	50%	
Wagle, Scal[627]	1970	58%	48%	14%
Skinner et al[631]	1971	65%	47%	51%
Ochsner et al[636]	1973	54%		47%
Katz, Davis[640]	1977	64%	56%	27%
Rochman et al[635]	1979	60%	71%	8%
Boxer et al[649]	1979	56%	100%	50%
Bellinger et al[644]	1979	72%	52%	18%
Waters Richie[650]	1979	51%	58%	
Oliver et al[645]	1979	82%	43%	37%
McNichols et al[779]	1981	67%	51%	33.5%
Fuhrman et al[655]	1982	47%	40%	
Tomera et al[662]	1983	69.8%*		
Selli et al[663]	1983	93%	63%	80%
Petersen†	1984	71%	0%	31%

Blanks denote lack of information; ‡ denotes data that pertain to grouped stages (combined stages II to IV).

* Study limited to grade 1 clear cell carcinoma

† Personal observations

on the radiologist to detect metastatic tumor in distant sites (*e.g.,* lung, bone, brain, liver) and the surgical pathologist to examine thoroughly and accurately radical nephrectomy specimens containing this malignancy. Extra care in the evaluation of the renal capsule and perirenal adipose tissue, the hilar vascular pedicle, and included lymph nodes is obligatory. The tumor grade must be determined and, importantly, the selected grading system applied in a consistent manner in all cases.

I further suggest the evaluation of specimens for possible tumor invasion of intrarenal tributaries of the renal venous system. The current controversy referable to the prognostic significance of (extra-)renal vein invasion may be resolved by the study of large numbers of patients staged by the TNM protocol comparing patients of stages T3a, T3c, and T3ac, with perirenal invasion, renal vein invasion, and concurrent renal vein and perirenal invasion. Such a study is not possible if the Robson protocol continues to be the basis of staging. Finally, studies focusing on the detection of intrarenal vascular invasion may further clarify why some "stage I" patients' tumors behave in an aggressive manner following nephrectomy. The relative risk of dissemination from tumors invading intrarenal tributaries may be only marginally lower than that associated with tumors within the extrarenal segments of the renal vein.

5-Year Survival				10-Year Survival						
III A	III B	III C	IV	I	II	III	III A	III B	III C	IV
27%			10%							
			5%	48%	14%	25%				0%
			0%							
			11%	60%	17%	31%				14%
			5%							
	21%		0%							
			11%	51%	38%	8%				3%
			8%	56%	20%	37%				7%
			0%							
			2.5%							
			8%	20%	66%	25%				0%
			2%	27%	38%	8%				3%
53%			0%							
			12%	72%	42%	24%				3%
			13.5%	56%	28%	20%				3%
			10%							
75%*‡				63.5%*			39.5%*‡			
			13%							
			19%	35%	0%	11%				0%

Metastatic Renal Cell Carcinoma

As previously noted, 25% to 57% of patients with renal cell carcinoma have detectable metastases at the time of initial presentation (see Table 1-22). Among these patients presenting with stage IV disease, metastases are most commonly identified in the lungs, bones, and brain, in order of decreasing frequency.[822,829] At the time of initial presentation, multiple-site metastases are more frequent than single-site metastases.[808,833]

Patients presenting with an undetected renal cell carcinoma but with signs and symptoms referable to a site of metastasis comprise a diagnostically challenging subset of stage IV cases. A wide spectrum of metastatic sites with an equally diverse spectrum of clinical presentations has been reported (see Table 1-17). In most instances, the single clinically dominant metastatic site is a reflection of widely disseminated disease as reflected by the overall poor survival of this group of patients (see Table 1-17).

Also among patients presenting with stage IV renal cell carcinoma are those who evidence apparent spontaneous regression of metastatic tumor foci followng surgical excision of the renal primary tumor.[781–786,815] Fairlamb (1981) collected 67 such cases reported in the literature to that time.[785] The majority of these patients have pulmonary metastases that are observed to regress on sequential chest x-ray films. Because only a few of these reported patients have histologic documentation of the alleged metastases, the true frequency of this phenomenon remains unknown. The rarity of spontaneous regression has been generally interpreted as an insufficient basis to warrant an aggressive surgical approach to the primary tumor in patients with multiple metastases at the time of presentation.[808,848] The value of surgical therapy of apparently single metastases to the lung, liver, or elsewhere is controversial and currently unsettled.[774,797,822,831,833]

Table 1-22   Renal Cell Carcinoma Stage Distribution at Time of Diagnosis

Author	Year	No. of Patients	Stages*			
			I	II	III	IV
Kaufman, Mims[620]	1966	100	56%	7%	24%	21%
Robson et al[625]	1969	87	38%	17%	31%	14%
Bottinger[630]	1970	91	34%	13%	18%	35%
Skinner et al[631]	1971	309	33%	7%	35%	25%
Mancilla-Jimenez et al[639]	1976	224	49%	9%	38%	3%
Katz, Davis[640]	1977	164	42%	11%	9%	38%
Patel, Lavengood[642]	1978	166	47%	4%	13%	36%
Waters, Richie[650]	1979	130	28%	20%	28%	24%
Boxer et al[649]	1979	96	36%	9%	20%	35%
Rochman et al[646]	1979	89	9%	20%	21%	49%
McNichols et al[654]	1981	506	35%	11%	42%	11%
Fuhrman et al[655]	1982	103	58%	15%	6%	21%
Fuselier et al[660]	1983	161	40.4%	7%	29%	24%
Petersen†	1984	80	36%	15%	20%	29%

* According to staging protocol of Robson (1969)

† Personal observations

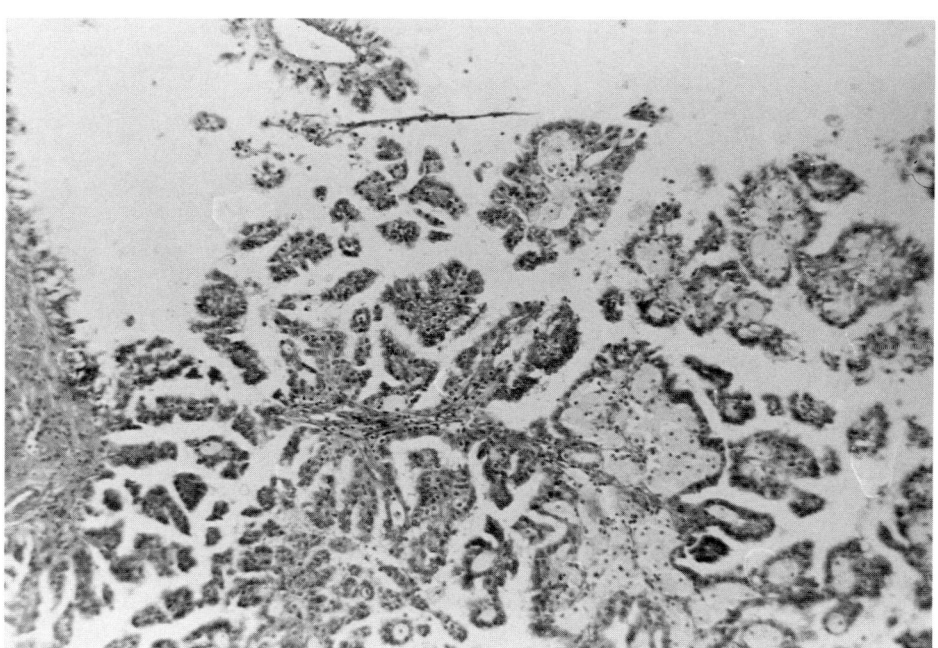

Figure 1-63 *Renal cell carcinoma, papillary-cystic type. Delicate papillary projections of the tumor extend from the wall of the cystic mass. Fragments of papillary fronds lie free in the cyst lumen. The central core of several papillae contains histiocytes (foam cells).*

Following the initial presentation and primary therapy, recurrent renal cell carcinoma most commonly manifests as metastatic tumor in the lungs, bones, brain, and liver. Uncommonly, recurrent tumors may manifest as metastases in the breast, skin, penis, ear, nasal cavities, and adrenal glands (Fig. 1-64).[659,802,804,805,813,842,843]

An interesting phenomenon, generally attributable only to breast and renal carcinoma, is the recurrence of the malignancy several years following diagnosis of the primary tumor (Fig. 1-65). Table 1-23 details 23 reported cases of renal cell carcinoma recurrent 10 years or longer after the original diagnosis. The longest recorded recurrence-free intervals of 36 years and 37 years were reported by Walter and Gillespie (1960) and Takats and Csapo (1966) respectively.[773,798] In rare instances, prolonged survival is recorded following surgical excision of the recurrence (metastasis) (see Table 1-23).

At autopsy, the pattern of metastases of renal cell carcinoma shows the same relative frequencies, with the exception of significantly higher lymph node involvement (66%), than observed clinically.[851-856] In order of decreasing frequency, metastases are observed in the lungs, lymph nodes (para-aortic), bones, brain, liver, contralateral kidney, and multiple other sites, all with frequencies less than 20%.[807,840,851-856] Saitoh (1982) observed the same distribution frequencies of metastatic sites in patients with and without prior nephrectomies.[844] The relatively high frequencies of lung, lymph node, and bone metastases are independent of the patient's age.[845] Liver and lymph node (other than retroperitoneal node) metastases are observed less frequently with increasing age.[845] These patterns suggest that hematogenous metastases are not affected by increasing age, in contrast to the decreased frequency of lymphatic dissemination in older patients.[845]

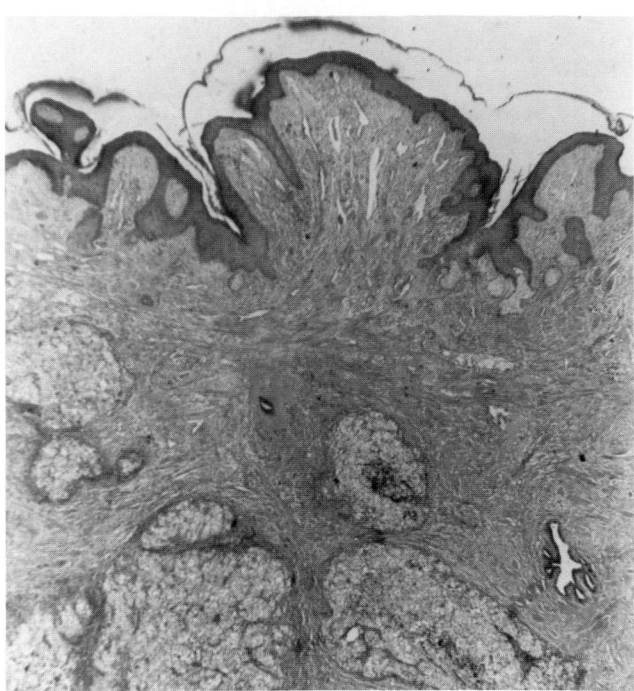

Figure 1-64   *Metastatic renal cell carcinoma in the breast. The nests of metastatic clear cell carcinoma from the kidney are present in the deep dermis intermingled with lactiferous ducts of the breast.*

Carcinoid

Nine documented renal carcinoid tumors were found in the literature.[857-865] Patients ranged in age from 20 years to 65 years; however, five of the nine cases occurred in the seventh decade. There is no sex predilection. The right and left kidneys are affected with approximately equal frequency. Most patients presented with a flank mass, commonly associated with pain. The largest tumor recorded to date measured 30 cm in diameter. The first example of renal carcinoid reported by Gleason and co-workers (1971) and Bloom (1972) was associated with alterations of small intestinal motility and absorption due to secretion of enteroglucagon by the tumor.[857,858] Radiologic findings have been nonspecific, demonstrating nonvisualization of the affected kidney, with mass displacement of the renal pelvis and ureter. No consistent arteriographic findings have been reported.

With two exceptions, the reported renal carcinoids have been well circumscribed, solid tumors. Hemorrhage and necrosis are common. Toker (1974) reported a carcinoid arising in a renal teratoma that was predominantly cystic.[859] Invasion of the renal vein and metastases to the hilar lymph nodes have been observed at the time of surgery. Microscopic features typical of carcinoids, including anastomosing columns and cords of cells or solid large nests with peripheral palisading of cells, are observed. Hemorrhage and necrosis are present in multifocal sites. The tumor cells show minimal pleomorphism, with round to oval nuclei and variable amounts of eosinophilic cytoplasm. Argentaffin-positive cells (Fontana-Masson stain) have been reported in only one case.[863] More fre-

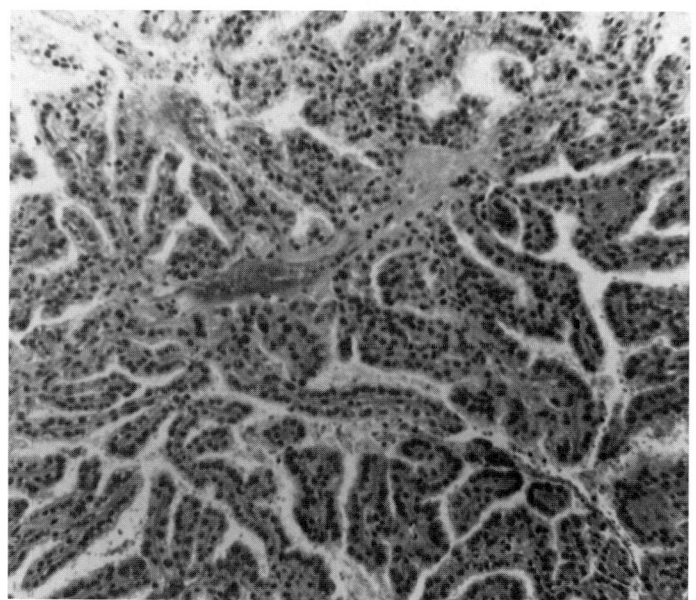

A

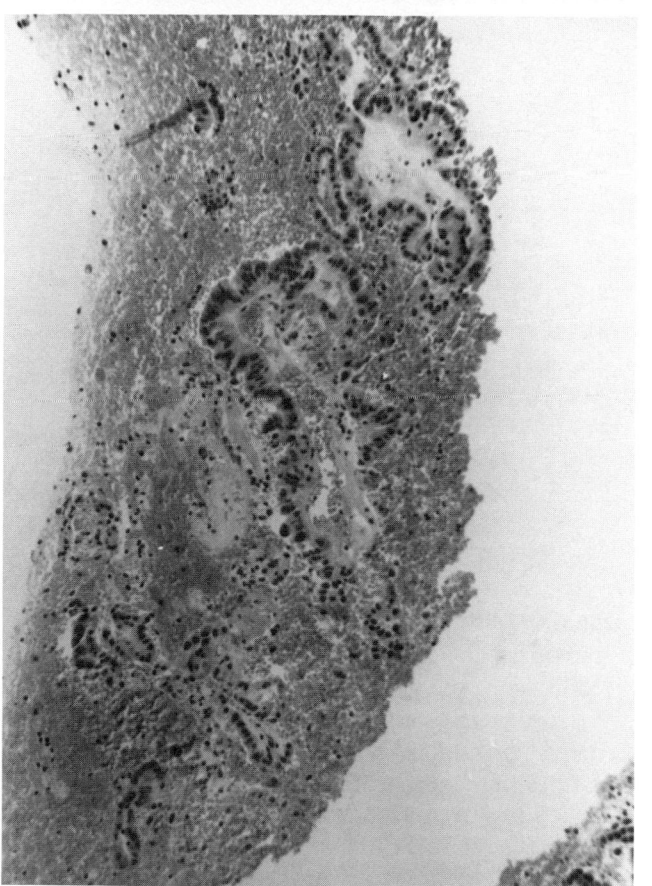

B

Figure 1-65   *Renal cell carcinoma with late recurrence.* (A) *The papillary pattern predominates in this primary renal cell carcinoma.* (B) *It is found in the retroperitoneal recurrence 23 years later as diagnosed by CT scan-directed thin needle biopsy.*

Table 1-23   *Reported Cases of Late Recurrence of Renal Cell Carcinoma*

Author	Year	Time of Recurrence (years)	Location of Recurrence	Survival Following Recurrence
Clairmont[761]	1904	10	Trachea	D§
Graves, Mabrey[762]	1935	20	Surgical scar	D, 1 yr
Caylor, Caylor[763]	1936	11	Thyroid	A, 1 yr
Starr, Miller[734]	1952	20	Jejunum	NI
Morton, Morton[765]	1953	16*	Thigh	A, 8 yr
Badenoch[766]	1958	24	Clavicle	NI
Kilnani, Wolf[767]	1960	13†	Duodenum	NI
Kilnani, Wolf[767]	1960	14‡	Lung	D, 1 wk
Walter, Gillespie[798]	1960	36	Lung	D, 10 yr
Rosof, Rubin[768]	1960	20	Lung, femur, scapula	D, "several months"
Eneroth, et al[769]	1961	13	Nasal cavity	A, 4 yr
Sklaroff, Moon[770]	1962	22	Multiple sites	D, 1.5 yr
Tandon et al[771]	1963	20	Surgical scar	A, 1 yr
Kradjian, Bennington[772]	1965	31	Surgical scar	A, 8 mo
Takats, Csapo[773]	1966	37	Multiple sites	D, 37
Middleton[774]	1967	14	Brain	A, 17 yr
Wilmore, Smith[775]	1969	19	Lung	NI
Weigensberg[776]	1972	15	Vertebra	NI
Lieguarda[777]	1973	15	Lung	A, 2 yr
Donaldson et al[778]	1976	20	Lung	D, 2 yr
Bloom et al[780]	1981	19	Renal fossa	A, 1 yr
Mc Nichols et al[779]	1981	13	Lung	D, 2 yr
Mc Nichols et al[779]	1981	12	Lung	A, 9 yr
Mc Nichols et al[779]	1981	14	Lung	A, 6 yr

* Case No. 4
† Case No. 2
‡ Case No. 3
§ D, dead; A, alive

quently, argyrophil cells (Bodian stain, Grimelius stain) are observed.[860-862,864,865] Electron microscopic demonstration of neurosecretory granules has been reported in six of the nine reported renal carcinoids.[857,859,862-865]

Follow-up information is not provided in half of the reported cases. Toker's patient was alive, without evidence of tumor, 7 years following nephrectomy.[863] Zak and colleagues reported survivals of 4 years and 6 years; however, the latter patient evidenced tumor metastases.[864]

The histogenesis of renal carcinoids has not been clarified. Origin from cells migrating from the neural crest, as postulated for intestinal carcinoids, or from resident renal parenchymal cells demonstrating carcinoid differentiation (as demonstrated in the prostate gland) has been considered.

Small-Cell Undifferentiated Carcinoma (Oat Cell Carcinoma)

Capella and associates (1984) have reported the only primary renal small-cell carcinoma.[866] The neoplasm was a 12-cm solid mass arising in the left kidney of a 68-year-old woman.[866] The patient died following surgery. At autopsy, widespread nodal metastases were found. Morphologically, the neoplasm demonstrated the typical light microscopic features of small-cell undifferentiated carcinoma. Argyrophil granules were found with the Grimelius stain, and electron microscopy demonstrated neurosecretory granules.[866] The kidney thus joins the prostate and urinary bladder as one of the primary genitourinary sites of this malignant neoplasm.

Neuroectodermal Neoplasms

Pheochromocytoma

A single case of intrarenal pheochromocytoma has been reported by Simon and co-workers (1979) in a 27-year-old woman presenting with systemic hypertension.[869] The 2.5-cm cystic and hemorrhagic mass was shelled out of the left kidney. The patient was normotensive and had a normal IVP 1 month after surgery.

Approximately 10% of pheochromocytomas are extra-adrenal (refer to Chap. 11). In addition to the single intrarenal case noted above, two additional cases, intracapsular and attached to the capsule, have been reported.[867,868]

Mesenchymal Neoplasms

Renomedullary Interstitial Cell Tumor

The term *renomedullary interstitial cell tumor* was introduced by Lerman and associates (1972) to identify more appropriately an interesting tumor of the renal medulla formerly known as renal medullary fibroma.[875]

Renomedullary interstitial cell tumors are common incidental findings at autopsy, with frequencies ranging from 16% to 41.8% in three reported series.[870,875,878] There is no sex predilection. These lesions are not seen in children and young adults, but thereafter they tend to increase with age.[596,870] Multiple lesions are not uncommon. The typical example appears as a gray-tan, well-defined, round nodule in the mid-medulla. The lesions vary in size from less than 1 mm to 1 cm. The smallest renomedullary interstitial cell tumors appear sharply circumscribed but those larger, although retaining the overall round configuration, have an irregular margin. None is encapsulated.

Microscopically, the nodule is composed of a variably myxoid to densely fibrous stroma, frequently with hyalinized collagen in a "brush-stroke" pattern (Figs. 1-66 and 1-67). Within this background are scattered spindle cells and entrapped, compressed, atrophic tubules. The irregular border observed on gross examination is confirmed microscopically. The abundant acid mucopolysaccha-

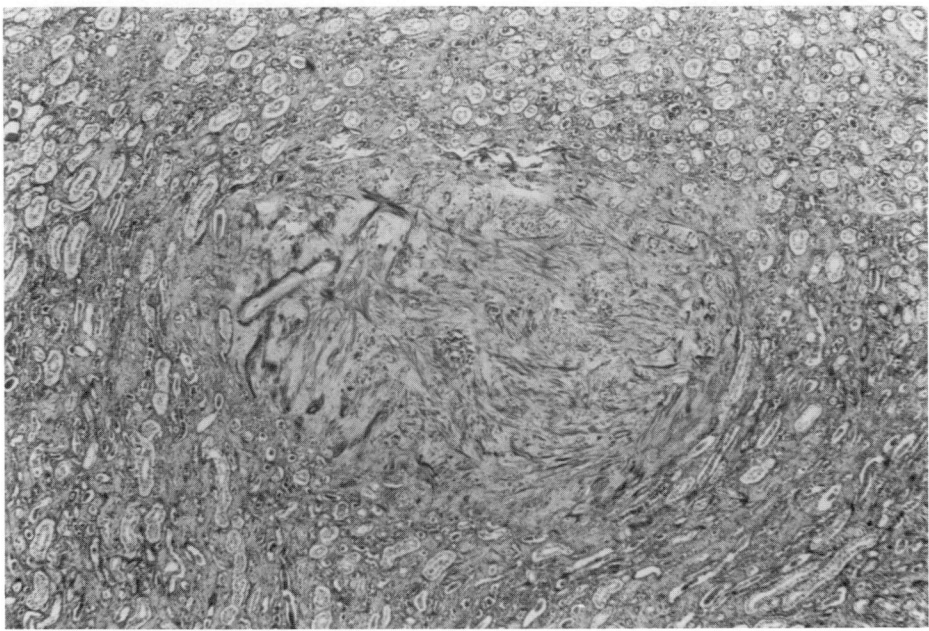

Figure 1-66   *Medullary interstitial cell tumor. The well-demarcated fibrous nodule contains scattered fibroblast-like cells and occasional entrapped renal tubules near the periphery.*

rides of the stroma are demonstrated by alcian blue and PAS stains. In addition, lipid droplets are detected in intra- and extracellular locations by oil red-O stain.

The original ultrastructural studies reported by Lerman and associates disclosed that the spindle cells dispersed throughout the stroma possessed the features of the medullary interstitial cells and not those of fibroblasts.[875] Lipid secretory ability of medullary interstitial cells was suggested by numerous intracellular osmophilic droplets and associated with cytoplasmic cisternae. Elongated cell processes were characteristic. The cell population, with features as described above, prompted the authors to propose the name *renomedullary interstitial cell tumor* to replace the former appellation, *medullary fibroma*. Furthermore, the uniformity of the cell population suggested that this lesion was a true neoplasm and not a hamartoma as previously thought.

Two clinical aspects of renal medullary interstitial cell tumors deserve comment. During the 1960s and early 1970s, interest in a possible antihypertensive endocrine effect of these neoplasms was expressed.[876] The basis for this speculation rested on work demonstrating an antihypertensive effect of autotransplants of renal medulla in experimental hypertension.[876] Two studies published in 1976 failed to demonstrate any correlation between the presence of these tumors and either heart weight or systemic blood pressure.[878,879] The absence of further efforts to associate these minute renal tumors and hypertension probably reflects the conclusion that the previous studies cited have put the matter to rest.

Finally, the relationship of renomedullary interstitial cell tumor to rare cases of clinically significant tumors reported as medullary fibroma, adenofibroma, renomedullary fibroma, myxoma, and fibroepithelial polyp requires clarification.[871–874,877,880–882] The same examples of all of these neoplasms were included in recently published literature reviews of fibroepithelial polyps of the renal pelvis

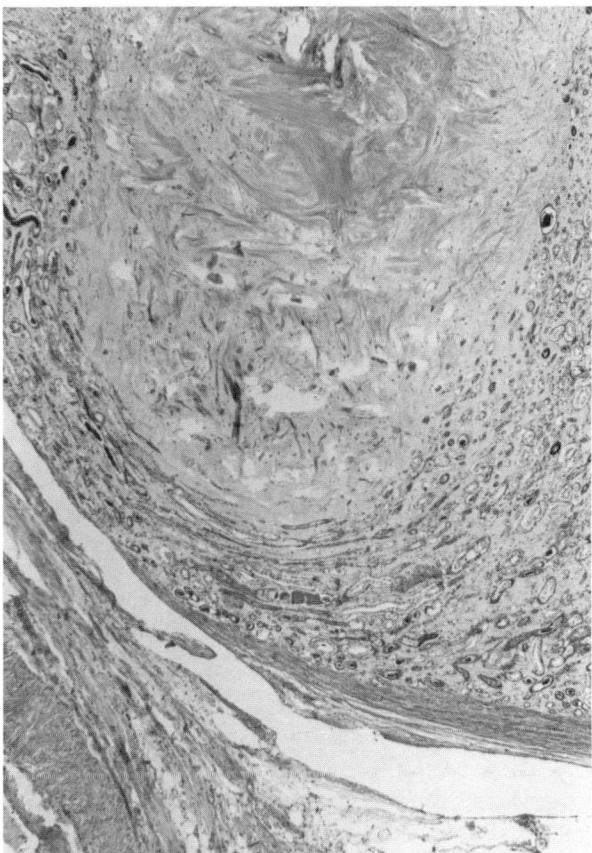

Figure 1-67   *Medullary interstitial cell tumor. This example is virtually acellular. The absence of a capsule is apparent at the periphery.*

and renomedullary fibromas.[881,882] Indeed, one example of "renomedullary fibroma" was a case of a fibrous tumor taking origin from the extrarenal pelvic wall.[872] Such tumors are not renomedullary fibromas and most definitely not clinically significant examples of renomedullary interstitial cell tumors. Such neoplasms are best regarded as fibroepithelial polyps of the renal pelvis (refer to the discussion of fibroepithelial polyps in Chap. 2). Histologically similar polyp-oid tumors taking origin from the renal pyramids and projecting into the renal pelvis remain difficult to classify. In spite of the fact that some of these tumors contain entrapped renal collecting tubules in a fibrous or myxoid stroma, there is no evidence currently available to justify regarding them as rare, large, and therefore clinically significant, examples of renomedullary interstitial cell tumors. The first published example of such a neoplasm examined by electron and light microscopy will clarify whether true renomedullary interstitial cell tumors ever attain such large size. Alternatively, these tumors may represent neoplasms of fibroblast origin or inflammatory pseudotumors that can be equated to fibroepithelial polyps. The relatively young age (mean age in the fourth decade) and marked female preponderance among the reported patients with intrapelvic fibrous tumors are in marked contrast to the age and sex of patients with renomedullary interstitial cell tumors.

Renal Capsule Neoplasms (Capsulomas)

Benign mesenchymal neoplasms taking origin from the renal capsule are common incidental findings at autopsy. Colvin (1942) reported finding 144 examples in 2634 consecutive autopsies for an incidence of 5.5%.[883] Their frequency increased with age, with none observed below the age of 19 years. Approximately 10% of patients older than 60 years had "capsulomas" at autopsy. In contrast, reported cases of clinically significant neoplasms of renal capsule origin are extremely rare.[884,886,887] Both benign and malignant mesenchymal tumors have been reported.[883–888]

The histogenesis of the small capsulomas found at autopsy is unresolved. These tumors are most commonly mixtures of proliferating smooth muscle, fibroblasts, and lipocytes in varying proportions (Fig. 1-68).[883,885] Less frequently, they are composed of only one cell type. The mixed composition of the majority of these tumors has suggested various histogenetic explanations, including neoplasms originating from renal blastema, multipotential primitive mesenchymal cells, and wolffian structures. The absence of these tumors in the kidneys of patients in the first two decades and the progressive increase in their frequency thereafter tends to support the theory of neoplastic development from multipotential mesenchymal cells of the renal capsule. The alternative possibility, choristoma, is favored by Bennington and Beckwith (1975), who draw an analogy between these mixed forms of capsuloma and angiomyolipomas.[885]

Clinically significant renal capsular tumors reported in the literature include leiomyomas, fibromas, and neurofibromas.[884–886,888] Rare examples of enormous benign mesenchymal neoplasms, weighing up to 43 lb, have been reported.[884] In such instances, the exact origin, renal capsule or parenchyma, is undetermined.[884] A malignant fibrous histiocytoma and a liposarcoma have been reported to take origin from the renal capsule.[887,888]

Angiomyolipoma

History

The term *angiomyolipoma,* introduced by Morgan and associates in 1951, described a renal tumor containing prominent thick-walled blood vessels with variable amounts of admixed smooth muscle and adipose tissue (Fig. 1-69).[891] The association of such mixed tumors with the cerebral lesions and the cutaneous manifestations of the tuberous sclerosing complex (Bourneville's disease) had been recognized for more than a half century.[889,890] Relatively little attention had been devoted to the pathology of this complex tumor, and as a result, many angiomyolipoms were incorrectly reported during the first half of the 20th century as examples of renal leiomyomas, leiomyosarcomas, and lipomas.[890–892] Other examples, reflecting recognition of the tumor's mixed composition, were reported under a wide variety of descriptive names, all basically permutations of the name now generally accepted, *angiomyolipoma*. The mixed composition has been generally regarded as evidence that angiomyolipomas represent hamartomas of the kidney, or a benign mesenchymoma.[890,894,895,898] Approximately 200 cases of angiomyolipoma have been reported to this time.[891–913]

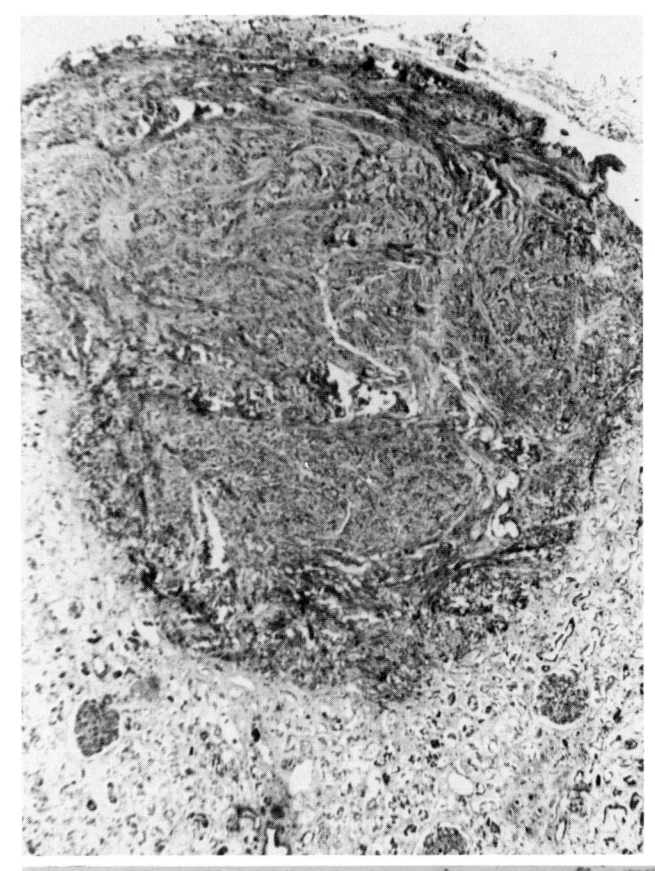

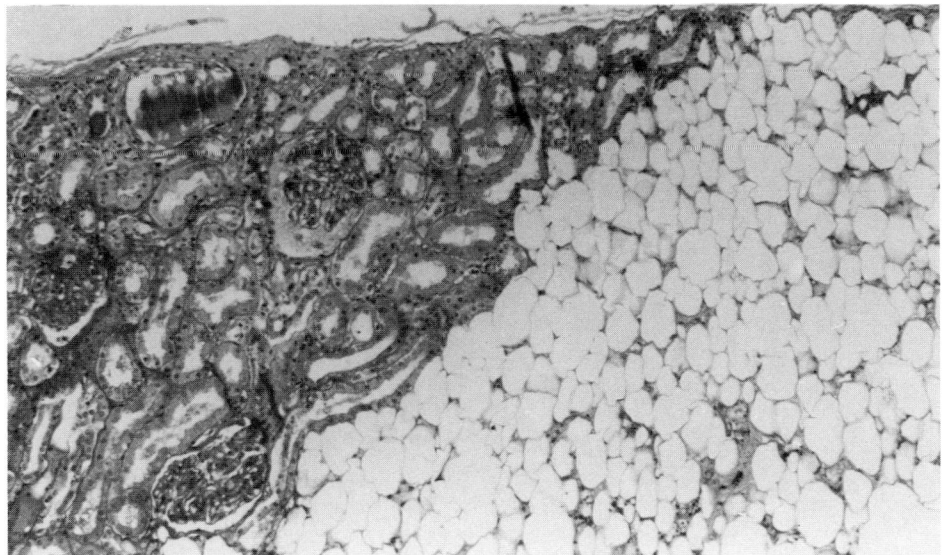

Figure 1-68 **Capsuloma.** (A) *The 2-mm capsular neoplasm is composed of interlacing bundles of smooth muscle cells and collagen fibers. (B) This capsuloma is composed exclusively of lipocytes present in the subcapsular cortex.*

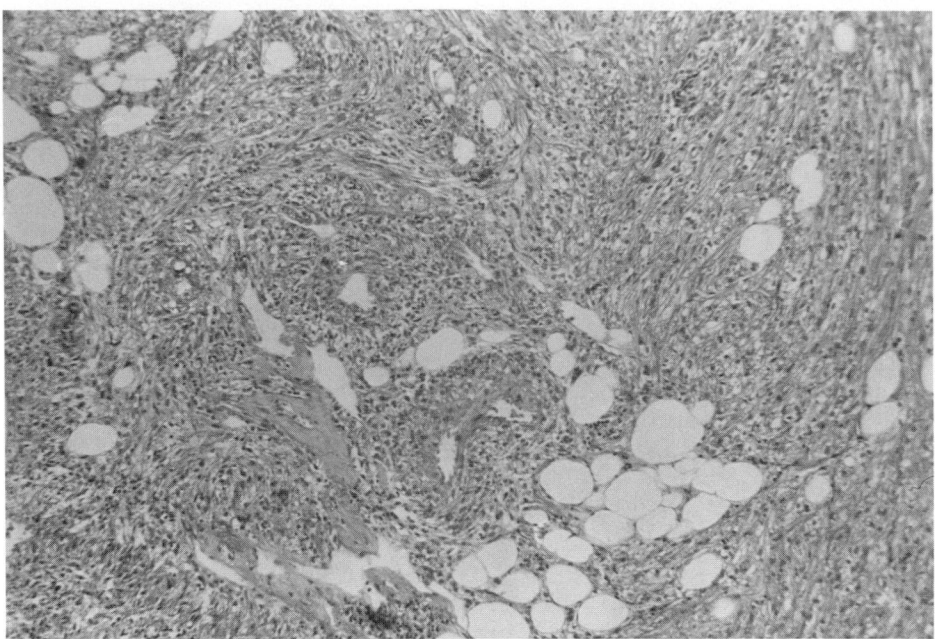

Figure 1-69   ***Angiomyolipoma.*** *The neoplasm is composed of randomly oriented smooth muscle fibers with interspersed clusters and single adipose cells. Characteristic thick-walled blood vessels are scattered among the smooth muscle fibers and fat.*

Clinical Features

Angiomyolipomas occurring in the absence of stigmata of the tuberous sclerosis complex most frequently involve women between the ages of 35 and 60 years. Such cases are more apt to be single large lesions that are symptomatic, in which the patient presents with flank pain and a palpable mass. Several cases of massive hemorrhage within the tumor resulting in a surgical emergency have been recorded.[896,899] When associated with tuberous sclerosis, renal angiomyolipomas are more commonly incidental findings discovered during the radiologic examination of a patient with the neural disorder or at the time of autopsy. Such patients tend to be younger adults than those patients with isolated angiomyolipomas.

Radiologically, there is the presence of a mass that is characteristically hypervascular and sharply demarcated from the uninvolved kidney. An onion-peel appearance has been described during the venous phase of renal angiography. Shawker and associates have described ultrasound and CT scan findings that are very suggestive of renal angiomyolipoma.[909] The principal lesions to be radiologically differentiated from angiomyolipoma are renal cell carcinoma and polycystic disease (both lesions have been observed on occasion to occur with angiomyolipomas).[147,904]

Pathologic Features

When found in a patient with tuberous sclerosis, angiomyolipomas tend to be small and multiple and frequently bilateral. This contrasts with the tendency of isolated angiomyolipomas to be unilateral, single, and large, with examples recorded to 20 cm in diameter.[895] The cut surface of the tumor has a variable appearance reflecting the relative proportions of smooth muscle and fat within the lesion. Although generally well demarcated, they do not exhibit a capsule, and some show local infiltration of the adjacent kidney parenchyma. On occasion, the infiltrating tumor may penetrate the renal capsule and extend into the perirenal adipose tissue. Hemorrhage and necrosis are common and may result in focal cystic degeneration. On rare occasion, the hemorrhage may be massive and extend into the adjacent uninvolved kidney parenchyma.

Histologically, the tumor exhibits a mixture of fat; smooth muscle cells in poorly organized fascicles; and prominent, thick-walled blood vessels. The relative proportions of the fat and smooth muscle cells show great variation from case to case and within the same tumor, undoubtedly contributing to earlier misdiagnoses as either lipomas or leiomyomas. The smooth muscle appears to take origin from the peripheral muscle of the blood vessel walls. Such muscle cells tend to "spin off" in a tangential manner from the periphery of the vessel wall and extend into the adjacent background of intermingled fat and smooth muscle bundles (Fig. 1-70). Electron microscopic study of an angiomyolipoma confirmed the smooth muscle and adipose cell components of this tumor.[907] Isolated renal tubules are commonly entrapped at the periphery of the tumor. Although the adipose cells within the lesion are uniformly mature in their morphologic features, the smooth muscle cells can show variation of nuclear size and staining, prompting concern about their biologic potential. Occasional mitoses in the smooth muscle component may add to this disturbing histologic picture. The sole importance of these findings rests with their misleading contribution to a misdiagnosis of leiomyosarcoma. The clinical behavior of these tumors bears no relationship to the relative proportions of fat and smooth muscle or to the extent of pleomorphism of the smooth muscle cells.

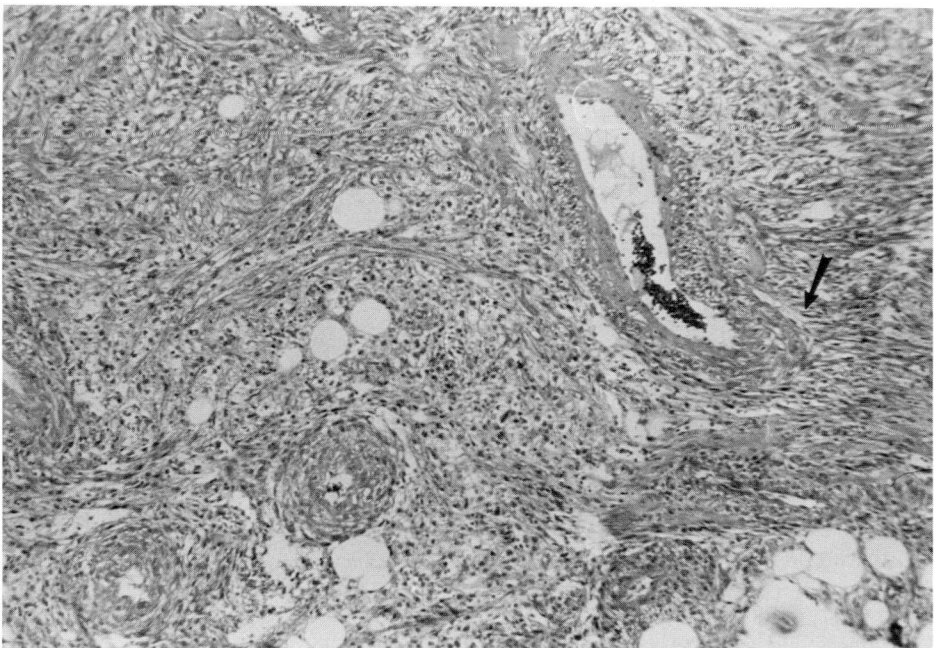

Figure 1-70   **Angiomyolipoma.** *The smooth muscle of the vascular walls merges with the smooth muscle cells dispersed throughout the lesion* (arrow).

A single case reported by Harveit and Halleraker (1960), interpreted as an example of angiolipomyosarcoma, showed invasion of the renal vein and capsule with "tumor tissue similar in all respects . . . " in the contralateral kidney.[897] This case was regarded by the authors as an example of metastatic behavior, but in retrospect it most probably represents bilateral angiomyolipomas with associated locally aggressive invasion of the renal vein. In the two decades since this report, no similar case has been reported. However, mention should be made of 11 reported examples of renal angiomyolipomas with associated hilar lymph nodes showing similar "metastases" or "inclusions" of angiomyolipomatous tissue.[912,913] Dissemination with subsequent tumor-related ontoward events have never been reported in such cases. The prevailing opinion is that these cases represent examples of multicentricity.[912] The findings of angiomyolipoma in the spleen of a patient with the renal lesion is interpreted in a similar manner.[913]

The diagnosis of angiomyolipoma requires thorough histologic examination to ensure the detection of all three components: smooth muscle, mature fat, and the characteristic vasculature. Treatment of unilateral, symptomatic angiomyolipomas requires nephrectomy, which is curative.

Hemangioma

Renal hemangiomas are more common than lymphangiomas, with approximately 150 documented cases in the literature.[914-928] These benign vascular neoplasms have been reported at ages ranging from 4 days to 72 years. Seventy percent of the cases are diagnosed in the third to fifth decades, with intermittent hematuria being the most common presenting symptom (95%). There is no significant side or sex predilection. The angiographic appearance of this vascular neoplasm in the kidney has been variously observed to be hypervascular, hypovascular, or normal.[922-924] The correct preoperative diagnosis reported in rare examples in the past was based on suggestive angiographic patterns combined with the clinical finding of unilateral hematuria in a relatively young adult.

Grossly, the typical renal angioma is well demarcated, and on cut surface it shows a cluster of blood-filled vascular channels. Thrombus formation in these channels has been observed. Summers (1977) has reported the finding of a typical renal angioma occurring as a nodule in the wall of a renal cortical cyst.[925] Microscopically, the majority of the reported cases conform to the features typical of cavernous hemangiomas with variably large blood-filled vascular tributaries in a disorganized tangle. The vascular walls vary in thickness and structure indicative of arterial and venous components. The cytologic features of the flat lining endothelial cells are benign, allowing for differentiation of this lesion from the rare malignant counterpart, angiosarcoma (refer to the discussion of angiosarcoma, later in this chapter).

Lymphangioma

Approximately twenty renal lymphangiomas have been reported.[925-930] These benign neoplasms have been reported at all ages (4 months – 76 years), with 70% occurring in patients older than 30 years.[929] The mean age of the reported patients is 32 years. Lymphangioma affects the right and left kidneys with equal frequency. Sixty-five percent of cases have been reported in female patients. Hematuria, commonly with an associated mass, is the most frequent clinical presentation. Radiologic examination discloses an avascular mass without specific identifying features and thus has not allowed differentiation of lymphangiomas from other benign renal mass lesions.[929] All reported cases have been diagnosed at the time of postoperative pathologic examination.

These neoplasms are well demarcated and show a honeycomb appearance on cut surface. Cysts range in size from microscopic to 1 cm to 2 cm. In contrast to hemangiomas, the neoplastic vessels do not contain blood. Microscopically, the lining endothelial cells are flat and evidence no cytologic features, nuclear enlargement, papillary tufting, or malignancy. The neoplastic vascular channels commonly have a faint eosinophilic proteinaceous substance in the lumen. Variable amounts of collagenous stroma separate the vessels. The presence of smooth muscle in the stroma is inconstant.[929]

There is no report of recurrence or metastases following nephrectomy in any of the recorded cases. Improvements in radiologic diagnostic techniques, possibly coupled with needle biopsy procedures, may enable preoperative diagnosis and less radical surgical therapy in the future.

Leiomyoma

Clinically significant leiomyomas are rare, with 27 cases found in the literature.[931-937] The number of authentic leiomyomas is most probably lower, because some of the cases found in the older literature may represent examples of angiomyolipoma. Renal leiomyomas have been reported in ages ranging from the newborn to 68 years.[933,935] The peak frequency is the fourth and fifth decades. A marked predilection for females is observed, with only five cases reported in males. Patients most frequently present with abdominal or flank pain and a palpable mass. An avascular renal mass, devoid of features suggesting the specific diagnosis, is observed on radiologic evaluation. The correct diagnosis is made only at the time of pathologic examination.

As is common to all benign smooth muscle neoplasms regardless of origin, renal leiomyomas are well-circumscribed solid masses with a pink-tan to ivory color and a whorled appearance on cut surface. These neoplasms are typically 5 cm to 10 cm in diameter but can grow to gigantic dimensions. Clinton-Thomas (1956) reported the successful surgical removal of an 82-lb renal leiomyoma, measuring 57.5 cm × 40 cm × 20 cm, from a 23-year-old man.[934] The microscopic features of renal leiomyomas are typical of this neoplasm in other locations. Leiomyoma is to be distinguished from its malignant counterpart, leiomyosarcoma, and from angiomyolipoma and congenital mesoblastic nephroma (so-called leiomyomatous hamartoma).

Lipoma

Benign lipomatous renal neoplasms of clinical significance are rare. Robertson and Hand collected 12 previously cited cases and reported 2 new cases in 1941.[938] Beadles and Urich (1952) again reviewed the literature, bringing the total number of reported cases to 15.[940] In contrast, clinically significant perirenal lipomas, some of enormous size, have been reported in approximately 200 patients.[939] Lipomatous neoplasms of renal capsular origin are a very common incidental finding at autopsy. Frequently these are neoplastic admixtures of smooth muscle, fibroblasts, and fat, prompting the designation *capsulomas* by

Colvin (1942) (refer to the preceding discussion of renal capsule neoplasms). The exact number of true lipomas among the rare examples reported as such is unknown, but some most probably represent angiomyolipomas, a judgment that can also be made referable to some of the reported cases of renal leiomyomas in the older literature.

Renal lipomas (and perirenal lipomas) grow slowly, frequently attaining large size. Examples weighing 2200 g were noted in the review by Robertson and Hand (1942).[938] The majority of patients present clinically with flank pain, sometimes associated with a palpable mass. These tumors exhibit all the gross and microscopic features of typical lipomas found in more common sites. The uniform cytologic appearance of the mature lipocytes and the absence of local invasion and secondary changes of hemorrhage and necrosis serve to differentiate lipoma from its malignant counterpart, liposarcoma (refer to the liposarcoma discussion, below). Renal lipomas are to be differentiated from angiomyolipomas.

The origin of lipomas within the kidney, which normally contains no fat, is unknown. Lipomatous differentiation of primitive mesenchymal cells is the most plausible explanation.

Leiomyosarcoma

The most frequently encountered primary renal sarcoma is leiomyosarcoma.[941-943] Three extensive literature reviews of this malignancy have been published by Bazaz-Malik and Gupta (1966), Loomis (1972), and Niceta and colleagues (1974).[952,961,963] Additional cases not included in these reviews and published later than 1974 bring the total number of reported cases to approximately 100.[944-951,953-960,962,964,965] Fewer than 10 additional cases reported to originate from the renal pelvis and one case arising from the renal vein have been reported. (Refer to the discussion of leiomyosarcoma in Chap. 2). One patient with bilateral renal leiomyosarcomas has been reported.[948]

Renal leiomyosarcomas have been reported in patients ranging from 10 to 86 years old, with the peak frequency in the fifth and sixth decades.[948,958] Approximately 75% of cases occur in patients older than 40 years. The neoplasm is more common in women, with a 2:1 female to male ratio. A flank mass, commonly associated with flank pain, is the most frequent clinical presentation. Hematuria has been reported in some cases. The large neoplasms frequently distort the renal pelvis as outlined in an IVP. No characteristic angiographic features have been reported for leiomyosarcoma.[960,962]

The gross and microscopic features of renal leiomyosarcomas are similar to those manifested by this neoplasm in more common locations. Renal and perirenal infiltration are frequent. Vascular invasion and metastases are more common than regional lymph node involvement.[963] Hematogenous dissemination to the lungs and liver is frequently reported. This neoplasm is to be differentiated from renal leiomyoma, angiomyolipoma, mesoblastic neophroma, and the one malignant mesoblastic nephroma reported in the literature.

The principal therapy of this neoplasm is radical nephrectomy, with radiation and chemotherapy reported only in the most recently cited cases.[962,963,965] Few reports of patients surviving 5 years could be found in the limited literature.[944,949]

Liposarcoma

Approximately 45 examples of renal liposarcomas have been reported in the literature.[966-974] I suspect that a significant number of these cases are actually renal angiomyolipomas (refer to the preceding discussion of angiomyolipoma). This is especially true of cases reported in the first half of the 20th century, approximately one third of which were associated with clinical evidence of tuberous sclerosis and among which none evidenced metastases either clinically or at autopsy. (Refer to the review by Williams and Savage, 1958.[966]) This is distinctly different from the observed clinical behavior of liposarcomas of the kidney not associated with tuberous sclerosis in the more recent literature.[967-974] Most cases involve young and middle-aged adults, with a female preponderance.

Grossly, these neoplasms tend to be large fatty masses that are apparently well demarcated but that commonly replace much of the renal parenchyma and extend through the renal capsule. The characteristic histologic and cytologic features atypical of liposarcomas elsewhere are found in examples taking origin within the kidney. This neoplasm is to be differentiated from both its benign counterpart, the lipoma, and angiomyolipoma.

Fibrosarcoma

Twenty-seven reported cases of renal fibrosarcoma could be found in the literature.[975-986] Patients range in age from 34 years to 74 years, with 80% older than 50 years. Clinical presentation is nonspecific, with hematuria, flank mass, flank pain, or absence of all symptoms and signs reported among the 27 cases. Radiologic evidence of a renal mass frequently led to nephrectomy. Only two patients have survived longer than 2 years.[976,986]

These neoplasms are solid, fleshy, firm masses invading the kidney and frequently the renal capsule and perirenal adipose tissue. Hemorrhage and necrosis within the tumor are uncommon. Microscopically, the typical histologic features of fibrosarcoma are observed. Adequate sectioning of such neoplasms may not definitively differentiate fibrosarcoma from renal leiomyosarcoma. Ultrastructural studies have been helpful in such cases. The typical mesoblastic nephroma involves younger patients and typically does not have the malignant cytologic features of fibrosarcoma. One important exceptional case is discussed in the section on mesoblastic nephroma, earlier in this chapter.

Hemangiopericytoma

Hemangiopericytoma, taking origin from the pericytes of Zimmermann, was first described by Stout and Murray in 1942.[987] It arises most commonly in the lower extremity and retroperitoneum of adults in the third to sixth decades, but it has been reported in the soft tissue of virtually all sites and in all age groups.[987,994,1002] Rare examples of hemangiopericytomas arising in visceral organs have been reported. Twenty examples involving the kidney were found in the literature.[988-993,995-1001,1003] Of these 20 cases, approximately half take origin from the kidney or invade the kidney parenchyma, the remaining cases described as taking origin from, or being attached to, the renal capsule or renal pelvis, without intrarenal involvement.

The age range of renal hemangiopericytomas is similar to that observed in other locations. Thirteen of the reported cases provided information on the patient's gender. Of these thirteen, nine occurred in women. Patients present with flank pain, with or without a palpable mass. Occasionally, patients present with hematuria. Three of the reported patients had accompanying tumor-related hypoglycemia.[991,992,999] Both hypo- and hypervascular angiographic patterns have been described.[996,999,1000,1003]

The majority of these renal and perirenal hemangiopericytomas are large, primarily solid masses, frequently with multiple foci of hemorrhage and cystic degeneration. The cut surface varies from gray-pink to yellow-brown. The mass is nonencapsulated but is characteristically well demarcated, with compression of the uninvolved kidney. Microscopically, densely cellular areas are mixed with areas of hemorrhage, cyst formation, and fibrosis. Within the cellular portion, the typical perivascular groups of round to spindle-shaped nuclei are found in the background of thin-walled vascular channels. The vessels show no endothelial proliferation, and many are compressed to thin slits, their presence made more apparent with the reticulin stain. Mitoses are not prominent. Ordonez and associates (1982) reported frequent mitoses in a tumor that clinically demonstrated lung metastases.[1000]

Ultrastructural features of hemangiopericytomas include (1) interdigitating cell processes, (2) basal lamina surrounding cells, (3) separation of the vascular tributaries from the tumor cells by well-developed basal lamina, (4) intracytoplasmic filaments and pinocytotic vacuoles, and (5) occasional desmosomes.[999,1000,1002,1003] Electron microscopy assists in the differentiation of hemangiopericytoma from sarcomatoid renal cell carcinoma, juxtaglomerular tumor, renal malignant fibrous histiocytoma, and leiomyosarcoma.[1000,1002,1003]

Among the twenty perirenal and renal hemangiosarcomas, six patients died of tumor-related causes, four within 3 years. Seven patients were alive at the time of publication for periods ranging from 10 months to 11 years. Only five of the twenty patients survived 5 years or more.

Malignant Fibrous Histiocytoma

Malignant fibrous histiocytoma (MFH) was initially recognized as a separate entity and described by Ozello and colleagues (1963) and O'Brien and Stout (1964).[1004,1005] This sarcoma was differentiated from pleomorphic examples of fibrosarcoma, rhabdomyosarcoma, liposarcoma, Hodgkin's disease, and nonneoplastic disorders such as xanthogranulomatous pyelonephritis. This differential diagnosis, on occasion, still remains a diagnostic challenge.

MFH has been classified into five histologic subtypes: (1) storiform pleomorphic, (2) myxoid, (3) giant cell, (4) inflammatory, and (5) angiomatoid.[1017] Common to all histologic subtypes are cytologically malignant spindle cells admixed with histiocytic-type cells. Variable features include multinucleated giant cells, myxomatous stromal change, chronic inflammatory cells including xanthoma cells, and vascular neogenesis. Hemorrhage and necrosis are common and may be extensive.

As suggested by its name, this sarcoma displays histologic evidence of dual differentiation to fibroblasts and histiocytes with collagen production and phagocytic activity. Whether the neoplasm involves a specialized fibroblast, histiocyte, or primitive precursor capable of this dual differentiation is unresolved. Ozzello and colleagues favored origin from histiocytes, which demonstrated morphologic changes resembling fibroblasts in tissue culture.[1004] This histogenetic explanation has not been uniformly accepted.[1017]

The cumulative experience with MFH during the past decades allows that it is the most frequent soft-tissue sarcoma in the elderly.[1009,1010,1017] The sites of predilection are the lower extremity and retroperitoneum, but it has been described in virtually all locations. Fourteen cases of primary renal MFH are reported in the literature.[1006-1009,1011-1016,1018-1021] The recognition of this sarcoma in the kidney, or perhaps its true frequency, seems to be increasing; nine of the recorded cases have been reported since 1980.[1013-1016,1018-1021] Meares and Kempson (1973) mention another case without details provided.[1007] Habib and Gislason (1965) report a "malignant histiocytic tumor" in a 9-year-old boy that may be an example of an angiomatoid MFH.[1006]

Renal MFH is most common in men (3 : 1) and during the sixth and seventh decades. The left kidney has been involved more frequently than the right (7 : 4). The presence of a mass, commonly with pain, is the most frequent clinical presentation. No characteristic radiologic picture of renal MFH has been described.

The neoplasm is solid and infiltrative at the margins, and it commonly shows hemorrhage and necrosis on cut surface. Focal calcification has been reported.[1008] The microscopic features of renal MFH are highly variable, as is true of this sarcoma in all locations. The storiform, pleomorphic variety is the most frequently described in renal MFH cases reported to this time. Renal MFH must be differentiated from the sarcomatoid form of renal cell carcinoma, xanthogranulomatous pyelonephritis, malakoplakia, and other primary and metastatic pleomorphic sarcomas.

Of the reported cases, six patients have died of tumor-related causes 2 months to 34 months following nephrectomy. Five patients were alive without evidence of disease 3 months to 9 years following surgery. The role of radiation and chemotherapy has not been defined in the treatment of renal MFH.

Osteosarcoma

Extraskeletal osteogenic sarcomas are rare in all sites.[1024,1030,1033] Ten osteosarcomas arising within the kidney have been reported.[1022,1023,1025,1027-1029,1031,1032,1034,1035] Their histogenesis is unknown, but most authors have accepted osseous differentiation of strombal fibroblasts with pluripotentiality as the explanation of renal osteosarcomas. In contrast to osteosarcomas arising within bone, which typically affect patients in the first two decades, extraskeletal osteosarcomas, including those of the kidney, involve patients in the fifth decade and older. The age range of the reported patients with renal osteosarcomas is 43 to 82 years, with an even distribution during that age span. There is no sex predilection. Most patients have presented with a painful flank mass. The right kidney has been involved in six of the ten reported cases. Characteristically, intrarenal calcification is observed on abdominal x-ray films. A "sunburst" appearance has been described in more recent reports.[1031,1032,1034] When present, this pattern may help in differentiating this neoplasm from more common causes of intrarenal calcification including cysts, inflammatory disorders, and other neoplasms.[1026] Independent of the therapy provided in these reported cases, this sarcoma has proved highly lethal, with only one patient living longer than 1 year following diagnosis.[1029]

The size of the reported cases of renal osteosarcomas ranges from 5 cm to 23 cm, with reported weights up to 2300 g.[1032] These neoplasms have variable consistency, from soft to bone hard, depending on the relative proportions of hemorrhagic necrosis and neoplastic bone formation, respectively. Local infiltration of the kidney and perirenal fat is extensive. Microscopically, the typical histologic picture is of osteosarcomas with pleomorphic spindle cells showing multifocal differentiation into neoplastic osteoblasts, with osteoid and bone formation. Vascular invasion is common and is the characteristic mode of metastases. Metastases to regional lymph nodes is uncommon but has been reported.[1027]

This neoplasm is to be distinguished from MFH, malignant mesenchymoma, and renal carcinosarcoma, all of which can have osteoid and have on rare occasions been reported in the kidney.

Rhabdomyosarcoma

The existence of a renal rhabdomyosarcoma as a nosologic entity has not been uniformly accepted. Alternative histogenetic theories maintain that these neoplasms are examples of Wilms' tumors with exclusive differentiation to skeletal muscle (refer to the earlier section on Wilms' tumor). Bennington and Beckwith (1975) have proposed that rhabdomyosarcomas arise from primitive pluripotential mesenchymal cells within the kidney.[1041]

Ten renal rhabdomyosarcomas have been reported in the literature.[1036-1040,1042-1044] The patients range in age from 1 year to 62 years. Seven of the ten patients are adults. There is no side or sex predilection. One case of bilateral renal rhabdomyosarcomas was reported by Constance (1947).[1038] Sparse clinical information is available for summary, but presentation with flank pain and a palpable mass is recorded most commonly. No characteristic radiologic findings unique to renal rhabdomyosarcoma have been described. Nephrectomy, with or without radiation, and chemotherapy have failed to produce survivals longer than 18 months in any of the recorded cases.[1036-1040,1042-1044] Widespread metastases to lungs and bone are observed.

Nine of the ten reported examples were interpreted as pleomorphic rhabdomyosarcoma. Kotecha (1977) reported the only embryonal rhabdomyosarcoma.[1042] Grossly, the neoplasms are poorly demarcated, solid, and gray-white to brown, with variable amounts of necrosis and hemorrhage. Focal calcification has been reported.[1042] Extension beyond the kidney is common. Metastases to hilar lymph nodes and gross involvement of the renal vein have been reported.

The diagnosis rests on the finding of typical rhabdomyoblast cells with cross striations, apparent in routine stained sections or demonstrated with the phosphotungstic acid hematoxylin (PTAH) stain. Alternative demonstration of the muscle nature of the malignancy can be achieved by the demonstration of Z-bands with electron microscopy. Adequate sectioning of the specimen will allow differentiation of renal rhabdomyosarcoma from other renal malignancies, especially the rhabdomyomatous variant of Wilms' tumor when the patient is young (refer to the earlier section on Wilms' tumor).

Angiosarcoma

Two examples of renal angiosarcoma have been documented in the literature.[1045,1047] Clinical presentation with hematuria and flank pain was recorded in both patients, 51- and 67-year-old men. Nephrectomy was carried out in both cases. At the time of publication, one patient was alive without evidence of disease at 3 months and the second had died of widespread metastases 2 months following surgery.

In 1980, Askari and colleagues reported an angiosarcoma encasing the external iliac vein anastomosis in a renal allograft recipient 4 years after transplantation.[1046] The kidney was free of tumor at the time of nephrectomy. Tumor metastases and death occurred 4 months after surgery.

The histologic feature of renal angiosarcoma, as exemplified by the two reported cases, is identical to examples reported elsewhere. Anastomosing vascular channels lined by cytologically malignant endothelial cells are characteristic. The endothelial nature of the lining cells can be verified by the application of immunoperoxidase staining for Factor VIII. The neoplastic cells of hemangiopericytoma are proliferating adjacent to, and not within, the vascular channels present in this neoplasm (refer to the discussion of hemangiopericytoma, earlier in this chapter).

Malignant Mesenchymoma

In 1948, Stout described a group of sarcomas that evidenced differentiation of two or more mesenchymal tissue types in addition to the fibrosarcomatous component.[1048] He termed these unique sarcomas *malignant mesenchymomas*.[1048] These neoplasms are uncommon, with most observed in the retroperitoneal and thigh soft tissues in the elderly.[1053] Only four examples of renal origin of this neoplasm could be found in the literature.[1049–1052] The most common combinations include fibrosarcoma with chondrosarcoma and osteosarcoma, but leiomyosarcomatous foci have also been reported.[1049–1052] Interestingly, two of these four cases had independent epithelial malignancies of the renal pelvis and thus qualify as examples of collision tumors involving malignant mesenchymomas with independent, noninvasive renal pelvic carcinomas.[1050,1051]

The patients included two in the third decade and two in the eighth decade. Three patients died with tumor within 1 year.[1049–1051] The fourth patient was alive at 14 months but showed evidence of tumor recurrence.[1052]

Plasmacytoma

Renal involvement in multiple myeloma is common and is characterized in most cases by microscopic infiltration of the renal interstitium by the malignant plasma cells, with or without associated evidence of renal amyloid.[1055] Within the spectrum of plasma cell disorders, uncommon examples of extraosseous plasmacytomas have been observed, most commonly (70%) involving the upper respiratory tract and oral cavity.[1062] Rarely, plasmacytomas are diagnosed in the kidney. The first renal plasmacytoma was reported by Knudson in 1939, and seven additional cases have been found in the literature.[1054,1056–1061,1063] Seven of the eight patients were men. The age range of the eight reported cases was from 22 to 64 years, with six of the eight cases occurring in the sixth and seventh decades. Most patients presented with a renal mass; however, one patient exhibited painless hematuria. Three patients demonstrated Bence Jones protein in the urine.[1058,1060,1063] The radiologic changes are nonspecific and include hypervascularity and palisading tumor vessels.[1057,1060] The preoperative diagnosis has not been made in any of the eight reported cases treated with nephrectomy.

Gross features of the reported cases include poor circumscription with massive replacement of renal parenchyma in half of the cases. The tumor is firm and tan. Capsular penetration, renal vein invasion, and hilar lymph node metastases have been observed in some cases. Microscopically, cytologically malignant plasma cells diffusely infiltrate the renal parenchyma. Amyloid deposition has been observed in one case.[1063]

As all extraosseous plasmacytomas may be either isolated or accompany multiple myeloma, radiologic evidence disclosed that three of the renal plasmacytomas had disseminated disease with bone and liver involvement.[1057,1058,1061] Of the eight reported cases, 5-year follow-up is provided in only one report.[1056]

Malignant Lymphoma

Renal lymphomatous involvement at autopsy is common and well documented.[1066] However, the clinical diagnosis of renal involvement is uncommon, and renal involvement as the initial presentation of the malignant lymphoma is distinctly rare.[1069,1074]

Richmond and co-workers (1962) reported that 34% of 696 patients dying of malignant lymphoma had evidence of renal involvement at autopsy.[1066] Similarly high frequencies of terminal renal involvement by lymphoma were noted in previous autopsy studies cited by Richmond and co-workers.[1066] Antemortem diagnosis of lymphomatous renal involvement was made in only 14% of the 142 patients in whom the diagnosis was made at autopsy. Bilateral involvement was found in 74% of the cases; however, uremia secondary to lymphomatous infiltration of the kidneys was found in only 0.5% of the total group.[1066]

All studies indicate a higher frequency of renal involvement by non-Hodgkin's lymphoma than by Hodgkin's disease.[1066,1067] Only scattered case reports describe the acute onset of uremia in patients with known malignant lymphoma.[1070,1072,1073] Dramatic improvement in renal function has been reported following radiation and chemotherapy.[1069,1070,1073,1074] Three cases of bilateral renal infiltration presenting with uremia of unknown cause are presented in the recent literature.[1069,1074]

Lymphomatous infiltration of the kidney may have a nodular or diffuse distribution throughout the organ or may take the form of a poorly demarcated single mass (Fig. 1-71).[1064,1066,1067] Concentric compression of the kidney has been observed in instances of retroperitoneal lymphomas massively infiltrating the perirenal space.[1064,1066,1067,1071] Microscopically, the lymphomatous infiltrate is observed within the interstitium, producing variable compression and obliteration of the tubules with apparently less destructive results on the glomeruli (Fig. 1-72). The monotonous cellular composition of the infiltrate allows distinction of lymphoma from a chronic inflammatory cell infiltrate commonly coexisting within the renal stroma.

Two reports in the literature purport to describe examples of primary renal

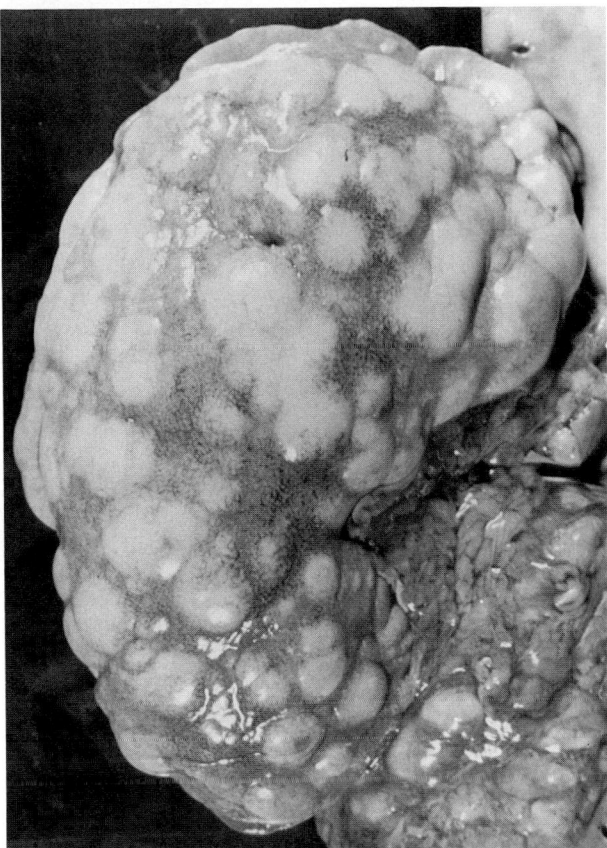

Figure 1-71 *Malignant lymphoma. Widespread multiple nodules of lymphoma are present on the cortical surface of the kidney.*

lymphoma occurring in patients without evidence of systemic extrarenal involvement.[1065,1068] Nephrectomy resulted in disease-free intervals of 1 and 5 years at the time of publication of these cases, respectively. Similar "primary" lymphomas have been reported in other urinary tract organs, including the ureter and urinary bladder (see Chaps. 3 and 4).

Leukemia

Leukemic infiltration of the kidneys, like malignant lymphoma, is rarely diagnosed prior to death but is observed in approximately two thirds of cases examined at autopsy.[1075] Sternby (1955) could find only three previously reported cases of uremia due to leukemic infiltration of the kidneys.[1075] Renal involvement by leukemia is apparently demonstrated more frequently by lymphocytic leukemias than by those of myelogenous origin.[1075]

The extent of leukemic infiltration of the kidneys has been reported to bear no relationship to either the size of these organs as determined radiologically or the presence or degree of impaired renal function.[1075–1078] Indeed, renal enlargement occurs in the apparent absence of leukemic infiltration without current explanation in about 20% of cases.[1075,1078] Conversely, massive leukemic infiltration can occur without impaired renal function.[1077]

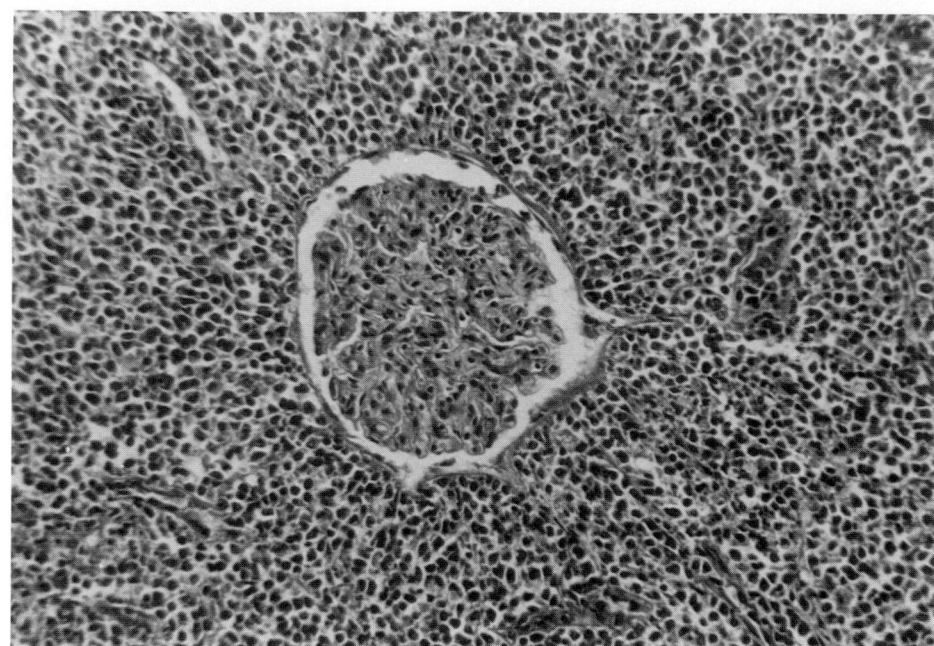

Figure 1-72   *Malignant lymphoma in the kidney. The interstitium of the cortex contains a massive infiltrate of lymphoma cells with destruction of renal tubules and apparent sparing of the glomerulus in the center.*

Pathologically, leukemic infiltrations of the kidney range from microscopic focal or confluent interstitial collections to grossly apparent, ill-defined, geographically confluent or patchy, pink-white infiltrates showing a predilection for the outer cortex.[1075] Focal areas of recent hemorrhagic necrosis are not uncommon and reflect terminal bleeding dyscrasias.

Carcinosarcoma

Malignant neoplasms with histologic evidence of both epithelial and mesenchymal differentiation are uncommon, and their histogenesis remains unresolved. Reflecting the presence of both malignant components within the same tumor, the term *carcinosarcoma* was introduced in the 19th century. Initial attempts to classify these interesting neoplasms on histogenetic grounds were published in 1920 by Meyers, who recognized three categories of carcinosarcomas: (1) composition tumors, (2) combination tumors, and (3) collision tumors.[1080] Composition tumors had malignant stromal and epithelial components, each derived from separate cell lines by malignant transformation in proximity in such manner as to give a single neoplasm. Combination tumors resulted from the malignant transformation and dual epithelial and mesenchymal differentiation of a single stem, or undifferentiated cell. Collision tumors, representing two independent neoplasms, one epithelial and the other mesenchymal, took origin in proximity to each other and demonstrated fusion at the sites of their nearest borders.

Willis (1967), recognizing that the collision tumors of Meyers bore no histogenetic relationship to "true carcinosarcomas" but rather represented the chance development of two independent neoplasms, introduced a new classification.[1085] Willis recognized two histogenetic types: (1) tumors representing neoplastic transformation in two distinct tissues (equivalent to the composition tumors of Meyers) and (2) tumors representing consequent sarcomatous change in the stroma of a carcinoma. Curiously, Willis did not recognize the histogenetic possibility of dual differentiation of an undifferentiated cell along both epithelial and mesenchymal lines.

There are thus two classifications of these interesting neoplasms, each incomplete, or conceptually in error, or both. In this background, numerous examples of so-called carcinosarcomas appear in the literature that represent examples included in either of these two classifications.

I employ a histogenetic classification that represents the combined and modified schemata of Meyers (1920) and Willis (1967).[1080,1085] This classification outlines the histogenetic possibilities of tumors correctly regarded as carcinosarcomas. Following malignant transformation, carcinosarcomas can develop by any of the following:

1. Undifferentiated cell differentiating along both epithelial and mesenchymal lines
2. Concomitant differentiation of a transformed stromal cell and a transformed epithelial cell within close proximity, producing a single neoplasm
3. An established carcinoma inducing a malignant transformation in the adjacent stroma with subsequent dual proliferation of both neoplastic components

A distinct phenomenon, superficially resembling carcinosarcoma, is the example of epithelial malignancy changing its morphologic features from a "well-differentiated squamous cell carcinoma or adenocarcinoma" to a less differentiated form, assuming a spindle cell configuration and on occasion showing apparent mesenchymal differentiation in the form of chondroid, osteoid, and so on. Well-documented examples of such neoplasms have been reported in the oral cavity and breast. Rarely, such malignancies arise in the kidney, where they are termed the *sarcomatoid type* of renal cell carcinoma. The epithelial origin of such sarcomatous foci is determined by extensive sampling of the tumor with resultant detection of transitions of epithelial cells to spindle cell areas. In addition, electron microscopic study of such cases may detect ultrastructural features characteristic of epithelial cells. Histochemical studies may assist in this distinction in the future (refer to the discussion of the sarcomatoid variant of renal cell carcinoma, earlier in this chapter).

In the final analysis, it must be stated that we are currently only at the stage of compiling criteria and making diagnoses accordingly. This is not the same as having a true understanding of the histogenetic events underlying these neoplasms. Fibroblasts, chondroblasts, or more accurately cells with morphologic features that fit the working definition of these cells may be derived (1) from a single cell with dual differentiation, giving rise to these cells and epithelial cells; (2) from a previously "committed mesenchymal cell"; or (3) from a malignant epithelial cell that has altered its genetic expression. The end result, as evaluated by current means of analysis, is the same. In more practical terms, this is translated into the current inability to distinguish carcinosarcomas taking origin from

Table 1-24   *Reported Cases of Renal Carcinosarcoma*

Author	Year	Age	Sex	Carcinoma	Sarcoma	Follow-Up
Fisher, Davis[1083]	1962	68	M	RCC*	Fibrosarcoma	D, 2 mo‡
Fisher, Davis[1083]	1962	61	M	RCC*	Rhabdomyosarcoma	D, 4 mo
Fisher, Davis[1083]	1962	43	M	RCC*	Fibrosarcoma	D, 3 mo
Hou, Willis[1084]	1963	77	M	TCC†	Malignant mesenchymoma	D, unknown duration
Ridolphi, Eggleston[1088]	1978	65	M	TCC†	Rhabdomyosarcoma	D, 1 mo
Chatelanat[1089]	1981	74	M	RCC*	Fibrosarcoma	A — NED, 5 mo
Tarry et al[1090]	1982	63	F	TCC†	Giant cell sarcoma	A — NED, 20 mo

* Renal cell carcinoma
† Transitional cell carcinoma
‡ D — dead; A, NED — alive, no evidence of disease

any of the previously outlined three histogenetic routes of development. At present, we are capable of identifying most examples of collision tumors and probably most examples of sarcomatoid variants of carcinomas. These neoplasms must be distinguished from acceptable cases of carcinosarcomas.

Most of the reported examples of "renal carcinosarcoma" appearing in the literature represent collision tumors. Excluding these collision tumors, only six acceptable cases of renal carcinosarcoma were identified (Table 1-24). Patients range in age from 43 years to 77 years. There is a male preponderance. Five of the patients died from their tumor 1 to 4 months after diagnosis. The most recently reported patient by Tarry and associates (1982) was alive without evidence of disease 20 months following nephrectomy.[1088] The epithelial component in half of these cases was renal cell carcinoma; the remainder took origin from the renal pelvis with invasion of the renal parenchyma. Fibrosarcoma is the most frequent component, but rhabdomyosarcoma and "giant cell sarcoma" have also been reported (Table 1-24). The case reported by Hou and Willis (1983) showed diverse sarcomatous differentiation including fibrosarcoma, osteochondrosarcoma, and areas "resembling malignant osteoclastoma," findings unique among renal carcinosarcomas.[1083]

Table 1-25   *Reported Cases of Renal Collision Tumors*

Author	Year	Age	Sex	Carcinoma
Kay[1081]	1957	62	F	RCC*
Fauci et al[1082]	1961	61	F	TCC†
Fisher, Davis[1083]	1962	68	M	RCC*
Elliott et al[1086]	1973	70	M	*In situ* SCC‡
Gallagher et al[1087]	1974	75	M	*In situ* TCC†

* Renal cell carcinoma
† Transitional cell carcinoma
‡ Squamous cell carcinoma

Carcinosarcomas, as noted above, are to be differentiated from (1) collision tumors, (2) sarcomatoid variants of epithelial malignancies, and (3) malignant mesenchymomas, examples of each having been incorrectly reported as carcinosarcomas in the past.

Collision Tumors

Five examples of collision tumors arising within the kidney have been reported, only one of which accurately indicates the true nature of the neoplasms (Table 1-25).[1081-1083,1086,1087] The epithelial neoplasm was renal cell carcinoma in two of the cases, with the remaining three cases comprising renal pelvic neoplasms. Gallagher and colleagues (1974) correctly regarded their case as not representing a carcinosarcoma, because the epithelial neoplasm showed no evidence of invasion of the renal parenchyma, the site of coexisting sarcoma.[1087] In contrast, an identical case, reported as renal carcinosarcoma, had a noninvasive squamous cell carcinoma of the renal pelvis in association with a renal sarcoma[1086] The combination of these epithelial neoplasms with the concurrent renal sarcomas must be regarded as independent and the result of chance, however improbable the occurrence of a second malignancy (the carcinomas) with the sarcoma in the kidney. The improbability reaches new heights in the case of Gallagher and associates' report, in which the sarcomatous neoplasm showed differentiation toward chondrosarcoma, osteosarcoma, and leiomyosarcoma, technically qualifying the tumor as a malignant mesenchymoma.[1087] This case thus qualifies as a renal malignant mesenchymoma with an independent noninvasive papillary transitional cell carcinoma.

Among the five patients with renal collision tumors, all patients were in the seventh and eighth decades. Of these patients, one died in the postoperative period and two died 2 months and 1 year following nephrectomy, respectively. There was no follow-up information provided on one patient, and the fifth patient died with tumor metastases, exclusively sarcomatous, 5 months following onset of symptoms. The collision tumors were diagnosed at autopsy in this case. These neoplasms must be differentiated from carcinosarcomas and the sarcomatoid type of renal cell carcinoma.

Sarcoma	Author's Diagnosis	Follow-Up
Leiomyosarcoma	Reported as malignant mixed mesodermal tumor	D, Postop
Leiomyosarcoma	Carcinosarcoma	No information
Fibrosarcoma	Reported as carcinosarcoma	D, Postop
Osteosarcoma, Chondrosarcoma, & fibrosarcoma	Reported as carcinosarcoma	D, w/tumor, 1 year
Osteosarcoma, Chondrosarcoma	Reported as coexistent chondrosarcoma & transitional cell carcinoma	5 mo from SES to death; diagnosis at autopsy

Teratoma

Intrarenal teratomas have been reported in six patients ranging in age from newborn to 59 years.[860,1091,1093-1095] An additional 41 cases of extrarenal retroperitoneal teratomas were reported in a review by Arnheim (1951).[1092] The gross and microscopic features of renal teratomas are typical of this neoplasm in more common locations (gonads), and with the exception of one case, were histologically and clinically benign. Kojiro and associates (1976) reported the exceptional example of a carcinoid developing in an otherwise typical teratoma of the kidney.[860] The histogenesis of renal teratomas, as with all other teratomas in extragonadal sites, is regarded to involve aberrant migration of germ cells during embryogenesis and subsequent neoplastic transformations.

Metastatic Neoplasms

The frequency of metastatic neoplasms involving the kidney at autopsy is exceeded only by the frequency of metastatic involvement in the liver, lungs, adrenal glands, and brain.[1106,1112] The frequency of renal metastases observed at autopsy is presented in Table 1-26.

The clinical diagnosis of metastatic tumor in the kidney is uncommon, with only 34 cases reported in the literature. Primary neoplasms giving origin to renal metastases clinically diagnosed include those of the lung, thyroid, breast, and larynx and liposarcoma of the leg.[1103,1104,1107-1109,1116,1117,1120,1121] In 8 of the 34 cases, the symptomatic renal metastases were the first clinical manifestation of the nonrenal primary tumors.[1102,1103,1105,1110,1118] Neoplasms presenting in this manner include lung (4 cases), esophagus, cervix, hepatoma, and choriocarcinoma of undetected primary source (1 case each).[1102,1103,1105,1110,1118]

Most patients with clinically diagnosed renal metastases present with hematuria; less frequently they present with a palpable mass or flank pain. Radiologic examination of the kidneys demonstrates single or multiple solid tumors, characteristically avascular in angiographic studies.[1108,1111,1114,1122] The correct diag-

Table 1-26 *Metastatic Neoplasms in Kidney: Reported Frequency at Autopsy*

Author	Year	No. of Autopsies	Number of Renal Metastases
Klinger[1098]	1951	5000*	118(2.3%)†
Willis[1106]	1967	500‡	38(7.6%)§
Wagle et al[1113]	1975	4413*	81(1.8%)§
Bracken et al[1115]	1979	11328‡	816(7.2%)§
Pascal[1119]	1980	314‡	25(8.0%)§
Petersen‖	1980	576‡	68(11.8%)§

* Consecutive autopsies on all hospital patients

† Includes hematopoietic malignancies

‡ Consecutive autopsies on patients with known cancer

§ Excludes hematopoietic malignancies

‖ Personal observations

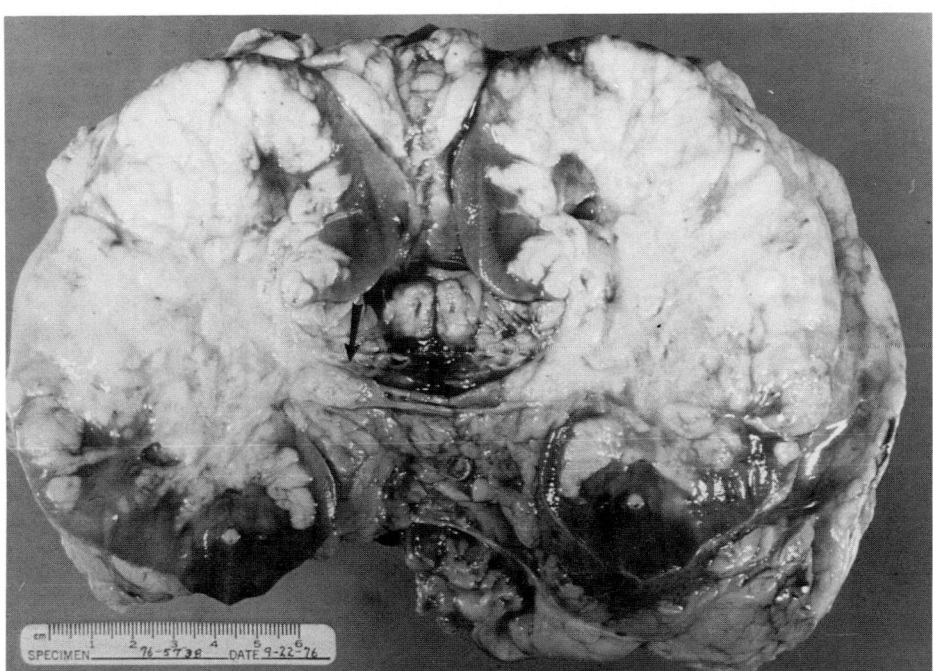

Figure 1-73 *Metastatic squamous cell carcinoma. The tumor shows widespread infiltration of the kidney with invasion of the renal vein (arrow). The primary site of the metastatic tumor was the larynx.*

nosis should be suspected in patients who have a documented history of a nonrenal malignancy and who present with sudden onset of hematuria and have radiologic findings compatible with metastatic neoplasm. Finally, the development of renal cell carcinoma in patients with a previously diagnosed nonrenal primary is well documented and must be considered when encountering the above described clinical dilemma. Urine cytology is rarely helpful in the diagnosis of metastatic neoplasms to the kidney.[1117] Alternatively, the CT scan—

Table 1-27 **Metastatic Neoplasms in Kidney: Frequency From Selected Primary Sites Based on Autopsy Studies**

Site	Willis[1106] (1967)	Bracken[1115] (1979)	Petersen* (1980)
Lung	15%	17.8%	29%
Breast	15.5%	8.3%	13%
Melanoma (skin)	25%	35.5%	40%
Kidney (contralateral)	40%	13.3%	17%
Esophagus	6%	10%	19%
Stomach	0%	5.8%	3%
Colon/rectum	5%	13.9%	8%
Pancreas	0%	16.2%	9%
Ovary	0%	3.8%	36%
Testis	NI	22.8%	20%

* Personal observations

directed needle aspiration biopsies of kidney masses is a useful diagnostic technique.

Gross examination of kidneys bearing small metastatic tumors reveals a predilection for the cortex, a feature commonly obscured by large metastatic lesions capable of significant renal destruction. Metastases are generally well demarcated, irregular, solid nodules. Bilateral metastases are present in the majority of cases.[1112,1113,1115] Penetration of the renal capsule and both intra- and extrarenal branches of the renal vein is common (Fig. 1-73). Invasion of the renal pelvis is relatively uncommon. Histologic evidence of both hematogenous and lymphatic routes of metastases has been presented in the literature. The majority of renal metastases reflect hematogenous spread to these organs.

At autopsy, the most common nonrenal primary malignancies metastasizing to the kidney are lung and breast carcinomas and malignant melanoma (Table 1-27). A wide variety of malignancies of other primary sites metstasize to the kidneys with a lower frequency (Table 1-27).

References

Normal Kidney

1. Parker AE: Studies on the main posterior lymph channels of the abdomen and their connections with the lymphatics of the genito-urinary system. Am J Anat 56:409, 1935
2. Graves FT: The anatomy of the intrarenal arteries and its application to segmental resection of the kidney. Br J Surg 42:132, 1954
3. Emery JL, Methol A: The weights of kidneys in late intra-uterine life and childhood. J Clin Pathol 13:490, 1960
4. Oliver JT, Rubenstein M, Meyer R et al: Congenital abnormalities of the urinary system. III. Growth of the kidney in childhood. Determination of normal weight. J Pediatr 61:256, 1962
5. Osathanondh V, Potter EL: Development of human kidney as shown by microdissection. II. Renal pelvis, calyces, and papillae. Arch Pathol 76:277, 1963
6. Osathanondh V, Potter EL: Development of human kidney as shown by microdissection. III. Formation and interrelationship of collecting tubules and nephrons. Arch Pathol 76:290, 1963
7. Meyers MA, Friedenberg RM, King MC et al: The significance of the renal capsular arteries. Br J Radiol 40:949, 1967
8. Potter EL: Normal development of the kidney. In Potter EL (ed): Normal and Abnormal Development of the Kidney, p 3. Chicago, Year Book Medical Publishers, 1972
9. Amin M, Blandford AT, Polk HC Jr: Renal fascia of Gerota. Urology 7:1, 1976
10. Marshall FF, Powell KC: Lymphadenectomy for renal cell carcinoma: Anatomical and therapeutic considerations. J Urol 128:677, 1982
11. Heptinstall RH: Anatomy. In Heptinstall RH (ed): Pathology of the Kidney, vol I, 3rd ed, p 1. Boston, Little, Brown & Co., 1983
12. Kissane JM: Development of the Kidney. In Heptinstall RH (ed): Pathology of the Kidney, vol. 1, 3rd ed, p 61. Boston, Little, Brown & Co., 1983

Agenesis

13. Potter EL: Bilateral renal agenesis. J Pediatr 29:68, 1946
14. Potter EL: Facial characteristics of infants with bilateral renal agenesis. Am J Obstet Gynecol 51:885, 1946

15. Davidson WM, Ross GIM: Bilateral absence of the kidneys and related congenital anomalies. J Pathol Bacteriol 68:459, 1954
16. Campbell MF: Congenital absence of one kidney. Unilateral renal agenesis. Ann Surg 88:1039, 1928
17. Collins DC: Congenital unilateral renal agenesis. Ann Surg 95:715, 1932
18. Ashley DJB, Mostofi FK: Renal agenesis and dysgenesis. J Urol 83:211, 1960
19. Doroshow LW, Abeshouse BS: Congenital unilateral solitary kidney: Report of 37 cases and a review of the literature. Urol Survey 11:219, 1961
20. Thompson DP, Lynn HB: Genital anomalies associated with solitary kidney. Mayo Clin Proc 41:538, 1966
21. Emanuel B, Nachman R, Aronson N et al: Congenital solitary kidney: A review of 74 cases. J Urol 111:394, 1974
22. Beeby DI: Seminal vesicle cyst associated with ipsilateral renal agenesis: Case report and review of literature. J Urol 112:120, 1974

Hypoplasia

23. Boissonnat P: What to call hypoplastic kidney? Arch Dis Child 37:142, 1962
24. Bernstein J: Developmental abnormalities of the renal parenchyma — renal hypoplasia and dysplasia. Pathol Ann 3:213, 1968

Segmental Hypoplasia (Ask-Upmark Kidney)

25. Ask-Upmark E: Uber juvenile maligne nephrosklerose und ihr verhaltnis zu storungen in der nierenent-wicklung. Acta Pathol Microbiol Scand 7:383, 1929
26. Zjungqvist A, Lagergren C: The Ask-Upmark kidney. A congenital renal anomaly studied by micro-angiography and histology. Acta Pathol Microbiol Scand 56:277, 1962
27. Risdon RA: Renal dysplasia. Part I. A clinicopathological study of 76 cases. J Clin Pathol 24:57, 1971
28. Dein RW, Walker D, Hackett RL: The Ask-Upmark kidney. A case report. Arch Pathol 96:10, 1973
29. Arant BS Jr, Sotelo-Avila C, Bernstein J: Segmental "hypoplasia" of the kidney (Ask-Upmark). J Pediatr 95:931, 1979.
30. Valderrama E, Berkman JI: The Ask-Upmark kidney in a premature infant. Clin Nephrol 11:313, 1979
31. Amat D, Camilleri JP, Phat VN et al: Renin localization in segmental renal hypoplasia. Immunohistochemical localization in two cases. Virchows Arch [A] 390:193, 1981
32. Shindo S, Bernstein J, Arant BS: Evolution of renal segmental atrophy (Ask-Upmark kidney) in children with vesicoureteric reflux: Radiographic and morphologic studies. J Pediatr 102:847, 1983

Renal Hypoplasia With Oligomeganephronia

33. Royer P, Habib R, Methieu H et al: L'hypoplasie renale bilaterale congenitale avec reduction du nombre et hypertrophie des nephrons chez e'enfant. Ann Pediatr 38:753, 1962
34. Habib R, Courtecuisse V, Mathiew H et al: Un type anatomo-clinique particulier d'insuifisance renale chronique de l'enfant: L'hypoplasie oligonephronique congenitale bilaterale. J Urol Nephrol 68:139, 1962
35. Fetterman GH, Habib R: Congenital bilateral oligonephronic renal hypoplasia with hypertrophy of nephrons (oligomeganephronie). Am J Clin Pathol 52:199, 1969
36. Van Acker KJ, Vincke H, Quatacker J et al: Congenital oligonephronic renal hypoplasia with hypertrophy of nephrons (oligonephronia). Arch Dis Child 46:321, 1971

37. Elfenbein IB, Baluarte HJ, Gruskin AB: Renal hypoplasia with oligomeganephronia. Arch Pathol 97:143, 1974
38. Berthoux FC, Khalil S, Sabatier JC et al: Diagnostic de l'hypoplasie renale avec oligomeganephronie chez l'adulte jeune: Valeur de l'angiographie renale avec agrandissement. J Urol Nephrol 84:872, 1978
39. Ng WL, Cheung MF, Chan CW et al: Oligomeganephronic renal hypoplasia. Pathology 12:639, 1980
40. Detre Z, Miltenyi M: Oligomeganephronic renal hypoplasia. Pathol Res Pract 178:416, 1984
41. Moerman Ph, van Damme B, Proesmans W et al: Oligomeganephronic renal hypoplasia in two siblings. J Pediatr 105:75, 1984

Malposition

Ectopia

42. Abeshouse BS: Crossed ectopia with fusion. Review of literature and a report of four cases. Am J Surg 73:658, 1947
43. Hawes CJ: Congenital unilateral ectopic kidney: A report of two cases. J Urol 64:453, 1950
44. Ward JN, Nathanson B, Draper JW: The pelvic kidney. J Urol 94:36, 1965
45. Tanenbaum B, Silverman N, Weinberg SR: Solitary crossed renal ectopia. Arch Surg 101:616, 1970
46. Malek RS, Kelalis PP, Burke EC: Ectopic kidney in children and frequency of association with other malformations. Mayo Clin Proc 46:461, 1971
47. Malter IJ, Stanley RJ: The intrathoracic kidney: With a review of the literature. J Urol 107:538, 1972
48. Marshall FF, Freedman MT: Crossed renal ectopia. J Urol 119:188, 1978

Supernumerary Kidney

49. Kretschmer HL: Supernumerary kidney. Report of a case with review of the literature. Surg Gynecol Obstet 49:818, 1929
50. Lintz RM: Bilateral double kidney with duplication of ureters. Ann Intern Med 5:924, 1932
51. Carson WJ: Supernumerary kidney. Ann Surg 99:796, 1934
52. Geisinger JF: Supernumerary kidney. J Urol 38:331, 1937
53. Exley M, Hotchkiss WS: Supernumerary kidney with clear cell carcinoma. J Urol 51:569, 1944
54. Bacon SK: Large hydronephrosis of a true supernumerary kidney. J Urol 57:459, 1947
55. Carlson HE: Supernumerary kidney: A summary of fifty-one reported cases. J Urol 64:224, 1950
56. Burgess SB: Supernumerary kidney. Report of a case. Arch Pathol 69:154, 1960
57. Antony J: Complete duplication of female urethra with vaginal atresia and supernumerary kidney. J Urol 118:877, 1977
58. Tada Y, Kokado Y, Hashinaka Y et al: Free supernumerary kidney: A case report and review. J Urol 126:231, 1981
59. N'Guessan G, Stephens FD: Supernumerary kidney. J Urol 130:649, 1983

Horseshoe Kidney

60. Foley FEB: Surgical correction of horseshoe kidney. JAMA 115:1945, 1940
61. Palumbo LT: Horseshoe kidney: Report of a case with right hydronephrosis and ptosis. Urol Cutan Rev 54:395, 1950
62. Lowsley OS: Surgery of the horseshoe kidney. J Urol 67:565, 1952
63. Culp OS, Winterringer JR: Surgical treatment of horseshoe kidney: Comparison of results after various types of operations. J Urol 73:747, 1955

64. Glenn JF: Analysis of 51 patients with horseshoe kidney. N Engl J Med 261:684, 1959

65. Culp OS, Rusche CF, Johnson SH III et al: Hydronephrosis and hydroureter in infancy and childhood: A panel discussion. J Urol 88:443, 1962

66. Dajani AM: Horseshoe kidney: A review of twenty-nine cases. Br J Urol 38:388, 1966

67. Blackard CE, Mellinger GT: Cancer in a horseshoe kidney. A report of two cases. Arch Surg 97:616, 1968

68. Kolln CP, Boatman DL, Schmidt JD et al: Horseshoe kidney: A review of 105 patients. J Urol 107:203, 1972

69. Albert PS, D'Anna J: Papillary cystadenocarcinoma in horseshoe kidney. Urology 2:296, 1973

70. Buntley D: Malignancy associated with horseshoe kidney. Urology 8:146, 1976

71. Ney E, Friedenberg RM: Congenital Anomalies of the Kidney. In Ney E, Friedenberg RM (eds): Radiographic Atlas of the Genitourinary System, vol. I, 2nd ed, p 104. Philadelphia, JB Lippincott, 1981

72. Ware SM, Shulman Y: Transitional cell carcinoma of renal pelvis in horseshoe kidney. Urology 21:76, 1983

73. Weiner M, Sarma D, Rao M: Renal cell carcinoma in a horseshoe kidney. J Surg Oncol 26:77, 1984

Renal Dysplasia

74. Bernstein J: Developmental abnormalities of the renal parenchyma — Renal hypoplasia and dysplasia. Pathol Annu 3:213, 1968

75. Risdon RA: Renal dysplasia. Part I. A clinicopathologic study of 76 cases. J Clin Pathol 24:57, 1971

76. Potter EL. Type II cystic kidney. Early ampullary inhibition. In Potter EL (ed). Normal and Abnormal Development of the Kidney, p 154. Chicago, Year Book Medical Publishers, 1972

Cystic Disease of the Kidneys

77. Virchow R: Uber Hydnops renum cysticus congenitus. Arch Pathol Anat 46:506, 1869

78. Hildebrand: Weiterer Beitrag zur pathologischen Anatomie der Nierengeschroulste. Arch Klin Chir 48:343, 1894

79. Herxheimer G: Uber cystenbildungen der Niere und abfuhrenden Harnwege. Arch Pathol Anat 185:52, 1906

80. Staemmler M: Ein Betrag zur Lehre von der Cystenniere. Beitr Pathol Anat 68:22, 1921

81. Kampmeier OF: A hitherto unrecognized mode of origin of congenital renal cysts. Surg Gynecol Obstet 36:208, 1923

82. Norris RF, Herman L: The pathogenesis of polycystic kidneys: Reconstruction of cystic elements in four cases. J Urol 46:147, 1941

83. Lambert PP: Polycystic disease of the kidney. A review. Arch Pathol 44:34, 1947

84. Osathanondh V, Potter EL: Pathogenesis of polycystic kidneys. Historical survey. Arch Pathol 77:459, 1964

85. Osathanondh V, Potter EL: Pathogenesis of polycystic kidneys. Type 1 due to hyperplasia of interstitial portions of collecting tubules. Arch Pathol 77:466, 1964

86. Osanthanondh V, Potter EL: Pathogenesis of polycystic kidneys. Type 2 due to inhibition of ampullary activity. Arch Pathol 77:474, 1964

87. Osanthanondh V, Potter EL: Pathogenesis of polycystic kidneys. Type 3 due to multiple abnormalities of development. Arch Pathol 77:485, 1964

88. Osanthanondh V, Potter EL: Pathogenesis of polycystic kidneys. Type 4 due to urethral obstruction. Arch Pathol 77:502, 1964

89. Osanthanondh V, Potter EL: Pathogenesis of polycystic kidneys. Survey of results of microdissection. Arch Pathol 77:510, 1964

90. Kendall AR, Pollack HM, Karafin L: Congenital cystic disease of kidney. Urology 4:635, 1974

91. Kissane JM: Congenital malformations. In Heptinstall RH (ed): Pathology of the Kidney, 3rd ed, p 83. Boston, Little, Brown, 1983

92. Wakeley CPG: A case of unilateral polycystic kidney in a child, age one year and eight months. Br J Surg 18:162, 1931

93. Schwartz J: An unusual unilateral multicystic kidney in an infant. J Urol 35:259, 1936

94. Ravitch MM, Sanford MC: Unilateral multicystic kidney in infants. Pediatrics 4:769, 1949

95. Spence HM: Congenital unilateral multicystic kidney: An entity to be distinguished from polycystic kidney disease and other cystic disorders. J Urol 74:693, 1955

96. Gutter W, Hermanek P: Malignant tumor in the kidney region simulating a "lump-kidney" (renal cystic blastoma). Urol Int 4:164, 1957

97. Fine MG, Burns E: Unilateral multicystic kidney: Report of six cases and discussion of the literature. J Urol 81:42, 1959

98. Ashley DJB, Mostofi FK: Renal agenesis and dysgenesis J Urol 83:211, 1960

99. Vellios F, Garrett RA: Congenital unilateral multicystic disease of the kidney. Am J Clin Pathol 35:244, 1961

100. Staubitz WJ, Jewett TC Jr, Pletman RJ: Renal cystic disease in childhood. J Urol 90:8, 1963

101. Pathak IG, Williams DI: Multicystic and cystic dysplastic kidneys. Br J Urol 36:318, 1964

102. Griscom NT: The roentgenology of neonatal abdominal masses. Am J Roentgenol 93:447, 1965

103. Persky L, Izant R, Bolande R: Renal dysplasia. J Urol 98:431, 1967

104. Raffensperger J, Abousleiman A: Abdominal masses in children under one year of age. Surg 63:514, 1968

105. Schroder FH, Fiedler U, Goodwin WE: Die multizystische dysplasie der niere — ein kninisches syndrom. Z Urol Nephrol 63:631, 1970

106. Greene LF, Feinzaig W, Dahlin DC: Multicystic dysplasia of the kidney: With special reference to the contralateral kidney. J Urol 105:482, 1971

107. Kyaw MM, Newman H: Adult multicystic renal disease. Br J Radiol 44:881, 1971

108. Newman L, Simms K, Kissane J et al: Unilateral total renal dysplasia in children. Am J Roentgenol 116:778, 1972

109. Fisher C, Smith JF: Renal dysplasia in nephrectomy specimens from adolescents and adults. J Clin Pathol 28:879, 1975

110. Ambrose SS: Unilateral multicystic renal disease in adults. Birth Defects 13:349, 1977

111. De Klerk DP, Marshall FF, Jeffs RD: Multicystic dysplastic kidney. J Urol 118:306, 1977

112. Summer T, Friedland GW, Parker B et al: Preoperative diagnosis of unilateral multicystic kidney with hydropelvis. Urology 11:519, 1978

113. Bloom DA, Brosman S: The multicystic kidney. J Urol 120:211, 1978

114. Okayasu I, Kajita A: Histopathological study of congenital cystic kidneys with special reference to the multicystic, dysplastic type. Acta Pathol Jpn 28:427, 1978

115. Barrett DM, Wineland RE: Renal cell carcinoma in multicystic dyplastic kidney. Urology 15:152, 1980

116. Marsidi PJ, Lin WI, Pilloff B: Congenital multicystic dysplastic kidney in the adult. Urology 16:511, 1980

117. Ambrose SS, Gould RA, Trulock TS et al: Unilateral multicystic renal disease in adults. J Urol 128:366, 1982

Infantile Type

118. Dalgaard OZ: Bilateral polycystic disease of the kidneys. Acta Med Scand [suppl] 328:1, 1957
119. Hooper JW Jr: Cystic disease of the kidney in infants J Urol 79:917, 1958
120. Kerr DNS, Harrison CV, Sherlock S et al: Congenital hepatic fibrosis. Q J Med 30:91, 1961
121. McCarthy LJ, Baggenstoss AH, Logan GB: Congenital hepatic fibrosis. Gastroenterology 49:27, 1965
122. Heggo O, Natvig JB: Cystic disease of the kidneys. Acta Pathol Microbiol Immunol [A] Scand 64:459, 1965
123. Becker SM, Finkel J, Amboy P, et al: Polycystic kidney disease type 1. Involvement of three of four siblings with postmortem findings. Arch Pathol 88:265, 1969
124. Lieberman E, Salinas-Madrigal L, Gwinn JL et al: Infantile polycystic disease of the kidneys and liver: Clinical, pathological and radiological correlations and comparison with congenital hepatic fibrosis. Medicine 50:277, 1971
125. Blyth H, Ockenden BG: Polycystic disease of kidneys and liver presenting in childhood. J Med Genet 8:257, 1971
126. Murray-Lyon IM, Ockenden BG, Williams R: Congenital hepatic fibrosis — Is it a single clinical entity? (Editorial) Gastroenterology 64:653, 1973
127. Sommerschild HC, Langmark F, Maurseth K: Congenital hepatic fibrosis: Report of two new cases and review of the literature. Surgery 73:53, 1973
128. Bernstein J, Kissane JM: Hereditary disorders of the kidney. Perspect Pediatr Pathol 1:117, 1973

Adult Type

129. Walters W, Braasch WF: Surgical aspects of polycystic kidney. Surg Gynecol Obstet 58:649, 1934
130. Melicow MM, Gile HH: An hypernephroma in a polycystic kidney: Review of literature and report of a case. J Urol 43:767, 1940
131. Fergusson JD: Observations on familial polycystic disease of the kidney. Proc R Soc Med 42:806, 1949
132. Poutasse EF, Gardner WJ, McCormack LJ: Polycystic kidney disease and intracranial aneurysm. JAMA 154:741, 1954
133. Bricker NS, Patton JF: Cystic disease of the kidneys. A study of dynamics and chemical composition of cyst fluid. Am J Med 18:207, 1955
134. Mehrizi A, Rosenstein BJ, Pusch A et al: Myocardial infarction and endocardial fibroelastosis in children with polycystic disease. Bull Johns Hopkins Hosp 115:92, 1964
135. Gardner KD Jr: Composition of fluid in twelve cysts of a polycystic kidney. N Engl J Med 281:985, 1969
136. Howard RM, Young JD Jr: Two malignant tumors in a polycystic kidney. J Urol 102:162, 1969
137. Blyth H, Ockenden BG: Polycystic disease of kidneys and liver presenting in childhood. J Med Genet 8:257, 1971
138. Roberts PF: Bilateral renal carcinoma associated with polycystic kidneys. Br Med J 3:273, 1973
139. Posso M, Safadi D, Van Dyk OJ: Unilateral polycystic or multicystic kidney associated with focal musal renal cell carcinoma: Presentation of a case. J Urol 109:559, 1973

140. Ross DG, Travers H: Infantile presentation of adult-type polycystic kidney disease in a large kindred. J Pediatr 87:760, 1975

141. Tan TH, Donner R, Oe PL: Renal carcinoma associated with polycystic kidneys: Occurrence after chronic hematuria and hypertension. J Urol 118:322, 1977

142. Manes JL, Kissane JM, Valdes AJ: Congenital hepatic fibrosis, liver cell carcinoma and adult polycystic kidneys. Cancer 39:2619, 1977

143. Cuppage FE, Huseman RA, Grantham JJ: Ultrastructural and functional correlation of cysts from human polycystic kidneys. Kidney Int 12:511, 1977

144. Segal AJ, Spataro RF, Barbaric ZL: Adult polycystic kidney disease: A review of 100 cases. J Urol 118:711, 1977

145. Trebbin WM, Newhouse JH, Whitmore E et al: Polycystic kidneys without radiologic enlargement. Urology 11:96, 1978

146. Baert L: Hereditary polycystic kidney disease (adult form): A microdissection study of two cases at an early stage of the disease. Kidney Int 13:519, 1978

147. Barbour GL, Casali RE: Bilateral angiomyolipomas and renal cell carcinoma in polycystic kidney. Urology 12:694, 1978

148. Milutinovic J, Fialkow PJ, Rudd TG et al: Liver cysts in patients with autosomal dominant polycystic kidney disease. Am J Med 68:741, 1980

149. Milutinovic J, Agodoa LCY, Cutler RE et al: Autosomal dominant polycystic kidney disease. Early diagnosis and consideration of pathogenesis. Am J Clin Pathol 73:740, 1980

150. Ney C, Friedenberg RM: Radiographic Atlas of the Genitourinary System, vol I, 2nd ed, p 100. Philadelphia, JB Lippincott, 1981

151. Kossow AS, Meek JM: Unilateral adult polycystic kidney disease. J Urol 127:297, 1982

Medullary Cystic Disease and Juvenile Nephronophthisis

152. Smith CH, Graham JB: Congenital medullary cysts of the kidneys with severe refractory anemia. Am J Dis Child 69:369, 1945

153. Fanconi G, Hanhart E, Atbertini Av et al: Die familiare juvenile Nephronophthise. (Die idiopathische parenchymatose Schrumpfniere.) Helv Paediatr Acta 6:1, 1951

154. Strauss MB: Clinical and pathological aspects of cystic disease of the renal medulla. An analysis of eighteen cases. Ann Intern Med 57:373, 1962

155. Winberg J: Congenital cysts (letter). Am D Dis Child 108:566, 1964

156. Mangos JA, Opitz JM, Lobeck CC et al: Familial juvenile nephronophthisis. Pediatrics 34:337, 1964

157. Faigel HC: Congenital cysts of the renal medulla. A case with severe refractory anemia. Am J Dis Child 107:277, 1964

158. Herdman RC, Good RA, Vernier RL: Medullary cystic disease in two siblings. Am J Med 43:335, 1967

159. Strauss MB, Sommers SC: Medullary cystic disease and familial juvenile. N Engl J Med 277:863, 1967

160. Castleman B, McNeely BU: Case records of the Massachusetts General Hospital. Case 15-1970. Presentation of case. N Engl J Med 282:799, 1970

161. Gardner KD: Evolution of clinical signs in adult-onset cystic disease of the renal medulla. Ann Intern Med 74:47, 1971

162. Rayfield RJ, McDonald FD: Red and blonde hair in renal medullary cystic disease. Arch Intern Med 130:72, 1972

163. Betts PR, Forrest-Hay I: Juvenile nephronophthisis. Lancet 2:475, 1973

164. Boichis H, Passwell J, David R et al: Congenital hepatic fibrosis and nephronophthisis. A family study. Q J Med 165:221, 1973

165. Avasthi PS, Erickson DG, Gardner KD: Hereditary renal-retinal dysplasia and the

medullary cystic disease-nephronophthisis complex. Ann Intern Med 84:157, 1976

166. Delaney V, Mullaney J, Bourke E: Juvenile nephronophthisis, congenital hepatic fibrosis and retinal hypoplasia in twins. Q J Med 186:281, 1978

167. Witzleben CL, Sharp AR: Nephronophthisis — Congenital hepatic fibrosis. Hum Pathol 13:728, 1982

Medullary Sponge Kidney

168. Lenarduzzi: Reperto pielografico poco comune (dilatazione delle vie urinarie intrarenali) (Abstract). Radiol Med (Torino) 26:346, 1939

169. Cacchi R, Ricci V: Sur une rare maladie kystique multiple des pyramides renales le "rein en epone." J Urol (Paris) 55·497, 1949

170. Vermooten V: Congenital cystic dilatation of the renal collecting tubules. A new disease entity. Yale J Biol Med 23:450, 1951

171. Mulvaney WP, Collins WT: Cystic disease of the renal pyramids. J Urol 75:776, 1956

172. Abeshouse BS, Abeshouse GA: Sponge kidney: A review of the literature and a report of five cases. J Urol 84:252, 1960

173. Pennisi SA, Bunts RC: Sponge kidney. J Urol 84:246, 1960

174. Murphy WK, Palubinskas AJ, Smith DR: Sponge kidney: Report of seven cases. J Urol 85:866, 1961

175. Felts JH, Headley RN, Whitley JE et al: Medullary sponge kidneys. Clinical appraisal. JAMA 188:233, 1964

176. Logie NJ: Medullary sponge kidney. Br J Urol 36:482, 1964

177. Deck MDF: Medullary sponge kidney with renal tubular acidosis: A report of 3 cases. J Urol 94:330, 1965

178. Morris RC, Yamauchi H, Palubinskas AJ et al: Medullary sponge kidney. Am J Med 38:883, 1965

179. Pyrah LN: Medullary sponge kidney. J Urol 95:274, 1966

180. Levine AS, Michael AF Jr: Ehlers-Danlos syndrome with renal tubular acidosis and medullary sponge kidneys. J Pediatr 71:107, 1967

181. Popa M, Stanescu V: Renal tubular acidosis and hypergammaglobulinaemic purpura in a 10 year old girl with roentgenographic signs suggesting medullary sponge kidney. Case report. Acta Paediatr Scand 58:290, 1969

182. Harrison AR, Williams JP: Medullary sponge kidney and congenital hemihypertrophy. Br J Urol 43:552, 1971

183. Spence HM, Singleton R: What is sponge kidney disease and where does it fit in the spectrum of cystic disorders? J Urol 107:176, 1972

184. Levitt MH, McCoy RC, Fetter BF: Glomerulopathy in medullary sponge kidneys: Case presentation and review of the literature. J Urol 112:710, 1974

185. Waseda N, Ogawa H, Sano M et al: Medullary sponge kidney, renal tubular acidosis. A case of Sjögren's syndrome associated with renal tubular acidosis, medullary sponge kidney and multiple immunological abnormalities. J Jpn Soc Intern Med 64:552, 1975

186. Modarelli RO, Wettlaufer JN: Surgically documented segmental medullary sponge kidney: Case report. J Urol 117:244, 1977

187. Baert L: Microdissection findings of medullary sponge kidney. Urology 11:637, 1978

188. Kumagai I, Matsuo S, Kato T: A case of incomplete renal tubular acidosis (type 1) associated with medullary sponge kidney followed by nephrocalcinosis. J Urol 123:250, 1980

189. Maynard JF: Case profile: Nephrocalcinosis with ureterocalcinosis secondary to medullary sponge kidney Urology 15:310, 1980

Glomerulocystic Disease

190. Roos A: Polycystic kidney. Report of a case studied by reconstruction. Am J Dis Child 61:116, 1941
191. Baxter TJ: Cysts arising in the renal corpuscle. A microdissection study. Arch Dis Child 40:455, 1965
192. Taxy JB, Filmer RB: Glomerulocystic kidney. Report of a case. Arch Pathol Lab Med 100:186, 1976
193. Krous HF, Richie JP, Sellers B: Glomerulocystic kidney. A hypothesis of origin and pathogenesis. Arch Pathol Lab Med 101:462, 1977
194. Dosa S, Thompson AM, Abraham A: Glomerulocystic kidney disease. Report of an adult case. Am J Clin Pathol 82:619, 1984

Multilocular Cyst and Benign Multilocular Cystic Nephroma

195. Meland EL, Braasch WF: Multilocular cysts of the kidney. J Urol 29:505, 1933
196. Burrell NL: Multilocular cysts of the kidney: Report of a case. J Urol 43:656, 1940
197. Powell T, Shackman R, Johnson HD: Multilocular cysts of the kidney. Br J Urol 23:142, 1951
198. Frazier TH: Multilocular cysts of the kidney. J Urol 65:351, 1951
199. Boggs LK, Kimmelstiel P: Benign multilocular cystic nephroma: Report of two cases of so-called multilocular cyst of the kidney. J Urol 76:530, 1956
200. Attwood HD, Grieve J: Solitary multilocular cyst of the kidney. Br J Urol 30:78, 1958
201. Arey JB: Cystic lesions of the kidney in infants and children. J Pediatr 54:429, 1959
202. Uson AC, Rosario CD, Melicow MM: Wilms' tumor in association with cystic renal disease: Report of two cases. J Urol 83:262, 1960
203. Gibson TE: Multilocular cyst of the kidney: Case report. Trans Am Assoc Genitourinary Surg 53:53, 1961
204. Dainko EA, Dammers WR, Economou SG: Multilocular cysts of the kidney in children. J Pediatr 63:249, 1963
205. Uson AC, Melicow MM: Multilocular cysts of kidney with intrapelvic herniation of a "daughter" cyst: Report of 4 cases. J Urol 89:341, 1963
206. Christ ML: Polycystic nephroblastoma. J Urol 98:570, 1968
207. Kawamura J, Miyakawa M: Multilocular cyst of the kidney in a male infant: Report of a case. Acta Urol Jpn 15:759, 1969
208. Fowler M: Differentiated nephrobalstoma: Solid, cystic or mixed. J Pathol 105:215, 1971
209. Felman AH, Hawkins IF Jr, Hackett RL et al: Multilocular cyst of the kidney. A case report with angiographic findings. Radiology 106:629, 1973
210. Austin SR, Castellino RA: Multilocular cysts of kidney. Urology 1:546, 1973
211. Behr G, Duari M: Cystic nephroblastoma in an adult. Br J Urol 47:268, 1975
212. Brown JM: Cystic partially differentiated nephroblastoma. J Pathol 115:175, 1975
213. Datnow B, Daniel WW Jr: Polycystic nephroblastoma. JAMA 236:2528, 1976
214. Davides KC, King LM, Siconolfi E et al: Multilocular kidney disease: Unusual angiographic appearance. J Urol 116:246, 1976
215. Baldauf MC, Schulz DM: Multilocular cyst of the kidney. Report of three cases with review of the literature. Am J Clin Pathol 65:93, 1976
216. Gallo GE, Penchansky L: Cystic nephroma. Cancer 39:1322, 1977
217. Joshi VV, Banerjee AK, Yadav K et al: Cystic partially differentiated nephroblastoma. Cancer 40:789, 1977
218. Epstein L, Wacksman J, Daughtry J et al: Multilocular cysts of kidney: A diagnostic dilemma. Urology 11:573, 1978
219. Fobi M, Mahour GH, Isaacs H Jr: Multilocular cyst of the kidney. J Pediatr Surg 14:282, 1979

220. Geller RA, Pataki KI, Finegold RA: Bilateral multilocular renal cysts with recurrence. J Urol 121:808, 1979
221. Hunt JB, Rao RN, Vanderzalm T et al: Abdominal mass in young child. J Urol 121:482, 1979
222. Dias R, Fernandes M: Multilocular cystic disease of kidney. Urology 13:58, 1979
223. Keegan GT, Peterson RF, Studki WJ et al: Case report: Cystic partially differentiated nephroblastoma (Wilms' tumor). J Urol 121:362, 1979
224. Abt AB, Demers LM, Shochat SJ: Cystic nephroma: An ultrastructural and biochemical study. J Urol 122:539, 1979
225. Coleman M: Multilocular renal cyst. Case report, ultrastructure and review of the literature. Virchows Arch [A] 387:207, 1980
226. Gonzalez-Crussi F, Kidd JM, Hernandez RJ: Cystic nephroma: Morphologic spectrum and implications. Urology 20:88, 1982
227. Andrews MJ Jr, Askin FB, Fried FA et al: Cystic partially differentiated nephroblastoma and polycystic Wilms' tumor: A spectrum of related clinical and pathologic entities. J Urol 129:577, 1983

Simple Cysts

228. Hepler AB: Solitary cysts of the kidney. A report of seven cases and observations of the pathogenesis of these cysts. Surg Gynecol Obstet 50:668, 1930
229. Chalkley TS, Sutton LE Jr: Infected solitary cyst of the kidney in a child, with a review of the literature. J Urol 50:414, 1943
230. Braasch WF, Hendrick JA: Renal cysts, simple and otherwise. J Urol 51:1, 1944
231. Travers EH: Solitary cysts of the kidney: Report of a case in an infant. J Urol 71:253, 1954
232. Gibson TE: Interrelationship of renal cysts and tumors: Report of three cases. J Urol 71:241, 1954
233. Christeson WW: Simple renal cysts in the newborn: Report of two cases. J Urol 72:1137, 1954
234. Clarke BG, Hurwitz IS, Dubinsky AB et al: Solitary serous cysts of the kidney: Biochemical cytologic and histologic studies. J Urol 75:772, 1956
235. Limjoco UR, Strauch AE: Infected solitary cyst of the kidney: Report of a case and review of the literature. J Urol 96:625, 1966
236. Lang EK: Coexistence of cyst and tumor in the same kidney. Radiology 101:7, 1971
237. Varma KR, Tiamson E, Goldman SM et al: Papillary carcinoma in wall of simple renal cyst. Urology 3:762, 1974
238. Sufrin G, Etra W, Gaeta J et al: Hypernephroma arising in wall of simple renal cyst. Urology 6:507, 1975
239. Ambrose SS, Lewis EL, O'Brien DP III et al: Unsuspected renal tumors associated with renal cysts. J Urol 117:704, 1977
240. Anderson JD, Lieber M, Smith RB: Latent adenocarcinoma in renal cysts. J Urol 118:861, 1977
241. Nelson RP: Letter. J Urol 119:145, 1978
242. Patel NP, Pitts WR Jr, Ward JN: Solitary infected renal cyst. Report of 2 cases and review of literature. Urology 11:164, 1978

Acquired Cysts in Renal Dialysis Patients

243. Matas AJ, Kjellstrand CM, Simmons RL et al: Increased incidence of malignancy during chronic renal failure. Lancet 1:883, 1975
244. Dunnill MS, Millard PR, Oliver D: Acquired cystic disease of the kidneys: A hazard of long-term intermittent maintenance haemodialysis. J Clin Pathol 30:868, 1977
245. Editorial: Acquired cystic disease of the kidney. Lancet 2:1063, 1977

246. Elliott HL, MacDougall AI, Buchanan WM: Acquired cystic disease of kidney (letter). Lancet 2:1359, 1977

247. Hughson MD, Hennigar GR, McManus JFA: Atypical cysts, acquired renal cystic disease, and renal cell tumors in end stage dialysis kidneys. Lab Invest 42:475, 1980

248. Ishikawa I, Saito Y, Onouchi Z et al: Development of acquired cystic disease and adenocarcinoma of the kidney in glomerulonephritic chronic hemodialysis patients. Clin Nephrol 14:1, 1980

249. Chung-Park M, Ricanati E, Lankerani M et al: Acquired renal cysts and multiple renal cell and urothelial tumors. Am J Clin Pathol 79:238, 1983

Endometriosis

250. Marshall VF: The occurrence of endometrial tissue in the kidney. Case report and discussion. J Urol 50:652, 1943

251. Maslow LA, Learner A: Endometriosis of kidney. J Urol 64:564, 1950

252. Fruhling L, Blum E: Endometriose renale contribution a l'etude de l'origine metaplasique de l'endometriose. J Urol (Paris) 57:151, 1951

253. Fruhling L, Hurter E, Blum E: A propos d'une nouvelle observation d'endometriome renal par metaplasie du parenchyme renal. Gynecol Obst 51:271, 1952

254. Komaev MF, Vigorski UP: Renal endometriosis. Urol Nefrol (Mosk) 28:56, 1963

255. Miles HB, Falconer KW:Renal endometriosis associated with hematuria. J Urol 102:291, 1969

256. Hajdu SI, Koss LG: Endometriosis of the kidney. Am J Obstet Gynecol 106:314, 1970

257. Bazaz-Malik G, Saraf V, Rana BS: Endometrioma of the kidney: Case report. J Urol 123:422, 1980

Renal Tuberculosis

258. Medlar EM: Cases of renal infection in pulmonary tuberculosis. Evidence of healed tuberculous lesions. Am J Pathol 2:401, 1926

259. Kretschmer HL: Tuberculosis of the kidney. A critical review based on a series of two hundred twenty-one cases. N Engl J Med 202:660, 1930

260. Greenberger ME, Wershub LP, Auebabach O: The incidence of renal tuberculosis. JAMA 104:726, 1935

261. Jameson EM: Renal tuberculosis in patients with active pulmonary tuberculosis. Surg Gynecol Obstet 67:56, 1938

262. Baggenstoss AH, Greene LF: Healed tuberculosis of the kidney. J Urol 45:165, 1941

263. Steyn JH, Logie NJ: Coincident tuberculous perinephric abscess and carcinoma of the kidney. Br J Urol 38:7, 1966

264. Gow JG: Genitourinary tuberculosis: A study of short course regimens. J Urol 115:707, 1976

265. Wisnia LG, Kukolj S, De Santa Maria JL, Camuzzi F: Renal function damage in 131 cases of urogenital tuberculosis. Urology 11:457, 1978

266. Flechner SM, Gow JG: Role of nephrectomy in the treatment of non-functioning or very poorly functioning unilateral tuberculous kidney. J Urol 123:822, 1980

267. Narayana AS: Overview of renal tuberculosis. Urology 24:231, 1982

Pyelonephritis

268. Weiss S, Parker F Jr: Pyelonephritis: Its relation to vascular lesions and to arterial hypertension. Medicine 18:221, 1939

269. Keefer CS: Pyelonephritis—Its natural history and course. Bull Johns Hopkins Hosp 100:107, 1957

270. Vivaldi E, Cotran R, Zangwill DP et al: Ascending infection as a mechanism in pathogenesis of experimental non-obstructive pyelonephritis. Proc Soc Exp Biol Med 102:242, 1959

271. Rosenheim ML: Discussion on pyelonephritis. Proc R Soc Med 52:669, 1959

272. Neumann CG, Pryles CV: Pyelonephritis in infants and children. Am J Dis Child 104:215, 1962

273. Kunin CM, Deutscher R, Paquin A Jr: Urinary tract infection in school children: An epidemiologic, clinical and laboratory study. Medicine 43:91, 1964

274. Vosti KL, Goldberg LM, Monto AS et al: Host-parasite interaction in patients with infections due to Escherichia coli. I. The serogrouping of E. coli from intestinal and extraintestinal sources. J Clin Med 43:2377, 1964

275. Freedman LR: Chronic pyelonephritis at autopsy. Ann Intern Med 66:697, 1967

276. Carter MJ, Ehrenkranz J, Burns J et al: Serologic responses to heterologous Escherichia serogroups in women with pyelonephritis. N Engl J Med 279:1407, 1968

277. Angell ME, Relman AS, Robbins SL: "Active" chronic pyelonephritis without evidence of bacterial infection. N Engl J Med 278:1303, 1968

278. Aoki S, Imamura S, Aoki M et al: "Abacterial" and bacterial pyelonephritis. Immunofluorescent localization of bacterial antigen. N Engl J Med 281:1375, 1969

279. Rocha H, da Silva Teles E, de Oliveira MMG et al: Experimental pyelonephritis: Enhancement of infection after delivery of Escherichia coli into the arterial supply of the kidney. J Infect Dis 120:119, 1969

280. Heptinstall RH: The enigma of chronic pyelonephritis. J Infect Dis 120:104, 1969

281. Kunin CM: Epidemiology of bacteriuria and its relation to pyelonephritis. J Infect Dis 120:1, 1969

282. Zinner SH, Kass EH: Long-term (10 to 14 years) follow-up of bacteriuria of pregnancy. N Engl J Med 285:820, 1971

283. Schwartz MM, Cotran RS: Common enterobacterial antigen in human chronic pyelonephritis and interstitial nephritis. An immunofluorescent study. N Engl J Med 289:830, 1973

284. Bailey RR: The relationship of vesico-uroteric reflux to urinary tract infection and chronic pyelonephritis—reflux nephropathy. Clin Nephrol 1:132, 1973

285. Murray T, Goldberg M: Chronic interstitial nephritis: Etiologic factors. Ann Intern Med 82:453, 1975

286. Uldall P, Frokjaer O, Ibsen KK: Intrarenal reflux. Acta Paediatr Scand 65:711, 1976

287. Lindberg U, Claesson I, Hanson LA: Asymptomatic bacteriuria in schoolgirls. J Pediatr 92:194, 1978

288. Svanborg-Eden C, Jodal U: Attachment of Escherichia coli to urinary sediment epithelial cells from urinary tract infection-prone and healthy children. Infect Immun 26:837, 1979

289. Kallenius G, Mollby R, Hultberg H et al: Structure of carbohydrate part of receptor on human uroepithelial cells for pyelonephritogenic Escherichia coli. Lancet 2:604, 1981

290. Winberg J, Bollgren I, Kallenius G et al: Clinical pyelonephritis and focal renal scarring. A selected review of pathogenesis, prevention, and prognosis. Pediatr Clin North Am 29:801, 1982

291. Roberts JA: Pathogenesis of pyelonephritis. J Urol 129:1102, 1983

292. Heptinstall RH: Urinary tract infection, reflux and pyelonephritis. In Heptinstall RH (ed): Pathology of the Kidney, 3rd ed, p 1257. Boston, Little, Brown & Co., 1983

293. Heptinstall RH: Pyelonephritis: Pathologic features. In Heptinstall RH (ed): Pathology of the Kidney, 3rd ed, p 1323. Boston, Little, Brown & Co., 1983

Papillary Necrosis

294. Edmondson HA, Martin HE, Evans N: Necrosis of renal papillae and acute pyelonephritis in diabetes mellitus. Arch Intern Med 79:148, 1947

295. Zollinger HU, Spuhler O: Die nicht-eitrige, chronische interstitielle Nephritis. Schweiz Z Allg Pathol Bacteriol 13:807, 1950

296. Garrett RA, Norris MS, Vellios F: Renal papillary necrosis: A clinicopathologic study. J Urol 72:609, 1954

297. Heppleston AG: Renal papillary necrosis associated with necrotising angiitis and tubular necrosis. J Pathol Bacteriol 70:401, 1955

298. Lagergren C, Ljungqvist A: The intrarenal arterial pattern in renal papillary necrosis. A micro-angiographic and histologic study. Am J Pathol 41:633, 1962

299. Harrow BR, Sloane JA, Liebman NC: Roentgenologic demonstration of renal papillary necrosis in sickle-cell trait. N Engl J Med 268:969, 1963

300. Harvald B: Renal papillary necrosis. A clinical survey of sixty-six cases. Am J Med 35:481, 1963

301. Burry AF: The evolution of analgesic nephropathy. Nephron 5:185, 1967

302. Gault MH, Blennerhassett B, Muehrcke RC: Analgesic nephropathy. A clinicopathologic study using electron microscopy. Am J Med 51:740, 1971

303. Pandya KK, Koshy M, Brown N et al: Renal papillary necrosis in sickle cell hemoglobinopathies. J Urol 115:497, 1976

304. Murray TG, Goldberg M: Analgesic-associated nephropathy in the U.S.: Epidemiologic, clinical and pathogenetic features. Kidney Int 13:64, 1978

305. Tomashefski JF Jr, Abramowsky CR: Candida-associated renal papillary necrosis. Am J Clin Pathol 75:190, 1981

306. Ney C, Friedenberg RM: Radiographic Atlas of the Genitourinary System, vol I, 2nd ed, p 294. Philadelphia, JB Lippincott, 1981

307. Watanabe T, Nagafuchi Y, Yoshikawa Y et al: Renal papillary necrosis associated with Wegener's granulomatosis. Hum Pathol 14:551, 1983

Xanthogranulomatous Pyelonephritis

308. Schlagenhaufer F: Uber eigentumliche staphylomykosen der nieren und des pararenalen bindegewebes. Frankfurt Z Pathol 19:139, 1916

309. Putschar W: Die entzundlichen Erkrankungen der ableitenden Harnwege und der Nierenhullen einschliesslich der Pyelonephritis und der Pyonephroses. In Lubarsh O, Henke F (eds): Handluch der Speziellen Pathologischen Anatomie und Histologie, vol 6, p 333. Berlin, Julius Springer, 1934

310. Osterlind S: Uber pyelonephritis xanthomatosa. Acta Chir Scand 90:369, 1944

311. Barrie HJ: Foam-cell granuloma in chronic pyonephrosis simulating tuberculosis. Br J Surg 36:316, 1949

312. Mack FG, Mador ML: Pyogenic (foam cell) granuloma in a case of pyonephrosis. J Urol 67:258, 1952

313. Ghosh H: Chronic pyelonephritis with xanthogranulomatous change. Am J Clin Pathol 25:1043, 1955

314. Selzer DW, Dahlin DC, DeWeerd JH: Tumefactive xanthogranulomatous pyelonephritis. Surgery 42:874, 1957

315. Hooper RG, Kempson RL, Schlegel JU: Xanthogranulomatous pyelonephritis. J Urol 88:585, 1962

316. Saeed SM, Fine G: Xanthogranulomatous pyelonephritis. Am J Clin Pathol 39:616, 1963

317. Smout MS, McAninch FN, Wyatt JK: Tumefactive xanthogranulomatous pyelonephritis. Br J Urol 35:129, 1963

318. Avnet NL, Roberts TW, Goldberg HR: Tumefactive xanthogranulomatous pyelonephritis. Am J Roentgenol 90:89, 1963

319. Friedenberg MJ; Spjut HJ: Xanthogranulomatous pyelonephritis. Am J Roentgenol 90:97, 1963

320. McKenzie KR: Xanthogranulomatous pyelonephritis: Confusion with renal carcinoma. J Urol 92:261, 1964

321. Hatch CS, Cockett ATK: Xanthogranulomatous pyelonephritis. J Urol 92:585, 1964

322. Rios-Dalenz J, Peacock RC: Xanthogranulomatous pyelonephritis. Cancer 19:289, 1966

323. Ravel R: Megalocytic interstitial nephritis. An entity probably related to malakoplakia. Am J Clin Pathol 47:781, 1967

324. Rossi P, Myers DH, Furey R et al: Angiography in bilateral xanthogranulomatous pyelonephritis. Case report. Radiology 90:320, 1968

325. Noyes WE, Palubinskas AJ: Xanthogranulomatous pyelonephritis. J Urol 101:132, 1969

326. Ceccarelli FE Jr, Wurster JC, Chandor SB: Xanthogranulomatous pyelonephritis in an infant. J Urol 104:755, 1970

327. Anhalt MA, Cawood CD, Scott R Jr: Xanthogranulomatous pyelonephritis: A comprehensive review with report of 4 additional cases. J Urol 105:10, 1971

328. Butnick R: Xanthogranulomatous pyelonephritis: An unusual case. J Urol 106:815, 1971

329. Povysil C, Konickova L: Experimental xanthogranulomatous pyelonephritis. Invest Urol 9:313, 1972

330. Malek RS, Greene LF, DeWeerd JH et al: Xanthogranulomatous pyelonephritis. Br J Urol 44:296, 1972

331. Graivier L, Vargas MA: Xanthogranulomatous pyelonephritis in childhood. Am J Dis Child 123:156, 1972

332. Mering JH, Kaplan GW, McLaughlin AP: Xanthogranulomatous pyelonephritis. Unusual clinical presentations. Urology 1:338, 1973

333. Gammill S, Rabinowitz JG, Peace R et al: New thoughts concerning xanthogranulomatous pyelonephritis (X-P). Am J Radiol 125:154, 1975

334. Abbate AD, Meyers J: Xanthogranulomatous pyelonephritis in childhood. J Urol 116:231, 1976

335. Schulman CC, Denis R: Re: Xanthogranulomatous pyelonephritis in childhood by Abbate AD, and Myers J (J Urol 116:231, 1976). (Letter) J Urol 117:398, 1977

336. Bagley FH, Stewart AM, Jones PF: Diffuse xanthogranulomatous pyelonephritis in children: An unrecognized variant. J Urol 118:434, 1977

337. Klugo RC, Angerson JA, Reid R et al: Xanthogranulomatous pyelonephritis in children. J Urol 117:350, 1977

338. Malek RS, Elder JS: Xanthogranulomatous pyelonephritis: A critical analysis of 26 cases and of the literature. J Urol 119:589, 1978

339. Shapiro SR, Adelman RD, Link D et al: Renal mass in an infant. J Urol 120:485, 1978

340. Jander HP, Pujara S, Murad TM: Tumefactive megalocytic intersitital nephritis. Radiology 129:635, 1978

341. Goodman M, Curry T, Russell T: Xanthogranulomatous pyelonephritis (XGP): A local disease with systemic manifestations. Medicine 58:171, 1979

342. Moller JC, Kristensen IB: Xanthogranulomatous pyelonephritis. A clinico-pathological study with special reference to pathogenesis. Acta Pathol Microbiol Scand 88:89, 1980

343. Ballesteros JJ, Faus R, Gironella J: Preoperative diagnosis of renal xanthogranulomatosis by serial urinary cytology: Preliminary report. J Urol 124:9, 1980

344. Tolia BM, Iloreta A, Freed SZ et al: Xanthogranulomatous pyelonephritis: Detailed analysis of 29 cases and a brief discussion of atypical presentations. J Urol 126:437, 1981

345. Yazaki T, Ishikawa S, Ogawa Y et al: Xanthogranulomatous pyelonephritis in childhood: Case report and review of English and Japanese literature. J Urol 127:80, 1982

346. Danielli L, Zaidel L, Raviv U et al: Xanthogranulomatous pyelonephritis in an infant. J Urol 127:304, 1982

Malakoplakia

347. Michaelis L, Gutmann C: Ueber einschlusse in Blasentumoren. Ztschr F Klin Med (Berlin) 47:208, 1902

348. McDonald S, Sewell WT: Malakoplakia of the bladder and kidneys. J Pathol Bacteriol 18:306, 1913

349. Ferrari E, Nicolich G: Malacoplachia della vescica (Hansemann). Folia Urol (Leipzig) 8:644, 1914

350. Bennett WH: Malacoplakia of the urinary tract: Report of three cases. J Urol 70:84, 1953

351. Gibson TE, Bareta J, Lake GC: Malakoplakia. Report of a case involving the bladder and one kidney and ureter. Urol Int 1:5, 1955

352. Scott EVZ, Scott WF Jr: A fatal case of malakoplakia of the urinary tract. J Urol 79:52, 1958

353. Purpon I, Tamayo RP: Malacoplakia of the kidney. J Urol 84:231, 1960

354. Cederqvist LL: Malacoplakia of the urinary tract. A theory of pathogenesis. Arch Pathol 80:495, 1965

355. Smith BH: Malacoplakia of the urinary tract. A study of twenty-four cases. J Urol 43:409, 1965

356. Ravel R: Megalocytic interstitial nephritis. An entity probably related to malakoplakia. J Urol 47:781, 1967

357. Angell JC, Smith I: Renal malakoplakia with perinephric extension. Br J Urol 40:429, 1968

358. Lambird PA, Yardley JH: Urinary tract malakoplakia: Report of a fatal case with ultrastructural observations of Michaelis-Gutmann bodies. Johns Hopkins Med J 126:1, 1970

359. Miller OS, Finck FM: Malacoplakia of the kidney: The great impersonator. J Urol 103:712, 1970

360. Rao NR: Malacoplakia: Report of a case with observations on experimental production of the lesion. J Urol 105:611, 1971

361. Bowers JH, Cathey WJ: Malakoplakia of the kidney with renal failure. Am J Clin Pathol 55:765, 1971

362. Galian Ph, Boccon-Gibod L: Localisations renales et ureterales de la malakoplakie (Etude anatomo-clinique d'une observation). Ann Anat Pathol (Paris) 16:271, 1971

363. Gupta JK, Schuster RA, Christian WD: Autopsy findings in a unique case of malacoplakia. Arch Pathol 93:42, 1972

364. Scullin DR, Hardy R: Malacoplakia of the urinary tract with spread to the abdominal wall. J Urol 107:908, 1972

365. Aikat BK, Radhakrishnan VV, Rao MS: Malakoplakia — A report of two cases with review of the literature. Indian J Pathol Bacteriol 16:64, 1973

366. Csapó Z, Bartók I, Kahán IL et al: Malakoplakia of the kidney. A light microscopic, fine structural and chromatographic study. Beitr Pathol 148:407, 1973

367. Arvis G, Franc B, Lecharpentier Y et al: Malakoplakie renale d'aspect tumoral. J Urol Nephrol 80:192, 1974

368. Sunshine B: Malacoplakia of the upper urinary tract. J Urol 112:362, 1974

369. Michielsen JP, Gigase P: Malacoplasie du rein. Acta Urol Belg 42:336, 1974

370. Scheiner C, Dor A-M, Basbous D et al: La malacoplasie: Formes anatomo-cliniques. Revue de la litterature, a propos de 15 observations personnelles. Arch Anat Pathol 23:199, 1975

371. L'Hermite J, Colombel P, Guillemin P: Malacoplasie renale et vesicale d'aspect tumoral. J Urol Nephrol 81:213, 1975
372. Clarke AJ, Korbel EI, Maher PO: Malakoplakia of kidney and bladder with large bowel invasion. Br J Urol 47:376, 1975
373. Osborn DE, Castro JE, Ansell ID: Malakoplakia in a cadaver. Renal allograft: A case study. Hum Pathol 8:341, 1977
374. Trillo A, Lorentz WB, Whitley NO: Malakoplakia of kidney simulating renal neoplasm. Urology 10:472, 1977
375. Cavins JA, Goldstein AMB: Renal malacoplakia. Urology 10:155, 1977
376. Deridder PA, Koff SA, Gikas PW et al: Renal malacoplakia. J Urol 117:428, 1977
377. Lamb GHR, Ayers AB: Ultrasound findings in a case of renal malacoplakia. Br J Radiol 50:753, 1977
378. McClure J, Hadden DR, Mudd DG et al: Adrenocortical hyperactivity with disseminated malacoplakia. J Clin Pathol 30:206, 1977
379. Arnesen E, Halvorsen S, Skjorten F: Malacoplakia in a renal transplant. Report of a case studied by light and electron microscopy. Scand J Urol Nephrol 11:93, 1977
380. Trojani M, Lacaze J, Mascarel A et al: La malacoplasie: Pseudo-tumeur inflammatoire. Une observation de localisation renale. Bordeaux Med 10:1073, 1977
381. Galla JH, Bhathena D: Malacoplakia of the kidney: apparent improvement following medical management. Clin Nephrol 9:35, 1978
382. Mullan H, Hesse VE: Malacoplakia of a cadaveric renal allograft: A case report. J Surg Oncol 10:197, 1978
383. Raymond G, Toubol J, Pastorini P et al: La malacoplasie renale. A propos d'un case. J Urol Nephrol 84:254, 1978
384. Cadnapaphornchai P, Rosenberg BF, Taher S et al: Renal parenchymal malakoplakia. An unusual cause of renal failure. N Engl J Med 299:1110, 1978
385. Ho K-L, Rassekh ZS, Nam SH: Bilateral renal malakoplakia. Urology 13:321, 1979
386. Hartman DS, Davis CJ Jr, Lichtenstein JE et al: Renal parenchymal malacoplakia. Radiology 136:33, 1980
387. Charpin C, Andrac L, Monier MCF et al: Tumor-like malacoplakia of the kidney. Arch Pathol Lab Med 104:611, 1980
388. Griggs WP, Hemstreet GP III: Pathologic and immunologic considerations in malakoplakia. Urology 16:638, 1980
389. Hillion D, Felsenheld C, Bergue A et al: Bilateral renal malakoplakia: One case and a review of the literature. Kidney Int 17:702, 1980
390. Carney GM, Faure JJ, Price SK: Malakoplakia. A case report and review of the renal manifestations and immunopathology. S Afr Med J 60:824, 1981
391. Benjamin E, Fox H: Malakoplakia of the adrenal gland. J Clin Pathol 34:606, 1981
392. Moller J Chr, Gerdes U: Renal malakoplakia. Report of a case with giant Michaelis-Gutmann bodies. Virchows Arch [A] 392:241, 1981
393. Katske FA, Bloom DA, Lupu AN: Renal malakoplakia. Acute onset of renal failure due to bilateral upper tract involvement. Urology 17:88, 1981
394. Stanton MJ, Maxted W: Malacoplakia: A study of the literature and current concepts of pathogenesis, diagnosis and treatment. J Urol 125:139, 1981
395. Garrett IR, McClure J: Renal malakoplakia. Experimental production and evidence of a link with interstitial megalocytic nephritis. J Pathol 136:111, 1982
396. Moussu J, Gauthe, De Cussac JB et al: Malacoplakie a localisation bilaterale renale. A propos d'un cas. J Urol (Paris) 88:399, 1982

Nodular Renal Blastema and Nephroblastomatosis

397. Hou LT, Holman RL: Bilateral nephroblastomatosis in a premature infant. J Pathol Bacteriol 82:249, 1961
398. Vlachos J, Tsakraklides V: A case of renal dysplasia and its relation to "bilateral nephroblastomatosis". J Pathol Bacteriol 95:560, 1968

399. Bove KE, Koffler H, McAdams AJ: Nodular renal blastema. Definition and possible significance. Cancer 24:323, 1969

400. Liban E, Kozenitzky IL: Metanephric hamartomas and nephroblastomatosis in siblings. Cancer 25:885, 1970

401. Bennington JL, Beckwith JB: In Tumors of the Kidney, Renal Pelvis, and Ureter, Atlas of Tumor Pathology, 2nd Series, Fascicle 12, p 31. Washington, D.C., AFIP, 1975

402. Rous SN, Bailie MD, Kaufman DB et al: Nodular renal blastema, nephroblastomatosis, and Wilms' tumor. Different points on the same disease spectrum? Urology 8:599, 1976

403. Bove KE, McAdams AJ: The nephroblastomatosis complex and its relationship to Wilms' tumor: A clinicopathologic treatise. Perspect Pediatr Pathol 3:185, 1976

404. Stambolis Chr: Benign epithelial nephroblastoma. A contribution to its histogenesis. Virchows Arch [A] 376:267, 1977

405. De Chaderevian J-P, Fletcher BD, Chatten J et al: Massive infantile nephroblastomatosis. A clinical, radiological, and pathological analysis of four cases. Cancer 39:2294, 1977

406. Cromie WJ, Engelstein MS, Duckett JW Jr: Nodular renal blastema, renal dysplasia and duplicated collecting systems. J Urol 123:100, 1980

407. Pichler E, Jurgenssen A, Balzar E et al: Massive bilateral nephroblastomatosis in a 13-year-old girl. Eur J Pediatr 138:231, 1982

Wilms' Tumor (Nephroblastoma)

408. Collins VP: The treatment of Wilms's tumor. Cancer 11:89, 1958

409. Lattimer JK, Melicow MM, Uson AC: Nephroblastoma (Wilms' tumor). Prognosis more favorable in infants under one year of age. JAMA 171:2163, 1959

410. Platt BB, Linden G: Wilms' tumor—A comparison of 2 criteria for survival. Cancer 17:1573, 1964

411. Balsaver AM, Gibley CW Jr, Tessmer CF: Ultrasturctural studies in Wilms's tumor. Cancer 22:417, 1968

412. Ledlie EM, Mynors LS, Draper GJ et al: Natural history and treatment of Wilms's tumour: An analysis of 335 cases occurring in England and Wales 1962–6. Br Med J 4:195, 1970

413. Knudson AJ Jr, Strong LC: Mutation and cancer: A model for Wilms' tumor of the kidney. J Natl Can Inst 48:313, 1972

414. Jereb B, Sandstedt B: Structure and size versus prognosis in nephroblastoma. Cancer 31:1473, 1973

415. Perez CA, Kaiman HA, Keith J et al: Treatment of Wilms' tumor and factors affecting prognosis. Cancer 32:609, 1973

416. Ganguly A, Gribble J, Tune B et al: Renin-secreting Wilms' tumor with severe hypertension. Report of a case and brief review of renin-secreting tumors. Ann Intern Med 79:835, 1973

417. Aron BS: Wilms' tumor—A clinical study of eighty-one patients. Cancer 33:637, 1974

418. Kumar APM, Hustu O, Fleming ID et al: Capsular and vascular invasion: Important prognostic factors in Wilms' tumor. J Pediatr Surg 10:301, 1975

419. Bond JV: Prognosis and treatment of Wilms' tumor at Great Ormond Street Hospital for sick children—1960–1972. Cancer 36:1202, 1975

420. Lawler W, Marsden HB, Palmer MK: Wilms' tumor—Histologic variation and prognosis. Cancer 36:1122, 1975

421. Makinen J, Rapola J: Renal tumours in children. A histological evaluation. Acta Pathol Microbiol Scand [A] 83:237, 1975

422. D'Angio GJ, Evans AE, Brelow NE et al: The treatment of Wilms' tumor. Results of the National Wilms' Tumor Study. Cancer 38:633, 1976

423. Lemerle J, Tournade M-F, Gerard-Marchant R et al: Wilms' tumor: Natural history and prognostic factors. A retrospective study of 248 cases treated at the Institut Gustave-Roussy 1952–1967. Cancer 37:2557, 1976

424. Staff of the Royal Children's Hospital, Melbourne: Tumours of the kidney. In Jones PG, Campbell PE (eds): Tumours of Infancy and Childhood, p 495. Oxford, Blackwell Scientific Publications, 1976

425. Editorial: Wilms's tumour. Br Med J 15:1166, 1976.

426. Jenkin RDT: The treatment of Wilms' tumor. Pediatr Clin North Am 23:147, 1976

427. Ramsay NKC, Dehler LP, Coccia PF et al: Acute hemorrhage into Wilms' tumor. A cause of rapidly developing abdominal mass with hypertension, anemia, and fever. J Pediatr 91:763, 1977

428. Beckwith JB, Palmer NF: Histopathology and prognosis of Wilms tumor. Results from the first National Wilms' Tumor Study. Cancer 41:1937, 1978

429. Breslow NE, Palmer NF, Hill LR et al: Wilms' tumor: Prognostic factors for patients without metastases at diagnosis. Results of the National Wilms' Tumor Study. Cancer 41:1577, 1978

430. Kheir S, Pritchett PS, Moreno H et al: Histologic grading of Wilms' tumor as a potential prognostic factor: Results of a retrospective study of 26 patients. Cancer 41:1199, 1978

431. Leape LL, Breslow NE, Bishop HC: The surgical treatment of Wilms' tumor: Results of the National Wilms' Tumor Study. Ann Surg 187:351, 1978

432. Ehrlich RM, Bloomberg SD, Gyepes MT et al: Wilms' tumor, misdiagnosed preoperatively: A review of 19 National Wilms Tumor Study I cases. J Urol 122:790, 1979

433. Shah K, Wasan S, Lott S: Wilms' tumor in adolescence. J Urol 121:365, 1979

434. D'Angio GJ, Beckwith JB, Breslow NE et al: Wilms' tumor: An update. Cancer 45:1791, 1980

435. Jereb B, Tournade MF, Lemerle J et al: Lymph node invasion and prognosis in nephroblastoma. Cancer 45:1632, 1980

436. Gates GF, Miller JH, Stanley P: Necrosis of Wilms' tumors. J Urol 123:916, 1980

437. Ney C, Friedenberg RM: Tumors of the kidney. In Ney C, Friedenberg RM (eds): Radiographic Atlas of the Genitourinary System, vol I, 2nd ed, p 600. Philadelphia, JB Lippincott, 1981

438. Gonzalez-Crussi F, Hsueh W, Ugarte N: Rhabdomyogenesis in renal neoplasia of childhood. Am J Surg Pathol 5:525, 1981

439. Mahoney JP, Saffos RS: Fetal rhabdomyomatous nephroblastoma with a renal pelvic mass simulting sarcoma botryoides. Am J Surg Pathol 5:297, 1981

440. Grimes MM, Wolff M, Wolff JA et al: Ganglion cells in metastatic Wilms' tumor. Review of a histogenetic controversy. Am J Surg Pathol 6:565, 1982

441. Culp OS, Hartman FW: Mesoblastic nephroma in adults: A clinico-pathologic study of Wilms' tumors and related renal neoplasms. J Urol 60:552, 1948

442. Fruhling L, Blum E, Gal L: Les tumeurs du blasteme renal chez l'adulte a propos de 4 observations personnelles. J Urol (Paris) 60:192, 1954

443. Klapproth HJ: Wilms tumor: A report of 45 cases and an analysis of 1,351 cases reported in the world literature from 1940 to 1958. J Urol 81:633, 1959

444. Altug M, Carmichael FA, Henry CL et al: Wilms' tumor in an adult: Long-time survival with palliative resection of lung and brain metastases. J Urol 91:212, 1964

445. Robinson JJ, Jordan WP Jr: Some unusual adult male urogenital tumors with dysontogenetic features. Reports of mesonephroma, Mullerian carcinosarcoma, transitional cloacogenic carcinoma and nephroblastoma. J Urol 97:357, 1967

446. Olsen BS, Bischoff AJ: Wilms' tumor in an adult. Cancer 25:21, 1970

447. Francis D, Olsen NJ: Adult nephroblastoma. Scand J Urol Nephrol 11:305, 1977

448. Bard RH, Greenwald ES, Kalnicki S et al: Adult Wilms' tumor treated with radiotherapy and chemotherapy: A case report. J Urol 121:679, 1979

449. Toulouse J, Millon G, Bouddier B, et al: El nephroblastome de l'adulte. A propos d'un cas. J Urol (Paris) 88:395, 1982
450. Scott LS: Bilateral Wilms' tumour. Br J Surg 42:513, 1955
451. Abeshouse BS: The management of Wilms' tumor as determined by National Survey and review of the literature. J Urol 77:792, 1957
452. Snyder HE, Brockman SK, Grant BP et al: Bilateral Wilms' tumor. Am J Surg 110:492, 1965
453. Anderson EE, Harper JM, Small MP et al: Bilateral diffuse Wilms' tumor: A 5-year survival. J Urol 99:707, 1968
454. DeLorimier AA, Belzer RO, Kountz SL et al: Simultaneous bilateral nephrectomy and renal allotransplantation for bilateral Wilms' tumor. Surgery 64:850, 1968
455. Garrett RA, Battersby JS: Bilateral Wilms' tumor: 4-year survival. J Urol 106:942, 1971
456. Ragab AH, Vietti TJ, Crist W et al: Bilateral Wilms' tumor. A review. Cancer 30:983, 1972
457. Fay R, Brosman S, Williams DI: Bilateral nephroblastoma. J Urol 110:119, 1973
458. Ehrlich RM, Goldman R, Kaufman JJ: Surgery of bilateral Wilms' tumors: The role of renal transplantation. J Urol 111:277, 1974
459. David HS, Lavengood RW Jr: Bilateral Wilms' tumor. Treatment, management, and review of the literature. Urology 3:71, 1974
460. Bond JV: Bilateral Wilms' tumour. Age at diagnosis, associated congenital anomalies, and possible pattern of inheritance. Lancet 2:482, 1975
461. D'Angio GJ, Evans AE, Breslow NE et al: The treatment of Wilms' tumor. Results of the National Wilms' Tumor Study. Cancer 38:633, 1976
462. Garrett RA, Donohue JP: Bilateral Wilms' tumors. J Urol 120:586, 1978
463. Toudoire A, Neveux J-Y: Deux cas de nephroblastome de la loge renale chez l'adulte. J Urol (Paris) 66:448, 1960
464. Moyson Fr, Maurus-Desmarez R, Gompel Cl: Tumeur de Wilms mediastinale? Acta Chir Belg (suppl) 2:118, 1961
465. Bhajekar AB, Joseph M, Bhat HS: Unattached nephroblastoma. Br J Urol 36:187, 1964
466. Nicod J-L: Tumeur de Wilms dans l'ovaire. Bull Cancer (Paris) 52:173, 1965
467. Edelstein G, Webb RS Jr, Romsdahl MM et al: Extrarenal Wilms' tumor. Am J Surg 109:509, 1965
468. Malik TK, Malik GB, Diesh G: Retroperitoneal teratoma with nephroblastic tissue as the main component. Int Surg 47:246, 1967
469. Wu JP, Garcia J: Supernumerary kidney with Wilms' tumor. Wis Med J 70:211, 1971
470. Thompson MR, Emmanuel IG, Campbell MS et al: Extrarenal Wilms' tumors. J Pediatr Surg 8:37, 1973
471. Tebbi K, Ragab AH, Ternberg JL et al: An extrarenal Wilms' tumor arising from a sacrococcygeal teratoma. Clin Pediatr 13:1019, 1974
472. Ward SP, Dehner LP: Sacrococcygeal teratoma with nephroblastoma (Wilms' tumor): A variant of extragonadal teratoma in childhood. A histologic and ultrastructural study. Cancer 33:1355, 1974
473. Carney JA: Wilms' tumor and renal cell carcinoma in retroperitoneal teratoma. Cancer 35:1179, 1975
474. Akhtar M, Kott E, Brooks B: Extrarenal Wilms' tumor. Report of a case and review of the literature. Cancer 40:3087, 1977
475. Madanat F, Osborne B, Cangir A et al: Extrarenal Wilms tumor. J Pediatr 93:439, 1978
476. McCauley GK, Safaii H, Crowley CA et al: Extrarenal Wilms' tumor. Am J Dis Child 133:1174, 1979
477. Adam YG, Rosen A, Oland J et al: Extrarenal Wilms tumor. J Surg Oncol 22:56, 1983

478. Miller RW, Fraumeni JF Jr, Manning MD: Association of Wilms's tumor with aniridia, hemihypertrophy and other congenital malformations. N Engl J Med 270:922, 1964

479. Fraumeni JF Jr, Geiser CF, Manning MD: Wilms' tumor and congenital hemihypertrophy: Report of five new cases and review of literature. Pediatrics 40:886, 1967

480. Haichen BN, Miller DR: Simultaneous occurrence of congenital aniridia, hamartoma, and Wilms' tumor. J Pediatr 78:497, 1971

481. Perlman M, Levin M, Wittels B: Syndrome of fetal gigantism, renal hamartomas, and nephroblastomatosis with Wilms' tumor. Cancer 35:1212, 1975

482. Pendergrass TW: Congenital anomalies in children with Wilms' tumor. A new survey. Cancer 37:403, 1976

483. Stay EJ, Vawter G: The relationship between nephroblastoma and neurofibromatosis (von Recklinghausen's disease). Cancer 39:2550, 1977

484. Sheth KJ, Tang TT, Blaedel ME et al: Polydipsia, polyuria, and hypertension associated with renin-secreting Wilms' tumor. J Pediatr 92:921, 1978

485. Riccardi VM, Sujansky E, Smith AC et al: Chromosomal imbalance in the aniridia-Wilms' tumor association: 11p interstitial deletion. Pediatrics 61:604, 1978

486. Redman JF, Harper DL: Nephroblastoma occurring in a multilocular cystic kidney. J Urol 120:356, 1978

487. Dew H: Sarcomatous tumors of the testicle. Surg Gynecol Obstet 46:447, 1928

488. Rao PB: A metastatic Wilms' tumour in the nasopharynx. J Laryngol Otol 83:381, 1969

489. Movassaghi N, Leikin S, Chandra R: Wilms' tumor metastasis to uncommon sites. J Pediatr 84:416, 1974

Congenital Mesoblastic Nephroma

490. Kay S, Pratt CB, Salzberg AM: Hamartoma (leiomyomatous type) of the kidney. Cancer 19:1925, 1966

491. Bolande RP, Brough AJ, Izant RJ Jr: Congenital mesoblastic nephroma of infancy. Pediatrics 40:272, 1967

492. Favara BE, Johnson W, Ito J: Renal tumors in the neonatal period. Cancer 22:845, 1968

493. Wigger HJ: Fetal hamartoma of kidney. A benign, symptomatic, congenital tumor, not a form of Wilms' tumor. Am J Clin Pathol 51:323, 1969

494. Waisman J, Cooper PH: Renal neoplasms of the newborn. J Pediatr Surg 5:407, 1970

495. Walker D, Richard GA: Fetal hamartoma of the kidney: Recurrence and death of patient. J Urol 110:352, 1973

496. Bogdan R, Taylor DEM: Leiomyomatous hamartoma of the kidney. A clinical and pathologic analysis of 20 cases from the kidney tumor registry. Cancer 31:462, 1973

497. Fu Y-S, Kay S: Congenital mesoblastic nephroma and its recurrence. An ultrastructural observation. Arch Pathol 96:66, 1973

498. Block NL, Grabstald HG, Melamed MR: Congenital mesoblastic nephroma (leiomyomatous hamartoma): First adult case. J Urol 110:380, 1973

499. Wigger HJ: Fetal mesenchymal hamartoma of kidney. A tumor of secondary mesenchyme. Cancer 36:1002, 1975

500. Larson DM: Congenital mesoblastic nephroma. Am J Dis Child 132:318, 1978

501. Blank E, Neerhout RC, Burry KA: Congenital mesoblastic nephroma and polyhydramnios. JAMA 240:1504, 1978

502. Shen SC, Yunis EJ: A study of the cellularity and ultrastructure of congenital mesoblastic nephroma. Cancer 45:306, 1980

503. Gonzalez-Crussi F, Sotelo-Avila C, Kidd JM: Malignant mesenchymal nephroma

of infancy. Report of a case with pulmonary metastases. Am J Surg Pathol 4:185, 1980

504. Snyder HM III, Lack EE, Chetty-Baktavizian A et al: Congenital mesoblastic nephroma: Relationship to other renal tumors of infancy. J Urol 126:513, 1981

505. Ganick DJ, Gilbert EF, Beckwith JB et al: Congenital cystic mesoblastic nephroma. Hum Pathol 12:1039, 1981

506. Levin NP, Damjanov I, Depillis VJ: Mesoblastic nephroma in an adult patient. Recurrence 21 years after removal of the primary lesion. Cancer 49:573, 1982

Clear Cell Sarcoma

507. Marsden HB, Lawler W: Bone-metastasizing renal tumour of childhood. Br J Cancer 38:437, 1978

508. Marsden HB, Lawler W, Kumar PM: Bone metastasizing renal tumor of childhood. Morphological and clinical features, and differences from Wilms' tumor. Cancer 42:1922, 1978

509. Morgan E, Kidd JM: Undifferentiated sarcoma of the kidney. A tumor of childhood with histopathologic and clinical characteristics distinct from Wilms' tumor. Cancer 42:1916, 1978

510. Lawler W, Marsden HB: Bone metastases in children presenting with renal tumours. J Clin Pathol 32:608, 1979

511. Marsden HB, Lawler W: Bone metastasizing renal tumour of childhood. Histopathological and clinical review of 38 cases. Virchows Arch [A] 387:341, 1980

512. Novak RW, Caces JN, Johnson WW: Sarcomatous renal tumor of childhood. An electron microscopic study. Am J Clin Pathol 73:622, 1980

513. Gonzalez-Crussi F, Baum ES: Renal sarcomas of childhood. A clinicopathologic and ultrastructural study. Cancer 51:898, 1983

514. Beckwith JB: Wilms' tumor and other renal tumors of childhood: A selective review from the National Wilms' Tumor Study Pathology Center. Hum Pathol 14:481, 1983

515. Haas JE, Bonadio JF, Beckwith JB: Clear cell sarcoma of the kidney with emphasis on ultrastructural studies. Cancer 54:2978, 1984

Malignant Rhabdoid Tumor

516. Lemos LB, Hamoudi AB: Malignant thymic tumor in an infant (malignant histiocytoma). Arch Pathol Lab Med 102:84, 1978

517. Beckwith JB, Palmer NF: Histopathology and prognosis of Wilms' tumor. Results from the first National Wilms' Tumor Study. Cancer 41:1937, 1978

518. Haas JE, Palmer NF, Weinberg AG et al: Ultrastructure of malignant rhabdoid tumor of the kidney. A distinctive renal tumor of children. Hum Pathol 12:646, 1981

519. Schmidt D, Harms D, Zieger G: Malignant rhabdoid tumor of the kidney. Histopathology, ultrastructure and comments on differential diagnosis. Virchows Arch [A] 398:101, 1982

520. Gonzalez-Crussi F, Goldschmidt RA, Hsueh W et al: Infantile sarcoma with intracytoplasmic filamentous inclusions. Distinctive tumor of possible histiocytic origin. Cancer 49:2365, 1982

521. Rousseau-Merch M-F, Nogues C, Nezelof C et al: Infantile renal tumors associated with hypercalcemia. Arch Pathol Lab Med 107:311, 1983

522. Lynch HT, Shurin SB, Dahms BB et al: Paravertebral malignant rhabdoid tumor in infancy. In vitro studies of a familial tumor. Cancer 52:290, 1983

523. Beckwith JB: Wilms' tumor and other renal tumors of childhood: A selective review from the National Wilms' Tumor Study Pathology Center. Hum Pathol 14:481, 1983

524. Frierson HF Jr, Mills SE, Innes D Jr: Malignant rhabdoid tumor of the pelvis. Cancer 55:1963, 1985
525. Small EJ, Gordon GJ, Dahms BB: Malignant rhabdoid tumor of the heart in an infant. Cancer 55:2850, 1985

Oncocytoma

526. Jaffe RH: Adenolymphoma (onkocytoma) of parotid gland. Am J Cancer 16:1415, 1932
527. Zippel L: Zur Kenntnis der Onkocyten. Virchows Arch [A] 308:360, 1942
528. Hamperl H: Benign and malignant oncocytoma. Cancer 15:1019, 1962
529. Poroshin KK, Galil-Oglyi GA: Onccotsitarie Adenomi. Arkh Patol 27:43, 1965
530. Wasilkowski A, Dabrowski H: Gruczolak Kwasochlonny Nerki. Pol Przegl Chir 43:1051, 1971
531. Berger G, Clermont A, Pinet F et al: Oncocytome pluricentrique du rein etude microangiographique. Arch Anat Pathol 21:287, 1973
532. Blessing MH, Wienert G: Onkozytom der Niere (Klinische und pathologisch-anatomische Befunde). Zentralbl Allg Pathol 117:227, 1973
533. Sos TA, Gray GF Jr, Baltaxe HA: The angiographic appearance of benign renal oxyphilic adenoma. Am J Roentgenol 127:717, 1976
534. Klein MJ, Valensi QJ: Proximal tubular adenomas of kidney with so-called oncocytic features. A clinicopathologic study of 13 cases of a rarely reported neoplasm. Cancer 38:906, 1976
535. Milstoc M: Renal oncocytoma: A rare case of renal adenoma. J Urol 118:856, 1977
536. Weiner SN, Bernstein RG: Renal oncocytoma: Angiographic features of two cases. Radiology 125:633, 1977
537. Tessler AN, Kurusu S, Klein MJ et al: Proximal tubular adenoma of kidney. Urology 10:203, 1977
538. Sarkar K, Ejeckam GC, McCaughey WTE et al: Oncocytic tumors of the kidney (so called "renal oncocytomas"). Lab Invest 40:282, 1978
539. Ambos MA, Bosniak MA, Valensi QJ et al: Angiographic patterns in renal oncocytomas. Radiology 129:615, 1978
540. Pearse HD, Houghton DC: Renal oncocytoma. Urology 13:74, 1979
541. Akhtar M, Kott E: Oncocytoma of kidney. Urology 14:397, 1979
542. Landier JF, Desligneres S, Boccon-Gibod L et al: Les oncocytomes du rein. Ann Urol 13:9, 1979
543. Weedon D, Splatt AJ, Moore AWE: Proximal tubular adenoma of the kidney. Aust NZ J Surg 49:250, 1979
544. Chaudhry AP, Satchidanand SK, Gaeta JF et al: Light and ultrastructural studies of renal oncocytic adenoma. Urology 14:392, 1979
545. Johnson JR, Thurman AE, Metter JB et al: Oncocytoma of kidney. Urology 14:181, 1979
546. Ejeckam G, Tolnai G, Sarkar K et al: Renal oncocytoma. Study of eight cases. Urology 14:186, 1979
547. Morales A, Wasan S, Bryniak S: Renal oncocytomas: Clinical, radiological and histological features. J Urol 123:261, 1980
548. Yu GSM, Rendler S, Herskowitz A et al: Renal oncocytoma. Report of five cases and review of literature. Cancer 45:1010, 1980
549. Barth KH, Menon M: Renal oncocytoma. Further diagnostic observations. Diagn Imaging 49:259, 1980
550. Kendall AR, Pollack HM, Petersen RO et al: Incidentally found renal mass. J Urol 124:269, 1980
551. Morales A, Wasan S, Bryniak S: Renal oncocytomas: Clinical, radiological and histological features. J Urol 123:261, 1980

552. Rodriguez CA, Buskop A, Johnson J et al: Renal oncocytoma. Preoperative diagnosis by aspiration biopsy. Acta Cytol 24:355, 1980
553. Bono AV, Caresano A, Roggia A et al: A case of renal oncocytoma. Eur Urol 6:247, 1980
554. Bokinsky GB: Renal oncocytoma. Urology 17:364, 1981
555. Lieber MM, Tomera KM, Farrow GM: Renal oncocytoma. J Urol 125:481, 1981
556. Woodard BH, Tannenbaum SI, Mossler JA: Multicentric renal oncocytoma. J Urol 126:247, 1981
557. Lautin EM, Gordon PM, Friedman AC et al: Radionuclide imaging and computed tomography in renal oncocytoma. Radiology 138:185, 1981
558. Mitchell KM, Shilkin KB: Renal oncocytoma. Pathology 14:75, 1982
559. Moura ACF, Nascimento AG: Renal oncocytoma: Report of a case with unusual presentation. J Urol 127:311, 1982
560. Hara M, Yoshida K, Tomita M et al: A case of bilateral renal oncocytoma. J Urol 128:576, 1982
561. Merino MJ, Livolsi VA: Oncocytomas of the kidney. Cancer 50:1852, 1982
562. Warfel KA, Eble JN: Renal oncocytomatosis. J Urol 127:1179, 1982
563. Choi H, Almagro UA, McManus JT et al: Renal oncocytoma. A clinicopathologic study. Cancer 51:1887, 1983
564. Shah I, Parekh N, Nayak PK et al: Renal oncocytoma associated with diffuse lymphoma. Urology 22:314, 1983
565. Hunt HA, Tudball CF, Sutherland RC, et al: Bilateral renal oncocytomas: A case report. J Urol 129:1220, 1983
566. Barnes CA, Beckman EN: Renal oncocytoma and its congeners. Am J Clin Pathol 79:212, 1983
567. Wasserman NF, Ewing SL: Calcified renal oncocytoma. Am J Roentgenol 141:747, 1983
568. Levine E, Huntrakoon M: Computed tomography of renal oncocytoma. Roentgenology 141:741, 1983
569. Chen KTK: Multifocal renal oncocytoma. J Urol 130:546, 1983
570. Fairchild TN, Dail DH, Brannen GE: Renal oncocytoma—bilateral, multifocal. Urology 22:355, 1983
571. Eble JN, Hull MT: Morphologic features of renal oncocytoma: A light and electron microscopic study. Hum Pathol 15:1054, 1984
572. Maatman TJ, Novick AC, Tancinco BF et al: Renal oncocytoma: A diagnostic and therapeutic dilemma. J Urol 132:878, 1984
573. Zhang G, Monda L, Wasserman NF, Fraley EE: Bilateral renal oncocytoma: Report of 2 cases and literature review. J Urol 133:84, 1985.

Renal Cortical "Adenoma"

574. Judd ES, Simon HE: Benign adenoma of the kidney. Report of a case. Surg Gynecol Obstet 44:169, 1927
575. Kretschmer HL, Doehring C: Adenoma of the kidney. Surg Gynecol Obstet 48:629, 1929
576. Creevy CD: Adenoma of the kidney. Report of a case with a discussion of its relationship to carcinoma (hypernephroma). Am J Cancer 15:2309, 1931
577. Carver J: Renal adenoma. Br J Urol 7:229, 1935
578. Zangemeister W: Untersuchungen uber Alterverteilung, Haufigkeit und Morphologie der Nierenfibrome unter Mitberucksichtigung der ubrigen ausgereiften Tumoren. Beitr Pathol Anat 97:142, 1936
579. Newcomb WD: The search for truth, with special reference to the frequency of gastric ulcer-cancer and the origin of Grawitz tumors of the kidney. Proc Soc Med 30:113, 1936

580. Trinkle AJ: The origin and development of renal adenomas and their relation to carcinoma of the renal cortex (hypernephroma). Am J Cancer 27:676, 1936
581. Bailey OT, Harrison JH: Large benign renal neoplasms: Their pathology and clinical behavior, with report of five cases. J Urol 38:509, 1937
582. Bell ET: A classification of renal tumors with observations on the frequency of the various types. J Urol 39:238, 1938
583. Kozoll DD, Kirshbaum JD: Relationship of benign and malignant hypernephroid tumors of kidney. Clinical and pathological study of 77 cases in 12,885 necropsies. J Urol 44:435, 1940
584. Corwin WC: Multiple adenomas of the kidneys. Report of a case. J Urol 43:249, 1940
585. Hale NG, Burkland CE: Unrecognized renal tumors: A study of 54 cases, in 6,577 autopsies, and personal cases. J Urol 49:426, 1943
586. Apitz K: Die Geschwulste und Gewebsmissbildungen der Nierenrinde. III. Mitteilung Die Adenome. Virchows Arch [A] 311:328, 1944
587. Higgins CC: Adenoma of the kidney. Report of six cases. Am J Surg 65:3, 1944
588. Bell ET: Tumors of the kidneys. In Bell ET (ed): Renal Diseases, p 411. Philadelphia, Lea and Febiger, 1950
589. Cristol DS, Bothe AE, Grotzinger PJ: Renal adenoma: Survey of reported clinical cases and another case report. J Urol 64:58, 1950
590. Reese AJM, Winstanley DP: The small tumour-like lesions of the kidney. Br J Cancer 12:507, 1958
591. Largiader F: Morphologie, Histogenese und Klassification de Nierentumoren. Urol Int 6:273, 1958
592. Ellner HJ, Bergman H, Alfonso G: Two cases of solitary giant tubular adenoma of the kidney simulating carcinoma of the renal parenchyma. J Urol 84:706, 1960
593. Woods FM, Melvin PD, Coplan MM et al: Renal adenoma: Two cases requiring surgical intervention. J Urol 85:17, 1961
594. Shimshony Z, Merimsky E, Suprun H: Adenoma of the kidney. Br J Urol 35:256, 1963
595. Hajdu SI, Thomas AG: Renal cell carcinoma at autopsy. J Urol 97:978, 1967
596. Jasmin G, Cha JW: Renal adenomas induced in rats by dimethylnitrosamine. An electron microscopic study. Arch Pathol 87:267, 1969
597. Murphy GP, Mostofi FK: Histologic assessment and clinical prognosis of renal adenoma. J Urol 103:31, 1970
598. Xipell JM: The incidence of benign renal nodules (A clinicopathologic study). J Urol 106:503, 1971
599. Ghosh L, Dorfman HD: Papillary cystadenoma of the kidney—Report of a case exhibiting clinical symptomatology and a review of the literature. Mt Sinai J Med 39:170, 1972
600. Bennington J: Cancer of the kidney—Etiology, epidemiology, and pathology. Cancer 32:1017, 1973
601. Bennington JL, Beckwith JB: In Tumors of the Kidney, Renal Pelvis and Ureter, 2nd series, fascicle 12, p 94. Washington, DC, AFIP, 1975
602. Evins SC, Varner W: Renal adenoma—A misnomer. Urology 8:85, 1979
603. Cass AS: Large renal adenoma. J Urol 124:281, 1980
604. Pfannkuch F, Leistenschneider W, Nagel R: Problems of assessment in the surgery of renal adenomas. J Urol 125:95, 1981

Renal Cell Carcinoma

605. Hand JR, Broders AC: Carcinoma of the kidney: The degree of malignancy in relation to factors bearing on prognosis. J Urol 28:199, 1932
606. Priestley JT: Survival following removal of malignant renal neoplasm. JAMA 113:902, 1939

607. Griffiths IH, Thackray AC: Parenchymal carcinoma of the kidney. Br J Urol 21:128, 1949

608. Beare JB, McDonald JR: Involvement of the renal capsule in surgically removed hypernephroma: A gross and histopathologic study. J Urol 61:857, 1949

609. Flocks RH, Kadesky MC: Malignant neoplasms of the kidney: An analysis of 353 patients followed five years or more. J Urol 79:196, 1958

610. Chute R, Ireland EF Jr, Houghton JD: Solitary distant metastases from unsuspected renal carcinomas. J Urol 80:420, 1958

611. Greenberg BE, Young JM: Pulmonary metastasis from occult primary sites resembling bronchogenic carcinoma. Dis Chest 33:496, 1958

612. Petkovic SD: An anatomical classification of renal tumors in the adult as a basis for prognosis. J Urol 81:618, 1959

613. Claes G: Concerning the relationship between the morphology and the symptomatology of hypernephroma. Uro Int 15:265, 1963

614. Thackray AC: The pathology and spread of renal adenocarcinoma. In Riches E (ed): Tumors of Kidney and Ureter, p 72. Edinburgh, E & S Livingston, 1964

615. Riches E: The natural history of renal tumours. In Riches E (ed): Tumors of Kidney and Ureter, p 124. Edinburgh, E & S Livingston, 1964

616. Griffiths IH: Factors in prognosis of renal adenocarcinoma as indicated by published reports. In Riches E (ed): Tumors of Kidney and Ureter, p 347. Edinburgh, E & S Livingston, 1964

617. Arner O, Blanck C, von Schreeb T: Renal adenocarcinoma. Morphology — Grading of malignancy — Prognosis. A study of 197 cases. Acta Chir Scand [suppl] 346:11, 1965

618. Murphy GP, Mostofi FK: The significance of cytoplasmic granularity in the prognosis of renal cell carcinoma. J Urol 94:48, 1965

619. Ochsner MG: Renal cell carcinoma: Five year followup study of 70 cases. J Urol 93:361, 1965

620. Kaufman JJ, Mims MM: Tumors of the kidney. In Ravitch MM, Ellison EH, Julian DC et al (eds): Current Problems in Surgery, p 1. Chicago, Year Book Medical Publishers, 1966

621. Adolfsson G: Hypernephroma metastasis in the lung with no demonstrable primary tumor. J Urol 97:221, 1967

622. Myers GH Jr, Fehrenbaker LG, Kelalis PP: Prognostic significance of renal vein invasion by hypernephroma. J Urol 100:420, 1968

623. Kay S: Renal carcinoma. A 10-year study. Am J Clin Pathol 50:428, 1968

624. Silverberg SG, Evans RH, Koehler AL: Clinical and pathologic features of initial metastatic presentations of renal cell carcinoma. Cancer 23:1126, 1969

625. Robson CJ, Churchill BM, Anderson W: The results of radical nephrectomy for renal cell carcinoma. J Urol 101:297, 1969

626. Hulten L, Rosencrantz M, Seeman T et al: Occurrence and localization of lymph node metastases in renal carcinoma. Scand J Urol Nephrol 3:129, 1969

627. Wagle DG, Scal DR: Renal cell carcinoma — A review of 256 cases. J Surg Oncol 2, No. 1:23, 1970

628. Rafla S: Renal cell carcinoma. Natural history and results of treatment. Cancer 25:26, 1970

629. Cox CE, Lacy SS, Montgomery WG et al: Renal adenocarcinoma: 28-year review, with emphasis on rationale and feasibility of preoperative radiotherapy. J Urol 104:53, 1970

630. Bottiger LE: Prognosis in renal carcinoma. Cancer 26:780, 1970

631. Skinner DG, Colvin RB, Vermillion CD et al: Diagnosis and management of renal cell carcinoma. A clinical and pathologic study of 309 cases. Cancer 28:1165, 1971

632. Hansen JB, Thybo E: Long-term survival after nephrectomy for adenocarcinoma renis. Scand J Urol Nephrol 6:47, 1972

633. Kiely E, Greally M, Greally J: On the significance of lymphoid cell infiltration in hypernephromas. Ir J Med Sci 14:108, 1972

634. Lansigan NC Jr, Benisch BM, Sidoti JS: Renal carcinoma presenting as metastasis to uvula. Urology 2:449, 1973

635. Holland JM: Cancer of the kidney — Natural history and staging. Cancer 32:1030, 1973

636. Ochsner MG, Brannan W, Pond HS III, et al: Renal cell carcinoma: Review of 26 years of experience at the Ochsner Clinic. J Urol 110:643, 1973

637. Kirchner AK Jr, Braren V, Smith C et al: Renal carcinoma discovered incidentally by arteriography during evaluation for hypertension. J Urol 115:643, 1976

638. Van Veldhuizen D, Tiede JJ, Gilman LC: Hypernephroma A plea for earlier diagnosis. Minn Med 59:445, 1976

639. Mancilla-Jimenez R, Stanley RJ, Blath RA: Papillary renal cell carcinoma. A clinical, radiologic, and pathologic study of 34 cases. Cancer 38:2469, 1976

640. Katz SA, Davis JE: Renal adenocarcinoma. Prognostics and treatment reflected by survival. Urology 10:10, 1977

641. Novick AC, Daughtry JD, Stewart BH et al: Pulmonary embolus presenting as initial manifestation of renal cell carcinoma. Urology 12:707, 1978

642. Patel NP, Lavengood RW: Renal cell carcinoma: Natural history and results of treatment. J Urol 119:722, 1978

643. Dekernion JB, Ramming KP, Smith RB: The natural history of metastatic renal cell carcinoma: A computer analysis. J Urol 120:148, 1978

644. Bellinger MF, Koontz WW Jr, Smith MJV: Renal cell carcinoma: Twenty years of experience. Va Med 106:819, 1979

645. Oliver JA, Laplante MP, Reid EC et al: Results of radical nephrectomy in 178 cases of renal cell adenocarcinoma. Can J Surg 22:409, 1979

646. Rochman SC, Belis JZ, Kandzari SJ: Renal cell carcinoma. South Med J 72:11, 1979

647. Susan LP, Daughtry JD, Stewart BH et al: Palatal metastases in renal cell carcinoma. Urology 13:304, 1979

648. Mukamel E, Nissenkorn I, Avidor I et al: Spontaneous rupture of renal and ureteral tumors presenting as acute abdominal condition. J Urol 122:696, 1979

649. Boxer RJ, Waisman J, Lieber MM et al: Renal carcinoma: Computer analysis of 96 patients treated by nephrectomy. J Urol 122:598, 1979

650. Waters WB, Richie JP: Aggressive surgical approach to renal cell carcinoma: Review of 130 cases. J Urol 122:306, 1979

651. Talamo TS, Shonnard JW: Small renal adenocarcinoma with metastases. J Urol 124:132, 1980

652. Chica GA, Johnson DE, Ayala AG: Renal cell carcinoma presenting as breast carcinoma. Urology 15:389, 1980

653. Schoborg TW, Saffos RO, Urdaneta L et al: Xanthogranulomatous pyelonephritis associated with renal carcinoma. J Urol 124:125, 1980

654. McNichols DW, Segura JW, DeWeerd JH: Renal cell carcinoma: Long-term survival and late recurrence. J Urol 126:17, 1981

655. Fuhrman SA, Lasky LC, Limas C: Prognostic significance of morphologic parameters in renal cell carcinoma. Am J Surg Pathol 6:655, 1982

656. Marshall FF, Powell KC: Lymphadenectomy for renal cell carcinoma: Anatomical and therapeutic considerations. J Urol 128:677, 1982

657. Heney NM, Nocks BN: The influence of perinephric fat involvement on survival in patients with renal cell carcinoma extending into the inferior vena cava. J Urol 128:18, 1982

658. Lewis RH, Clark MA, Dobson CL et al: Multilocular cystic renal adenocarcinoma arising in a solitary kidney. J Urol 127:314, 1982
659. Carr BI: Renal carcinoma manifesting as breast mass. Urology 21:166, 1983
660. Fuselier HA Jr, Guice SL III, Brannan W et al: Renal cell carcinoma: The Ochsner Medical Institution experience (1945–1978). J Urol 130:445, 1983
661. Siminovitch JMP, Montie JE, Straffon RA: Prognostic indicators in renal adeno-carcinoma. J Urol 130:20, 1983
662. Selli C, Hishaw WM, Woodard BH et al: Stratification of risk factors in renal cell carcinoma. Cancer 52:899, 1983
663. Tomera KM, Farrow GM, Lieber MM: Well differentiated (Grade 1) clear cell renal carcinoma. J Urol 129:933, 1983
664. Singh EO, Benson RC Jr, Wold LE: Cancer-to-cancer metastasis. J Urol 132:340, 1984
665. Borovoy B, Rome P: Hypernephroma in a 10-year-old child. Am J Dis Child 105:85, 1963
666. Bennington JL, Laubscher FA: Epidemiologic studies on carcinoma of the kidney. I. Association of renal adenocarcinoma with smoking. Cancer 21:1069, 1968
667. Jasmin G, Cha JW: Renal adenomas induced in rats by dimethylnitrosamine. An electron microscopic study. Arch Pathol 87:267, 1969
668. Aron BS, Gross M: Renal adenocarcinoma in infancy and childhood: Evaluation of therapy and prognosis. J Urol 102:497, 1969
669. Palma LD, Kenny GM, Murphy GP: Childhood renal carcinoma. Cancer 26:1321, 1970
670. Steinberg SM, Brodovsky HS, Goepp CE: Renal carcinoma in mother and daughter. Cancer 29:222, 1972
671. Guirguis AB: Renal-cell carcinoma. Unusual occurrence in four members of one family. Urology 2:283, 1973
672. Ward JS, Middleton RG: Renal-cell carcinoma in children. Urology 2:50, 1973
673. Pratt-Thomas HR, Spicer SS, Upshur JK et al: Carcinoma of the kidney in a 15-year-old boy. Cancer 31:719, 1973
674. Castellanos RO, Aron BS, Evans AT: Renal adenocarcinoma in children: Incidence, therapy and prognosis. J Urol 111:534, 1974
675. Wynder EL, Mabuchi K, Whitmore WF Jr: Epidemiology of adenocarcinoma of the kidney. J Natl Can Inst 53:1619, 1974
676. Hamilton JM: Renal carcinogenesis. Adv Cancer Res 22:1, 1975
677. Kantor ALF, Meigs JW, Heston JF et al: Epidemiology of renal cell carcinoma in Connecticut, 1935–1973. J Natl Can Inst 57:495, 1976
678. Kantor AF: Current concepts in the epidemiology and etiology of primary renal cell carcinoma. J Urol 117:415, 1977
679. Cohen AJ, Li FP, Berg S et al: Hereditary renal-cell carcinoma associated with a chromosomal translocation. N Engl J Med 301:592, 1979
680. Abrams HJ, Buchbinder MI, Sutton AP: Renal carcinoma in adolescents. J Urol 121:92, 1979
681. Lieber MM, Tomera FM, Taylor WF et al: Renal adenocarcinoma in young adults: Survival and variables affecting prognosis. J Urol 125:164, 1981
682. Hartman DS, Davis CJ Jr, Madewell JE et al: Primary malignant renal tumors in the second decade of life: Wilms' tumor versus renal cell carcinoma. J Urol 127:888, 1982
683. Plimpton CH, Gellhorn A: Hypercalcemia in malignant disease without evidence of bone destruction. Am J Med 21:750, 1956
684. Stauffer MH: Nephrogenic hepatosplenomegaly. Gastroenterology 40:694, 1961
685. Gordon DA: The extrarenal manifestations of hypernephroma. Can Med Assoc J 88:61, 1963

686. Lemmon WT Jr, Holland PV, Holland JM: The hepatopaphy of hypernephroma. Am J Surg 110:487, 1965

687. Thomson WHF, Karat ABA: Hypercalcaemia associated with adenocarcinoma of kidney without demonstrable bone lesions. Br Med J 2:745, 1966

688. Walsh PN, Kissane JM: Nonmetastatic hypernephroma with reversible hepatic dysfunction. Arch Intern Med 122:214, 1968

689. Warren MM, Kelalis PP, Utz DC: The changing concept of hypernephroma. J Urol 104:376, 1970

690. Utz DC, Warren MM, Gregg JA et al: Reversible hepatic dysfunction associated with hypernephroma. Mayo Clin Proc 45:161, 1970

691. Chisholm GD, Roy RR: The systemic effects of malignant renal tumours. Br J Urol 43:687, 1971

692. Castleman B, Scully RE, McNeely BU: Case records of the Massachusetts General Hospital. Case 13-1972. Presentation of case. N Engl J Med 286:713, 1972

693. Warren MM, Utz DC, Kelalis PP: Concurrence of hypernephroma and hypercalcemia. Ann Surg 174:863, 1971

694. Ramos CV, Taylor HB: Hepatic dysfunction associated with renal carcinoma. Cancer 29:1287, 1972

695. Golde DW, Schambelan M, Weintraub BD et al: Gonadotropin-secreting renal carcinoma. Cancer 33:1048, 1974

696. Downing V, Levine S: Erythrocytosis and renal cell carcinoma with pulmonary metastases: Case report with 18-year followup and brief discussion of literature. Cancer 35:1701, 1975

697. Cronin RE, Kaehny WD, Miller PD et al: Renal cell carcinoma. Unusual systemic manifestations. Medicine 55:291, 1976

698. Gehring SH, Amin M, Eickenberg H U: Renal carcinoma-Experience at the University of Louisville Hospitals. J Ky Med Assoc 76:456, 1976

699. Scully FE, Galdabini JJ, McNeely BU: Case records of the Massachusetts General Hospital. Case 42-1980. Presentation of case. N Engl J Med 303:985, 1980

700. Pavelic K, Popovic M: Insulin and glucagon secretion by renal adenocarcinoma. Cancer 48:98, 1981

701. Goffman TE, Schechter GP, McKeen EA et al: Renal cell carcinoma causing a selective mineralocorticoid insufficiency. J Urol 128:370, 1982

702. Fan K, Smith DJ: Hypercalcemia associated with renal cell carcinoma: Probable role of neoplastic stromal cells. Hum Pathol 14:168, 1983

703. Vanatta PR, Silva FG, Taylor WE et al: Renal cell carcinoma and systemic amyloidosis: Demonstration of AA protein and review of the literature. Hum Pathol 14:195, 1983

704. Evans J: The accuracy of diagnostic radiology. Arteriography and nephrotomography. JAMA 204:223, 1968

705. Grumstedt B, Wahlqvist L: Prognostic significance of clinical, angiographic and histological findings in renal carcinoma. A study of 31 cases. Scand J Urol Nephrol 3:117, 1969

706. Lang EK: Arteriography in the diagnosis and staging of hypernephromas. Cancer 32:1043, 1973

707. McLaughlin AP III, Talner LB, Leopold GR et al: Avascular primary renal cell carcinoma: Varied pathologic and angiographic features. J Urol 111:587, 1974

708. Blath RA, Mancilla-Jimenez R, Stanley RJ: Clinical comparison between vascular and avascular renal cell carcinoma. J Urol 115:514, 1976

709. Krieger JN, Sniderman KW, Seligson GR et al: Calcified renal cell carcinoma: A clinical, radiographic and pathologic study. J Urol 121:575, 1979

710. Ney C, Friedenberg RM: Tumors of the kidney. In Ney C, Friedenberg RM (eds):

Radiographic Atlas of the Genitourinary System, vol I, 2nd ed, p 583. Philadelphia, JB Lippincott, 1981

711. Sengel FL, Bottone JJ, Murray GE: Bilateral hypernephroma: Case report. J Urol 57:106, 1947

712. Hanley HG: Discussion on partial nephrectomy. A collected review (abridged). Proc R Soc Med 43:1027, 1950

713. Bailey MK, Youngblood VH: Bilateral renal hypernephroma: Report of a case. J Urol 63:593, 1950

714. Borski AA, Kimbrough JC: Bilateral carcinoma in polycystic renal disease — A unique case. J Urol 71:677, 1954

715. Krumbach RW, Ansell JS: Partial resection of the right kidney and radical removal of the left kidney in a patient with bilateral hypernephroma. Surgery 45:585, 1959

716. Klotz PG: Hypernephroma in a solitary kidney treated by partial nephrectomy: A case report. J Urol 84:456, 1960

717. Meyer R, Dawson-Edwards P, Harrison JH: Surgery of the solitary kidney. J Urol 83:360, 1960

718. Bastable KRG: Bilateral carcinoma of the kidneys. Br J Urol 32:60, 1960

719. Kaplan C, Sayre GP, Greene LF: Bilateral nephrogenic carcinomas in Lindau-Von Hippel disease. J Urol 86:36, 1961

720. Fiorentini L, Sicari A: Su di un caso di neoplasia renale bilaterale. Urologie 30:440, 1963

721. Malament M: Bilateral renal cell carcinoma: A 14-year survival. J Urol 94:348, 1965

722. Small MP, Anderson EE, Atwill WH: Simultaneous bilateral renal cell carcinoma: Case report and review of the literature. J Urol 100:8, 1968

723. Grabstald H, Aviles E: Renal cell cancer in the solitary or sole-functioning kidney. Cancer 22:973, 1968

724. Steg A, Benassayag E, Draoui D et al: Cancer du rein bilateral nephrectomie elargie droite et nephrectomie partielle gauche en un temps. Ann Urol 3:211, 1969

725. Jochimsen PR, Braunstein PM, Najarian JS: Renal allotransplantation for bilateral renal tumors. JAMA 210:1721, 1969

726. Marchetti LJ, Gonick P, Ciavarra V: Partial nephrectomy in bilateral renal carcinoma: Discussion and case report. J Urol 106:818, 1971

727. Malek RS, Greene LF: Urologic aspects of Hippel-Lindau syndrome. J Urol 108:800, 1971

728. Kolln CP, Boldus RA, Brandon DNK et al: Bilateral partial nephrectomy for bilateral renal cell carcinoma: A case report. J Urol 105:45, 1971

729. Vermillion CD, Skinner DG, Pfister RC: Bilateral renal cell carcinoma. J Urol 108:219, 1972

730. Calne RY: Treatment of bilateral hypernephromas by nephrectomy, excision of tumour, and autotransplantation. Report of three cases. Lancet 2:1164, 1973

731. York WN, Mawn TJ: Aggressive surgical management of bilateral adenocarcinoma of the kidney. Cancer 31:1160, 1973

732. Hyman RA, Voges V, Finby N: Bilateral hypernephroma. Am J Roentgenol 117:104, 1973

733. Strout RF, Shearer JK, Traurig AR et al: Bilateral adenocarcinoma of the kidney treated by nephrectomy: A case report and review of the literature. J Urol 111:272, 1974

734. Lange D, Lange J: Cancer bilateral du rein. 7 observations. J Urol Nephrol 81:523, 1975

735. Morales JC, Pereira R, Napoles I: Tres carcinomas renales simultaneos en un mismo paciente. Rev Cub Cir 14:473, 1975

736. Wickham JEA: Conservative renal surgery for adenocarcinoma. The place of bench surgery. Br J Urol 47:25, 1975

737. Kuss R, Le Guillou M: Possibilites et limites de la chirurgie conservatrice dans le cancer du rein bilateral de l'adulte. Chirurgie ex vivo et hemodialyse. Ann Urol 10:217, 1976

738. Mullin EM, Whiter RD, Peterson LJ et al: Bilateral renal carcinoma in Von Hippel-Lindau disease. Urology 8:475, 1976

739. Beraha D, Block NL, Politano VA: Simultaneous surgical management of bilateral hypernephroma: An alernative therapy. J Urol 115:648, 1976

740. Finkbeiner A, Moyad R, Herwig K: Bilateral simultaneously occurring adenocarcinoma of the kidney. J Urol 116:26, 1976

741. Luciani L, Muraro GB, Pecori M et al: Il carcinoma de rene bilaterale simultaneo. Contributo casistico revisione della letteratura. Minerva Urol 29:289, 1977

742. Viets DH, Vaughan ED Jr, Howards SS: Experience gained from the management of 9 cases of bilateral renal cell carcinoma. J Urol 118:937, 1977

743. Novick AC, Stewart BH, Straffon RA et al: Partial nephrectomy in the treatment of renal adenocarcinoma. J Urol 118:932, 1977

744. Fetner CD, Barilla DE, Scott T et al: Bilateral renal cell carcinoma in Von Hippel-Lindau syndrome: Treatment with staged bilateral nephrectomy and hemodialysis. J Urol 117:534, 1977

745. Elkouss G, Gonick P: Extensive renal involvement by renal cell carcinoma. Urology 11:120, 1978

746. Johnson DE, Voneschenback A, Sternberg J: Bilateral renal cell carcinoma. J Urol 119:23, 1978

747. Palmer JM, Swanson DA: Conservative surgery in solitary and bilateral renal carcinoma: Indications and technical considerations. J Urol 120:113, 1978

748. Schiff M Jr, Bagley DH, Lytton B: Treatment of solitary and bilateral renal carcinomas. J Urol 121:581, 1979

749. Bokinsky GB, Goldman M: Multiple renal cell carcinoma in solitary kidney. Urology 15:391, 1980

750. Jacobs SC, Berg SI, Lawson RK: Synchronous bilateral renal cell carcinoma: Total surgical excision. Cancer 46:2341, 1980

751. Farrow GM, Harrison EG Jr, Utz DC: Sarcomas and sarcomatoid and mixed malignant tumors of the kidney in adults — Part III. Cancr 22:556, 1968

752. Fink H: Case #6. Metastatic renal cell carcinoma ('sarcoma-like' variant). Mo Med 69 (suppl 1):16, 1972

753. Piscioli F, Micoli G, Olivetti G: Differential morphologic criteria in sarcomatous-like renal carcinoma. Tumori 62:227, 1976

754. Matsuda M, Osafune M, Nakano E et al: Renal cell carcinoma having heterogeneous histological appearance and homogeneous enzymatic property. Cancer 45:528, 1980

755. Deitchman B, Sidhu GS: Ultrastructural study of a sarcomatoid variant of renal cell carcinoma. Cancer 46:1152, 1980

756. Tomera KM, Farrow GM, Lieber MM: Sarcomatoid renal carcinoma. J Urol 130:657, 1983

757. Robbins JK, Bonsib SM, Chiu LC et al: A large renal mass in a pregnant woman. J Urol 131:933, 1984

758. Oberling CH, Riviere M, Haguenau FR: Ultrastructure of the clear cell in renal carcinoma and its importance for the demonstration of their renal origin. Nature 186:402, 1960

759. Tannenbaum M: Ultrastructural pathology of human renal cell tumors. Pathol Annu 6:249, 1971

760. Fisher ER, Horvat B: Comparative ultrastructural study of so-called renal adenoma and carcinoma. J Urol 108:382, 1972

761. Clairmont P: Ueber ein Hypernephrom-Impfrecidiv in den Bronchiallynphdrusen. Arch Klin Chir 83:620, 1904

762. Graves RG, Mabrey RE: Adenocarcinoma of kidney recurrent after twenty years. N Engl J Med 212:416, 1935

763. Caylor HD, Caylor TE: Bizarre metastasis from a hypernephroma (report of a case). Urol Cutan Rev. 40:576, 1936

764. Starr A, Miller GM: Solitary jejunal metastasis twenty years after removal of a renal-cell carcinoma. N Engl J Med 246:250, 1952

765. Morton JJ Jr, Morton JH: Cancer as a chronic disease. Ann Surg 137:683, 1953

766. Badenoch AW: Adeno-carcinoma of the kidney (hypernephroma). Br J Clin Pract 12:601, 1958

767. Khilnani MT, Wolf BS: Late involvement of the alimentary tract by carcinoma of the kidney. Am J Dig Dis 5:529, 1960

768. Rosof BM, Rubin R: Metastasis from hypernephroma twenty years after nephrectomy. Report of a case. J Am Med Assoc 173:896, 1960

769. Eneroth C-M, Martonsson G, Thulin A: Profuse epistaxis in hypernephroma metastases. Acta Otolaryngol 53:546, 1961

770. Sklaroff DM, Moon CS: Delayed appearance of metastasis from hypernephroma of the kidney. Clin Med 69:1139, 1962

771. Tandon PL, Kumar M, Hafeez MA: Metastasis from renal-cell carcinoma twenty years after nephrectomy. A case report. Br J Urol 35:30, 1963

772. Kradjian RM, Bennington JL: Renal carcinoma recurrent 31 years after nephrectomy. Arch Surg 90:192, 1965

773. Takats LJ, Csapo Z: Death from renal carcinoma 37 years after its original recognition. Cancer 19:1172, 1966

774. Middleton RG: Surgery for metastatic renal cell carcinoma. J Urol 97:973, 1967

775. Willmore LJ Jr, Smith KR Jr: Intracerebral metastatic hypernephroma appearing 17 years postnephrectomy. Mo Med 66:883, 1969

776. Gerard FP, Sabety JS Jr: Latent lung metastasis of renal tumor. Ann Thorac Surg 7:27, 1969

777. Leiguarda R, Jost L, Turin M: Renal adenocarcinoma: Long survival (Letter). Ann Intern Med 78:311, 1973

778. Donaldson JC, Slease RB, DuFour R et al: Metastatic renal cell carcinoma 24 years after nephrectomy. JAMA 236:950, 1976

779. McNichold DW, Segura JW, DeWeerd JH: Renal cell carcinoma: Long-term survival and late recurrence. J Urol 126:17, 1981

780. Bloom DA, Kaufman JJ, Smith RB: Late recurrence of renal tubular carcinoma. J Urol 126:546, 1981

781. Bartley O, Hultquist GT: Spontaneous regression of hypernephromas. Acta Pathol Microbiol Scand 27:448, 1950

782. Hallahan JD: Spontaneous remission of metastatic renal cell adenocarcinoma: A case report. J Urol 81:522, 1959

783. Gartfield DH, Kennedy BJ: Regression of metastatic renal cell carcinoma following nephrectomy. Cancer 30:190, 1972

784. DeWeerd JH, Hawthorne J, Adson MA: Regression of renal cell hepatic metastasis following removal of primary lesions. J Urol 117:790, 1977

785. Fairlamb DJ: Spontaneous regression of metastases of renal cancer: A report of two cases including the first recorded regression following irradiation of a dominant metastasis and review of the world literature. Cancer 47:2102, 1981

786. Katz SE, Schapira HE: Spontaneous regression of genitourinary cancer—An update. J Urol 128:1, 1982

Metastatic Renal Cell Carcinoma

787. Scudder CL: The bone metastases of hypernephroma. A report from the Massachusetts General Hospital Clinic. Ann Surg 44:851, 1906

788. Beggs RC: Persistent priapism due to secondary carcinoma in the corpora cavervosa. Br Med J 2:10, 1928

789. Creevy CD: Confusing clinical manifestation of malignant renal neoplasms. Arch Intern Med 55:895, 1935

790. Maytum CK, Vinson PP: Pulmonary metastasis from hypernephroma, with ulceration into a bronchus simulating primary bronchial carcinoma. Report of a case. Arch Otolaryngol 23:101, 1936

791. Freid JR: Skeletal and pulmonary metastases from cancer of the kidney, prostate and bladder. Am J Roentgenol 55:153, 1946

792. Bandler CG, Roen PR: Solitary testicular metastasis simulating primary tumor and antedating clinical hypernephroma of the kidney: Report of a case. J Urol 55:663, 1946

793. Burrell NL: Priapism due to metastatic hypernephroma in corpora cavernosa penis. J Urol 60:636, 1948

794. McClanahan CW, Bonann LJ: Signal skeletal metastases from renal carcinoma. Am J Roentgenol 70:387, 1953

795. Castigliano SG, Rominger CJ: Metastatic malignancy of the jaws. Am J Surg 87:496, 1954

796. Burns JR, Edwards MH, Pessel JF et al: Epistaxis resulting from metastatic renal carcinoma. JAMA 161:226, 1956

797. Strauss FH, Scanlon EF: Five-year survival after hepatic lobectomy for metastatic hypernephroma. Arch Surg 72:328, 1956

798. Walter CW, Gillespie DR: Metastatic hypernephroma of fifty years' duration. An interesting report of a patient living fifty years with a hypernephroma and metastases. Minn Med 43:123, 1960

799. Eneroth C-M, Martensson G, Thulin A: Profuse epistaxis in hypernephroma metastases. Acta Otolaryngol 53:546, 1961

800. Sellstrom LG: Hypernephroma metastases in the ear and nose region. Acta Otolaryngol 55:545, 1962

801. Gerle R, Felson B: Metastatic endobronchial hypernephroma. Dis Chest 44:225, 1963

802. Connor DH, Taylor HB, Helwig EB: Cutaneous metastasis of renal cell carcinoma. Arch Pathol 76:339, 1963

803. Trinidad S, Lisa JR, Rosenblatt MB: Bronchogenic carcinoma simulated by metastatic tumors. Cancer 16:1521, 1963

804. Smith MJV, Bonacarti AF: Malignant priapism due to clear cell carcinoma: A case report and review of the literature. J Urol 92:297, 1964

805. Friedman I, Osborn DA: Metastatic tumours in the ear, nose and throat region. J Laryngol Otol 79:576, 1965

806. Bernstein JM, Balogh K Jr: Metastatic tumors to the maxilla, nose, and paranasal sinuses. Laryngoscope 76:621, 1966

807. Rosenblatt MB, Lisa JR, Trinidad S: Pitfalls in the clinical and histologic diagnosis of bronchogenic carcinoma. Dis Chest 49:396, 1966

808. Middleton RG: Surgery for metastatic renal cell carcinoma. J Urol 97:973, 1967

809. Hajdu SI, Thomas AG: Renal cell carcinoma at autopsy. J Urol 97:978, 1968

810. Weisman EB, Hardison JE, Burns JB: Priapism as the initial manifestation of renal carcinoma. Arch Intern Med 123:58, 1969

811. Hulten L, Rosencrantz M, Seeman T et al: Occurrence and localization of lymph node metastases in renal carcinoma. Scand J Urol Nephrol 3:129, 1969

812. Hajdu SI, Berg JW, Foote FW Jr: Clinically unrecognized, silent renal-cell carcinoma in elderly cancer patients. J Am Geriatr Soc 18:443, 1970

813. Arvis G, Aboulker P: Cancer metastatique du penis: a propos de 2 cas. J Urol Nephrol 76:92, 1970

814. Mulcahy JJ, Furlow WL: Vaginal metastasis from renal cell carcinoma: Radiographic evidence of possible route of spread. J Urol 104:50, 1970

815. Garfield DH, Kennedy BJ: Regression of metastatic renal cell carcinoma following nephrectomy. Cancer 30:190, 1972

816. Weigensberg IJ: Metastatic renal carcinoma: Unusual and deceptive presenting features. South Med J 65:611, 1972

817. Silverman EM, Oberman HA: Metastatic neoplasms in the breast. Surg Gynecol Obstet 138:26, 1974

818. Jackman SJ, Maher FT, Hattery RR: Detection of renal-cell carcinoma with 99m Tc polyphosphate imaging of bone. Mayo Clin Proc 49:297, 1974

819. Tallerman A, Kniestedt WF: Testicular tumor as the first manifestation of renal carcinoma. J Urol 111:584, 1974

820. Yamasaki M, Ueda G, Sato Y et al: A case of hypernephroma metastasis to the vagina. Acta Obstet Gynecol Jpn 22, No. 2:67, 1975

821. McCanse LRA, Moore JD, Markel L et al: Renal cell carcinoma presenting with nephrotic syndrome: A case report and review of the literature. J Urol 114:938, 1975

822. Johnson DE, Kaesler KE, Samuels ML: Is nephrectomy justified in patients with metastatic renal carcinoma? J Urol 114:27, 1975

823. Katz SA, Davis JE: Hypernephroma presenting as solitary metastasis to penis. Urology 7:206, 1976

824. Redman JF, Roman-Lopez JJ: Renal cell carcinoma and vaginal metastasis. Urology 10:148, 1977

825. Knight EL Jr, Kandzari SJ, Milam DF: Renal cell carcinoma presenting as vaginal bleeding. Urology 10:249, 1977

826. Narayana AS, Kelly DG, Duff FA: Malignant priapism. Br J Urol 49:326, 1977

827. Kagan AR, Steckel RJ: Metastatic carcinoma presenting as shoulder arthritis. Am J Roentgenol 129:137, 1977

828. Lang EK: Renal cell carcinoma presenting with metastases to pulmonary hilar nodes. J Urol 118:543, 1977

829. Montie JE, Stewart BH, Straffon RA et al: The role of adjunctive nephrectomy in patients with metastatic renal cell carcinoma. J Urol 117:272, 1977

830. DeWeerd JH, Hawthorne NJ, Adson MA: Regression of renal cell hepatic metastasis following removal of primary lesions. J Urol 117:790, 1977

831. Katzenstein A-L, Purvis R Jr, Gmelich J, Askin F: Pulmonary resection for metastatic renal adenocarcinoma. Pathologic findings and therapeutic value. Cancer 41:712, 1978

832. Dekernion JB, Ramming KP, Smith RB: The natural history of metastatic renal cell carcinoma. A computer analysis. J Urol 120:148, 1978

833. O'Dea MJ, Zincke H, Utz DC et al: The treatment of renal cell carcinoma with solitary metastasis. J Urol 120:540, 1978

834. Waters WB, Richie JP: Aggressive surgical approach to renal cell carcinoma: Review of 130 cases. J Urol 122:306, 1979

835. Sogani PC, Whitmore WF Jr: Solitary vaginal metastasis from unsuspected renal cell carcinoma. J Urol 121:95, 1979

836. Cihak RW, Haas R Jr, Koenen CT et al: Metastatic renal carcinoma to the prostate gland: Presentation as prostatic hypertrophy. J Urol 123:791, 1980

837. Nocks BN, Sacknoff EJ: Vaginal metastasis of renal carcinoma without renal vein involvement. Br J Urol 52:327, 1980

838. Talamo TS, Shonnard JW: Small renal adenocarcinoma with metastases. J Urol 124:132, 1980

839. Fairlamb DJ: Spontaneous regression of metastases of renal cancer: A report of two cases including the first recorded regression following irradiation of a dominant metastasis and review of the world literature. Cancer 47:2102, 1981

840. Saitoh H: Distant metastasis of renal adenocarcinoma. Cancer 48:1487, 1981

841. Taxy JB: Renal adenocarcinoma presenting as a solitary metastasis: Contribution of electron microscopy to diagnosis. Cancer 48:2056, 1981

842. Previte SR, Wiilscher MK, Burke CR: Renal cell carcinoma with solitary contralateral adrenal metastasis: Experience with 2 cases. J Urol 128:132, 1982

843. Neal PM, Leach GE, Kaswick JA et al: Renal cell carcinoma: Recognition and treatment of synchronous solitary contralateral adrenal metastasis. J Urol 128:135, 1982

844. Saitoh H, Nakayama M, Nakamura K et al: Distant metastasis of renal adenocarcinoma in nephrectomized cases. J Urol 127:1092, 1982

845. Saitoh H, Shiramizu T, Hida M: Age changes in metastatic patterns in renal adenocarcinoma. Cancer 50:1646, 1982

846. Ordonez NG, Ayala AG, Bracken RB: Renal cell carcinoma metastatic to penis. Urology 19:417, 1982

847. Ritch PS, Hansen RM, Collier BD: Metastatic renal cell carcinoma presenting as shoulder arthritis. Cancer 51:968, 1983

848. Appelqvist P: The role and value of surgery in metastatic renal adenocarcinoma: A retrospective clinical study of 106 nephrectomized cases. J Surg Oncol 26:138, 1984

849. Alexios G, Papadopoulou-Alexiou M, Karakousis CP: Renal cell carcinoma presenting as skeletal muscle mass. J Surg Oncol 27:23, 1984

850. Sarma DP, Woods AL III, Rodriguez FH Jr et al: Priapism as the presenting feature of renal cell carcinoma. J Surg Oncol 28:103, 1985

851. Hajdu SI, Thomas AG: Renal cell carcinoma at autopsy. J Urol 97:978, 1967

852. Kobayashi A, Hoshino H, Ohbe Y et al: Bilateral renal cell carcinoma. Arch Dis Child 45:141, 1970

853. Hajdu SI, Berg JW, Foote FW Jr: Clinically unrecognized, silent renal-cell carcinoma in elderly cancer patients. J Am Geriatr Soc 18:443, 1970

854. Saitoh H: Distant metastasis of renal adenocarcinoma. Cancer 48:1487, 1981

855. Saitoh H, Shiramizu T, Hida M: Age changes in metastatic patterns in renal adenocarcinoma. Cancer 50:1646, 1982

856. Saitoh H, Nakayama M, Nakamura K et al: Distant metastasis of renal adenocarcinoma in nephrectomized cases. J Urol 127:1092, 1982

Carcinoid

857. Gleeson MH, Bloom SR, Polak JM et al: Endocrine tumour in kidney affecting small bowel structure, motility, and absorptive function. Gut 12:773, 1971

858. Bloom SR: An enteroglucagon tumour. Gut 13:520, 1972

859. Toker C: Carcinoidal renal tumor. J Urol 111:10, 1974

860. Kojiro M, Ohishi H, Isobe H: Carcinoid tumor occurring in cystic teratoma of the kidney. A case report. Cancer 38:1636, 1976

861. Lanson Y, Bruant D, Benatre A et al: Tumeur carcinoide du rein. A propos d'un cas. J Urol (Paris) 84:47, 1978

862. Stahl RE, Sidhu GS: Primary carcinoid of the kidney. Light and electron microscopic study. Cancer 44:1345, 1979

863. Ghazi MR, Brown JS, Warner RS: Carcinoid tumor of kidney. Urology 14:610, 1979

864. Zak FG, Jindrak K, Capozzi F: Carcinoidal tumor of the kidney. Ultrastruct Pathol 4:51, 1983

865. McDonald EC, Mukai K, Burke BA et al: Primary carcinoid tumor of the kidney: A light and electron microscopic, and immunohistochemical study. J Urol 130:333, 1983

Small-Cell Undifferentiated Carcinoma (Oat Cell Carcinoma)

866. Capella C, Eusebi V, Rosai J: Primary oat cell carcinoma of the kidney. Am J Surg Pathol 8:855, 1984

Pheochromocytoma

867. Pengelly CDR: Phaeochromocytoma within the renal capsule. Br Med J 2:477, 1959

868. Preger L, Gardner RE, Kawala BO et al: Intrarenal pheochromocytoma. Preoperative angiographic diagnosis. Urology 8:194, 1976
869. Simon H, Carlson DH, Hanelin J et al: Intrarenal pheochromocytoma: Report of a case. J Urol 121:805, 1979

Renomedullary Interstitial Cell Tumor

870. Zangemeister W: VI. Untersuchungen uber Altersverteilung, Haufigkeit und Morphologie der Nierenfibrome unter Mitberucksichtigung der ubrigen ausgereiften Tumoren. Beitr Z Pathol Anat 97:142, 1936
871. Immergut S, Cottler ZR: Intrapelvic fibroma. J Urol 66:673, 1951
872. Schucksmith HS: Fibroma of the renal pelvis. Br J Urol 35:261, 1963
873. Bernier L, Bedard A, Narcisse R: Fibrome du Bassinet. Can J Surg 13:315, 1970
874. Cassimally KAI: Fibroma filling the renal pelvis: Report of a case. Can J Surg 14:350, 1971
875. Lerman RJ, Pitcock JA, Stephenson P et al: Renomedullary interstitial cell tumor (formerly fibroma of renal medulla). Hum Pathol 3:559, 1972
876. Muirhead EE, Brooks B, Pitcock JA et al: Renomedullary antihypertensive function in accelerated (malignant) hypertension. J Clin Invest 51:181, 1972
877. Lennox KW, Clark RE: Renal medullary fibroma: Report of a case presenting as a submucosal pelvic tumor. J Urol 113:288, 1975
878. Martin MR, Tiltman AJ: Incidence of renomedullary interstitial cell tumours and correlation with hypertension. S Afr Med J 50:2099, 1976
879. Stuart R, Salyer WR, Salyer DC et al: Renomedullary interstitital cell lesions and hypertension. Hum Pathol 7:327, 1976
880. Polga JP: Renal medullary fibroma presenting as a calcified mass with neovascularity. J Urol 116:105, 1976
881. Wolgel CD, Parris AC, Mitty HA et al: Fibroepithelial polyp of renal pelvis. Urology 19:436, 1982
882. Glover SD, Buck AC: Renal medullary fibroma: A case report. J Urol 127:758, 1982

Renal Capsule Neoplasms (Capsulomas)

883. Colvin SH Jr: Certain capsular and subcapsular mixed tumors of the kidney herein called "capsuloma." J Urol 48:585, 1942.
884. Foster DG: Large benign renal tumors: A review of the literature and report of a case in childhood. J Urol 76:231, 1956
885. Bennington JL, Beckwith JB: In Tumors of the Kidney, Renal Pelvis and Ureter, Atlas of Tumor Pathology, 2nd series, Fascicle 12, p 201. Washington, DC, AFIP, 1975
886. Fishbone G, Davidson AJ: Leiomyoma of the renal capsule. Radiology 92:1006, 1969
887. Osamura RY, Watanabe K, Yoneyama K et al: Malignant fibrous histiocytoma of the renal capsule. Virchows Arch [A] 380:327, 1978
888. Myerson D, Rosenfield AT, Itzchak Y: Renal capsular tumors: The angiographic features. J Urol 121:238, 1979

Angiomyolipoma

889. Critchley M, Earl CJC: Tuberose sclerosis and allied conditions. Brain 55:311, 1932
890. Moolten SE: Hamartial nature of the tuberous sclerosis complex and its bearing on the tumor problem. Report of a case with tumor anomaly of the kidney and adenoma sebaceum. Arch Intern Med 69:589, 1942
891. Morgan GS, Straumfjord JV, Hall EJ: Angiomyolipoma of the kidney. J Urol 65:525, 1951

892. Kerr JA: Gastric and renal leiomyosarcoma. Br J Surg 41:478, 1954

893. Tweeddale DN, Dawe CJ, McDonald JR et al: Angiolipoleiomyoma of the kidney. Report of a case with observations on histogenesis. Cancer 8:764, 1955

894. Lucke B, Schumberger HG: Tumors of the kidney, renal pelvis and ureter. In Atlas of Tumor Pathology, section VIII, Fascicle 30, p 21. Washington, DC, AFIP, 1957

895. Klapproth HJ, Poutasse EF, Hazard JB: Renal angiomyolipomas. Report of four cases. Arch Pathol 67:400, 1959

896. Perou ML, Gray PT: Mesenchymal hamartomas of the kidney. J Urol 83:240, 1960

897. Hartveit F, Halleraker B: A report of three angiolipomyomata and one angiolipomyosarcoma. Acta Pathol Microbiol Scand 49:329, 1960

898. Price EB Jr, Mostofi FK: Symptomatic angiomyolipoma of the kidney. Cancer 18:761, 1965

899. Vasko JS, Brockman SK, Bomar RL: Renal angiomyolipoma: A rare cause of spontaneous massive retroperitoneal hemorrhage. Ann Surg 161:577, 1965

900. Perkoff GT: The hereditary renal diseases. N Engl J Med 277:79, 1967

901. Farrow GM, Harrison EG Jr, Utz DC et al: Renal angiomyolipoma. A clinicopathologic study of 32 cases. Cancer 22:564, 1968

902. Hajdu SI, Foote FW Jr: Angiomyolipoma of the kidney: Report of 27 cases and review of the literature. J Urol 102:396, 1969

903. McCullough DL, Scott R Jr, Seybold HM: Renal angiomyolipoma (hamartoma): Review of the literature and report of 7 cases. J Urol 105:32, 1971

904. McCullough DL: Renal hamartoma. Current concepts of diagnosis and surgical management. Urology 4:235, 1974

905. Chonko AM, Weiss SM, Stein JH et al: Renal involvement in tuberous sclerosis. Am J Med 56:124, 1974

906. Bissada NK, White HJ, Sun CN et al: Tuberous sclerosis complex and renal angiomyolipoma. Collective review. Urology 6:105, 1975

907. Chalvardjian A, Kovacs K, Horvath E: Renal angiomyolipoma: Ultrastructural study. Urology 12:717, 1978

908. Eason AA, Cattolica EV, McGrath TW: Massive renal angiomyolipoma: Preoperative infarction by balloon catheter. J Urol 121:360, 1979

909. Shawker TH, Horvath KL, Dunnick NR et al: Renal angiomyolipoma: Diagnosis by combined ultrasound and computerized tomography. J Urol 121:675, 1979

910. Vetrani A, Palombini L, Vecchione R et al: L'angiomiolipoma relane. Pathologica 73:473, 1981

911. Vetrani A, Palombini L, Vecchione R et al: L'angiomiolipoma renale. Pathologica 73:473, 1981

912. Bloom DA, Scardino PT, Ehrlich RM et al: The significance of lymph nodal involvement in renal angiomyolipoma. J Urol 128:1292, 1982

913. Hulbert JC, Graf R: Involvement of the spleen by renal angiomyolipoma: Metastasis or multicentricity? J Urol 130:328, 1983

Hemangioma

914. Judd ES, Simon HE: Angioma of the kidney. Surg Gynecol Obstet 46:711, 1928

915. White EW, Braunstein LE: Cavernous hemangioma: A renal vascular tumor requiring nephrectomy: An unusual entity. J Urol 56:183, 1946

916. Lazarus JA, Marks MS: Renal hemangioma. Urol Cutan Rev 51:500, 1947

917. McCrea LE: Hemangioma of the kidney: Review of the literature. Urol Cutan Rev 55:670, 1951

918. Waller JI, Throckmorton MA, Barbosa E: Renal hemangioma. J Urol 74:186, 1955

919. Edward HG, DeWeerd JH, Woolner LB: Renal hemangiomas. Mayo Clin Proc 37:545, 1962
920. Hagen A: Renal angioma. Four cases of angioma of the renal pelvis. Acta Chir Scand 126:657, 1963
921. Peterson NE, Thompson HT: Renal hemangioma. J Urol 105:27, 1971
922. Summers JL, Keitzer WA: A radiographic clue to the diagnosis of hemangioma of the kidney. J Urol 108:852, 1972
923. Cubillo E, Hesker AE, Stanley RJ: Cavernous hemangioma of the kidney: An angiographic-pathologic correlation. J Can Assoc Radiol 24:254, 1973
924. Gordon R, Rosenmann E, Barzilay B et al: Correlation of selective angiography and pathology in cavernous hemangioma of the kidney. J Urol 115:608, 1976
925. Summers JL: Hemangioma in the wall of a cyst. J Urol 118:529, 1977
926. Ducassou J, Richard C, Duvinage JF: Angiome renal. 3 observations. J Urol Nephrol 83:460, 1977
927. Ferrer-Roda J, Sanjuan C, Vilar J et al: Hemangioma of the kidney. Eur Urol 9:189, 1983
928. Glintsov AG, Gurevich MN, Baitsova VV: Kravatechenya iz gemangiomi pochki, cimylirovavshee "ostriy zhivot." Klin Khir 5:27, 1983

Lymphangioma

929. Joost J, Schafer R, Altwein JE: Renal lymphangioma. J Urol 117:22, 1977
930. Singer DRJ, Miller JDB, Smith G: Lymphangioma of kidney. Scott Med J 28:293, 1983

Leiomyoma

931. Gordon MP Jr, Kimmelstiel P, Cabell CL: Leiomyoma of the kidney. Report of a case with review of the literature. J Urol 42:507, 1939
932. Crabtree EG: Leiomyoma of the kidney associated with hemorrhagic cyst. J Urol 52:480, 1944
933. Zuckerman IC, Kershner D, Laytner BD et al: Leiomyoma of the kidney. Ann Surg 126:220, 1947
934. Clinton-Thomas CL: A giant leiomyoma of the kidney. Br J Surg 43:497, 1956
935. McCune WR, Galleher EP, Wood C: Leiomyoma of the kidney in a newborn infant. J Urol 91:646, 1964
936. Palmer FJ, Tynan AP: Leiomyoma of the kidney. J Urol 112:22, 1974
937. Fisher KS, van Blerk PJP: Childhood leiomyoma of kidney. Urology 21:74, 1983

Lipoma

938. Robertson TD, Hand JR: Primary intrarenal lipoma of surgical significance. J Urol 46:458, 1941
939. Pfeiffer GE, Gandin MM: Massive perirenal lipoma with report of a case. J Urol 56:12, 1946
940. Beadles RO Jr, Urich RW: Intrarenal lipoma: Report of a case. J Urol 67:460, 1952

Sarcoma

941. Gupta OP, Dube MK: Rare primary renal sarcoma. Br J Urol 43:546, 1971
942. Gonzalez-Crussi F, Baum ES: Renal sarcomas of childhood. A clinicopathologic and ultrastructural study. Cancer 51:898, 1983
943. Srinivas V, Sogani PC, Hajdu SI et al: Sarcomas of the kidney. J Urol 132:13, 1984

Leiomyosarcoma

944. Tetelman MM, Lisa JR: Leiomyosarcoma of the kidney: Report of 2 cases. J Urol 54:225, 1945

945. Bagolan P: Su un caso raro di leiomiosarcoma bilaterale dei reni. Tumori 24:75, 1950

946. Blum E, Fruhling L: Deux observations anatomocliniques de sarcomes leiomyoblastiques du rein. J Urol Nefrol 57:46, 1951

947. Petkovic S: Myomatous tumors of the kidney. Urol Cutan Rev 55:730, 1951

948. Bhende YM: Plain muscle tumors of the kidney. Indian J Med Sci 6:747, 1952

949. Hava O, Herout V, Macik I: Pozdni metastasa sarkomu hilu ledvinneho do plic 16 let po odstraneni ledviny. Rozhl Chir 36:297, 1957

950. Dedola G, Rabitti V: Il leiomioma maligno (leiomiosarcoma) del rene (contributo casistico e rivista sintetica). Arch Ital Chir 85:496, 1959

951. Gupta JC, Nagrath C, Bhagwat AG: A leiomyosarcoma of kidney. Case report and brief review of literature. Indian J Pathol Bacteriol 6:66, 1963

952. Bazaz-Malik G, Gupta DN: Leiomyosarcoma of kidney: Report of a case and review of the literature. J Urol 95:754, 1966

953. Peach B: Smooth muscle tumours of the kidney (report on two cases). Br J Urol 38:382, 1966

954. Distasi AL: Il leiomioma maligno (leiomiosarcoma) del rene (rivista sintetica e contributo casistico). Rassegna Internazionale di Clinica e Terapia 47:175, 1967

955. Becker H, Gasteyer KH: Leiomyosarkom der Niere. Med Welt 16:1013, 1967

956. Hegemann G, Schmitz W: Nierentumoren bei tuberoser Hirnsklerose. Urol Int 22:406, 1967

957. Farrow GM, Harrison EG Jr, Utz DC et al: Sarcomas and sarcomatoid and mixed malignant tumors of the kidney in adults — Part I. Cancer 22:545, 1968

958. Islam MU, Talibi MA, Boyd PF et al: Leiomyosarcoma of kidney. JAMA 212:2266, 1970

959. Jenkins JD, Anderson CK, Williams RE: Renal sarcoma. Br J Urol 43:263, 1971

960. Ziter FMH Jr, Wieche DR, McAndrews JF: Renal leiomyosarcoma: A case report with angiographic findings. J Urol 105:776, 1971

961. Loomis RC: Primary leiomyosarcoma of the kidney: Report of a case and review of the literature. J Urol 107:557, 1972

962. Helmbrecht LJ, Cosgrove MD: Triple therapy for leiomyosarcoma of kidney. J Urol 112:581, 1974

963. Niceta P, Lavengood RW Jr, Fernandes M et al: Leiomyosarcoma of kidney. Review of the literature. Urology 3:270, 1974

964. Radhakrishanan J, Alrenga DP, Ghosh BC: Isolated hepatic metastasis from renal vein leiomyosarcoma. Arch Pathol Lab Med 102:606, 1978

965. Srinivas V, Sogani PC, Hajdu SI et al: Sarcomas of the kidney. J Urol 132:13, 1984

Liposarcoma

966. Williams JP, Savage PT: Liposarcoma of kidney. Br J Surg 46:225, 1958

967. McDermott EN, Kennedy JD: Liposarcoma of the kidney. Br J Urol 32:282, 1960

968. Maquinay CH, Muller P: Un cas de liposarcome du rein. Acta Urol Belg 33:525, 1965

969. Schmiedt E, Thurmayer R, Hruby E: Uber die sogenannten Liposarkome der Niere. Müncher Medizinische Wochenschrift 109:1433, 1967

970. Farrow GM, Harrison EG Jr, Utz DC et al: Sarcomas and sarcomatoid and mixed malignant tumors of the kidney in adults — Part I. Cancer 22:545, 1968

971. Rios JT: Renal liposarcoma with hypertension. Urology 1:246, 1973

972. Lien WM: Liposarcoma of the kidney. Postgrad Med J 49:660, 1973

973. Bennington JL, Beckwith JB: In Tumours of the Kidney, Renal Pelvis, and Ureter, Atlas of Tumor Pathology, 2nd series, Fascicle 12, p 217. Washington, DC, AFIP, 1975

974. Cano JY, D'Altorio RA: Renal liposarcoma: Case report J Urol 115:747, 1976

Fibrosarcoma

975. Mintz ER: Sarcoma of the kidney in adults. Ann Surg 105:521, 1937
976. Weisel W, Dockerty MB, Priestley JT: Sarcoma of the kidney. J Urol 50:564, 1943
977. Armstrong CP: Fibrosarcoma of the kidney. A case report. JSC Med Assoc 46:155, 1950
978. Moore TD: Unusual renal tumors. J Urol 66:533, 1951
979. Ruff TE: Fibrosarcoma of the adult kidney: Case report. J Urol 69:474, 1953
980. McNally A, Drinker H Jr: Spindle cell sarcoma of the kidney with associated eosinophilia. Q J Northwestern Univ Med School 33:12, 1959
981. Bignardi P: Il sarcoma fusocellulare del rene. Arch Ital Urol 33:149, 1960
982. Naib ZM, Young JD Jr, Philippidjis PJ: Exfoliative cytology of a primary fibrosarcoma of the kidney. J Urol 90:386, 1963
983. Gupta OP, Dube MK: Rare primary renal sarcoma. Br J Urol 43:546, 1971
984. Busuttil A, More IAR: Two malignant soft tissue tumors of the kidney: An ultrastructural appraisal. J Urol 112:24, 1974
985. Kansara V, Powell I: Fibrosarcoma of kidney. Urology 16:419, 1980
986. Srinivas V, Sogani PC, Hajdu SI et al: Sarcomas of the kidney. J Urol 132:13, 1984

Hemangiopericytoma

987. Stout AP, Murray MR: Hemangiopericytoma. A vascular tumor featuring Zimmerman's pericytes. Ann Surg 116:26, 1942
988. Black HR, Heinemann S: Hemangiopericytoma: Report of a case involving the kidney. J Urol 74:42, 1955
989. Berk LE, Ering AI, McManus RG: Hemangiopericytoma involving a kidney. Report of a case. N Engl J Med 263:1185, 1960
990. Lee HC, Kay S: Hemangiopericytoma: Report of a case involving the kidney with an 11-year follow up. Ann Surg 156:125, 1962
991. Simon R, Greene RC: Perirenal hemangiopericytoma. A case associated with hypoglycemia. JAMA 189:155, 1964
992. Farrow GM, Harrison EG Jr, Utz DC et al: Sarcomas and sarcomatoid and mixed malignant tumors of the kidney in adults — Part I. Cancer 22:545, 1968
993. Rifai GM: Renal and perirenal hemangiopericytoma. Urology 1:148, 1973
994. Enzinger FM, Smith BH: Hemangiopericytoma. An analysis of 106 cases. Hum Pathol 7:61, 1976
995. Tomik F, Vojacek K, Horvath A: Hemangiopericytoma. Neoplasma 24:445, 1977
996. Capek J, Ochova A, Bednar B: Hemangiopericytom v ramci smiseneho nadoru ledviny. Cas Lek Cesk 117:244, 1978
997. Klimenko AA, Karlashenko NI: Kombinirovannoe lechenie zlokachestvennykl opulholei pochki. Urol Nefrol 2:47, 1979
998. Susila M, Brezina L, Blaha V: Hemangiopericytom ledviny. Cesk Radiol 34:325, 1980
999. Asa SL, Bedard YC, Buckspan MB et al: Spontaneous hypoglycemia associated with hemangiopericytoma of the kidney. J Urol 125:864, 1981
1000. Ordonez NG, Bracken RB, Stroehlein KB: Hemangiopericytoma of kidney. Urology 20:191, 1982
1001. Chatterjee D, Powell A: Renal hemangioendothelioma. Int Surg 67:373, 1982
1002. Enzinger FM, Weiss SW: Hemangiopericytoma in Soft Tissue Tumors, p 463. St Louis, CV Mosby, 1983
1003. Weiss JP, Pollack HM, McCormick JF et al: Renal hemangiopericytoma: Surgical, radiological and pathological implications. J Urol 132:337, 1984

Malignant Fibrous Histiocytoma

1004. Ozzello L, Stout AP, Murry MR: Cultural characteristics of malignant histiocytomas and fibrous xanthomas. Cancer 16:331, 1963
1005. O'Brien JE, Stout AP: Malignant fibrous xanthomas. Cancer 17:1445, 1964

1006. Habib W, Gislason GJ: Malignant histiocytic tumor of the kidney. J Urol 94:208, 1965

1007. Meares EM, Kempson RL: Fibrous histiocytoma of the scrotum in an infant. J Urol 110:130, 1973

1008. Klugo RC, Farah RN, Cerny JC: Renal malignant histiocytoma. J Urol 112:727, 1974

1009. Bennington JL, Beckwith JB: In Tumors of the Kidney, Renal Pelvis, and Ureter, Atlas of Tumor Pathology, 2nd series, Fascicle 12, p 229. Washington, DC, AFIP, 1975

1010. Taxy JB, Battifora H: Malignant fibrous histiocytoma: A clinicopathologic and ultrastructural study. Cancer 40:254, 1977

1011. Osamura RY, Wetanabe K, Yoneyama K et al: Malignant fibrous histiocytoma of the renal capsule: Light and electron microscopic study of a rare tumor. Virchows Arch [A] 380:327, 1978

1012. Chen KTK: Fibroxanthosarcoma of kidney. Urology 13:439, 1979

1013. Raghavaiah NV, Mayer RF, Hagitt R et al: Malignant fibrous histiocytoma of the kidney. J Urol 123:951, 1980

1014. Chatelapat F: Sarcomatous tumors of the kidney. In Fenoglio CM, Wolff M (eds): Progress in Surgical Pathology, vol. III, p 181. New York, Masson Publishers, 1981

1015. Adophs H-D, Helpap B, Koischwitz D: Retroperitoneal and inguinal manifestation of malignant fibrous histiocytoma. Urology 20:639, 1982

1016. Singh EO, Barrett DM, Adams VI: Synchronously occurring malignant fibrous histiocytoma of the kidney with contralateral renal cell carcinoma. J Urol 128:586, 1982

1017. Enzinger FM, Weiss SW: Malignant fibrohistiocytic tumors. In Enzinger FM, Weiss SW (eds). Soft Tissue Tumors, p 166. St Louis, CV Mosby, 1983

1018. Scriven RR, Thrasher TV, Smith DC et al: Primary renal malignant fibrous histiocytoma: A case report and literature review. J Urol 131:948, 1984

1019. Chen KTK: Malignant fibrous histiocytoma of the kidney. J Surg Oncol 27:248, 1984

1020. Witz M, Bernheim J, Dinbar A et al: Kidney fibroxanthoma (malignant fibrous xanthoma): A rare tumor and an unusual cause of retroperitoneal hemorrhage. J Surg Oncol 26:146, 1984

1021. Srinivas V, Sogani PC, Hajdu SI et al: Sarcomas of the kidney. J Urol 132:13, 1984

Osteosarcoma

1022. Haining RB, Poole FE: Osteoblastoma of the kidney. Histologically identical with osteogenic sarcoma. Arch Pathol 21:44, 1936

1023. Hamer HG, Wishard N Jr: Osteogenic sarcoma involving the right kidney. J Urol 60:10, 1948

1024. Shaffer LW Jr: Extraskeletal osteochondrosarcoma. Review of the literature and report of a case. Am Surg 18:739, 1952

1025. Hudson HC: Osteogenic sarcoma involving the left kidney. J Urol 75:21, 1956

1026. Salik JO, Abeshouse BS: Calcification, ossification and cartilage formation in the kidney. Am J Roentgenol 88:125, 1962

1027. Soto PJ Jr, Rader ES, Martin JM et al: Osteogenic sarcoma of the kidney: Report of a case. J Urol 94:532, 1965

1028. Johnson LA, Ancona VC, Johnson T et al: Primary osteogenic sarcoma of the kidney. J Urol 104:528, 1970

1029. Dalinka MK, Fiveash AE, Aston JK: Metastatic extraosseous osteosarcoma to the liver: A case demonstrated by 85Sr and 99mTc-Colloid scanning. J Nucl Med 12:754, 1971

1030. Allan CJ, Soule EH: Osteogenic sarcoma of the somatic soft tissues. Clinicopathologic study of 26 cases and review of the literature. Cancer 27:1121, 1971

1031. Chambers A, Carson R: Primary osteogenic sarcoma of the kidney. Br J Radiol 48:316, 1975
1032. Axelrod R, Naidech HJ, Myers J et al: Primary osteosarcoma of the kidney. Cancer 41:724, 1978
1033. Rao U, Chang A, Didolkar MS: Extraosseous osteogenic sarcoma. Cancer 41:1488, 1978
1034. Biggers R, Stewart J: Primary renal osteosarcoma. Urology 8:674, 1979
1035. Micolonghi TS, Liang D, Schwartz S: Primary osteogenic sarcoma of the kidney. J Urol 131:1164, 1984

Rhabdomyosarcoma

1036. Messinger WJ, Jarman WD: Rhabdomyosarcoma of the kidney: Case report with autopsy findings. Surgery 2:26, 1937
1037. Herzog H: Nierengeschwulste mit quergestreifter Muskulatur. Z Krebsforsch 48:424, 1939
1038. Constance TJ: Bilateral rhabdomyoma of the kidney. J Pathol Bacteriol 59:492, 1947
1039. Seabury JC Jr: Renal rhabdomyosarcoma. JAMA 201:167, 1967
1040. Farrow GM, Harrison EG Jr, Utz DC et al: Sarcomas and sarcomatoid and mixed malignant tumors of the kidney in adults — Part I. Cancer 22:545, 1968
1041. Bennington JL, Beckwith JB: In Tumors of the Kidney, Renal Pelvis, and Ureter, Atlas of Tumor Pathology, 2nd series, Fascicle 12, p 216. Washington, DC, AFIP, 1975
1042. Kotecha NM: Embryonal rhabdomyosarcoma of the kidney. J Urol 118:325, 1977
1043. Lifschultz BD, Gonzalez-Crussi F, Kidd JM: Renal rhabdomyosarcoma of childhood. J Urol 127:309, 1982
1044. Srinivas V, Sogani PC, Hajdu SI et al: Sarcomas of the kidney. J Urol 132:13, 1984

Angiosarcoma

1045. Prince CL: Primary angio-endothelioma of the kidney: Report of a case and brief review. J Urol 47:787, 1942
1046. Askari A, Novick A, Braun W et al: Late ureteral obstruction and hematuria from de novo angiosarcoma in a renal transplant patient. J Urol 124:717, 1980
1047. Allred CD, Cathey WJ, McDivitt RW: Primary renal angiosarcoma: A case report. Hum Pathol 12:665, 1981

Malignant Mesenchymoma

1048. Stout AP: Mesenchymoma, the mixed tumor of mesenchymal derivatives. Ann Surg 127:278, 1948
1049. Jenkins JD, Anderson CK, Williams RE: Renal sarcoma. Br J Urol 43:263, 1971
1050. Elliott JT, Pontius EE, McCallum DC: Carcinosarcoma of kidney. Urology 1:151, 1973
1051. Gallagher JC, Winslow DJ, Grossman A: Coexistent chondrosarcoma and transitional-cell carcinoma in kidney. Urology 3:473, 1974
1052. Mead JH, Herrera GA, Kaufman MF et al: Case report of a primary cystic sarcoma of the kidney, demonstrating fibrohistiocytic, osteoid, and cartilaginous components (malignant mesenchymoma). Cancer 50:2211, 1982
1053. Enzinger RM, Weiss SW: Malignant Mesenchymoma in Soft Tissue Tumors, p 808. St Louis, CV Mosby, 1983

Plasmacytoma

1054. Knudsen O: Et tilfaelde af plasmocytoma renis. Nord Med 14:1493, 1937
1055. Hayes DW, Bennett WA, Heck FJ: Extramedullary lesions in multiple myeloma. Review of literature and pathologic studies. Arch Pathol 53:262, 1952

1056. Farrow GM, Harrison EG Jr, Utz DC: Sarcomas and sarcomatoid and mixed malignant tumors of the kidney in adults — Part II. Cancer 22:551, 1968

1057. Solomito VL, Grise J: Angiographic findings in renal (extramedullary) plasmacytoma. Case report. Radiology 102:559, 1972

1058. Catalona WJ, Biles JD III: Therapeutic considerations in renal plasmacytoma. J Urol 111:582, 1974

1059. Silver TM, Thornbury JR, Teears RJ: Renal peripelvic plasmacytoma: Unusual radiographic findings. Am J Radiol 128:313, 1977

1060. Siemers PT, Coel MN: Solitary renal plasmacytoma with palisading tumor vascularity. Radiology 123:597, 1977

1061. Morris SA, Vaughan ED Jr, Makoui C: Renal plasmacytoma. Urology 9:303, 1977

1062. Batasakis JG: Extramedullary plasmacytoma. In Batsakis JG (ed): Tumors of the Head and Neck: Clinical and Pathologic Considerations, 2nd ed, p 472. Baltimore, Williams & Wilkins, 1982

1063. Kandel LB, Harrison LH, Woodruff RD et al: Renal plasmacytoma: A case report and summary of reported cases. J Urol 132:1167, 1984

Malignant Lymphoma

1064. Gibson TE: Lymphosarcoma of the kidney. J Urol 60:838, 1948

1065. Knoepp LF: Lymphosarcoma of kidney. Surgery 39:510, 1956

1066. Richmond J, Sherman RS, Diamond HD et al: Renal lessions associated with malignant lymphomas. Am J Med 32:184, 1962

1067. Farrow GM, Harrison EG Jr, Utz DC: Sarcomas and sarcomatoid and mixed malignant tumors of the kidney in adults — Part II. Cancer 22:551, 1968

1068. Silber SJ, Chang CY: Primary lymphoma of kidney. J Urol 110:282, 1973

1069. Ellman L, Davis J, Lichtenstein NS: Uremia due to occult lymphomatous infiltration of the kidneys. Cancer 33:203, 1974

1070. Kanfer A, Vandewalle A, Morel-Maroger L et al: Acute renal insufficiency due to lymphomatous infiltration of the kidneys. Report of six cases. Cancer 38:2588, 1976

1071. Goswami AP: Metastatic cancer to the ureter and kidney from malignant lymphoma. A review of the literature. J Urol 117:381, 1977

1072. Dumbadze I, Crawford ED, Mulvaney WP: Lymphomatoid tumor infiltration of renal veins. J Urol 121:88, 1979

1073. Coggins CH: Renal failure in lymphoma. Kidney Int 17:847, 1980

1074. Randolph VL, Hall W, Bramson W: Renal failure due to lymphomatous infiltration of the kidneys. Cancer 52:1120, 1983

Leukemia

1075. Sternby NH: Studies in enlargement of leukaemic kidneys. Acta Haematol (Basel) 14:354, 1955

1076. Moell H: Size of normal kidneys. Acta Radiol 46:640, 1956

1077. Gilbert EF, Rice C, Lechaux PA: Renal function in children with leukemia. Am J Dis Child 93:150, 1957

1078. Besse BE Jr, Lieberman JE, Lusted LB: Kidney size in acute leukemia. Radiology 80:611, 1958

1079. Boggs DR, Wintrobe MM, Cartwright GE: The acute leukemias. Analysis of 322 cases and review of the literature. Medicine 41:163, 1962

Carcinosarcoma; Collision Tumors

1080. Meyer R: Beitrag zur Verstandigung uber die Namengebung in der Geschwulstlehre. Zentralbl Allg Pathol 30:291, 1920

1081. Kay S: Malignant mixed mesodermal tumor of the kidney. Am J Clin Pathol 28:655, 1957

1082. Fauci PA Jr, Therhag HG, Davis JE: Carcinosarcoma of the renal pelvis. J Urol 85:897, 1961

1083. Fisher ER, Davis ER: Carcinosarcoma of kidney. J Urol 87:109, 1962

1084. Hou LT, Willis RA: Renal carcino-sarcoma, true and false. J Pathol Bacteriol 85:139, 1963

1085. Willis RA: Carcino-Sarcoma in Pathology of Tumors, 4th ed, p 138. New York, Appleton-Century-Crofts, 1967

1086. Elliott JT, Pontius EE, McCallum DC: Carcinosarcoma of kidney. Urology 1:151, 1973

1087. Gallagher JC, Winslow DJ, Grossman A: Coexistent chondrosarcoma and transitional-cell carcinoma in kidney. Urology 3:473, 1974

1088. Ridolfi RL, Eggleston JC: Carcinosarcoma of the renal pelvis. J Urol 119:569, 1978

1089. Chatelanat F: Sarcomatous tumors of the kidney. In Feroglio CM, Wolff M (eds): Progress in Surgical Pathology, vol III, p 181. New York, Masson Publishers, 1981

1090. Tarry WF, Morabito RA, Belis JA: Carcinosarcoma of the renal pelvis with extension into the renal vein and inferior vena cava. J Urol 128:582, 1982

Teratoma

1091. McCrudy GA: Renal neoplasms in childhood. J Pathol Bacteriol 39:623, 1934

1092. Arnheim EE: Retroperitoneal teratomas in infancy and childhood. Pediatrics 8:309, 1951

1093. Bilger FR, Stoll G, Raiga JCL: Teratome kystique complexe de la loge renale. J Urol (Paris) 58:861, 1952

1094. Dehner LP: Intrarenal teratoma occurring in infancy: Report of a case with discussion of extragonadal germ cell tumors in infancy. J Pediatr Surg 8:369, 1973

1095. Aaronson IA, Sinclair-Smith C: Multiple cystic teratomas of the kidney. Arch Pathol Lab Med 104:614, 1980

1096. Glazier WB, Lytton B, Tronic B: Renal teratomas: Case report and review of the literature. J Urol 123:98, 1980

Metastatic Neoplasms

1097. Rawson AJ: Distribution of the lymphatics of the human kidney as shown in a case of carcinomatous permeation. Arch Pathol 47:283, 1949

1098. Klinger ME: Secondary tumors of the genito-urinary tract. J Urol 65:144, 1951

1099. Galluzzi S, Payne PM: Brondial carcinoma: A statistical study of 741 necropsies with special reference to the distribution of blood-borne metastases. Br J Cancer 9:511, 1955

1100. Lucke B, Schlumberger HG: In Tumors of the Kidney, Renal Pelvis and Ureter, Atlas of Tumor Pathology, Fascicle 30, p 136. Washington, DC, AFIP, 1957

1101. Onuigbo WIB: The spread of lung cancer to the kidneys. Cancer 11:737, 1958

1102. Payne RA: Metastatic renal tumours. Br J Surg 43:310, 1960

1103. Newsam JE, Tulloch WS: Metastatic tumours in the kidney. Br J Urol 38:1, 1966

1104. Ridlon HC, McAdams GB: Breast carcinoma metastatic to kidney. J Urol 98:328, 1967

1105. Patrick CE, Norton JH, Dacso MR: Choriocarcinoma in kidney: Case report. J Urol 97:444, 1967

1106. Willis RA: In Willis RA (ed): Pathology of Tumours, 4th ed, p 174. 1967

1107. Takayasu H, Kumamoto Y, Terawaki Y et al: A case of bilateral metastatic renal tumor originating from a thyroid carcinoma. J Urol 100:717, 1968

1108. Bosniak MA, Stern W, Lopez F et al: Metastatic neoplasm to the kidney. A report of four cases studied with angiography and nephrotomography. Radiology 92:989, 1969

1109. Silber I, Bowles WT: A case of epidermoid carcinoma of the larynx with metastases to the kidney. J Urol 102:549, 1969

1110. Roy JB, Walton KN: Secondary tumors of the kidney. J Urol 103:411, 1970

1111. Schreck WR, Holmes JH: Ultrasound as a diagnostic aid for renal neoplasms and cysts. J Urol 106:281, 1970

1112. Olsson CA, Moyer JD, Laferte RO: Pulmonary cancer metastatic to the kidney — A common renal neoplasm. J Urol 105:492, 1971

1113. Wagle DG, Moore RH, Murphy GP: Secondary carcinomas of the kidney. J Urol 114:30, 1975

1114. Ferrera DN, Vitenson JH, Siegel J: Computerized axial tomography scan in urology. Urology 10:212, 1977

1115. Bracken RB, Chica G, Johnson DE et al: Secondary renal neoplasms: An autopsy study. South Med J 72:806, 1979

1116. Davis RI, Corson JM: Renal metastases from well differentiated follicular thyroid carcinoma. A case report with light and electron microscopic findings. Cancer 43:265, 1979

1117. Chung HR: Bronchogenic squamous cell carcinoma metastatic to kidney. Detection by urine sediment cytology. Urology 13:561, 1979

1118. Marsan RE, Baker DA, Morin ME: Esophageal carcinoma presenting as a primary renal tumor. J Urol 121:90, 1979

1119. Pascal RR: Renal manifestations of extrarenal neoplasms. Hum Pathol 11:7, 1980

1120. Badlani G, Pillari G, Hajdu E et al: Primary renal or pulmonary tumor — A diagnostic dilemma. J Urol 125:721, 1981

1121. Johnson MW, Morettin LB, Sarles HE et al: Follicular carcinoma of the thyroid metastatic to the kidney 37 years after resection of the primary tumor. J Urol 127:114, 1982

1122. Weiner SN: Intraluminal renal vein thrombus secondary to metastatic disease to the kidney: A case report. J Urol 128:372, 1982

Renal Pelvis

2

Normal Structure

The mucosa of the calyceal system and renal pelvis is composed of transitional epithelium with two to three cell layers (Fig. 2-1). The epithelium is attached to a basement membrane covering the renal papillae continuous with the renal pelvis.

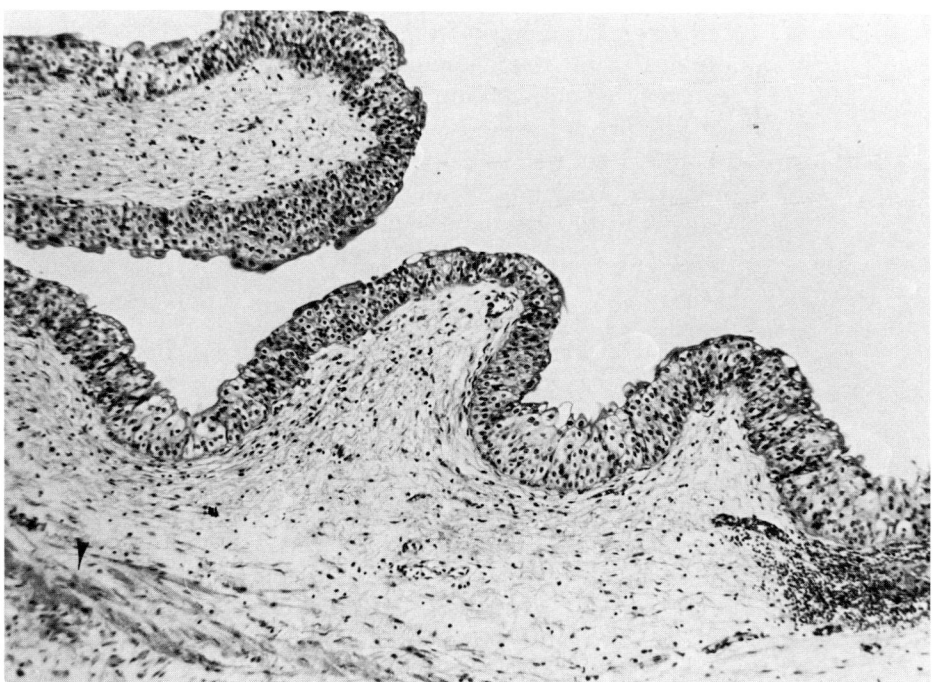

Figure 2-1   ***Normal renal pelvis.*** *Transitional cell urothelium covers a lamina propria composed of delicate collagen with scattered smooth muscle fibers* (arrowhead).

Subjacent to the basement membrane of both the calyces and the pelvis is smooth muscle, the organization of which is variable and unique to the site. The muscle of the renal pelvis is arranged in a spiral continuous with the muscularis of the ureter.[3,4] The configuration of the calyces is controlled by three groups of sphincteric muscles as described by Narath.[2]

The lymphatic drainage of the renal pelvis and kidney is to the regional para-aortic nodes (lateral lumbar nodes).[1]

Congenital Disorders

Calyceal Diverticulum

Calyceal diverticulum, variously called congenital hydrocalycosis, megacalycosis, calyceal cyst, and calyceal diverticulum, is characterized by a cystic dilatation of a single calyx of the kidney. The dilated calyx retains continuity with the uninvolved calyceal system through a narrow distal channel.[5-7] The affected calyx is most commonly (70% of cases) found in the upper pole of the kidney. A congenital defect in the embryologic formation of the calyx is the most probable underlying cause.

Calyceal diverticula are observed in both sexes with approximately equal frequency. The majority of the cases (89%) are diagnosed in patients 20 years to 59 years of age. Only rare examples of multiple calyceal diverticula have been reported, including examples of bilateral involvement.[6,7]

The size of the reported calyceal diverticula varies from a few millimeters to 7 cm, with the typical example averaging 2 cm to 3 cm. A calyceal diverticulum produces no symptoms unless complicated by associated infection or calculi. Many cases are detected as incidental findings during retrograde pyelography. In rare instances the enlarged cyst is of such magnitude that a flank mass is observed clinically as exemplified in Weyrauch and Fleming's case report involving a newborn female infant.[5]

Grossly, a calyceal diverticulum distorts the contour of the kidney, occasionally obliterating the overlying cortex when it extends to the renal capsule. The diverticulum retains continuity with the remainder of the calyceal system through an attenuated neck. Unless complicated by calculi and associated inflammation, the diverticular wall is thin.

Histologically, the diverticulum is lined by normal urothelium contiguous with urothelium lining the uninvolved calyceal system through the attenuated patent channel. Histologic evidence of acute and chronic inflammation in the adjacent renal parenchyma is observed commonly, especially in association with calculi. Calyceal diverticula are differentiated from retention cysts by the presence of the urothelial lining and communicating channel in the former.

Surgical treatment involving unroofing the diverticulum is required only for symptomatic, large examples of this congenital disorder.

Ureteropelvic Junction Obstruction

Ureteropelvic junction obstruction, an uncommon congenital disorder with resultant hydronephrosis of the affected kidney, is most frequently encountered in male infants younger than 6 months of age. The left kidney is involved more commonly than the right.[9] Twenty percent to thirty percent of cases are bilateral.[9,11]

Multiple causes have been identified. Murnaghan reported abnormal organization of the smooth muscle bundles at the ureteropelvic junction, with a predominance of longitudinal fibers in cases of ureteropelvic junction obstruction.[3] Excess collagen deposition within the intramural stroma between the muscle bundles was observed in an electron microscopy study by Hanna.[4] Extrinsic compression by aberrant renal vessels was observed in 25% of cases reported by Johnston.[9] Starer reported pelvic compression by normal renal vessels.[8] Finally, an abnormally high insertion of the ureter has been observed in some cases.[9] The disorder has been reported to have a familial occurrence.[10]

Amyloidosis

Selective deposition of amyloid in the wall of the renal pelvis has been reported in fewer than ten patients.[12-15] Similar deposits have been reported more frequently in the ureter and bladder. (Refer to Chap. 3 and 4.) In none of the reported cases has there been an accompanying plasma cell dyscrasia. The pathogenesis of these deposits remains unknown, and they are regarded as examples of primary amyloidosis.

When such deposits occur in the renal pelvis (or ureter), the clinical presentation is that of hematuria, or obstruction, resulting from the local accumulation of amyloid. Radiographic studies show distortion or filling defects in the renal pelvis.[12-15] Rare cases have admixed submucosal calcification, evident radiologically.[12,14]

Histologically, the amorphous eosinophilic material is deposited in the lamina propria. Mucosal erosions are associated with extensive deposition. Confirmation of the amyloid nature of the deposits is assisted by the observation of the light green birefringence with polarized light following staining with Congo red. Electron microscopy will demonstrate the characteristic extracellular fibrils.

Inflammatory Disorders

Malakoplakia

Malakoplakia involving the renal pelvis (and ureter) was first reported by Gibson in 1955.[16] Twelve additional cases have been located in the literature subsequent to Gibson's report[17-23] (Table 2-1). With the exception of the case reported by Sozer (1966), all other patients were women aged 36 years to 37 years.[21] Two cases had bilateral renal pelvic involvement.[17,19]

The lesions appear as discrete plaques, or ill-defined masses involving the renal pelvic mucosa. Associated renal parenchymal involvement is common. Evidence of malakoplakia elsewhere, especially the ipsilateral ureter, and bladder is reported in the majority of cases with renal pelvic involvement.

The diagnosis requires histologic review with demonstration of the pathognomonic Michaelis–Gutmann bodies by PAS and von Kossa stains.

A more complete discussion of this entity appears in Chapters 1 and 4. The occurrence of this inflammatory disorder in other sites of the urinary tract and genital system is recorded in each corresponding chapter.

Fungal Infection

Rare cases of renal pelvic fungal infections with *Candida albicans* and *Aspergillus* organisms have been reported.[24,25] Fungal growth of a magnitude sufficient to obstruct the ureteropelvic junction has been observed.[25]

Plasma Cell Granuloma

Two cases of plasma cell granulomas producing filling defects of the renal pelvis have been reported.[26,27] This lesion also has been observed in the urinary bladder. (Refer to Chap. 4.) This inflammatory lesion, characterized by a mixed chronic inflammatory cell infiltrate with a preponderance of mature plasma cells, has been reported most frequently in the lung.[28] The etiology is unknown. The greatest significance of this lesion is awareness of its occurrence in the urinary tract, which assists in differentiating such a lesion from a plasmacytoma. Plasmacytomas contain both mature and, importantly, atypical, immature plasma cells, without the admixture of lymphocytes and histiocytes present in plasma cell granulomas (see Figs. 4-58, 4-59).

Submucosal Hematoma (Antopol–Goldman Lesion)

Submucosal hematoma, which is a rare lesion, was described first by Antopol and Goldman in 1948. It has been reported in 13 patients.[29-32] The typical case involves a woman in the fourth to sixth decade of life, presenting with flank pain,

Table 2-1	*Malakoplakia*					
Author	*Year*	*Age*	*Sex*	*Side*	*Other Sites*	
Gibson et al[16]	1955	51	F	R	Pelvis, ureter	
Van Zile Scott, Scott[17]	1958	64	F	R, L	Ureter, kidney	
Lewis et al[18]	1961	67	F	R	None	
Cederqvist[19]	1965	44	F	R, L	Diagnosis at autopsy	
Smith[20]	1965	6 cases; no details			None	
Sozer[21]	1966	39	M	R	None	
Schneiderman, Simon[22]	1968	53	F	L	Ureter, kidney	
Sunshine[23]	1974	36	F	R	Ureter, bladder	

gross hematuria, and a renal pelvic filling defect detected radiologically.[29-32] All reported cases have been treated by nephrectomy or partial nephrectomy. Focal or diffuse subepithelial hematoma and intrapelvic blood clots are the characteristic features present in the excised kidney. Some cases have perirenal hemorrhage, and 5 of the 13 reported cases (39%) have independent congenital abnormalities of the renal vasculature or renal pelvis.[29,30]

Microscopically, old and recent hemorrhage is present beneath the suburothelium of the calyces and renal pelvis. Cortical infarcts of the affected kidney are reported in approximately half of the cases. No specific and consistent histologic abnormality of the intrarenal vasculature has been reported.

The cause of this lesion is unknown. Previous trauma was reported in two patients, anticoagulant therapy in one patient, and history of analgesic abuse recently was reported in a fourth patient.[29,31,32]

Submucosal Calcification

A single case of submucosal calcification was found in the literature.[33] The 48-year-old male patient had neither a history nor current evidence of urinary tract infection, abnormality of calcium metabolism, or renal pelvic amyloidosis. The etiology of the diffuse, radio-opaque, subepithelial calcification found in this patient was unknown.

Fibroepithelial Polyps

Fibroepithelial polyps of the renal pelvis have been reported in 12 patients.[34-43] Similar polyps are observed in the ureter, most commonly at the ureteropelvic junction, or the proximal third of the ureter (see discussion of fibroepithelial polyps of ureter, Chap. 3). Synonyms found in the literature include inflammatory polyp, fibroma, and hamartoma.[38] The various names reflect the unsettled pathogenesis of these tumors, which have been regarded variously as congenital, inflammatory, hamartomatous, or neoplastic lesions in the past.[34-43]

The youngest reported patient was a 4-year-old boy, and the oldest a 60-year-old man.[40] The peak frequency is in the third and fourth decades. A preponderance of cases involve the left kidney in women. Patients have flank pain with or without hematuria. One patient reportedly passed fragments of tissue through the urethra, retrospectively regarded as derived from such a lesion in the renal pelvis.[37]

These polypoid structures are smooth nodules or filiform projections varying in size from a few millimeters to several centimeters. Their exophytic growth produces smooth-contoured filling defects in the renal pelvis when examined by retrograde pyelography.

Histologically, normal or hyperplastic urothelium covers the central edematous stromal stalk containing collagen fibers, fibroblasts, and variable numbers of small blood vessels. Smooth muscle fibers have been observed in some cases. Acute and chronic inflammatory cells, focal hyalinization of the stroma, and calcification are inconstant features. Both the epithelial surface and the stromal cells are devoid of cytologic atypia.

The absence of both clinical and histologic evidence of inflammation in many cases does not support an inflammatory origin of these lesions. When inflammatory cells are present, they reflect a result of the polypoid growth with local irritation and obstruction. The presence of smooth muscle in some of these lesions suggests that they most probably represent hamartomatous proliferations rather than true neoplasms.

Metaplastic and Proliferative Variants

The metaplastic and proliferative variants of urothelium observed in the renal pelvis are outlined in Table 2-2. The recognition of these urothelial changes was first reported over 200 years ago, but their pathogenesis and clinical significance remains unsettled. (Refer to discussion of metaplastic and proliferative variants, Chap. 4.) Morgagni described minute mucosal cysts (pyelitis ureteritis, cystitis cystica) in 1761.[44] Von Limbeck (1887) and von Brunn (1893) described the histologic features of epithelial "buds" and "nests" capable of changing into the mucosal cysts.[46,47] These cysts, capable of enlarging to several millimeters, are undoubtedly the structures described earlier by Morgagni. Transformation of these urothelial mucosal cysts to mucus-secreting glandular structures (pyelitis, glandularis) was reported by Stoerk and Zuckerkandl in 1907 and 1911.[48,49] Transformation of the normal urothelium to a squamous mucosa was described first by Rokitansky in 1861.[45] The most recently recognized metaplastic change, currently termed "nephrogenic metaplasia" or "nephrogenic adenoma," was reported first by Davis in 1949.[60] These proliferative and metaplastic changes occur most frequently in the bladder, but are observed at all levels of the urinary tract including the renal pelvis.

Urothelial Hyperplasia
Simple Hyperplasia

Simple hyperplasia refers to an increase in the numbers of cell layers of the mucosal transitional epithelium. In the renal pelvis, the maximum number of cell layers is three to five, increasing to seven in the urinary bladder. This change

Table 2-2   **Urothelial Proliferative and Metaplastic Variants**

Urothelial hyperplasia	Simple hyperplasia
	Brunn's invaginations and nests
	Pyelitis cystica
Combined urothelial hyperplasia and metaplasia	Pyelitis glandularis
	Mucinous or "colonic" metaplasia
	Nephrogenic metaplasia (nephrogenic adenoma)
	Squamous metaplasia of surface epithelium (keratinizing desquamative squamous metaplasia)[76]
	Squamous metaplasia of Brunn's nests

has a flat configuration, with neither papillary features nor invaginations into the lamina propria (as is observed in Brunn's nests).

Simple hyperplasia can be seen in the apparent absence of associated urothelial abnormalities, but commonly is seen accompanying inflammatory disorders, and in association with renal pelvic urothelial neoplasms.[69,74] Its biological significance, beyond the empirical observations noted above, is not known.

Brunn's Nests

Bulbous invaginations of the surface epithelium encroaching into the lamina propia are characteristic of Brunn's nests (buds, invaginations). Alternately, solid, round nests of urothelial cells, apparently detached from the surface, are observed within the lamina propria. The cells within the buds and nests are cytologically similar to the surface epithelial cells; however, they do retain the surface urothelium's ability to undergo glandular or squamous metaplasia. Rare cases show both forms of differentiation within a single microscopic field.[52,56,64]

Pyelitis Cystica

Small slits or round spaces are commonly present in otherwise solid Brunn's nests or buds. The size of this central lumen varies as does the number of surrounding cell layers. Eosinophilic, proteinaceous material is commonly present within the lumen. The surrounding cells are flat, with the exception of the luminal layer cells, which may show a cuboidal configuration. These cysts occasionally achieve sufficient size to be apparent on gross examination.

Combined Urothelial Hyperplasia and Metaplasia
Pyelitis Glandularis

Pyelitis glandularis is characterized by glandular structures lined by mucin-secreting columnar epithelial cells. The glands are haphazardly arranged or are clustered within the lamina propria, and frequently in proximity to von Brunn's nests and pyelitis cystica. The latter structures differ from pyelitis glandularis only in the nature of the lining cells. Structures with cytologic features of both pyelitis cystica and pyelitis glandularis (incomplete metaplastic change) are not uncommon (see Fig. 2-5). Indeed, all gradations of this metaplastic change can be observed in a single specimen. Mucicarmine stain demonstrates both intracellular and luminal mucin. In most cases the overlying surface epithelium remains of the transitional cell type, but metaplastic squamous epithelium or mucus-secreting columnar cells similar to that observed in the underlying glandularis structures have been reported.[51,53,58,65,67]

Pyelitis glandularis is commonly focal, but rare cases of diffuse glandularis metaplasia have been reported.[51,53,58,65] When extensive, and demonstrating columnar cell metaplasia of the surface urothelium, its resemblance to colonic mucosa is striking. Paneth cells have been observed in rare cases.[66-68] The absence of a muscularis mucosa allows separating this extensive metaplastic change of the renal pelvis from colon mucosa.[65,67] Combined squamous metaplasia has been observed in a few cases.[65-67,77]

Nephrogenic Metaplasia

Nephrogenic metaplasia (so-called nephrogenic adenoma), the most recently described urothelial proliferative alteration, has not been described in the renal pelvis. It occurs most frequently in the bladder trigone, but rare cases have been reported in the urethra and in the ureter.[60,61,75,79] (Refer to nephrogenic metaplasia in Chap. 3.)

Squamous Metaplasia

Squamous metaplasia of the renal pelvic urothelium is uncommon, with less than 100 cases reported in the literature.[76] Here, as well as in the urinary bladder where it occures more frequently, it is commonly termed "leukoplakia" (Fig. 2-2). This term is both nonspecific and noninformative when applied to urinary tract alterations. Its literal meaning is "white plaque." The rationale of returning a pathologic diagnosis of leukoplakia to a clinician, whose concern about a white plaque prompted the biopsy in the first place, escapes me. The use of the term leukoplakia by surgical pathologists is discouraged.

Squamous metaplasia most commonly evidences no dysplastic changes, but if the latter feature is present, this should be noted in the pathology report. Concurrent inflammation and surface keratinization may or may not be present (Fig. 2-3). When the latter is present, the term "keratinizing, desquamative

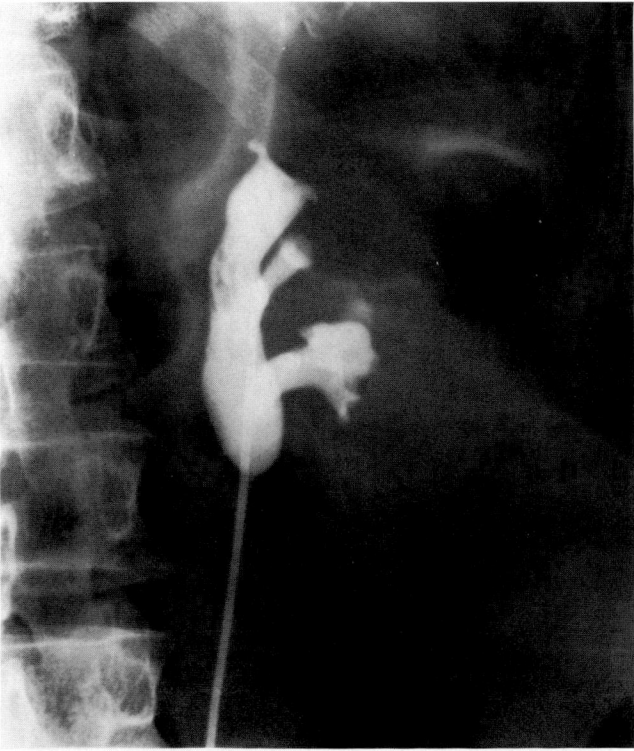

Figure 2-2 *Squamous metaplasia (leukoplakia). A retrograde pyelogram demonstrates linear mucosal striations in the renal pelvis. The diagnosis of leukoplakia was confirmed at surgery.*

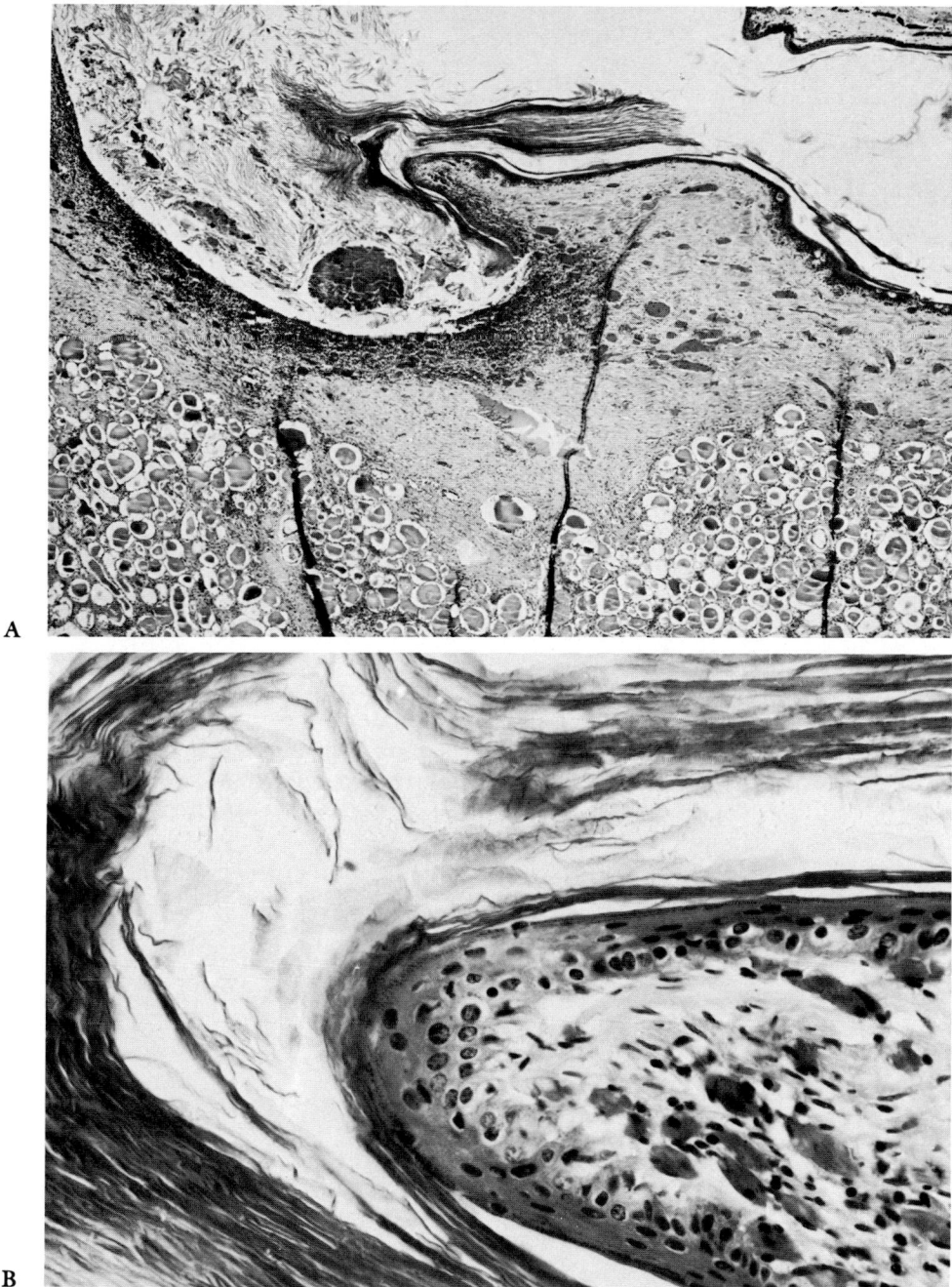

Figure 2-3   ***Squamous metaplasia of renal pelvis.*** (A) *Keratinizing squamous epithelium has replaced the normal transitional epithelium of the renal pelvis. Associated chronic pyelonephritis is present in the underlying renal medullary pyramid.* (B) *Granular layer with abundant keratin debris is present below corium.*

squamous metaplasia" has been suggested recently.[76] Senger reported one case of bilateral squamous metaplasia of the renal pelvis.[62]

Clinical Significance of the Proliferative and Metaplastic Variants

Brunn's Nests

Historically, Brunn's nests have been regarded as a microscopic hallmark of longstanding urinary tract inflammation, and the nests themselves as a local reaction of the urothelium to the inflammation. In 1928 Morse observed cell nests and cysts in 86% of cases examined in an autopsy study. Interestingly, in spite of the fact that only 58% of cases with these proliferative changes demonstrated associated inflammation, he concluded "epithelial buds and nests of von Brunn are inflammatory in nature."[52] Half a century later, a similar study by Koss and co-workers found associated inflammation in only 62% of cases.[71,72] They and others have concluded on the basis of these data that urothelial proliferations are proliferative variants of the urothelial mucosa, which can arise in the absence of any demonstrable associated abnormality. The etiology of this proliferative variant in otherwise normal urinary tracts is unknown.

There is general agreement that cystica and glandularis structures of the urothelium take origin from Brunn's nests and buds. There is also general agreement that glandularis structures are the result of metaplastic change, and not a reflection of embryonic nests of this type of epithelium.[49,50,52,63] The sequence of events transforming Brunn's nests to cystica and glandularis structures has received considerable attention, and remains unsettled.[47,54,55,59] (Refer to discussion in Chap. 4.)

In most cases Brunn's nests are focal urothelial changes (Fig. 2-4). Rare cases

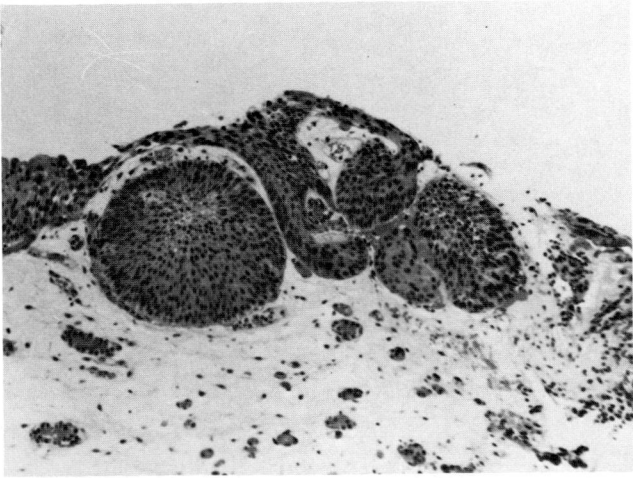

Figure 2-4   *Brunn's nests. Nests of cytologically normal urothelial cells are present below the urothelial surface. Scattered chronic inflammatory cells are present in the adjacent lamina propria.*

have been reported describing extensive involvement of the renal pelvis and entire length of the contiguous ureter.[57] Such diffuse involvement must not be misinterpreted as a malignant neoplasm. Alternatively, associated severe inflammation, with or without lithiasis, can alter the configuration of the nests and superficially suggest neoplastic invasion.[73]

The inherent capability of this nonneoplastic urothelial proliferation to undergo neoplastic change is currently unknown. Stern recently reported a localized, recurring proliferation of Brunn's nests within the bladder, which was interpreted as a benign tumor of Brunn nest origin.[70] No similar case could be found in the literature. The possibility that some inverted papillomas arise from Brunn's nests was recently suggested in a study by Kunze.[78]

Finally, although Brunn's nests in proximity to transitional cell carcinoma may show variable degrees of cytologic atypia, including carcinoma in situ, there is no evidence that the epithelium of Brunn's nests is at greater risk to undergo malignant change than the surface epithelium. Similarly, there is no evidence that the presence of Brunn's nests, per se, increases the risk of the surface epithelium to undergo malignant transformation.

Pyelitis Cystica

As noted in the discussion of Brunn's nests above, pyelitis cystica is commonly present in the context of inflammatory disorders within the urinary tract, but, importantly, is also found in the absence of any apparent associated urothelial disorder. There is general agreement that cystica structures are related to both Brunn's nests and glandularis structures.[47,52,54,55,59,63]

In spite of extensive study, it is unsettled whether cystica structures give origin to glandularis by means of metaplasia, or glandularis structures become cystica structures as a result of retention of secretion.[54,55,59] I favor the view that both mechanisms can occur and that the formation of glandularis structures with mucus-secreting columnar lining cells arise by metaplastic change of the urothelium originally within Brunn's nests.

The relationship of pyelitis cystica to neoplasms is similar to that of Brunn's nests. Both can be found in proximity to established urothelial malignancy, but there is no evidence that the epithelium of these structures, or their presence per se, contributed to the risk, or the origin of the established malignant neoplasm. The possible role of cystica structures in the histogenesis of inverted papillomas requires further study.[78]

Pyelitis Glandularis

The sparse literature about pyelitis glandularis suggests this metaplastic change is rare, but the true frequency is unknown.[76] Among the few studies reported, associated infection is common. It can be a focal change, or involve the renal pelvis diffusely (Fig. 2-5).

The relationship of pyelitis glandularis and its diffuse variant mucinous (or "colonic") metaplasia with renal pelvis adenocarcinoma has been the subject of much speculation. Among the 47 cases of adenocarcinoma of the renal pelvis reported in the literature, associated metaplastic change has been reported in 18 cases (58%) of the 31 cases providing this information (see Table 2-16). The absence of observed glandular metaplasia in the 13 reports specifically com-

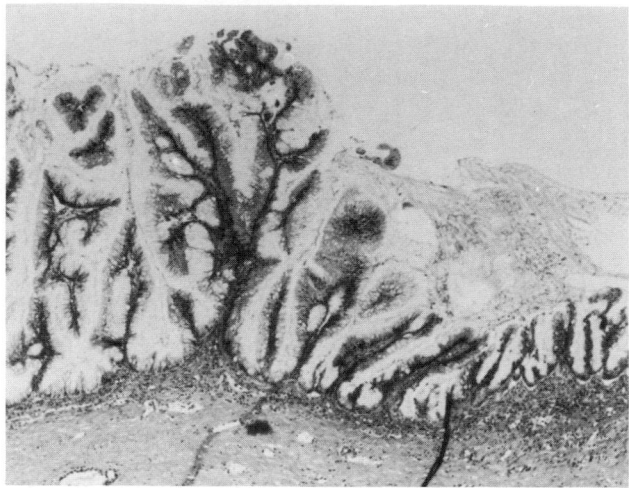

Figure 2-5   *Glandular metaplasia. The urothelium has been converted to mucus-secreting glandular epithelium by metaplasia. Brunn's nests and pyelitis cystica were present elsewhere in this renal pelvis. All were incidental findings at autopsy.*

menting on this feature is not particularly disturbing or mysterious. Tumor growth could possibly have obliterated any residue of the glandular metaplastic population from which it took origin. In summary, the association of glandular metaplasia with some urothelial adenocarcinomas allows only that the malignant neoplasm did indeed take origin from this metaplastic cell population. This speculation is not equatable to the conclusion that the glandular metaplastic cell population is inherently at greater risk of malignant transformation. The carcinogenic agent(s) and events are operative and occur at the site that happens to be populated by the metaplastic glandular epithelium. The documentation of progressively severe dysplastic changes within glandular metaplasia ultimately progressing to frank adenocarcinoma, as has been reported in rare cases in the bladder, does not demonstrate greater inherent risk of this change in the metaplastic population, as has been claimed. (Refer to discussion of adenocarcinoma in Chap. 4.)

Squamous Metaplasia

Squamous metaplasia of the upper urinary tract is rare. In a recent extensive review, Hertle and Audroulakakis outlined the cumulative experience gained from 80 published cases.[76] Thirty-two cases (41%) had no associated disorders of the urinary tract. Recurrent urinary tract infection and lithiasis were reported in 53% of the cases of squamous metaplasia (Fig. 2-6).[76] Thus, squamous metaplasia, as with Brunn's nests and cystica lesions, is observed in the context of established inflammation, but can develop spontaneously without identifiable injury to the urothelium.

The presenting clinical feature, which is flank pain in 73% of cases, relates to the accumulation of keratin debris, commonly with obstruction of the upper urinary tract.[76] Almost half of the patients report noting passage of this debris in the urine.[76]

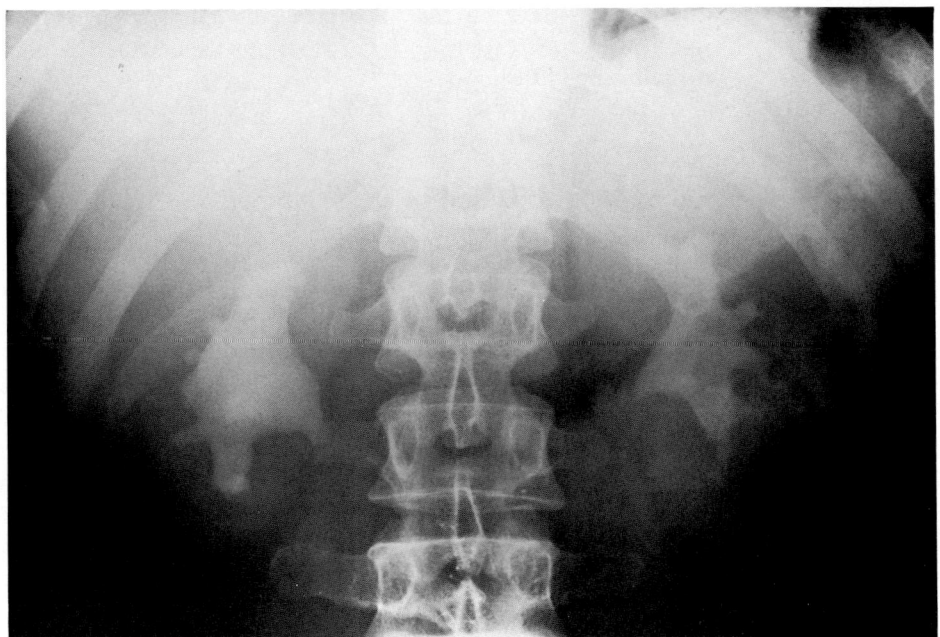

Figure 2-6   *Staghorn calculus. Bilateral staghorn calculi are seen in this scout film of the abdomen without contrast. Opacification of almost the entire intrarenal collecting system is present.*

Squamous metaplasia is associated with less than 10% of the reported renal pelvic squamous cell carcinomas. (Refer to section on squamous cell carcinoma later in this chapter.) Hertle and Androulakakis noted that no reported case of squamous metaplasia of the upper urinary tract has progressed to squamous cell carcinoma.[76]

In summary, the urothelium demonstrates a wide spectrum of proliferative and metaplastic changes that can occur spontaneously, but which also are observed commonly in the context of established urinary tract inflammation. These same changes may be observed in association with a similar spectrum of malignant epithelial neoplasms that most probably take origin from their metaplastic counterparts. There is no substantial evidence that these metaplastic populations are inherently at significantly greater risk of malignant transformation than the original urothelial cell population under similar circumstances.

Classification of Neoplasms of the Renal Pelvis

A classification of renal pelvic neoplasms is presented in Table 2-3. The most frequently observed neoplasms are epithelial and malignant, in particular, transitional cell carcinoma. Squamous cell carcinoma and adenocarcinoma are uncommon, with approximately 300 cases reported in the literature. All other neoplasms, benign epithelial, and both benign and malignant mesenchymal neoplasms, are rare. Neoplasms metastatic to the renal pelvis are limited to rare, scattered, anecdotal reports. Varying degrees of male predominance are exhibited by all renal pelvic neoplasms with the exception of smooth muscle tumors. There is no characteristic age predilection that would allow clinical distinction of epithelial and mesenchymal, benign and malignant neoplasms. All are most frequent in the fifth to seventh decades, but have been observed at virtually any age, including childhood.

Benign Epithelial Neoplasms
Papilloma

The working definition of *papilloma,* and therefore the attributed behavior, has not been constant through the past.[80-83,108,109] Uncertainty still persists as evidenced by perusal of several current urology and pathology textbooks. Some authors equate papilloma and grade 1 papillary transitional cell carcinoma.

Miller, strictly applying the histologic criteria of a papillary lesion of urothelium that has a mucosal covering of three to five cells morphologically indistinguishable from normal urothelium, reported no recurrences within 5 years in a series of cases (Fig. 2-7).[81] This is a clinical evolution quite different from that attributable to papillary transitional cell carcinoma, grade 1.

Greater cumulative experience with this lesion, with consistently applied diagnostic criteria, is required in the future to change the uncertainty to confidence in patient management.

Inverted Papilloma

Inverted papillomas are rare urothelial neoplasms most frequently observed in the trigone region of the urinary bladder. Less commonly it arises in the renal pelvis, ureter, or urethra in order of decreasing frequency. A marked male predilection (90%) is observed in all sites.[84-90] The characteristic downward proliferation of urothelial cells within the underlying lamina propria is of such magnitude as to result in an exophytic papillomatous tumor. Potts and Hirst introduced the descriptive term "inverted papilloma" in 1963.[84] Until recently it was regarded as a benign neoplasm without associated increased risk of malignant change. This was in contrast to inverted papillomas of the upper respiratory tract, which

Table 2-3   *Classification of Renal Pelvic Neoplasms*

Epithelial	Benign
	  Papilloma
	  Inverted papilloma

	Malignant
	  Transitional cell carcinoma
	  Squamous cell carcinoma
	  Adenocarcinoma
	  Mixed carcinoma
	  Undifferentiated carcinoma

Mesenchymal	Benign
	  Hemangioma
	  Leiomyoma

	Malignant Leiomyosarcoma
Malignant mixed neoplasms	Carcinocarcinoma

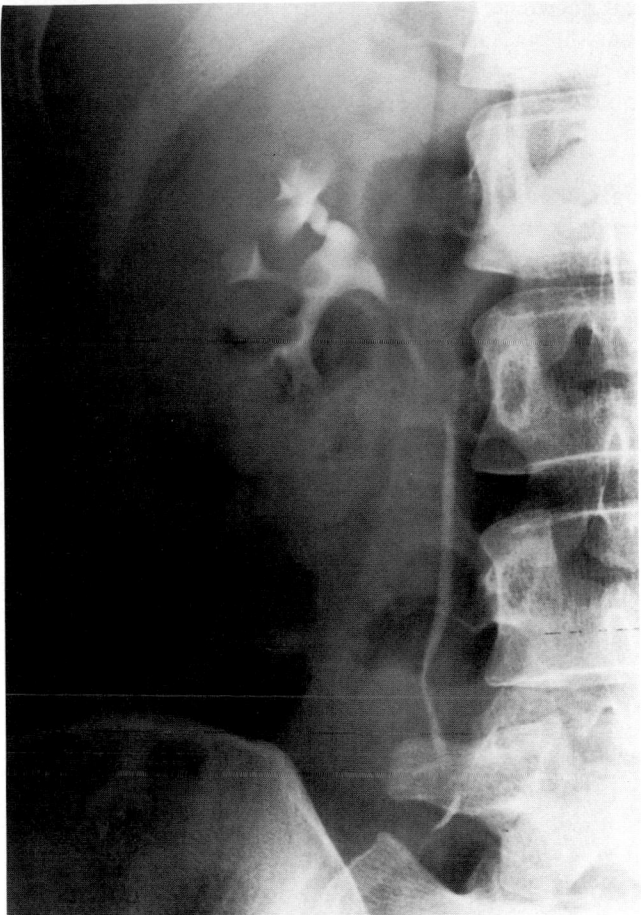

Figure 2-7   ***Papilloma of renal pelvis.*** *This intravenous urogram demonstrates a 6-mm intrinsic lesion of the renal pelvis, which at surgery was found to be a transitional cell papilloma. The patient was a 33-year-old woman who presented with hematuria.*

demonstrate a tendency to recur, and not uncommonly undergo malignant change. This same tendency is now being reported with inverted papillomas of the urinary tract, and therefore they are no longer regarded as innocuous benign neoplasms. (Refer to section on inverted papilloma, Chap. 4.)

Ten cases of inverted papilloma arising in the renal pelvis have been reported.[85-90] The age range is 49 years to 89 years with the peak incidence in the seventh decade. The right and left renal pelves are affected equally. No examples of multiple or bilateral inverted papilloma have been observed. Patients most commonly have flank pain, with or without hematuria. Retrograde pyelography detects the exophytic lesion in the renal pelvis.

The size of the reported lesions in the renal pelvis varies from 1 cm to 3 cm. The surface of the papilloma is smooth or nodular. Histologically, inverted papillomas show a urothelial cell proliferation taking origin from the surface mucosa, and organized in a trabecular pattern within the expanded lamina propria. Typically the peripheral urothelial basal cells show palisading with lesser degrees of organization in the centrally located cells. The trabeculae commonly show focal microcyst formation with associated expansion of the trabeculum. Focal squamous metaplasia may be observed. The surface mucosa may be normal, attenuated, or hyperplastic. Loose fibrovascular stroma intervenes between the branching trabeculae of epithelial cells. Kunze and co-workers recently have described a second histological variant: the glandular pattern in vesicle inverted papillomas.[78] The solid trabecular pattern has characterized all renal pelvic inverted papillomas reported to this time.

To date, no inverted papilloma of the renal pelvis has been diagnosed preoperatively. The consideration of this lesion in the differential diagnosis of renal pelvic masses increases the probability of more limited surgical excisions in the future. However, this judgment is tempered by the recent report of a transitional cell carcinoma found in association with a renal pelvic inverted papilloma, an association previously limited to examples arising in the urinary bladder.[89] (Refer to Chap. 4.) Determination of the true frequency of associated urothelial malignancies and malignant transformation of renal pelvic inverted papillomas must await greater cumulative experience with this neoplasm.

Malignant Epithelial Neoplasms
Staging Protocol

The proposed tumor staging protocol for renal pelvic neoplasms is an adaptation of that originally proposed for the urinary bladder by Jewett, Strong, and Marshall,[91–93] and the ureter as proposed by Heney and co-workers.[94] The staging protocol used here is presented in Table 2-4. Alternative staging protocols for renal pelvic malignancies have been proposed by Newman and co-workers,[113] Grabstald and colleagues,[116] Wagle and associates,[119] and Rubenstein and co-workers.[132]

Transitional Cell Carcinoma

Epidemiology and Etiology

The increased frequency of bladder urothelial neoplasms observed in dye industry workers by Rehn (1895) initiated the epidemiologic interest in environmental carcinogens causally related to this neoplasm.[95] In subsequent years similar observations were made referable to transitional cell carcinoma of the renal pelvis. MacAlpine (1947)[96] and Poole-Wilson (1969)[98] reported transi-

Table 2-4   **Staging Protocol for Renal Pelvic Carcinoma**

Stage	Extent of Invasion
O	Confined to mucosa, noninvasive
A	Invasion of lamina propria of extrarenal pelvis or focal superficial invasion of renal pyramids
B	Invasion of muscularis of extrarenal pelvis or diffuse microscopic invasion of renal pyramids
C	Gross invasion of kidney or gross or microscopic invasion of peripelvic adipose tissue
D	D1 — Lymph node metastases
	D2 — Distant metastases

tional cell carcinoma of the renal pelvis and ureter occurring among English dye industry workers. The consistently higher frequency of environmental carcinogen-induced urothelial neoplasms in the urinary bladder than observed in the pelvis and ureter may be due in part to the more rapid transit time of urine through the upper urinary tract.[97,101] The carcinogens to which these workers were exposed included alpha-naphthylamine, beta-naphthylamine, and benzidine.[98] Poole-Wilson reported a lag time averaging about one decade between exposure and diagnosis of tumor.[98]

In addition to the known association of phenacetin abuse and papillary necrosis, this analgesic now has been causally related to transitional cell carcinoma of the renal pelvis. This association was reported first by Hultengren and co-workers in six Swedish patients in 1965.[97] Rathert and colleagues collected 118 subsequently reported cases of renal pelvic transitional cell carcinoma in patients with a history of phenacetin abuse.[103] The duration of phenacetin abuse among these patients was 15 years to 20 years.[103] In contrast to the male predominance among patients with this neoplasm without prior phenacetin abuse, the sex ratio was virtually 1 : 1 among cases of renal pelvic transitional cell carcinoma with such an analgesic abuse history.[103] Bengtsson and associates (1978) identified potential carcinogens produced in the catabolic pathways of phenacetin, including N-hydroxy-p-phenetidine, p-nitroso-phenetidine, and 2-hydroxyphenetidine.[105] Calder and co-workers have reported the experimental production of neoplasms in rats administered N-hydroxy-phenacetin, a metabolic product of phenacetin.[104] In 1982, McCredie reported that regular consumption of analgesics was associated with a tenfold increased risk of renal pelvic carcinoma in women, and a four- to eightfold increased risk in men.[107] When analgesic consumption was associated with tobacco consumption, a synergistic effect was observed.[107]

Schmauz and Cole observed a relationship between tobacco and coffee consumption and the frequency of upper urinary tract carcinoma in Eastern Massachusetts.[102] A similar relatonship exists with the urothelial neoplasms of the bladder. The increased risk of renal pelvic and ureteral carcinoma was observed only when relatively high levels of consumption were recorded.[102]

Petkovic has reported an unusually high (9%) frequency of bilateral renal pelvic and ureteral transitional cell carcinomas observed in one clinic in Belgrade, Yugoslavia.[106] Petkovic noted the association of these neoplasms with Balkan nephropathy (Danubian endemic familial nephropathy), endemic in Yugoslavia, Bulgaria, and Rumania.[106] Because the cause of this nephropathy remains unknown, so does the nature of the relationship between Balkan nephritis and transitional cell carcinoma of the upper urinary tract.[98]

In 1973, Elliott and co-workers reported the identification of RNA viral particles in cases of renal pelvic transitional cell carcinoma.[101] This remains the only reported study linking viruses and urothelial neoplasms of the renal pelvis. A role, if any, in the causation of these tumors requires further study.

For the sake of completeness, mention should be made of 23 cases of renal pelvic carcinoma following exposure to Thorotrast included in a literature review by Grampa.[100]

Incidence

In 1933, Swift-Jolly culled 337 primary renal pelvic neoplasms reported to that time.[108] Sixty-four percent of these cases were regarded as malignant (transitional cell carcinoma, papillary carcinoma, squamous cell carcinoma), and 36% were regarded as "benign papillomata."

Approximately 20 years later, Riches and co-workers reported a series of 2314 neoplasms of the kidney, renal pelvis, and ureter diagnosed in the British Isles.[109] Renal pelvic primaries comprised 7% of the total. "Simple papillomata" constituted 23% of the renal pelvic neoplasms. These relatively high frequencies of benign urothelial papillary lesions (36% and 23%) reflect the different diagnostic criteria applied in early studies of urothelial neoplasms. Currently, papillary urothelial lesions regarded as benign are distinctly rare, and thus the relative frequency of the different histologic types of renal pelvic neoplasms reported in the early literature is limited to its historical value.

Table 2-5 presents the clinical and pathologic findings and overall survival rates of the 20 largest published series of renal pelvic transitional cell carcinoma. The combined series represents data on 1188 patients, the majority of whom were reported since 1970.

Demography

The age range of most reported series is the third to ninth decades with a peak frequency in the sixth and seventh decades. The mean age is 60 years to 65 years (Table 2-5). The youngest patient with a renal pelvic transitional cell carcinoma was a 4-month-old boy, reported by Koyanagi and co-workers in 1975.[126] Sixty-eight percent of the patients presented in this cumulative series were men. The right and left kidneys are equally affected.

Table 2-5   *Transitional Cell Carcinoma*

Author	Year	Cases	Sex	
			M	F
McDonald, Priestly[80]	1944	75	56	19
Riches et al[109]	1951	172	136	36
Kaplan et al[110]	1951	133	103	30
Taylor[111]	1959	32	23	9
Newman et al[113]	1967	59	40	19
Grace et al[114]	1968	32	27	10
Grabstald et al[116]	1971	70	48	22
Williams, Mitchell[118]	1973	43	33	10
Wagle et al[119]	1974	78	52	26
Johansson et al[120]	1974	62	29	33
Say, Hori[122]	1974	13	8	5
Cummings et al[123]	1975	35	24	11
Donnelly, Koontz[124]	1975	13	9	4
Rafla[125]	1975	28	16	12
Johansson et al[127]	1976	94	61	33
Leong et al[128]	1976	23	15	8
Strong, Pearse[131]	1976	50	44	6
Rubenstein et al[132]	1978	70	48	22
Johansson et al[133]	1979	38	17	21
Nocks et al[136]	1982	68	40	28

YSR, year survival rate; NI, no information.

* Five-year survival rate not available from information provided.

Clinical Presentation

Virtually all patients (approximately 90%) present with hematuria, most commonly painless.[109,111,113,114,124,137] Flank pain alone is recorded in 20% of patients, and hematuria with flank pain is noted in another 20%.[113,114,118,119,122, 123,136,139] A mass is palpable in only 10% of cases of transitional cell carcinoma of the renal pelvis.[114,118,119,124] Detection of a renal pelvic primary in asymptomatic patients accounts for approximately 10% of reported cases.[109,118,122,132,136] These incidental neoplasms frequently are discovered during follow-up diagnostic procedures in patients with previously diagnosed lower urinary tract neoplasms. Radiologic examination reveals a renal pelvic filling defect. Approximately 10% of patients have associated renal lithiasis.[80,109,116,118,119,124,128]

Rare patients with renal pelvic transitional cell carcinomas presenting with peripheral neuropathy, hypercalcemia, or distant metastases have been reported.[112, 129, 130, 132,136]

Pathology

Cytology Studies. The results of urine cytology studies in ten published series of renal pelvic carcinoma are presented in Table 2-6. Positive urine cytologies were found in only 38% of 195 cases.[114,115,117,119,122–124,128,136,139] The frequency of positive cytology correlates with the grade of the tumor: high grade transi-

Age		Side	Calculi	Hematuria	Bilateral	Follow-up Information
Range	Mean	L/R				
96% > 40	NI	42/33	12%	NI	0	30% 5-YSR
1st–9th	(50–69)	96/76	5%	90%	0	35% 5-YSR
25–79	57	NI	NI	NI	0	NI
32–81	6th decade	22/10	NI	90.4%	0	23.3% 5-YSR
4th–8th	63	32/26	NI	80%	0	17% 5-YSR
32–84	65	12/26	NI	92%	1	36% 5-YSR
21–83	58	29/36	7%	85%	5	*
31–76	60	L = R	5%	83%	0	*
37–86	61.5	42/35	6%	98.7%	1	5-YSR
37–79	58	26/33	NI	88%	3	44% 10-YSR
30–77	64	5/8	NI	67%	0	42.8% 5-YSR
29–83	6th, 7th decade	NI	NI	97%	0	*
NI	63	7/6	7%	77%	1	*
38–NI	5th, 6th decade	L = R	0%	NI	0	43% 5-YSR
29–85	66	NI	NI	88%	0	51% 5-YSR
26–84	56	NI	17%	69%	0	NI
41–88	64.2	27/33	NI	67%	0	NI
32–88	60	33/37	NI	79%	0	*
23–69	62	NI	NI	95%	0	14% 5-YSR
39–90	60	42/26	NI	72%	0	57% 5-YSR

Table 2-6   *Cytology Studies*

Author	Year	Number of Patients*	Results of Urine Cytology Examination		
			Positive	Suspicious	Negative
Grace et al[114]	1968	15	5 (33%)	3 (20%)	7 (47%)
Sarnacki[115]	1971	22	12 (59%)	0	9 (41%)
Cullen et al[117]	1972	7	5 (71%)	0	2 (38%)
Say, Hori[122]	1974	4	1 (25%)	1 (25%)	2 (50%)
Wagle et al[119]	1974	78	24 (31%)	0	NI
Donelly, Koontz[124]	1975	13	5 (37%)	0	8 (63%)
Cummings et al[123]	1975	9	2 (22%)	7 (78%)	0
Leong et al[128]	1976	8	2 (25%)	0	6 (75%)
Nocks et al[136]	1982	31	15 (48%)	0	16 (52%)
Mahadevia[139]	1983	8	4 (50%)	3 (38%)	0

* All patients had renal pelvic transitional cell carcinoma proven histologically subsequent to cytology studies.

tional cell carcinomas of the upper urinary tract are more frequently positive than low grade neoplasms.[136] Ureteral or ureteropelvic junction obstruction accounts in part for this low yield. Future application of retrograde brushing or thin needle biopsy may prove more consistently helpful. In my opinion, a truly reliable noninvasive diagnostic procedure will not emerge until a substantive technical change is developed, overcoming the inherent limitations of the Papanicolaou smear when applied to urine. (Refer to discussion of cytology of bladder neoplasms, Chap. 4.)

Gross Features.   The majority of renal pelvic transitional cell carcinomas are exophytic papillary lesions (Fig. 2-8). Fewer cases show both exophytic and infiltrative features, and the least common variety is predominantly infiltrative, frequently with associated surface necrosis and ulceration. These gross features are correlated with the tumor grade as subsequently observed on microscopic review: low grade neoplasms tend to be exophytic, whereas high grade neoplasms tend to be predominantly infiltrating. The extent of renal pelvic involvement varies. The majority arise from the extrarenal pelvis. Fewer cases originate from the calyces and intrarenal pelvis. Lesions located at the ureteropelvic junction, or larger exophytic neoplasms elsewhere in the pelvis, commonly produce obstruc-

Table 2-7   **Grade Distribution for Transitional Cell Carcinoma**

Author	Year	Number of Patients	Grade (%)			
			1	2	3	4
Cummings et al[123]	1975	35	11	34	29	26
Rubenstein et al[132]	1978	70	18	42	22	18
Johansson, Wahlqvist[133]	1979	108	5	42	39	15
Williams, Mitchell[118]	1973	43	46	35	19	
Nocks et al[136]	1982	68	7	44	49	

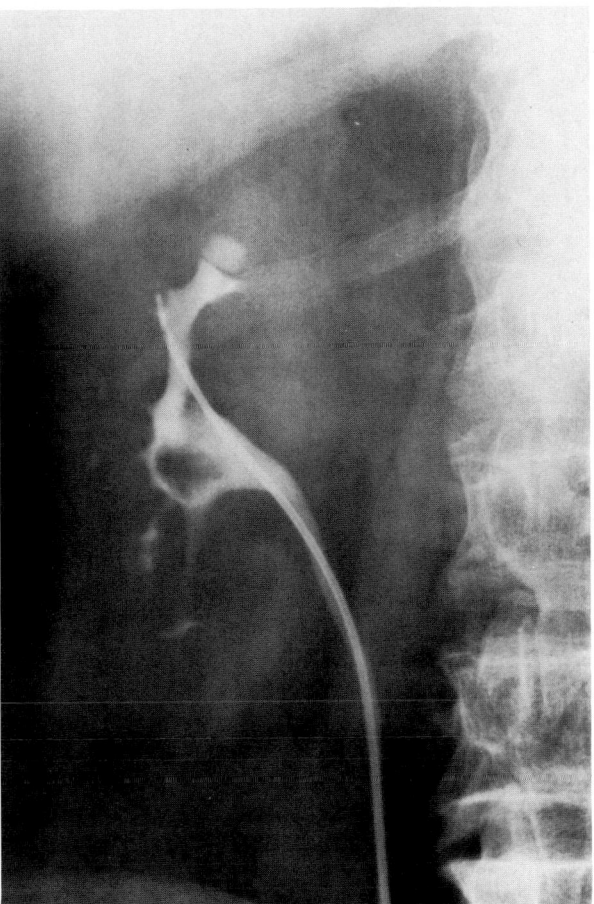

Figure 2-8   *Transitional cell carcinoma of the renal pelvis. A
retrograde pyelogram shows a 1.5-cm exophytic mass of the
renal pelvic wall. The lesion was found to be a transitional
cell carcinoma, confirming the radiologic diagnosis. The
differential diagnosis includes other intrinsic lesions of the
renal pelvis, such as nonopaque stone, sloughed papillae,
and benign epithelial or stromal neoplasms.*

tion and dilatation of the more proximal pelvocalyceal system. Invasion of the
wall of subjacent renal pelvic wall and adjacent peripelvic retroperitoneum or the
adjacent renal medullary parenchyma may be apparent on gross examination. On
occasion, more extensive invasion of the renal parenchyma or peripelvic peritoneum, or both, is readily apparent (Fig. 2-9).

Microscopic Features.   Table 2-7 presents the reported grade distribution of
renal pelvic transitional cell carcinomas. Both the traditional four-grade system
and the World Health Organization three-grade system have been used in the
studies published in the last decade. (Refer to discussion of tumor grading in
Chap. 4.) Because of the wide range of reported frequencies of the respective
grades in these studies, few generalized conclusions can be made from the data.
However, regardless of the grading system applied, the moderately differentiated

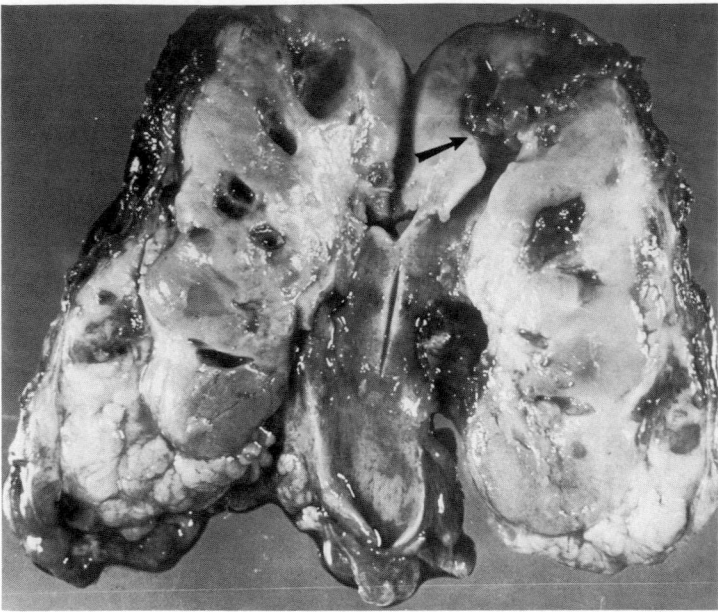

Figure 2-9   ***Transitional cell carcinoma of the renal pelvis.*** *The tumor protrudes into the pelvis and invades the kidney* (arrow).

papillary transitional cell neoplasms are most common, with fewer cases of very well differentiated (low grade) and poorly differentiated (high grade) tumors. Nocks and co-workers have demonstrated the correlation of tumor grade and tumor stage, with the majority of grade 1 and 2 tumors evidencing minimal or absence of invasion.[136] Conversely, most high grade neoplasms are found to be high stage at the time of diagnosis.

Tumor spread occurs along the pelvic mucosa with retrograde involvement of the renal collecting ducts commonly observed. In some cases extensive intratubular spread, occasionally reaching the cortex, is seen. This mucosal spread may be localized or extensive (Figs. 2-10 to 2-12). Recently published mapping studies have demonstrated hyperplasia and dysplasia in the urothelium adjacent to transitional cell carcinomas at this site.[74,139] Similar findings were documented previously in transitional cell carcinomas of the urinary bladder. (Refer to Chap. 4.)

On rare occasions carcinoma in situ is observed in the renal pelvis and ureter in the absence of accompanying papillary transitional cell carcinoma.[115,121,135] Microscopic hematuria is detected in the majority of reported patients. The clinical management of patients with positive urine cytology preparations, and neither radiologic nor biopsy evidence of accompanying neoplasms, is problematic. The cytologic features of carcinoma in situ are more evidently malignant than that observed in the cells shed from low grade papillary transitional cell carcinoma.[115,121,135]

Direct tumor invasion of the renal pelvic wall and contiguous renal parenchyma and peripelvic retroperitoneum is common, and its presence and extent should be documented in the final surgical pathology report.

Uncommonly, transitional cell carcinomas will show focal squamous differentiation. This is most frequently observed in high grade (3 and 4) tumors. The

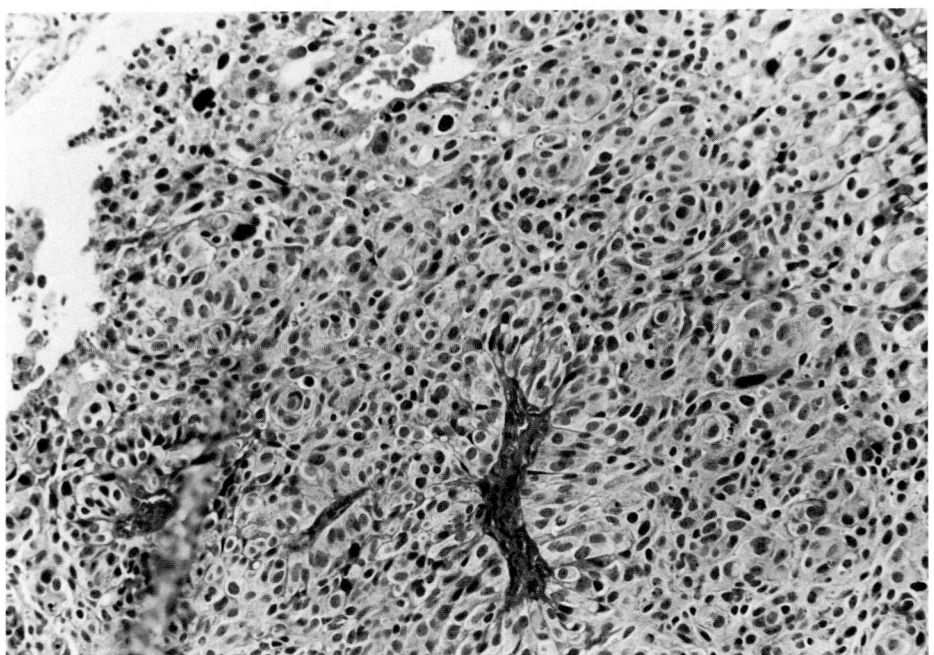

Figure 2-10 **Transitional cell carcinoma, grade 3.** *The papillary nature of the tumor was evident only by the scattered fibrovascular central cores, such as those present in the center. Individual papillary projections were not present but had merged into a single, irregular exophytic mass emanating from the renal pelvic mucosa.*

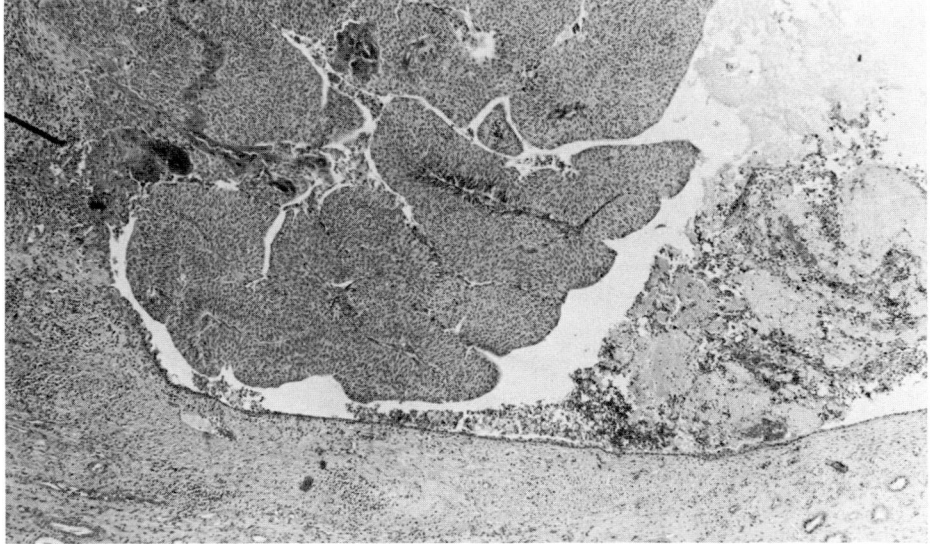

Figure 2-11 **Transitional cell carcinoma, grade 1.** *The papillary neoplasm arises from the renal pelvic urothelium, projects into the lumen, and invades the underlying renal pyramid.*

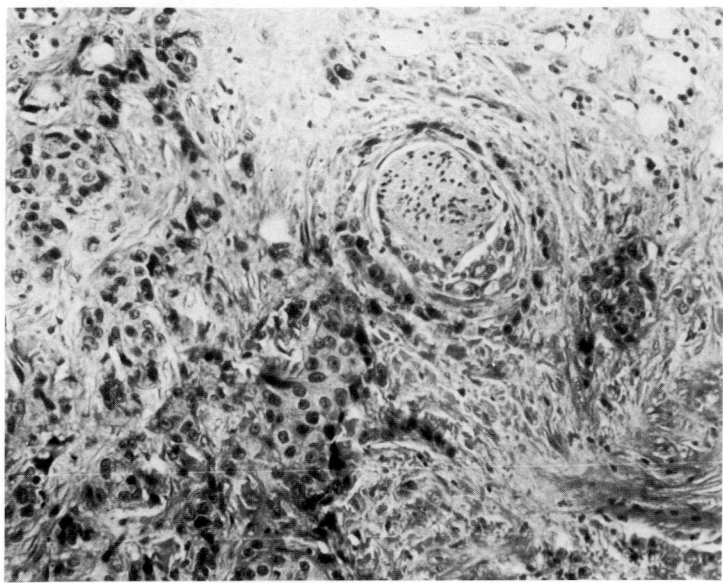

Figure 2-12   *Transitional cell carcinoma, grade 3. The tumor has invaded the hilar adipose tissue and shows perineural invasion.*

low grade tumors characteristically tend to be uniformly composed of transitional cells arranged in a papillary configuration. Invasion of the renal pelvic wall, renal parenchyma, and perirenal retroperitoneum is associated rather consistently with a disappearance of the papillary histologic configuration, and the invading tumors are disposed in nests, cords, and sheets of malignant cells with an accompanying desmoplastic response.

Vascular and lymphatic invasion may be present and should be included in the final report. The presence of any hilar lymph nodes accompanying the specimen should be determined and possible metastases from the renal pelvic primary evaluated. Although formal mapping studies of the pelvic and ureteral urothelium may be excessive in the routine study of these neoplasms, certainly additional sections of the ureter, most importantly of the ureteral resection margin, must be included in the complete review of each specimen received.

The extent of tumor dissemination of renal pelvic carcinoma recorded in four studies is presented in Table 2-8. As with tumor grade distribution, significant variation among the four studies is noted. Thirty percent to sixty percent of

Table 2-8   **Stage Distribution for Transitional Cell Carcinoma**

Author	Year	Number of Patients	Stage (%)			
			A	B	C	D
Wagle et al[119]	1974	78	14	27	28	31
Cummings et al[123]	1975	35	11	34	29	23
Rubenstein et al[132]	1978	70	39	27	20	14
Nocks et al[136]	1982	68	46	9	16	29

the cases reported have spread beyond the renal pelvic wall at the time of diagnosis. As outlined in Table 2-9, both tumor grade and tumor stage are closely correlated with patient survival at 5 years.

Natural History

The natural history of urothelial neoplasms, including renal pelvic transitional cell carcinoma, requires considerations of the evolution of the primary neoplasms, and attention to the significant frequency of associated urothelial neoplasms.

Survival

The survival rate of patients with diagnosed renal pelvic transitional cell carcinoma is correlated with both tumor grade and stage. The overall survival of patients with this tumor is presented in Table 2-5. The limited survival data available referable to tumor grade and tumor stage are recorded in Table 2-9. Over the past 40 years little progress has been achieved in the overall survival rate at 5 years. The reported 5-year survival rates ranges from 14% to 57%, with most studies recording overall survival rates of 20% to 45% (Table 2-5). These figures tend to mask the high survival rates achieved among patients with low grade and especially low stage neoplasms (Table 2-9). Tumors that have infiltrated beyond the renal pelvis (stage C) are associated with low survival (35% or less at 5 years). Virtually all patients with stage D neoplasms at the time of initial presentation succumb to their malignancy within 3 years. Regional and distant metastases are observed most commonly in the lungs, liver, para-aortic lymph nodes, and bone.[109,116,124,125] Uncommon sites reported include brain, heart, and vagina.[109,116,124,125]

RBC Adherence Studies

Limited studies of red cell adherence test applied to renal pelvic and ureteral transitional cell carcinomas have demonstrated a high overall correlation of the clinical behavior of these neoplasms and the presence or absence of these cell surface antigens.[137,138] The retention of the surface antigens is associated with absence of invasion, whereas their loss from the surface of the malignant cells is observed frequently in invasive tumors.

Table 2-9   *Grades and Stages of Transitional Cell Carcinoma Compared with 5-Year Survival Rates*

Author	Year	5-Year Survival (%)			
		Grade 1	*Grade 2*	*Grade 3*	*Grade 4*
Rubenstein et al[132]	1978	88	33	11	0
Nocks et al[136]	1982	100	90	23	0
		Stage I	*Stage II*	*Stage III*	*Stage IV*
Cummings et al[123]	1975	100	75	0	0
Rubenstein et al[132]	1978	63	43	0	0
Johansson, Wahlqvist[133]	1979	88	65	24	
Nocks et al[136]	1982	100	65	34	0

Multiple Neoplasms

In common with urothelial tumors throughout the urinary tract, transitional cell carcinomas of the renal pelvis demonstrate a significant frequency of associated urothelial neoplasms. This propensity for multicentricity has been recognized since the early part of this century. Lower found 18 cases of multiple tumors reported prior to 1914.[140] Additional cases subsequently were reported by Thomas, Regnier (1924), Scholl (1924), Hunt (1927), and others.[141-145] Kimball and Ferris found 74 multiple urothelial neoplasms in a review of the world literature in 1934.[150] Of these 74 cases, 48 involved patients with renal pelvic neoplasms in association with second tumors in the ureter or bladder. Approximately half of these cases involved metachronous tumors. Of the metachronous group, the second tumor was diagnosed within 3 years of the first diagnosed tumor in 85% of cases.[150]

Recognition of the occurrence and frequency of cases with multiple tumors initiated two debates that remain unresolved to this time. The first question centers around the pathogenesis of the multiple tumors, and the second relates to the determination of the most appropriate surgical procedure for upper urinary tract neoplasms. In summary, the pathogenesis of the multiple neoplasms has been interpreted variously as "drop metastases," or indications of a field effect, resulting from exposure of the entire urinary tract to carcinogens in the urine. Suffice it to say that an unequivocal case of "drop metastasis" has never been presented. The most substantive support for this hypothesis is indirect: the frequency of ipsilateral multiple tumors exceeds that of bilateral neoplasms. The question of appropriate surgical therapy addresses itself to the frequency and significance of second tumors (or drop metastases) in the ureteral stump when a nephrectomy is combined with an incomplete ureterectomy (as opposed to complete ureterectomy with bladder cuff removal). Although the relatively high frequency is not debated (refer to Table 2-11), the significance of these second neoplasms referable to ultimate patient survival remains controversial.

The frequency of multiple neoplasms associated with renal pelvic transitional cell carcinoma, as reported in the more recent literature, is summarized below.

Bilateral renal pelvic neoplasms. Forty-two cases of bilateral renal pelvic transitional cell carcinomas were found in the literature (Table 2-10). Eleven of these cases were synchronous and 19 were metachronous, with intervals of 6 months to 19 years separating the diagnoses of the tumors. The time of occurrence was not given in 12 cases. Associated ureteral and bladder tumors were recorded in 11 (26%) of these patients.

Simultaneous ureteral and bladder neoplasms. Synchronous transitional cell carcinoma of the ureter has been reported in an average of 20% of 9 reported series (range: 4% to 38%). Simultaneous bladder neoplasms were diagnosed in an average of 13% of 187 reported cases of renal pelvic transitional cell carcinomas (Tables 2-11 and 2-12).

Previous ureteral and bladder neoplasms. Ureteral and bladder carcinomas are diagnosed prior to the diagnosis of renal pelvic carcinoma in an average of 8% of cases with a reported range of 3% to 14% (Table 2-13).

Subsequent ureteral neoplasms. Twelve percent of 191 reported cases of renal pelvic patients whose renal pelvic primary tumors were treated with nephrec-

Table 2-10 **Bilateral Transitional Cell Carcinoma**

Author	Year	Age	Sex	Comments
Sanford[147]	1931	56	M	Synchronous
Macalpine[156]	1947	47	M	Synchronous*
Colston, Arcadi[159]	1955	57	F	Metachronous, 3 yr*
Colston[160]	1960	86	M	Metachronous, 14 yr
Potampa, Schneider[161]	1961	66	M	Metachronous, 19 yr
Harvard, Evans[163]	1964	75	F	Synchronous
Carroll[164]	1965	51	M	Metachronous, 13 yr*
Gibson[165]	1967	86	M	Metachronous, 12 yr
Grace et al[114]	1968	NI	NI	NI, 1 case of series
Grabstald et al[116]	1971	NI	NI	Metachronous, 25 mo*
Grabstald et al[116]	1971	NI	NI	Metachronous, 34 mo*
Grabstald et al[116]	1971	NI	NI	Synchronous*
Grabstald et al[116]	1971	NI	NI	Metachronous, 5 yr*
Grabstald et al[116]	1971	NI	NI	Metachronous, 14 mo*
Gillis et al[168]	1971	72	F	Metachronous†
Wagle et al[119]	1974	NI	NI	Synchronous
Johnson et al[120]	1974	NI	NI	Synchronous
Johnson et al[120]	1974	NI	NI	Synchronous
Johnson et al[120]	1974	NI	NI	Synchronous
Johnson et al[120]	1974	NI	NI	Metachronous, 18 mo
Johnson et al[120]	1974	NI	NI	Metachronous, 18 mo
Donnelly, Koontz[124]	1975	NI	NI	Metachronous, 6 mo
Bogaard, Goldstein[170]	1975	55	F	Synchronous
McLoughlin[171]	1975	35	M	Synchronous
Strong, Pearse[131]	1976	NI	F	Metachronous, 3 yr‡
Augspurger, Peterson[173]	1977	73	M	Metachronous, 14 yr*
Petkovic[106]	1978			See footnote§
Rubenstein et al[132]	1978	NI	NI	Metachronous, NI
Rubenstein et al[132]	1978	NI	NI	Metachronous, NI
Ross, Pressman[177]	1979	50	M	Metachronous, 6 mo
Murphy et al[178]	1980	NI	NI	Synchronous
Nocks et al[136]	1982	NI	NI	Metachronous, 2 yr

* Associated bladder TCC.

† Associated bladder and ureter TCC.

‡ Associated bladder TCC and renal adenocarcinoma.

§ Details of 12 cases of bilateral renal pelvic malignancies combined with 15 cases of bilateral ureteral neoplasms and 18 cases of renal pelvic and contralateral ureteral neoplasms. The combined 45 cases represent a 9% frequency of bilaterality of pelvic and ureteral neoplasms studied in one clinic in Belgrade, Yugoslavia. The association of these neoplasms with Balkan nephropathy, endemic in some areas of Yugoslavia, is noted by the author.

Table 2-11   **Transitional Cell Carcinoma and Associated Ureteral Neoplasms**

Author	Year	Frequency (%)	
Simultaneous Ureteral Neoplasms			
Cabot, Allen[148]	1933	17.8	
McDonald, Priestley[80]	1944	26.7	
Taylor[111]	1959	31.2	
Newman et al[113]	1968	18.8	99/499 (19.8%)*
Grace et al[114]	1968	8.1	
Wagle et al[119]	1974	38.5	
Donnally, Koontz[124]	1975	4.5	
Rubenstein et al[132]	1978	9.0	
Subsequent Ureteral Neoplasms: Nephrectomy			
Kinder, Wallace[162]	1963	56	22/44 (50%)*
Strong, Pearse[131]	1974	42	
Subsequent Ureteral Neoplasms: Nephrectomy with Incomplete Ureterectomy			
Cabot, Allen[148]	1933	3.8	
Kinder, Wallace[162]	1963	33.0	
Strong, Pearse[131]	1974	6.6	22/191 (11.5%)*
Rubenstein et al[132]	1978	16.0	
Johansson, Wahlqvist[133]	1979	4.0	
Nocks et al[136]	1982	18.0	

* Cumulative frequency (all studies).

Table 2-12   **Transitional Cell Carcinoma and Associated Bladder Neoplasms**

Author	Year	Frequency (%)	
Simultaneous Bladder Neoplasms			
Taylor[111]	1959	15.6	
Williams, Mitchell[118]	1973	6.9	
Donnelly, Koontz[124]	1975	18.2	26/204 (13%)*
Leong et al[128]	1976	35.3	
Johansson, Wahlqvist[133]	1979	7.4	
Subsequent Bladder Neoplasms			
Cabot, Allen[148]	1933	8.9	
McDonald, Priestly[80]	1944	22.7	
Taylor[111]	1959	22.0	
Williams, Mitchell[118]	1973	46.0	86/421 (20%)*
Rubenstein et al[132]	1978	20.0	
Johansson, Wahlqvist[133]	1979	15.0	
Nocks et al[136]	1982	21.0	

* Cumulative frequency (all studies).

Table 2-13   ***Frequency of Previous Ureteral or Bladder Carcinoma***

Author	Year	Frequency (%)	
Grace et al[114]	1968	14 ⎫	
Cummings et al[123]	1975	9 ⎪	17/210 (8%) *
Johansson, Wahlqvist[133]	1979	3 ⎬	
Nocks et al[136]	1982	10 ⎭	

* Cumulative frequency (all studies).

tomy and incomplete ureterectomy, subsequently developed transitional cell carcinoma in the ureteral stump. Twenty percent of patients with renal pelvic primaries subsequently have a bladder transitional cell carcinoma (Table 2-11).

Transitional cell carcinomas of the ureter and bladder demonstrate this same tendency of multicentricity with an even greater frequency. (Refer to Chap. 3 and 4.)

Finally, mention is made of 21 reported cases of renal pelvic transitional cell carcinoma occurring in kidneys harboring a concurrent renal cell carcinoma (Table 2-14). The same combination of tumors, involving opposite kidneys has been reported on five occasions.[152,166,172,176]

Table 2-14   ***Simultaneous Renal Pelvic Transitional Cell Carcinoma and Renal Cell Carcinoma in the Same Kidney***

Author	Year	Age	Sex	Side Affected
Graves, Templeton[141]	1921	52	M	Left
Patch, Rhea[144]	1924	68	M	Left
deVries[146]	1930	57	M	Left (horseshoe kidney)
Wildbolz[149]	1933	NI	NI	NI
Balch[151]	1935	63	M	Left
Dick[153]	1942	51	F	Left
Melicow[154]	1945	65	M	Right
McAlpine[156]	1947	72	F	Left
Rupel, Sutton[157]	1950	58	F	Left
Kline et al[158]	1955	47	NI	Left
Walker, Jordan[167]	1968	70	F	Left
Gillis et al[168]	1971	72	F	Left
Grabstald et al[116]	1971	NI	NI	NI
Wagle et al[119]	1974	NI	NI	NI
Fallon, Schellhammer[169]	1975	58	M	Left
Strong, Pearse[131]	1976	NI	NI	NI
Strong, Pearse[131]	1976	NI	NI	NI
Strong, Pearse[131]	1976	NI	NI	NI
Voneschenbach et al[174]	1977	61	M	Right
Anseline, Howarth[175]	1977	68	F	Left
Lundell et al[179]	1982	73	M	Left

Squamous Cell Carcinoma

Squamous cell carcinoma of the renal pelvis, the second most frequent primary epithelial malignancy of this site, has been reported in approximately 250 patients (Table 2-15). Gahagan and Reed presented three cases and found 103 cases reported prior to 1949.[182] The largest series was reported by Riches and co-workers (69 cases) in 1951.[109] Table 2-15 reflects the recorded experience with this uncommon neoplasm in the recent literature. Squamous cell carcinomas of the renal pelvis are approximately six times more frequent than in the ureter, where it has been reported 43 times. (Refer to squamous cell carcinoma in Chap. 3.)

This neoplasm occurs most frequently in males (55%) during the sixth and seventh decades (see Table 2-15). The youngest and oldest recorded patients are 3 years and 92 years, respectively.[182,197] The right and left kidneys are equally affected. Bilateral squamous cell carcinoma has been reported once, and two reported cases occurring in horseshoe kidneys appear in the literature.[190,194,197] Associated calculus disease is observed in 14% to 57% of reported cases (see Table 2-15).

The patients commonly have a palpable mass (75%), with hematuria and flank pain reported in 50% to 100% and 45% of cases, respectively. Hypercalcemia has been reported rarely in association with renal pelvic squamous cell carcinomas.[194,198]

The majority of reported cases have invaded the pelvic wall, and contiguously into the adjacent peripelvic adipose tissue when first diagnosed. Gross examination of the nephrectomy specimen discloses that the exophytic component is overshadowed by the local infiltration of the kidney, peripelvic tissues, or both. Areas of necrosis are common.

Histologically, the typical case is a moderately to poorly differentiated squamous cell malignancy. The squamous differentiation must not be focal, but rather present diffusely throughout the neoplasm to justify the diagnosis of squamous cell carcinoma. Focal squamous cell differentiation of transitional cell carcinomas, particularly high grade examples, is not rare. (This is true of transitional cell carcinomas regardless of site of origin.) Such tumors should be classified as transitional cell carcinomas with focal squamous differentiation, and not

Table 2-15   **Squamous Cell Carcinoma**

Author	Year	Cases	Sex	
			M	F
Gahagan, Reed[182]	1949	106(3)	55%	45%
Oberkircher et al[184]	1951	15	6%	9%
Utz, McDonald[189]	1957	23	86%	14%
Seth-Smith[191]	1959	25	48%	52%
Wagle et al[196]	1974	12	67%	33%
Latham, Kay[197]	1974	8	75%	25%
Donnelly, Koontz[124]	1974	9	77%	23%
Rafla[125]	1975	14	64%	36%
Johansson et al[127]	1976	8	12%	88%

squamous cell carcinoma, conceding that the natural history of renal pelvic squamous cell carcinomas, and high grade transitional cell carcinomas, with focal squamous change, has not been shown to be significantly different. The presence of associated squamous metaplasia of the adjacent pelvic urothelium has been reported in 7% to 33% of cases (see Table 2-15). The true frequency of this change is unknown, because comment on this feature is found in only a small percentage of available studies.

The aggressive behavior of this tumor (compared to renal pelvic transitional cell carcinomas as a group) is reflected in the higher frequency of local and regional dissemination (high stage), and the significantly lower survival rate: only 12 patients are reported to have survived 5 years.[125,127,181,189,192,196,199]

The cause of this neoplasm is unknown. The etiologic and epidemiologic factors identified referable to transitional cell carcinoma, including industrial exposure to "dyes," phenacetin abuse, and Balkan nephritis have not been found associated with squamous cell carcinoma. A recent case report describes a right renal pelvic squamous cell carcinoma developing in a patient who received external radiation to a hepatic hemangioma on two occasions, 20 and 12 years previously.[200] A higher frequency of associated chronic inflammation and lithiasis is observed with renal pelvic squamous cell carcinomas than that observed with transitional cell carcinoma (see Tables 2-5, 2-15). The role of these factors in the causation of squamous cell carcinoma, if any, is currently unknown. No reported case of clinically diagnosed squamous metaplasia of the renal pelvis has ever undergone malignant change.[76]

Adenocarcinoma

Adenocarcinoma, which is a rare neoplasm, was first described in the renal pelvis by Grohe in 1901.[201] Ackerman reported the first case in the American literature 45 years later (1946).[203] Aufderheide and Streitz reported two cases and reviewed the literature in 1974.[226] Additional cases have appeared subsequent to their review.[227-236] A total of 46 cases were found in the literature to 1984 (Table 2-16). This number compares with 15 adenocarcinomas reported in the ureter. (Refer to adenocarcinoma, Chap. 3.) The sex distribution among the recorded cases is equal in contrast to the male predominance observed with both transi-

(Text continues on p. 214.)

Age		Side	Calculi (%)	Metaplasia (%)	Follow-Up
Range	Mean	L/R			
3–79	55	L = R	48	8	0% 5-YSR; 50% 6-MSR
43–81	62	7/8	26	7	27% 1-YSR; 0% 5-YSR
42–70	54	10/13	57	17	21% 5-YSR
35–77	59	8/13	28		0% 5-YSR; (NI—9 cases)
48–86	67	6/6	33	33	33% 1-YSR; 8.3% 5-YSR
35–92	64	4/4	43		12% 2-YSR
	64	3/6	33		22% 2-YSR
		L = R	14		14% 5-YSR
			37		20% 5-YSR

Table 2-16 *Adenocarcinoma*

Author	Year	Age	Sex
Grohe[201]	1901	58	F
Grohe[201]	1901	60	M
Pachkis[202]	1909	47	M
Ackerman[203]	1946	66	M
Ragins, Rolnick[204]	1950	51	F
Anderson[205]	1955	63	F
Arcadi[206]	1956	68	M
Stone, Baer[226]	1957	57	M
Kennedy, Fidler[207]	1958	70	F
Kennedy, Fidler[207]	1958	74	M
Seth-Smith[208]	1959	49	F
Hasebe et al[209]	1960	60	M
Emson[210]	1962	45	F
Ashley, Hickey[212]	1964	38	F
Ashley, Hickey[212]	1964	40	M
Lopez Engelking et al[211]	1964	50	F
Schrodt[213]	1964	72	F
Suzuki, Siminovich[214]	1965	52	F
Saxena et al[215]	1966	40	M
Wahal[216]	1966	52	M
Jain[217]	1967	44	F
Suzuki, Milan[218]	1967	87	F
Hayahara et al[220]	1968	30	M
Quattelbaum, Shirley[219]	1968	61	M
Quattelbaum, Shirley[219]	1968	69	M
Toyoda, Hirakata[221]	1969	55	F
Murphy, Stevenson[222]	1970	42	F
Kataria, Shanker[223]	1973	45	F
Solov, Martines[225]	1974	74	M
Aguilo, Furlow[224]	1974	47	M
Aguilo, Furlow[224]	1974	65	M
Aguilo, Furlow[224]	1974	61	F
Aufderheide, Streitz[226]	1974	40	M
Aufderheide, Streitz[226]	1974	49	M
Guha[227]	1975	45	F
Liwnicz et al[228]	1975	62	F
Filimon et al[229]	1977	34	F
Bhargava et al[230]	1979	60	M
O'Brien et al[232]	1980	13	F
Brawer, Waisman[233]	1980	37	M
Pujari et al[231]	1980	32	F
Kulkarni et al[234]	1981	50	M
Kutscher et al[235]	1982	58	F
Kobayashi et al[236]	1983	57	M
Kobayashi et al[236]	1983	64	F

Lithiasis, Inflammation	Mucin Stain	Associated Metaplasia	Stage	Follow-up Information
O	NI	O	NI	NI
O	NI	O	NI	NI
O	+	+	2	Alive, NED, 7 mo
+	+	+	NI	Dead with tumor, 6 yr
+	+	NI	3	Dead with tumor, 11 mo
+	+	+	NI	Alive, NED, 14 mo
+	+	+	3	Alive, NED, 16 mo
+	+	NI	3	Dead with tumor, 6 mo
+	+	+	2, ?3	Dead with tumor, 5 mo
O	+	O	3	Alive, NED 25 mo
O	+	O	4	Dead with tumor, 4 yr
+	O	NI	NI	Dead with tumor, 10 yr
+	+	+	4	Alive, NED, 7 mo
+	+	+	2	Alive, NED, 5 yr
+	+	NI	NI	Alive, NED, 5 yr
+	+	NI	NI	NI
+	+	+	4	Dead with tumor, 1 yr
O	+	+	4	Dead with tumor, 7 mo
O	+	+	2	Dead; postoperative
O	+	+	2	Alive, 5 mo
+	+	O	4	Postoperative death
O	+	NI	4	Dead with tumor, 7 mo
O	NI	+	NI	NI
O	+	NI	NI	Alive, NED, 2 yr
O	+	NI	NI	Alive, NED, 6 mo
+	+	NI	4	Dead with tumor
+	+	NI	4	Lost to follow-up, 2 mo
+	+	NI	3	Dead with tumor
O	+	NI	2	At post
+	+	NI	4	Dead with tumor, 6 mo
O	+	NI	4	Dead with tumor, 8 mo
O	+	NI	3	Alive, NED, 4 mo
+	+	O	4	Dead with tumor, 4 mo
+	+	O	1	Alive, NED, 20 mo
+	+	NI	NI	NI
+	+	+	3	Dead postoperatively, 1 day
O	+	NI	2	Alive with tumor 1 yr
+	+	+	3	NI
+	O	+	2, ?3	Alive, NED, 7 mo
O	+	+	4	Dead with tumor, 4 mo
NI	+	NI	NI	Alive, NED, 1.5 yr
+	O	O	NI	NI
+	+	O	4	Alive with tumor, 5+ yr
O	+	+	3	Dead with tumor, 3 mo
+	+	+	4	Alive, NED, 2 yr

+, present; O, not present; NI, no information; NED, no evidence of disease.

tional cell carcinoma and squamous cell carcinoma of the renal pelvis. The mean age is 60 years, with the peak frequency in the sixth and seventh decades (48%). Thirty-nine percent of cases have been reported in patients younger than 50 years, the youngest being 13 years old.[232] The right and left kidneys are equally affected.

Hematuria is significantly less frequent (33%) than that observed with transitional cell carcinomas (90%). Fifty percent of the reported patients complain of flank pain, while 33% have a detectable mass.

The neoplasm is characteristically mucinous. Lithiasis is observed in 60% of cases, a frequency far exceeding that reported with transitional cell carcinoma of the same site. The majority of the reported cases demonstrate invasion of the pelvic wall and adjacent peripelvic adipose tissue at the time of surgery.

Histologically, renal pelvic adenocarcinomas show a papillary, glandular–papillary or signet-ring cell pattern. The similarity of many of these neoplasms to colonic adenocarcinomas is striking. The mucin production varies among tumors and in different areas of the same neoplasm. Mucin may be scant and may be detected only with appropriate staining, or alternatively may be present in pools in which signet-ring cells are observed. Intracellular mucin can be so abundant that the neoplastic nature of the lesion is determined with difficulty if reliance is placed only on evaluation of nuclear features. The presence of invasion and complex gland-in-gland formation are histologic features indicating malignancy (Figs. 2-13, 2-14). Associated glandular metaplasia has been reported in the adjacent pelvic mucosa in 50% of cases. The true frequency of glandular metaplasia is probably higher, because no reference was made to this feature in many reports. Occasional cases have noted foci of squamous metaplasia in the uninvolved renal pelvic mucosa. Histologic evidence of chronic inflammation of the renal pelvis and parenchyma is common.

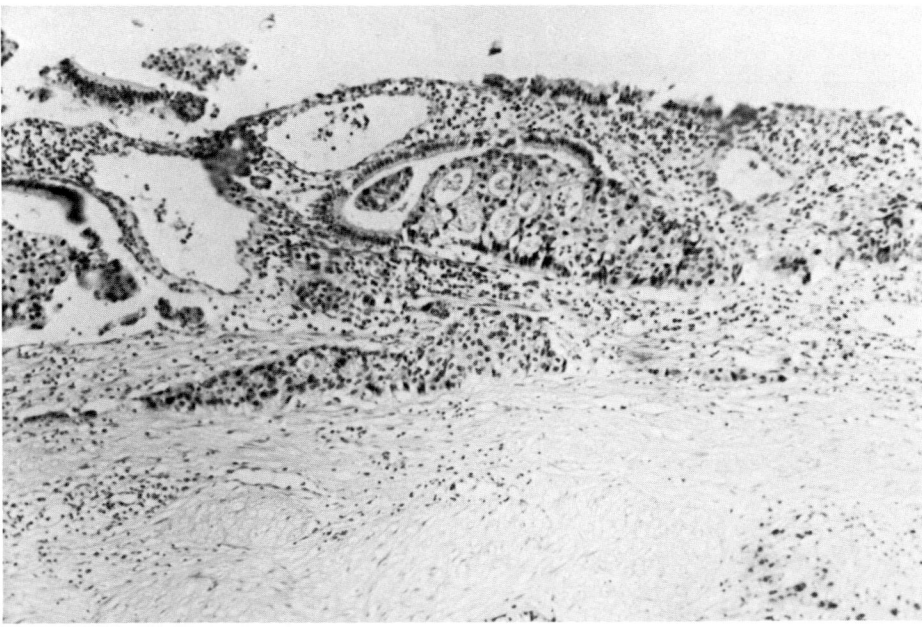

Figure 2-13   *Adenocarcinoma of the renal pelvis. Neoplastic glands, some showing cribiform pattern, are invading the wall of renal pelvis.*

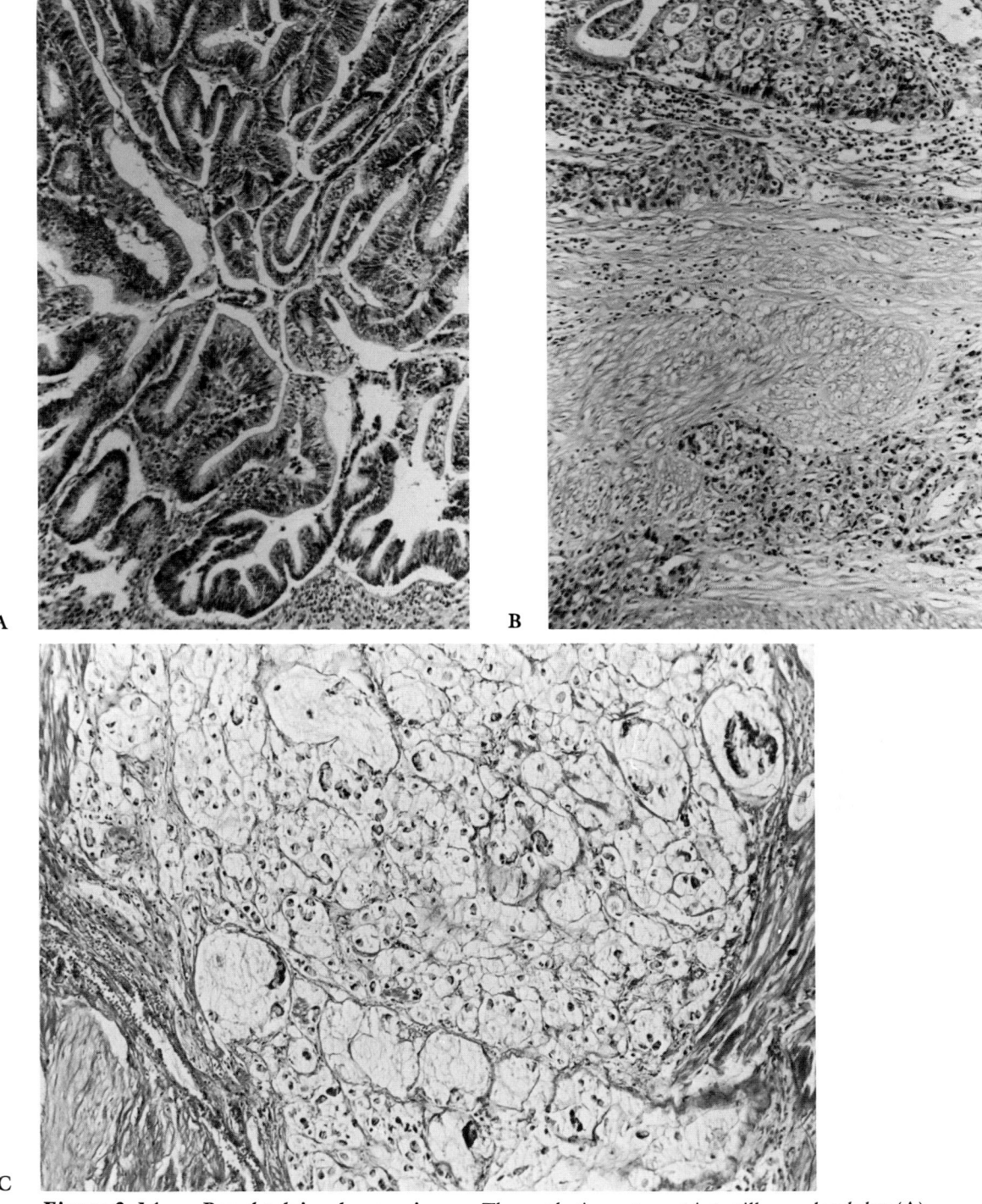

Figure 2-14 **Renal pelvic adenocarcinoma.** *The exophytic component is papillary–glandular* (A), *which changes to a glandular pattern in the invasive nests with the wall of the renal pelvis* (B). *Other areas show prominent mucin production by tumor cells in solid nests* (C).

Reflecting the higher frequency of palpable mass observed with renal pelvic adenocarcinoma than with transitional cell carcinomas, the majority of the former are found to be stage III and IV. Follow-up information is limited in many reported cases. Five of the 47 patients found in the literature survived 5 years.[203,209,212,235]

Malignant Epithelial Neoplasms with Mixed Differentiation and Undifferentiated Carcinoma

Urothelial neoplasms on occasion show variable differentiation.[237,238] Most commonly this takes the form of focal areas of squamous differentiation in an otherwise uniformly high grade transitional cell carcinoma. Mixtures of transitional cell carcinoma with focal gland formation, with evident mucin production, are observed uncommonly. This is to be differentiated from the more common pseudogland formation present in transitional cell carcinomas of high grade.

Alternatively, some malignant epithelial neoplasms are neither recognizable as transitional cell carcinomas nor do they show glandular or squamous differentiation. These undifferentiated carcinomas tend to be uniformly aggressive high stage neoplasms.

Mesenchymal Neoplasms

Hemangioma

Hemangioma, which is a benign vascular neoplasm, has been reported in 17 patients. Lazarus and Marks collected 11 cases in the literature prior to 1947.[239] Six cases have been reported subsequently.[240-243]

Right and left kidneys are equally affected, and there is no sex predilection. The reported age range is 8 years to 62 years, but approximately half of the patients are in the fourth and fifth decades. Hematuria is the most common presenting complaint.

Microscopically, multiple thin-walled vascular channels of varying size located immediately beneath the pelvic mucosa account for the dark red–blue blebs observed macroscopically. Flattened endothelial lining cells are characteristic.

The majority of reported cases are correctly diagnosed only at the time of postoperative examination. Andersen and Rasmussen reported the preoperative radiologic diagnosis of a renal hemangioma utilizing selective renal angiography.[243]

Leiomyoma

Benign smooth muscle neoplasms taking origin in the renal pelvis have been reported in four women between the ages of 24 years and 50 years.[244-247] Female preponderance is observed in both benign and malignant smooth muscle neoplasms not only of the renal pelvis but also of the ureter and urethra. The opposite is true of bladder smooth muscle neoplasms where they are more common in males. (Refer to Chap. 4.)

Flank pain is the most common clinical presentation. Radiologic procedures detect the intrapelvic mass, commonly in association with renal pelvic dilatation. The neoplasm is well demarcated.

Histologically, the neoplasm is characterized by interlacing fascicles of cytologically benign smooth muscle cells. Rare, or no, mitotic figures are present. The neoplasm is differentiated from the malignant counterpart by absence of invasion, low mitotic activity, absence of numerous bizarre cells, and presence of relatively uniform spindle nuclei.

Leiomyosarcoma

Eight renal pelvic leiomyosarcomas could be found in the literature.[248-252] This compares with 11 cases recorded in the ureter. (Refer to Chap. 3.) The sex of the patient was indicated in three of the eight reported cases, all female.[248,251,252] The age range of the reported cases is 23 years to 61 years.[248,251,252] Flank pain with or without associated hematuria is the most common clinical presentation. The neoplasm can produce a filling defect detectable on IVP, but this is not a constant finding.[248,249,251]

Microscopically, the malignant nature of the tumor is associated with increased cellularity, nuclear pleomorphism, and hyperchromaticity, numerous mitoses, tumor necrosis, and local invasion.

The reported cases have been surgically excised. I am unaware of any patients surviving five years.

Malignant Mixed Neoplasms

Carcinosarcoma

Simultaneous epithelial and stromal malignancies occurring in the renal pelvis have been reported in five patients.[254-258] Only two of these cases represent carcinosarcomas.[257,258] The cases reported by Fauci and co-workers,[254] Elliott and colleagues,[255] and Gallagher and associates[256] are examples of the chance occurrence of a renal sarcoma and a transitional cell carcinoma arising independently in the same renal pelvis. The diagnosis of carcinosarcoma requires the exclusion of cases showing (1) an independent carcinoma and sarcoma as exemplified by the case cited above; (2) anaplastic spindle cell change of a high grade transitional cell carcinoma; and (3) benign metaplastic stromal changes (chondroid, osteoid) in association with an epithelial malignancy.[253] The two cases appropriately regarded as carcinosarcomas involved patients (one female and one male) in the seventh decade.

References

Normal Structure

1. Parker AE: Studies on the main posterior lymph channels of the abdomen and their connections with the lymphatics of the genito-urinary system. Am J Anat 56:409, 1935
2. Narath PA: The hydromechanics of the calyx renalis. J. Urol 43:145, 1940

3. Murnaghan GF: The dynamics of the renal pelvis and ureter with reference to congenital hydronephrosis. Br J Urol 30:321, 1958
4. Hanna MK, Jeffs RD, Sturgess JM et al: Ureteral structure and ultrastructure. Part II. Congenital ureteropelvic junction obstruction and primary obstructive megaureter. J Urol 116:725, 1976

Calyceal Diverticulum

5. Weyrauch HM, Fleming AE: Congenital hydrocalycosis: Hydrocalycosis of a single renal calyx in a newborn infant with complete destruction of the kidney. J Urol 63:582, 1950
6. Abeshouse BS, Abeshouse GA: Calyceal diverticulum: A report of sixteen cases and review of the literature. Urol Int 15:329, 1963
7. Williams G, Blandy JP, Tresiddes GC: Communicating cysts and diverticula of the renal pelvis. Br J Urol 41:163, 1969

Ureteropelvic Junction Obstruction

8. Starer R: Partial hydronephrosis due to pressure from normal renal arteries. Br Med J 1:98, 1968
9. Johnston JH, Evans JP, Glassberg KI et al: Pelvic hydronephrosis in children: A review of 219 personal cases. J Urol 117:97, 1977
10. Cohen B, Goldman SM, Kopilnick et al: Ureteropelvic junction obstruction: Its occurrence in 3 members of a single family. J Urol 120:361, 1978
11. Marshall FF, Jeffs RD, Smolev JK: Neonatal bilateral ureteropelvic junction obstruction. J Urol 123:107, 1980

Amyloidosis

12. Chisholm GD, Cooter NBE, Dawson JM: Primary amyloidosis of the renal pelvis. Br Med J 1:736, 1967
13. Tripathi VNP, Desautels RE: Primary amyloidosis of the urogenital system: A study of cases and brief review. J Urol 102:96, 1969
14. Gardner Jr KD, Castellino RA, Kempson R et al: Primary amyloidosis of the renal pelvis. N Engl J Med 284:1196, 1971
15. Dias R, Fernandes M, Patel RC et al: Amyloidosis of renal pelvis and urinary bladder. Urol 14:401, 1979

Malakoplakia

16. Gibson TE, Bareta J, Lake GC: Malakoplakia. Report of a case involving the bladder and one kidney and ureter. Urol Int 1:5, 1955
17. Van Zile Scott E, Scott WF: A fatal case of malakoplakia of the urinary tract. J Urol 79:52, 1958
18. Lewis JA, Vieralves G, Landes RR et al: Malakoplakia of the renal pelvis, calyces and upper ureter: Case report. J Urol 85: 243, 1961
19. Cederqvist LL: Malacoplakia of the urinary tract. Arch Pathol 80:495, 1965
20. Smith BH: Malacoplakia of the urinary tract. A study of twenty-four cases. J Urol 43:409, 1965
21. Sozer IT: A rare localization of malakoplakia: Renal pelvis. J Urol 95:746, 1966
22. Schneiderman C, Simon MA: Malakoplakia of the urinary tract. J Urol 100:694, 1968
23. Sunshine B: Malacoplakia of the upper urinary tract. J Urol 112:362, 1974

Fungal Infection

24. Boldus RA, Brown RC, Culp DA: Fungus balls in the renal pelvis. Radiology 102:555, 1972

25. Eisenberg RL, Hedgcock MW, Shanser JD: Aspergillus mycetoma of the renal pelvis associated with uretero–pelvic junction obstruction. J Urol 118:466, 1977

Plasma Cell Granuloma

26. Davides KC, Johnson III SH, Marshall Jr M et al: Plasma cell granuloma of the renal pelvis. J Urol 107:938, 1972
27. Itoh H, Namiki M, Yoshioka T et al: Plasma cell granuloma of the renal pelvis. J Urol 127:1177, 1982
28. Tchertkoff V, Lee BY, Wagner BM: Plasma cell granuloma of the lung. Case report and review of the literature. Chest 44:440, 1963

Hematoma

29. Antopol W, Goldman L: Subepithelial hemorrhage of renal pelvis simulating neoplasm. Urol Cutan Rev 52:189, 1948
30. Labay GR, Orkin LA: Subepithelial hemorrhage of renal pelvis simulating neoplasm (Antopol–Goldman lesion). Mt Sinai J Med 39:178, 1972
31. Viamonte M, Roen SA, Viamonte Jr M et al: Subepithelial hemorrhage of renal pelvis simulating neoplasm (Antopol–Goldman lesion). Urol 16:647, 1980
32. Levitt S, Waisman J, de Kernion J: Subepithelial hematoma of the renal pelvis (Antopol–Goldman lesion): A case report and review of the literature. J Urol 131:939, 1984

Submucosal Calcification

33. Firstater M, Farkas, A: Submucosal renal pelvic calcification simulating a pelvic stone. J Urol 126:802, 1981

Fibroepithelial Polyps

34. Boross E, Puhr L: Fibroma of renal pelvis. Orv Hetil 73:1055, 1929
35. Husch P: Uber einen fall von myxom des nierenbeckens. Z Urol 42:286, 1949
36. Immergut S, Cottler ZR: Intrapelvic fibroma. J Urol 66:673, 1951
37. Le Brun HI, Kellet HS, Macalister CLO: Renal hamartoma. Br J Urol 27:394, 1955
38. Evans AT, Stevens RK: Fibroepithelial polyps of ureter and renal pelvis: A case report. J Urol 86:313, 1961
39. Shucksmith HS: Fibroma of the renal pelvis. Br J Urol 35:261, 1963
40. Bernier L, Bedard A, Narcisse R: Fibrome du bassinet. Can J Surg 13:315, 1970
41. Cassimally KAI: Fibroma filling the renal pelvis: Report of a case. Can J Surg 14:350, 1971
42. Bennington JL, Beckwith JB: Tumors of the kidney, renal pelvis, and ureter, p 320. In Atlas of Tumor Pathology, Second Series, Fascicle 12. Washington, DC, AFIP, 1975
43. Wolgel CD, Parris AC, Mitty HA et al: Fibroepithelial polyp of renal pelvis. Urol 19:436, 1982

Proliferative and Metaplastic Variants

44. Morgagni JB: De sedibus et causis morborum per anatomen indagatis libri quinque. William Cooke Translation, London, 2:316, 1822
45. Rokitansky C: Manual of pathological anatomy. London, 2:216, 1861
46. von Limbeck R: Zur kenntsniss der epithelcysten der harnblase und der ureteren. Z Hielk 8:55, 1887
47. von Brunn A: Uber drusenahnliche bildungen in der schleimhaut des nierenbeckens des ureters und der harnblase beim menschen. Arch f Mikro Anat 41:294, 1893
48. Stoerk O, Zuckerkandel O: Ueber cystitis glandularis und den drusenkrebs der harnblase. Z Urol 1:1, 1907

49. Zuckerlandl O: Umwandlung des blasenepithels in sezernierendes zylinderepithel. Z Urol 5:622, 1911

50. Formiggini B: Lavori e contributi originali. Riforma Med 36:352, 1920

51. Brutt H: Uber pyelitis glandularis. Z Urol Chir 14:157, 1924

52. Morse HD: The etiology and pathology of pyelitis cystica, ureteritis cystica and cystitis cystica. Am J Pathol 4:33, 1928

53. Plaut A: Diffuses dickdarmahnliches adenom des nierenbeckens mit geschwulstartiger wucherung von gefassmuskulatur. Z Urol Chir 26:562, 1929

54. Patch FS, Rhea LJ: The genesis and development of Brunn's nests and their relation to cystitis cystica, cystitis glandularis, and primary adeno-carcinoma of the bladder. Can Med Assoc J 33:597, 1935

55. Stirling C, Ash JE: Chronic proliferative lesions of the urinary tract. J Urol 45:342, 1941

56. Foot NC: Glandular metaplasia of the epithelium of the urinary tract. South Med J 37:137, 1944

57. Everett HS, Wayburn GJ: A unique case of submucosal epithelial nests in the ureter and renal pelvis. J Urol 56:310, 1946

58. Torassa GL: Pyelitis glandularis. J Urol 60:393, 1948

59. Fagerstrom DP: Proliferative tumors of the ureter and renal pelvis, with further observations on the significance of "epithelial cell nests": Six case reports. J Urol 59:333, 1948

60. Davis TA: Hamartoma of the urinary bladder. Northwestern Med 48:182, 1949

61. Freidman NB, Kuhlenbeck H: Adenomatoid tumors of the bladder reproducing renal structures (nephrogenic adenomas). J Urol 64:657, 1950

62. Senger FL, Bottone JJ, Kelleher JH: Bilateral leukoplakia of the renal pelvis. J Urol 65:528, 1951

63. Mostofi FK: Potentialities of bladder epithelium. J Urol 71:705, 1954

64. Aiken D: Pyelitis glandularis. Br J Surg 42:412, 1955

65. Krag DO, Alcott, DL: Glandular metaplasia of the renal pelvis: Report of a case. Am J Clin Pathol 29:672, 1957

66. Gordon A: Intestinal metaplasia of the urinary tract epithelium. J Pathol Bact 85:441, 1963

67. Salm R: Combined intestinal and squamous metaplasia of the renal pelvis. J Clin Pathol 22: 187, 1969

68. Davis EL, Goldstein AMB, Morrow JW: Unusual bladder mucosal metaplasia in a case of chronic prostatitis and cystitis. J Urol 111:767, 1974

69. Goldstein AMB, Fauer RB, Chinn M, Kaempf MJ: New concepts on formation of Brunn's nests and cysts in urinary tract mucosa. Urol 11:513, 1978

70. Stern JB: Unusual benign bladder tumor of Brunn nest origin. Urol 14:288, 1979

71. Wiener DP, Koss LG, Sablay B et al: The prevalence and significance of Brunn's nests, cystitis cystica and squamous metaplasia in normal bladders. J Urol 122:317, 1979

72. Koss LG: Mapping of the urinary bladder: Its impact on the concepts of bladder cancer. Hum Pathol 5:533, 1979

73. Selli C, Dini S, Fiorelli C et al: Chronic inflammation of the ureter with urothelial ingrowth simulating inverted papilloma. Br J Urol 53:80, 1981

74. Chasko SB, Gray GF, McCarron Jr JP: Urothelial neoplasia of the upper urinary tract. Pathol Annu (part II) 16:127, 1981

75. Navarre RJ, Loening SA, Platz C et al: Nephrogenic adenomas: A report of 9 cases and review of the literature. J Urol 127:775, 1982

76. Hertle L, Androulakakis P: Keratinizing desquamative squamous metaplasia of the upper urinary tract: Leukoplakia–cholesteatoma. J Urol 127:631, 1982

77. Blacklock ARE, Geddes JR, Black JW: Mucinous and squamous metaplasia of the renal pelvis. J Urol 130:544, 1983

78. Kunze E, Schauer A, Schmitt M: Histology and histogenesis of two different types of inverted urothelial papillomas. Cancer 51:348, 1983
79. Lugo M, Petersen RO, Elfenbein IB et al: Nephrogenic metaplasia of the ureter. Am J Clin Pathol 80:92, 1983

Papilloma

80. McDonald JR, Priestley JT: Carcinoma of renal pelvis. Histopathologic study of seventy-five cases with special reference to prognosis. J Urol 51:245, 1944
81. Miller A, Mitchell JP, Brown NJ: The Bristol bladder tumor registry. Br J Urol 41(suppl):1, 1969
82. Bennington JL, Beckwith JB: Tumors of the kidney, renal pelvis, and ureter, p. 264. In Atlas of Tumor Pathology, Second Series, Fascicle 12. Washington, DC, AFIP, 1975
83. Koss LG: Tumors of the urinary bladder, p. 19. In Atlas of Tumor Pathology, Second Series, Fascicle 11. Washington, DC, AFIP, 1975

Inverted Papilloma

84. Potts, IF, Hirst E: Inverted papilloma of the bladder. J Urol 90:173, 1963
85. Matz LR, Wishart VA, Goodman MA: Inverted urothelial papilloma. Pathol 6:37, 1974
86. Assor D: Inverted papilloma of the renal pelvis. J Urol 116:654, 1976
87. Di Cello V, Brischi G, Durval A et al: Inverted papilloma of the ureteropelvic junction. J Urol 123:110, 1980
88. Thoret G, Paquin F, Shick E et al: Inverted papilloma of urinary tract. Urol 16:149, 1980
89. Uyama T, Moriwaki S: Inverted papilloma with malignant change of renal pelvis. Urol 17:200, 1981
90. Anderstrom C, Johansson S, Pettersson S: Inverted papilloma of the urinary tract. J Urol 127:1132, 1982

Carcinoma

91. Jewett HJ, Strong GH: Infiltrating carcinoma of the bladder: Relation of depth of penetration of the bladder wall to incidence of local extension and metastases. J Urol 55:366, 1946
92. Jewett HJ: Carcinoma of the bladder: Influence of depth of infiltration on the 5-year results following complete extirpation of the primary growth. J Urol 67:672, 1952
93. Marshall VF: The relation of the preoperative estimate of the pathologic demonstration of the extent of vesicle neoplasms. J Urol 68:714, 1952
94. Heney NM, Nocks BN, Daly JJ et al: Prognostic factors in carcinoma of the ureter. J Urol 125:632, 1981

Transitional Cell Carcinoma

Epidemiology, Etiology

95. Rehn L: Uber Basentumoren bei Fuchsinarbeitern. Arch Klin Chir 50:588, 1895
96. MacAlpine JB: Papilloma of the renal pelvis in dye workers. Two cases, one of which shows bilateral growths. Br J Surg 35:137, 1947
97. Hultengren N, Lagergren C, Ljungqvist A: Carcinoma of the renal pelvis in renal papillary necrosis. Acta Chir Scand 130:314, 1965
98. Poole-Wilson DB: Occupational tumors of the renal pelvis and ureter in the dye-making industry. Proc R Soc Med 62:93, 1969
99. Cracium EC, Roscullescu I: On Danubian endemic familial nephropathy (Balkan nephropathy). Am J Med 49:774, 1970

100. Grampa G: Radiation injury with particular reference to thorotrast. Pathol Annu 6:147, 1971
101. Elliott AY, Fraley EE, Cleveland P et al: Isolation of an RNA virus from papillary tumors of the human renal pelvis. Science 179:393, 1973
102. Schmauz R, Cole P: Epidemiology of cancer of the renal pelvis and ureter. J Natl Can Inst 52:1431, 1974
103. Rathert P, Melchior H, Lutzeyer W: Phenacetin: A carcinogen for the urinary tract? J Urol 113:653, 1975
104. Calder IC, Goss DE, Williams PJ et al: Neoplasia in the rat induced by N-hydroxy-phenacetin, a metabolite of phenacetin. Pathology 8:1, 1976
105. Bengtsson U, Johannson S, Angervall L: Malignancies of the urinary tract and their relation to analgesic abuse. Kidney Int 13:107, 1978
106. Petkovic SD: Treatment of bilateral renal pelvic and ureteral tumors. A review of 45 cases. Eur Urol 4:397, 1978
107. McCredie M, Ford JM, Taylor JS et al: Analgesics and cancer of the renal pelvis in New South Wales. Cancer 49:2617, 1982

Clinical – Pathologic Studies

108. Swift-Jolly J: Proceedings of the 5th International Congress of Urology. Br J Urol 5:327, 1933
109. Riches EW, Griffiths IH, Thackray AC: New growths of the kidney and ureter. Br J Urol 23:297, 1951
110. Kaplan JH, McDonald JR, Thompson GJ: Multicentric origin of papillary tumors of the urinary tract. J Urol 66:792, 1951
111. Taylor, WN: Tumors of the kidney pelvis. J Urol 82:452, 1959
112. Bourne HH, Tremblay RE, Ansell JS: Stupor, hypercalcemia and carcinoma of the renal pelvis. N Engl J Med 271:1005, 1964
113. Newman DM, Allen LE, Wishard Jr WN et al: Transitional cell carcinoma of the upper urinary tract. J Urol 98:322, 1967
114. Grace DA, Taylor WN, Taylor JN et al: Carcinoma of the renal pelvis: A 15-year review. J Urol 98:566, 1968
115. Sarnacki CT, McCormack LJ, Kiser WS et al: Urinary cytology and the clinical diagnosis of urinary tract malignancy: A clinicopathic study of 1400 patients. J Urol 106:761, 1971
116. Grabstald H, Whitmore WF, Melamed MR: Renal pelvic tumors. J Am Med Assoc 281:845, 1971
117. Cullen TH, Pepham RR, Voss HJ: Urine cytology and primary carcinoma of the renal pelvis and ureter. Aust NZ J Surg 41:230, 1972
118. Williams CB, Mitchell JP: Carcinoma of the renal pelvis: A review of 43 cases. Br J Urol 45:370, 1973
119. Wagle DG, Moore RH, Murphy GP: Primary carcinoma of the renal pelvis. Cancer 33:1642, 1974
120. Johansson S, Angervall L, Bengtsson U et al: Uroepithelial tumors of the renal pelvis associated with abuse of phenacetin-containing analgesics. Cancer 33:743, 1974
121. Murphy WM, von Buedingen RP, Poley RW: Primary carcinoma in situ of renal pelvis and ureter. Cancer 34:1126, 1974
122. Say CC, Hori JM: Transitional cell carcinoma of the renal pelvis: Experience from 1940 and 1972 and literature review. J Urol 112:438, 1974
123. Cummings KB, Correa RJ, Gibbons RP et al: Renal pelvic tumors. J Urol 113:158, 1975
124. Donnelly JD, Koontz WW: Carcinoma of the renal pelvis: A ten-year review. South Med J 68:943, 1975
125. Rafla S: Tumors of the upper urothelium. Am J Roentgen 123:540, 1975

126. Koyanagi T, Sasaki K, Arikado D et al: Transitional cell carcinoma of renal pelvis in an infant. J Urol 113:114, 1975

127. Johansson S, Angervall L, Bengstsson U et al: A clinicopathologic and prognostic study of epithelial tumors of the renal pelvis. Cancer 37:1376, 1976

128. Leong CH, Lim TK, Wong KK et al: Carcinoma of the renal pelvis: An analysis of the diagnostic problems in 23 cases. Br J Surg 63:102, 1976

129. Fawcett DP, McBrien MP: Transitional cell carcinoma of the renal pelvis presenting with peripheral neuropathy. Br J Urol 49:202, 1977

130. Mandell J, Magee MC, Fried FA: Hypercalcemia associated with uroepithelial neoplasms. J Urol 119:844, 1978

131. Strong DW, Pearse HD: Recurrent urothelial tumors following surgery for transitional cell carcinoma of the upper urinary tract. Cancer 38:2178, 1976

132. Rubenstein, MA, Walz BJ, Bucy JG: Transitional cell carcinoma of the kidney: 25-year experience. J Urol 119:594, 1978

133. Johansson S, Wahlqvist L: A prognostic study of urothelial renal pelvic tumors. Cancer 43:2525, 1979

134. Khan AU, Farrow GM, Zincke H et al: Primary carcinoma in situ of the ureter and renal pelvis. J Urol 121:681, 1979

135. Stragier M, Desmet R, Denys H et al: Primary carcinoma in situ of renal pelvis and ureter. Br J Urol 52:401, 1980

136. Nocks BN, Heney NM, Daly JJ et al: Transitional cell carcinoma of renal pelvis. Urol 19:472, 1982

137. Hall L, Faddoul A, Saberi A et al: The use of the red cell surface antigen to predict the malignant potential of transitional cell carcinoma of the ureter and renal pelvis. J Urol 127:23, 1982

138. Gruber MB, Becker SN, Warren MM et al: Specific red cell adherence test applied to tumors of ureter and renal pelvis. Urol 19:361, 1982

139. Mahadevia PS, Karwa GL, Koss LG: Mapping of urothelium in carcinomas of the renal pelvis and ureter. A report of nine cases. Cancer 51:890, 1983

Multiple Urothelial Neoplasms, Associated Neoplasms

140. Lower WE: Neoplasms of the renal pelvis with especial reference to transportation in the ureter and bladder. Surg Gynecol Obstet 18:151, 1914

141. Graves RC, Templeton ER: Combined tumors of the kidney. J Urol 5:517, 1921

142. Thomas GJ, Regnier EA: Tumors of the kidney, pelvis, and ureter. J Urol 11:205, 1924

143. Scholl AJ: Papillary tumors of the renal pelvis. Surg Gynecol Obstet 38:186, 1924

144. Patch FS, Rhea LJ: Papillary cystadenoma of kidney associated with papillomatous growths in pelvis, ureter and bladder. J Urol 7:671, 1924

145. Hunt VC: Papillary epithelioma of the renal pelvis. J Urol 18:225, 1927

146. de Vries JK: Hypernephroma, papilloma and stone occurring in horseshoe kidney. Am J Surg 10:487, 1930

147. Sanford HL: Carcinoma of both kidneys. Report of a case with review of the literature on multiple primary malignant tumors. Surg Gynecol Obstet 53:360, 1931

148. Cabot H, Allen RB: Epithelioma primary in the renal pelvis. Report of forty-five cases. Lancet 2:1301, 1933

149. Wildboltz H: Discussion. Br J Urol 5:338, 1933

150. Kimball FN, Ferris HW: Papillomatous tumor of the renal pelvis associated with similar tumors of the ureter and bladder. J Urol 31:257, 1934

151. Balch JF: Papillary carcinoma and hypernephroma occurring in the same kidney. J Urol 33:138, 1935

152. Camerer J: Simultaneous occurrence of the medullary carcinoma of pelvis of one kidney and hypernephroma of other kidney. Z fur Path 54:313, 1940

153. Dick VS: Papilloma of the renal pelvis associated with an early renal cell carcinoma. Lahey Clin Bull 2:231, 1942
154. Melicow MM: Tumors of the urinary drainage tract: Urothelial tumors. J Urol 54:186, 1945
155. MacAlpine JB: Papilloma of the renal pelvis in dye workers. Two cases, one of which shows bilateral growths. Br J Surg 35:137, 1947
156. MacAlpine JB: A case in which two dissimilar growths, an adenoma (adenocarcinoma) and a papillo-carcinoma, occurred in the same kidney. Br J Surg 35:134, 1947
157. Rupel E, Sutton WE: Carcinoma of renal parenchyma: One case with metastases to opposite kidney, bladder and ureteral wall; the other associated with papillary carcinoma of same kidney and metastases to skin. J Urol 63:487, 1950
158. Kline DW, Marshall Jr M, Johnson III SH et al: Concurrent dissimilar malignancies of the urinary tract. J Urol 73:964, 1955
159. Colston JAC, Arcadi JA: Bilataral renal papillomas: Transpelvic electro-resection with preservation of kidney. Contralateral nephrectomy; four-year survival. J Urol 73:460, 1955
160. Colston JAC: Followup report on a case of bilateral papillary carcinoma of the renal pelvis. J Urol 83:355, 1960
161. Potampa PB, Schneider IJ: Bilateral true primary papillary carcinoma of the kidneys. J Urol 86:522, 1961
162. Kinder CH, Wallace DM: Recurrent carcinoma in the ureteric stump. Br J Surg 50:202, 1963
163. Harvard BM, Evans JS: Simultaneous bilateral transitional cell carcinoma of the renal pelvis. J Urol 91:14, 1964
164. Carroll G: Bilateral transitional cell carcinoma of the renal pelvis. J Urol 93:132, 1965
165. Gibson TE: Local excision in transitional cell tumors of the upper urinary tract. J Urol 97:619, 1967
166. Villegas AC: Bilateral primary malignant renal tumors of dissimilar histogenesis: Report of two cases and review of the literature. J Urol 98:450, 1967
167. Walker D, Jordan Jr WP: Renal carcinoma and transitional cell carcinoma in the same kidney. South Med J 61:829, 1968
168. Gillis DJ, Finnerty P, Maxted WC: Simultaneous occurrence of hypernephroma and transitional cell carcinoma with development of transitional cell carcinoma in the opposite kidney: Case report. J Urol 106:646, 1971
169. Fallon B, Schellhammer PF: Transitional cell carcinoma and renal cell adenocarcinoma in single kidney. Urol 6:774, 1975
170. Bogard TP, Goldstein AMB: Bilateral transitional cell carcinoma of the renal pelvis with unilateral non-functioning kidney. J Urol 113:565, 1975
171. McLoughlin MG: The treatment of bilateral synchronous renal pelvic tumors with bench surgery. J Urol 114:463, 1975
172. Jozsi BP, Wise HA, Quilter TN et al: Bilateral simultaneous tumors of dissimilar cell type: A case report with emphasis on operative approach. J Urol 116:655, 1976
173. Augspurger RR, Peterson NE: Transitional cell carcinoma replacing the intrarenal pelvis of a solitary kidney. J Urol 118:677, 1977
174. Voneschenbach AC, Johnson DE, Ayala AG: Simultaneous occurrence of renal adenocarcinoma and transitional cell carcinoma of the renal pelvis. J Urol 118:105, 1977
175. Anseline P, Howarth VS: A case of transitional cell carcinomas of the renal pelvis, clear cell renal carcinoma, and analgesic nephropathy. Aust NZ J Surg 47:521, 1977
176. McDonald MW, Konnak JW: Simultaneous, contralateral hypernephroma and renal transitional cell carcinoma. Urol 14:509, 1979
177. Ross LS, Presman D: What about the other kidney? J Urol 122:394, 1979

178. Murphy DM, Zincke H, Furlow WL: Primary grade 1 transitional cell carcinoma of the renal pelvis and ureter. J Urol 123:629, 1980
179. Lundell C, Kadir S, Engel R et al: Concurrent renal cell and transitional cell carcinoma in a single kidney: A case report. J Urol 127:761, 1982

Squamous Cell Carcinoma

180. Gilbert JB, Macmillan SF: Cancer of the kidney. Squamous-cell carcinoma of the renal pelvis with special reference to etiology. Ann Surg 100:429, 1934
181. Higgins CC: Squamous cell carcinoma of the kidney pelvis. Trans Am Assoc Genitourinary Surg 30:13, 1937
182. Gahagan HQ, Reed WK: Squamous cell carcinoma of the renal pelvis: Three case reports and review of the literature. J Urol 62:139, 1949
183. Atkinson RL: Calculus pyonephrosis associated with squamous cell carcinoma of the renal pelvis. J Urol 63:61, 1950
184. Oberkircher OJ, Staubitz WJ, Blick MS: Squamous cell carcinoma of the renal pelvis. J Urol 66:551, 1951
185. Higgins CC: Tumors of the renal pelvis. Ann Surg 137:195, 1953
186. O'Conor VJ: The diagnosis of tumors of the renal pelvis and ureter. Trans Am Assoc Genitourinary Surg 47:66, 1955
187. Dees JE: Prognosis of primary tumors of renal pelvis and ureter. Trans Am Assoc Genitourinary Surg 47:113, 1955
188. MacLean JT: Pathology of tumors of the renal pelvis and ureter. J Urol 75:384, 1956
189. Utz DC, McDonald JR: Squamous cell carcinoma of the kidney. J Urol 78:540, 1957
190. Thompson IM, Schneider J, Kavan LC: Bilateral squamous cell carcinoma of the kidneys. J Urol 79:807, 1958
191. Seth-Smith AB: Tumours of the renal pelvis: Review of sixty-four cases. Br J Urol 31:265, 1959
192. Carlson HE: Squamous cell carcinoma of the renal pelvis: A five year cure. J Urol 83:813, 1960
193. Charlton CAC, Richardson WW: Squamous cell carcinoma of an ectopic kidney with staghorn calculus: Case report. Br J Urol 38:428, 1966
194. Dean ACB, Lambie AT, Shivas AA: Hypercalcaemic crisis and squamous carcinoma of the renal pelvis. Br J Urol 56:375, 1969
195. McCullough DL, McLaughlin AP: Squamous cell carcinoma of the renal pelvis. Am J Surg 124:416, 1972
196. Wagle DC, Moore RH, Murphy GP: Squamous cell carcinoma of the renal pelvis. J Urol 111:453, 1974
197. Latham HS, Kay S: Malignant tumors of the renal pelvis. Surg Gynecol Obstet 138:613, 1974
198. Pigadas A, Chang J, McGowan AJ et al: Squamous cell carcinoma of the renal pelvis presenting with hypercalcemia. J Urol 119:126, 1978
199. Kinn A-C: Squamous cell carcinoma of the renal pelvis. Scand J Urol Nephrol 14:77, 1979
200. Weschler Z: Squamous cell carcinoma of the renal pelvis as a late complication of hepatic irradiation: A case report. J Surg Oncol 22:84, 1983

Adenocarcinoma

201. Grohe B: Unsere nierentumoren in therapeutischer, klinischer, und pathologisch-anatomischer beleuchtung. Deutsche Z Chir 60:1, 1901
202. Paschkis R: Zur kasuistik der nierenbeckengeschwulste. Z Urol 3:681, 1909
203. Ackerman LV: Mucinous adenocarcinoma of the pelvis of the kidney. J Urol 55:36, 1946

204. Ragins AB, Rolnick HC: Mucus producing adenocarcinoma of the renal pelvis. J Urol 63:66, 1950

205. Anderson CK: Metaplasia in the epithelium of the urinary tract. Proc R Soc Med 48:699, 1955

206. Arcadi JA: Mucus-producing cystadenocarcinoma of the renal pelvis and ureter. Arch Pathol 61:264, 1956

207. Kennedy JS, Fidler HK: Primary adenocarcinoma of the renal pelvis. J Urol 80:208, 1958

208. Seth-Smith AB: Tumours of the renal pelvis: Review of sixty-four cases. Br J Urol 31:265, 1959

209. Hasebe M, Serizawa S, Chino S: Uber einen fall von papillarzysto-adenokarzinom infolge maligner entartung des papilladenoms im nierenbecken. Yokolama Med Bull 11:491, 1960

210. Emson HE, Estey HW: Primary mucigenic adenocarcinoma of the renal pelvis: Report of a case. J Urol 88:604, 1962

211. Lopez Engelking RL, Morales EA, Maldonado ME: Adenocarcinoma mucinoso primario de la pelvis renal. Rev Mex Urol 23:301, 1964

212. Ashley DJB, Hickey BB: Adenocarcinoma of the renal pelvis. Br J Urol 36:309, 1964

213. Schrodt GR, Bickers E, Howerton L: Primary adenocarcinoma of the renal pelvis. Report of a case. Am J Clin Pathol 41:517, 1964

214. Suzuki H, Siminovitch M: Primary mucus-producing adenocarcinoma of the renal pelvis: Report of a case. J Urol 93:562, 1965

215. Saxena O, Sanghal BC, Bhargava KN: Primary adenocarcinoma of renal pelvis. Review of literature with first case report from India. Indian J Path Bact 9:344, 1966

216. Wahal KM, Rastogi BL, Mehrotra RML et al: Mucus producing adenocarcinoma of renal pelvis. Report of a case and review of the literature. Indian J Path Bact 9:352, 1966

217. Jain BJ: Adenocarcinoma of the renal pelvis. J Urol 97:55, 1967

218. Suzuki H, Milam DF: Primary mucus-producing adenomatous tumor: Adenocarcinoma of renal pelvis. Arch Pathol 84:468, 1967

219. Quattlebaum RB, Shirley SW: Adenocarcinoma of the renal pelvis. J Urol 99:384, 1968

220. Hayahara N, Maekawa M, Shin T: Primary mucinous adenocarcinoma of renal pelvis and ureter: A case report and review of literature. Acta Urol Jap 14:433, 1968

221. Toyoda H, Hirakata Y: An autopsy case of adenocarcinoma of renal pelvis with vertebral metastasis. Jap J Cancer Clin 15:1093, 1969

222. Murphy TE, Stevenson JE: Primary adenocarcinoma of the renal pelvis: Report of a case. J Urol 104:62, 1970

223. Kataria PN, Shanker KG: Adenocarcinoma of renal pelvis. J Indian Med Assoc 61:91, 1973

224. Aguilo JJ, Furlow WL: Mucus-producing adenocarcinoma of renal pelvis. Urol 4:488, 1974

225. Solov K, Martines D: Gelatinous adenocarcinoma of the renal pelvis. Folia Medica 16:179, 1974

226. Aufderheide AC, Streitz JM: Mucinous adenocarcinoma of the renal pelvis. Report of two cases. Cancer 33:167, 1974

227. Guha T, Datta BN, Aikat BK et al: Tumours of renal pelvis. Indian J Path Bact 18:21, 1975

228. Liwnicz BH, Lepow H. Schutte H et al: Mucinous adenocarcinoma of the renal pelvis: Discussion of possible pathogenesis. J Urol 114:306, 1975

229. Filimon C, Stancu N, Bucur ST et al: Adenocarcinome pyelique. A propos d'un cas. J Urol Nephrol 83:549, 1977

230. Bhargava S, Tandon V, Sharma KC et al: Papillary mucoid adenocarcinoma of renal pelvis. Report of a case with review of literature. Indian J Cancer 16:78, 1979

231. Pujari BD, Deshpande MS, Phansopkar M: Adenocarcinoma of the pelvis of a horseshoe kidney. Br J Urol 52:63, 1980

232. O'Brien PK, Bedard YC: A papillary adenocarcinoma of the renal pelvis in a young girl. A light- and electron-microscopic study. Am J Clin Pathol 73:427, 1980

233. Brawer BK, Waisman J: Mucinous adenocarcinoma probably arising in the renal pelvis and ureter: A case report. J Urol 123:424, 1980

234. Kulkarni SH, Kohlatkar RM, Ranabhise AM et al: Adenocarcinoma of the renal pelvis with associated tuberculosis of the kidney. Indian J Cancer 18:229, 1981

235. Kutscher HA, Trainer TD, Fagan Jr WT: Mucinous adenocarcinoma of renal pelvis. Urol 20:94, 1982

236. Kobayashi S, Ohmori M, Akaeda T et al: Primary adenocarcinoma of the renal pelvis. Report of two cases and brief review of literature. Acta Pathol Japan 33:589, 1983

Mixed Carcinomas

237. MacLean JT, Fowler VB: Pathology of tumors of the renal pelvis and ureter. J Urol 75:384, 1956

238. Kennedy JS, Fiddler HK: Primary adenocarcinoma of the renal pelvis. J Urol 80:208, 1958

Mesenchymal Neoplasms

Hemangioma

239. Lazarus JA, Marks MS: Renal hemangioma. Urol Cutan Rev 51:500, 1947

240. Raff LG, Podolsky WG: Hemangioma of the kidney. New York J Med 51:1536, 1951

241. Anderson JB, Lee JJ, Hancock RZ, Black SR: Hemangioma of the kidney pelvis. J Urol 70:869, 1953

242. Edward HG, Deweerd JH, Woolner LB: Renal hemangiomas. Proc Staff Meet Mayo Clin 37:545, 1962

243. Andersen JB, Rasmussen T: Renal haemangioma diagnosed preoperatively by selective renal angiography. Report of a case. Acta Radiol 2:201, 1964

Leiomyoma

244. Litzky GM, Seidel RF, O'Brien JE: Leiomyoma of the renal pelvis. J Urol 105:171, 1971

245. Bennington JL, Beckwith JB: Tumors of the kidney, renal pelvis, and ureter, p. 312. In Atlas of Tumor Pathology, Second Series, Fascicle 12. Washington, DC, AFIP, 1975

246. Belis JA, Post GJ, Rochman SC et al: Genitourinary leiomyomas. Urol 13:424, 1979

247. Uchida M, Watanabe H, Mishina T et al: Leiomyoma of the renal pelvis. J Urol 125:572, 1981

Leiomyosarcoma

248. Crosbie AH, Pinkerton H: Malignant leiomyoma of the kidney. J Urol 27:27, 1932

249. Dockerty MB, Priestley JT: Sarcoma of the kidney. J Urol 50:564, 1943

250. Farrow GM, Harrison EG, Utz DC et al: Sarcomas and sarcomatoid and mixed malignant tumors of the kidney in adults: Part I. Cancer 22:545, 1968

251. Loomis RC: Primary leiomyosarcoma of the kidney: Report of a case and review of the literature. J Urol 107:557, 1972

252. Tolia BM, Hajdu SI, Whitmore Jr WF: Leiomyosarcoma of the renal pelvis. J Urol 109:974, 1973

Malignant Mixed Neoplasms

Carcinosarcoma

253. Willis RA: In Pathology of Tumors, 4th ed, p 138. New York, Appleton – Century – Crofts, 1967
254. Fauci Jr PA, Therhag HG, Davis JE: Carcinosarcoma of the renal pelvis. J Urol 85:897, 1961
255. Elliott JT, Pontius EE, McCallum DC: Carcinosarcoma of kidney. Urol 1:151, 1973
256. Gallagher JC, Winslow DJ, Grossman A: Coexistent chondrosarcoma and transitional-cell carcinoma in kidney. Urol 3:473, 1974
257. Ridolfi RL, Eggleston JC: Carcinosarcoma of the renal pelvis. J Urol 119:569, 1978
258. Tarry WF, Morabito RA, Belis JA: Carcinosarcoma of the renal pelvis with extension into the renal vein and inferior vena cava. J Urol 128:582, 1982

Ureter

3

Normal Structure

The transitional cell epithelium of the ureter is composed of three to five cell layers. No basement membrane is apparent by light microscopy, but it is readily demonstrated by electron microscopy.[2] Loose collagen fibers, thin-walled vessels, and unmyelinated nerves are present in the underlying lamina propria.[2,3] Historically, the ureteral smooth muscle has been described in two layers: the inner longitudinal and the outer circular. More recent studies with serial cross sectioning of the abdominal ureter describe the muscles organized in interlacing spirals without layers.[2,3] The originally described layers were found only in the distal ureter. At this level an additional longitudinal muscle layer was observed between the circular muscle bundle and the adventitia.[3] Contraction of the circumferential muscle produces the stellate lumen characteristic of cross sections of the ureter (Figs. 3-1, 3-2). External to the muscularis, the adventitia is well-vascularized, loose, fibroadipose tissue of the retroperitoneum.

The ureteral arterial supply is from branches of the renal, gonadal, common iliac, and vesical arteries, which have numerous anastomoses.[1] The corresponding veins receive the venous drainage from the ureter. The proximal ureteral lymphatic drainage is to the para-aortic lymph nodes, and that of the distal ureter is to the internal iliac lymph nodes.

Embryology

The ureter, along with the renal pelvis and the kidney, has three stages of embryologic development.[4,5] In the first stage at 3 weeks, multiple pronephric tubules develop in the mesoderm. Ultimately, they connect with the pronephric duct, which grows caudally to connect with the cloaca. In humans, the pronephric tubules never attain a functional state and quickly regress, with the pronephric duct becoming the mesonephric duct.

229

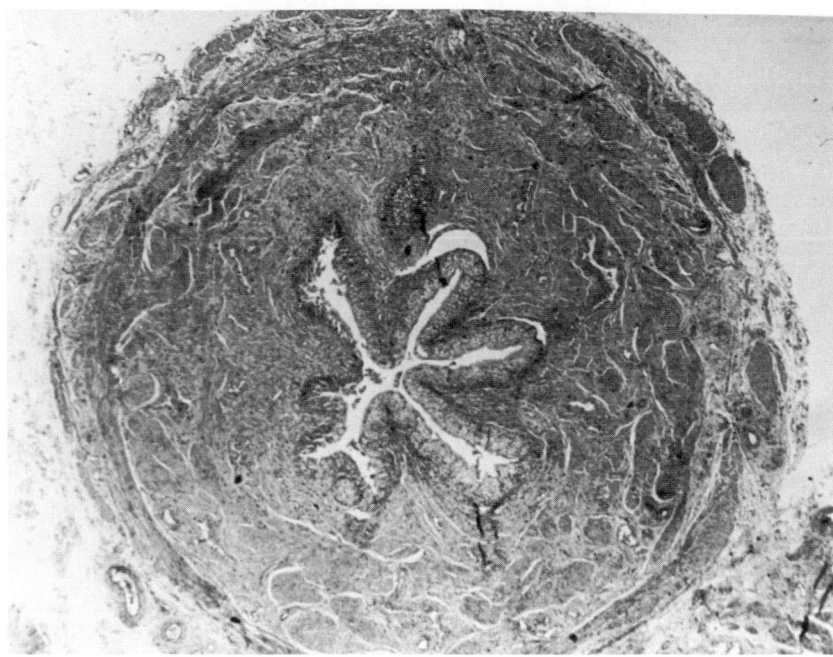

Figure 3-1   *Normal ureter. The cross section shows the stellate lumen lined by transitional cell urothelium. The inner longitudinal muscle layer is surrounded by the outer circumferential muscle layer.*

At 4 weeks, mesonephric tubules emerge, initially at the cephalad end, and grow to connect with the mesonephric duct (formerly, the pronephric duct). As more caudal tubules develop, the cephalad tubules regress. The mesonephric kidney and ductal system function briefly, and attain their maximum size at 8 weeks. Subsequently, the mesonephric system regresses. This occurs most completely in the female, where the only vestiges in the adult are remnants of Gartner's duct found in the wall of the fallopian tubes and uterus to the level of lateral vagina. In the male, the mesonephric duct system evolves, under the influence of androgens, to become the testicular adnexa. The mesonephric tubules become the efferent ductules of the epididymis, and the mesonephric duct ultimately becomes the epididymis, vas deferens, seminal vesicle, and ejaculatory duct. Nonfunctional vestigial structures such as the appendix epididymis originate in the regressed mesonephric tubules.

The third phase of the embryologic development of the urinary tract is the outgrowth of the metanephric duct from the distal mesonephric duct at a point near the latter's entrance into the cloaca. The metanephric duct, beginning as the metanephric diverticulum, grows cephalad after a mass of mesenchyme (metanephrogenic mesenchyme) envelops its blind end (sixth week). The metanephric duct induces the development of nephrons (glomeruli, and tubules from proximal convoluted tubule to distal convoluted tubule) in this metanephric mesenchyme. As a unit, the metanephric duct, in association with the differentiating metanephric mesenchyme, migrates cephalad. In turn, the metanephric mesenchyme induces the blind end of the metanephric duct to subdivide, progressively forming the major calyces and minor calyces. The latter gives rise to the collecting tubules, which ultimately connect with the tubular system of the nephron.

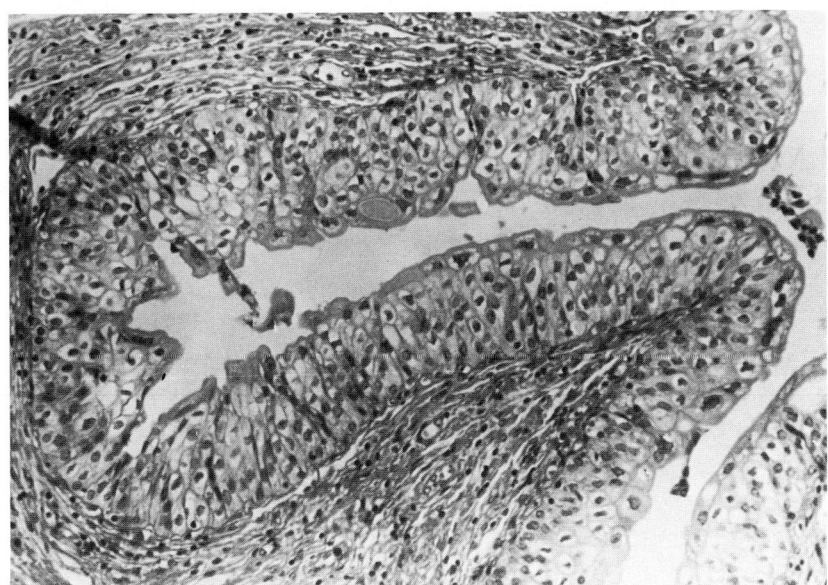

Figure 3-2 *Normal ureter. The transitional cell urothelium rests on a lamina propria composed of fibromuscular tissue.*

At the distal end, the cloaca is subdivided into the urogenital sinus and the rectum. The distal mesonephric duct is partially absorbed into the lateral wall of the urogenital sinus, thus separating the ostia of the metanephric duct (the future ureter) and the mesonephric duct (the future male ejaculatory duct system). Ureteral muscle appears at 12 weeks, and is present throughout the length of the ureter at 18 weeks.

Congenital Disorders

Developmental Anomalies

Agenesis of a ureter results from the failure of the metanephric diverticulum to develop from the mesonephric duct. It is associated with agenesis of the ipsilateral kidney, which is related, in turn, to the absence of the inducer for the metanephric mesenchyme.

Ureteral duplication is among the most common anomalies of the urinary system; in contrast, ureteral triplication is a very rare anomaly. They may result either from formation of multiple metanephric buds, or premature bifurcation of a single bud.[6-11] The former results in complete duplication (or triplication), and the latter results in incomplete duplication (or triplication). The majority of such anomalies are unilateral.

Ectopic ureters are the result of anomalous development of the distal mesonephric duct as it is absorbed into the lateral urogenital sinus with the metanephric duct. Because the distal mesonephric duct ultimately forms part of the proximal urethra, ejaculatory duct, seminal vesicle, and vas deferens, any abnormal juxtaposition of the ostium of the metanephric duct (the future ureter) may result in future termination of the ureter into any of these mesonephric structures.[11,12] There is a similar explanation for ureters terminating in the lateral fallopian tube, uterus, or vagina of the female. Such ectopic terminations frequently are associated with multiple ipsilateral ureters (complete or incomplete). All forms of ureteral ectopia are more common in females.

Ureterocele is a dilatation of the terminal ureter, frequently ectopic, due to stenosis of the ureteral ostium. There is evidence that it is due to a delayed rupture of Chwalla's membrane.[13-16]

Congenital Ureteral Valves

Congenital ureteral valves are rare. Seitzman and co-workers, in a review of the literature, found 13 cases reported during the years 1926 to 1969.[18] They added one additional case. Wall and Wachter (1952) proposed criteria to distinguish congenital ureteral valves from acquired valves present in dilated, tortuous ureters usually secondary to distal ureteral obstruction.[17] Congenital ureteral valves show (1) transverse folds of ureteral mucosa containing smooth muscle; (2) ureteral obstructive changes above the valve and normal ureteral structure below the valve; and (3) no other associated obstructive abnormalities of the ureter.[17]

The patients in Seitzman's report range in age from 4 years to 94 years.[18] There is no age, sex, or side predilection. Only one case evidenced bilateral involvement. Sixty-four percent of the congenital ureteral valves are located in the distal ureter, and the remainder are in the proximal ureter.[18] The resultant hydronephrosis, observed consistently, predisposes the patients to upper urinary tract infection, which was observed in most of the patients.[18] The diagnosis in the past has been made most commonly at the time of surgery, or at autopsy.

Congenital Megaureter

The term *congenital megaureter* is a description applied to many distinct entities that have only recently been classified on the basis of etiology and pathogenesis.[19-21] Regardless of underlying cause, the resultant hydronephrosis progresses to renal function impairment if left uncorrected.

There is no single pathologic abnormality observed, and the underlying causes are diverse. The diagnosis is made on the basis of clinical, radiologic, and histologic evidence, the last obtained from both light microscopy and ultrastructural features.[19-21]

Diverticulum

Ureteral diverticulum is rare and its cause remains unsettled. In a review of the literature, Culp (1947) accepted only 10 of 52 previously reported cases as ureteral diverticula.[22] He excluded all cases of hydronephrosis and hydroureter proximal to ureteral strictures, ureteroceles, bladder diverticula located at the ureteral orifice, fusiform dilatated terminal ends of ureters at the vesicle wall, and incomplete bifid ureters with a blind end. True ureteral diverticula (1) contain all components of the ureteral wall, including the muscularis in the wall of the diverticulum; and (2) are round to oval extraureteral sacs that communicate with the ureteral lumen through a stoma.[22] Culp considered all such examples as congenital. Those ureter outpouchings lacking all structural components of the ureteral wall (*i.e.,* muscle) were regarded as acquired defects associated with prior trauma, infection, calculi, or distal strictures.

Although most subsequent studies have reflected an acceptance of Culp's criteria, some authors have raised criticisms that remain unanswered. Rank and co-workers observed that the structure of blind-end bifid ureter segments contain all layers of the ureteral wall and differ only in their configuration (*i.e.,* their length exceeds their width), as opposed to the round to oval configuration required by Culp.[22,24] Rank and others point out that intraluminal pressure may be capable of altering the configuration of a bifid ureteral blind-end limb to conform to the required shape of a "true diverticulum." In addition, other cases diagnosed in adults with a history or current evidence of infection fulfill Culp's criteria of true congenital diverticulum.[26] The possibility that all cases except incomplete bifid ureters are of an acquired nature cannot be dismissed.[26,28]

Separated from cases of single ureteral diverticula are examples of ureteral diverticulosis, first reported by Holly and Sumcad.[23] These are commonly bilateral. Among the unilateral examples, this variant shows a predilection for the left side.[25,27,29] A history of urinary tract infection and obstruction is common. Most cases are reported in males, frequently older than 50 years.[25,27,29] Histologic studies of such cases with multiple diverticula are limited to three cases.[25,27] Thus, even less is known about this entity than the limited understanding of etiology and pathogenesis of examples of single diverticulum of the ureter.

It should be mentioned that one reported case of transitional cell carcinoma developing in a ureteral diverticulum was reported in 1983 by Harrison.[30]

Amyloidosis

Localized deposits of amyloid in the ureteral wall with resultant ureteral obstruction have been reported in 21 patients.[31-51] Of the reported cases, 13 involved women, and 15 of the 21 cases were located in the distal ureter. Ages of the patients ranged from the second to the eighth decades, with a peak frequency in the sixth and seventh decades. Two cases had bilateral involvement.[37,44] Renal pelvic involvement was found concomitantly in two cases.[32,34]

The clinical presentation in most cases is nonspecific. Flank pain with hematuria (frequently microscopic) leads to a radiologic diagnosis of ureteral obstruction. The distal ureter is the most common location for both amyloid tumors and primary ureteral neoplasms, and thus both entities are among the differential diagnoses. The definitive diagnosis is made during microscopic examination. A frozen section diagnosis may contribute to unnecessary radical surgery.

The affected ureter shows an ill-defined segmental firm thickening, frequently with proximal ureteral dilatation. Histologically, the amorphous amyloid is deposited in the interstitium of the ureteral wall. Associated plasma cells and lymphocytes are commonly present in the background. The picture is similar to localized amyloid deposits found in other organs. One case reported by Higbee and Millett contained calcified bone in association with the amyloid deposits, a finding reported in occasional cases of amyloidosis involving the renal pelvis.[33,43]

Endometriosis

Involvement of the ureter by endometriosis was first reported by Cullen in 1917.[52] Subsequently, approximately 100 cases have been reported in the literature.[53-78] The disorder is most common in the fourth and fifth decades, but it has been reported in a 21-year-old woman and in three postmenopausal women aged 56 years, 59 years, and 63 years.[66-69] Unilateral involvement is most common but bilateral ureteral endometriosis has been reported in rare cases.[52,57,66,69,78] The lower one third of the ureter is the most frequently involved site (Fig. 3-3).[53,55,58,60-62,64,70-78] Frequently, there is associated endometriosis of other organs of the urinary system (bladder, kidney) and the genital organs (ovaries, fallopian tubes, and uterus).[52,55,56,58,62,70,74]

Ureteral endometriosis is classified as extrinsic or intrinsic. Extrinsic endometriosis of the ureter, which constitutes 80% of reported cases, is characterized by involvement in the periureteral retroperitoneal adventitia in a focal or concentric manner.[55,60,65,66] Intrinsic endometriosis is characterized by involvement of the muscular layer, the lamina propria, and on occasion, the mucosa of the ureter. Whether extrinsic or intrinsic, endometriosis contains endometrial stroma with or without demonstrable endometrial glands, in association with variable amounts of collagenous fibrosis (Fig. 3-4). Evidence of recent and old hemorrhage as demonstrated by the presence of hemosiderin in the endometrial stroma is observed frequently.[52,59,61,62,65,67,69,74,76] The fibrosis is in part the cause of the ureteral stricture, and is the result of the inflammatory response to the repetitive local hemorrhage.

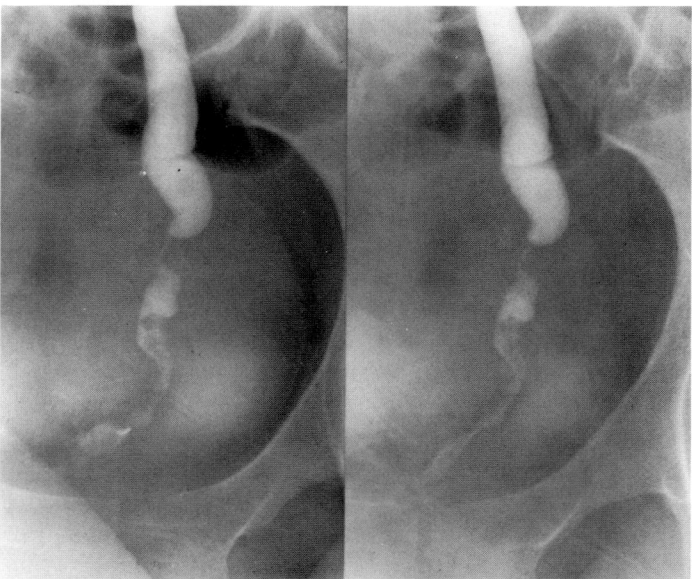

Figure 3-3   *Endometriosis. Antegrade ureterogram following percutaneous nephrostomy demonstrates obstruction in the lower one third of ureter. The excised lesion demonstrated periureteral endometriosis with only focal muscular involvement. The differential diagnosis must include other neoplastic and inflammatory disorders capable of constricting the distal ureter.*

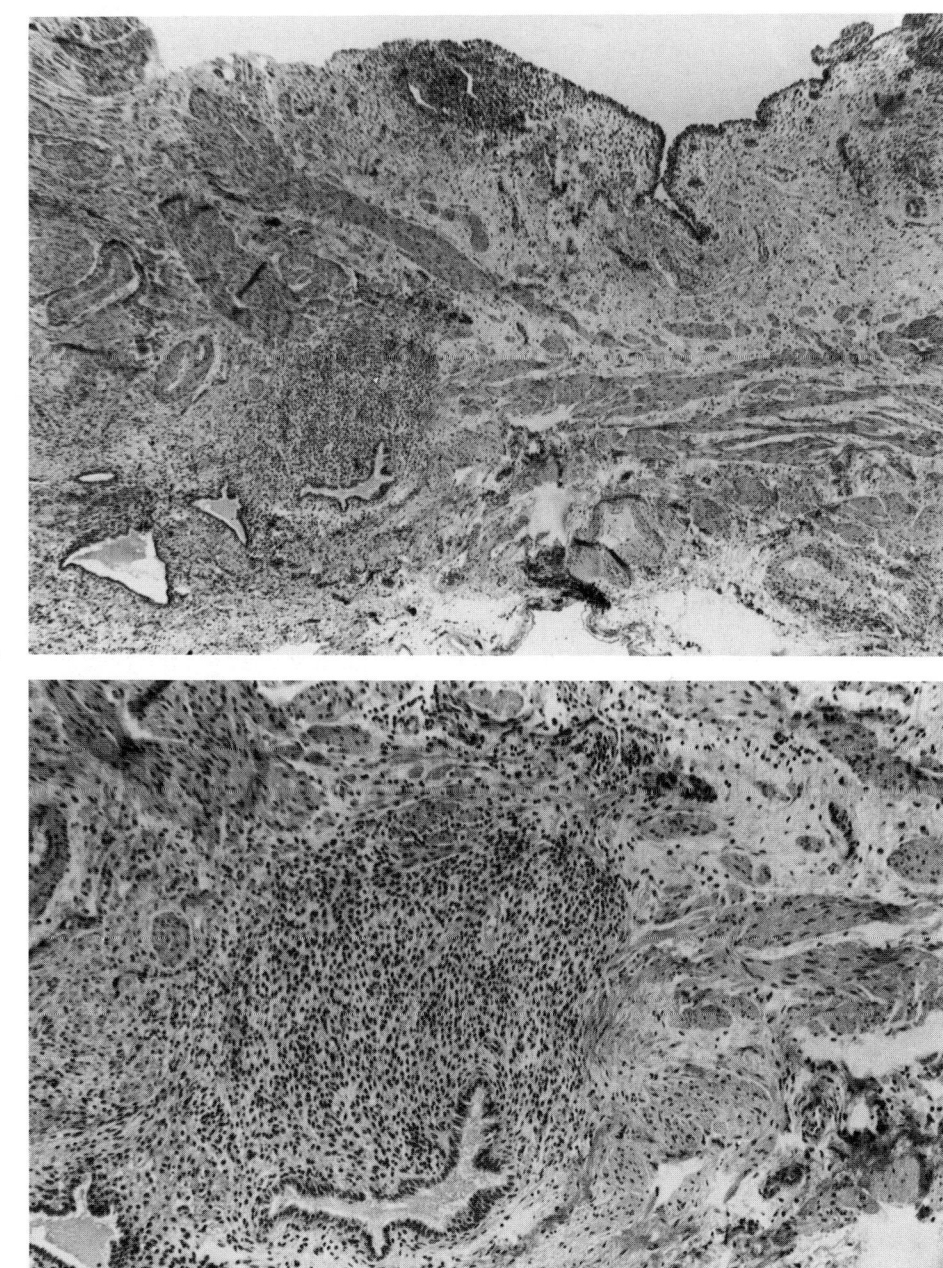

A

B

Figure 3-4 ***Endometriosis.*** *(A) The focus of endometriosis is present in the outer muscularis and adventitia. (B) The characteristic stroma surrounds the endometriotic gland.*

Secondary changes of hydroureter, hydronephrosis, and pyelonephritis are observed commonly in the ipsilateral ureter and kidney.[60-63,65,74]

In 1972 Yates-Bell and co-workers reported one case (case 3) of "poorly differentiated adenocarcinoma" arising in endometriosis involving the ureter. The malignancy was not described further or illustrated, and the patient was observed for 17 years without evidence of recurrent tumor.[67] No other case with malignant change of ureteral endometriosis has been reported, although this has been reported in other locations.[56]

Malakoplakia

Ureteral malakoplakia has been reported in 13 cases (Table 3-1).[79-90] Concurrent renal, renal pelvic, and bladder involvement is common among these cases. Ureteral malakoplakia has not been observed in males to this time and has been reported only in middle-aged and elderly women. Most cases are unilateral, but bilateral involvement has been observed in two patients.[80,87] Ureteral obstruction is a common feature in all cases. Both segmental and diffuse ureteral involvement have been reported. The clinical presentation of patients with ureteral obstruction, whether due to amyloidosis, endometriosis, malakoplakia, or malignancy is nonspecific, and the diagnosis is made at the time of histologic review.

Malakoplakia is to be differentiated from granulomatous inflammation of specific etiology and from retroperitoneal fibrosis. The diagnosis is made histologically, and requires finding the typical Michaelis–Gutmann bodies either within histiocytes or in extracellular locations within the characteristically dense background of mixed chronic inflammatory cells.

The historical, etiologic, pathogenetic and epidemiologic aspects of malakoplakia are discussed in the chapter on the urinary bladder.

Table 3-1   *Malakoplakia*

Author	Year	Age	Sex	Side	Other Sites
Gibson et al[79]	1955	51	F	R	Kidney, bladder
Van Zile Scott, Scott[80]	1958	64	F	R, L*	Kidney
Lewis et al[81]	1961	69	F	R	Renal pelvis
Kalodny[82]	1966	48	F	L	None
Schneiderman, Simon[83]	1968	53	F	L	Kidney, renal pelvis
Elliott et al[84]	1972	2 cases; no details			NI
Halpern et al[85]	1974	42	F	L	None
Sunshine[86]	1974	36	F	R	Renal pelvis, bladder
O'Dea et al[87]	1977	51	F	R	Bladder
O'Dea et al[87]	1977	NI	NI	R, L†	Bladder
Nieh, Althausen[88]	1979	55	F	L	Kidney
Sexton et al[89]	1982	62	F	L	Renal pelvis, bladder
Rudd, Mathews[90]	1982	39	F	R	None

NI, no information.
* Metachronous
† Synchronous

Radiation Injury

Radiation injury, resulting in stricture and ureteral obstruction or fistula formation, is commonly encountered subsequent to radiation therapy for cervical carcinoma in women.[91-94] Localized ureteral injury with fibrosis has been reported in one patient following radiation therapy for prostatic carcinoma.[96] Radiation-induced transitional cell carcinoma of the ureter has been reported in one patient, occurring 39 years after retrograde pyelography with a contrast solution containing Thorotrast.[95] The characteristic α particle tracks were observed in tumor autoradiographs.

Clinical evidence of unilateral or bilateral ureteral obstruction has been observed as early as 1 month or as much as 29 years following radiation therapy.[91-94] It is most common within 2 years of the radiation treatment.

Intramural and periureteral fibrosis with ureteral stricture is observed in surgical specimens. Histologic findings include atypical fibroblasts with enlarged, hyperchromatic nuclei associated with variable amounts of fibrosis. The characteristic subintimal collections of histiocytes also may be present. A nonspecific chronic inflammatory cell infiltrate and stromal edema are inconstant findings. The preoperative differential diagnosis must include recurrent or metastatic tumor, especially when the known primary tumor is a cervical squamous cell carcinoma.[91-94] Because metastatic tumors in the ureter commonly produce a desmoplastic response, the true nature of the ureteral stricture may not be apparent at surgery. Frozen section consultation will clarify the cause of the obstruction.

Fungal and Helminthic Infections

Candidiasis

Candidiasis involving the ureter was reported by Cohen in 1973.[97] Both intraluminal fungal colonies (fungal balls) and exophytic, intramural fungal lesions were visualized radiologically. Similar fungal balls have been reported in the renal pelvis, on occasion resulting in obstruction at the ureteropelvic junction. (Refer to section about fungal infections in Chap. 2.) Whether predominantly manifesting in the renal pelvis or the ureter, candidal pyelonephritis is invariably present and serves as the focus for downstream dissemination.

Schistosomiasis

In endemic areas, bilharzial involvement of the ureter is common due to the ureteral venous anastomoses and with the portal venous system. The ureteral lesions of schistosomiasis include strictures, polyps, calcification, and diffuse urothelial metaplastic changes including squamous metaplasia and ureteritis cystica.[98,99]

Fibroepithelial (Hamartomatous) Polyps

Fibroepithelial polyps are grossly and histologically similar to those occurring in the renal pelvis. (See discussion of fibroepithelial polyps of the renal pelvis in Chap. 2.) Approximately 50 cases have been reported in the ureter.[100–119]

When observed in the ureter, the unsettled pathogenesis is reflected in the numerous synonyms for this lesion that appear in the literature. The following terms are the most frequently used synonyms for *ureteral polyp.*

Polyp[103]

Benign polyp[111]

Stromal polyp[102]

Fibrous polyp[106,109,113,118]

Benign fibrous polyp[109]

Fibroma[103]

Angiofibromatous polyp[107]

Fibromuscular hamartoma[112]

Polypoid hamartoma[108]

Fibroepithelial polyp[116,117,119]

Fibroepithelioma[114]

Xanthomatous ureteral polyp[115]

Ureteral polyposis (Peutz–Jeghers syndrome)[110]

These ureteral polyps are most probably hamartomatous proliferations and not true neoplasms. The presence of multiple components in variable proportions, including smooth muscle, collagen, and thin-walled vessels, supports this interpretation. The frequent absence of both clinical and histologic evidence of inflammation, both past and current, precludes considering that all represent inflammatory polyps.

Patients most commonly present with flank pain and hematuria, associated with radiologic evidence of ureteral obstruction.[117] Seventy percent of reported cases are in the age range of 10 years to 40 years.[117] In contrast to the lesion in the renal pelvis, it is more common in males and in the left ureter.[117] Approximately 60% are present at the ureteropelvic junction, and at the proximal one third of the ureter (Figs. 3-5 to 3-7). Twenty percent are found in the distal ureter. Most examples are single polyps, but cases with multiple polyps within the renal pelvis and ureter have been observed.[110,105,109,113] One patient had multiple ureteral polyps associated with colonic polyps of the Peutz–Jeghers syndrome.[110] Polyp-induced intussusception of the ureter has been reported in six patients.[107,119]

Recognition of this entity, awareness of the characteristic age of the patients (10 years to 40 years), and predilection for the proximal ureter will assist in differentiating these lesions from malignant epithelial neoplasms of the ureter. It is hoped that the frequency of excessively radical surgical procedures will be reduced.

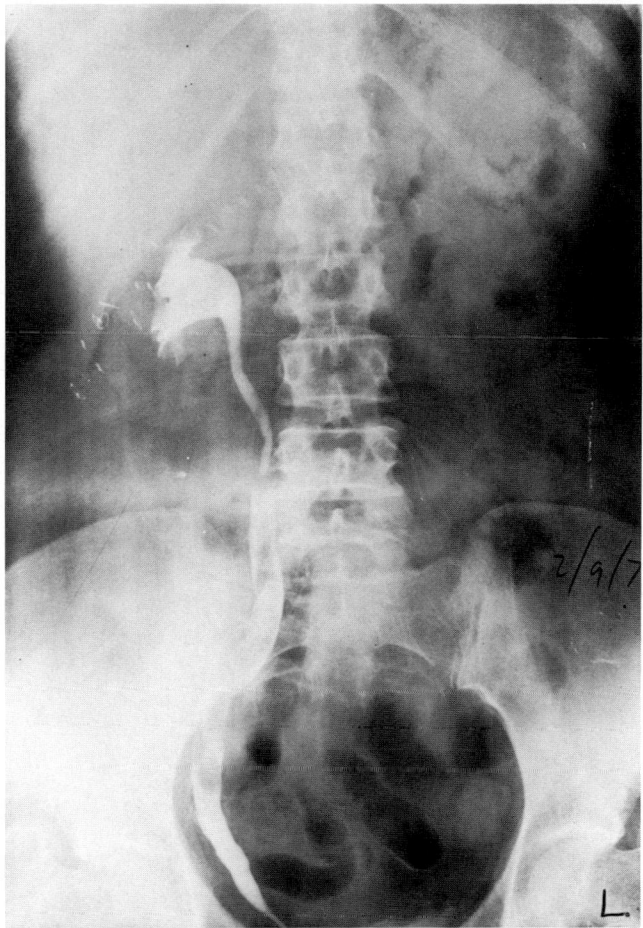

Figure 3-5   *Fibroepithelial polyp. Retrograde ureterogram demonstrates a*
long polypoid filling defect (13 cm) arising in the proximal
ureter and extending down to the pelvic ureter. The differential
diagnosis includes blood clot, inflammatory debris, and
nonopaque calculus.

Proliferative and Metaplastic Variants

Brunn's Nests and Ureteritis Cystica (Glandularis)

The original description of Brunn's nests and ureteritis cystica is attributed to
Morgagni (1761) who noted the cystic lesions of the ureter later to be called
ureteritis cystica. (Refer to discussion of urothelial proliferative variants in Chap.
2.) The distribution of these urothelial alterations was reported by Morse (1928)
in an autopsy series.[120] They were observed most commonly in the bladder, renal
pelvis, and upper ureter.

Although commonly associated with chronic inflammation, 42% of the

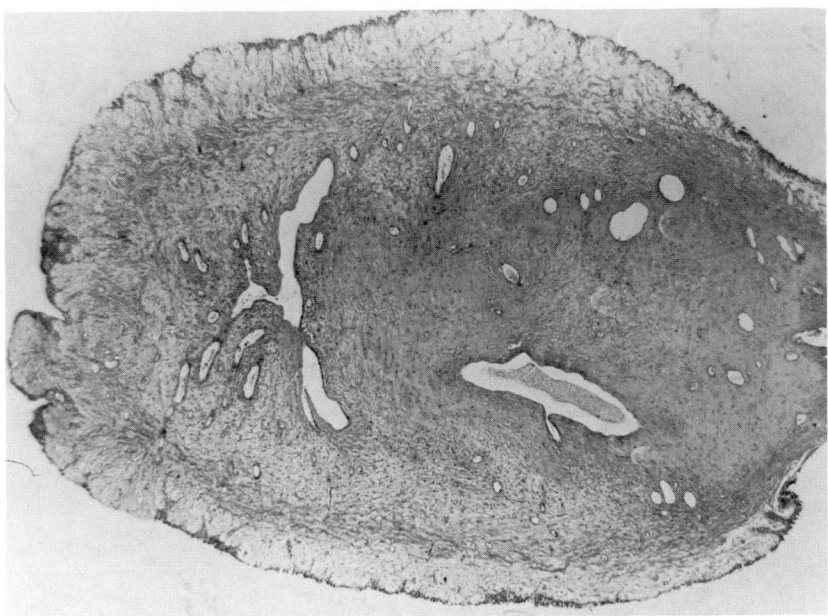

Figure 3-6   *Fibroepithelial polyp. A thin urothelial lining covers the fibrovascular core of the polypoid structure.*

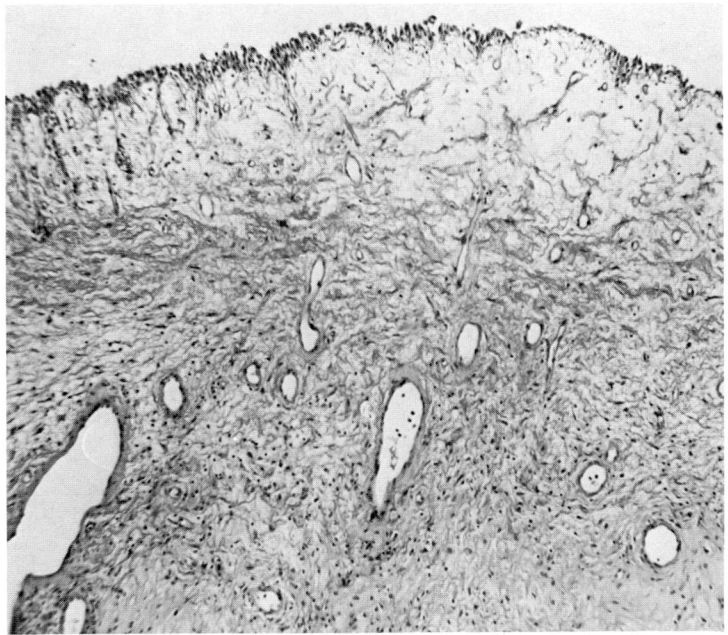

Figure 3-7   *Fibroepithelial polyp. The fibrous tissue immediately beneath the urothelium is edematous. Several thin-walled blood vessels are present in the deeper fibrous stroma.*

cases studied by Morse showed no inflammation.[120] The pathogenesis of these alterations became the subject of numerous studies in subsequent years. (Refer to discussion in Chap. 2.)

The clinical significance of these urothelial proliferative alterations centers around their possible relationship to urothelial neoplasms. In rare instances, the exuberance of the urothelial proliferation in the form of Brunn's nests in the renal pelvis and ureter histologically may suggest invasive transitional cell carcinoma.[121,131] The cytologically benign features of the cells in the nests are the critical feature that distinguishes them from a urothelial neoplasm. There is no evidence that these proliferative changes, Brunn's nests, and the cystic or glandular variants, are premalignant or have premalignant potential (whatever that is), regardless of location in the urinary tract (Figs. 3-8 to 3-11). The same is true for squamous metaplasia and nephrogenic metaplasia.

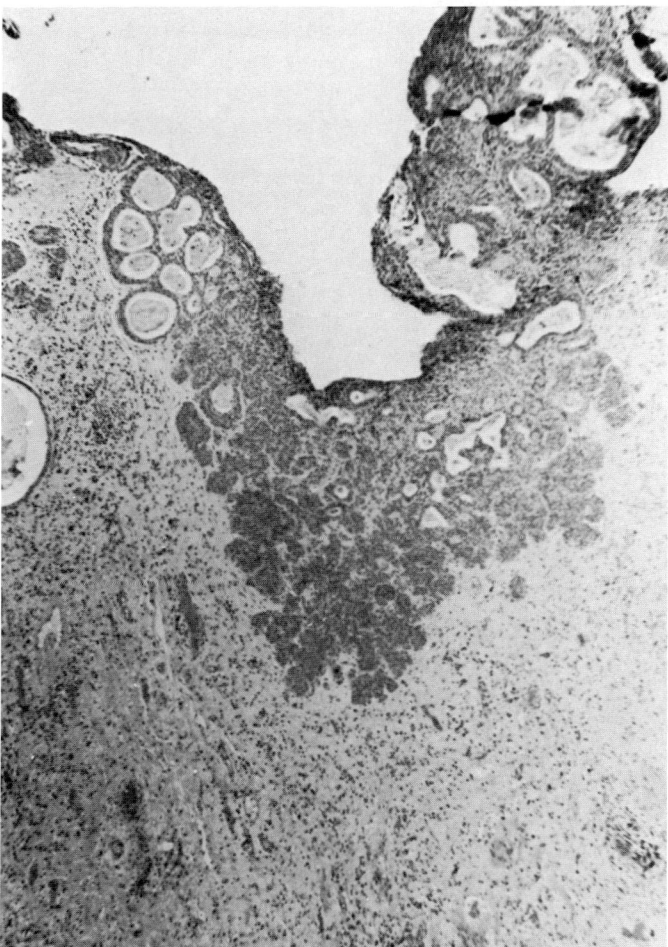

Figure 3-8 **Brunn's nests and ureteritis cystica.** *Adjacent to the multiple solid Brunn's nests in the ureteral wall are scattered cystica structures with a central lumen containing eosinophilic secretions. The cytologic features of the surface urothelium were identical to those seen in the proliferative variance encroaching in the lamina propria.*

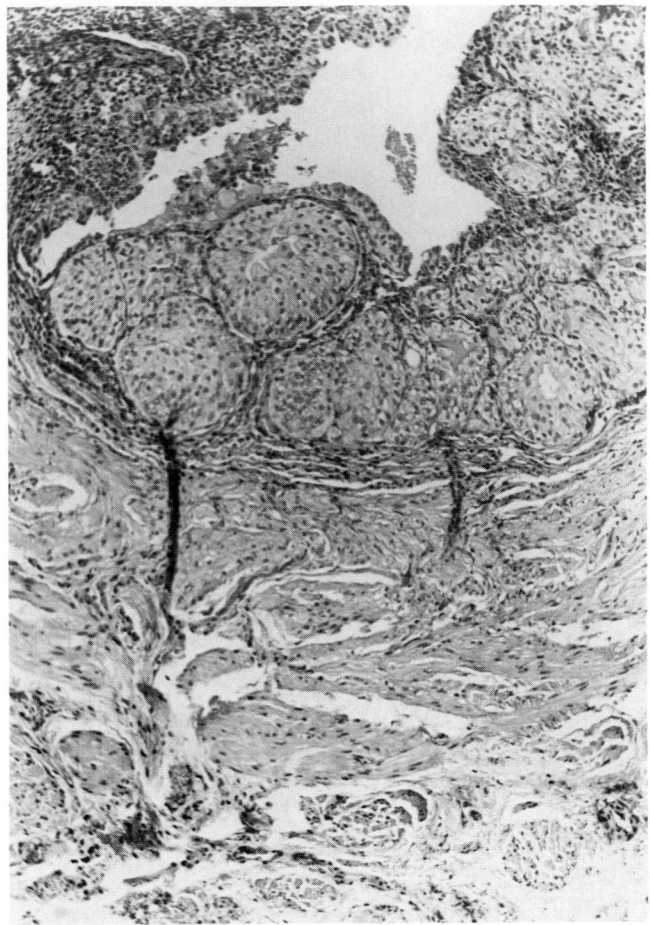

Figure 3-9   *Multiple Brunn's nests, some with early, centrally located clefts, are present in the lamina propria of the ureter.*

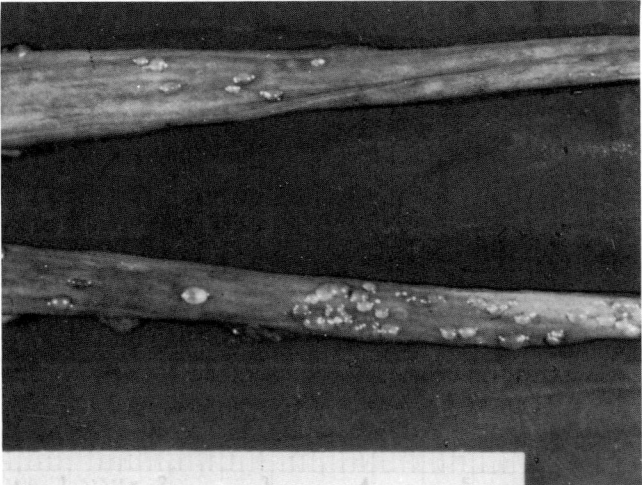

Figure 3-10   ***Ureteritis cystica.*** *The typical mucosal blebs of ureteritis cystica are demonstrated in this segment of upper ureter.*

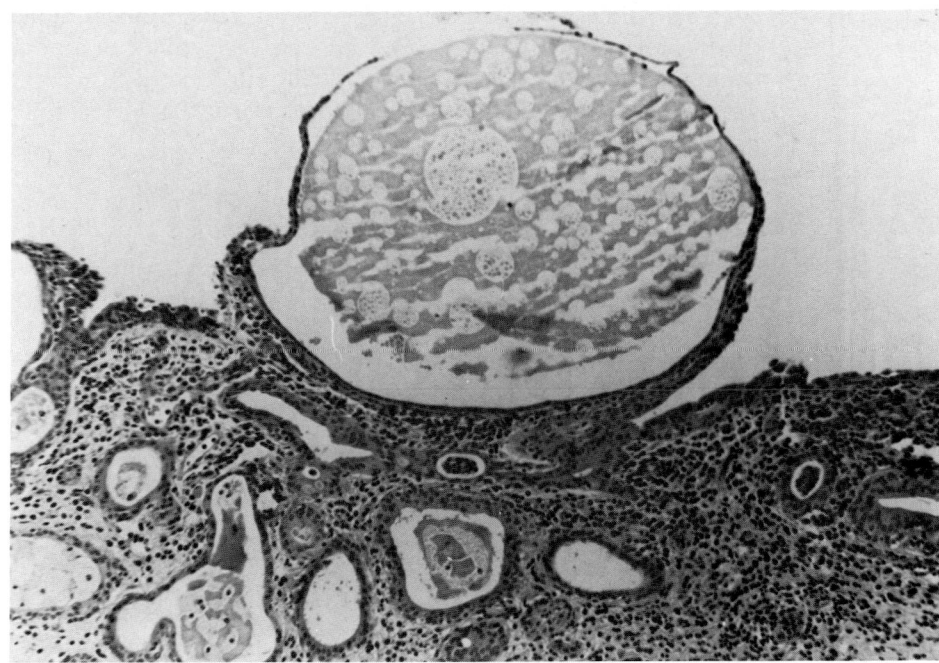

Figure 3-11   *Ureteritis cystica. The markedly dilated cystica structure protrudes into the lumen of the ureter. Smaller, similar ureteritis cystica structures are present in the subjacent lamina propria.*

Squamous Metaplasia

Urothelial squamous metaplasia has been referred to as *cholesteatoma* and *leukoplakia* in the urologic literature.[122,123] The two terms are descriptive and histogenetically vague. Recently, Hertle and Androulakakis, in a critical review, detailed the variable and imprecise understanding of this metaplastic change as reflected in the available literature.[123] These authors suggested the term *keratinizing desquamative squamous metaplasia* (KDSM) for this urothelial alteration. This metaplastic change most frequently is observed in the bladder, but it also is observed in the upper urinary tract. Hertle and Androulakakis reviewed 78 published cases, four of which involved the ureter.[123] Of all the cases reviewed by these authors, only 62% were associated with urinary tract inflammation. Importantly, 48% were not associated with any other pathologic process. Thus, the pathogenesis of squamous metaplasia of the urinary tract remains unresolved in spite of the inflammatory changes associated with some cases. There is no evidence that squamous metaplasia in any location in the urinary tract is associated with an increased risk of subsequent malignancy.[123] Their clinical significance relates to the accumulation of keratin debris and resulting potential for renal pelvic or ureteral obstruction. The clinical presentation relates to the urinary tract obstruction, and 35% of the reported cases evidence a filling defect on IVP.[123] The majority of patients are in the fourth to the sixth decade, and 60% of the patients are men.[123]

Histologically, the urothelial surface is transformed to squamous epithelium with or without evidence of keratinization. Absence of any cytologic atypia is characteristic, but if it is present, it should be noted in the formal pathology report. The biologic significance of this is yet to be determined.

Nephrogenic Metaplasia (Adenoma)

Three cases of nephrogenic adenoma of the ureter were reported recently.[124-126] One case, involving a 32-year-old man with a history of recurrent urinary tract infections, showed metachronous bilateral involvement.[124] The lesions resulted in partial ureteral obstruction. Surgical segmental resection of the involved portions of the ureters was curative.

The microscopic features are identical to examples observed in the bladder,

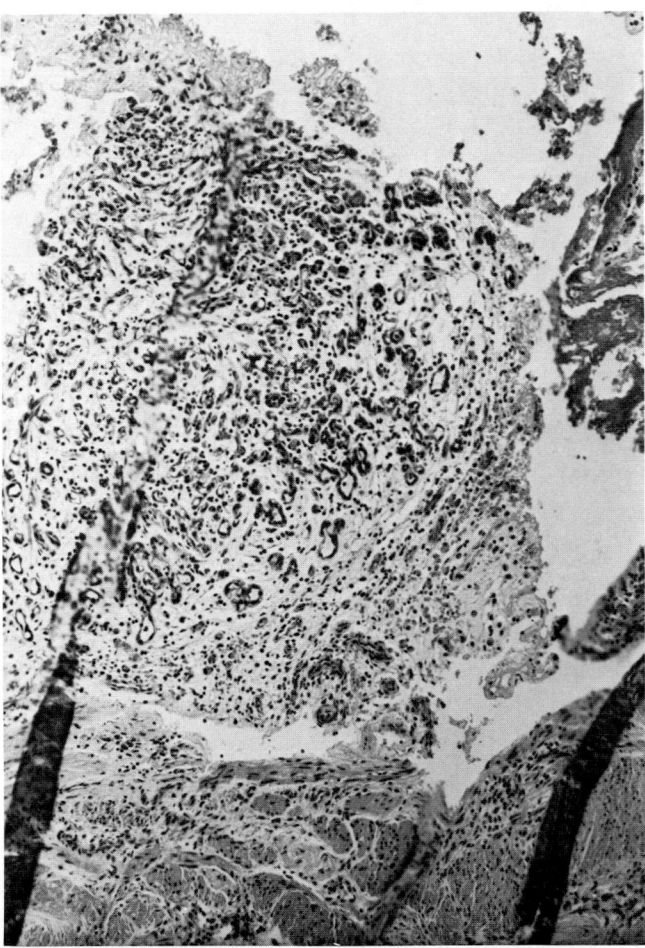

Figure 3-12   *Nephrogenic metaplasia. The expanded mucosa projecting into the ureteral lumen is composed of the proliferating nephrogenic tubules within an edematous stroma. Chronic inflammatory cells are scattered throughout the stroma. The overlying urothelium is denuded. The entire lesion is limited to the lamina propria.*

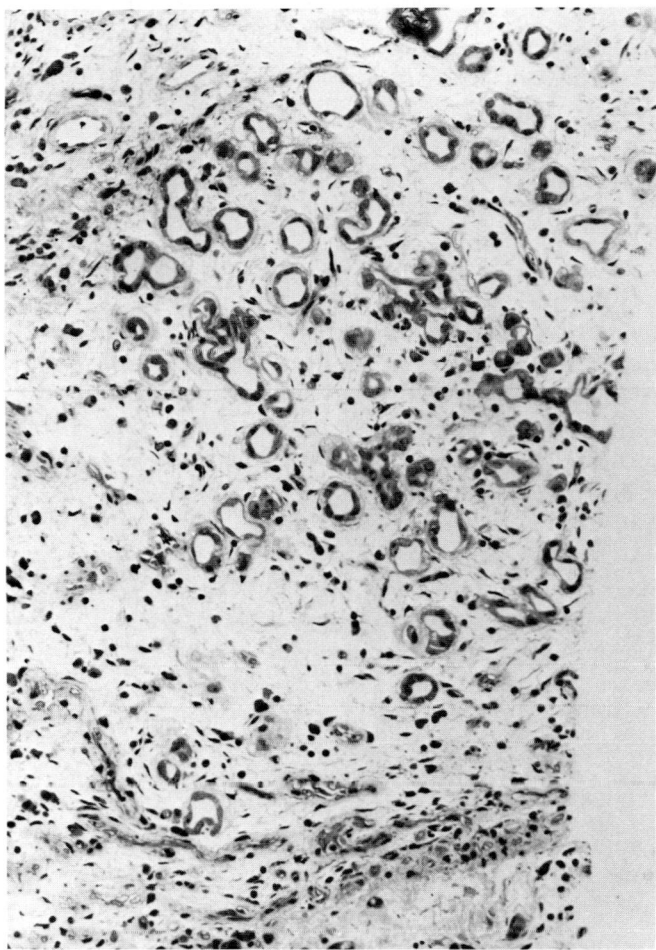

Figure 3-13 *Nephrogenic metaplasia. The simple tubules, which indeed resemble renal tubules, show peritubular stromal condensation, and a well-defined basement membrane when stained with PAS. The tubular pattern and the variation of nuclear chromaticity and overall size have been misdiagnosed as adenocarcinoma in the past.*

the most common location for this metaplastic change. (Refer to section on nephrogenic metaplasia in the chapter about the urinary bladder.) The tubules formed in nephrogenic metaplasia are surrounded by a well-defined basement membrane, and are confined to the lamina propria without evidence of encroachment of the muscularis (Fig. 3-12). The basement membrane is clearly demonstrated by the PAS stain (Fig. 3-13). These features assist in distinguishing this metaplastic change from adenocarcinoma, which it superficially resembles.

Primary Ureteral Neoplasms

With the exception of ureteral carcinoma and in particular transitional cell carcinoma, all other ureteral neoplasms — benign and malignant, epithelial and mesenchymal — are uncommon to rare. Transitional cell carcinoma, with approximately 2000 cases reported in the literature, constitutes more than 90% of all ureteral neoplasms.

Historically, the term *papilloma* was applied to many urothelial neoplasms now regarded as low grade transitional cell carcinomas. In my experience, and that reflected in the more recent literature, true urothelial papillomas are rare. A distinct benign urothelial neoplasm, the inverted papilloma, has been reported recently in the ureter.

Ureteral mesenchymal neoplasms of all types are rare. Both benign and malignant smooth muscle tumors have been reported primary in the ureter, and are more common than all the other varieties of stromal tumors combined.

Metastatic neoplasms involving the ureter are being recognized clinically with greater frequency, but are still silent until discovered at autopsy in the majority of cases. When diagnosed clinically, appropriate therapy can be instituted with reports of dramatic improvement in renal function. This can be accomplished only if there is high index of suspicion suggesting the diagnosis.

The presence of a ureteral neoplasm commonly is suggested by the clinical presentation of hematuria (frequently only microscopic) and flank pain, with or without a palpable mass. Radiologic studies are frequently helpful in the differential diagnosis of a filling defect involving the upper urinary tract. Urine cytology studies in the diagnosis of upper urinary tract epithelial malignancies are unreliable in the majority of cases. Thin needle biopsy procedures guided by computed tomography (CT scan) are potentially of greater value in the future.

Although the etiology of ureteral carcinoma is unknown, epidemiologic studies have implicated environmental carcinogens. Similar evidence has emerged about transitional cell carcinoma involving all sites of the urinary tract from the renal pelvis to the urethra. (Refer to section about multiple urothelial neoplasms in Chap. 2.) Clinical experience strongly suggests that the urothelium throughout the urinary tract is a "target organ," and multicentric urothelial malignancies in individual patients is the rule, not the exception. This characteristic of the urothelium has a significant influence on the natural history of urothelial malignancies, and should form the basis for appropriate definitive therapy and subsequent clinical observation of patients.

Staging of Ureteral Carcinoma

Many staging protocols for ureteral carcinoma have been proposed in the urologic literature, all of which are variations on the original theme proposed by Jewett, Strong, and Marshall for bladder carcinoma.[147,151,158,161,163,164,166] (Refer

Table 3-2   *Suggested Staging Protocol for Ureteral Carcinoma*

Stage	Extent of Tumor
O	Noninvasive; limited to mucosal surface
A	Invasion limited to lamina propria
B	Invasion limited to muscularis
C	Invasion into periureteral adventitia
D1	Metastases to regional lymph nodes
D2	Metastases to distant sites

to Chap. 4 on bladder carcinoma.) Some of these variations are significant, underscoring the need for a uniformly accepted staging protocol for ureteral carcinoma. Because the ureter has no submucosa (there is no muscularis mucosa), and there is no apparent reason to include a benign neoplasm (papilloma) in the staging protocol of ureteral carcinoma, those protocols including such terminology are not accepted.[158,166] The staging protocol presented in Table 3-2 is suggested for ureteral carcinoma.

Benign Epithelial Neoplasms
Inverted Papilloma

Inverted papillomas of the ureter have been observed only recently (1979).[129] Thirteen patients ranging in age from 19 years to 77 years have been reported.[129,130,132–137] Eighty-five percent of patients are in the sixth to the eighth decades. It is more common in males (9 : 4). There is no characteristic location in the ureter, and both the left and the right ureters are affected approximately equally. Clinical evidence of ureteral obstruction with associated flank pain is the most common presentation. The lesions are grossly and microscopically identical to those described elsewhere. (See discussion of inverted papilloma in Chaps. 2 and 4.) Selli and co-workers caution against misinterpreting marked urothelial proliferation of Brunn's nests, in the context of ureteritis, as inverted papilloma.[131]

Treatment requires surgical excision. None of the cases reported taking origin in the ureter have been associated with independent malignancies or malignant transformation.

Malignant Epithelial Neoplasms
Transitional Cell Carcinoma
Incidence

Wising and Blix (1878) and Davy (1884) are credited with the first reports of histologically documented carcinomas of the ureter.[127,138] Scott collected 59 cases reported prior to 1934, a number that increased to 153 in the 1956 review by Abeshouse.[127,138] In subsequent years, the number has increased to approximately 2000.[139–166] (Summarized data of 20 of the largest series reported from 1955 to 1983 appear later in Table 3-4.) Thirty-eight cases of bilateral transitional cell carcinomas of ureters were found in the literature (Table 3-3). Five cases of simultaneous renal cell carcinoma and ipsilateral ureteral transitional cell carcinoma have been reported.[155,185–188]

Epidemiology and Etiology

The cause(s) are unknown. Because I regard the urothelium of the entire urinary tract as a single "target organ," the reviews of the epidemiologic, etiologic, and experimental data presented in Chapter 2 on renal pelvis and Chapter 4 on urinary bladder apply to transitional cell carcinoma of the ureter.

Studies specifically relating ureteral carcinoma and prior exposure to (1) industrial aniline dyes, (2) uroradiologic procedures employing contrast material, (3) cigarettes, and (4) coffee have been reported.[127,154] (Refer to section on etiology of renal pelvic carcinoma in Chap. 2.) Petkovic has reported an increased frequency of bilateral renal pelvic and ureteral tumors observed in a Belgrade, Yugoslavia clinic that treats patients who have Balkan nephritis, an endemic disease.[182] Recently the first case of ureteral carcinoma occurring subsequent to cyclophosphamide therapy was reported by Schiff and co-workers.[165]

Demography

The reported age range of patients with ureteral transitional cell carcinoma is 29 years to 93 years, with a peak frequency observed in the sixth and seventh decades.

Table 3-3

Bilateral Transitional Cell Carcinomas

Author	Year	Age	Sex
Ratliff et al[167]	1949	60	M
Felber[168]	1953	58	F
Gracia, Bradfield[169]	1958	44	M
Crassweller[170]	1958	60	M
Gaca[171]	1960	54	M
Utz et al[172]	1962	69	M
Viek et al[173]	1963	71	M
Perlmutter et al[174]	1965	64	M
Gillenwatter et al[175]	1966	81	M
Barroso et al[176]	1966	NI	M
Newman et al[173]	1967	NI	NI
Scarzella, McDonald[143]	1967	55	M
Barber[178]	1968	55	M
Talavera et al[179]	1970	68	M
Talavera et al[179]	1970	63	M
Sozer[180]	1974	72	M
Batata et al[156]	1975	NI	M
Levine, Airhart[181]	1977	59	M
Levine, Airhart[181]	1977	61	M
Petkovic[182]	1978	*	*
Werth et al[164]	1981	NI	M
Gonzalez, Zoretic[183]	1982	56	M
Mills, Vaughan[166]	1983	NI	NI
Mills, Vaughan[166]	1983	NI	NI

A-NED, alive with no evidence of disease; NI, no information; TCC, transitional cell carcinoma.

* Details of 15 cases of bilateral ureteral malignancies combined with 30 cases of bilateral renal pelvic neoplasms. The combined 45 cases represent a 9% frequency of bilaterality of pelvic and ureteral neoplasms studied in one clinic in Belgrade, Yugoslavia. The association of these neoplasms with Balkan nephropathy, endemic in some areas of Yugoslavia, is noted by the author. Twenty-four of the 45 cases were synchronous.

† Death due to disseminated bladder transitional cell carcinoma.

The sex distribution varies among different studies only in the extent of male predominance. Overall figures show that approximately 70% of patients are male (Tables 3-4 and 3-5). The right and left sides are affected equally.

Clinical Presentation

At the time of diagnosis, 6% to 26% (average 12%) of patients are asymptomatic.[149,158,160,161,164] The existence of the tumor in such patients is discovered commonly as incidental radiologic findings during follow-up evaluations of previously diagnosed bladder neoplasms.[147,152,153,156,161,184]

The majority of patients have signs and symptoms that ultimately lead to the preoperative radiologic diagnosis. Hematuria is observed in 75%, flank pain in

Synchronous/ Metachronous	Location		Associated GU Neoplasms	Follow Up
	Right	Left		
Synchronous	Mid	Mid	None	A-NED, 2 mo
Meta (8 yr)	Mid	Mid	TCC, ureter stump, and TCC, bladder (subsequent)	A-Bladder TCC, 2 yr
Synchronous	Low	Low	None	A-NED, 2 yr
Synchronous	Mid	Low	None	A-NED, 16 mo
Meta (3 yr)	Upper	Upper	None	A-NED, 6 mo
Meta (5 mo)	Mid	Low	TCC, bladder (subsequent)	A-NED, 21 mo
Synchronous	Low	Mid	None	NI
Synchronous	Mid	Entire	None	A-NED, 13 mo
Synchronous	Low	Low	None	A-NED, 6 mo
Synchronous	Low	Mid	None	A-NED, 2 yr
Meta (14 yr)	NI	NI	NI	NI
Meta (7 yr)	Low	Low	None	Lost to follow up
Meta (4 mo)	Low	Low	None	A-NED, 3 yr
Synchronous	Upper	Low	None	A-NED, 12 mo
Synchronous	Mid	Low	TCC, bladder (subsequent)	A-NED, 4.5 yr
Synchronous	Low	Low	None	A-NED, 19 mo
Meta (2 yr)	NI	NI	TCC, bladder (subsequent)	Dead, 6 yr†
Synchronous	Low	Mid	TCC, bladder (prior, subsequent)	A-NED, 6 yr
Synchronous	Upper	Mid	None	A-NED, 1 yr
*	*	*	*	*
Synchronous	NI	NI	NI	D-pneumonia, 2 yr
Synchronous	Mid	Mid	TCC, bladder (prior)	A-NED, 22 mo
Synchronous	NI	NI	NI	NI
Synchronous	NI	NI	NI	NI

Table 3-4   **_Transitional Cell Carcinoma_**

Author	Number of Cases	Year	Sex M/F	Age Range
Whitlock et al[141]	33	1955	27/45	37–8 dec.
Ochsner, Brannan[142]	15	1960	10/5	41–77
Meyer[144]	21	1969	15/5	49–84
Beck et al[146]	40	1969	NI	NI
Mackinney[145]	16	1969	11/5	36–90
Bloom et al[147]	102	1970	3/1	38–93
Hawtrey[149]	52	1971	5.5/1	44–82
Arger, Stolz[210]	21	1972	14/7	49–82
Kim et al[151]	29	1972	22/7	4–9 dec.
Almgard et al[152]	45	1973	30/15	45–82
Williams, Mitchell[153]	34	1973	23/11	43–79
Burger, Spjut[155]	22	1974	19/3	35–71
Batata et al[156]	41	1975	29/12	29–79
Mazeman[157]	377	1976	3.4/1	*
Batata, Grabstald[158]	63	1976	48/15	NI
Ghazi[160]	25(27)	1979	21/6	42–83
Babian, Johnson[161]	40(44)	1980	26/18	33–77
Heney[163]	60	1981	45/15	43–86
Werth et al[164]	35	1982	28/7	14–88
Mills, Vaughn[166]	53	1983	NI	NI

* 65% of tumors occurred in patients 50 years to 70 years of age.

30%, and a palpable mass in 7% of patients found to have a ureteral transitional cell carcinoma (Table 3-5). At the time of diagnosis, 2% to 16% (average 10%) of patients give a history or have concurrent evidence of lithiasis.[127,158,166]

Pathology

The risk of neoplastic change of the ureteral mucosa is not uniform throughout its length. This is true of all histologic types of ureteral carcinoma. The lower one

Table 3-5   **_Clinical Features of Epithelial Malignancies_**

Histological Type	Number of Cases (>1970)*	Sex Distribution	Hematuria (%)	Flank Pain (%)	Mass (%)	Lithiasis (%)	Location (Distal 1/3) (%)
Transitional cell carcinoma†	2000(1800)	70% male	75	30	7	10	63
Squamous cell carcinoma‡	43(12)	70% male	90	56	44	25	65
Adenocarcinoma§	15(8)	72% male	27	>90	20	40	45

* Figure in parentheses denotes cases reported after 1970.
† References 127, 142, 146–149, 157, 158, 160, 161, 163, 164, 166
‡ References 127, 139, 142, 147, 156, 160, 161, 189–201
§ References 142, 156, 164, 202–213

Mean	L/R	Hematuria (%)	Location (%)			Other GU Neoplasms (%)	Follow up, 5-Year Survival Rate (%)
			U1/3	M1/3	L1/3		
NI	21/12	NI	15	27	58	41	38.8
61	NI	80		58 in L1/2		NI	NI
64	7/8	NI	NI			28.5	NI
NI	NI	70	NI			5	NI
NI	4/12	75	NI			NI	37
65.8	NI	82	NI			7	42
66	24/27	81	19	17	64	48	25
66	9/8	61	5	NI	NI	NI	20
7 dec.	R = L	83	NI	NI	66	24	35
R = L	NI	NI	NI			55	NI
64	NI	91	20	18	56	37	NI
65	15/7	NI	36	18	45	27	41
60	24/17	76	25	25	50	36	41
*	200/177	83	NI	NI	NI	27	31
6–7 dec.	NI	82	NI			40	38.4
5–7 dec.	16/9	44	NI	NI	70	33	NI
61	26/18	59	3	24	73	25	67
65	NI	NI	NI			48	NI
60	16/18	81	25	6	69	64	NI
NI	NI	62	NI			36	48

third of the ureter is the site of transitional cell carcinoma in 50% to 73% (mean 63%) of reported cases (Tables 3-4 and 3-5). The least frequent site of the neoplasm is the proximal one third of the ureter.

The gross and microscopic appearances of ureteral transitional cell carcinomas are similar to those in the renal pelvis and the more distal urinary tract. The exophytic component results in variable degrees of luminal obstruction with proximal hydroureter and hydronephrosis (Figs. 3-14 to 3-16). Neoplasms demonstrating invasion of the ureteral wall further compromise the lumen with stricture production. The distribution of tumor grades reported in six recently published series of ureteral transitional cell carcinomas is presented in Table 3-6. The traditional tumor grading system (grades 1 to 4) or the World Health Organization grading system (grades 1 to 3) is utilized in these studies. Grade 1 constitutes 8% to 20% of all cases regardless of the grading system employed. The majority of all cases are grades 1 and 2. Grades 3 and 4 constitute 33% to 48% of all cases, compared to grade 3 cases that constitute approximately 40% when the WHO system is employed. Progressive decrease in survival is observed with increasing tumor grade (Table 3-7).

Natural History and Survival

The distribution of tumor stage reported in seven studies of ureteral carcinoma is presented in Table 3-8. Tumors confined to the mucosa (stage O) without evidence of invasion constitute 9% to 58% (mean 27%) of all ureteral transi-

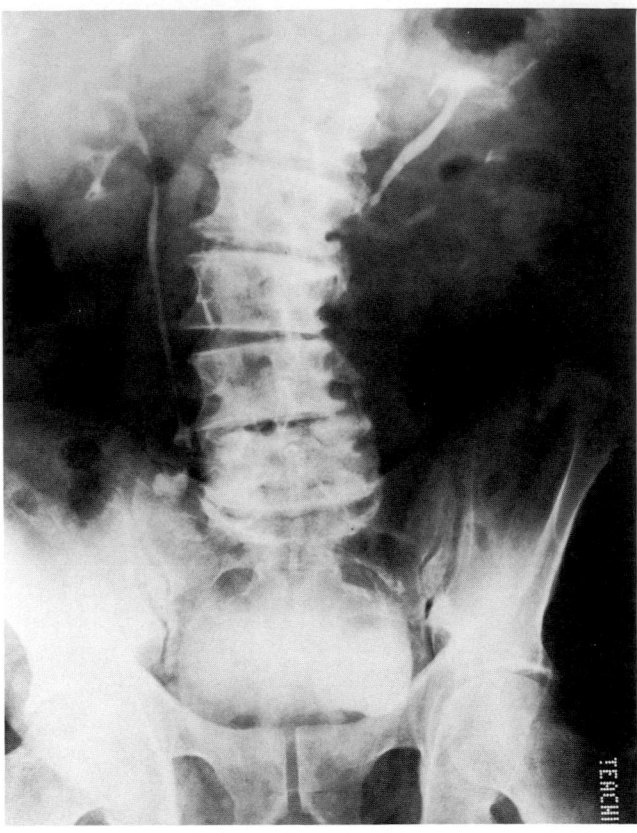

Figure 3-14   *Transitional cell carcinoma of the ureter. A filling defect*
(1.5 cm) in the distal right ureter is demonstrated by IVP. The
ureteral dilatation distal to the defect is more suggestive of a
slowly evolving neoplasm than other causes such as blood clot,
sloughed renal papillae, fungus ball, and nonopaque calculus.

tional cell carcinomas. Invasion limited to the lamina propria (stage A) is observed in 18% to 43% (mean 30%) of cases, whereas an additional 6% to 30%
(mean 16%) of cases have invasion of the muscularis (stage B). Of all tumors,
approximately two thirds are confined to the ureteral wall (stages O, A, B) and
one third have spread beyond the ureter (stages C, D) at the time of surgery.

Tumor grade and tumor stage are correlated closely.[147,156,163] Virtually all
grade 1 tumors are found to be stage O or A. Conversely, the majority (70% to
80%) of grade 4 tumors have spread beyond the ureter (stages C, D).

Both grade and stage are correlated closely with 5-year survival (Tables 3-7
and 3-9). Tumors with regional or distant metastases (stage D) are associated
with a 0% to 7% survival rate at 5 years. If spread is limited to direct invasion of
the periureteral soft tissue (stage C), the survival rate increases to 17% to 33% at 5
years. If the invasion is confined to the muscularis of the ureter (stage B), 25% to
82% (mean 47%) of patients survive 5 years. Although Bloom and co-workers
(1971) reported a 62% 5-year survival rate among noninvasive (stage O) ureteral
carcinomas, and Kim and co-workers (1972) observed a 40% 5-year survival rate
among patients with neoplasms invasive to the lamina propria (stage A), several

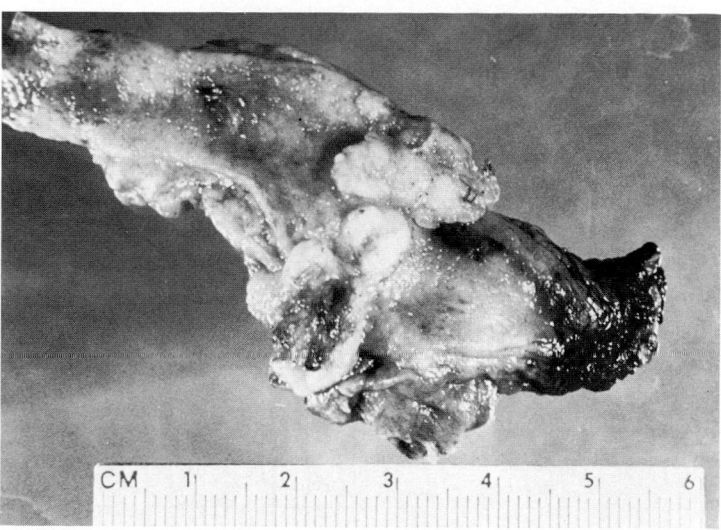

Figure 3-15   *Transitional cell carcinoma of the ureter. The neoplasm is an irregular raised lesion with central ulceration.*

more recent studies report significantly better survival rates.[147,151,161,163,166] No cancer-related deaths were found among the patients with noninvasive tumors in three studies published from the Massachusetts General Hospital, M.D. Anderson Hospital, and Cornell University.[161,163,166] In these same series, cases showing invasion limited to the lamina propria (stage A) have a 5-year survival rate of 80% to 100% (Table 3-9).

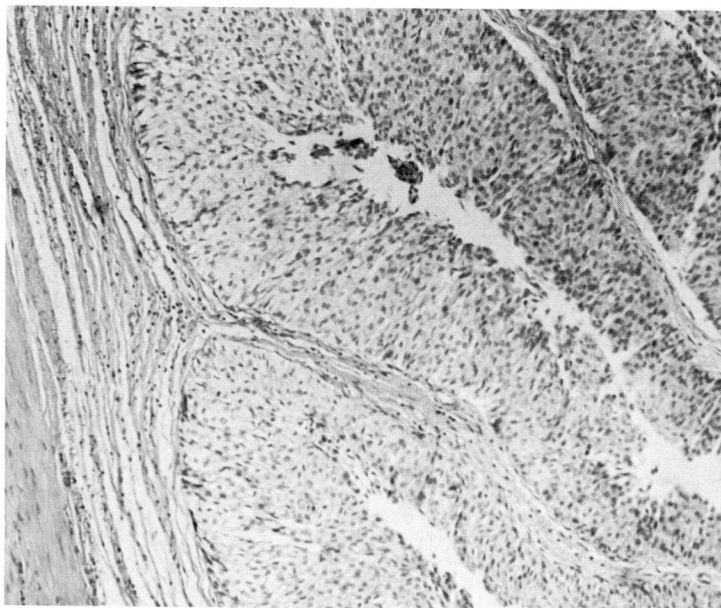

Figure 3-16   *Transitional cell carcinoma, grade 2. The typical papillary structure of this low grade transitional cell carcinoma is evident. No invasion of the ureter wall is present in this section.*

Table 3-6   *Grade Distribution of Transitional Cell Carcinoma*

Author	Year	Number of Patients	Grade (%)			
			1	2	3	4
Bloom et al[147]	1970	102	9.8	47	31	12
Hawtrey[149]	1971	52	20	37	28	15
Burger, Spjut[155]	1974	22	14	54	27	4
Babian, Johnson[161]	1980	40	10	52	39	
Werth et al[164]	1981	28	8	54	21	17
Heney et al[163]	1981	60	15	43	40	

Table 3-7   *Grade Compared with 5-Year Survival Rate for Transitional Cell Carcinoma*

Author	Year	Number of Patients	Grade (%)			
			1	2	3	4
Bloom et al[147]	1970	102	83	52	18	12
Hawtrey[149]	1971	52	89	41	31	0
Babian, Johnson[161]	1980	40	100	78	37	
Heney et al[163]	1981	60	100	81	29	

Table 3-8   *Stage Distribution of Transitional Cell Carcinoma*

Author	Year	Stages (%)				
		O	A	B	C	D
Bloom et al[147]	1970	58		6	11	22
Kim et al[151]	1973		43	30	26*	
Burger, Spjut[155]	1974	32	23	18	18	9
Batata, Grabstald[158]	1975		28	18	31	23
Babian, Johnson[161]	1981	14	18	16	14	9
Heney et al[163]	1981	28	22	15	15	20
Mills, Vaughn[166]	1982	9	37	13	11	28

* Includes cases with regional node metastases.

Table 3-9   *Stage Compared with 5-Year Survival Rate for Transitional Cell Carcinoma*

Author	Year	Stages				
		O	A	B	C	D
Bloom et al[147]	1970	62		25	33	0
Kim et al[151]	1973		40	33	28*	
Batata, Grabstald[156]	1975		90	43	17	0
Babian, Johnson[161]	1981	100	100	50	50	0
Heney et al[163]	1981	100	95	82	29	0
Mills, Vaughn[166]	1982	100	80	50	33	7

* Includes cases with regional node metastases.

Associated Urothelial Neoplasms

The risk of developing multiple urothelial neoplasms is well demonstrated in patients with ureteral transitional cell carcinomas in several studies. Concurrent and subsequent bladder tumors are diagnosed in patients with ureteral carcinoma with average frequencies of 10% and 27%, respectively (Table 3-10). Previous urothelial bladder carcinomas are observed in 20% of these patients. The risk of subsequent bladder carcinoma appears to be (1) greatest during the 2 months to 3 years following diagnosis of the ureteral tumor, and (2) independent of the grade of the ureteral tumor.[147,153,156,161,162,164] The extent of surgical therapy for ureteral carcinoma and risk of subsequent bladder neoplasms is unsettled. Bloom and co workers and Williams and Mitchell reported an increased frequency of subsequent bladder neoplasms following nephrectomy and incomplete ureterectomy operations for the ureteral primary compared with patients who had a nephrectomy and complete ureterectomy including bladder cuff.[147,153] This difference was not found in the series reported by Abeshouse.[127]

The pathogenetic considerations of multiple urothelial neoplasms observed in patients with ureteral carcinoma are the same as those of transitional cell

Table 3-10   **Bladder Neoplasms Associated with Transitional Cell Carcinoma**

Author	Year	Frequency (%)	
Previous Bladder Neoplasms			
Bloom et al[147]	1971	7	
Almgaard et al[152]	1973	42	
Williams, Mitchell[153]	1973	36	62/310 (20%)*
Batata et al[156]	1975	26	
Ghazi et al[160]	1979	11	
Babian, Johnson[161]	1980	16	
Simultaneous Bladder Neoplasms			
Williams, Mitchell[153]	1973	7	
Babian, Johnson[161]	1980	10	10/105 (10%)*
Kakizoe et al[162]	1980	18	
Subsequent Bladder Neoplasms			
Whitlock et al[141]	1955	42	
Abeshouse[127]	1956	27	
Bloom et al[147]	1971	16	
Almgaard et al[152]	1973	16	
Williams, Mitchell[153]	1973	50	
Burger, Spjut[155]	1974	23	138/512 (27%)*
Batata et al[156]	1975	32	
Ghazi et al[160]	1979	22	
Babian, Johnson[161]	1980	35	
Kakizoe et al[162]	1980	36	
Werth et al[164]	1981	20	

* Cumulative frequency (all studies).

carcinoma of the renal pelvis. (Refer to section on this subject in Chap. 2.) The increasing application of tumor mapping of both renal pelvic and ureteral primaries may clarify this currently unsettled question.

Although the extent of surgery has a demonstrated bearing on the risk of ureteral stump recurrences as noted above, there is little evidence that this factor influences the ultimate outcome significantly.[156,161,166] Appropriate follow up of all patients with diagnosed urothelial malignancies requires periodic cystoscopic examinations at close intervals, especially during the first 3 years after diagnosis and primary treatment. Metachronous neoplasms then will be detected and treated appropriately. Of paramount importance to survival is tumor stage and grade as determined at primary treatment. Low stage, low grade neoplasms are associated with excellent survival rates, and high grade, high stage neoplasms are associated with low survival rates, independent of the extent of surgery in each circumstance.[158,159,163,166]

The extent of surgery for ureteral carcinoma and its effect on the risk of subsequent ureteral stump neoplasms has received much attention in the urologic literature. By definition, no stump recurrences are observed among patients treated with a complete ureterectomy and bladder cuff excision. The frequency of ureteral stump recurrences among all patients treated with nephrectomy and incomplete ureterectomy is 8% (Table 3-11).

Metastases

The pattern of metastases from ureteral primary carcinomas is regional lymph nodes, lung, bone, and liver in order of decreasing frequency.[127,156,161] Of the metastases not apparent at the time of surgery, the majority become clinically manifest within the first 2 postoperative years.[156,161]

Squamous Cell Carcinoma

Squamous cell carcinoma of the ureter has been reported in 43 patients, 70% of whom are men.[189-201] The reported age range is 22 years to 82 years with the highest frequency in the sixth and seventh decades (Table 3-12). Ninety percent of patients present with hematuria, and half with flank pain, a palpable mass, or both.[189-201] Renal pelvic or ureteral lithiasis is reported in 25% of patients. The

Table 3-11   *Nephrectomy and Incomplete Ureterectomy: Ureteral Stump Recurrences*

Author	Year	Frequency (%)
Abeshouse[127]	1956	12
Strong, Pearse*	1976	25
Bloom et al[147]	1971	4
Batata et al[156]	1975	5
Ghazi et al[160]	1979	7
Babian, Johnson[161]	1980	4
Werth et al[164]	1981	6

* Refer to References for Chapter 2.

Table 3-12   Squamous Cell Carcinoma

Case No.	Author	Year	Age	Sex	Side	Location	Follow Up
1	Rundle*	1896	46	M	R	distal 1/3	D/T
2	Jona*	1894	NI	M	L	distal 1/3†	D/T
3	Adler*	1905	69	M	L	distal 1/3	D/T, 1 mo
4	Zironi*	1909	36	F	R	mid 1/3	D/T
5	Butler*	1914	53	M	R	mid 1/3	D/T, 2 mo
6	Ascher*	1922	38	M	R	prox. 1/3	NI
7	Rousselot, Lamon[189]	1930	48	F	L	prox. 1/3	D/T
8	Spampinato[190]	1932	NI	NI	R	distal 1/3	Diagnosed at autopsy
9	von Sauer[191]	1932	57	M	NI	prox. 1/3	D/NI
10	Sargent, Marquardt[194]	1933	54	F	R	prox. 1/3	A/NED at discharge
11	Lownes[192] (Case 1)	1933	50	F	L	distal 1/3	D/T, 5 mo
12	McAlpine[193]	1933	NI	NI	NI	mid 1/3	D/T, 1 yr
13	Colston[195]	1934	62	F	L	distal 1/3‡	D/?T, 1 yr
14	Gilbert[196]	1937	68	M	L	distal 1/3	Diagnosed at autopsy
15	Foord, Ferrier[139] (Case 1)	1939	69	F	R	distal 1/3‡	D/?T, 1 yr
16	Foord, Ferrier[139] (Case 2)	1939	82	M	L	distal 1/3	D/T (inop), 6 days
17	Foord, Ferrier[139] (Case 3)	1939	65	M	L	distal 1/3	Diagnosed at autopsy
18	Foord, Ferrier[139] (Case 4)	1939	22	F	L	mid 1/3	Diagnosed at autopsy
19	Foord, Ferrier[139] (Case 5)	1939	72	F	R	distal 1/3	Diagnosed at autopsy
20	Foord, Ferrier[139] (Case 6)	1939	69	M	R	distal 1/3	Diagnosed at autopsy
21	Riches et al[197]	1951	1 case; no details			NI	A/NED, 6 mo
22	Loef, Casella[198]	1952	66	M	R	distal 1/3‡	D/T, 2 mo
23	Baker, Graf[199] (Case 4)	1953	61	M	R	distal 1/3‡	D/T, 2 mo
24	Baker, Graf[199] (Case 6)	1953	57	M	L	mid 1/3	D/T, 1 yr
25	Baker, Graf[199] (Case 15)	1953	65	M	R	distal 1/3	D/T, 15 mo
26	Baker, Graf[199] (Case 16)	1953	53	M	L	distal 1/3	D/T, 3 yr
27	Abeshouse[127]	1954	70	M	L	distal 1/3‡	D/T, 4 mo
28–29	Ochsner, Brannan[142]	1960	2 cases; no details			NI	NI
30	Amar[200]	1964	62	M	L	distal 1/3‡	D/T, 8 mo
31	Sozer[201]	1968	46	M	L	distal 1/3‡	NI
32–39	Bloom[147]	1970	8 cases; no details			NI	NI
40–41	Batata[156]	1975	2 cases; no details			NI	D/T, <3 yr
42	Ghazi et al[160]	1979	1 case; no details			NI	NI
43	Babian, Johnson[161]	1980	1 case; no details			NI	NI

NI, no information; A/NED, alive, no evidence of disease; D/T, dead with tumor.

* Cited in review by Scott.[138]   † Arising in ureteral diverticulum.   ‡ Arising in ureteral stump.

right and left ureters are affected equally. Sixty-five percent of these neoplasms are found in the distal one third of the affected ureter.

The gross and histologic features of ureteral squamous cell carcinoma are similar to those observed elsewhere in the urinary tract. Invasion beyond the ureter (stages III and IV) is recorded in most of the published cases.

Survival information is available about only 21 of the reported patients. The diagnosis was made initially at autopsy in five patients. The longest recorded survival is 3 years, with most patients succumbing within 1 year of diagnosis.[199]

Adenocarcinoma

Adenocarcinoma, which is the rarest primary malignant epithelial neoplasm of the renal pelvis, is even rarer in the ureter. A total of 15 cases have been reported since the first case reported by Metcalf and Sanford in 1906.[202-213] This compares with 33 reported adenocarcinomas in the renal pelvis. Noteworthy is the fact that 8 of the 15 cases of ureteral adenocarcinoma have been reported since 1970 (Table 3-13).

The peak age frequency is the sixth and seventh decades with a reported age range of 29 years to 73 years (Table 3-13). Seventy-two percent of patients have been males, the highest male predominance demonstrated by any type of renal pelvic or ureteral epithelial malignancy. Of the 15 cases, 67% involved the left side, and 45% were located in the distal ureter. A history or concurrent evidence

Table 3-13   Adenocarcinoma

Author	Year	Age	Sex	Location	Lithiasis	Metaplasia	Other Gu Neoplasms	Follow-up Information
Metcalf, Safford[202]	1905	47	M	L, dist 1/3	+	+	O	D/T, 3 mo
Lazarus[203]	1934	66	M	L, dist 1/3	O	NI	O	NI
Kittredge et al[204]	1947	41	M	R, mid 1/3	NI	NI	O	NI
Kojen, Petkovic[205]	1949	36	F	L, prox 1/3	O	O	O	NI
Jacob, Mau (Case 2)[206]	1951	57	M	L, prox 1/3	+	+	O	NI
Ochsner, Brannan[142]	1960	NI	NI	NI	NI	NI	NI	NI
Richmond, Robb[207]	1967	63	F	R, dist 1/3	O	+	O	Dead, post-op; mets +
Arger, Stoltz[210]	1971	49	M	L, NI	NI	NI	NI	D/T, 3 yr
Thomas et al[208]	1971	61	M	L, entire	NI	NI	+(*)	Dead, ? with tumor, 3 yr
Ray, Lingard[209]	1971	73	F	R, dist 1/3	NI	NI	O	NI
Batata et al[156]	1975	29	M	L, entire	O	O	O	D/T, 34 mo
Adolphs, Stephens[211]	1977	66	F	L, NI	+	NI	O	NI
Brawer, Waisman[212]	1980	37	M	L, prox 1/3	O	+	+(†)	D/T, 5 mo
Werth et al[164]	1981	65	M	NI, dist 1/3	O	NI	O	A/NED, 4 yr
Brawer, Waisman[213]	1982	62	M	L, uret stump	+	NI	+(‡)	D/T,§ 2 mo

NI, no information; A/NED, alive, no evidence of disease; D/T, dead with tumor.

* Associated renal pelvic adenocarcinoma, and bladder adenocarcinoma.

† Associated renal pelvic adenocarcinoma.

‡ Associated bladder squamous cell carcinoma and transitional cell carcinoma.

§ Death resulting from metastatic squamous cell carcinoma of bladder.

of lithiasis was recorded in 40% of patients. Two of the reported cases had concurrent renal pelvic adenocarcinomas, and one of these patients had an additional adenocarcinoma of the bladder.[208,212] An additional patient had an associated bladder squamous cell carcinoma and transitional cell carcinoma.[213] No examples of bilateral ureteral adenocarcinomas have been reported.

Hematuria was found in 27% of patients, which is significantly less frequent than observed with transitional cell carcinomas of both the renal pelvis and ureter (75% to 90%) (Table 3-5). Flank pain and a palpable mass, in contrast, are three times more frequent than observed with renal pelvic or ureteral transitional cell carcinomas (Table 3-5).

The majority of the reported cases evidence invasion beyond the ureter at surgery. Proximal ureteral obstruction is common but not invariable. Histologically, moderately well-differentiated adenocarcinomas showing papillary configuration are typical. Many evidence mucin production. Glandular metaplasia of the adjacent ureteral urothelium has been recorded in four cases.[202,206,207,212] The true frequency is undoubtedly higher, because this feature usually has received no attention in the reports available.

Survival data is limited to only 9 of the 15 reported cases. Among the nine cases with follow-up information provided, the longest reported survival is 4 years.[164] Tumor-related deaths were recorded in six patients (Table 3-13).

Benign Mesenchymal Neoplasms

For historical reviews of benign mesenchymal neoplasms, see References 214 to 216.

Leiomyoma

Five acceptably documented cases of ureteral leiomyomas were found in the literature.[217-221] Kao discusses other reported, but inadequately documented, cases.[219]

Ureteral leiomyomas most commonly arise in the mid or proximal right ureter in women in the fourth to sixth decades. One exceptional case involved the left ureter of 4-year-old boy.[220] The patients had flank pain and hematuria. Ureteral obstruction and hydroureter are common.

The gross and microscopic features are typical of this benign smooth muscle neoplasm as seen in more common sites. All reported cases involved the proximal or mid-ureter. Ureteral leiomyomas are firm, spherical, intramural masses that have varied from 2.0 cm to 5 cm. One example, measuring 10 cm in length, was exophytic, and extended through the ureteral lumen.[218] Stout interpreted this neoplasm as leiomyoblastoma (epithelioid leiomyoma), in contrast to the others that revealed the characteristic interlacing bundles of cytologically benign spindle cells.[220] No recurrences have been reported following surgical excision.

Lymphangioma

Jeppesen reported the only case of ureteral lymphangioma resulting in obstruction of the ureter in a 79-year-old woman.[222] The neoplasm was located in the distal one third of the left ureter. With a preoperative diagnosis of primary ureteral tumor, a nephroureterectomy was performed.

Histologically, the lesion was characterized by numerous dilated endothelial-lined vascular channels containing stainable protein interpreted as "coagulated lymph."[222] The lymphatic channels were located in the lamina propria of the ureter wall with denudation of the overlying urothelial mucosa. The malignant counterpart, lymphangiosarcoma, has not been reported in the ureter.

Neurofibroma

The only case of primary ureteral neurofibroma was reported in 1935 by Ravich.[223] In contrast, this lesion has a higher frequency of occurrence in the bladder, especially in the context of neurofibromatosis. The gross and histologic characteristics are identical to those observed in this neoplasm elsewhere, and are described in Chapter 4.

Hemangioma

Primary ureteral hemangiomas have been reported in six patients.[224-228] The neoplasm is more common in the kidney and the urinary bladder. Virtually all cases have hematuria. Five of the six patients had lesions in the lower one third of the ureters. The ages of the patients range from 21 years to 60 years, and there is no sex predominance.

Characteristic highly vascular periureteral or intraureteral exophytic masses have been described. The typical case is composed of numerous dilated thin-walled vascular channels, lined by flat endothelial cells and filled with blood. Hemangiosarcoma has not been reported to take origin from the ureter.

Malignant Mesenchymal Neoplasms

In 1956 Abeshouse recorded six previously reported ureteral sarcomas in a literature review.[127] Two examples of leiomyosarcoma, two "neurogenic sarcomas," and one "round cell sarcoma" constituted the total recorded experience to that

Table 3-14   *Leiomyosarcoma*

Author	Year	Age	Sex	Side	Follow Up
Rademaker[229]	1943	59	F	L	A/NED 14 mo
Rossien, Russel[230]	1946	55	F	R	D/T 2 yr
Alznauer[231]	1955	60	F	R	D/T 8 mo
Werner et al[232]	1959	66	F	L	D/T 6 mo
Hoger[233]	1965	77	F	L	Diagnosed at autopsy
Shah, Kothari[234]	1971	60	F	L	No information
Giraud, Rouge[235]	1975	34	F	L	A/NED 5 yr
Kolhatkar et al[236]	1979	50	M	R	Lost to follow up
Roemer et al[237]	1980	79	F	L	D/T 15 mo
Werth et al[238]	1981	NI	M	NI	A/NED 5 yr
Rushton et al[239]	1983	53	F	R	A/NED 7 mo

NI, no information; A/NED, alive, no evidence of disease; D/T, dead with tumor.

time. There has been no significant increased frequency in the years subsequent to this review.

Leiomyosarcoma

Acceptable examples of malignant smooth muscle neoplasms originating in the ureteral wall have been reported in 11 patients (Table 3-14). Three additional cases cited in previous reviews contain insufficient detail to support the diagnosis. Nine of the reported 11 ureteral leiomyosarcomas occurred in women (82%). The peak frequency is the sixth and seventh decades with an age range of 34 years to 79 years. Most patients have flank pain with or without a palpable mass.

The reported ureteral leiomyosarcomas show no predilection for either side, or for level of the ureter. Most of the neoplasms are 5 cm to 10 cm in diameter at the time of diagnosis, but some as small as 2 cm have been reported. The cut surface of this solid mass shows the characteristic whorled appearance. The color is affected by the presence and extent of hemorrhage and necrosis within the tumor. Areas away from these changes are white-pink to white-tan. The proximal ureter and renal pelvis frequently show evidence of ureteral obstruction by the neoplasm. The predominant histologic pattern is one of interlacing fascicles of spindle cells with elongated nuclei with rounded ends. The cellularity, frequency of mitosis, areas of hemorrhage, necrosis, and pleomorphic, bizarre cells are all more prominent than observed in leiomyoma, the benign counterpart, and serve as the criteria supporting the diagnosis of malignancy. The ultrastructural features of one ureteral leiomyosarcoma have been described in one case report.[238]

Of this limited number of cases (11), two patients were known to live 5 years, one case was found incidentally at autopsy, and four patients died with tumor metastases. The follow-up data were incomplete in the remaining four patients (Table 3-14).

Carcinosarcoma

One example of ureteral carcinosarcoma was reported by Renner in 1931.[239] This neoplasm is more common in the renal pelvis and the urinary bladder. (Refer to Chaps. 2 and 4.)

The patient reported by Renner was a 71-year-old man who died 6 weeks after the diagnosis and removal of a neoplasm in the bladder that had been interpreted as sarcoma. It was found at autopsy to represent contiguous spread from a carcinosarcoma primary in the right mid-ureter. In addition to the carcinomatous component, malignant stroma showing myxoid and cartilagenous areas were present.

Neoplasms Metastatic to the Ureter

Rarely are neoplasms metastatic to the ureter. Ureteral metastases have been the subject of several reviews since the first reported case by Stow in 1909 (malignant lymphoma).[240] Pressman and Ehrlich collected 35 cases and added 2 more in 1948.[242] Cohen and co-workers found 111 and added 31 new cases from their autopsy study in 1974.[245] Fitch and colleagues collected 160 from the literature.[246] Subsequent reports bring the current number to approximately 200 reported cases.[240-309] The distribution of recorded primary sites with metastatic involvement of the ureter(s) is presented in Table 3-15. Metastatic involvement of the ureter, originating in breast, stomach, bladder, colon, cervix, and prostate primary sites (in decreasing order of frequency), accounts for 80% of the reported cases.

To differentiate true metastatic (discontinuous) dissemination to the ureter from cases representing direct (continuous) invasion, MacKenzie and Ratner (1931) and later Pressman and Ehrlich (1948) suggested specific criteria to justify the diagnosis of tumor metastatic to the ureter.[241,242] Pressman and Ehrlich required the demonstration of malignant cells in the ureteral wall with the absence of a neoplasm in adjacent organs.[242] MacKenzie and Ratner's more rigid criteria which require the demonstration of tumor cells in vascular or lymphatic channels of the ureteral wall, is more precise, but impractical.[241]

The frequency of ureteral metastases observed at autopsy, although relatively low, is significantly higher than clinical diagnoses. The majority of ureteral metastases are clinically silent. Clinical suspicion of ureteral metastases (usually late in the course of a malignancy) is raised when a patient with a known malignancy has flank pain with or without clinical and radiologic evidence of ureteral obstruction. Bilateral metastases with obstruction are not uncommon among these cases. Thin needle biopsy has been employed to clarify the cause of ureteral obstruction under these circumstances.[247]

Specific Urogenital Malignancies Metastatic to the Ureter
Renal Cell Carcinoma

Renal cell carcinoma has been reported metastatic to the ipsilateral ureter in 37 patients.[248-265] Renal cell carcinoma metastatic to the contralateral ureter has been recorded in five patients.[266-270] Approximately half of such metastases were diagnosed in the ureteral stump 2 months to 7 years subsequent to a nephrectomy and incomplete ureterectomy for the renal primary. The majority of such recurrences are diagnosed within the first 2 years postoperatively. Alternatively, spread to the ureter may take the form of a contiguous cast in the ureter, discovered at the time of surgery, extending from the primary renal neoplasm.[264]

The pathogenesis of metastases to the ipsilateral ureter from renal cell carcinoma has been the focus of considerable debate. The evolution and current hypothesis of these metastases can be summarized as follows. Early studies considered ureteral spread of renal cell carcinoma to be the result of downstream implants of viable tumor cells that had invaded the more proximal collecting system (intrarenal or renal pelvis). Prior retrograde instrumentation injury to the ureteral mucosa may increase the ureter's susceptibility to such drop implants.[258] Case presentations and literature review of such implant metastases were published by Macalpine (1948) and Hovenian (1950).[251,253] Alternatively, others have favored lymphatic or hematogenous metastatic spread through the left gonadal vein (Abeshouse, 1956).[256] Circumstantially supporting hematogenous dissemination to the ureter (and other sites including the bladder, testis, penis, and vagina) is the observation that the majority of the primary renal neoplasms were located on the left side. Incontrovertible proof of metastases by intraureteral transplant and implantation has not been presented to date. Most cases with ureteral metastases evidence extensive local perirenal invasion or widespread systemic dissemination, or both, suggesting that the ureter simply represents one of many locations of lymphatic or retrograde hematogenous venous metastases.

Renal Pelvis

I regard simultaneous, subsequent transitional cell carcinomas in the renal pelvis and ureter as manifestations of multicentricity of tumors involving a urothelial cell population evidently at greater risk. The possibility that concurrent or subsequent neoplasms in the more distal urinary tract are true implant metastases has been favored, suggested, and diagnosed for years but never has been proven. Simultaneous and subsequent ureteral neoplasms are observed in a minimum of 20% and 12% of patients with diagnosed renal pelvic transitional cell carcinomas, respectively. (See Table 2-11 in Chap. 2.) Similarly, 10% and 18% of these patients demonstrate simultaneous or subsequent transitional cell carcinomas in the urinary bladder.[271-274]

Bladder and Urethra

Retrograde spread of bladder carcinoma to involve the distal ureter is more frequent than discontinuous spread (metastases). Thomas and Regnier (1924), Carson (1925), Kirschbaum (1933), and Freiman and co-workers (1978) reported examples of clinically apparent, true metastases to the ureter from transitional cell carcinomas of the urinary bladder.[247,275-277] A total of 17 cases diagnosed either clinically or at autopsy were recorded by Fitch and co-workers.[246] Metastatic spread from urethral transitional cell carcinoma has been observed in only one patient (a woman) reported by Shaw (1935).[278]

Table 3-15 **Distribution of Primary Sites of Neoplasms Metastatic to Ureter***

Primary Site	Number of Cases
Malignant lymphoma	150
Breast	42
Stomach	27
Cervix	18
Rectum	18
Bladder	17
Colon	13
Prostate	13
Melanoma	12
Ovary	10
Lung	6
Testis	5
Pancreas	4
Urethra	1
Other	9

* References 240–309

Testis

Klinger reported two cases of ureteral metastases from the testis in an autopsy series at the Henry Ford Hospital in 1948.[279] Lucke and Schlumberger (1956) cited one case without details.[280] Saubidet and Castria (1963) recorded a testicular seminoma metastatic to the left ureter.[281] Cohen, Freed, and Hasson (1974) cited one case in an autopsy study without further details.[245] Johnson and co-workers reported a clinically diagnosed testicular seminoma metastatic to the ureter.[282] Taking origin in the left testis, this germ cell tumor metastasized to the ipsilateral ureter.

Prostate

Giordano and Bumpus (1922) reported the first case of prostate carcinoma metastatic to the ureter.[283] Twelve additional cases have been found in the literature.[241,247,275-277,284-286] Only three of these cases had been diagnosed before death.[247,284,286] Bilateral involvement by prostate metastases has been reported only at autopsy.[241,277]

Ovary

Seven cases of ovarian carcinoma metastatic to the ureter have been reported.[279,287,288] Five of these cases were reported in one autopsy study by Klinger.[279] Two cases, each diagnosed before death, were reported by Lazarus (1941) and Alexander and co-workers (1973).[287,288]

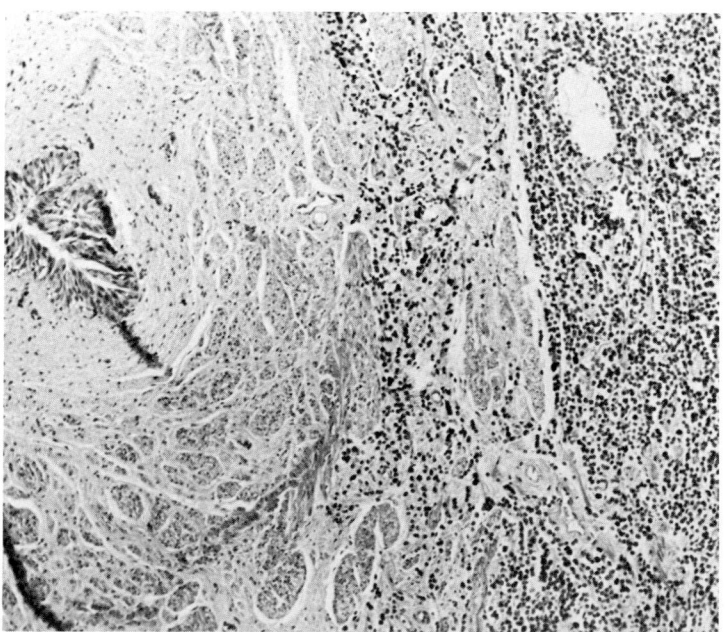

Figure 3-17   *Malignant lymphoma invading the ureter. The lymphoma cells surrounding the ureter infiltrate the outer circular muscle bundles.*

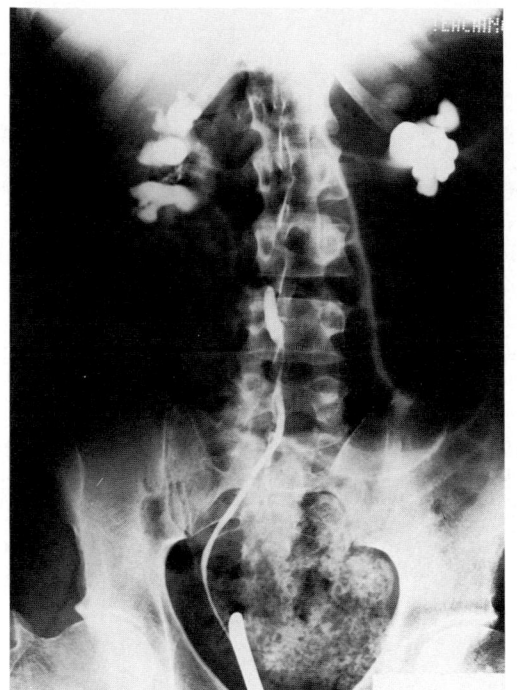
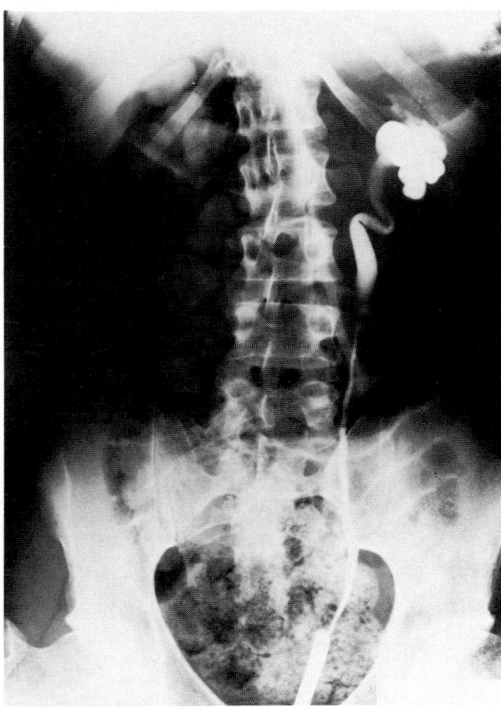

A B

Figure 3-18 **Retroperitoneal fibrosis.** *(A, B) Bilateral retrograde pyelography demonstrates bilateral obstructed ureters at levels L4 and L5. There is also medial deviation of the right ureter (A). Bilateral ureteral obstruction in the lower lumbar region is highly suggestive of retroperitoneal fibrosis.*

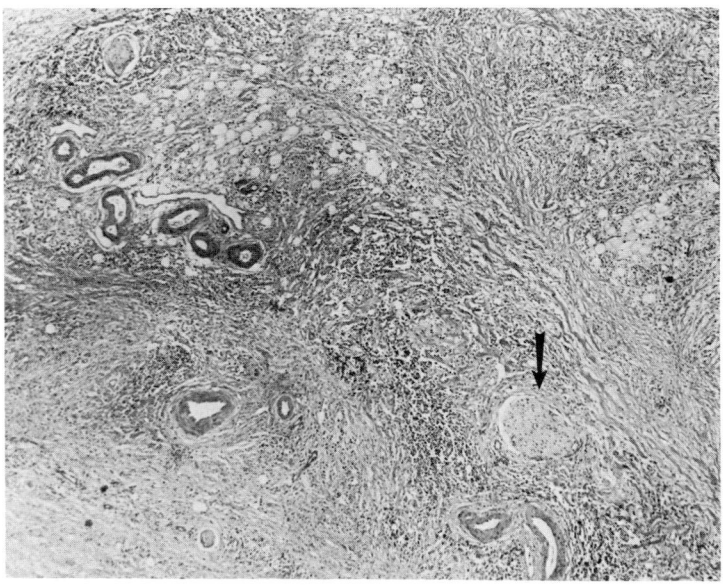

Figure 3-19 *Idiopathic retroperitoneal fibrosis. Collagenous fibrous tissue infiltrates the retroperitoneal fat and around a nerve segment (arrow) accompanied by chronic inflammatory cells including histiocytes, lymphocytes, and plasma cells.*

Malignant Lymphoma

Ureteral involvement by malignant lymphoma is uncommon at autopsy, and rare prior to death. Ureteral obstruction may result from either extrinsic ureteral compression by enlarged periaortic lymph nodes, periureteral retroperitoneal invasion by lymphoma, or by lymphomatous infiltration of the ureteral wall (Fig. 3-17). Extrinsic ureteral compression produced by malignant lymphoma must be differentiated from that produced by other retroperitoneal neoplasms, endometriosis, and retroperitoneal fibrosis (Figs. 3-18, 3-19).

Lymphomatous involvement of the ureter was first reported by Stow in 1909.[240] To date, approximately 150 cases have been reported, most of these in autopsy studies.[301–309] Fewer clinical reports of lymphomatous ureteral obstruction appear in the literature.

The histologic type of lymphoma has a bearing on the frequency of ureteral involvement. Ureteral obstruction by lymphoma is more common in non-Hodgkin's lymphoma than in Hodgkin's disease, 8.8% versus 5.5% of clinically detected cases.[305] The overall frequency of clinically detected lymphomatous obstruction varies from 0.86% to 8.8%.[302,305] This compares to a reported range of 9% to 16% observed at autopsy.[303,309]

References

Normal Structure

1. Daniel O, Shackman R: Blood supply of the human ureter in relation to ureterocolic anastomosis. Br J Urol 24:334, 1952
2. Hanna, MK, Jeffs RD, Sturgess JM et al: Ureteral structure and ultrastructure. Part I. The normal human ureter. J Urol 116:718, 1976
3. Notley RG: Ureteral morphology. Anatomic and clinical considerations. Urol 12:8, 1978
4. Crelin ES: Normal and abnormal development of ureter. Urol 12:2, 1978
5. Moore KL: The Urogenital System in the Developing Human, 3rd ed, pp 255–297. Philadelphia, WB Saunders, 1982

Congenital Disorders

6. Kretschmer HL: Duplication of the ureter at their distal ends, one pair ending blindly. J Urol 30:61, 1933
7. Campbell MF: Anomalies of the ureter. In Campbell MF, Harrison JH (eds): Urology, 3rd ed, pp 1487–1542. Philadelphia, WB Saunders, 1970
8. Lenaghan D: Bifid ureters in children: An anatomical, physiological, and clinical study. J Urol 87:808, 1962
9. Smith I: Triplicate ureter. Br J Surg 34:182, 1946
10. Parker RM, Pohl DR, Robinson JR: Ureteral triplication with ectopia. J Urol 103:727, 1970
11. Tessler AN, Mahmood P: Blind-ending duplications of ureter. Urol 1:46, 1973
12. Williams DI, Royle M: Ectopic ureters in the male child. Br J Urol 41:421, 1969
13. Ayyat F, Palmer MD, Tingley JO: Ectopic vas deferens communicating with lower ureter. Urol 19:423, 1982
14. Chwalla R: The process of formation of cystic dilatation of the vesical end of the ureter and of diverticula at the ureteral ostium. Urol Cutan Rev 31:499, 1927

15. Johnston JH, Johnston LM: Experiences with ectopic ureteroceles. J Urol 41:61, 1969
16. Snyder HM, Johnston JH: Orthotopic ureteroceles in children. J Urol 119:543, 1978
17. Wall B, Wachter HE: Congenital ureteral valve: Its role as a primary obstructive lesion: Classification of the literature and report of an authentic case. J Urol 68:684, 1952
18. Seitzman DM, Montero GG, Miele AJ: Congenital ureteral valves. J Urol 101:152, 1969
19. Mackinnin KJ, Foote JW, Wiglesworth FW et al: The pathology of the adynamic distal ureteral segment. J Urol 103:134, 1970
20. Hanna MK, Jeffs RD, Sturgess JM et al: Ureteral structure and ultrastructure. Part III. The congenitally dilated ureter (megaureter). J Urol 117:24, 1977
21. Lockhart JL, Singer AM, Glenn JF: Congenital megaureter. J Urol 122:310, 1979

Diverticulum

22. Culp OS: Ureteral diverticulum: Classification of the literature and report of an authentic case. J Urol 58:309, 1947
23. Holly II LE, Sumcad B: Diverticular ureteral changes. A report of four cases. Am J Roentgenol 78:1053, 1957
24. Rank WB, Mellinger GT, Spiro E: Ureteral diverticula: Etiologic considerations. J Urol 83:566, 1960
25. Williams JL, Goodwin WE: Congenital multiple diverticula of the ureter. Br J Urol 37:299, 1965
26. Crumplin KH, Jones SM: A further case of ureteric diverticulum — congenital or acquired? Br J Urol 44:91, 1972
27. Lester PD, Kyaw MM: Ureteral diverticulosis. Roentgenologic manifestation of ureteritis. Radiology 106:77, 1973
28. Barrett DM, Malek RS: Ureteral diverticulum. J Urol 114:33, 1975
29. Schoborg TW, Florence TJ: Ureteral diverticulosis. J Urol 116:107, 1976
30. Harrison GSM: Transitional cell carcinoma in a congenital ureteral diverticulum. J Urol 129:1231, 1983

Amyloidosis

31. Lehman G: Ueber ortliche amyloidablagerung (lokales amyloid) in der wand des harnleiters. Zentralbl Allg Pathol 68:209, 1937
32. Gilbert LW: Primary amyloidosis of the renal pelvis and ureter: Report of a case. J Urol 68:137, 1952
33. Higbee DR, Millett WD: Localized amyloidosis of the ureter: Report of a case. J Urol 75:424, 1956
34. Sato S: Primary amyloidosis of the renal pelvis and ureter: Report of a case. Acta Medica et Biologica 5:15, 1957
35. Andreas BF, Oosting M: Primary amyloidosis of the ureter. J Urol 79:929, 1958
36. Konrath M, Mobius G: Uber tumorformige paraamyloidose des ureter. Zentralbl Allg Pathol 101:195, 1961
37. Johnson HW, Ankenman GJ: Bilateral ureteral primary amyloidosis. J Urol 92:275, 1964
38. Yalowitz PA, Kelalis PP: Primary amyloidosis of the ureter. J Urol 96:668, 1966
39. Magri J, Atkinson EA: Primary amyloidosis of the ureter. Br J Urol 42:37, 1970
40. Takada M, Nagata H, Sonoda T: Localized amyloid tumor of the ureter: Report of a case. J Urol 105:502, 1971
41. Klotz PG: Primary amyloidosis of the ureter: Case report. Br J Urol 47:518, 1975
42. Lee KT, Deeths TM: Localized amyloidosis of the ureter. Radiology 120:60, 1976

43. Thomas SD, Sanders III PW, Pollack H: Primary amyloidosis of urinary bladder and ureter. Cause of mural calcification. Urol 9:586, 1977
44. Mariani AJ, Barrett DM, Kurtz SB et al: Bilateral localized amyloidosis of the ureter presenting with anuria. J Urol 120:757, 1978
45. Willen H: Primary amyloidosis of the ureter simulating malignancy. Acta Pathol Microbiol Scand 86A:357, 1978
46. Krakowski J, Szcudrawa J: Obstruction of a ureter by isolated primary focal amyloidosis. Eur Urol 5:53, 1979
47. Yazaki T, Lizumi T, Ogawa Y et al: Renal autotransplantation for localized amyloidosis of the ureter. J Urol 128:119, 1982
48. Willen R, Willen H, Lindstedt E et al: Localized primary amyloidosis of the ureter. Scand J Urol Nephrol 17:385, 1983
49. Farrands PA, Tribe DR, Slade N: Localized amyloid of the ureter: Case report and review of the literature. Histopathology 7:613, 1983
50. Miller R, Bowley NB: Localized amyloidosis of the ureter. J Urol 131:112, 1984
51. Robinson CR, Fowler Jr JE: Localized amyloidosis of the ureter. J Urol 131:110, 1984

Endometriosis

52. Cullen TS: Adenomyoma of the recto-vaginal septum. Bull Johns Hopkins Hosp 28:343, 1917
53. Randall A: Endometrioma of the ureter. J Urol 46:419, 1941
54. Frank IL, Geist SH: Postmenopausal endometriosis. A case report and review of the literature. Am J Obstet Gynecol 44:652, 1942
55. Ratliff RK, Crenshaw WB: Ureteral obstruction from endometriosis. Surg Gynecol Obstet 100:414, 1955
56. Ferreira HP, Clayton SG: Three cases of malignant change in endometriosis including two cases arising in the recto-vaginal septum. J Obstet Gynecol Br Commonw 65:41, 1958
57. Simon HB, Zimet RR, Schneider E et al: Bilateral ureteral obstruction due to endometriosis. JAMA 183:487, 1963
58. Lasio E, Marcelli G: L'endometriosi delle vie urinare. Arch Ital Urol Nefrol 37:255, 1964
59. Bulkley GL, Carrow LA, Estensen RD: Endometriosis of the ureter. J Urol 93:139, 1965
60. Kerr Jr WS: Endometriosis involving the urinary tract. Clin Obstet Gynaecol 9:331, 1966
61. Sen SK, Treherne CA, Perry FA et al: Endometriosis of the ureter in a post-hysterectomy patient. J Natl Med Assoc 59:327, 1967
62. Rising JA, Hasen HB: Obstructive ureteral endometriosis: Case report. J Urol 98:77, 1967
63. Ochsner T, Markland C: Endometriosis obstructing the ureter. J Urol 98:462, 1967
64. Brooks Jr RT, Fraser WE, Lucas WE: Endometriosis involving the urinary tract: A report of 2 cases with ureteral obstruction. J Urol 102:184, 1969
65. Bates JS, Beecham CT: Retroperitoneal endometriosis with ureteral obstruction. Obstet Gynecol 34:242, 1969
66. Stiehm WD, Becker JA, Weiss RM: Ureteral endometriosis. Radiology 102:563, 1972
67. Yates-Bell AJ, Molland EA, Pryor JP: Endometriosis of the ureter. Br J Urol 44:58, 1972
68. Dick AL, Lang DW, Bergman RT et al: Postmenopausal endometriosis with ureteral obstruction. Br J Urol 45:153, 1973
69. Reddy AN, Evans AT: Endometriosis of the ureters. J Urol 111:974, 1974

70. Langmade CF: Pelvic endometriosis and ureteral obstruction. Am J Obstet Gynecol 122:463, 1975
71. Way S, Young JR: Ureteric invasion by endometriosis. Short case report. Br J Urol 48:38, 1976
72. Lavelle KJ, Melman AW, Cleary RE: Ureteral obstruction owing to endometriosis: Reversal with synthetic progestin. J Urol 116:665, 1976
73. Fujita K: Endometriosis of the ureter. J Urol 116:664, 1976
74. Klein RS, Cattolica EV: Ureteral endometriosis. Urol 13:477, 1979
75. Rosenberg SK, Jacobs H: Endometriosis of upper ureter. J Urol 121:512, 1979
76. Rosner N, Boger A: Endometriosis of the ureter. Eur Urol 5:294, 1979
77. Kokotas N, Kontogeorgos L, Kalis E et al: Intrinsic endometriosis of the ureter. Int Urol Nephrol 13:127, 1981
78. Slutsky JN, Callahan D: Endometriosis of the ureter can present as renal failure: A case report and review of endometriosis affecting the ureters. J Urol 130:336, 1983

Malakoplakia

79. Gibson TE, Bareta J, Lake GC: Report of a case involving the bladder and one kidney and ureter. Urol Int 1:5, 1955
80. von Zile Scott E, Scott WF: A fatal case of malakoplakia of the urinary tract. J Urol 79:52, 1958
81. Lewis JA, Vieralves G, Landes RR, Powell LW: Malakoplakia of the renal pelvis, calyces and upper ureter: Case report. J Urol 85:243, 1961
82. Kalodny GM: Ureteral dilatation with pyuria. JAMA 197:577, 1966
83. Scheiderman C, Simon MA: Malakoplakia of the urinary tract. J Urol 100:694, 1968
84. Elliott GB, Moloney PP, Clement JG: Malacoplakia of the urinary tract. Am J Roentgen 116:830, 1972
85. Halpern GN, Kalies DW, Factor S et al: Malacoplakia causing bilateral ureteropelvic junction obstruction. Urol 3:628, 1974
86. Sunshine B: Malakoplakia of the upper urinary tract. J Urol 112:362, 1974
87. O'Dea MJ, Malek RS, Farrow GM: Malacoplakia of the urinary tract: Challenges and frustrations with 10 cases. J Urol 118:739, 1977
88. Nieh PT, Althausen AF: Malacoplakia of the ureter. J Urol 122:701, 1979
89. Sexton CC, Lowman RM, Nyongo AO et al: Malacoplakia presenting as complete unilateral ureteral obstruction. J Urol 128:139, 1982
90. Rudd EG, Matthews MD: Malacoplakia: An unusual etiology of ureteral obstruction. Obstet Gynecol 60:134, 1982

Radiation Injury

91. Sotto LS, Graham JB, Pichren JW: Postmortem findings in cancer of the cervix: An analysis of 180 autopsies in the past 5 years. Am J Obstet Gynecol 80:791, 1960
92. Graham JB, Abad RS: Ureteral obstruction due to radiation. Am J Obstet Gynecol 99:409, 1967
93. Shingleton HM, Fowler WC, Pepper FD et al: Ureteral stricture following therapy for carcinoma of the cervix. Cancer 24:77, 1969
94. Slater JM, Fletcher JH: Ureteral strictures after radiation therapy for carcinoma of the uterine cervix. Am J Roentgen 111:269, 1971
95. Mihatsch MJ, Rutishauser G: Thorotrast induced transitional cell carcinoma in a residual ureter after nephrectomy. Cancer 32:1346, 1973
96. Jacobs JA, Rosenthal RS, Shaw JL: Localized ureteral fibrosis: An unrecognized complication of radiation therapy for prostatic carcinoma. J Urol 115:610, 1976

Candidiasis

97. Cohen GH: Obstructive uropathy caused by ureteral candidiasis. J Urol 110:285, 1973

Schistosomiasis

98. Maged A, Soliman LAM: Bilharzial pseudo-calculus of the ureter. J Urol 99:30, 1968
99. Saad HS, Hanafy HM: Bilharzial (schistosomal) ureteritis cystica. Urol 4:261, 1974

Hamartomatous Polyps

100. Johnson CM, Smith DR: Benign polyps of the ureter. J Urol 47:448, 1942
101. Cooney CJ: Fibroma of the ureter. J Urol 47:651, 1942
102. Vest SA: Conservative surgery in certain benign tumors of the ureter. J Urol 53:97, 1945
103. Abeshouse BS: Primary benign and malignant tumors of the ureter. A review of the literature and report of one benign and twelve malignant tumors. Am J Surg 91:237, 1956
104. Howard TL: Giant polyp of ureter. J Urol 79:397, 1958
105. Compere DE, Begley GF, Isaacks HE et al: Ureteral polyps. J Urol 79:209, 1958
106. Brock DR: Benign polyp of ureter. J Urol 83:572, 1960
107. Gerdes G, Nordquist L: Intussusception of the ureter caused by a primary benign tumour. Acta Chir Scand 132:397, 1966
108. Auerback S, Lewis HY, McDonald JR: Recurrent polypoid hamartoma and epithelial cell nests in the ureter and renal pelvis of an adolescent. J Urol 95:691, 1966
109. Crum PM, Sayegh ES, Sacher EC et al: Benign ureteral polyps. J Urol 102:678, 1969
110. Sommerhaug RG, Mason T: Peutz–Jeghers syndrome and ureteral polyposis. JAMA 211:120, 1970
111. Vastola JW, Hajdu SI, Grabstald H: Benign ureteral polyps. NY State J Med 71:2679, 1971
112. Hudson HC, Howland Jr RL: Primary benign ureteral tumor of mesodermal origin. J Urol 105:794, 1971
113. Al Hussaini MA, Marden Jr HE, Woodruff MW: Multiple fibrous polyps of ureter. Urol 2:563, 1973
114. Pinto RS, Fauver E, Anderson Jr: Benign fibroepithelioma of ureter. Urol 3:747, 1974
115. Elson EC, McLaughlin AP: Xanthomatous ureteral polyp. Urol 4:214, 1974
116. Bennington JL, Beckwith JB: Tumors of the kidney, renal pelvis, and ureter, pp 243–245. In Atlas of Tumor Pathology, Second Series, Fascicle 12. Washington, DC, AFIP, 1975
117. Stuppler SA, Kandzari SJ: Fibroepithelial polyps of ureter. A benign ureteral tumor. Urol 5:553, 1975
118. Davides KC, King LM: Fibrous polyps of the ureter. J Urol 115:651, 1976
119. Fiorelli C, Durval A, Di Cello V et al: Ureteral intussusception by a fibroepithelial polyp. J Urol 126:110, 1981

Proliferative and Metaplastic Variants

Brunn's Nests, Ureteritis Cystica

120. Morse HD: The etiology and pathology of pyelitis cystica, ureteritis cystica and cystitis cystica. Am J Pathol 4:33, 1928
121. Everett HS, Wayburn GJ: A unique case of submucosal epithelial nests in the ureter and renal pelvis. J Urol 56:310, 1946

Squamous Metaplasia

122. Shrader DA, Bergreen PW: Cholesteatoma of ureter masquerading as ureteral tumor. Urol 9:556, 1977
123. Hertle L, Androulakakis P: Keratinizing desquamative squamous metaplasia of the upper urinary tract: Leukoplakia – cholesteatoma. J Urol 127:631, 1982

Nephrogenic Metaplasia

124. Lugo M, Petersen RO, Elfenbein IB et al: Nephrogenic metaplasia of the ureter. Am J Clin Pathol 80:92, 1983
125. Jakse G, Mikuz G: Nephrogenic adenoma of the ureter. Eur Urol 9:60, 1983
126. Satodate R, Koike H, Sasou S et al: Nephrogenic adenoma of the ureter. J Urol 131:332, 1984

Benign Epithelial Neoplasms

Papilloma

127. Abeshouse BS: Primary benign and malignant tumors of the ureter. A review of the literature and report of one benign and twelve malignant tumors. Am J Surg 91:237, 1956
128. Bennington JL, Beckwith JB: Tumors of the kidney, renal pelvis, and ureter, p. 264. In Atlas of Tumor Pathology, Second Series, Fascicle 12. Washington, DC, AFIP, 1975

Inverted Papilloma

129. Vicini D, Ravasi S, Castello A: Il papilloma invertito dell'urotelio. Contributo di 4 casi. Urologia 46:753, 1979
130. Geisler CH, Mori K, Leiter E: Lobulated inverted papilloma of the ureter. J Urol 123:270, 1980
131. Selli C, Dini S, Fiorelli C et al: Chronic inflammation of the ureter with urothelial ingrowth simulating inverted papilloma. Br J Urol 53:80, 1981
132. Fromowitz FB, Steinbook ML, Lautin EM et al: Inverted papilloma of the ureter. J Urol 126:113, 1981
133. Silverstein SV, Carlton Jr CE: Inverted papilloma of ureter. Urol 17:160, 1981
134. Ajrawat HS, Skogg DP, Asirwatham JE et al: Lobulated inverted papilloma of ureter. Urol 20:290, 1982
135. Pluot M, Prawerman S, Leclerc PH et al: Papillome inverse de l'uretere. Etude histochimique et ultrastructurale. Discussion histogenetique. Arch Anat Cytol Pathol 30:39, 1982
136. Jacobellis U, Resta L, Ruotolo G: Inverted papilloma of the ureter. Eur Urol 9:370, 1983
137. Naito S, Minoda M, Hirata H: Inverted papilloma of ureter. Urol 22:290, 1983

Malignant Epithelial Neoplasms

Transitional Cell Carcinoma

138. Scott WW: Primary carcinoma of the ureter. Surg Gynecol Obstet 58:215, 1934
139. Foord AG, Ferrier PA: Primary carcinoma of the ureter. With report of seven cases. JAMA 112:596, 1939
140. Mortensen H, Murphy L: Primary epithelial tumours of the ureter. A report of six cases and a review of the recent literature. Br J Urol 22:103, 1950
141. Whitlock GF, McDonald JR, Cook EN: Primary carcinoma of the ureter: A pathologic and prognostic study. J Urol 73:245, 1955
142. Ochsner SF, Brannan W: Primary neoplasms of the ureter. South Med J 53:497, 1960

143. Newman DM, Allen LE, Wishard Jr WN et al: Transitional cell carcinoma of the upper urinary tract. J Urol 98:322, 1967

144. Meyer PC: The histological grading of primary epithelial neoplasms of the ureter. J Urol 102:30, 1969

145. Mackinney CC, Kohler FP, Uhle CAW: Primary tumors of the ureter. J Urol 101:33, 1969

146. Beck AD, Heslin JE, Milner WA et al: Primary tumors of the ureter: Diagnosis and management. J Urol 102:683, 1969

147. Bloom NA, Vidone RA, Lytton B: Primary carcinoma of the ureter: A report of 102 new cases. J Urol 103:590, 1970

148. Washida H, Ueda K: Primary carcinoma of the ureter: Report of a case and a survey of 294 cases reported in Japan. Acta Urol Jap 17:755, 1971

149. Hawtrey CE: Fifty-two cases of primary ureteral carcinoma: A clinical – pathologic study. J Urol 105:188, 1971

150. Lull Jr GF, Cohen SL: Incidence of primary carcinoma of the ureter: A report of five cases. Milit Med 136:629, 1971

151. Kim KH, Leiter E, Brendler H: Primary tumors of the ureter. J Urol 107:955, 1972

152. Almgard LE, Freedman D, Ljungqvist A: Carcinoma of the ureter. With special reference to malignancy grading and prognosis. Scand J Urol Nephrol 7:165, 1973

153. Williams CB, Mitchell JP: Carcinoma of the ureter: A review of 54 cases. Br J Urol 45:377, 1973

154. Schmauz R, Cole P: Epidemiology of cancer of the renal pelvis and ureter. J Natl Can Inst 52:1431, 1974

155. Burger R, Spjut HJ: Primary ureteral carcinoma. Urol 4:40, 1974

156. Batata MA, Whitmore Jr WF, Hilaris BS et al: Primary carcinoma of the ureter: A prognostic study. Cancer 35:1626, 1975

157. Mazeman E: Tumours of the upper urinary tract calyces, renal pelvis and ureter. Eur Urol 2:120, 1976

158. Batata M, Grabstald H: Upper urinary tract urothelial tumors. Urol Clin N Am 3:79, 1976

159. Johnson DE, Babaian RJ: Conservative surgical management for noninvasive distal ureteral carcinoma. Urol 13:365, 1979

160. Ghazi MR, Morales PA, Al-Askari S: Primary carcinoma of ureter. Report of 27 new cases. Urol 14:18, 1979

161. Babaian RJ, Johnson DE: Primary carcinoma of the ureter. J Urol 123:357, 1980

162. Kakizoe T, Fujita J, Murase T et al: Transitional cell carcinoma of the bladder in patients with renal pelvic and ureteral cancer. J Urol 124:17, 1980

163. Heney NM, Nocks BN, Daly JJ et al: Prognostic factors in carcinoma of the ureter. J Urol 125:632, 1981

164. Werth DD, Weigel JW, Mebust WK: Primary neoplasms of the ureter. J Urol 125:628, 1981

165. Schiff HI, Finkel M, Schapira HE: Transitional cell carcinoma of the ureter associated with cyclophosphamide therapy for benign disease: A case report. J Urol 128:1023, 1982

166. Mills C, Vaughan Jr D: Carcinoma of the ureter: Natural history, management and 5-year survival. J Urol 129:275, 1983

Bilateral Transitional Cell Carcinoma

167. Ratliff RK, Baum WC, Butler WJ: Bilateral primary carcinoma of the ureter. A case report. Cancer 2:815, 1949

168. Felber E: Papilloma of the ureter with subsequent cancer of the ureteral stump, bladder and vagina. J Med Assoc Georgia 42:198, 1953

169. Gracia V, Bradfield EO: Simultaneous bilateral transitional cell carcinoma of the ureter: A case report. J Urol 79:925, 1958

170. Crassweller PO: Bilateral primary carcinoma of the ureter with use of ileal graft for ureteral replacement: Case report. Br J Urol 30:152, 1958

171. Gaca VA: Das doppelseitige papillare harnleiterkarzinom. Z Urol 53:261, 1960

172. Utz DC, Brunsting CD, Harrison Jr EG: Bilateral ureteral and vesical carcinomas occurring asynchronously: Report of a case. J Urol 88:488, 1962

173. Viek NF, Uhlman RC, Verrilli R: Simultaneous bilateral transitional cell carcinoma of the ureters. J Urol 89:49, 1963

174. Perlmutter AD, Retik AB, Harrison JH: Simultaneous bilateral carcinoma of the ureter present for five years before surgery. J Urol 93:582, 1965

175. Gillenwater JY, Howard RS, Paquin Jr AJ: Bilateral primary carcinoma of the ureter. JAMA 197:1040, 1966

176. Barroso Jr CH, Florence TJ, Scott Jr C: Bilateral papillary carcinomas of the ureters: Presentation of a case and 2-year followup report. J Urol 96:451, 1966

177. Scarzella GI, Macdonald GR: Asynchronous bilateral primary epithelial tumors of the ureters: Report of a case. J Urol 97:464, 1967

178. Barber JW: Bilateral simultaneous primary carcinoma of the ureter. Radiology 90:318, 1968

179. Talavera JM, Carney JA, Kelalis PP: Bilateral, synchronous, primary transitional cell carcinoma of the ureter: Report of 2 cases and review of literature. J Urol 104, 679, 1970

180. Sozer IT: Simultaneous bilateral carcinoma of the ureter. Urol 4:217, 1974

181. Levine RL, Airhart RA: Bilateral synchronous transitional ureteral carcinoma: Two additional cases. South Med J 70:1418, 1977

182. Petkovic SD: Treatment of bilateral renal pelvic and ureteral tumors. A review of 45 cases. Eur Urol 4:397, 1978

183. Gonzalez JA, Zoretic SN: Bilateral synchronous transitional cell ureteral carcinoma. Urol 20:300, 1982

184. Zincke H, Garbeff PJ, Beahrs JR: Upper urinary tract transitional cell cancer after radical cystectomy for bladder cancer. J Urol 131:50, 1984

Associated Renal Cell Carcinoma

185. McAlpine JB: Implantation of secondaries from a renal carcinoma ('hypernephroma') within the ureteric lumen. Br J Surg 36:164, 1948

186. Marshall F, Johnson AJ: Double primary tumors: Case report. J Urol 85:724, 1961

187. Richardson EJ, Woodburn RL: Dissimilar primary tumors in the right upper urinary tract: Case report. J Urol 90:253, 1963

188. Wilenius R, Mattila K: Simultaneous occurrence of renal adenocarcinoma and primary transitional cell carcinoma of the ureter. Ann Chir Gynaecol Fenn 59:108, 1970

Squamous Cell Carcinoma

189. Rousselot LM, Lamon JD: Primary carcinoma of the ureter. Report of a case and a review of the literature. Surg Gynecol Obstet 50:17, 1930

190. Spampinato C: Tumori primitivi dell'uretere. Arch Ital Urol 9:347, 1932

191. von Sauer H: Zur klink und pathologic der primaeren uretertumoren. Z Urol Chir 34:165, 1932

192. Lownes JB: Primary carcinoma of the ureter. Penn Med J 36:587, 1933

193. Macalpine JB: Discussion. Br J Urol 5:331, 1933

194. Sargent JC, Marquardt CR: Primary carcinoma of the ureter. J Urol 30:625, 1933

195. Colston JAC: Primary tumor of the ureter. A new method for complete nephro-ureterectomy. Bull Johns Hopkins Hosp 55:361, 1934

196. Gilbert JB: Studies of the natural history of genitourinary tumors. I: Primary cancer of ureter. Autopsy study with review of the literature. Am J Surg 36:711, 1937

197. Riches EW, Griffiths IH, Thackray AC: New growths of the kidney and ureter. Br J Urol 23:297, 1951
198. Loef JA, Casella PA: Squamous cell carcinoma occurring in the stump of a chronically infected ureter many years after nephrectomy. J Urol 67:159, 1952
199. Baker WJ, Graf EC: Tumors of the ureter. J Urol 70:390, 1953
200. Amar AD: Squamous cell carcinoma of ureteral stump 40 years after nephrectomy. J Urol 91:337, 1964
201. Sozer IT: Squamous cell carcinoma and calculi in ureteral stump: 12 years postnephrectomy. J Urol 99:264, 1968

Adenocarcinoma

202. Metcalf WF, Safford HE: A case of carcinoma of the ureter apparently induced by a calculus lodged in its juxtavesical portion. Am J Med Sci 129:50, 1905
203. Lazarus JA: Primary tumors of the ureter with special reference to the malignant tumors. Report of three cases. Ann Surg 99:769:1934
204. Kittredge WE: Primary tumors of the ureter with special reference to the malignant tumors. Ann Surg 99:769, 1934
205. Kojen L, Petkovic S: A clinical review of ureteral tumors. Urol Cutan Rev 53:275, 1949
206. Jacob Jr NH, Mau W: Metaplasia of ureteral epithelium resulting in intestinal mucosa and adenocarcinomatous transformation: Report of two cases. J Urol 65:20, 1951
207. Richmond WG, Robb WAT: Adenocarcinoma of the ureter secondary to ureteritis cystica. Br J Urol 39:359, 1967
208. Thomas DG, Ward AM, Williams JL: A study of 52 cases of adenocarcinoma of the bladder. Br J Urol 43:4, 1971
209. Ray P, Lingard WF: Primary adenocarcinoma of the ureter. J Urol 106:655, 1971
210. Arger PH, Stolz JL: Ureteral tumors. The radiologic evaluation of a differential diagnosis "throw-in". Am J Roentgenol 116:812, 1972
211. Adolphs HD, Steffens L: Primare harnllitertumoren. Med Klin 72:414, 1977
212. Brawer MK, Waisman J: Mucinous adenocarcinoma probably arising in the renal pelvis and ureter: A case report. J Urol 123:424, 1980
213. Brawer MK, Waisman J: Papillary adenocarcinoma of ureter. Urol 19:205, 1982

Benign Mesenchymal Neoplasms

Historical Reviews

214. Melicow MM, Findlay HV: Primary benign tumors of the ureter. Review of literature and report of a case. Surg Gynecol Obstet 54:680, 1932
215. Rusche C, Bacon SK: Primary ureteral neoplasms. Report of two cases and review of literature. J Urol 39:319, 1938
216. Edelstein JM, Marcus SM: Primary benign neoplasm of the ureter. J Urol 61:409, 1948

Leiomyoma

217. Leighton KM: Leiomyoma of the ureter. Br J Urol 27:256, 1955
218. de Jager H: Bizarre smooth-muscle tumour of the ureter. J Pathol Bact 87:424, 1964
219. Kao VCY, Graff PW, Rappaport H: Leiomyoma of the ureter. A histologically problematic rare tumor confirmed by immuno-histochemical studies. Cancer 24:535, 1969
220. Mondschein LJ, Sutton AP, Roghfeld SH: Leiomyoma of the ureter in a child: The first reported case. J Urol 116:516, 1976
221. Sekar N, Nagrani B, Yadav RVS: Ureterocele with leiomyoma of ureter. Br J Urol 52:400, 1980

Lymphangioma

222. Jeppesen FB: Lymphangioma of the ureter. J Urol 70:410, 1953

Neurofibroma

223. Ravich A: Neurofibroma of the ureter. Report of a case with operation and recovery. Arch Surg 30:442, 1935

Hemangioma

224. Caulk JR: Haemangiomata of the bladder and ureter. Surg Gynecol Obstet 41:49, 1925
225. Galbraith WW: Pedunculated vascular tumour of the ureter. Br J Urol 22:195, 1950
226. Woller A: Homangiom des ureters. Z Urol 46:668, 1953
227. Brodny ML, Hershman H: Pedunculated hemangioma of the ureter. J Urol 71:539, 1954
228. Uhlir K: Hemangioma of the ureter. J Urol 110:647, 1973

Malignant Mesenchymal Neoplasms

Leiomyosarcoma

229. Rademaker L: Primary sarcoma of the ureter. Case report and review of the literature. Am J Surg 62:402, 1943
230. Rossien AX, Russell TH: Leiomyosarcoma involving the right ureter. Arch Pathol 41:655, 1946
231. Alznauer RL: Leiomyosarcoma of right ureter. Report of a case. Arch Pathol 59:94, 1955
232. Werner JR, Klingensmith W, Denko JV: Leiomyosarcoma of the ureter: Case report and review of literature. J Urol 82:68, 1959
233. Hoger PMH: Leiomyosarkom des ureters. Z Urol 58:701, 1965
234. Shaw JP, Kothari AB: Leiomyosarcoma of the ureter. J Urol 105:505, 1971
235. Girard B, Rouge M: Les sarcomes primitifs de l'uretere. J Urol Nephrol 81:563, 1975
236. Kolhatkar RK, Kulharni SH, Phansopkar MA et al: Leiomyosarcoma of ureter presenting as acute renal failure. Br J Urol 51:326, 1979
237. Roemer CE, Pfister RC, Brodsky G et al: Primary leiomyosarcoma of ureter. Urol 16:492, 1980
238. Rushton HG, Sens MA, Garvin AJ et al: Primary leiomyosarcoma of the ureter: A case report with electron microscopy. J Urol 129:1045, 1983

Carcinosarcoma

239. Renner MJ: Primary malignant tumors of the ureter. Surg Gynecol Obstet 52:793, 1931

Metastatic Malignancies

240. Stow B: Fibrolymphosarcomata of both ureters metastatic to a primary lymphosarcoma of the anterior mediastinum of thymus origin. Ann Surg 50:901, 1909
241. MacKenzie DW, Ratner M: Metastatic growth of ureter. Brief review of literature, and report of 3 cases. Trans Amer Assoc Genito–Urin Surg 24:165, 1931
242. Presman D, Ehrlich L: Metastatic tumors of the ureter. J Urol 59:312, 1948
243. McCrea LE, Peale AR: Metastatic carcinoma to the ureter. Urol Cutan Rev 55:11, 1951
244. Scott WW, McDonald DF: Tumors of the ureter. In Campbell MF, Harrison JH (eds): Urology, 3rd ed, pp. 977–1002. Philadelphia, WB Saunders, 1970
245. Cohen WM, Freed SZ, Hasson J: Metastatic cancer to the ureter: A review of the literature and case presentations. J Urol 112:188, 1974

246. Fitch WP, Robinson JR, Radwin HM: Metastatic carcinoma of the ureter. Arch Surg 111:874, 1976
247. Freiman DB, Ring EJ, Oleaga JA et al: Thin needle biopsy in the diagnosis of ureteral obstruction with malignancy. Cancer 42:714, 1978

Ipsilateral Renal Cell Carcinoma

248. Schacht FW: Hypernephroma: Extension to the ureter. Surg Gynecol Obstet 53:102, 1931
249. Kozoll DD, Kirshbaum JD: Relationship of benign and malignant hypernephroid tumors of kidney. Clinical and pathological study of 77 cases in 12,885 necropsies. J Urol 44:435, 1940
250. Nalle Jr BC: Distant metastases of 58 renal neoplasms: A case report of secondary metastatic pulsations from a renal tumor. J Urol 57:662, 1947
251. Macalpine JB: Implantation of secondaries from a renal carcinoma ('hyper-nephroma') within the ureteric lumen. Br J Surg 36:164, 1948
252. Stepita CT, Newman HR: Empyema of the ureteral stump with surgical excision: Report of 15 cases. J Urol 63:500, 1950
253. Hovenanian MS: Implantation of renal parenchymal carcinoma. J Urol 64:188, 1950
254. Howell RD: Ureteral implantation of renal adenocarcinoma. J Urol 66:561, 1951
255. Heslin JE, Milner WA, Garlick WB: Lower urinary tract implants or metastases from clear cell carcinoma of the kidney. J Urol 73:39, 1955
256. Abeshouse BS: Metastasis to ureters and urinary bladder from renal carcinoma. Report of two cases. J Int Coll Surg 25:117, 1956
257. Sargent JW: Ureteral metastasis from renal adenocarcinoma presenting a bizarre urogram. J Urol 83:97, 1960
258. Ostenfeld J: Hypernephroma with implantation-metastasis. Urol Int 11:253, 1961
259. Young IS: Ureteral implant from renal adenocarcinoma: Report of a case and review of the literature. J Urol 98:661, 1968
260. Chordia ML, Ockuly EA, Ockuly JJ et al: Ureteral and vesical metastases from parenchymal renal carcinoma: Case report and review of literature. J Urol 102:298, 1969
261. Seppanen J, Willenius R: Implant metastases to the ureteral stump from hyper-nephroma. Report of a case. Scand J Urol Nephrol 4:81, 1970
262. Gross M, Minkowitz S: Ureteral metastasis from renal adenocarcinoma. J Urol 106:23, 1971
263. Hook G, Scheinman LJ: Ureteral stump metastasis from renal adenocarcinoma. Urol 3:352, 1974
264. Roller MF, Stuppler SA, Kandzari SJ et al: Hypernephroma and associated ureteral involvement. Urol 8:575, 1976
265. Bissada NK, Finkbeiner AE: Ureteral stump metastases from renal adenocarcinoma. J Urol 118:327, 1977

Contralateral Renal Cell Carcinoma

266. Wechsler H, Spivack LL: Metastasis in ureter from adenocarcinoma of the contralateral kidney. NY State J Med 57:1942, 1957
267. Melicow MM, Uson AC: Nonurologic symptoms in patients with renal cancer. JAMA 172:146, 1960
268. Leblanc GA: Contralateral metastasis from renal adenocarcinoma. J Urol 86:316, 1961
269. Hudson HC, Windsor JL: Ureteral metastasis from hypernephroma of the contralateral kidney. South Med J 64:618, 1971
270. Hughes MA, Arkell DG, Dawson-Edwards P et al: Contralateral ureteric metastasis from renal carcinoma. Short case report. Br J Urol 48:402, 1976

Renal Pelvis

271. Kimball FN, Ferris HW: Papillomatous tumor of the renal pelvis associated with similar tumors of the ureter and bladder. Review of literature and report of two cases. J Urol 31:257, 1934
272. Kinder CH, Wallace DM: Recurrent carcinoma in the ureteric stump. Br J Surg 50:202, 1962
273. Latham HS, Kay L: Malignant tumors of the renal pelvis. Surg Gynecol Obstet 138:613, 1974
274. Strong DW, Pearse HD, Tank Jr ES et al: The ureteral stump after nephroureterectomy. J Urol 115:654, 1976

Bladder and Urethra

275. Thomas GJ, Regnier EA: Tumors of the kidney, pelvis and ureter. J Urol 11:205, 1924
276. Carson WJ: Metastatic carcinoma in the ureter. Report of additional cases. Ann Surg 86:549, 1927
277. Kirshbaum JD: Metastatic tumors of the ureters. J Urol 30:665, 1933
278. Shaw EC: Primary tumor of the female urethra with metastasis to each ureter. J Urol 34:244, 1935

Testis

279. Klinger ME: Secondary tumors of the genito-urinary tract. J Urol 65:144, 1951
280. Lucke B, Schlumberger HG: Secondary tumors of the ureter, p. 202. In Tumors of the Kidney, Renal Pelvis, and Ureter, AFIP Fascicle 30. Washington, DC, AFIP, 1957
281. Saubidet JA, Castria MA: Carcinoma indiferenciado. Rev Argent de Urol y Nefrol 32:157, 1963
282. Johnson RD, Johnson FR, Bannayan GA: Seminoma metastatic to ureter. Urol 17:281, 1981

Prostate

283. Giordano A, Bumpus Jr HC: Carcinoma in the ureteropelvic juncture metastatic from the prostate. Report of a case. J Urol 8:445, 1922
284. Brotherus JV, Westerlund RM: Metastatic carcinoma of the ureter. A report of three cases. Scand J Urol Nephrol 5:86, 1971
285. Babaian RJ, Johnson DE, Ayala AG et al: Secondary tumors of ureter. Urol 14:341, 1979
286. Kost LV, Leberman PR: Metastatic carcinoma to the ureter: A case report. J Urol 93:367, 1965
287. Lazarus JA: Metastatic urethral obstruction following carcinoma of the ovary. Report of an unusual case of pyonephrosis resulting from a metastatic carcinoma of the ureter. J Urol 45:527, 1941
288. Alexander S, Kim K, Pinck BD et al: Metastatic ureteral tumors. J Urol 110:288, 1973

Nongenitourinary Primary Sites

289. Fergusson JD: Ureteral stricture with perinephric urinary extravasation, caused by metastases from a silent carcinoma of the stomach. Br J Surg 31:283, 1944
290. Kniseley RM, Baggenstoss AH: Primary melanoma of the adrenal gland. Arch Pathol 42:345, 1946
291. Robbins JJ, Lich Jr R: Metastatic carcinoma of the ureter. J Urol 75:242, 1952
292. Reuter UH: Zur kasuistik des metastatischen ureterkarzinoms. Z Urol 48:256, 1955

293. Abeshouse BS: Primary and secondary melanoma of the genitourinary tract. Southern Med J 51:994, 1958

294. Neuberg HJ: Doppelseitige uretermetastasen mit ureterstenose beiderseits bei magenkarzinom. Z Urol 52:580, 1959

295. Samellas W, Marks AR: Metastatic melanoma of the urinary tract. J Urol 82:21, 1961

296. Judd RL: Melanoma of the ureter: A case report. J Urol 87: 805, 1962

297. Williams DF, Chaffey BT: Metastatic adenocarcinoma of the sigmoid colon masquerading as bilateral intraluminal ureteral papillomas. Br J Urol 38:563, 1966

298. McKenzie DJ, Bell R: Melanoma with solitary metastasis to ureter. J Urol 99:399, 1968

299. Grabstald H, Kaufman R: Hydronephrosis secondary to ureteral obstruction by metastatic breast cancer. J Urol 102:569, 1969

300. Kopelson G, Munzehrider JE, Kelley RM et al: Radiation therapy for ureteral metastases from breast carcinoma. Cancer 47:1976, 1981

Malignant Lymphomas

301. MacLean JT, Fowler VB: Pathology of tumors of the renal pelvis and ureter. J Urol 75:384, 1956

302. Rosenberg SA, Diamond HD, Jaslowitz B et al: Lymphosarcoma: A review of 1269 cases. Med 40:31, 1961

303. Richmond J, Sherman RS, Diamond HD et al: Renal lesions associated with malignant lymphomas. Am J Med 32:184, 1962

304. Kaufman JJ: Unusual causes of extrinsic ureteral obstruction, Part II. J Urol 87:328, 1962

305. Abeloff MD, Lenhard Jr RE: Clinical management of ureteral obstruction secondary to malignant lymphoma. Johns Hopkins Med J 134:34, 1974

306. Leoning S, Carson III CC, Faxon DP et al: Ureteral obstruction from Hodgkin's disease. J Urol 111:345, 1974

307. Williams G, Peet TND: Bilateral ureteral obstruction due to malignant lymphoma. Urol 7:649, 1976

308. Goswami AP: Metastatic cancer to the ureter and kidney from malignant lymphoma. A review of the literature. J Urol 117:381, 1977

309. Scharifker D, Chalasani A: Ureteral involvement by malignant lymphoma. Ten years' experience. Arch Pathol Lab Med 102:541, 1978

Urinary Bladder

4

Normal Structure

Embryologic Development

The urinary bladder of the newborn developed in two stages from the cloaca and urogenital sinus. The urogenital sinus results from the partitioning of the cloaca into the dorsal rectum and the more ventral urogenital sinus.[4,5] The urogenital sinus ultimately is continuous with the allantois cranially and terminates caudally at the urogenital membrane. The urogenital sinus serves as the origin of what ultimately evolves into the urachus, urinary bladder, and proximal urethra. The progressive attenuation of the urachus forms the umbilical ligament in the adult, with retained attachment to the bladder dome. The caudal urogenital sinus makes contact with an ectodermal invagination (glandular plate) at the urogenital membrane (which normally disappears), thus forming the complete urethral lumen. Thus, the bladder and urethral urothelium are of endodermal origin, with the exception of the most distal segment, which is of ectodermal origin. The incorporation of the mesonephric duct into the bladder wall in the region of the trigone transiently results in a localized mesonephric contribution to bladder mucosa. Gyllensten has reported that this mesonephric urothelium is replaced by urothelium of endodermal derivation from the urogenital sinus.[2] Each ureter, originating from the mesonephric duct in the form of a metanephric diverticulum, is of mesodermal origin. With growth and enlargement of the bladder, the mesonephric duct is absorbed into the wall of the urogenital sinus at a location that ultimately becomes the proximal urethra. Thus, the ureters (the metanephric duct) come to open into the bladder, and the ejaculatory duct (mesonephric duct) enters more caudally, in the proximal urethra. The stromal muscular investments of the ureters, bladder, and urethra are of mesodermal origin.

Anatomy and Histology

The mucosal lining of the urinary bladder is composed of urothelial cells (transitional epithelium) with five to seven layers from basal cells to the surface (Fig. 4-1). The urothelium is continuous with that of the ureters and the urethra,

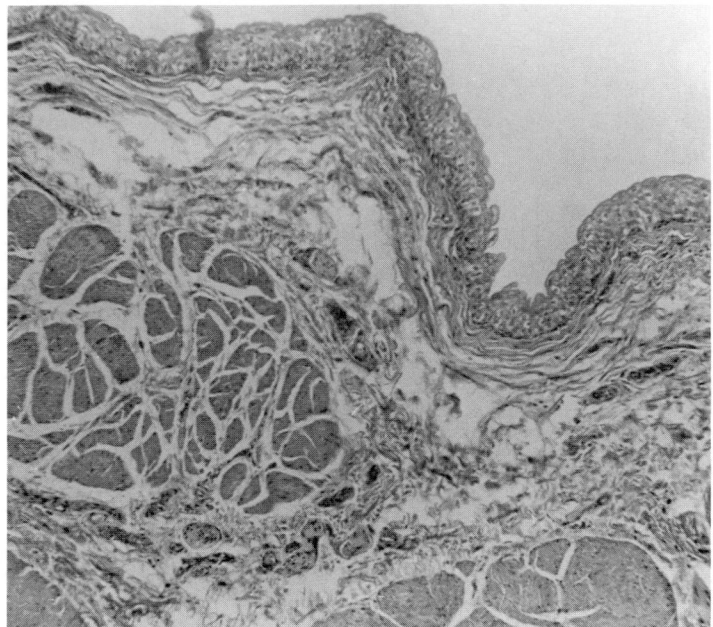

A

B

Figure 4-1   ***Normal bladder.*** (A) *The bladder mucosa overlies loose collagenous fibrous tissue of the lamina propria. The muscularis is organized in bundles of smooth muscle with variable orientation in the plane of section. Blood vessels, lymphatics, and nerves are present in the fibrous stroma of the lamina propria and muscularis. (B) The urothelium is composed of transitional cells five to eight layers thick. The configuration of the bladder transitional cells, here reflecting a flaccid bladder, is variable.*

which tend to have fewer layers. A basal lamina is present beneath the urothelium, separating it from the richly vascularized subjacent lamina propria stroma. The histologic appearance of the urothelium is dependent on the degree of distention at the time of fixation. The most superficial cells, the so-called "umbrella cells," are relatively large in the distended bladder and drop over adjacent smaller cells in the intermediate layer. In the past, the presence of these surface umbrella cells has been equated to an indication of normal urothelial structure, and proliferative kinetics. However, umbrella cells may be observed on the surface of low grade papillary malignancies of the urothelium, and thus attribution of normalcy to these cells is not justified.

The lamina propria, composed of loose collagen, vessels, lymphatics, and nerves, is interspersed between the mucosa and the deeper muscularis layer. The latter is composed of interlacing bundles of smooth muscle fibers.[1,3] Adipose tissue and peritoneum cover the muscularis. Occasional lymphoid aggregates are present in the subserosal adipose tissue. The anatomical areas of the bladder include the dome, anterior and posterior walls, lateral walls, trigone region, and bladder neck. Urachal remnants are commonly observed in the bladder wall most frequently in the region of the dome, and less frequently in the anterior wall.

The urinary bladder lies anterior to the uterus in the female, and superior to the prostate, and anterior and superior to the seminal vesicles in the male. Neoplasms arising in these organs may spread by direct invasion to involve the bladder wall. Alternatively, mucosal neoplasms, including the flat carcinoma in situ, originating in the bladder may be associated with similar histologic changes in the ureter or distal urethra, and on occasion, the contiguous distal prostatic ducts.

Congenital Malformations

Congenital malformations of the urinary bladder are uncommon to rare and include agenesis, incomplete and complete duplication, hourglass deformity, and diverticulum.[6-9] With the exception of agenesis, most are of little clinical significance and are most frequently detected during radiologic procedures or at autopsy.

Two congenital disorders — exstrophy of the bladder and complications of persistent urachus — are clinically important and will be discussed separately.

Exstrophy

Exstrophy is a congenital vesical-cutaneous fistula that is the result of incomplete closure of the anterior abdominal wall and the underlying anterior bladder wall (Fig. 4-2). It is now regarded as the result of overgrowth of the cloacal membrane.[9] The normal mesodermal structures thus develop around this central diversion, which ultimately ruptures and exposes the bladder mucosa to the exterior.[9] Associated anomalies are common and include epispadias, failure of fusion of the labia, and lack of fusion of the symphysis pubis.[9] The bladder mucosa is exposed to the exterior around and through the defect in the anterior abdominal wall. Resulting abrasion by clothing and continuous escape of urine results in chronic infection of the involved area. The disorder is a noninherited

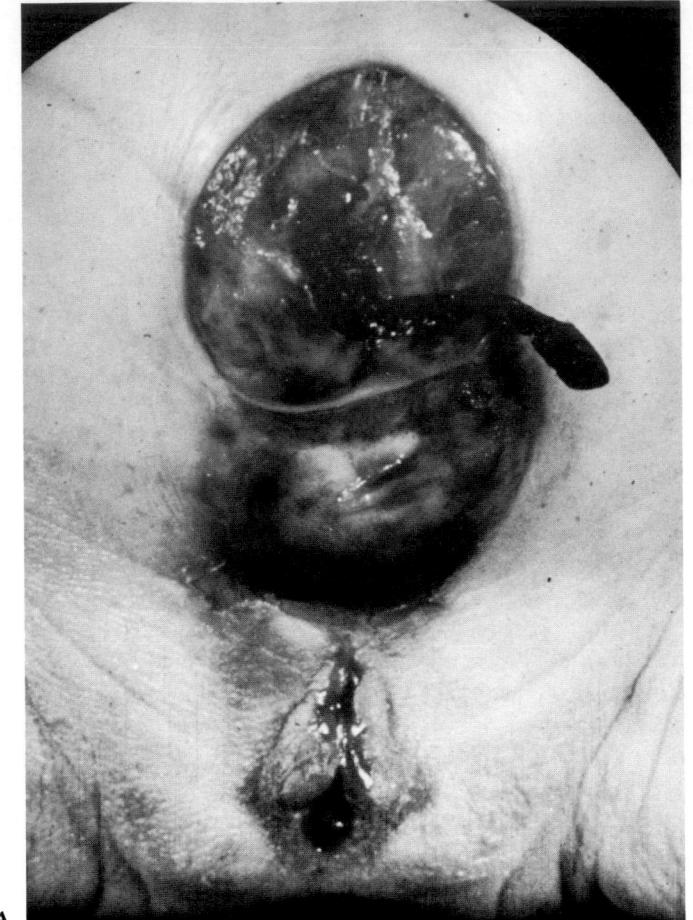

A

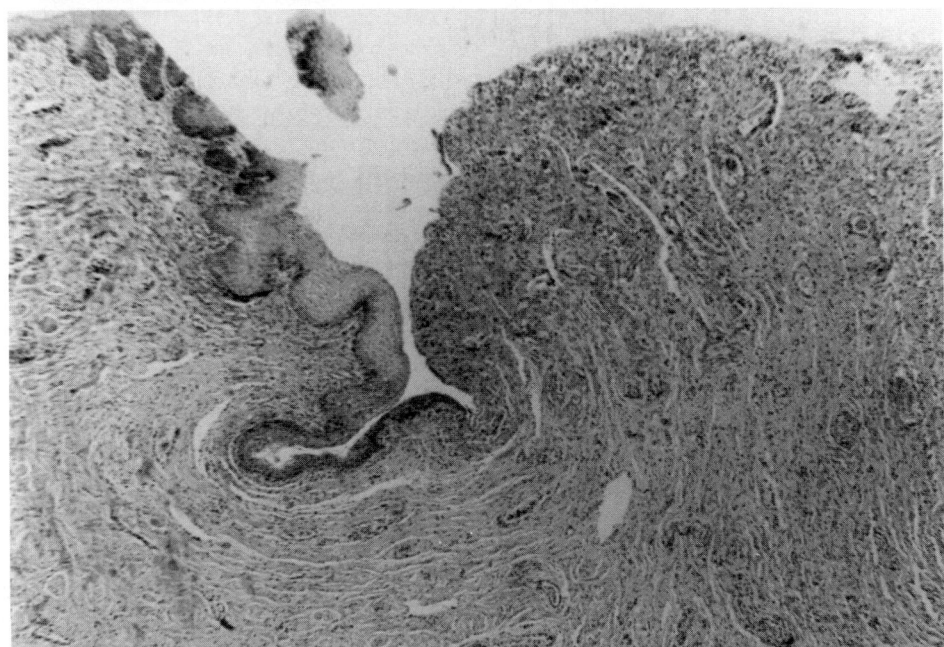

B

Figure 4-2   **(A) *Exstrophy and omphalitis.*** *The defect in the anterior abdominal wall with exstrophy of the urinary bladder is seen in this 2-month-old infant girl.* **(B) *Exstrophy.*** *The exstrophic urinary bladder on the right is contiguous with the skin epidermis on the left. Abundant inflammation and fibrosis are present in the lamina propria of the exstrophic urinary bladder.*

congenital defect more common in males than females.[18] The estimated frequency is 1/50,000 births.[8,13]

The histologic changes occurring in the externalized bladder mucosa have been the subject of numerous studies.[10,11,13] Evidence of acute and chronic inflammation is present in the mucosa of exstrophied bladders of patients in all age groups. Metaplastic changes are invariably found, including squamous and glandular metaplasia in association with mucosal proliferation, including Brunn's nests, cystitis cystica, and cystitis glandularis. A histologically normal bladder mucosa is rare.[11,13] The metaplastic changes have been observed in infants as young as 2 weeks, and tend to become more frequent and widespread with increasing age.[11,13] Increasing fibrosis and chronic inflammation is present in the muscularis in all patients older than 1 year.[11,14] Reflecting the high frequency of persistent infection of bladder following surgical closure as reported by Lattimer and Smith, Rudin and associates observed persistence of the mucosal metaplastic changes and chronic inflammation in sequential biopsies of treated patients. Histologic improvement was observed in only 25% of patients subsequent to surgical procedures to close the bladder defect.[12,14]

The uncorrected exstrophic bladder carries with it a lamentable existence for the patient. There is continual leakage of urine, with persistent or recurrent local infection, and increased risk of ascending urinary tract infection with renal involvement. Superimposed on this dilemma is the increasing risk of neoplastic transformation of the metaplastic urothelium, with resultant adenocarcinoma, squamous cell carcinoma, and least frequently, transitional cell carcinoma (refer to separate discussions).

Neoplasms Complicating Exstrophy

Uncorrected exstrophy, with persistence of the bladder wall defect and external exposure, carries a significant risk of neoplastic development in adulthood. The risk begins in the third decade and increases thereafter. Infection, invariably present in uncorrected exstrophy, is undoubtedly important in the pathogenesis of these malignancies.

Seventy-three cases of malignancy complicating exstrophy are reported in the literature.[15-45] McCown thoroughly reviewed the early literature in 1940 and compiled 24 previously reported cases and added a personally encountered case.[16] The patient reported by Montpellier was not included in McCown's review[15] (Table 4-1).

The reported patients range in age from 21 years to 73 years.[24,26] A unique case of a vesical rhabdomyosarcoma occurring in repaired exstrophic bladder of a 4-year-old boy is recorded.[41] The median age of all patients is in the fifth decade, with 74% of patients aged 30 years to 59 years. Seventy-five percent of the reported cases providing information on gender involved males. The development of local pain and bleeding, occasionally associated with a mass, prompts patients to seek medical attention, at which time the neoplasm is diagnosed by biopsy. One patient, a 52-year-old man, developed vesical adenocarcinoma 21 years after a successful surgical procedure to correct the congenital abnormality.[40]

The neoplasms complicating longstanding uncorrected exstrophy have been treated by a wide variety of radical surgical procedures. Usually, the neoplasm involves the urinary bladder mucosa extensively and is not limited to the orifice

Table 4-1   *Reported Cases of Malignancy Complicating Bladder Exstrophy*

Author(s)	Year	Age	Sex	Histologic Type*	Follow up†
Montpellier et al[15]	1935	40	M	AC	D; surgery Rx
McCown[16]	1940	23–66	‡	AC	‡
McCown[16]	1940	62	M	AC	Death during operation
Graham[17]	1942	48	M	AC	A-NED, 8 mo
Graham[17]	1942	53	M	AC	A-NED, 4 yr
Abeshouse[18]	1943	58	M	AC	Post operative death, 3 wk
Etherington-Wilson[19]	1945	59	M	AC	Post operative death, 7 wk
Reid et al[20]	1948	63	M	AC	Post operative death, 2 wk
Lange[21]	1948	53	M	AC	NI
Comar[22]	1950	50	M	AC	Post operative death
Davidson[23]	1950	52	M	NI	NI
Davidson[23]	1950	47	M	NI	NI
Davidson[23]	1950	47	F	AC	NI
Goyanna et al[24]	1951	38	F	AC	D w/tumor, 15 yr
Goyanna et al[24]	1951	65	F	AC	A-NED, 16 yr
Goyanna et al[24]	1951	21	F	AC	D w/tumor, 10 mo
Goyanna et al[24]	1951	49	M	AC	A-NED, 6 mo
Bunge[25]	1952	53	M	AC	NI
Sanchez[26]	1952	21	M	AC	A-NED, 2 yr
Sanchez[26]	1952	40	F	AC	A-NED, 1 yr
Wheeler, Hill[27]	1954	41	M	AC	A-NED, 4 mo
Wheeler, Hill[27]	1954	56	M	AC	A w/tumor, 1 yr
Martinez-Pinero[28]	1954	54	M	AC	A-NED, 2.5 yr
Mostofi et al[29]	1955	47	M	AC	D w/tumor, 7 yr, 9 mo
Mostofi et al[29]	1955	56	M	AC	A-NED, 4.5 yr
McIntosh, Worley[30]	1955	36	M	AC	D w/tumor, 2 yr
McIntosh, Worley[30]	1955	35	M	AC	A-NED, 1 yr
Scott, Sorbie[31]	1956	58	M	AC	A-NED, 8 mo
Staubitz et al[32]	1956	66	M	AC	A-NED, 15 mo
Wattenberg et al[33]	1956	36	M	AC	D w/tumor, 7 mo
Wattenberg et al[33]	1956	55	M	AC	D w/tumor, 11 mo
Sayegh, Ishak[34]	1957	52	M	AC	Post operative death
Cordonnier, Spjut[35]	1957	52	M	TCC	NI
Stuart[36]	1962	68	F	SCC	D w/tumor, 6 mo
Marshall, Muecke[37]	1962	NI	F	AC	NI
Chelloul et al[38]	1967	35	M	AC	A, 3 yr
Chelloul et al[38]	1967	38	F	AC	A, 6 mo
O'Kane, Megaw[39]	1968	38	M	AC	A-NED, 1 yr
Engell, Wilkinson[40]	1970	35	M	AC	A-NED, 6 yr
Engell, Wilkinson[40]	1970	41	M	AC	Post operative death
Engell, Wilkinson[40]	1970	52	M	AC	D w/tumor, 2 yr
Semerdjian et al[41]	1972	4	M	RS	A-NED, 13 mo

Table 4-1
(continued)

Author(s)	Year	Age	Sex	Histologic Type*	Follow up†
Kanzari et al[42]	1974	70	M	AC	NI
Daroca et al[43]	1976	48	M	AC	A-NED, 3 mo
Jacobo et al[44]	1977	65	M	AC	NI
Allen[45]	1977	50	F	AC	NI

* AC, adenocarcinoma; TCC, transitional cell carcinoma; SCC, squamous cell carcinoma; RS, rhabdomyosarcoma; NI, no information

† D, dead; A-NED, alive-no evidence of disease; A, alive; NI, no information

‡ McCown reported one case and tabulated 24 previously reported malignancies complicating exstrophy.[16] The patients included 14 males and 9 females, ranging in age from 23 years to 66 years. The histologic form of these malignancies included 19 adenocarcinomas and 2 squamous cell carcinomas. Details of histologic type were not provided in three reports. McCown's review did not include the case report of Montpellier and associates.[15]

of the bladder defect. Sixty-two, or 85%, of all reported malignancies are adeno-carcinomas, with fewer numbers of squamous cell carcinomas. Transitional cell carcinoma has been reported in only one patient.[35] The involved exstrophied bladder is consistently chronically inflamed and evidences variably extensive glandular metaplasia with or without squamous metaplasia.

Definitive follow-up information is available for only about one half of the reported patients with malignancy complicating exstrophy. No information was provided in the reports of 20 patients. Nine patients died in the postoperative period, and an additional seven patients received no therapy. Twenty-three patients were alive 2 months to 16 years after surgical treatment at the time of publication. Nine patients had died, five with known tumor recurrence. Of the total of 73 patients, only 5 patients (7%) were known to survive more than 5 years.[16,24,29,40]

Diverticulum

Bladder diverticula are relatively common clinical disorders. They require surgical excision only infrequently, and therefore the surgical pathologist does not commonly encounter them. In spite of their relatively common occurrence, their cause remains unsettled. Some studies indicate that all are the result of increased intravesical pressure secondary to some form of outlet obstruction.[47,52] Others disagree, and regard some as being of congenital origin.[50] Bladder diverticula are observed in patients of all ages with the majority observed in men older than 50 years, invariably with obstruction secondary to prostatism.[47,51] They are observed less frequently in infants and children, and in some studies, in young patients without evidence of obstruction.[50,52] Regardless of age, the most common location is in the vicinity of the ureteral orifices, frequently immediately superior.[52] In this location, enlargement of the diverticulum can result in secondary obstruction or vesical reflux.[52] Small saccules and diverticula are without symptoms and clinical significance. Progressive enlargement, rarely to enormous proportions with volumes exceeding that of the urinary bladder itself, is associated with stagnation of urine, infection, and calculus formation.[46,48] Only when urine stagnation is present is there a significant frequency in the complications noted, and thus a need for surgical intervention. In addition to these frequently occurring complications, 2% to 7% of patients develop neoplasms within the diverticulum (refer to discussion of neoplasms in bladder diverticula).

The excised bladder diverticulum will show a relatively narrow orifice opening into a larger cavity evidently distorting the outside contour of the bladder. The narrow intramural neck is found between bundles of the inner layer of bladder muscle. The distended wall of the diverticulum contains attenuated muscle fibers most commonly in young patients. This observed difference in frequency of smooth muscle has led to the impression that congenital diverticula are identified by the presence of this structural component, and those of acquired nature have no muscle within the diverticular wall. In practice, all diverticula with evidence of longstanding chronic inflammation tend to show fibrosis of the wall that may have replaced the original resident muscle. This observation is independent of patient age. As noted previously, muscle can be found in diverticula in elderly men with evident outlet obstruction. When present, the muscle is attenuated bundles of the outer two layers; the thicker bundles of the inner layer do not participate in this investment.[47] Superimposed chronic inflammation, with or without squamous metaplasia, is observed in the majority of excised specimens.[51] Fibrosis is common and variable in extent. Less than 20% of diverticula are histologically normal.[51]

Table 4-2   *Reported Cases of Neoplasms Arising in Diverticulum*

Author(s)	Year	Age	
		Range	*Mean*
Abeshouse, Goldstein[53]	1943	40–83	57.9
Pearlman, Bobbitt[54]	1948		76
Boylan et al[55]	1951	38–86	61.8
Thomas, Abernathy[56]	1952		67
Mayer, Moore[57]	1954	53–72	NI
Ward[58]	1958		76
Knappenberger et al[59]	1960	44–78	66
Fox et al[60]	1962	NI	NI
Shawdon et al[61]	1965	39–67	57.5
Kelalis, McLean[62]	1967	44–84	64
Ostroff et al[63]	1973	21–90	57
Siegel[64]	1974	60–78	69
Montague, Boltuch[65]	1976	56–81	66.7
Ramthor[66]	1980		61
Shirai et al[67]	1984	66–84	75
Totals		21–90	57–75

Neoplasms Arising in Diverticula

Neoplasms are a rare complication supervening in bladder diverticula. There are 197 examples in the literature, 10% reported since the extensive review of Abeshouse and Goldstein.[53-67] The details of these reported cases are summarized in Table 4-2. Shirai and associates cited an additional 100 cases published in the Japanese literature.[67] The age range of the reported patients is 21 years to 90 years, with mean ages varying from 57 years to 75 years in the cited studies. Only eight cases (4%) have occurred in women. Transitional cell carcinomas and squamous cell carcinomas are the most frequently encountered histologic types, together accounting for 65% of all cases. Ten sarcomas and one carcinosarcoma have been reported.

The clinical presentation of patients with neoplasms in diverticula is not specific to this complication. Symptoms most commonly relate to urinary tract infection, calculi, or the diverticulum itself. Hematuria may be found. Cystoscopic detection of the neoplasm within the diverticulum may be difficult because of the relative sizes of the diverticulum and the tumor. "Blind biopsies" within the diverticulum frequently are performed when clinical suspicion is high. The detection of the neoplasm within the diverticulum may be based on positive urine cytologies, and filling defects observed on cystogram. A spectrum of surgical and

| Sex | | No. of Cases | Histologic Diagnosis* | | | | | | |
Male	Female		TCC	SCC	AC	UC	S	B	NI
92	3	95†	21	16	1	35	6	16	
1	0	1	1						
25	0	25	16	7	1	1			
1	0	1				1			
7	1	8	7				1		
0	1	1					1		
17	1	18	14	2					2
4	0	4	1	3					
4	0	4	3	1					
19	0	19	12	6			1		
4	0	4	1	1			2‡		
3	1	4	4						
10	0	10	8	2					
0	1	1		1					
2	0	2	1§	1‡		1			
189 (96%)	8 (4%)	197	89 (45%)	40 (20%)	2	38	11‡	16	2

* TCC, transitional cell carcinoma; SCC, squamous cell carcinoma; AC, adenocarcinoma; UC, undifferentiated carcinoma, carcinoma of unspecified type; S, sarcoma; B, benign neoplasm; NI, no information.

† Ninety-one cases found in literature review and four personal cases added.

‡ One case was carcinosarcoma.

§ Two separate neoplasms in diverticulum, one transitional cell carcinoma and one squamous cell carcinoma.

adjunct forms of therapy has been reported in the literature. Survival rates cited in the literature are poor, and most probably reflect the relatively long period before diagnosis and treatment because of the occult location of growth, and the relative ease of deep invasion of the attenuated bladder wall thickness in the diverticulum. Undoubtedly, stasis of urine and chronic inflammation, on occasion associated with calculus disease, play a role in the development of neoplasia with a vesical diverticulum.

Urachus

The urachus is a tapered cephalad extension of the urogenital sinus (later to become the urinary bladder) that is contiguous with the allantois. Following birth, this tubular structure normally undergoes progressive atrophy as it descends caudally with the urinary bladder, to which it remains attached. The point of attachment most commonly is found at the vesical dome. The regressive changes, which result in closure of both the cephalad end at the umbilicus and the caudal end at the bladder wall, obliterate the intervening segment and convert it to a solid cord of fibrous tissue.[68-70]

Careful dissection of the midline anterior abdominal wall, including the bladder dome, discloses microscopic tubular remnants of the urachus in 32% to 70% of adults at autopsy.[69,70] These microscopic remnants are lined most commonly by transitional epithelium. One third demonstrate columnar cell metaplasia.[69,70] The configuration of the urachal remnant within the bladder wall varies from a uniform narrow tube, to those showing random microcystic dilatations or irregular lateral pouches.[70]

These microscopic vestiges are of no clinical significance, but knowledge of their presence and structure has important implications referable to those anomalies of the urachus that have clinical importance. The disorders of the urachus having their origin in persistence of the urachal lumen include fistula or cyst formation, associated infection with or without concomitant calculus formation, and neoplasia of either the epithelial lining or the supporting stroma.

The clinical disorders associated with persistent urachus relate to the extent and location of the urachus that remains patent. Persistence of the entire urachus from the bladder to the umbilicus results in drainage of urine from the umbilicus, and supervening infection is common. Alternatively, incomplete persistence of the urachus may result in blind pouches open either to the skin at the umbilicus, or to the urinary bladder. Segmental persistence of lumen with closure at both ends results in a urachal cyst. Drainage of urine from the umbilicus, associated infection, or the gradual enlargement of a midline mass resulting from the accumulation of secretion with urachal cysts all bring these disorders to clinical attention. Appropriate culture and sensitivity testing will indicate appropriate antibiotic therapy, and commonly will accompany surgical excision of the anomalous segment responsible for the symptoms. These complications are observed in patients of all ages. The most severe is persistence of the entire urachus, which is most common in infants.

The least common, but most serious, complication of persistent urachal segments is the development of neoplasia.

Neoplasms

The first description of urachal structures persistent into adulthood giving origin to a malignant neoplasms is attributed to Hue and Jacquin in 1863.[71,73] The neoplasm described by these authors was a mucinous adenocarcinoma in a 45-year-old man.[45] The cases reported in the later literature have been catalogued in numerous reviews by Begg, Slater and Torassa, Wheeler and Hill, and Raatzsch and Wehnert.[68,72-99] In 1971, Ohman and co-workers compiled a total of 130 reported cases.[100] An additional 70 cases are detailed in case studies reported to 1985 for a total of 200.[101-113]

Yu and Leong reported that urachal malignancies constitute 0.34% of bladder neoplasms.[103] Table 4-3 summarizes the sex and age distribution of the reported urachal malignancies. Overall, 75% of the 200 reported neoplasms involved men. Approximately 65% involve patients in the fifth to seventh decades, with cited mean ages of 48 years to 64 years. Exceptions to the age distribution demonstrated by urachal carcinomas are the nine reported patients with urachal sarcomas with a mean age of 22 years.

Patients with malignancies of the urachus most commonly have hematuria and abdominal mass.[99,112] Umbilical discharge or mucus in the urine may be observed in the minority of patients with urachal mucinous adenocarcinomas.[112] With the exception of discharge of pus, blood, or mucus from the umbilicus, all other clinical features are nonspecific and may be exhibited by disorders primary in the urinary bladder. Radiologic signs of calcific stippling and a filling defect in the region of the bladder dome are very suggestive of urachal neoplasms and are most helpful in the preoperative evaluation of patients.[99,109] Because the surgical approach to urachal malignancies is significantly different than that for primary neoplasms of the bladder, accurate preoperative diagnosis is critical. Cystoscopy may or may not disclose a mucosal lesion in the bladder dome. Intramucosal urachal malignancies are apparent and accessible to biopsy at cystoscopy. Intramuscular and supravesical neoplasms are less accessible, and not uncommonly produce a mass of extrinsic features in the bladder dome. Less commonly, no abnormality whatever is evident. Mucosal biopsies in the region of the bladder dome, regardless of the cystoscopic appearance of the mucosa, provide valuable

Table 4-3   **Reported Cases of Urachal Malignancies**

Histologic Type	No. of Cases	Sex		Age (Years)	
		Male	*Female*	*Range*	*Mean*
Adenocarcinoma	168 ⎫ (90%)	129 (78%)	39	20–84	54
Adenocarcinoma, signet-ring type	12 ⎭	9	3	30–71	48
Transitional cell carcinoma	4	4	0	44–73	64
Squamous cell carcinoma	3	2	1	32–62	51
Undifferentiated carcinoma	2	0	2	15–76	45
Carcinoma, NOS	2	1	1	48–49	48
Sarcoma	9 (5%)	5	4	4 mo–51 yr	22
Totals	200	150 (75%)	50		

information. If the urachal orifice is patent in the vesical mucosa, manual expression of urachal contents may provide diagnostic tissue fragments.

Pathologic Features

The distribution of histologic types of urachal malignancies reported in the literature appears in Table 4-3. Approximately 95% of all neoplasms of the urachus are epithelial and the remainder (nine cases) are sarcomas. Ninety percent of all urachal malignancies are adenocarcinomas, commonly demonstrating mucin production. Rarely, signet-ring type mucinous adenocarcinomas are observed. Metaplasia of the urachal mucosa to columnar epithelium or squamous epithelium and subsequent neoplastic transformations explain the varied histologic spectrum of the neoplasms.

The similarity of the histologic spectrum of urachal and vesical neoplasms, their markedly different frequency distribution notwithstanding, consistently presents a diagnostic challenge when the physician is dealing with neoplasms involving the dome of the bladder. Urachal neoplasms in a supravesical location, without apparent gross or microscopic continuity with the bladder wall, offer no major problem. However, when the neoplasm is intramuscular, and especially if it is intramucosal, distinction from a primary bladder neoplasm may be difficult, and on occasion may be practically impossible to determine with certainty. Intramural neoplasms with ulceration of the overlying urothelial mucosa significantly accentuate the difficulty of origin determination.

Wheeler and Hill[85] and Mostofi and associates[29] outlined the following minimal diagnostic criteria to support the urachal origin of a malignancy:

1. Tumor located in dome or anterior wall of bladder;
2. Bulk of the tumor located in muscularis rather than in lamina propria;
3. Tumor infiltration of the bladder wall, with contiguous spread through space of Retzius in the anterior abdominal wall;
4. Urachal remnant associated with tumor;
5. A sharp demarcation between the tumor and the overlying bladder mucosa of the bladder dome;
6. Absence of glandular or polypoid proliferations of bladder mucosa (in region of dome).

The practical application of these criteria to distinguish neoplasms of urachal origin from those of vesical origin has proved frustrating on several occasions, especially when encountering large tumors with extensive vesical mucosal ulceration in addition to extensive intramural infiltration. Incomplete resections and inadequate sectioning of specimens compound the difficulty in attempting to arrive at a confident diagnosis. It must be stated that a reliable diagnosis cannot be made on review of the neoplasm's histologic features alone, independent of the diagnostic criteria outlined above.

Following surgical excision, the most common course in the natural history of these malignancies is local recurrence involving the paravesical tissue, the bladder wall, and the anterior abdominal wall, in order of decreasing frequency.[112] Distant metastases are usually late, and most frequently involve the lung and varous intra-abdominal sites, including the liver.[112] Urachal carcinomas have consistently demonstrated a poorer survival rate than the corresponding histologic type of vesical malignancy.[112]

Proliferative and Metaplastic Variants

A spectrum of urothelial proliferative changes of hyperplastic and metaplastic nature are observed commonly in the urinary bladder. Indeed, these same mucosal changes are observed throughout the urinary tract and have been discussed in detail in Chapter 2.

The hyperplastic urothelial changes include simple hyperplasia of the surface urothelium, and the focal proliferative mucosal invaginations traditionally termed Brunn's buds or Brunn's nests, and cystitis cystica. The metaplastic proliferations include cystitis glandularis, squamous metaplasia, and nephrogenic metaplasia. In spite of extensive study of these proliferative changes since the late 19th century, their cause(s), histogenesis, and clinical significance remain problematic. They have been regarded variously as normal proliferative variants, or alternatively as reactive urothelial proliferations with established, or potential, premalignant qualities.[117,125,141] Each will be discussed briefly with reference to their occurrence within the bladder.

Simple Hyperplasia

The normal urothelial mucosa of the urinary bladder has seven to eight cell layers.[138] Vesical urothelium with thickness in excess of this normal baseline is termed *simple hyperplasia*. This proliferative change is typically flat, but is also commonly present in examples of polypoid cystitis. By definition, simple hyperplasia is without a dysplastic component; however, urothelial dysplasia may involve hyperplastic urothelium, most commonly in proximity to transitional cell carcinomas (refer to discussion of carcinoma in situ). Full-thickness dysplasia, or carcinoma in situ, has no characteristic number of cell layers, and therefore may be observed in an attenuated or hyperplastic urothelium. The clinical significance of simple hyperplasia is unknown, beyond its recognized association with inflammatory disorders, including lithiasis, and vesical neoplasms.

Brunn's Buds and Nests

Proliferative invaginations of urothelium retaining continuity with the surface are termed *Brunn's buds* (Fig. 4-3). Well-defined solid nests of urothelial cells within the superficial lamina propria are termed *Brunn's nests*. Typically, both buds and nests are observed in proximity, suggesting a histogenetic relationship. Indeed, origin of these nests from the mucosal invaginations has been generally accepted.[117,125] More recently, Goldstein and associates reported migration of surface urothelial cells into the lamina propria and subsequent proliferation with resultant cell nests beneath the mucosal surface.[139] The significance of this experimental model to clinical Brunn's nests is currently unknown.

Historically, these nests and buds of von Brunn have been regarded as reactive proliferations associated with intravesical inflammation.[117,119,124] This interpretation was based on multiple studies, most importantly that of Morse in 1928, who reported evidence of chronic inflammation in 58% of bladders with

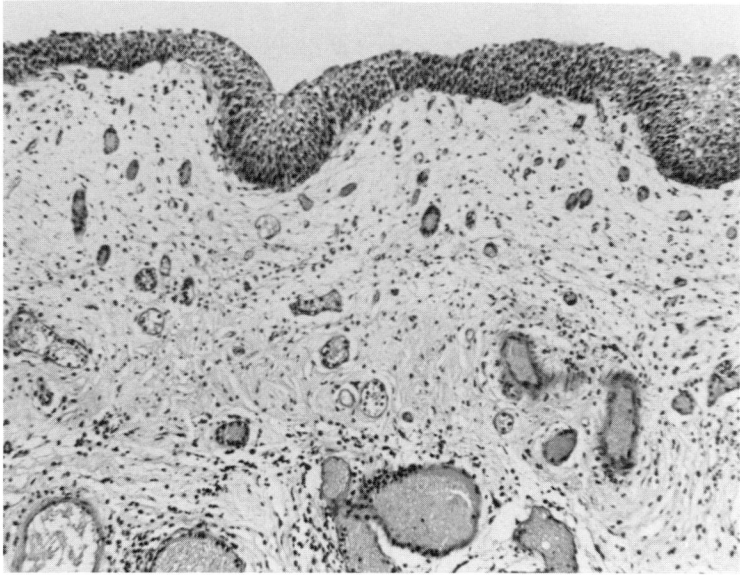

Figure 4-3   *Brunn's buds. The lamina propria is focally penetrated by a solid bud of urothelial cells similar to the surface epithelium. Scattered chronic inflammatory cells and vascular dilatation are noted in the deep lamina propria.*

epithelial buds and nests.[117] The regularity with which these proliferative changes are observed in inflamed bladders provides anecdotal support for Morse's conclusion. The inflammatory basis of these proliferative lesions is not supported by the cases with Brunn's nests unaccompanied by chronic inflammation, which amounted to 42% of Morse's cases.[117] More recent studies of these urothelial proliferative lesions have recorded the high frequency of these lesions in normal bladders (89%).[140,141] These findings suggest that Brunn's buds and nests may represent urothelial proliferative variants, which may arise spontaneously, or may reflect one of a limited number of reactions to injury demonstrated by this cell population.

In a typical case, randomly scattered Brunn's buds invaginate into the underlying lamina propria. These invaginations are sharply delimited by the basement membrane continuous with the surface urothelium. The cytologic features of the bud-invaginated urothelium are identical with those of the adjacent surface mucosa. Brunn's nests, apparently having lost their contiguity with the surface urothelium, commonly accompany the buds. The nests tend to occur in clusters, and tend to be round and equally as well delimited as the Brunn's buds. Commonly, the otherwise solid nests show a slit or circular lumen that may contain eosinophilic, PAS-positive, and mucicarmine-positive secretions.[126,133] Brunn's nests with this feature commonly have a layer of luminal cells that are cuboidal or low columnar in contrast to the surrounding peripheral layers of more typical urothelial cells. This histologic change reflects an early phase in a gradation that ultimately transforms the previously solid nest to a cystic or glandular structure (cystitis cystica and cystitis glandularis).

Cystitis Cystica and Cystitis Glandularis

The historical evolution of our understanding of cystitis cystica and cystitis glandularis closely parallels our knowledge of the buds and nests of von Brunn. Morse interpreted these urothelial proliferations to be of inflammatory origin, similar to the origin of Brunn's buds and nests.[117] This conclusion was generally accepted in most studies until recent years. Cystitis cystica and cystitis glandularis are observed commonly in circumstances characterized by urothelial inflammation including urinary tract infections, calculus disease, neurogenic bladders, and exstrophy.[117,132]

Experimental bladder exstrophy procedures demonstrate similar proliferative changes.[136] Alternative causes of cystitis cystica and cystitis glandularis offered in the early literature included infection, allergy, hormonal imbalance, vitamin deficiency, or origin in embryonic nests.[117,119,124] However, the finding of cystitis cystica in 60% of normal bladders suggests that, along with Brunn's nests, it may represent a spontaneous normal proliferative variant of urothelium (Fig. 4-4).[140,141]

The genesis of cystitis glandularis from Brunn's nests has been generally accepted, but the sequence of events constituted a major controversy during the 1920s to 1940s.[114,115,117,118] Origin of cystitis glandularis from von Brunn's nests by degeneration of the central cells, or by metaplastic change of the urothelium,

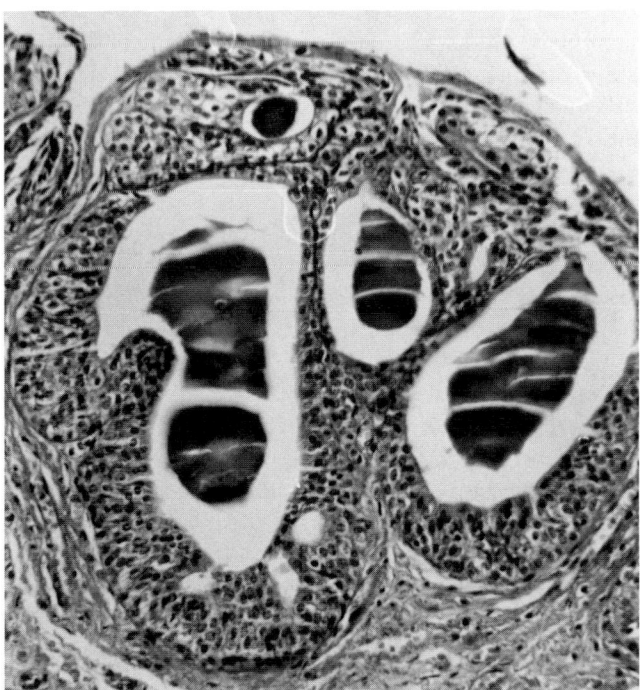

Figure 4-4   *Cystitis cystica. Urothelial cell nests with a central lumen that contains secretions are present beneath the surface, here devoid of urothelial cells. Step sections revealed continuity of the lining urothelial cells of the cysts with the surface.*

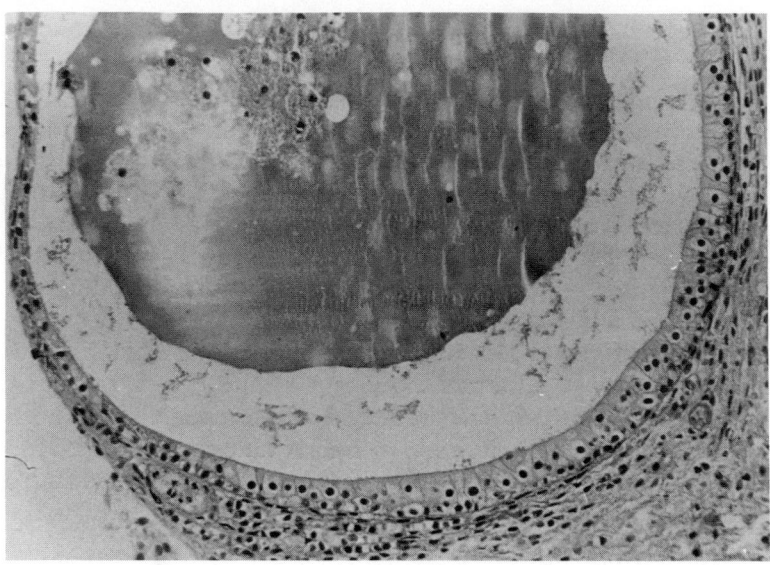

Figure 4-5   *Cystitis glandularis. Secretions markedly distend the glandular structure lined by metaplastic mucus-secreting columnar cells of urothelial origin.*

was debated. Alternatively, the cysts were the result of duct obstruction of a glandularis structure with accumulation of secretions within the lumen.[119,124] The bulk of evidence suggests that cystitis cystica or Brunn's nests undergoes metaplasia, creating a cystitis glandularis structure characterized by a goblet cell lining with evident mucin production (Figs. 4-5 and 4-6).[116,118] On occasion, cystitis cystica with variably extensive but incomplete metaplastic goblet cell metaplasia is observed, demonstrating transition forms between cystica and glandularis structures.

The metaplastic change occasionally can create glands that recapitulate colonic epithelium to an amazing degree. Rare examples demonstrating argentaffin and Paneth's cells admixed with the goblet cells have been reported.[129,131,137] Such mucosal changes may be focal or extensive with rare reported examples involving the entire bladder.[121,123,130,142] Under such circumstances differentiation from vesical adenocarcinoma may prove a diagnostic challenge.[120,122,123,130]

The clinical significance of cystitis glandularis relates to the risk of neoplastic transformation occurring in bladder demonstrating this metaplastic change. In five large series of vesical adenocarcinomas, metaplastic cystitis glandularis was found in 10% to 42% of the reported cases (see Table 4-14). Examining the association of cystitis glandularis and vesical adenocarcinoma from another perspective, a review of the literature uncovered only three reported cases of adenocarcinoma arising in urinary bladders previously determined by biopsy to exhibit cystitis glandularis.[127,134,135] These three neoplasms were diagnosed 5 years, 7 years, and 15 years following the detection of cystitis glandularis. An increased risk of developing a vesical malignancy associated with cystitis glandularis may exist, as suggested by these data. This must not be equated to granting cystitis glandularis the status of a "premalignant lesion," as some have concluded.[118,125,127] The persistence of causal factor(s) related to the development of the cystitis glandularis are to be implicated in the neoplastic transformation

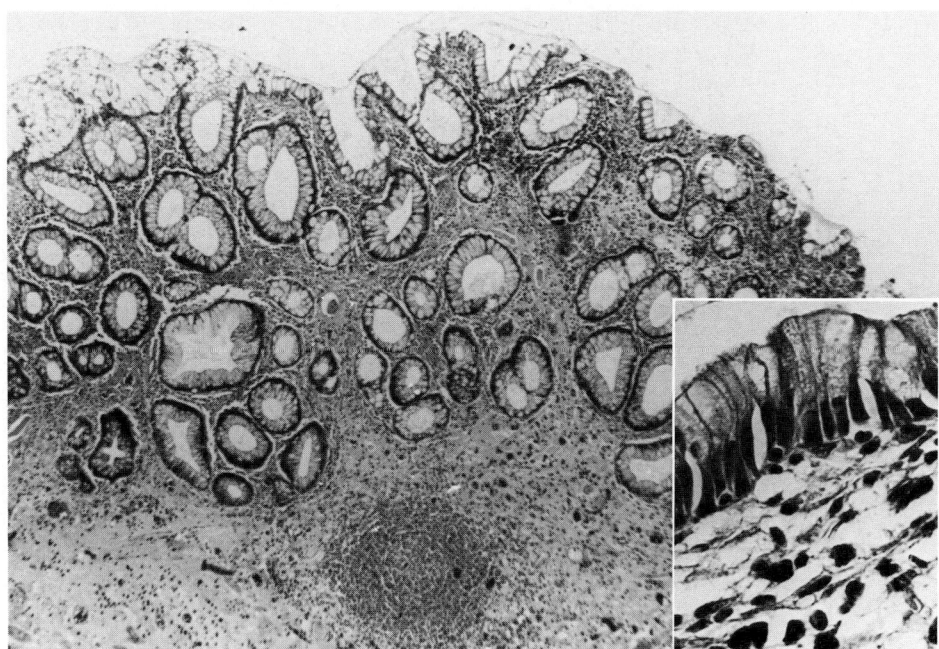

Figure 4-6   *Cystitis glandularis. Numerous gland structures, present in the lamina propria, are lined by mucus-secreting cells* (inset) *identical to those present on the surface. A variably dense chronic inflammatory cell infiltrate is present in the interstitium with a lymphoid follicle present in the deep lamina propria.*

resulting in the adenocarcinoma. There is no evidence that the metaplastic urothelium (cystitis glandularis) per se possesses a unique propensity to undergo neoplastic transformation. From a practical perspective, the patient with cystitis glandularis must be regarded at risk, and prolonged close follow up is obligatory.

Squamous Metaplasia (Leukoplakia)

The ability of the urothelial mucosa of the urinary tract to undergo metaplastic change is further demonstrated by examples of squamous metaplasia, or leukoplakia, as it is termed in the clinical literature. Approximately 400 cases have been reported in multiple studies, exclusive of the single study of 450 patients reported by Widran and co-workers.[143-152] Vesical squamous metaplasia (leukoplakia) has been reported at all ages, but the majority of patients are middle-aged or older.[145,151,152] With the exception of the study by Widran and co-workers, males are more commonly affected (56% to 78%).[145,151,152] Patients almost invariably seek medical attention for symptoms related to urinary tract infection or calculus disease, at which time squamous metaplasia (leukoplakia) is detected on cystoscopy (Fig. 4-7).[151] The vesical mucosa contains patchy white opacified, shaggy, or glistening areas.[144,145,152]

Bladder biopsies show squamous replacement of the urothelial transitional epithelium (Figs. 4-8 and 4-9). The squamous cell mucosa shows normal maturation with or without hyperkeratosis. Traditional diagnostic criterion—

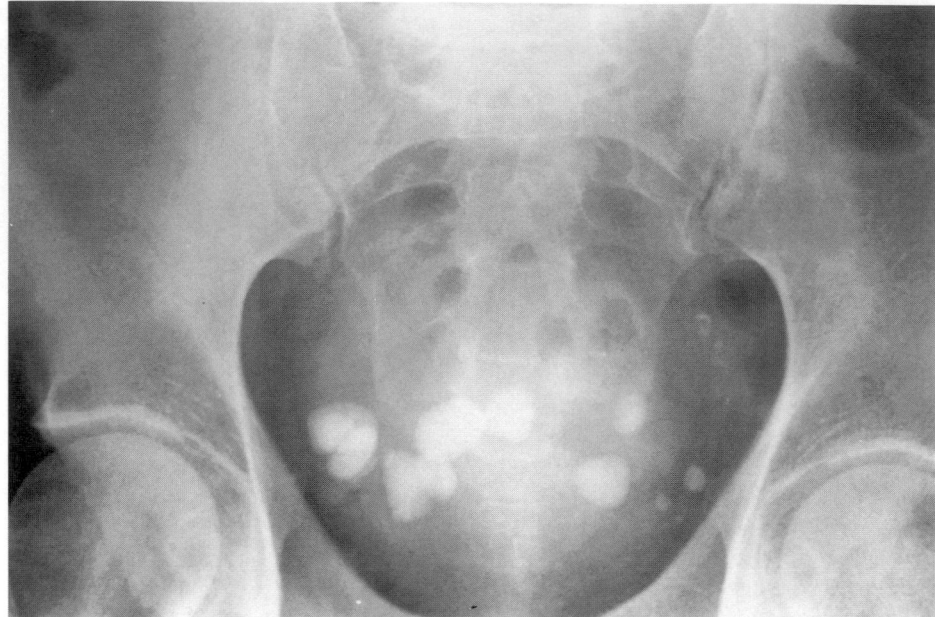

A

B

Figure 4-7   ***Bladder calculi.*** *(A) A preliminary film shows several opaque densities in the region of the urinary bladder. (B) Intravenous urographic contrast material identifies the calculi within the urinary bladder.*

cornification of a noncornifying membrane — is attributed to McDonald.[143] Two histologic types of squamous metaplasia are observed: the nonkeratinizing form and the keratinizing form. Recently, Benson and co-workers, equating the keratinizing form of squamous metaplasia to leukoplakia, outlined diagnostic criteria including the following: squamous metaplasia with keratinization; downward growth of rete pegs; and dysplastic squamous maturation.[152] The suggested criteria are regarded as unhelpful from two perspectives: the perpetua-

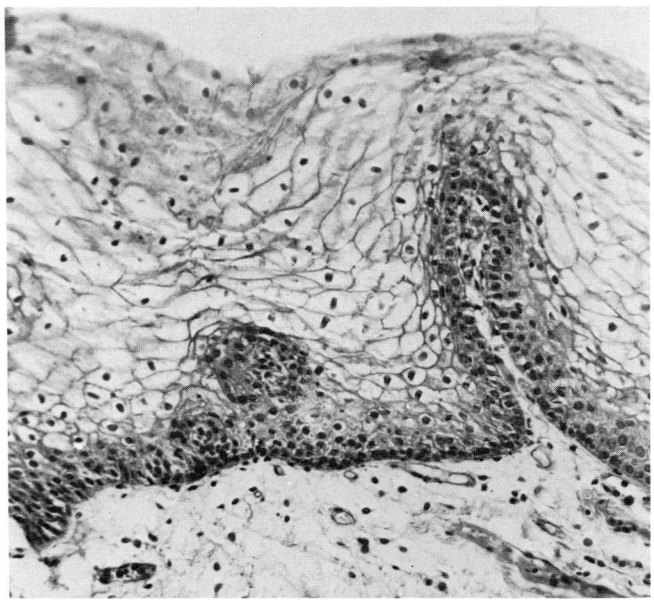

Figure 4-8   ***Squamous metaplasia.*** *The typical transitional urothelium has been replaced by squamous epithelium. No atypia is present.*

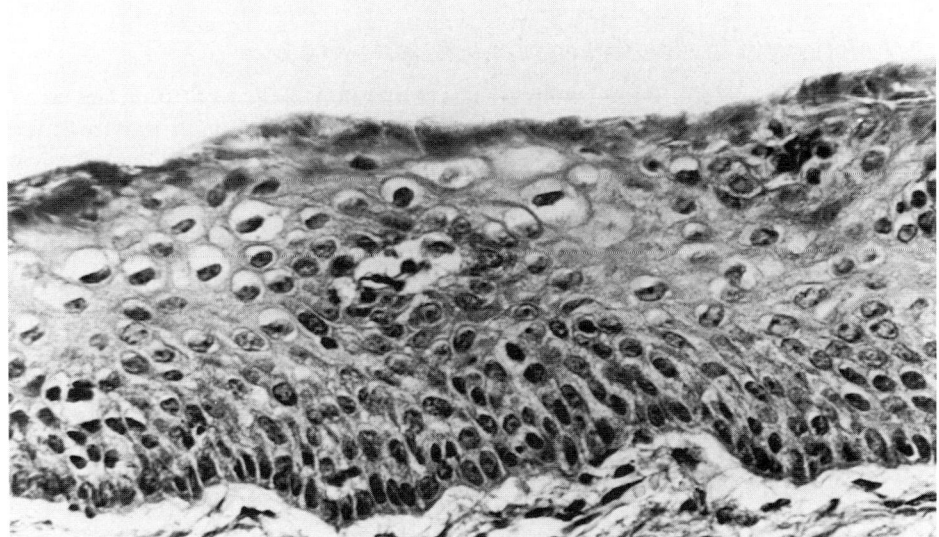

Figure 4-9   ***Squamous metaplasia.*** *This example of squamous metaplasia contains scattered atypical (dysplastic) cells with irregular nuclear outline and a mildly prominent nucleolus. Squamous cell carcinoma was present elsewhere in the bladder.*

tion of the use of the term *leukoplakia,* an imprecise clinical term that is to be discouraged in pathologic diagnoses of urologic lesions (and elsewhere); and the introduction of the criterion of dysplasia, which would disqualify the vast majority of examples of squamous metaplasia, keratinizing or not, because they typically show no dysplastic changes. Uncommonly, dysplasia of varying severity may be present, and its presence should be noted in the final diagnosis. To my knowledge, no studies have been reported evaluating the clinical behavior of vesical squamous metaplasia demonstrating dysplasia.

The clinical significance of squamous metaplasia in the urinary bladder relates to the frequently associated (possibly causal) urinary tract infection with or without lithiasis. As with Brunn's nests, cystitis cystica, and cystitis glandularis, squamous metaplasia traditionally has been attributed to the reactive urothelial proliferations not commonly associated with inflammation. However, apparent spontaneous squamous metaplasia has been found in 7% of adult males and 46% of females.[140,141] Thus, its presence may not be equated to established cystitis.

The relation of squamous metaplasia with or without keratinization to vesical neoplasms, in particular to squamous cell carcinoma, has received much attention. Reported series of squamous cell carcinomas of the urinary bladder indicate that 17% to 25% are associated with squamous metaplasia in the affected bladders (see Table 4-13). Nine percent to 22% of cases of vesical leukoplakia are associated with a bladder malignancy at the time of diagnosis, and another 10% to 20% subsequently are reported to develop carcinoma of the bladder.[145,151,152] The interpretation of this cumulative experience has been variously interpreted to indicate that squamous metaplasia of the urinary bladder is a premalignant, potentially premalignant, or non-premalignant change of the urothelium.[143-152] From the clinical perspective, the patient is at greater risk of bladder malignancy, and therapeutic efforts to eliminate a cause of inflammation if present, coupled with prolonged follow up, are obligatory.

Nephrogenic Metaplasia (Adenoma)

Nephrogenic metaplasia is a urothelial lesion of unknown etiology and uncertain pathogenesis. It occurs most frequently in the urinary bladder, and is characterized by numerous small tubules clustered in the lamina propria producing an exophytic nodule (Fig. 4-10). It is commonly found in the clinical context of chronic inflammation. The lesion originally was described by Davis.[153] Friedman and Kuhlenbeck reported seven cases, and coined the term *nephrogenic adenoma*.[154] A total of 64 cases have been reported in the bladder.[153-179] Extravesical examples of this lesion were first reported by Peterson and Matsumoto, who observed an example in a urethral diverticulum[168] (refer to discussion of nephrogenic metaplasia in Chap. 5). The first examples of nephrogenic metaplasia occurring in the ureter were reported in three separate case studies in 1983 (refer to discussion of nephrogenic metaplasia in Chap. 3). In all locations — ureter, bladder, and urethra — the recognition of this distinctive lesion is relatively recent, with 85% of all cases reported since 1970.

Clinical Features

Nephrogenic metaplasia (adenoma) is most commonly encountered in the bladders of males (74%). Reported patients range in age from a 3-week-old infant (Ritchey and associates) to the eighth decade (Berger and associates; Navarre and co-workers).[172,176,178] Approximately 40% of cases are observed in patients younger than 30 years of age, 20% in patients between 30 years and 49 years of age, and 40% in patients older than 50 years of age.

The diagnosis of nephrogenic metaplasia (adenoma) is almost invariably

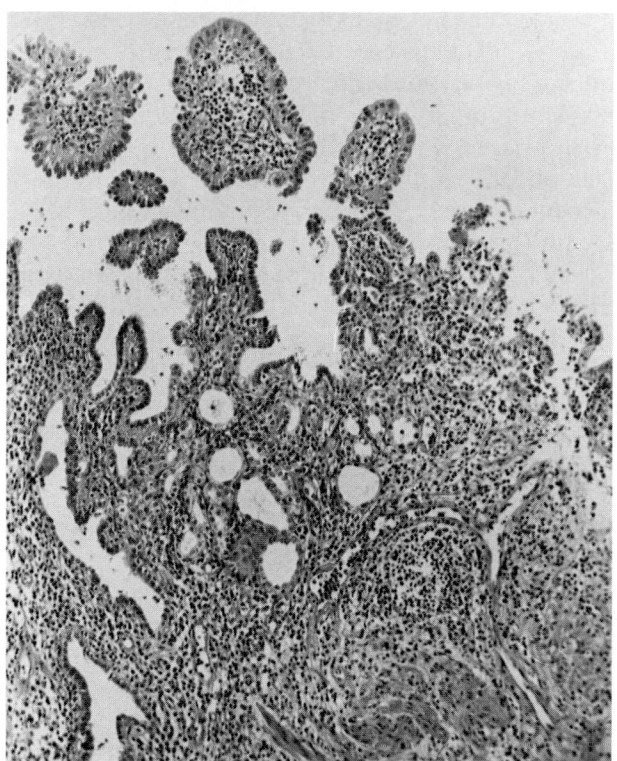

Figure 4-10   *Nephrogenic adenoma. Papillary and simple tubular structures located in the mucosa and superficial lamina propria and lined by epithelium similar to renal tubular epithelium characterized this lesion. Numerous acute and chronic inflammatory cells infiltrate the adjacent lamina propria.*

made in the clinical context of chronic bladder infection, with calculus disease, prior instrumentation, surgery, trauma, or catheterization recorded in the patient's medical history.[171,174,176-178] Clinical presentation commonly is prompted by irritative bladder symptoms, occasionally with hematuria, mulberry-like or shaggy exophytic lesions in the background of an inflamed bladder are observed at cystoscopy. These lesions are most common in the trigone region, but have been observed in all locations within the bladder. Transurethral resection constitutes the most common form of therapy. Recurrences are common.

Pathologic Features

The basic microscopic features of nephrogenic metaplasia (adenoma) are multiple tubular structures within the lamina propria in association with variably intense acute and chronic inflammation (see Fig. 4-10). Plasma cells and lymphocytes predominate, but surface ulceration may produce a localized predominance of neutrophils. Eosinophils and histiocytes may be observed in some examples, but they are not prominent. The surface urothelium is frequently ulcerated, or may show focal hyperplasia. There is no cytologic atypia. The tubular structures are lined by flat or low cuboidal epithelium and are surrounded by a well-defined basement membrane, effectively demonstrated by PAS or silver stains.[174,177] The epithelial cells have lightly eosinophilic cytoplasm, occasional enlarged nuclei, and absence of both mitotic activity and prominent nucleoli.[172,176] The tubular configuration is predominantly round, but occasional tubules show elongation, rarely demonstrating direct continuity with the surface urothelium.[174,177] Tubular lining cells and intraluminal secretions stain positively with mucicarmine, PAS, and alcian blue.[174,177]

Ultrastructural studies confirm the epithelial nature of the tubular lining cells.[165,169,173,174,177] Microvilli, complex intercellular interdigitations, and tight junctions are observed.

The diagnosis is based on the histologic features described previously. The lack of significant cytologic atypia, associated inflammation, uniform circumscription of the tubules by a basement membrane, and localization of the lesion to the lamina propria, in combination, allow differentiation from other lesions, in particular adenocarcinoma.

Pathogenesis

The variable names found in the literature applied to nephrogenic metaplasia (including nephrogenic adenoma, nephrogenic metaplasia, adenomatoid tumor, and adenomatoid metaplasia) reflect the unsettled state of the lesion's histogenesis.[154,161,165,177,180] The invariable association of this lesion with inflammation of the urinary tract, the occasional demonstration of continuity of the tubular epithelium with the surface, and the occasional foci of squamous metaplasia all support the mechanism of metaplasia as the underlying pathogenesis, as originally proposed by Mostofi.[180] The reported localization of this lesion in the ureter, urethra, and urinary bladder diminishes the probability that embryonic mesodermal rests are involved. Their superficial resemblance to adenomatoid tumors as observed in genital adnexal structures does not justify applying the term to these lesions of the urothelium of the ureter, bladder, and urethra. The ultrastructural features have been variously interpreted as recapitulating various segments of the renal tubules, including proximal convoluted tubules, thin limb of Henle's loop, or collecting tubules.[174] It is hoped that future histochemical studies will provide additional information of the precise nature of the tubular epithelium, most probably representing a metaplastic phenomenon.

Finally, it should be mentioned that nephrogenic metaplasia has been found in the bladder of one patient with vesical adenocarcinoma of the mesonephric or clear cell type (refer to discussion of clear cell carcinoma). The relationship of nephrogenic metaplasia to adenocarcinoma of this type within the urinary bladder is currently unknown.

Inflammatory Disorders

The high frequency of inflammatory disorders of the urinary bladder encountered by urologists is not experienced by the surgical pathologist. The relative infrequency of biopsy confirmation of the clinical impression obtained at cystoscopy accounts for this discrepancy. The vast majority of acute and chronic cystitis cases are caused by coliform bacteria, and are treated successfully after culture and sensitivity procedures identify the specific bacterial offender.

Under circumstances of recurrent cystitis that is refractory to standard antibiotic treatment, or when cystoscopic findings are not typical, biopsy may be performed. Bladder biopsies also may be taken under other specific clinical circumstances.

The causes of cystitis are numerous and include bacterial, viral, fungal, and protozoan agents. Gram-negative organisms, especially *E. coli,* are the most frequent offenders. Less commonly, mixed gram-negative and gram-positive organisms are encountered. Specific gas-forming gram-negative organisms are associated with emphysematous cystitis, a unique form. Tuberculosis of the urinary bladder is now distinctly uncommon and invariably is associated with tuberculous infection of the kidneys. Schistosomiasis is distinctly rare in the United States, contrasting with the high frequency of its occurrence in the Middle East. Papilloma virus infection of the bladder urothelium in the form of condyloma acuminatum is distinctly rare throughout the world. It is invariably associated with similar lesions of the urethra and perineum. Among nonbiologic agents implicated in occasional cases of cystitis are physical trauma (instrumentation, catheterization), radiation, and chemotherapeutic agents. Bladder calculi frequently have associated bacterial contamination of vesical urine with resultant cystitis. Finally, a number of histologically distinctive forms of cystitis are of unknown etiology: interstitial cystitis, eosinophilic cystitis, malakoplakia, eosinophilic granuloma, and plasma cell granuloma. The roles of vascular compromise, nutritional disturbances, and altered immune status in the cause and evolution of some forms of cystitis are currently being studied.

Cystitis may be classified according to cause, duration (acute or chronic), and finally according to histologic appearance. The majority of cases of both acute and chronic cystitis evidence histologic features characteristic of acute and chronic inflammatory responses, but in all other respects are nonspecific. Exceptions to this histologically nonspecific picture include cases of tuberculosis, gas-forming bacterial infections (cystitis emphysematosa), schistosomiasis, papilloma virus infections (condyloma acuminatum), eosinophilic cystitis, gangrenous cystitis, hemorrhagic cystitis, malakoplakia, plasma cell granuloma, and eosinophilic granuloma.

The forms of cystitis distinguished by clinical or pathologic features, whether or not the specific etiology is known, will be discussed separately.

Polypoid Cystitis

Polypoid cystitis is a reversible inflammatory lesion of the bladder mucosa characterized by papillary and polypoid exophytic mucosal projections, histologically associated with vascular congestion, stromal edema, and an inflammatory cell infiltrate involving the lamina propria cores of the excrescences (Figs. 4-11 and 4-12).[180,183-185] When these mucosal elevations are broad-based, wider than they are tall, they are described as *bullous cystitis.*[182] The basic histologic features of the lamina propria are qualitatively identical, and differ only in the apparent greater stromal edema present in bullous cystitis than in polypoid cystitis.

Most cases are associated with indwelling catheters, which explains this lesion's predilection for the posterior wall and dome of the bladder.[181,183,184] Ekelund and associates observed spontaneous disappearance of the majority of these polyps within 10 weeks of removal of the inciting catheter.[184] Some polyps

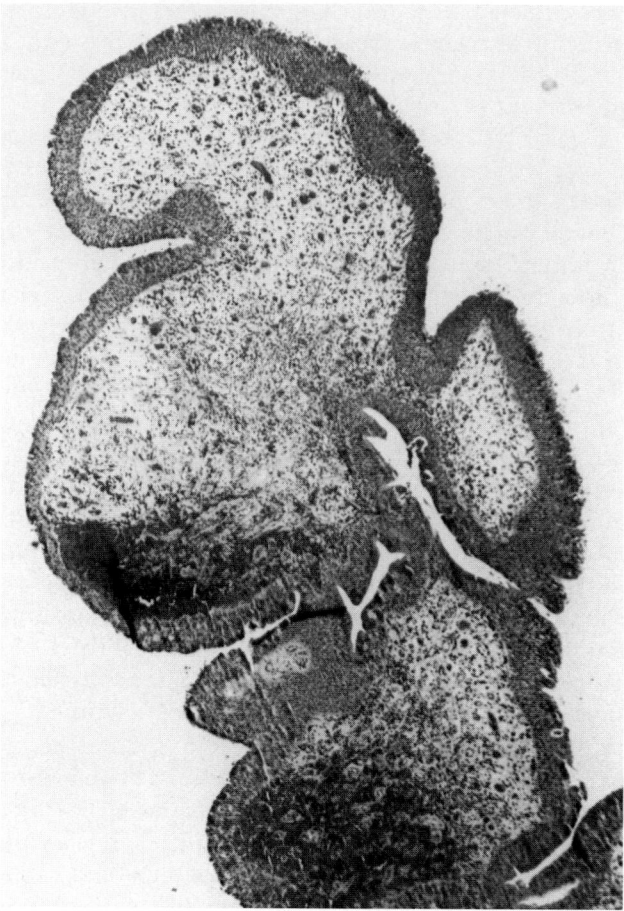

Figure 4-11   *Polypoid cystitis. The polypoid structure is lined by a focally hyperplastic urothelial surface devoid of dysplastic changes. The underlying lamina propria has a chronic inflammatory cell infiltrate of variable density in the background of marked stromal edema.*

were observed to persist for longer periods of time. Under such circumstances, microscopic examination disclosed pronounced stromal fibrosis. The histologic picture resembles that described under the entity *fibrous polyps* as seen in the ureter, urethra, and less commonly in the urinary bladder (refer to Chaps. 3 and 5). The deposition of collagen within the stalk of these polypoid lesions transforms an initially reversible lesion of the mucosa into a permanent lesion.

Although these lesions are clearly related to indwelling catheters in a causal manner, and are familiar to urologists as catheter cystitis, the infrequency with which biopsies are done may contribute to lack of familiarity on the part of surgical pathologists. These inflammatory polyps must not be misinterpreted as papillary neoplasms.[185] Several features allow differentiation from papillomas and papillary carcinomas. The urothelium of inflammatory polyps shows focal ulceration, microabscesses, focal atrophy, and occasionally marked hyperplasia. A tangential cut of these mucosal excrescences can markedly exaggerate the apparent extent of the urothelial hyperplasia. There is no cytologic atypia, surface

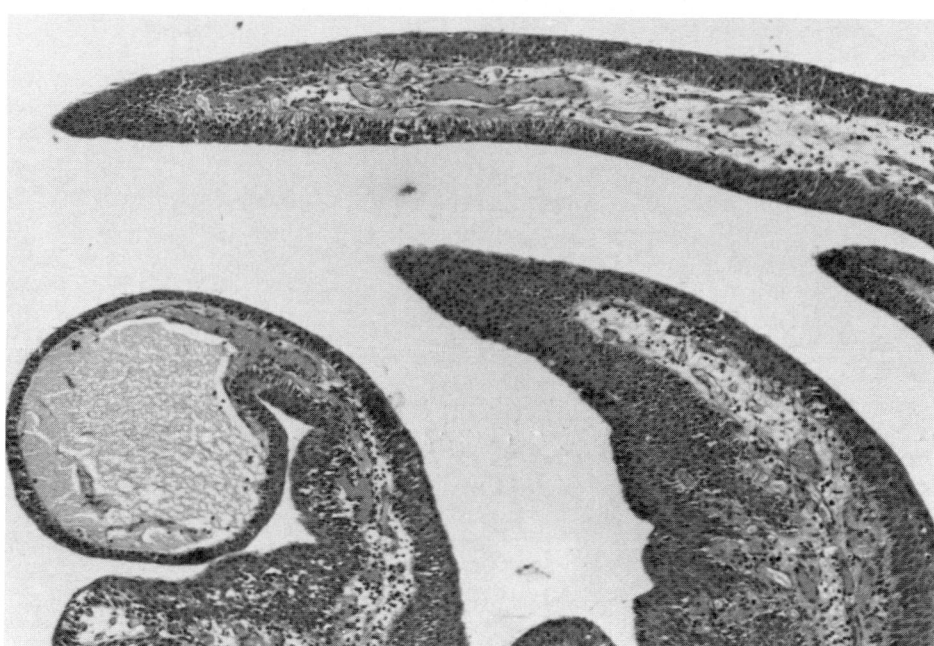

Figure 4-12   *Polypoid cystitis. The urothelium shows focal hyperplasia and papillary folds, some of which are tapered. Stromal edema is present in the fibrovascular cores producing the bulbous enlargement of the papillary structure* (lower left).

umbrella cells are retained, and the number of cell layers is generally fewer than seven to eight cells. In contrast to neoplastic papillary structures composed principally of the proliferating urothelial cells supported by an attenuated fibrovascular stalk, the opposite is characteristic of polypoid cystitis with dominance of the edematous stromal core.

In summary, these inflammatory reactive lesions of urothelium, commonly but not invariably associated with longstanding indwelling catheters, span a morphologic spectrum as shown by the *papillary cystitis, polypoid cystitis,* and *bullous cystitis.* They are all potentially reversible, as noted previously. Fibrosis of the lamina propria stroma may result in a permanent papillary fibrous polyp. These lesions are occasionally associated with pronounced hemorrhage confined to the polyp structure, and a clinical presentation with hematuria.[181] The importance of distinguishing these lesions from neoplastic papillary lesions both at the time of cystoscopy and microscopic review cannot be understated.

Eosinophilic Cystitis

The term *eosinophilic cystitis* accurately describes the predominant cell in the inflammatory infiltrate of this enigmatic form of cystitis. The lesion was independently described in 1960 by Brown and Palubinskas.[186,187] In subsequent years, approximately 50 cases have been reported in the literature.[188-195] The cause or causes are unknown. Patients frequently, but not invariably, have clinical evidence of allergic diatheses involving the lungs or gastrointestinal tract.[187] A peripheral eosinophilia may accompany this bladder lesion. Eosinophilic cys-

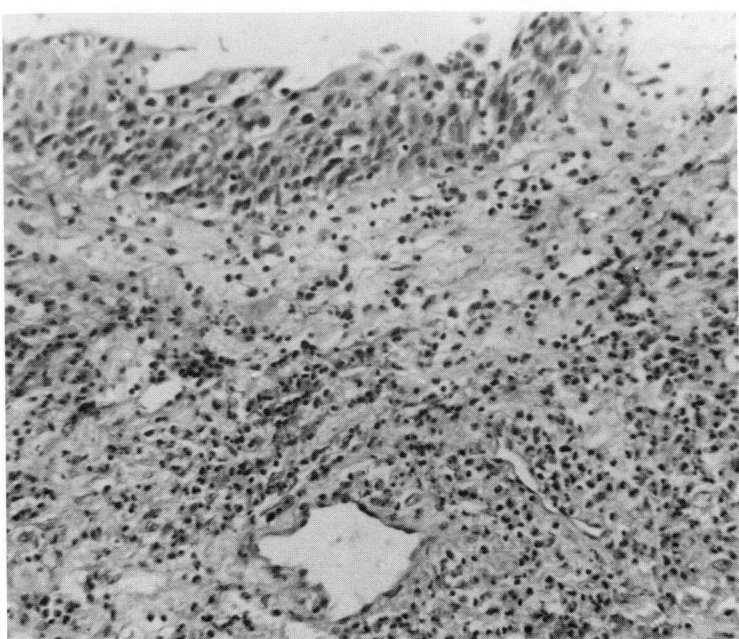

Figure 4-13   *Eosinophilic cystitis. The lamina propria and bladder mucosal cells contain a dense infiltrate composed almost exclusively of eosinophils.*

titis is regarded as an allergic reaction involving the bladder mucosa based on the cumulative evidence of sterile urine cultures, prominence of eosinophils, and response to antihistaminic and steroid therapy in some patients.[189,190] Alternatively, the identical lesion can be observed in elderly male patients with bladder outlet obstruction, frequently with history of previous surgical therapy.[194] The disease is most common in middle-aged adults, but has been observed in a 5-day-old infant and a 75-year-old man.[191,193] Patients present with dysuria, frequency, and less commonly hematuria. The bladder appears inflamed at cystoscopy but has no features specific for this form of cystitis. The disease characteristically has frequent exacerbations.[189]

Microscopically, the lamina propria shows a dense infiltrate of eosinophils with variable associated stromal edema (Fig. 4-13). The infiltrate may involve all layers of the bladder wall, including the muscularis, but is typically most pronounced in the lamina propria. Associated intramural fibrosis may be extensive.[194] Focal mucosal ulceration is common. The biopsy features reflect the clinical picture, with fewer eosinophils, stromal edema, and greater numbers of lymphocytes present as the recurrence subsides. The diagnosis requires close correlation of clinical and pathologic features.

Chronic Interstitial Cystitis (Hunner's Ulcer)

Chronic interstitial cystitis is an inflammatory disorder of unknown etiology of the urinary bladder. It was first described by Hunner.[196] The classic Hunner ulcer is commonly present in longstanding cases, but it is not invariable, and is not required for the diagnosis.[199] Some investigators propose that the diagnosis should be based on the combination of characteristic clinical features supported with cystoscopy and biopsy findings consistent with the diagnosis of chronic interstitial cystitis.[199]

The typical case involves a middle-aged adult woman, but the lesion has been observed in adult men, and uncommonly, even in children.[197] The most common symptoms are suprapubic pain, frequency, urgency, and nocturia, with or without hematuria. All are constant, and are commonly of several months' duration.[197,199] Bladder capacity is commonly, but not invariably, decreased, as determined by cystoscopy under anesthesia. At cystoscopy mucosal edema, focal petechia or irregular hemorrhagic stains, and the characteristic but inconstant ulcers are observed. These lesions are most prevalent in the dome, posterior wall, and lateral wall, and only rarely are present in the trigone region. The negative urine cultures are both characteristic and confounding when considering the underlying cause.[198,199] Cultures may be positive for coliform bacteria, but this is regarded as a superimposed infection.[197] Various forms of therapy have been employed in interstitial cystitis, but none has been entirely satisfactory. The chronicity of the disorder is typical.

Pathologic Features

The specificity of the microscopic features of chronic interstitial cystitis, as claimed by Smith and Dehner, has been questioned more recently by Messing and Stamey.[197,199] The mucosa may be entirely normal or show nonspecific proliferative variants such as Brunn's nests, cystitis cystica and so forth. As noted previously, ulcers may be absent, especially in early cases.[197] When present they are nonspecific with typical acute inflammatory reactive changes in the ulcer crater. The mere presence of urothelial ulcers does not by itself justify the diagnosis of chronic interstitial cystitis (Hunner's ulcer). The predominant findings in the lamina propria are vascular dilatation, marked stromal edema, and a

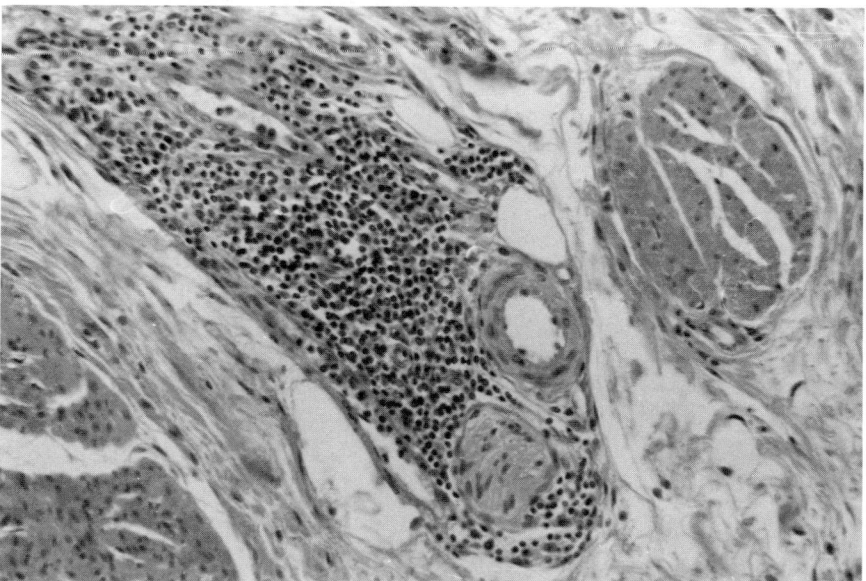

Figure 4-14   *Interstitial cystitis. The inflammatory infiltration of lymphocytes, plasma cells, and occasional neutrophils is present deep in the muscularis of the bladder. The overlying mucosa (not shown) was extensively ulcerated.*

variably dense chronic inflammatory cell infiltrate. These changes are most marked in the superficial lamina propria. The cell infiltrate is composed primarily of lymphocytes and plasma cells, with fewer neutrophils and inconstant eosinophils and histiocytes (Fig. 4-14). In addition, mast cells may be observed, but the constancy of this finding is unsettled.[197,199] The muscularis layer shows interstitial edema, chronic inflammatory cell infiltrate, and commonly fibrosis. Smith and Dehner observed a tendency for perineural infiltration by lymphocytes, but this was not observed by Messing and Stamey.[197,199] In sum, although the aggregate of histologic features in all layers of the bladder wall as described previously constitute the findings in recorded cases, these are nonspecific when viewed individually, and the diagnosis should be rendered only when combined with all available clinical and cystoscopic information. As the absence of ulcers should not militate against the diagnosis, so too should it be realized that the amalgam of microscopic features described previously can be observed in occasional cases of severe cystitis of bacterial origin in patients devoid of any of the clinical features of chronic interstitial cystitis. Thus, the etiology, pathogenesis, and effective therapy of this ill-defined disorder remain unknown.

Gangrenous Cystitis

Gangrenous cystitis is a serious and extensive form that is currently uncommon. However, one gains the impression that it was more frequent in the past.[200–202] In 1934, Stirling and Hopkins reviewed 207 cases reported in the literature.[200]

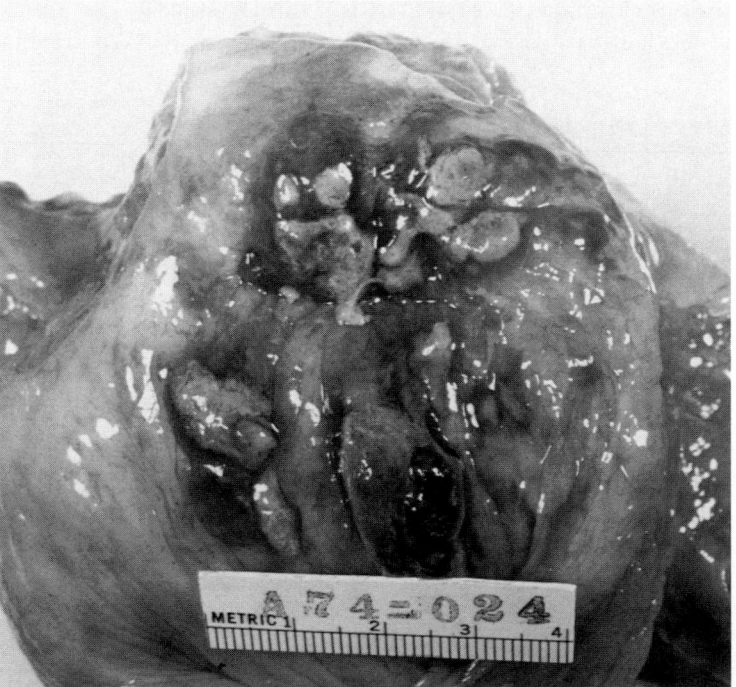

Figure 4-15   *Gangrenous cystitis. The bladder mucosa is covered, and in many sites is replaced by, adherent inflammatory exudate.*

Underlying contributory factors among these cases included extrinsic pressure (such as pregnant uterus), complications of labor, chronic cystitis, urethral obstruction, and systemic infections, in order of decreasing frequency.[200,201] Sixty percent of these patients died of the bladder disorder.[200] The cystoscopic appearance prompted numerous descriptive names, including exfoliative cystitis, membranous cystitis, and diphtheritic cystitis, among others enumerated by Cristol and Greene.[201]

Currently, this form of cystitis is most typically encountered in debilitated, elderly patients, frequently with the background of compromised circulation and with systemic infection.[202] Any or all of these factors may accompany a urinary tract infection that ultimately develops into a diffuse gangrenous cystitis. No specific pathogen has been identified as preponderantly responsible for this serious disorder.[202] Most probably, the ischemia of variable severity or duration combines with other pathogenetic factors noted previously to produce gangrenous cystitis.

Characteristically, all or virtually all of the bladder urothelium is necrotic and ulcerated, and in association with blood clot and acute inflammatory exudate, forms a membranous cast of the bladder lumen (Figs. 4-15 and 4-16). The depth of necrosis of the bladder wall is variable, but not uncommonly extends

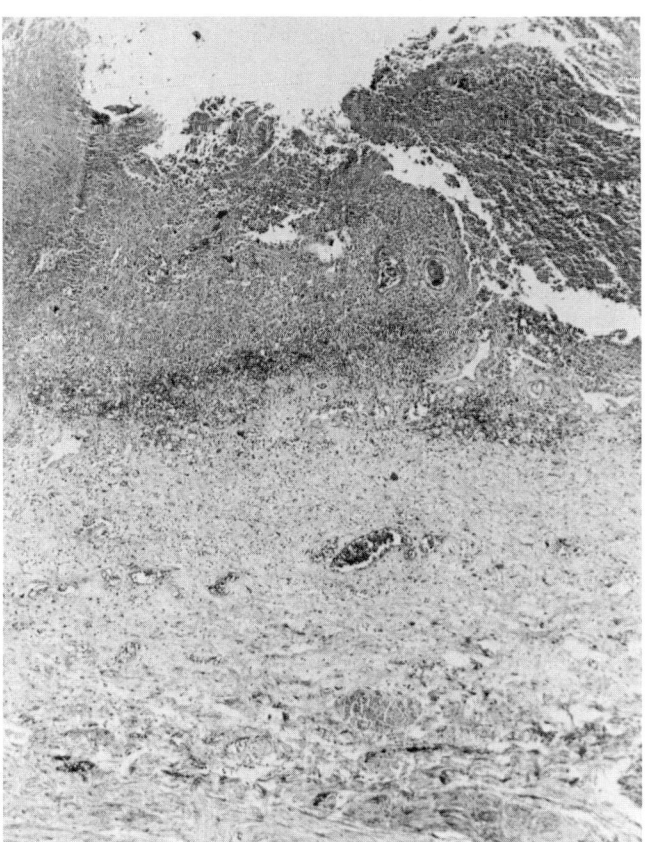

Figure 4-16   *Gangrenous cystitis. The mucosal destruction is accompanied by a dense infiltrate of acute inflammatory cells with fibrin deposition in the superficial lamina propria.*

into the muscularis. The histologic features are those of extensive necrosis, acute inflammation, and ulceration. The features are most intensive in the superficial portions of the bladder wall, but focal extension involves the muscularis, as noted previously. Necrosis of blood vessels results in intramural and intraluminal hemorrhage.

Follicular Cystitis

The diagnosis of follicular cystitis rests on the microscopic identification of lymphoid follicles with germinal centers located in the lamina propria of the bladder (Fig. 4-17).[203-206] In 1970, Sarma wrote, "Cystitis follicularis is a condition of indefinite etiology and obscure pathogenesis. Diagnosis is histologic, treatment is empirical, and prognosis is speculative."[206] A decade and a half later, nothing more can be added to Sarma's summary. Attempts to associate follicular cystitis with specific etiologic agents have failed, and the characteristic histologic features have been observed in bladder biopsies in the absence of any evidence of urinary tract infection.[206] Thus, the term *follicular cystitis* is a misnomer, because it is not equatable to an inflammatory lesion.[206] Similar lymphoid aggregates are observed in the upper urinary tract, also in the absence of clinical or other pathologic evidence of infection. (These lymphoid aggregates are reported to have a characteristic cystoscopic appearance.[203])

Emphysematous Cystitis

Emphysematous cystitis is a rare inflammatory disorder characterized by the intramural accumulation of gas produced by bacteria, most commonly *E. coli* and *A. aerogenes*.[208,209] Numerous other bacterial organisms, including *C. perfringens,* are responsible less frequently.[209,210] The gas-forming organisms produce mucosal blebs with characteristic radiologic and cystoscopic appearance.[207,210]

Affected patients are most frequently elderly, debilitated, and commonly diabetic.[208-210] Less frequently, clinical disorders of vesical diverticula, traumatic bladder injury, various vesical fistulae, bladder outlet obstruction, and sepsis are recorded.[208-210]

The essential pathologic features are numerous gas-filled intramural cysts apparent on the mucosal surface. Microscopically, the surrounding lamina propria is compressed by the expanding gas-filled cyst, which appears as a hole in the section. Occasionally, inflammatory cells, including multinucleated giant cells, are present in the adjacent stroma (Figs. 4-18 and 4-19).

Therapy consists of appropriate antibiotic administration following microbiologic identification of the offending organism.

Eosinophilic Granuloma

Eosinophilic granuloma is an uncommon disorder occurring either as a multicentric or unicentric lesion most frequently involving bones or lung. The precise nature of eosinophilic granuloma is uncertain, and the cause is unknown. Histor-

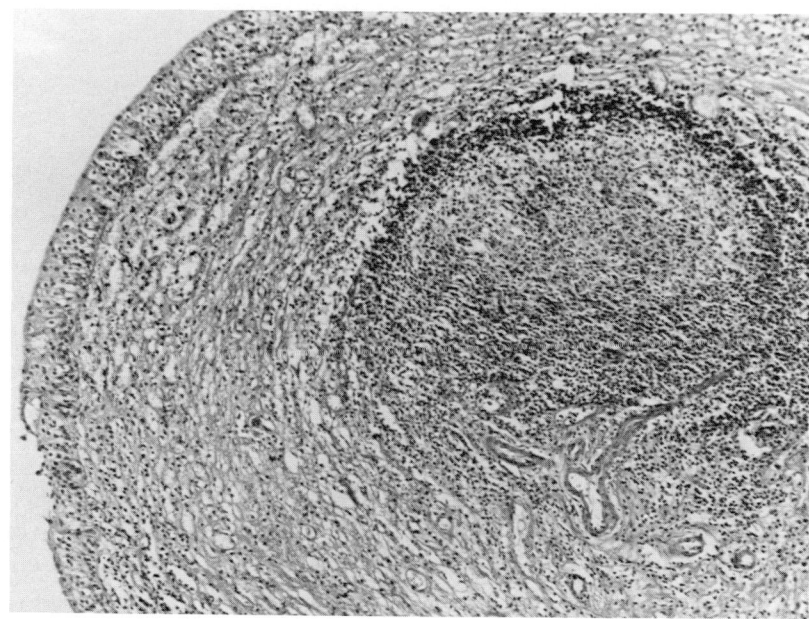

Figure 4-17 *Follicular cystitis. The intact urothelium overlies a lamina propria containing a lymphoid aggregate with a germinal center. Scattered lymphocytes are present throughout the lamina propria.*

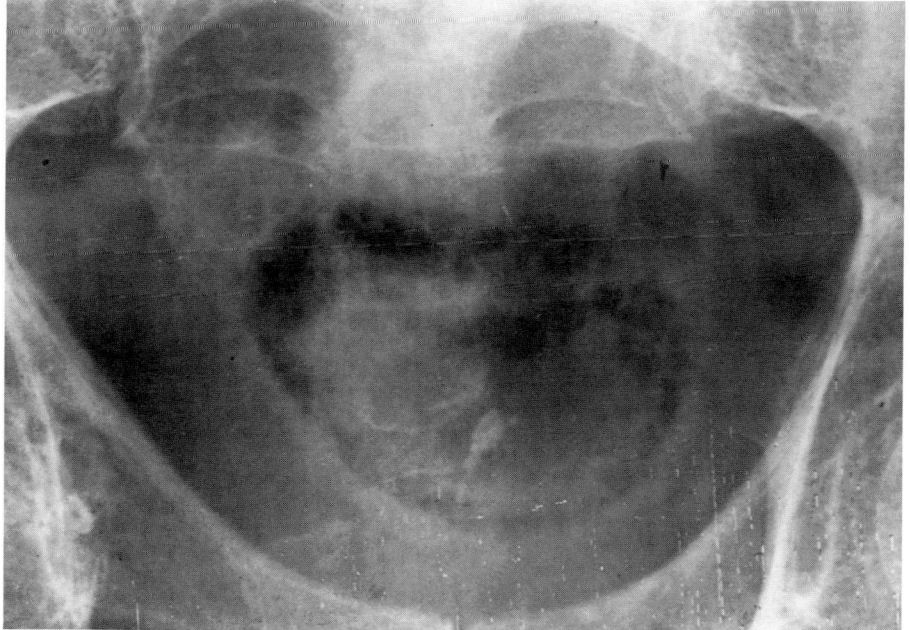

Figure 4-18 *Emphysematous cystitis. Air is present throughout the wall of the bladder in this preliminary film of the pelvis. The identified organism was* E. coli.

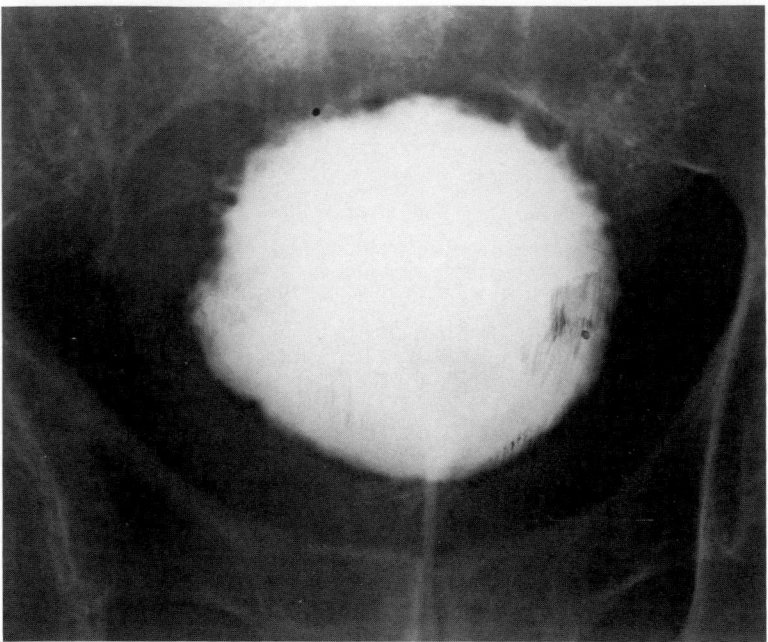

Figure 4-19   *Emphysematous cystitis. The emphysematous, air-filled mucosal folds are well outlined following injection of contrast medium.*

ically, eosinophilic granuloma has been included with Hand – Schüller – Christian disease and Letterer – Siwe disease, which are collectively called histiocytosis – X diseases.[211,212,214] The lesions of these disorders are characterized by dense collections of histiocytes and fewer lymphocytes and plasma cells.[211,214] The histologic features of eosinophilic granuloma are further characterized by an admixture of numerous eosinophils. Unicentric eosinophilic granuloma offers the best prognosis. Examples of apparent spontaneous resolution of lung lesions have been reported, suggesting a reactive non-neoplastic disorder.[212,214] A single case of eosinophilic granuloma involving the urinary bladder was found in the literature.[213] This lesion has not been reported in any organ of the genitourinary (GU) tract.

Plasma Cell Granuloma

Plasma cell granulomas are distinctive inflammatory lesions of unknown etiology, most commonly reported in the lung.[215–217] The characteristic histologic feature of this lesion is the mixed cell infiltrate composed predominantly of mature plasma cells with fewer histiocytes and lymphocytes.[216,217] Fibrous tissue, within and surrounding the inflammatory cell infiltrate, is variable. The lesions, both those occurring more commonly in the lung, and demonstrated by the one case reported arising in the bladder, can attain large size. The one example recorded in the urinary bladder involved a 47-year-old man who presented with gross hematuria.[217] A 9-cm mass removed at surgery demonstrated all the histologic hallmarks of plasma cell granuloma. The non-neoplastic nature of the lesion was further demonstrated by its substance, supported by the polyclonal results demonstrated with immunoperoxidase stains for IgA, IgG, and IgM immunoglobulins, all of which were positive.[217] This single case of vesical plasma cell granuloma accompanies only two other reports of this lesion in the urinary tract, both involving the renal pelvis (refer to discussion of plasma cell granuloma in Chap. 2).

Malakoplakia

Malakoplakia is an inflammatory disorder of unknown cause. It was described originally in the urinary tract, but in recent years, it has been reported in a wide variety of non-GU sites.[222,224,231] The inflammatory lesions are characterized by a predominance of histiocytes, the so-called von Hansemann cells, with the diagnostic intracytoplasmic inclusions, Michaelis–Gutmann bodies.

This histiologically distinct inflammatory lesion is commonly associated with urinary tract infections of *E. coli* bacteria. A direct causal relationship between these bacteria and malakoplakia is doubted, primarily because of the high frequency of urinary tract infections caused by these bacteria, and the rarity of the lesions of malakoplakia.

The urinary bladder is the single most common site of occurrence of this enigmatic inflammatory disorder in the urinary tract, with approximately half of all reported cases occurring in this organ (Table 4-4). One hundred and forty cases could be found in the literature beginning with the first description by Michaelis and Gutmann in 1902.[218] Melicow collected 65 reported cases, and Smith collected 110 cases from the literature.[219,221] Cases reported after Smith's review in 1965 bring the total to 140.[220,222,224,232]

Malakoplakia is found in all age groups, from infants to the tenth decade, with the peak frequency occurring in the fifth to seventh decades.[221] There is a marked female preponderance among all cases, regardless of the site of occurrence. A clinical background of intercurrent disease including immunosuppression, chronic infectious disorders, or malignancy is not uncommon.[231] When this disorder involves the urinary bladder, the presenting symptoms are nonspecific (frequency, dysuria, and hematuria), suggesting cystitis. At cystoscopy, the

Table 4-4   ***Malakoplakia of Genitourinary Organs***

Organ Site	No. of Reported Cases (%)*
Kidney	53 (18%)
Renal pelvis	13 (4%)
Ureter	14 (5%)
Urinary bladder	140 (49%)
Urethra	3 (1%)
Testis	30 (10%)
Epididymis	12 (4%)
Prostate	21 (7%)
Total	286

* Multiple organ involvement is common among reported cases of malakoplakia.

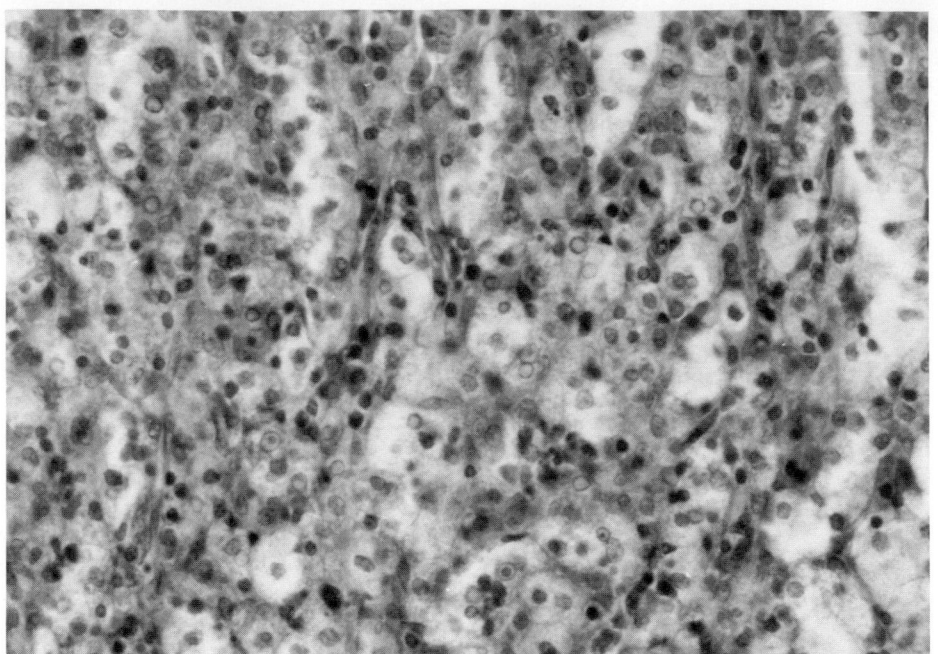

Figure 4-20   **Malakoplakia.** *Numerous Michaelis–Gutmann bodies are seen as well-defined spherical structures, some of which have a central inclusion. The background inflammatory cells are composed principally of histiocytes with fewer lymphocytes.*

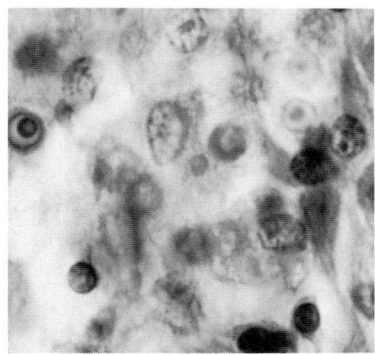

A

B

Figure 4-21   **Malakoplakia.** *(A) Michaelis–Gutmann bodies are seen at high magnification following staining with PAS stain. (B) Michaelis–Gutmann bodies are identified by von Kossa's stain.*

typical lesions are yellow-tan plaques, or nodules, a few millimeters to 2.5 cm in diameter.[221,222,230] They are frequently multiple. Some reported examples have central umbilication.[221,222] Less commonly, they have superficial ulcers.[221,222,230] There is no site of predilection within the bladder.[221,222] The diagnosis requires microscopic examination of biopsy specimens.

Pathologic Features

The histologic features of malakoplakia are temporally related to the stage of lesion production, as originally fully described by Smith.[221] Three phases were identified: the early (prediagnostic) phase; the classic phase; and the final fibrosing phase. The early or prediagnostic phase is characterized by stromal edema and a plasma cell and lymphocyte infiltrate that is gradually replaced by a predominance of histiocytes. This histologic picture emerges to the classic lesion of malakoplakia typified by the numerous large histiocytes (von Hansemann cells) with fewer lymphocytes and plasma cells. Numerous intracellular and extracellular Michaelis–Gutmann bodies (MG) are identified, allowing the specific diagnosis of malakoplakia (Fig. 4-20). The Michaelis–Gutmann bodies stain positively with PAS, Prussian blue, and von Kossa's stains (Fig. 4-21). Variable staining results are obtained with oil red–0.[221,222,230] The MG bodies are mucicarmine negative. X-ray diffraction studies identify calcium phosphate within the MG bodies.[223] Ultrastructural studies disclose characteristic concentric crystalline laminations, with a dense inner zone and thin outer zone (Fig. 4-22).[229,230]

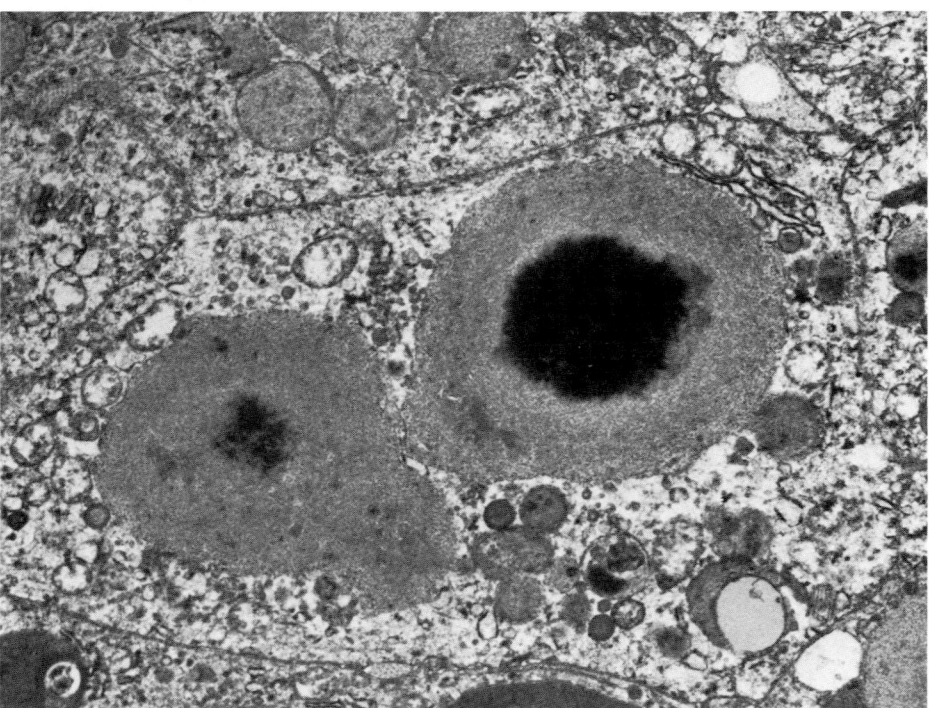

Figure 4-22   *Malakoplakia. The ultrastructural characteristics of the Michaelis–Gutmann bodies are illustrated by these two intracellular examples found within the cytoplasm of a histiocyte (original magnification ×9,280).*

The final fibrosing phase is typified by a progressive decrease in the number of inflammatory cells and a concomitant increase in fibrosis. Scattered extracellular MG bodies may be detected in the fibrous stroma, disclosing the true nature of this cicatrix.[221]

When it occurs in the urinary bladder, malakoplakia is less commonly confused with other disorders than when it involves such organs as the kidney (differentiate from xanthogranulomatous pyelonephritis) or the prostate (requiring differentiation from adenocarcinoma and granulomatous prostatitis). (Refer to discussions malakoplakia in Chaps. 1 and 8.) Rarely, malakoplakia will contain multinucleated histiocytic giant cells, suggesting granulomatous inflammation, and thus requiring differentiation from tuberculosis. Familiarity with the variable histologic phases and the wide spectrum of possible sites of occurrence will contribute to the recognition of this lesion in biopsy specimens.

Etiology and Pathogenesis

As stated at the outset, the cause of malakoplakia is currently unknown. Early investigators regarded malakoplakia as either a reflection of a neoplastic process, or an infectious disorder of tuberculous, fungal, or viral etiology.[221,231] Regarding malakoplakia as an inflammatory lesion of an infectious nature, specifically due to *E. coli,* does not explain the disparity of frequencies of *E. coli* urinary tract infections and malakoplakia. Lewin and associates have demonstrated that the strains of *E. coli* detected in patients with malakoplakia developing in the background of urinary tract infections, are not unusual, and reflect those strains cultured in the absence of malakoplakia.[224] The high frequency of depressed immune status in patients with malakoplakia has recently received attention.[225–227,232] Abdou and associates and Schreiber have detected decreased monocyte capacity to kill *E. coli* in patients with malakoplakia.[225,227] An acquired functional deficit of monocytes in malakoplakia is currently receiving the greatest attention in attempts to understand the etiology and pathogenesis of this interesting disorder. Therapeutic benefit has been reported with the use of cholinergic agents, which are known to increase intracellular cyclic GMP, which in turn stimulates microtubule formation and lysosomal activity.[225,227] The ultrastructural identification of fragments of bacteria within the histiocytes of malakoplakia lesions may reflect an acquired defect in lysosomal degradation of the bacteria.[224,229,230] Future studies should clarify the nature of the defect and possibly may elucidate the circumstances and underlying causes of malakoplakia.

Radiation Injury

Radiation injury to the urinary bladder is associated with radiation therapy of uterine, colonic, and prostatic neoplasms. The clinical presentation of an acute cystitis typically begins 4 weeks to 6 weeks following radiation therapy, but late reaction may appear months to years following cessation of radiation exposure.[234,237] As observed in association with cyclophosphamide, the injury to the bladder resulting from radiation exposure can manifest with an inflammatory component, and cytologic atypia of the urothelium. (Refer to discussion of cytology in bladder carcinoma later in the chapter.)

The histologic features of radiation cystitis are time- and dose-dependent.[233-235,237] Intravesical radiation in therapeutic doses prior to cystectomy is invariably associated with radiation-induced inflammation and necrosis, as determined by examination of the specimen following subsequent surgery. External radiation delivered to malignancies in adjacent pelvic organs is substantially less frequent.[237] Warren described an initial transient phase of hyperemia within 24 hours of radiation exposure, followed weeks later by a more pronounced reaction characterized by extensive vascular dilatation, stromal edema, and focal ulcerations.[233] The edematous lamina propria produces a nodular mucosal surface, which Koss has termed *bullous cystitis.*[236] (Refer to discussion of polypoid cystitis earlier in this chapter.)

Diagnostically challenging cytologic atypia of the urothelial mucosa is common at this time and requires a differential diagnosis including carcinoma in situ. The resemblance of such radiation atypia to carcinoma in situ is striking. Koss suggests that radiation atypia tends to disappear within 3 months, an event not expected when dealing with true carcinoma in situ of bladder urothelium.[236]

The acute changes of radiation injury described previously are followed by more permanent footprints of radiation exposure. These include scattered atypi-

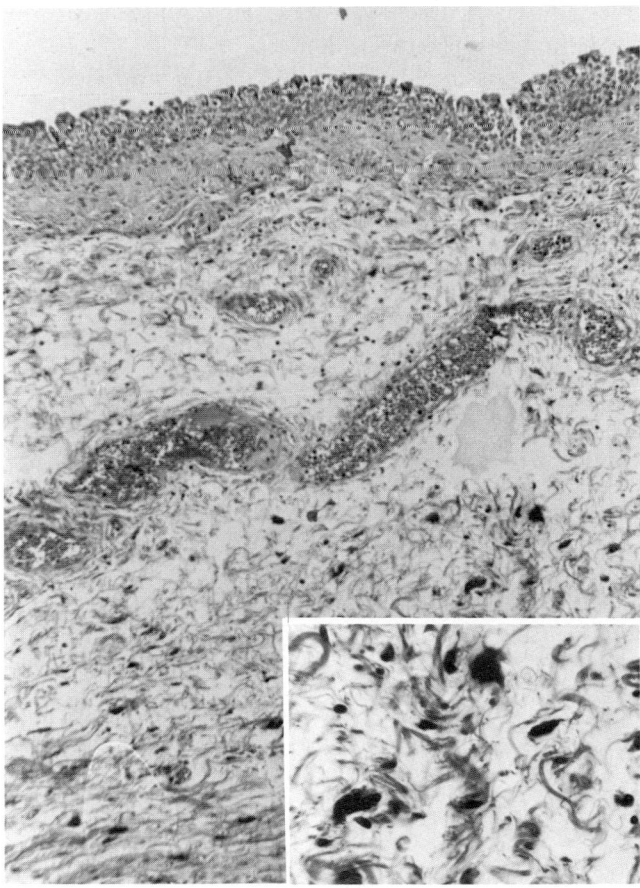

Figure 4-23   **Radiation cystitis.** *The presence of numerous enlarged, hyperchromatic fibroblasts* (inset) *with increased collagenous fibrosis in the lamina propria is characteristic of radiation injury.*

cal fibroblasts in the intramural stroma; stromal edema and variably dense fibrosis within the lamina propria and muscularis; and hyalinization of the vascular changes, including hyalinization of the media, and either intimal fibrosis or collections of foamy histiocytes in subendothelial locations (Fig. 4-23). The vascular lesions and atypical fibroblasts are reasonably specific for radiation injury and persist at the site for years. Superimposed on these features of chronic injury are mucosal ulcerations with associated necrosis, acute inflammation, hemorrhage, and fibrinous exudate on the surface.

Chemotherapy-Induced Hemorrhagic Cystitis

Cyclophosphamide was introduced in 1957 as an effective form of chemotherapy in certain cases of leukemia. Shortly thereafter, there were reports of hemorrhagic cystitis occurring in patients receiving this agent. Typically patients noted a sudden onset of dysuria and hematuria. On occasion, the hematuria was reported to be massive and intractable.[239,242] Repeated confirmation of this complication of cyclophosphamide therapy was reported from multiple medical centers.[241,242] Lawrence and associates reported an observed frequency of 8% among 314 patients receiving the drug.[242] The occurrence of hemorrhagic cystitis appears to be independent of the administered dose.[240,242]

Studies of the possible mechanism of tissue injury were reported by Philips and associates. They observed bladder lesions after instilling urine from dogs receiving the drug into the bladders of recipient dogs.[238] The direct instillation of

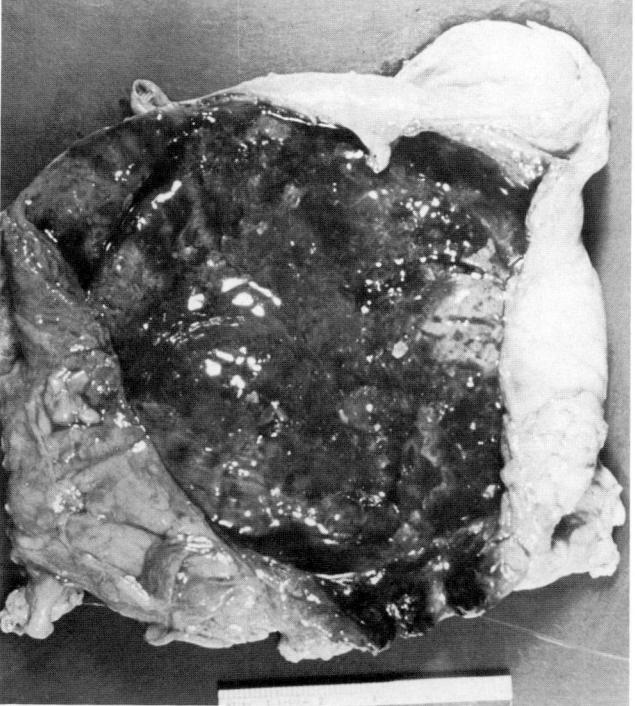

Figure 4-24   *Hemorrhagic cystitis. The bladder mucosa is intact but reflects diffuse hemorrhage throughout the lamina propria.*

cyclophosphamide into the bladder urine of recipient dogs failed to produce mucosal lesions. These findings suggested that the observed mucosal lesions in patients experiencing cyclophosphamide-induced hemorrhagic cystitis resulted from metabolic breakdown products of the chemotherapeutic agent excreted in the glomerular filtrate.[238]

The histologic changes observed in cases of hemorrhagic cystitis related to cyclophosphamide-induced severe edema and hemorrhage within the lamina propria associated with mucosal ulcerations (Figs. 4-24 and 4-25).

In 1964, Forni and associates reported a related but independent lesion, namely, a reversible cytologic atypia, of the bladder mucosal cells in such patients.[240] These findings have been confirmed.[245] Cyclophosphamide-induced changes of urothelial cytologic features include marked but variable cell enlargement involving both nucleus and cytoplasm; nuclear hyperchromaticity and irregularity of outline; even distribution of coarse chromatin; and cytoplasmic vacuolization.[240,248] The degree of cytologic atypia showed no relationship to the dose of drug received.[240] These cytologic changes tended to revert to normal or disappear totally within weeks of cessation of the drug.[240] However, of greater concern are the occasional reports of patients developing transitional cell carcinoma subsequent to cyclophosphamide therapy (refer to discussion of carcinoma of the bladder in this chapter).

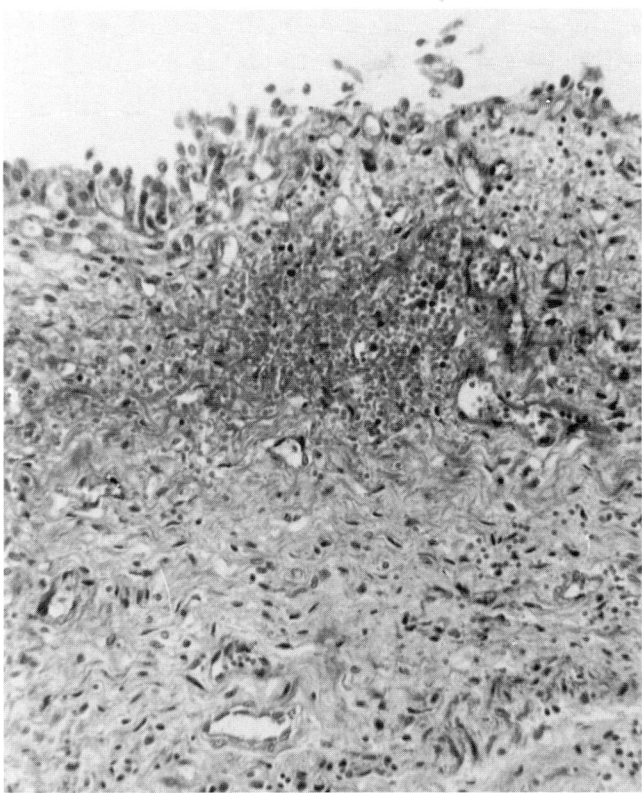

Figure 4-25   *Hemorrhagic cystitis. Dilated and congested vessels with extensive extravasation of red blood cells within the lamina propria are the prominent features. The urothelium shows focal ulceration and extensive sloughing.*

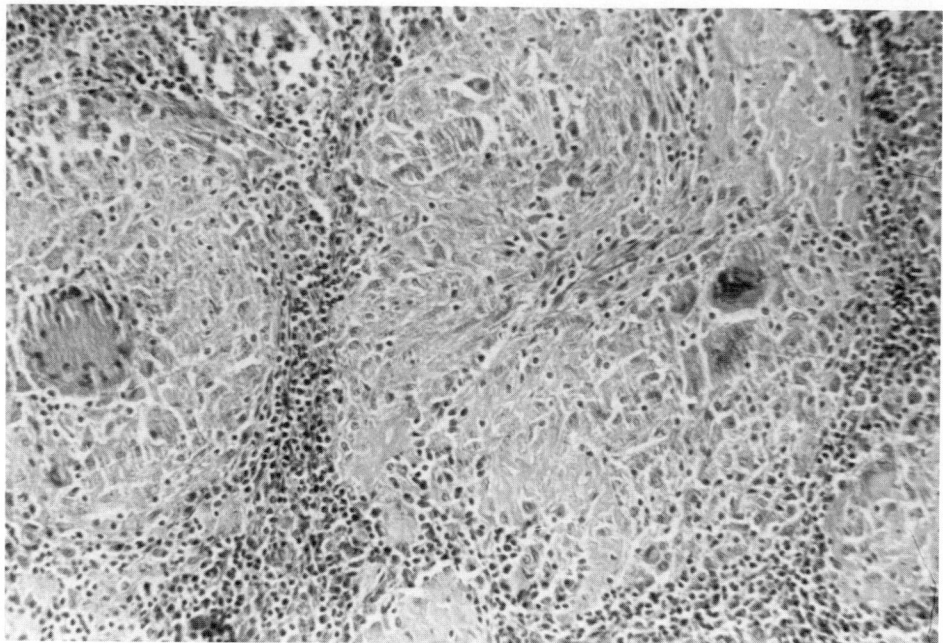

Figure 4-26   *Tuberculosis. Two adjacent granulomas with central necrosis and giant cells are present. Acid-fast organisms were present in appropriately stained sections. Numerous lymphocytes and histiocytes surround the granulomas.*

Significantly less frequent is the association of hemorrhagic cystitis with busulfan therapy, first reported in 1978.[243,246] Only two such patients could be found in the literature.[243,246]

Tuberculosis

Coincident with the overall decrease in frequency of tuberculosis in the United States, tuberculous infection of the urinary tract including the urinary bladder is now rarely encountered. When encountered, it is invariably located in the trigone region as a result of downstream infection from an infected kidney. The microscopic features of a vesical tuberculous lesion are identical with the classic caseating granulomas associated with tuberculosis wherever encountered (Fig. 4-26). Definitive diagnosis requires demonstration of the organisms in biopsies by appropriate special stains or culture techniques. Dissemination of the tubercle bacilli to organs of the male genital tract is not uncommon in cases of established vesical tuberculosis. (Refer to Chaps. 6 to 8.)

Schistosomal Cystitis

Inflammation of the urinary bladder in schistosomiasis is most frequently due to *S. haematobium* with fewer cases caused by *S. mansoni*.[247,251] The disease is endemic in the Middle East and North Africa, with only rare cases encountered in

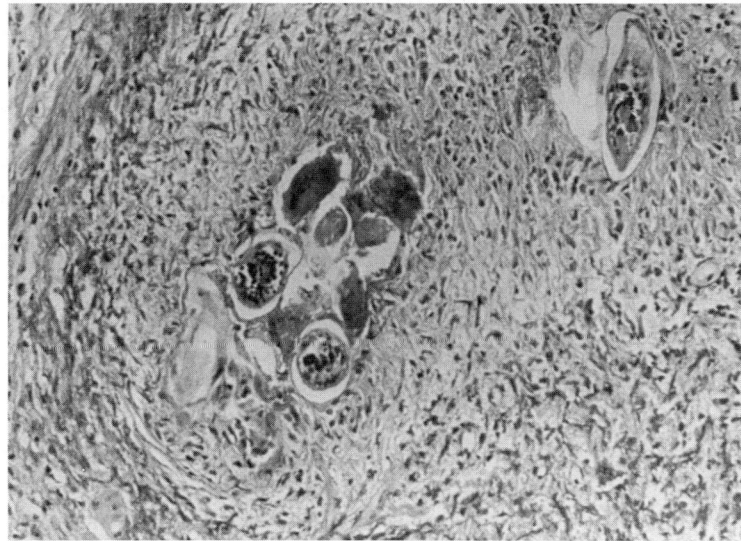

Figure 4-27   *Schistosomiasis. The ova of the schistosome organisms are surrounded by reactive fibrosis and chronic inflammatory cells.*

the United States. I have two cases in my files; both patients were immigrants from the Middle East.

Patients are infected by the cercariae penetrating the skin subsequent to their release from the intermediate host, snails.[252] The cercariae enter the venous system, and mature into adults after passing through the lungs. The adults pass by means of the vasculature to the bladder wall, where eggs are deposited in perivascular locations of the lamina propria and muscularis. The intense inflammatory response results in mucosal ulceration with release of the eggs into the urine.

The acute inflammatory reaction progresses to chronic inflammation characterized by abundant neutrophils, eosinophils, lymphocytes, and foreign body-type histiocytic multinucleated giant cells. In time, abundant fibrosis accompanies the entrapped ova, commonly with associated dystrophic calcification (Fig. 4-27). The latter feature serves as a diagnostic radiologic finding of vesical and ureteral schistosomiasis. The chronicity of the inflammatory response is commonly associated with mucosal changes, including polypoid cystitis and hyperplasia, and with metaplastic changes, including squamous metaplasia and cystitis glandularis.[248] Patients with longstanding schistosomal infection of the urinary bladder are at significantly greater risk of carcinoma.[249,250] Vesical carcinomas associated with schistosomiasis are most frequently of the squamous variety, with fewer cases of transitional cell carcinoma, adenocarcinoma, and verrucous carcinoma observed.[249,250] (Refer to discussion of squamous cell carcinoma.)

Condyloma Acuminatum

Condyloma acuminatum of the urinary bladder is distinctly rare. The first cases were reported independently by Kleiman and Lancaster and by Lewis and associates.[253,254] Subsequently reported cases bring the total to nine, including six women and three men (Table 4-5). Patients range in age from 34 years to 76 years. Concurrent involvement of the urethra was observed in seven patients, and a cystostomy stroma in one patient. With the exception of one patient, all the women had involvement of the vulva or vagina in association with the bladder lesion. The bladder involvement typically occurred months to years after the initial diagnosis. Multiple recurrences of perineal or urethral condylomatous lesions occurred frequently. Six of the nine patients ultimately required cystectomy after reported failures with more conservative therapy, including podophyllin, fluorouracil, transurethral resection, or fulguration. Conservative surgical procedures proved successful in three patients, all of whom had small lesions involving the bladder.

The gross and microscopic features of vesical condyloma are identical to the lesions in more common locations (*i.e.,* penis, perineum, and urethra; refer to Chaps. 5 and 9). The large size of some of the bladder lesions (refer to Table 4-5) is somewhat unusual. Such lesions, whether arising in the bladder or in the penis, require differentiation from verrucous carcinoma, a neoplasm that only rarely occurs in the bladder. (Refer to discussions of verrucous carcinoma in this chapter and in Chap. 9.)

Amyloidosis

Amyloid deposits within the wall of the urinary bladder are rare. Their principal significance is their ability clinically and cystoscopically to mimic malignancy, and their capacity to cause gross life-threatening hematuria. Most cases of vesical amyloidosis are of the localized type, with fewer cases of the secondary variety (Table 4-6).

Clinically significant amyloid deposits have been reported in 58 patients (Table 4-6). Vesical deposits of this substance were diagnosed at autopsy in two additional patients.[273] In 1961, Kinzel and associates reported five cases and extensively reviewed the previously reported 16 cases.[263] An additional 37 cases were found in the literature, virtually all in the form of case studies (Table 4-6).[264-291]

Amyloidosis involving the urinary bladder affects men and women equally,

Author(s)	Year	Age	Sex	Bladder Location	Other Sites
Kleiman, Lancaster[253]*	1962	NI	M	Entire bladder	Cystostomy stoma
Lewis et al[254]	1962	34	F	Multifocal	Urethra
Lewis et al[254]	1962	34	F	R wall of bladder	Vagina
Hotchkiss, Rouse[255]	1968	41	F	Entire bladder	Vagina, vulva, urethra, ureters
Bissada et al[256]	1974	31	M	"Extensive"	Penis, urethra
Petterssen et al[257]	1976	53	F	Trigone	Vulva, urethra
Petterssen et al[257]	1976	36	F	Trigone	Vulva, urethra
Masse et al[258]	1981	76	M	Anterior wall	None
Keating et al[259]	1985	56	F	Entire bladder	Vulva, vagina, urethra, distal ureters†

Table 4-5   *Condyloma Acuminatum*

* An additional case was brought to authors' attention and briefly discussed by Kleiman and Lancaster.[253]

† Histologic evidence of associated carcinoma in situ involving vulva noted.

most commonly in the fifth to seventh decades (72% of reported cases) (Table 4-6). The youngest reported case was a 28-year-old woman and the oldest was an 80-year-old woman.[275,281] Gross hematuria is the most frequent clinical presentation (88% of cases), but occasional patients experience dysuria as the prominent symptom. Among the 58 reported cases of vesical amyloidosis, six patients had established diagnoses of rheumatoid arthritis, Crohn's disease, or familial Mediterranean fever.[271,273,275,277,284] These six cases are examples of secondary amyloidosis with bladder involvement, in contrast to the other 52 cases, which all were of the localized type. Radiologic findings are not diagnostic. Similar to occasional cases of amyloid deposition in the renal pelvis, rare cases of vesical amyloid will show calcifications within the affected area of the bladder wall.[263,284,285] There is no site of predilection within the bladder, and several cases have demonstrated multifocal areas of amyloid deposition. The cystoscopic appearance is likewise nonspecific with impressions ranging from carcinoma to cystitis with ulceration. Massive hemorrhage has been described in rare cases.[284] The magnitude and persistence of the bleeding has required surgical resection of the lesions by transurethral resection, fulguration, and partial or complete resection of the bladder, depending on the extent of bladder involvement (Table 4-6). The correct preoperative diagnosis has been made only in scattered reported cases (Table 4-6).

The gross lesions vary in size, configuration, and number. Single plaques, nodules, or masses, frequently with surface ulceration, are encountered. The diagnosis requires the microscopic detection of the characteristic amorphous eosinophilic interstitial deposits of amyloid fibrils. These deposits are most abundant within the lamina propria, but commonly are also present within the muscularis. Deposition within the vascular walls may be observed. The surrounding interstitium contains variable numbers of chronic inflammatory cells, including plasma cells, and acute inflammatory cells in association with the secondary mucosal ulcerations. Confirmation of the amyloid nature of the deposits is achieved by special staining with crystal violet, Congo red, and thioflavine-T. Each one possesses shortcomings of sensitivity or specificity, but when they are used in concert, they give reliable results.[286,289] Ultrastructural studies will disclose the diagnostic β-pleated fibrils typical of amyloid.[279,286]

Subsequent to conservative surgical therapy, approximately 20% of the reported patients experienced recurrent episodes of hematuria (Table 4-6). The true frequency of recurrent hematuria because of vesical amyloidosis is not known because approximately half of the patients reported without recurrence had follow-up durations less than 2 years when their case studies were published. Among those patients who evidenced recurrent episodes of hematuria, 50% did so 2 years or longer after the original surgical therapy.

Understanding of the diverse chemical nature of amyloid proteins has advanced significantly in the last decade.[288] However, the underlying cause of amyloid deposition involving the urinary bladder remains unknown.

Endometriosis

The urinary bladder is the most common site of endometriosis of the urinary tract. Fewer cases are reported involving the ureter, kidney, and urethra, in order of decreasing frequency (refer to corresponding chapters). Vesical endometriosis was first described by Judd.[292] Nixon found 35 reported cases, and Abeshouse

(Text continues on p. 324.)

Table 4-6   *Amyloidosis*

Author(s)	Year	Sex	Age	Presentation
Houtappel, Lauwers[260]	1960	F	60	Gross hematuria
Werner[261]	1961	F	61	Gross hematuria
Nagel[262]	1961	F	67	Gross hematuria
Kinzel et al[263]	1961	M	48	Gross hematuria
Kinzel et al[263]	1961	M	36	Gross hematuria
Kinzel et al[263]	1961	M	43	Gross hematuria
Kinzel et al[263]	1961	M	48	Gross hematuria
Kinzel et al[263]	1961	M	48	Gross hematuria
Nagel[264]	1962	M	73	Gross hematuria
Grace, Walton[265]	1964	F	58	Gross hematuria
Grace, Walton[265]	1964	M	56	Gross hematuria
Krzeski[266]	1964	F	37	Renal colic
Hudson, Tingley[267]	1965	F	59	Gross hematuria
Narwani, Lingard[268]	1966	M	31	Gross hematuria
Sinkevichis, Lyutkus[269]	1966	M	39	Gross hematuria
Lerut, Lerut[270]	1967	F	67	Gross hematuria
Bender, Kelly[271]	1969	M	40	Gross hematuria
Tripathi, Desautels[272]	1969	M	41	Gross hematuria
Tripathi, Desautels[272]	1969	M	42	Gross hematuria
Gerami et al[274]	1970	M	60	Gross hematuria
Missen, Tribe[273]	1970	M	41	Gross hematuria
Missen, Tribe[273]	1970	F	54	Gross hematuria
Malek et al[275]	1971	F	80	Gross hematuria
Malek et al[275]	1971	M	40	Gross hematuria
Malek et al[275]	1971	F	50	Dysuria
Malek et al[275]	1971	F	40	Gross hematuria
Bergqvist, Westermark[276]	1971	F	70	Gross hematuria
Montie, Stewart[277]	1973	M	39	Micro hematuria
Strong et al[278]	1974	M	32	Gross hematuria
Hofer et al[279]	1974	F	53	Gross hematuria
Au, Gilbaugh[280]	1975	F	77	Gross hematuria
Robertson et al[281]	1975	F	28	Dysuria
Blath, Bucy[282]	1976	F	70	Dysuria, hematuria
Blath, Bucy[282]	1976	F	71	Dysuria, hematuria
Thomas et al[285]	1977	F	64	Gross hematuria
Ambrovici et al[284]	1977	F	46	Gross hematuria
Akhtar et al[286]	1978	F	54	Gross hematuria
Kampehl et al[287]	1979	M	63	Gross hematuria
Caldamone et al[289]	1980	M	46	Gross hematuria
Caldamone et al[289]	1980	M	49	UTL, lithiasis
Nakajima et al[290]	1980	M	65	Gross hematuria
Mead et al[291]	1982	M	61	Polyuria, nocturia
Mead et al[291]	1982	M	66	Hematuria, dysuria

Preoperative Diagnosis	Treatment	Follow up
Carcinoma	Partial cystectomy	NI
Carcinoma	Biopsy	1 Recurrence — 4 yr
Carcinoma	Biopsy	1 Recurrence — 4 yr
Benign tumor	Partial cystectomy	2 Recurrences — 6, 8 yr
Carcinoma	Complete cystectomy	No recurrence — 24 yr
Amyloidosis	Partial cystectomy	No recurrence — 24 yr
Amyloidosis	TUR	No recurrence — 19 yr
Amyloidosis	TUR	No recurrence — 7 yr
Carcinoma	TUR	1 Recurrence — 4 yr
Cystitis	TUR	NI
Granular excrescence	Biopsy	D/8 yrs; no recurrence
Cystitis glandularis	Fulguration	No recurrence — 4 mo
Carcinoma	Complete cystectomy	D/2 yr; unrelated causes
Carcinoma	TUR; fulguration	Multi recurrences — 5 yr
Carcinoma	Partial cystectomy	No recurrence — 2 mo
Tumor	TUR; fulguration	No recurrence — 11 mo
Cystitis	TUR; fulguration	No recurrence — 10 mo
NI	TUR; fulguration	No recurrence — 15 yr
Carcinoma	TUR; fulguration	Occasional hematuria — 10 yr
NI	Partial cystectomy	No recurrence
Petechial hemorrhage	None	D/6 mo (recur. hematuria)
Gangrenous cystitis	None	D/5 day (recur. hematuria)
Amyloidosis	TUR	D/1 yr (heart disease)
Carcinoma	TUR	No recurrence — 7 yr
TB	TUR	No recurrence — 8 yr
Ulcerative cystitis	TUR	D/2 yr (multi recurrences)
Carcinoma	Subtotal cystectomy	No recurrence — duration NI
NI	Biopsy	D — Crohn's disease
Nonspecific ulcer	Partial cystectomy	No recurrence 16 mo later
NI	TUR	Recurrent hematuria
Inflammatory tumor	TUR	No recurrence, 3 mo
Carcinoma	TUR/partial cystectomy	Recurrent hematuria
NI	TUR	No recurrence, 6 mo
Chronic cystitis	Reimplantation of uterers	No recurrence, 6 mo
NI	Ureteral resection, reimplantation	D — recurrent hematuria, 15 yr
Hemorrhagic cystitis	Partial cystectomy, cystectomy	D/5 mo
NI	Partial cystectomy	Recurrences, multiple
NI	Cystectomy	Recurrences, multiple
Probable carcinoma	TUR	Recurrence, 7 mo
NI	Biopsy	Lost to follow up
NI	TUR	No recurrence, 8 mo
NI	Reimplantation of ureters	No recurrence, 6 mo
Vascular tumor	Partial cystectomy	No recurrence, 6 mo

TUR, transuretheral resection; UTI, urinary tract infection; NI, no information.

and Abeshouse accumulated 127 in the literature.[294-301] Fein and Horton found an additional 23 reported cases, but did not include 19 cases reported by Stanley and co-workers.[302-306] Twenty-five cases were found in the literature since 1966, bringing the total to approximately 200.[307-317]

The reported patients range in age from the second decade to the fifth decade, with the peak frequency observed in the fourth decade.[306] Endometriosis has been observed in only two postmenopausal women, each of whom were

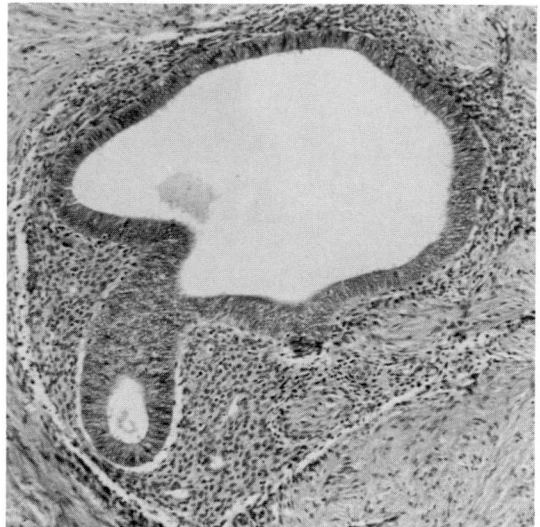

A

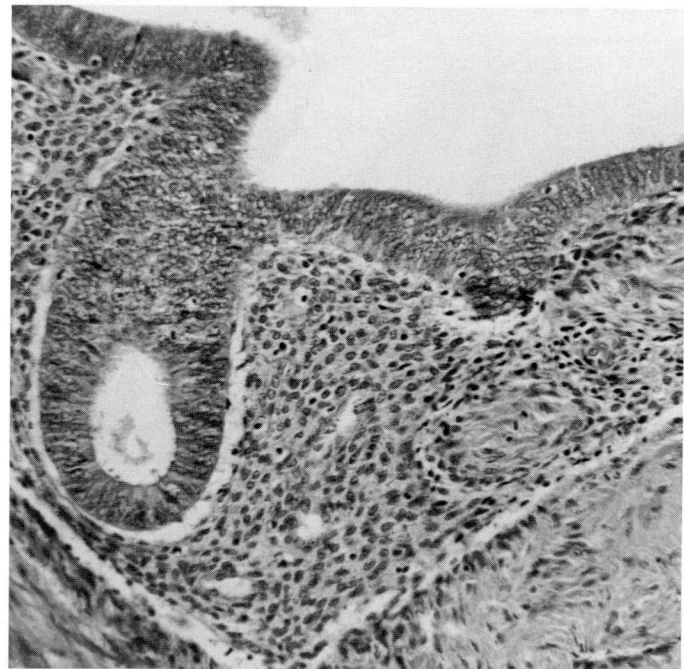

B

Figure 4-28   *Endometriosis of the urinary bladder.* (A) *Endometrial glandular epithelium with associated endometrial stromal cells within the vesical muscularis layer are diagnostic.* (B) *The endometrial gland epithelium is surrounded by typical endometrial stromal cells.*

receiving exogenous estrogen at the time of diagnosis.[309,310] Vesical endometriosis has occurred in three men, all of whom were receiving exogenous estrogen for therapy of prostatic carcinoma.[308,314,315]

Patients most commonly present with pelvic pain or pressure, associated with frequency and urgency.[306] Hematuria is reported in about one fourth of the patients.[306] A suprapubic mass is palpable in about half of the patients.[306] Approximately 60% of the patients have a history of pelvic surgery, including hysterectomies, cesarean sections, and other procedures capable of disseminating fragments of endometrium.[306,316,317] This historical information strongly suggests an implantation pathogenesis in such cases.[293,311] The pathogenesis of endometriosis in the absence of prior surgery has remained unsettled for almost a century.[306,317] Embryonal nests and Müllerian metaplasia have been suggested in addition to the implantation theory.[306,317]

The appearance of vesical endometriosis at cystoscopy is highly suggestive only when the endometriotic lesion is located in the lamina propria. Lesions deep in the muscle or subserosa may not be apparent or suggest extrinsic compression. Bladder biopsies at the time of cystoscopy have correspondingly been less than uniformly successful in detecting the lesion.[306,307] Radiologic evaluation of such lesions includes cystograms, echography, and computed tomographic (CT) scan, which can disclose intramural lesions and allow a presumptive diagnosis of endometriosis. Therapy has included partial cystectomy for large lesions with more recent hormonal therapy providing regression of the lesions.[301,306,310,313,317]

The pathologic features reflect the hormonal responsiveness of the endometrial tissue in the extrauterine site. Evidence of recent and old hemorrhage within the tissue is a characteristic feature. With minimal past hemorrhage the lesions are well defined, a feature obscured when the hemorrhage has infiltrated adjacent bladder wall stroma beyond the endometrial tissue. Endometrial glands and investing stroma, both with histologic evidence of past hemorrhage, are characteristic (Fig. 4-28). To date, no reported cases of vesical endometriosis have been associated with malignant change.

Neoplastic Disorders

The urinary bladder is the site of origin of both epithelial and mesenchymal neoplasms of either benign or malignant nature. Benign epithelial neoplasms, and all mesenchymal neoplasms, are uncommon to rare. Epithelial neoplasms constitute greater than 98% of all primary tumors, virtually all represented by transitional cell carcinoma. The metaplastic potential of urothelium contributes a mechanism for epithelial neoplasms other than transitional cell malignancies. A working classification of vesical epithelial malignancies is as follows:

Transitional cell carcinoma

Squamous cell carcinoma

   Verrucous carcinoma

Adenocarcinoma

   Mucinous carcinoma

   Signet-ring cell carcinoma

   Clear cell carcinoma

Carcinoma with mixed differentiation

Carcinoid

Small cell undifferentiated carcinoma

Malignant melanoma

The term *transitional cell carcinoma in situ* is reserved for flat urothelial cell proliferations exhibiting full-thickness dysplastic cytologic features without evidence of invasion of the underlying basement membrane. Increasing evidence implicates this flat lesion rather than the papillary form of transitional cell carcinoma as the principal origin of invasive bladder cancer.

Papillary lesions of the urinary bladder regarded as benign include transitional cell papilloma and inverted papilloma.

Inverted Papilloma

Inverted papillomas are unique and rare neoplasms of the urothelial mucosa. These typically exophytic proliferations appear grossly as bald papillomas. They are characteristically covered by histologically normal urothelium from which endophytic cords originate and grow into the subjacent lamina propria in a manner reminiscent of exaggerated Brunn's nests. The localized nature of these endophytic columns or cords of urothelium produces the cumulative effect of an exophytic mass. When arising in the urinary bladder, they are most common in the trigone region. A total of 160 examples of inverted papilloma has been reported arising in the urinary bladder, with fewer numbers reported in the ureter, renal pelvis, and urethra, in order of decreasing frequency.[318-360] (Refer to Chapters 2, 3, and 5.)

Until recently, inverted papillomas reported in the urinary tract were uniformly benign in histologic appearance and clinical behavior. In contrast, the identical lesion in the nasopharynx typically has a high frequency of recurrence, and may evidence malignant histologic features and clinical behavior.[320] As experience with urothelial inverted papillomas increases, these differences may very well disappear. Recent reports of apparent malignant change have appeared in the literature.[336,347,351,355,358,360] The true frequency of this phenomenon is currently unknown. I have observed three cases of papillary transitional cell carcinoma arising in or adjacent to a typical inverted papilloma of the urinary bladder.

The general recognition of inverted papilloma of the urinary tract is relatively recent, with approximately 90% of all reported cases appearing in the literature in the last 10 years. This lesion was originally described in the urinary bladder by Paschkis in 1927, and was "rediscovered" by Potts and Hirst in 1963, who apparently were unaware of the previous description 36 years before.[318,319] The name *inverted papilloma* was introduced by Potts and Hirst, and is accurately descriptive and generally accepted in later publications.

This neoplasm is most commonly observed in the urinary bladder (75% of reported cases), but has now been observed in the renal pelvis by Matz, the ureter by Vicini, the urethra by Trites (refer to discussions of inverted papilloma in corresponding chapters).[322,329] The distribution of 194 reported cases of inverted papillomas by site of origin is as follows:

Renal pelvis, 12 cases;

Ureter, 13 cases;

Bladder, 160 cases,

Urethra, 9 cases.

Inverted papilloma arising in the bladder most frequently occurs in men, with only 21% of the reported cases observed in women. The ages affected patients ranges from 14 years (reported by Francis) to 94 years (reported by Stein and co-workers).[349,360] The peak frequency is the sixth and seventh decades, with approximately 60% recorded between ages 50 years and 79 years. Hematuria of recent onset is the most common clinical presentation. Some examples by virtue of their location (*i.e.,* low bladder neck) have produced outlet obstruction. Dysuria and frequency have been recorded but are uncommon in patients with inverted papilloma of the bladder. Cystogram discloses an exophytic lesion, most commonly in the trigone region.[327]

At cystoscopy, inverted papillomas appear as smooth or nodular polypoid structures. They may be sessile or pedunculated with a short stalk.[319,336] Most are 1 cm to 2 cm in diameter, but examples smaller than 1 cm to 3 cm have been reported.[331,334,356] The most common location is the bladder neck, followed by other locations in the trigone area and region of the ureteral ostia.[331,336,356,359] They are uncommon elsewhere in the bladder. Only rarely are the lesions multiple. Most reported cases have been treated by transurethral resection resulting in a variably fragmented specimen submitted for histologic review.

The characteristic microscopic features of inverted papilloma include a relatively smooth surface contour covered by histologically and cytologically normal urothelium. The surface urothelium shows randomly scattered invaginations producing double cords or columns of urothelial cells of variable diameter. The basement membrane investing the endophytic cords of urothelium is continuous with that underlying the surface urothelium (Figs. 4-29 and 4-30). Bulbous enlargements of the epithelial cords commonly are observed randomly scattered along their length. These bulbous enlargements may show focal squamous metaplasia or cystic change with a lumen reminiscent of cystitis cystica. The relative proportion of stroma to epithelial component of these exophytic lesions varies from case to case and within the same lesion. Commonly the stroma is minimal, and is compressed between numerous endophytic columns of urothelial cells. The smooth contour of the individual columns, the absence of significant atypia, and the continuity of the endophytic columns with normal urothelial cells on the surface assist in distinguishing the inverted papilloma from a superficially invasive transitional cell carcinoma.

Two important variations on the above features are, in aggregate, the "classic microscopic appearance." In an excellent recent study of the histogenesis of these neoplasms, Kunze and associates illustrated examples of a glandular type of inverted papilloma.[359] These lesions were characterized by numerous structures morphologically equivalent to cystitis glandularis, rather than by endophytic solid columns or trabeculae filling the exophytic mass. On the basis of the two histologic patterns observed, Kunze and associates proposed a histogenesis in which the trabecular (column) pattern originated from the basal cell proliferation followed by neoplastic transformation. The origin of the glandular pattern was neoplastic transformation of cystitis cystica or glandularis that arise from

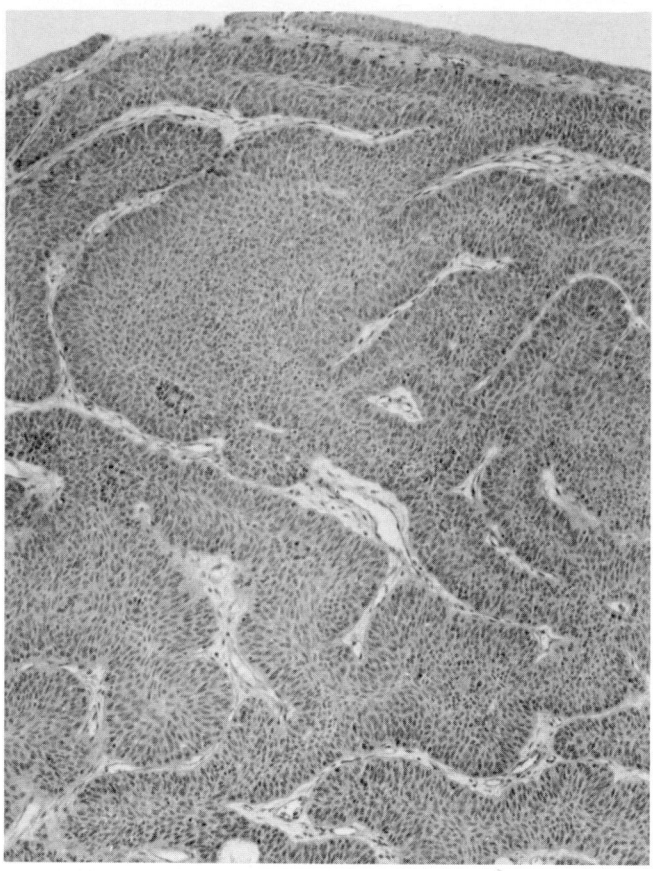

Figure 4-29   *Inverted papilloma. Interweaving cords of transitional epithelium originating from the surface mucosa dominate the exophytic bladder lesion. The surface mucosa is histologically unremarkable. The lamina propria is limited to the fibrovascular septae separating the invading cords of urothelial cells.*

Brunn's nests (refer to discussion of proliferative variants and metaplastic changes of urothelium).

The second microscopic variation from the typical features of inverted papillomas are those indicating malignancy. As mentioned previously, malignancy occurring within or associated with inverted papilloma is an observation reported only recently. To date, this has taken the form of either papillary transitional cell carcinomas separate from the inverted papilloma;[330] or papillary transitional cell carcinoma arising in, or in continuity with, an inverted papilloma.[336,347,358,360] Alternatively, Uyama and Altaffer and associates have reported inverted papillomas with frankly malignant cytologic features.[351,355] The ultimate clinical behavior of these morphologically malignant inverted papillomas is not provided in the limited follow-up details provided.

The true frequency of inverted papilloma most likely is higher than reflected in the number of reported cases. This frequency curve reflects the belated growing recognition of the entity. Inverted papillomas continue to be misinterpreted as low grade transitional cell carcinomas. The frequency of this misdiagnosis is

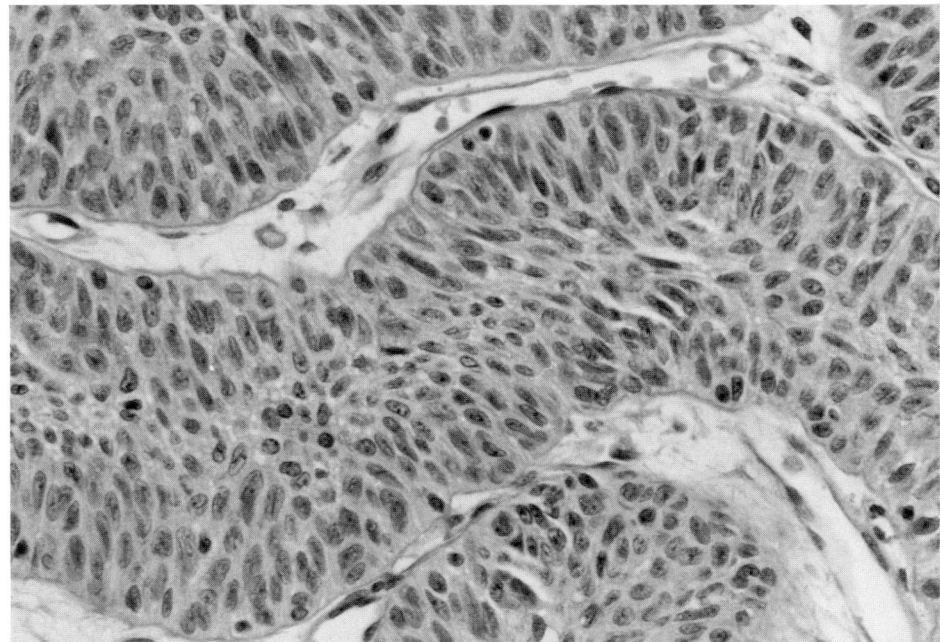

A

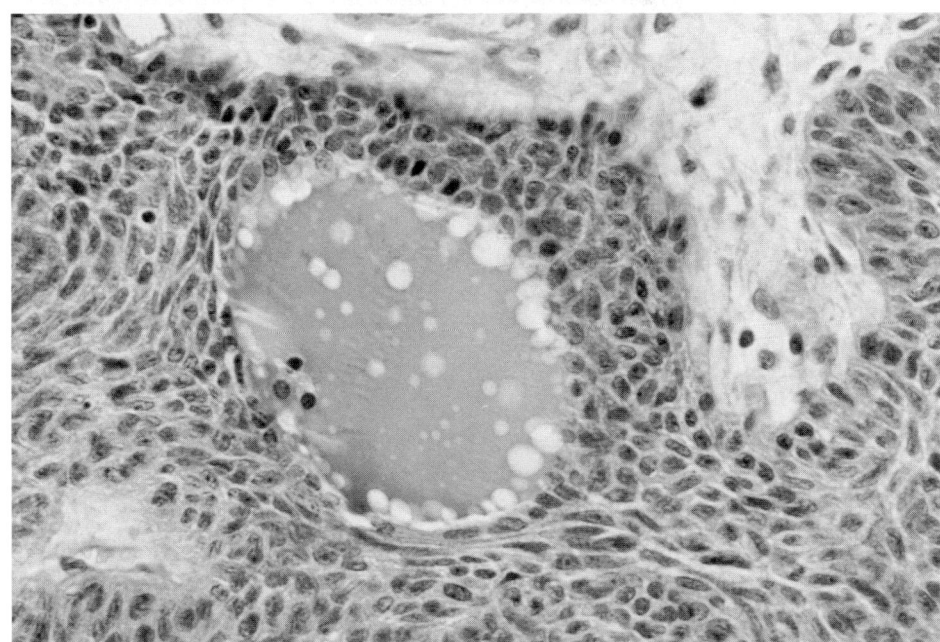

B

Figure 4-30   *Inverted papilloma.* (A) *The higher magnification of the solid epithelial cords shows the*
well-defined basement membrane separating the intervening attenuated stroma of the
lamina propria from the cords of urothelium. (B) *Randomly scattered microcystic spaces are*
commonly found in the otherwise solid cords of urothelium of inverted papillomas.

increased when inverted papillomas occur in association with a true exophytic, papillary transitional cell carcinoma. Thus, the true frequency of inverted papillomas, their association with transitional cell carcinoma, the frequency of malignant change with retention of the endophytic morphology of inverted papillomas, and the clinical behavior of morphologically malignant examples all must await future detailed studies with prolonged follow up. The repetitive reporting of these unusual vesical lesions before the patient is discharged from the hospital is pointless.

Transitional Cell Papilloma

Papillary neoplasms of the urinary bladder characterized by histologically and cytologically normal urothelial mucosal epithelium seven or fewer layers thick are termed *transitional cell papillomas* (Fig. 4-31).[363,366,367,369] Papillary neoplasms meeting these criteria are uncommon to rare, and their general acceptance as papillomas, rather than low grade transitional cell carcinomas, has occurred only in the last 15 years.[368,369] This acceptance was preceded by decades of debate about their existence and biologic behavior. This historical debate may in time prove to have been a question of minor importance in our understanding of the genesis of invasive bladder cancer. It is ironic that the general acceptance of transitional cell papillomas as a pathologic entity occurred at the same time that evidence emerged implicating the flat carcinoma in situ as the source of invasive bladder cancer, and not the papillary lesions, papillomas, or carcinomas.

The origins of the papilloma debate are historically based, and arose when diagnostic criteria for papillary transitional cell neoplasms were neither clearly outlined nor uniformly applied. Knowledge of the pathogenesis of bladder neoplasms was similarly limited, with neoplasms emerging during follow up generally regarded as recurrences, a property not typical of benign tumors. Further complicating those historical limitations were studies, the conclusions of which were based on the gross features as determined by cystoscopy.[362,364,365] Attitudes during this time ranged from denying the existence of benign papillary lesions, to accepting their reality but conceding an inability to recognize them reliably, to an

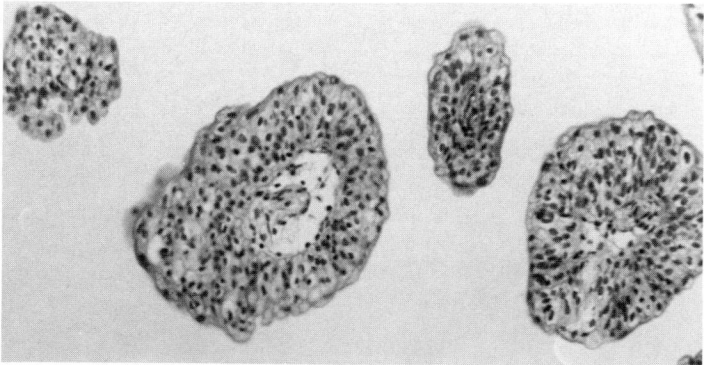

Figure 4-31   *Papilloma. The thin papillary structures have a central fibrovascular core covered by transitional epithelium with normal cytologic features. The number of cell layers is not greater than normal bladder urothelium.*

acceptance of rigidly defined papillary lesions as papillomas.[361,365] Ash clarified the use of the term *recurrence,* stating that in most instances recurrences actually represent new neoplasms developing elsewhere in the bladder.[361] This has been generally accepted and is supported by accumulated experience and the mapping studies applied to urothelial neoplasms.[369]

Among many studies of bladder papillomas, the most important are the limited number that apply the rigid criteria outlined above: Deming, Melicow, Mostofi, and Koss.[363,366,367,369] These studies describe neoplasms constituting approximately 2% to 3% of bladder tumors, most frequently occurring in males older than 50 years who present with painless hematuria.[363] The majority of cases are single lesions 2 cm to 5 cm in diameter, but multiple lesions are not uncommon.[363] Recurrence is common (approximately 70%), and ultimate development of invasive carcinoma is observed in 7%.[363] Thus, although there is no evidence that the papillomas are clinically malignant, they arise in a urothelial mucosa that is not at rest, and subsequently evolving neoplasms can be detected only by cystoscopic follow-up evaluation over prolonged periods of time. Approximately one third of patients will show no recurrence or new neoplasms following removal of the original papilloma.[363]

Transitional Cell Carcinoma in Situ

The concept of carcinoma in situ (CIS) was originally applied to the vesical urothelium by Melicow.[371] Current conventional use of this appellation is limited to full-thickness dysplastic changes present in flat, or nonpapillary, urothelium, which is historically consistent with Melicow's original description.[376,383,389] The term *carcinoma in situ* is not applied (by further convention) to noninvasive papillary transitional cell carcinoma in spite of the fact that the lesion is by definition confined to the mucosal surface.

The histologic and cytologic features of CIS have been described in numerous studies. The summarized criteria include the following.[376,384,389,392,398]

1. Urothelium of variable thickness (3 to 20 or more cell layers) with cytologic abnormalities involving the entire mucosa from basal layer to surface, including the following:
2. Nuclear enlargement, hyperchromaticity, irregular shape, and variable polarity;
3. Prominent nucleoli (variable) and coarse chromatin;
4. Occasional multinucleated cells; and
5. Variation of amount of cytoplasm, which, with the variable nuclear polarity, produces a disorganized appearance in the urothelium.

Some authors have called urothelial lesions with these features *severe atypia, atypical hyperplasia,* and *grade III dysplasia.*[384,389,398] No formal grading system has been adopted for dysplasia involving less than the full thickness of the urothelial mucosa. I have found that classifying flat urothelium into four categories is the most consistently reproducible method: normal; simple hyperplastic; dysplasia (with or without hyperplasia); and carcinoma in situ. Hyperplasia describes a urothelial mucosa that has more than seven cell layers, and is devoid of dysplastic cytologic changes (Fig. 4-32). Dysplastic lesions involving urothelium of variable thickness are characterized by surface maturation, including umbrella

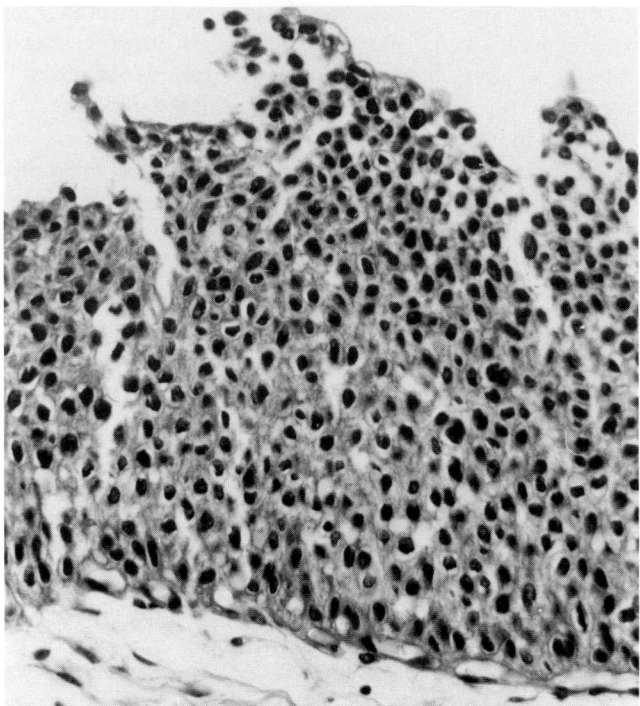

Figure 4-32   *Hyperplasia with atypia. The epithelium is significantly thickened and contains mild atypical (dysplastic) features, including focal loss of nuclear polarity and variation of nuclear size and shape.*

cells overlying the cytologically abnormal cells (Fig. 4-33). The cytologic abnormalities include nuclear enlargement, irregularity of outline, and nuclear crowding. The chromatin granularity and nucleolar prominence are less than observed in CIS lesions (Fig. 4-34).[397,398]

The original observations of CIS by Melicow occurred during a study designed to explain the tendency of urothelial neoplasms to recur following surgical therapy.[371] The finding of various proliferative changes, including those he termed carcinoma in situ, in the flat urothelium in the vicinity of exophytic papillary carcinomas suggested a possible origin for bladder carcinoma recurrence.[371] He correctly suggested that the development of new tumors originating in the flat proliferative lesions could explain the recurrences of bladder cancer.[371] The association of carcinoma in situ with clinically apparent papillary transitional cell carcinoma was studied extensively in the next two decades. CIS was found most frequently adjacent to the cystoscopically apparent papillary tumors, but could be demonstrated at sites distant from such tumors.[384,387] Mapping studies confirmed investigations employing multiple biopsies of tumor-bearing bladders and showed that the CIS lesions could be remarkably widespread.[392,395,396] The frequency of CIS was more common with high grade transitional cell carcinomas than with those of lower grades. In addition to the proposed role of CIS lesions in the development of bladder tumor recurrences proposed by Melicow, their association with papillary transitional cell carcinomas bestowed increased aggressive behavior on all respective grades of these

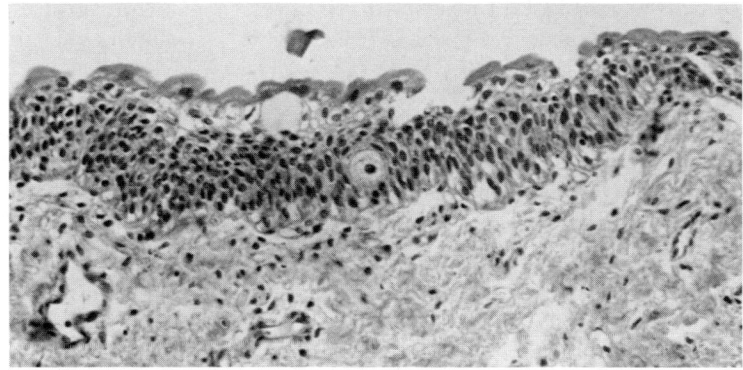

Figure 4-33   *Dysplasia of bladder urothelium. Scattered atypical nuclei with loss of polarity and variability of size and shape are present. The superficial layers, with the exception of focal interruptions, are preserved. The basement membrane is intact.*

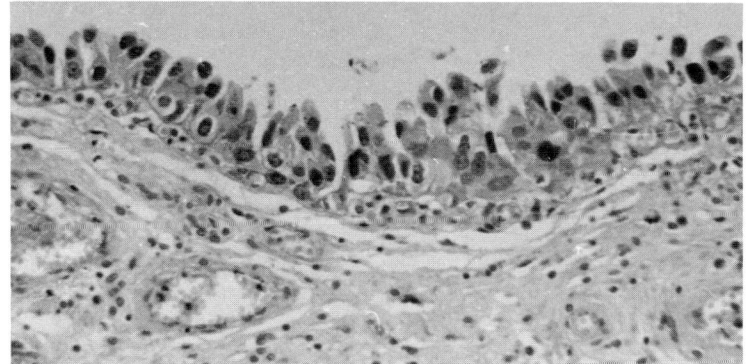

Figure 4-34   *Carcinoma-in-situ of the bladder. The atypical urothelial cells have hyperchromatic nuclei which vary in size, shape, and orientation. Focal areas with loss of intercellular cohesion are present. The basement membrane is intact.*

neoplasms.[373,390,393] Later studies demonstrated that CIS lesions could be found in 8.5% to 57% of distal ureters of cystectomy specimens.[377,379,380,387,392] Similar studies observed CIS in 12% to 62% of urethral segments included in cystectomy specimens.[387,391,392,394] Extension into, or multifocal involvement of, distal prostatic ducts by CIS in patients with bladder cancer treated by radical cystectomy was reported.[372,386,388,392,399] In all extravesical sites, the frequency of concomitant involvement by CIS was correlated with the extent of CIS within the bladder. Advocacy of urethrectomy at the time of cystectomy for bladder cancer is based on observed invasive recurrences developing in retained urethras previously determined to harbor CIS.[374,375,391]

The previously cited studies demonstrated directly and indirectly the potential role of CIS as a source of clinically significant, invasive carcinoma. Beginning in 1964 with a study reported by Melamed, respect for carcinoma in situ took a quantum leap.[376] Melamed demonstrated that vesical carcinoma in situ occurring alone was associated with the subsequent development of invasive bladder carcinoma in 32% of a series of 25 cases.[376] Multiple studies confirmed these findings, frequently reporting even higher frequencies of subsequent invasive carcinoma (50% to 83%).[378,381,385]

Typically, the patient with CIS of the urinary bladder occurring in the absence of a cystoscopically apparent tumor, was a man over 50 years of age (80% of cases), presenting with dysuria, frequency, and urgency of variable duration.[376,378,381,382,392,393] Seventy percent of such patients showed multifocal CIS.[378] The development of invasive carcinoma occurred within 3 years of the diagnosis of CIS in the majority of reported patients.[376,381] Because transitional cell carcinoma in situ has cytologic abnormalities similar to high grade papillary transitional cell carcinoma, and has a tendency of decreased intercellular cohesion with shedding of cells, its detection by urine cytology has been repeatedly demonstrated (Figs. 4-35 to 4-37).[380,382,392]

Thus, in the 30 years since the original description of vesical CIS by Melicow, we have progressed from the speculated role of this lesion in the development of new tumors (recurrences) to its demonstrated role in the genesis of invasive bladder cancer, and recognition of its role in invasive urethral and intraprostatic recurrences. This concern is appropriately applied to the evaluation of frozen ureteral resection margins at the time of cystectomy for bladder carcinoma. The extent of vesical CIS in the spatial association of hyperplasia, dysplasia, and carcinoma in situ has been demonstrated repeatedly in mapping studies of renal pelvic, ureteral, and vesical invasive transitional cell carcinomas.[396,395] (Refer to Chaps. 2 and 3.) The role of carcinoma in situ in the genesis of the majority of invasive bladder carcinomas is yet to be clarified. Two separate histogenetic routes potentially lead to invasive carcinoma of the bladder: (1) invasion following multiple recurrences of low grade noninvasive papillary transitional cell

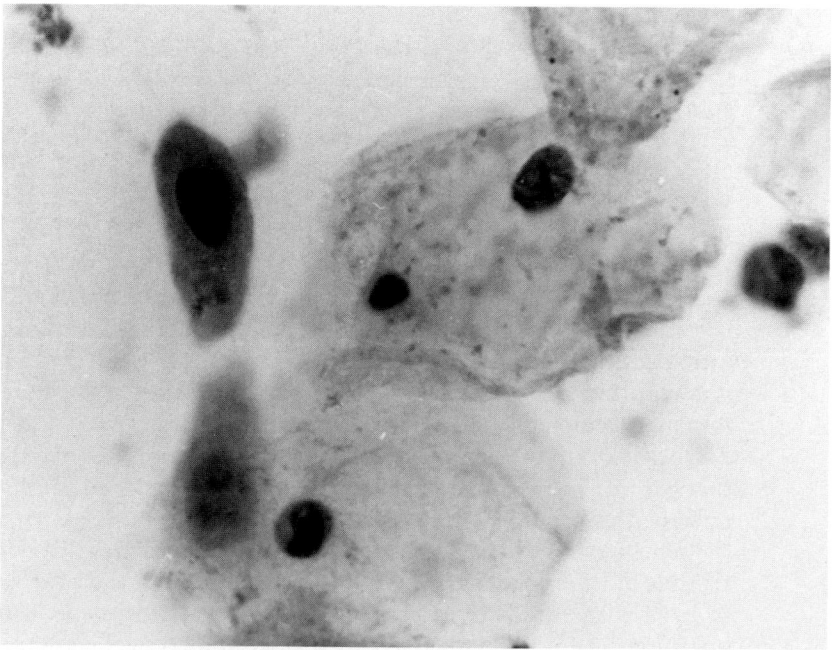

Figure 4-35   *Urine cytology. Normal urothelial cells and squamous cells are present.*

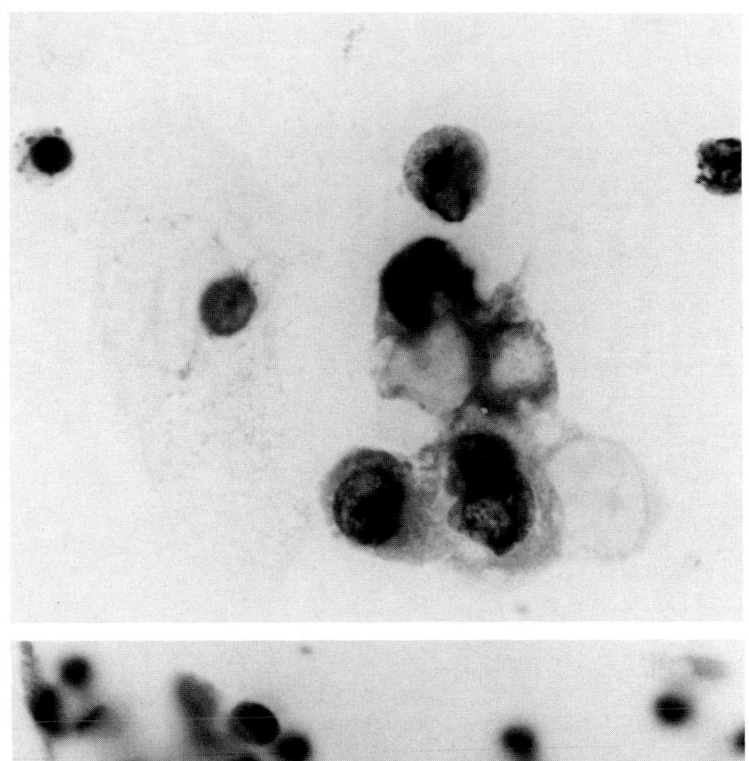

A

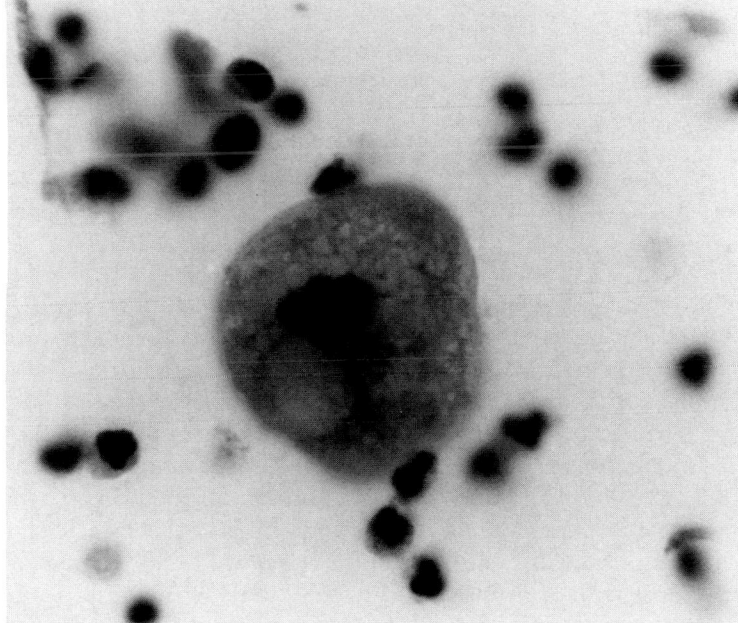

B

Figure 4-36 ***Urine cytology.*** (A, B) *Exfoliated urothelial cells demonstrating cytologic features of chemotherapy effect.*

carcinoma; or (2) invasion without a history of preceding noninvasive neoplasms (which is the more common route). The past preoccupation with the clinically apparent exophytic papillary neoplasms may prove to be a major error in identifying the enemy, if the aggressive clinical behavior of invasive bladder carcinoma originates in flat carcinoma in situ. (Refer to discussion of natural history of transitional cell carcinoma.)

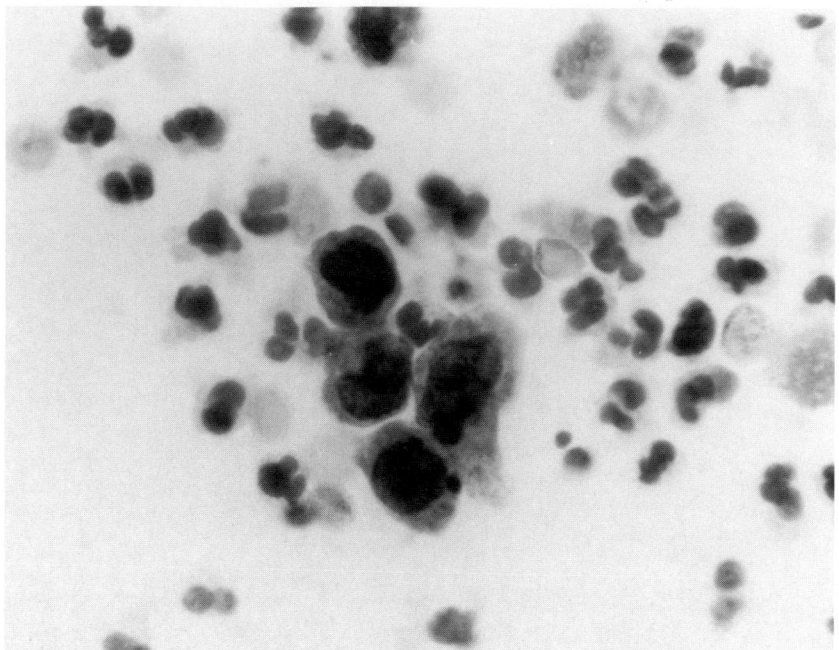

Figure 4-37   *Urine cytology. Urothelial cells with irregular, hyperchromatic enlarged nuclei from a vesical transitional cell carcinoma, grade III (carcinoma in-situ).*

Transitional Cell Carcinoma

Epidemiology and Etiology

The incidence of bladder carcinoma shows significant geographic and racial differences throughout the world. The highest frequencies are recorded in the United States and Western Europe, with low frequencies observed in Japan and among blacks in the United States.[422]

The age and sex distribution of patients with bladder cancer is presented in Table 4-7. Males consistently are affected more frequently than females in a ratio of 3 : 1 to 4 : 1. The male predominance is observed in all age groups. The age range of patients with bladder carcinoma is the first to the tenth decades. Most patients (80%) fall within the age range of 50 years to 79 years.[459,469] The mean patient age in most studies is 59 years to 65 years. Bladder carcinoma in young patients is rare, with only one example occurring within the first decade, and fewer than 100 cases reported in patients aged 30 years or younger.[406,409,414,416,419] The occurrence of malignant neoplasms in association with bladder exstrophy, diverticulum, and those originating in urachal remnants have demographic, clinical, and pathologic features unique to each of these circumstances, and are discussed separately (refer to discussions of bladder exstrophy and diverticulum, and urachus).

The association of bladder cancer with occupational exposure to certain organic chemicals has been known since the original observation published in 1895 by Rehn.[400] The increased frequency of bladder malignancy observed among workers in the German dye industry reported by Rehn was subsequently confirmed by Gehrman and by Gay among dye industry workers in the United States.[401-403] The experimental production of bladder carcinoma in dogs by the administration of betanaphthylamine, one compound to which the dye industry workers were exposed, was reported by McDonald and Lund.[405] These experiments proved the bladder carcinomas were initiated by the exposure of the bladder mucosa to urine containing the carcinogen. In subsequent years, occupational exposure to bladder carcinogens with increased risk of bladder cancer has been identified in the leather, rubber, paint, and organic chemical industries.[408,424]

Social habits, including cigarette, pipe, and cigar smoking, have been associated with an increased frequency of bladder cancer.[407,412,424] Conflicting data about the risk associated with coffee consumption have been reported, with an increased risk found by Miller and by Weinberg, which was not confirmed in the recent study by Gonzalez and co-workers.[412,421,424] The risk associated with artificial sweeteners remains unresolved.[413,418] There is no evidence that either viruses or radiation are etiologically linked to bladder cancer.[420]

The events of the chemical carcinogenesis involved in bladder malignancies have been investigated extensively during the past three decades. Epidemiologic studies of occupational risk of bladder cancer led to the implication of the naphthylamines. The experimental work of McDonald and Lund confirmed the carcinogenic properties of betanaphthalamines in the production of bladder cancer.[405] Importantly, they also demonstrated that the route of exposure to the carcinogen was not the bloodstream, but the urine.[405] Elucidation of the metabolic pathways of the naphthylamines clarified the organ specificity of their carcinogenic action. Major advances in understanding these events can be summarized as follows. The arylamines are oxidized and conjugated with glucuronic acid in the liver.[411] The glucuronic acid conjugates of the naphthylamines have been detected in the urine.[410] The bladder epithelium synthesizes beta-glucuronidase, an enzyme capable of hydrolizing the glucuronic acid conjugate at acidic pH of the urine.[411] Kadlubar and co-workers demonstrated the hydrolysis of the glucuronic acid conjugate of N-hydroxy-arylamine with the production of arylinitrenium ions, which are capable of binding to the guanine moiety of DNA of

Table 4-7   ***Age and Sex Distribution of Bladder Carcinoma***

Author(s)	Year	No. of Cases	Sex		Age		Peak Incidence
			Male	Female	Range	Mean	
Royce, Spjut[451]	1959	130	76%	24%	22–85	59.8	
Francis[453]	1961	326	86%	14%	1–89		7th–8th decades
Stone, Hodges[458]	1966	37	78%	22%	44–82	61.2	
Maltry[459]	1968	153	*	*	21–85	65	6th–8th decades
Long et al[463]	1972	205	75%	25%	24–91	69	
Richie et al[468]	1975	141	75%	25%	37–80	59	
Wajsman et al[469]	1975	92	80%	20%	30–80		5th–6th decades
Pearse et al[476]	1978	52	75%	25%	44–82	59.5	
Kishi et al[500]	1981	87	78%	22%	33–79	64	

* Study based on Veterans Administration Hospital patients with male predominance.

the bladder mucosal cells.[415] These investigations have thus clarified the metabolic events underlying the organ-specific carcinogenic action of the naphthylamines, or more specifically, their metabolic breakdown product acting as the ultimate carcinogen.

The role of pharmaceutical agents in the development of urothelial malignancies was first reported in reference to phenacetin (refer to discussion of transitional cell carcinoma of the renal pelvis in Chap. 2). In recent years reports implicating an increased risk of bladder malignancies in patients receiving the alkylating agent, cyclophosphamide, have appeared in the literature.[425–432]

Clinical Features

The presence of a vesical transitional cell carcinoma is most frequently announced by the onset of hematuria (70% to 95% of cases), and less frequently by dysuria (20% of cases).[437,453,459,468,500,507,511] The vesical neoplasm may be detected incidentally during routine follow up of patients previously treated for transitional cell carcinoma of the upper urinary tract. As discussed in Chapters 2 and 3, subsequent bladder carcinomas are diagnosed in 20% and 27% of patients treated for renal pelvic and ureteral transitional cell carcinomas, respectively (refer to Tables 2-12 and 3-10). Rarely, patients present with complaints referable to distant metastases from a previously undetected bladder malignancy.[502]

Cystograms reveal a filling defect confirmed at cystoscopy (Figs. 4-38, 4-39). Twenty-five percent to 36% of patients exhibit multiple tumors.[467,475,500] Transitional cell carcinomas are observed in all sites within the bladder; however, the lateral walls, followed by the posterior wall, are the most frequent sites of origin.[459,467,500] These neoplasms vary from a few millimeters to several centimeters

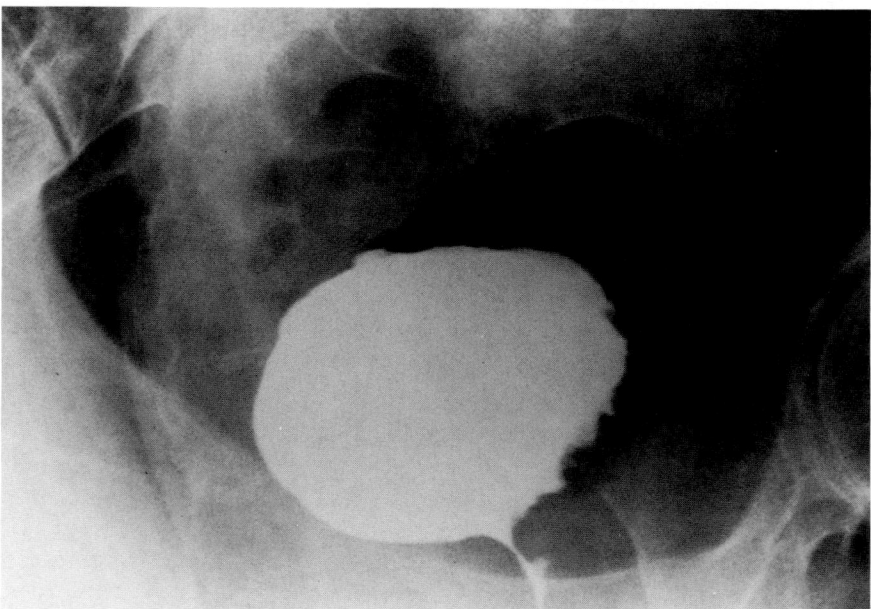

Figure 4-38   *Transitional cell carcinoma. An irregular margin along the left lateral wall of the bladder is observed on cystography. This radiographic appearance is characteristic of invasive transitional cell carcinoma of the bladder.*

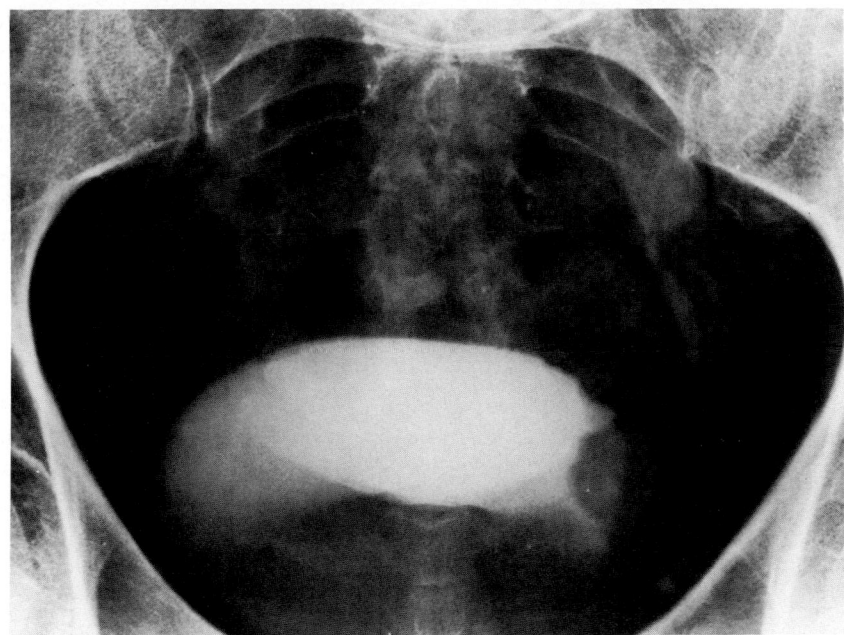

Figure 4-39 *Transitional cell carcinoma. A filling defect is seen arising from the left wall of the bladder in this cystogram. The localized lesion measured 2 cm in diameter at the base.*

in diameter. The papillary structure evident on histologic examination is apparent at the time of cystoscopy among low grade neoplasms (refer to discussion of pathologic features). Gross characteristics demonstrated by these neoplasms range from delicate, small, papillary lesions apparently limited to the surface, to larger, more solid invasive masses, frequently showing surface ulceration.

The cumulative impressions obtained by palpation and cystoscopy formulate the basis of clinical staging of such neoplasms. Radiologic procedures, radionucleotide scans, and bone marrow biopsies evaluate the possibility of distant metastases. Accurate staging is achieved in only 39% to 58% of cases, with 21% to 44% of cases understaged, and 4% to 37% of cases clinically overstaged.[445,468,469,473] The tendency to understage increases with increasing pathologic stage and tumor grade.[468,473]

Pathologic Features

Transitional cell carcinomas show growth patterns that are either exophytic and papillary, infiltrating, or both papillary and infiltrating. The lower grade neoplasms tend to be predominantly, if not exclusively, papillary and exophytic, whereas the predominantly infiltrating neoplasms are more typically high grade (Fig. 4-40). An increase in histologic grade is associated with a diminution of the papillary feature and an increased tendency to solid growth. High grade neoplasms with an exophytic and infiltrating pattern are typically solid bulky masses with variably extensive surface ulceration. These lesions lack the surface desquamation of keratin characteristic of squamous cell carcinoma and the mucinous features commonly observed in adenocarcinomas. A fourth growth pattern, nonpapillary and noninfiltrating, is characteristic of flat transitional cell carcinoma in situ lesions (refer to discussion of carcinoma in situ).

The grading of transitional cell carcinomas reported in the literature shows the application of many available protocols and a corresponding lack of uniformity. Table 4-8 presents some of the grading schemes suggested in the past. The World Health Organization grading protocol contains three grades that are characterized by the least anaplastic (grade 1), the most anaplastic (grade 3), and all others in between (grade 2) (Figs. 4-41 to 4-45).[465] What the system provides in simplicity, it lacks in objectivity, because no specific histologic or cytologic

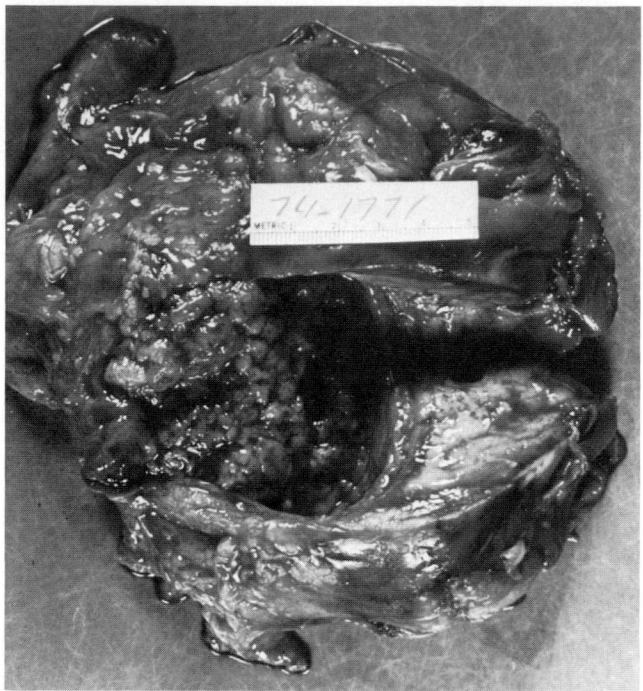

Figure 4-40   *Transitional cell carcinoma of the bladder.* The extensive papillary neoplasm is present in the center.

Table 4-8   **Grading Protocols for Bladder Carcinoma**

Ash[361]	*Bergkvist*[457]	*WHO*[465]
Transitional cell carcinoma, grade 1	Transitional cell carcinoma, grade 0	Papilloma
Transitional cell carcinoma, grade 2	Transitional cell carcinoma, grade 1	Transitional cell carcinoma, grade 1
	Transitional cell carcinoma, grade 2	Transitional cell carcinoma, grade 2
Transitional cell carcinoma, grade 3	Transitional cell carcinoma, grade 3	Transitional cell carcinoma, grade 3
Transitional cell carcinoma, grade 4	Transitional cell carcinoma, grade 4	Undifferentiated carcinoma

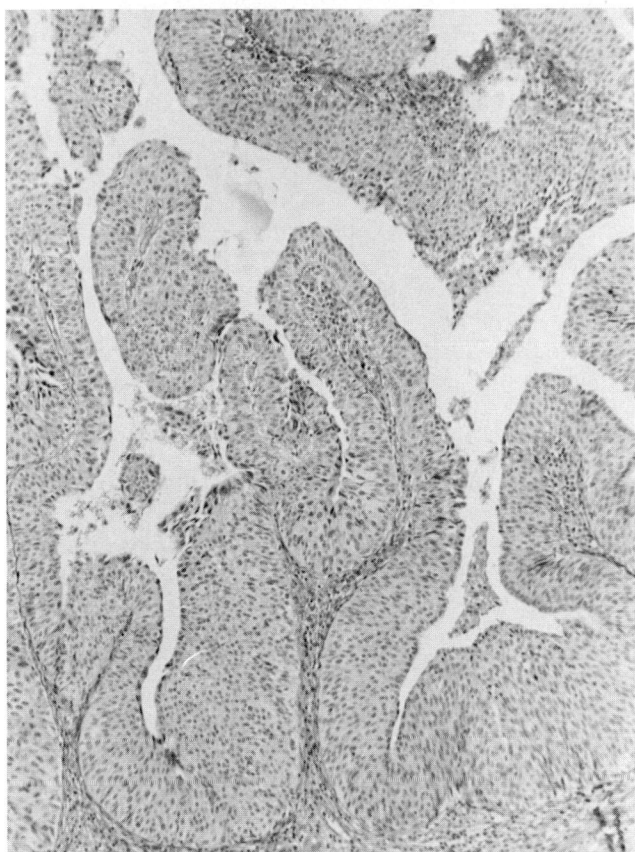

Figure 4-41 *Transitional cell carcinoma, grade 1. The papillary structures are covered by a thickened urothelium demonstrating only slight nuclear atypical features. Mitotic figures were rare in this neoplasm.*

criteria regarded as characteristic of the respective grades are provided. Among the alternative grading protocols, including Ash and Bergkvist, the latter has been found (with modification) to be the clearest outline of histologic criteria.[438,457] I utilize Berkvist's grade 0 to define the rare transitional cell papilloma, and his grade IV criteria detail the features of undifferentiated carcinomas of the bladder. Thus, I recognize the transitional cell papilloma, grades 1 to 3 transitional cell carcinoma, and undifferentiated carcinoma in the urinary bladder. Undifferentiated carcinomas of the urinary bladder are usually of the large cell type, and commonly have focal or predominating spindle cell features. Typical small cell undifferentiated carcinoma (oat cell carcinoma) of the urinary bladder is distinctly rare (refer to discussion of small cell undifferentiated carcinoma).

As discussed in the section dealing with carcinoma in situ, the flat urothelium adjacent to grossly apparent neoplasms may be hyperplastic and variably dysplastic. The same cytologic changes may be found at sites distant from the obvious neoplasm, as disclosed in mapping studies of bladder carcinoma.[479,494] The presence of dysplastic changes in urothelium adjacent to papillary neoplasms

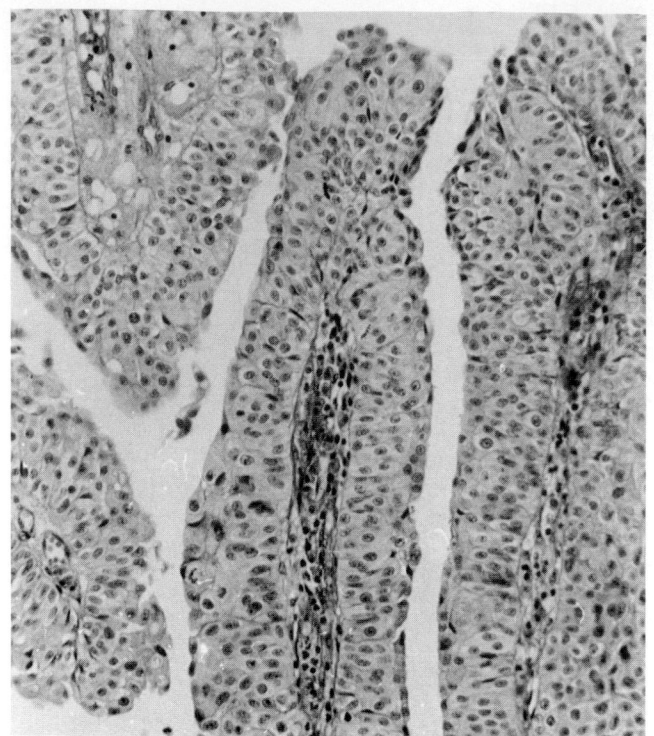

Figure 4-42 *Transitional cell carcinoma, grade 2. This papillary neoplasm is characterized by nuclear pleomorphism and uncommon to rare mitoses. Most tumor cells have prominent nucleoli.*

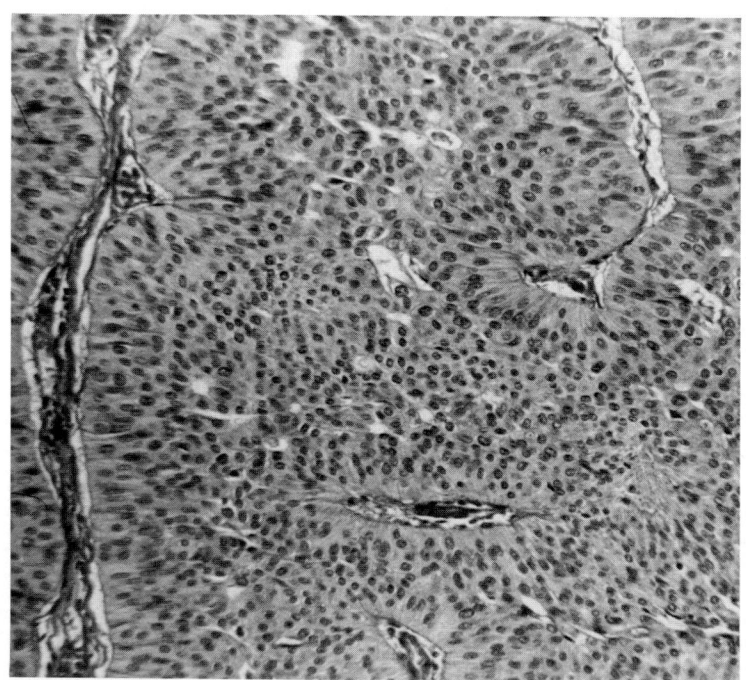

Figure 4-43 *Transitional cell carcinoma, grade 2. Fused papillary projections of transitional cell carcinoma with moderate variation of nuclear size and shape are present. (Compare with Fig. 4-42.)*

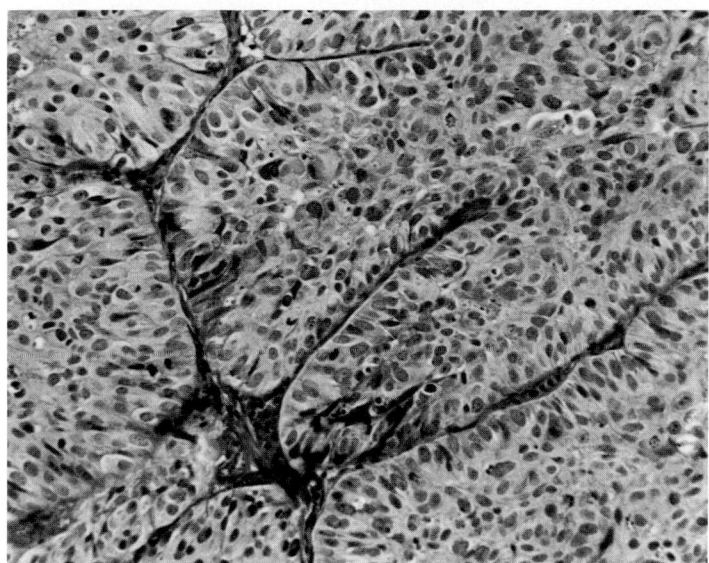

Figure 4-44 *Transitional cell carcinoma, grade 3. Marked nuclear pleomorphism and frequent mitoses associated with blunting and fusing of the papillae are present.*

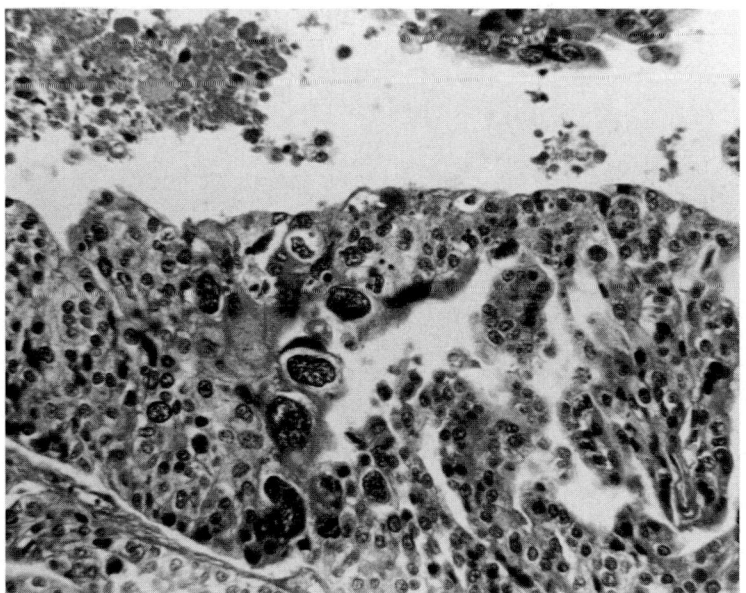

Figure 4-45 *Transitional cell carcinoma, grade 3. A focus of marked nuclear pleomorphism in the center is present in a background of more uniform malignant transitional cells.*

in cystoscopic biopsies should be noted in the final pathology report, for reasons discussed in the sections on carcinoma in situ and natural history. Importantly, these dysplastic changes may be found at the ureteral and urethral resection margins of cystectomy specimens. When found in such locations, the probability of local recurrence at these sites is increased. Dysplastic changes may involve Brunn's buds and nests and must be distinguished from early invasion of the lamina propria. This differential may be difficult in occasional cases, but generally is readily accomplished. The well-defined solid Brunn's nests differ from most infiltrating tumor nests, which tend to be more irregular in outline, less well demarcated, and associated with a localized stromal edema, or alternatively, fibroblastic response. The identification of true tumor invasion is not to be based on anticipated cytologic features more anaplastic than those characterizing the cells in the surface papillary component. Typically, no such cytologic difference is observed. Both vascular and lymphatic invasion are possible once a neoplasm has invaded the stroma of the lamina propria (Fig. 4-46). The identification of small vascular and lymphatic tributaries, difficult in routinely stained sections, may be accomplished by appropriate special stains.[435,442,462,490]

Cystectomy specimens subjected to preoperative radiation characteristically show morphologic changes attributable to acute radiation injury. Necrosis of tumor is variable, and may be apparently complete. In such cases extensive step-sectioning of the entire area previously occupied by tumor fails to disclose viable tumor cells. More frequently, the preoperative radiation achieves a reduction in stage: that is, tumors evidencing muscle invasion (stage B) in previous biopsies show viable tumor cells only in the lamina propria (stage A) in the cystectomy specimen.[490] The radiation-induced tumor necrosis is associated with an intense acute and chronic inflammatory cell infiltration, frequently in association with foreign body giant cells. Variable dysplasia of the surface urothelium may be present, but is most frequently found in cases demonstrating this change in the previous biopsies, and therefore it is not to be attributed to the effects of radiation administered shortly before the cystectomy procedure. Unfortunately, the microscopic review of cystectomy specimens more commonly reveals a higher stage than determined either clinically or by prior biopsy. The limited

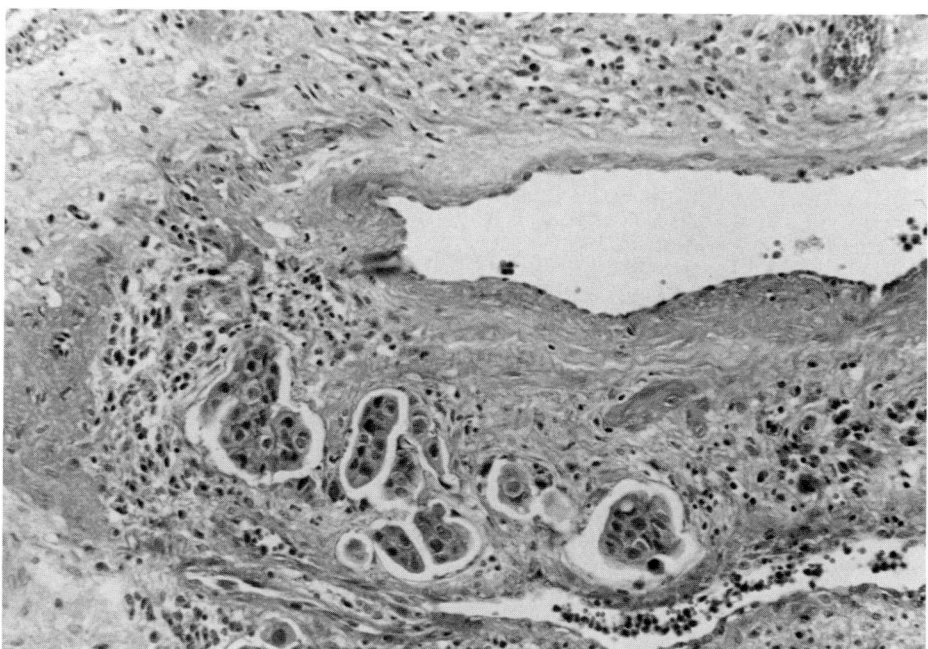

Figure 4-46   *Transitional cell carcinoma. Tumor cells are readily apparent in the dilated intramural lymphatics.*

ability to detect microscopic metastases to regional nodes accounts for many of these understaged cases.

Transitional cell carcinomas commonly show divergent cytologic features including clefts or round holes in the tumor nests (pseudoglands), true glandular or squamous differentiation, or spindle cell configuration (Fig. 4-47). Pseudogland formation can be observed in all grades of invasive transitional cell carcinoma, whereas focal glandular, squamous, and spindle cell change are typical only of high grade neoplasms. When such variant forms of differentiation are prominent throughout the tumor, it is designated as a neoplasm of mixed differentiation (refer to discussion of mixed cell type neoplasms).

The diagnosis of low grade transitional cell carcinoma requires differentiation from transitional cell papillomas, inverted papillomas, and polypoid cystitis, each of which are discussed in their respective sections.

Papanicolaou and Marshall first reported the diagnostic value of urine cytology in 1945.[439] The cumulative experience of the subsequent 40 years has both confirmed the value and clarified the limitations of this diagnostic technique.[446,452,454,460,461,470,474,481,485]

The sensitivity of cytologic examination of urine in detecting low grade papillary transitional cell carcinoma is unacceptably low (50% to 75%). Because of this high frequency of false-negative interpretations, urine cytology screening programs have been less successful than studies utilizing this diagnostic technique to detect recurrences of high grade carcinomas. This inability to detect low grade papillary lesions reliably may prove of lesser overall significance than its success with high grade lesions, including carcinoma in situ. In view of the recent clarification of the importance of CIS in the development of invasive bladder carcinoma, screening programs of selected patient groups may provide earlier detection and thereby reduce the mortality from this malignancy.[511] The cytolo-

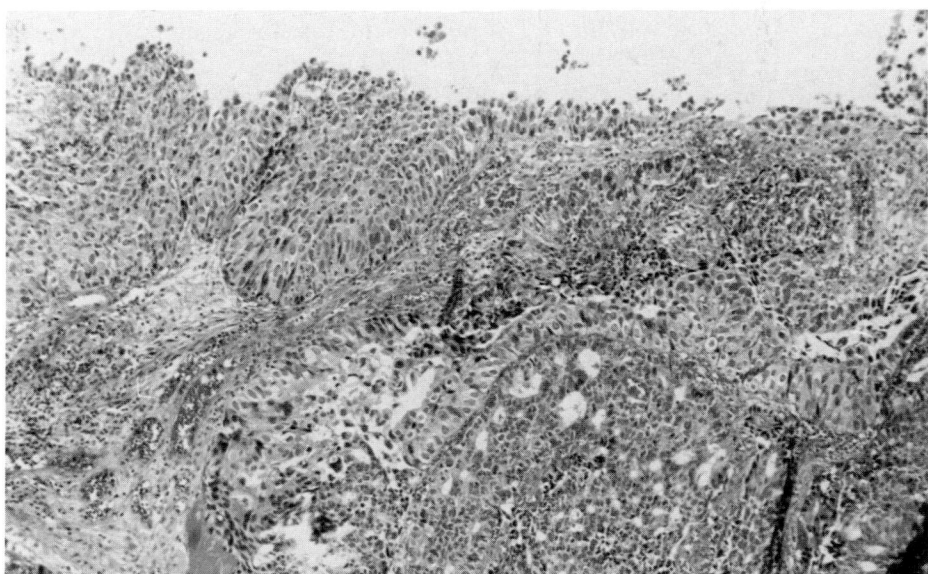

Figure 4-47   ***Bladder carcinoma with mixed differentiation.*** *This predominantly transitional cell carcinoma, here evident on the surface and invading the lamina propria, showed focal areas of glandular differentiation* (lower right).

gic detection of the flat lesions of CIS in the face of negative cystoscopic findings has been reported.[472,483]

The major diagnostic challenges to urine cytology specificity are the changes produced by inflammation, especially when associated with lithiasis, and radiation and chemotherapy (see Figs. 4-35 to 4-37).

Natural History

The earliest attempts to relate the pathologic features of bladder neoplasms to prognosis were reported by Aschner in 1928.[433] Aschner proposed a combined histologic, grade, and stage classification that recognized prognostic value in the presence or absence of invasion of the bladder wall. This modest beginning was followed by the formal tumor staging protocols of Jewett and Strong, Jewett, and the modification introduced by Marshall (Table 4-9).[440,444,445] These studies, relating the depth of tumor infiltration and the survival probability following surgical therapy, detailed the increasing frequency of lymph node metastases associated with progressively deeper bladder wall invasion.[440,441,445,503] The Marshall modification of the Jewett staging protocol became generally accepted. More recently, the American Joint Committee introduced a TNM staging protocol for bladder cancer (Table 4-10),[509] which may be compared to the Jewett–Strong–Marshall staging protocol shown in Table 4-9.

Both staging protocols may be applied to either clinical or pathologic staging of bladder neoplasms, the latter reflecting the more accurate determination of extent of tumor spread. Historically, the clinical staging of bladder tumor is fraught with a high frequency of error, ranging from 15% to 61% when subsequently compared to the pathologic stage determined after microscopic review of the cystectomy specimen.[445,467–469,473] The greatest tendency is to clinically understage bladder neoplasms, especially among stage B1, B, and C tumors.[445,467–469,473] Recent improvements in diagnostic procedures including echography and CT scans may increase the accuracy of the preoperative clinical staging.[487,495,508]

At the time of initial presentation, 85% of patients have tumor confined to the urinary bladder (stages 0 to C) whereas 15% have regional or distant metastases (stages D1, D2).[504] Approximately half of patients at the initial presentation have neoplasms confined to the mucosa or lamina propria. The remaining patients show muscle invasion, perivesical fat or nodal dissemina-

Table 4-9　Staging Protocols for Bladder Carcinoma

Extent of Invasion/Dissemination	Jewett, Strong[440]	Jewett[444]		Marshall[445]
Mucosa		Noninfiltrating		Stage 0
Lamina propria	Group A	Group A	Superficial	Stage A
Superficial muscle		Group B1		Stage B1
Deep muscle	Group B	Group B2		Stage B2
Perivesical tissue	Group C	Group C	Deep	Stage C
Pelvic lymph nodes				Stage D1
Distant metastases				Stage D2

tion.[459,463,471,510,511] Thus, at least two patient groups are apparent: those with advanced (deeply infiltrating or disseminated neoplasms) at the outset; and those patients who present with noninvasive or superficially invasive neoplasms fully capable of progression in time.

Noninvasive and Superficially Invasive Papillary Transitional Cell Carcinoma

The diagnosis of noninvasive and superficially invasive papillary transitional cell neoplasms occurs at cystoscopy and is confirmed by biopsy. The generally accepted therapy for stage 0 and A tumors is transurethral resection (TUR). Subsequent to surgical eradication by TUR, the natural history is characterized by one of three clinical patterns: (1) apparent cure without recurrence or development of new vesical neoplasms; (2) recurrence or development of new neoplasms of similar low grade and stage; or (3) recurrence or development of new neoplasms evidencing progression to higher stage (muscle invasion), and frequently, higher grade. Of all such initially stage 0 and A cases, 57% to 85% recur, and 4% to 30% demonstrate tumor progression with muscle invasion.[467,471,510] In the latter circumstance, the ultimate survival rate of the patients is significantly reduced from an average 74% at 5 years (50% to 90%) for stage 0 and A patients, to an average

Table 4-10 **TNM Staging Protocol for Bladder Carcinoma**

Stage	Extent of Invasion
T: Primary	
Tis	Carcinoma in situ, "flat tumor"
Ta	Papillary noninvasive carcinoma
T0	No evidence of primary tumor
T1	Invasion limited to lamina propria
T2	Invasion limited to superficial muscle
T3a	Invasion limited to deep muscle
T3b	Invasion through bladder wall
T4	Contiguous spread to adjacent organs
T4a	Uterus, vagina, prostate
T4b	Pelvic or abdominal wall
TX	Extent of invasion cannot be determined
N: Regional and Juxtaregional Lymph Nodes	
N0	No evidence of regional node involvement
N1	Metastases to single ipsilateral regional node
N2	Metastases to contralateral, bilateral, or multiple lymph nodes
N3	Metastatic involvement of fixed regional lymph nodes on the pelvic wall
N4	Metastases to juxtaregional lymph nodes
NX	Lymph node metastases cannot be determined
M: Distant Metastases	
M0	No evidence of distant metastases
M1	Evidence of distant metastases
MX	Distant metastases cannot be determined

Table 4-11   *Relation of Bladder Carcinoma Tumor Stage to 5-Year Survival Rate*

Author(s)	Year	No. of Patients	Stage* 0	A	B1	B2	C	D	Treatment
Francis[453]	1961	326		93%	59%	1.9%	0%		TUR,† or segmental resection
Whitmore, Marshall[433A]	1962	230	←— 47% —→			17%	13%	4%	Radical cystectomy
Jewett[455]	1964	71		50%	50%	16%	12%		Cystectomy
Jewett[455]	1964	133		58%	58%	16%	16%		Partial cystectomy
Stone, Hodges[458]	1966	37	←—80%—→			←— 36% —→		12%	Cystectomy
Cordonnier[459B]	1968	126		53.7%	52.6%	28.6%	17.9%	0%	Simple cystectomy
Maltry[459]	1968	153	50%	53%	64%	19%	12%	0%	Variable surgery, radiation, other
Utz et al[465A]	1973	199		68%	47%	40%	29%	1%	Segmental resection
Scott et al[465B]	1973	73	←—59%—→			←—12%—→		0%	Surgery, with or without radiation
Richie et al[468]	1975	141	66%	86%	39.9%	40.4%	19.7%	6.2%	Cystectomy
Wajsman et al[469]	1975	92	←—50%—→			←—31.7%—→		0%	Cystectomy
Whitmore et al[473]	1977	137	←—63%—→			←—20%—→		6%	Radical cystectomy
Whitmore et al[473]	1977	109	←—60%—→			←—27%—→		8%	6000-R radiation, radical cystectomy 1 yr
Whitmore et al[473]	1977	119	←—58%—→			←—38%—→		11%	4000-R radiation, radical cystectomy 4 wk
Whitmore et al[473]	1977	86	←—56%—→			←—57%—→		14%	2000-R radiation, radical cystectomy 1 wk
Pearse[476]	1978	52	←—64%—→			50%	20%	18%	Radical cystectomy
Brannan et al[477A]	1978	45	100%	68.8%	54.5%	62.5%	33.3%	0%	Partial cystectomy

* Arrows indicate reported survival of patients in combined stages.

† Transurethral resection.

54% for patients with superficial muscle invasion and 30% for patients showing deep muscle invasion (refer to Table 4-11).

Factors related to the frequency of both tumor recurrence and progression have been the subject of extensive study. Referable to the probability of recurrences or new neoplasms, the frequency is higher among those examples showing multiplicity, large size, and associated dysplasia of the adjacent urothelium at the time of initial presentation.[464,471,492,510,512] Neither tumor grade nor stage (0 to A) is predictive of future recurrences.[467,474,477,492] The majority of recurrences are detected within 12 months following diagnosis of the first neoplasm.[451,492]

An increased probability of tumor progression in subsequent recurrences is associated with large tumor size, high stage, high grade, the presence of multiple tumors, vascular or lymphatic invasion, and urothelial dysplasia, including carcinoma in situ.[471,475,490,491,510,512,513] The disappearance or absence of ABO antigens on tumor cell surfaces, as detected by the specific red cell adherence test (SRCA), is associated with aggressive future behavior.[478,480,496,497,505,506] The value of DNA and RNA flow cytometry in separating nonaggressive from aggressive bladder carcinomas is currently being evaluated.[514,515] Thus, the complete evaluation of TUR excisions of bladder neoplasms requires determination of the tumor grade, presence and depth of tumor invasion, lymphatic or vascular invasion, and presence of atypia of the adjacent non-neoplastic urothelium. The major therapeutic decisions, including the appropriateness and timing of cystectomy, rests on the combined clinical information obtained at cystoscopy, and the pathologic findings diagnosed and reported by the surgical pathologist.

Invasive Bladder Carcinoma

The term *invasive bladder carcinoma* as applied in this discussion refers to cancer showing muscle or perivesical fat invasion. The recent literature has more clearly defined the clinical evolution of bladder cancer with muscle invasion.[501] Eighty percent to 91% of all patients with stage B1 and B2 bladder tumors demonstrated this muscle invasion at the time of initial presentation.[501,507,511] The remaining

Table 4-12   ***Distribution of Metastatic Sites of Bladder Carcinoma***

Author(s)	Year	No. of Cases	Liver	Lungs	Bone	Lymph Nodes	Other
Smith, Mintz[434]	1933	34	7%	7%	13%	32%	*
Spooner[435]	1934	163	28%	18%	2%	69%	*
Colston, Leadbetter[436]	1936	98	42%	29%	18%	40%	*
Jewett, Strong[440]	1946	52	50%	35%	21%	63%	*
Royce, Ackerman[443]	1951	21	43%	28%	14%	85%	*
Fetter et al[450]	1959	55	13%	40%	37%	51%	*
Cooling[449]	1959	77	51%	39%	22%	88%	*
Maltry[459]	1968	51	40%	36%	32%	40%	*
Melicow[466]	1974	87	17%	18%	15%	41%	*
Whitmore et al[473]	1977	113	20%	32%	34%	31%	*
Babaian et al[488]	1980	107	38%	36%	27%	78%	*
Kishi et al[500]	1981	125	30%	30%	24%	38%	*

* Multiple other sites, all less than 10%.

9% to 20% of patients have a history of noninvasive transitional cell carcinoma that recurred and progressed with ultimate demonstration of invasion of muscle. As noted previously, such progression is observed in 4% to 30% of patients who initially present with superficially invasive or noninvasive neoplasms.[467,471,510] The significantly lower survival rates of clinical stage B1 and B2 bladder cancer is in part attributed to the significant increase in regional lymph node metastases associated with tumors that have invaded to the level of the muscularis.[445,468,469,493] Hopkins and associates have reported that 60% of these patients will have regional lymph node metastases and a median survival of 11 months.[511] Those patients whose tumors are confined to the bladder as determined by pathologic review have a median survival of 23 months. The overall 5-year survival for stages B1 to D is presented in Table 4-11. The majority of these high stage tumors diagnosed at initial presentation are also high grade. This observation raises the possibility that cytology screening of appropriate age groups would afford the opportunity to detect these occult neoplasms at an earlier stage with attendant increased survival probability.

Metastases of bladder carcinomas recorded in several studies are presented in Table 4-12. Regional lymph nodes and para-aortic lymph nodes, liver, lung, and bone, in order of decreasing frequency, are the most common metastatic sites. Multiple other sites, all with a frequency of less than 10%, have been observed.[466,473,500] The immediate causes of death in patients with bladder carcinoma are attributable to uremia, carcinomatosis, and pneumonia, in order of decreasing frequency.[500]

Squamous Cell Carcinoma

The frequency of squamous cell carcinoma is significantly higher in the Middle East, which is related directly to the prevalence of schistosomiasis in that area of

Table 4-13   *Squamous Cell Carcinoma of the Bladder*

Author(s)	Year	No. of Patients	Sex		Age		Invasion at Presentation	Squamous Metaplasia	Follow up
			Male	Female	Range	Mean			
Sakkas[517]	1966	47	72%	28%	45–75		86%	NI	NI
Newman et al[518]	1968	63 (84)*	67%	33%	30–90	80% (40–69)	96%	NI	8% — 5 YSR
Sarma[519]	1970	72	66%	34%			100%	†	NI
Bessette et al[520]	1974	75	60%	40%	32–70+	50% (51–70)	98%	17%	7% — 5 YRS
Johnson et al[521]	1976	90	56%	44%	37–86	66.6	100%	17%	10.6% — 5 YSR
Richie et al[522]	1976	33	42%	58%	37–84	72% (50–70)	100%	25%	48% — 5 YSR
Rous[523]	1978	17	35%	35%	NI	58	100%	NI	8% — 5 YSR
Faysal[525]	1981	46	66%	44%	45–86	NI	91%	NI	20% — 5 YSR

* Twenty-one cases were mixed TCC or AC with SCC.

† Present, but not quantitated.

NI, no information; YSR, year survival rate

the world. Squamous cell carcinoma constitutes 3% to 7% of urothelial malignancies of the urinary bladder.[467,469,500,519,523] The clinical and pathologic features of 443 cases of this malignancy reported in eight series are presented in Table 4-13. Patients range in age from 30 years to 90 years, with a peak frequency in the fifth to seventh decades. With the exception of the series reported by Richie and co-workers, in which only 42% of cases involved males, all other studies show male predominance ranging from 56% to 72%. Patients present with hematuria and dysuria. A history of urinary tract infection is common. Associated lithiasis has been reported in 10% to 20% of patients. Voiding cystogram is abnormal in 37% to 78% of cases.

Pathologic Features

Squamous cell carcinoma of the bladder, if not differing significantly from the more frequent transitional cell carcinoma from a clinical perspective, has distinctive gross and microscopic features. The malignancy tends to be infiltrative and ulcerating, rather than forming an exophytic papillary mass as observed in typical transitional cell carcinomas (Fig. 4-48). At the time of initial presentation, 86% to 100% of squamous cell carcinomas demonstrate invasion of the bladder wall (see Table 4-13). The extent of invasion and dissemination is commonly significantly greater (the pathologic stage higher) than appreciated clinically.[522] Associated squamous metaplasia has been observed in 17% to 25% of cases. The grading of squamous cell carcinomas of the urinary bladder has not been formalized, and most studies express tumor grade as well differentiated, moderately differentiated, and poorly differentiated. The majority of vesical squamous cell carcinomas are moderately well differentiated. Vascular, lymphatic and perineural invasion are observed frequently. Regional lymph node metastases are commonly found on microscopic review.

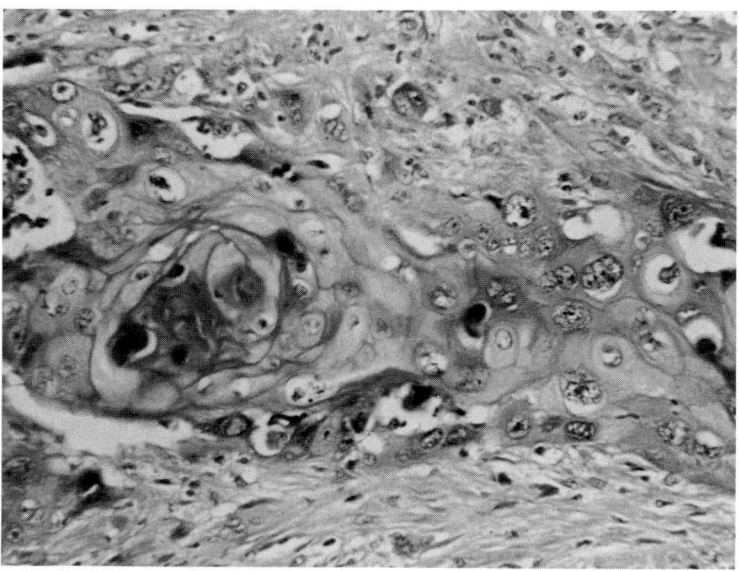

Figure 4-48 *Squamous cell carcinoma. Squamous differentiation was present uniformly throughout this invasive bladder neoplasm.*

Natural History

The low 5-year survival rate (7% to 20%) associated with bladder squamous cell carcinoma in most studies, is directly related to the high stage manifested at presentation (see Table 4-13).[522,525] The studies of Richie and associates and Faysal clearly demonstrate the high frequency of elevated stage at presentation, and the close correlation of survival with 50% to 70% of stage B case, 13% to 33% of stage C cases, and 0 to 20% of stage D cases surviving 5 years. The standard therapy is cystectomy. The therapeutic value of chemotherapy and radiation therapy requires further evaluation, but currently are not acceptable primary forms of therapy.

The role of squamous metaplasia, or leukoplakia, in the evolution of squamous cell carcinoma is unresolved. Long-term follow-up studies of vesical leukoplakia demonstrate that 15% to 28% of patients ultimately develop carcinoma.[516,524,526] The most common form of the carcinomas developing in the historical background of leukoplakia is squamous cell carcinoma, with fewer examples of transitional cell carcinoma.[516,524,526] To regard squamous metaplasia or leukoplakia as premalignant, however, is unjustified. Most probably both the leukoplakia and the malignancy are independently related to an underlying unidentified, causally related stimulus.

Verrucous Carcinoma

Verrucous carcinoma, first described in the oral cavity by Ackerman in 1948, has been observed subsequently in the cervix, vagina, anal region, penis, skin of the leg, and the bladder.[528] (Refer to discussion of verrucous carcinoma in Chap. 9.) This interesting neoplasm is uncommon in all locations, and is distinctly rare in the urinary bladder. El Sebai and associates reported a series of 22 cases involving the urinary bladder of Egyptian patients, all of whom had a history of schistosomal cystitis.[531] In their series of 655 bladder neoplasms, squamous cell carcinoma accounted for 483 (73.7%), and the 22 cases of verrucous carcinoma constituted 3.4% of the total series.[531] With an entirely different epidemiologic background, verrucous carcinoma of the urinary bladder has been observed in only one patient in North America. Wyatt and Craig described a typical example in a 72-year-old man.[532] Additional cases, reported as condyloma acuminatum, are probably examples of vesical verrucous carcinoma (refer to discussion of condyloma acuminatum).

The gross and microscopic features and clinical behavior of verrucous carcinoma are characteristic, regardless of the site of origin. The typical lesion is a warty, exophytic squamous cell neoplasm that invades underlying tissues with a pushing margin, showing little tendency to metastasize to regional lymph nodes or distant sites. Prior to the original description of verrucous carcinoma by Ackerman, Buschke and Löwenstein described a similar, if not identical, lesion which was called giant condyloma.[529] This lesion was referred to as *Buschke– Löwenstein's tumor* in the subsequent literature. In the ensuing decades considerable controversy existed about the nosologic identity or dissimilarity of these lesions (refer to discussion of verrucous carcinoma in Chap. 9). In summary, although not universally accepted, most investigators currently regard the lesions of Buschke–Löwenstein and verrucous carcinoma, in all locations of origin, as synonymous.[533,535]

Beyond this historical controversy surrounding verrucous carcinoma, two recent facets of this neoplasm have emerged. In the 1960s, the adverse effect on the clinical behavior of verrucous carcinoma induced by radiation therapy was reported.[529,530] Radiation-induced cytologic anaplasia associated with an increased tendency to metastasize was described. These findings, based on small numbers of patients, were generally accepted, but have been challenged recently in the literature.[535] This aggressive clinical behavior, originally attributed to radiation, has been observed in the absence of radiation.

Related to this phenomenon (*i.e.,* aggressive behavior of verrucous carcinoma) are the recent reports of foci of typical squamous cell carcinoma detected in the course of extensive sectioning of lesions otherwise characteristic of verrucous carcinoma.[534] The presence of such foci, possibly overlooked in previous cases of verrucous carcinoma examined in a routine manner, may account for the pathologic and clinical features previously attributed to radiation.

Referable to verrucous carcinoma originating in the urinary bladder, none of the cases reported by El Sebai and associates and Wyatt and Craig exhibited metastases.[531,532] The patients present most commonly with dysuria. Hematuria is observed, but is uncommon. El Sebai and associates reported that patients commonly reported "passing white encrusted fragments of tissue," undoubtedly representing keratin debris from the lesion.[531] A shaggy, exophytic white mucosal lesion is observed at cystoscopy.[532]

Pathologic Features

The characteristic microscopic features of verrucous carcinoma, regardless of site of origin, include the following: (1) marked acanthosis, hyperkeratosis, and

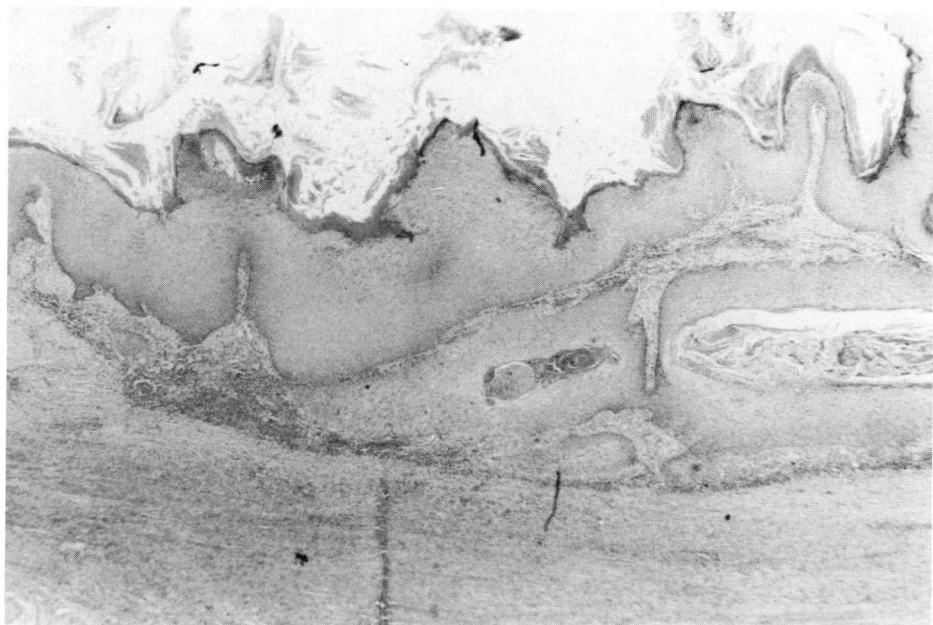

Figure 4-49   *Verrucous carcinoma. This squamous cell neoplasm present on the surface with abundant keratinization is also observed to be encroaching within the lamina propria in large, well-defined cords of tumor cells. An accompanying chronic inflammatory cell infiltrate is present in the stroma of the lamina propria.*

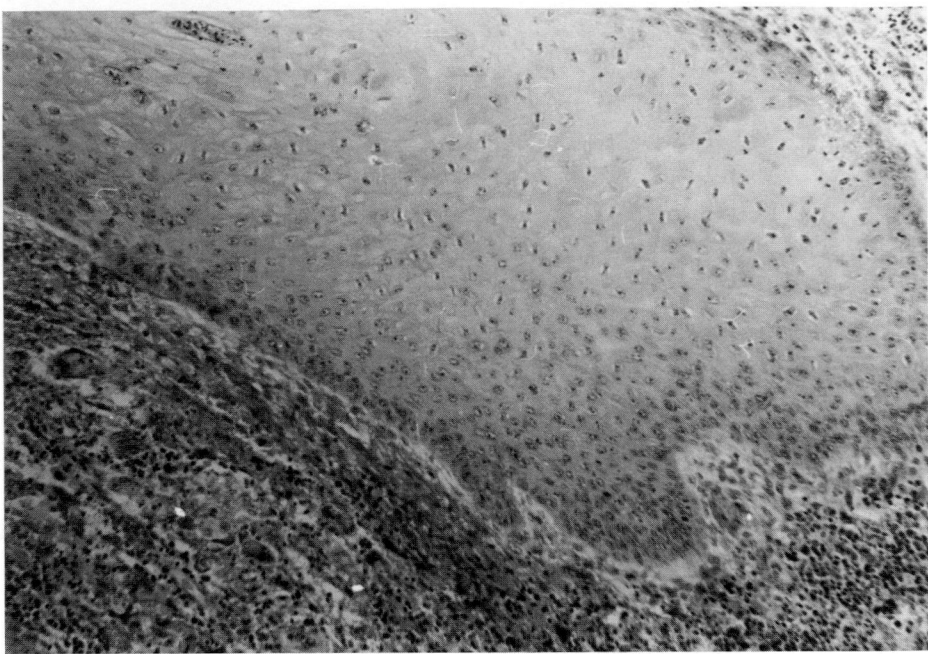

Figure 4-50   *A higher magnification of the tumor encroaching in the lamina propria shows the extremely well-differentiated cytologic features typical of verrucous carcinoma.*

typical bulbous papillomatosis; (2) minimal or absent cytologic atypia of the squamous cells; (3) mitotic activity limited to the basal region; (4) crowding or confluent papillary downgrowths advancing on or encroaching on a broad front in association with a variably dense chronic inflammatory cell infiltrate in the underlying stroma with fewer numbers of acute inflammatory cells in the underlying stroma (Figs. 4-49, 4-50).

The diagnostic features of verrucous carcinoma are principally located in the deeper levels of the lesion. The more superficial layers, exhibiting nonspecific histologic changes, in association with the banal cytologic features of verrucous carcinoma, are of little diagnostic value in superficial biopsies. Biopsies of diagnostic value include the full thickness of the mucosal lesion. Examination of the specimen, whether from the bladder or from other anatomical sites, requires extensive sectioning to aid in detecting foci of more typical squamous cell carcinoma, as noted in recent studies cited previously.

Adenocarcinoma

Adenocarcinoma is the third most frequent histologic type of bladder carcinoma. Excluding examples arising in association with exstrophy and urachal remnants, and the signet-ring cell variant of vesical adenocarcinoma (all discussed elsewhere in this chapter), 321 cases of adenocarcinoma of the urinary bladder were culled from the literature.[536-560] Of these 321 cases, 208 were presented in 8 collected series of this malignancy, and the remainder as case reports (Table 4-14). Prior to 1970, the collective experience with bladder adenocarcinoma was limited, but has substantially increased in subsequent years. Approximately 80% of all reported vesical adenocarcinomas have appeared in the literature since 1970.

Clinical Features

Patients range in age from 6 years to 92 years, with peak frequencies and mean ages reported in the sixth decade (see Table 4-14). Approximately 70% of reported cases are found in men. The presenting symptoms are not specific for vesical adenocarcinoma, with most patients experiencing hematuria, with or without dysuria. Rarely, the passage of mucous material at micturition is found to be associated with a mucin-producing adenocarcinoma.[551,556,559] Radiologic features of adenocarcinoma of the bladder are not specific. The diagnosis is made on biopsy material obtained at the time of cystoscopy.

Pathologic Features

Adenocarcinomas are most frequently single lesions, with a predilection for the trigone region and bladder dome in most reported series.[551] Less frequently, multiple tumors are present. When involving the dome, or the anterior–superior wall of the bladder, consideration of urachal origin is obligatory (refer to discussion of urachal malignancies in this chapter). The necessity of excluding origin from a nonvesical primary site is necessary in all cases of adenocarcinoma involving the bladder. The most frequent gland-forming neoplasms involving the urinary bladder by direct extension or metastases include prostate, colorectal, uterine, stomach, and breast adenocarcinomas (refer to discussion of metastatic tumors in this chapter). The gross features range along a spectrum of ulcerative, papillary, or nodular-ulcerative. Virtually all cases evidence invasion of the blad-

Table 4-14   Selected Published Studies of Adenocarcinoma*

Author(s)	Year	No. of Cases	Sex		Age		Metaplasia	Stage	Survival 5 Years
			Male	Female	Range	Mean (Peak Frequency)			
Mostofi et al[537]	1955	24†	17	6	18–77	(6th decade)	42%	NI	29%
Thomas et al[544]	1971	28	25	3	54–78	(7th decade)	14%	50% > stage B	7%
Johnson et al[545]	1972	17‡	14	3	38–78	55	18%	53% > stage B	17%
Jacobo et al[550]	1977	19§	12	7	36–80	62	NI	75% > stage B	0%
Kramer et al[551]	1979	34	25	9	38–80	59	26%	53% > stage B	19%
Jones et al[552]	1980	10	8	2	48–65	59	10%	40% > stage B	40%
Nocks et al[560]	1983	12	NI	NI	38–86	60	NI	17% > stage B	27%
Anderstrom et al[558]	1983	64‖	40	24	30–93	(7th decade)	NI	62% > stage B	18%

* The included eight studies comprise all published series containing ten or more patients.

† The sex of one patient was unknown.

‡ Includes four cases of signet-ring cell carcinoma.

§ Includes one case arising in exstrophic bladder.

‖ Data indicate frequency of associated glandular metaplasia (cystitis glandularis).

NI, no information

der wall at the time of cystectomy, with 17% to 75% demonstrating pathologic stage C or greater (see Table 4-14).

The histologic patterns encountered in vesical adenocarcinomas include papillary, glandular, mucinous (with large pools of mucin), adenoid cystic, signet-ring cell, and clear cell types (Figs. 4-51, 4-52). Mixtures of these patterns are very common. In addition, focal areas of transitional cell carcinoma, with or without squamous cell carcinomatous foci, are not uncommon.[558,560] Rarely, foci of undifferentiated malignant cells showing no evidence of differentiation of squamous, glandular, or transitional epithelial cells are found. Adenocarcinomas have been described as well differentiated, moderately differentiated, or poorly differentiated, or grades I to III, generally based on the predominant differentiation according to WHO classification.[465] The resemblance of some examples to colon carcinoma is remarkable, including the presence of Paneth's cells in one instance.[554]

The association of cystitis cystica and cystitis glandularis has been observed in 10% to 50% in six reported series (see Table 4-14). Case reports have described longstanding cystitis cystica and cystitis glandularis temporally preceding, and associated with, vesical adenocarcinoma.[538,543,546,553] In three such reports progression of cystitis glandularis has been observed, prompting some authors to unjustifiably regard cystitis glandularis as a premalignant lesion.[538] That adenocarcinomas arise in the background of cystitis glandularis, and squamous cell carcinomas occur in bladders demonstrating squamous metaplasia (so-called leukoplakia), should neither be a surprise nor serve as a rationale for regarding the preceding and accompanying lesions as premalignant. The noxious influence underlying the metaplastic change to cystitis glandularis most probably is responsible for the temporally later event, neoplasia.

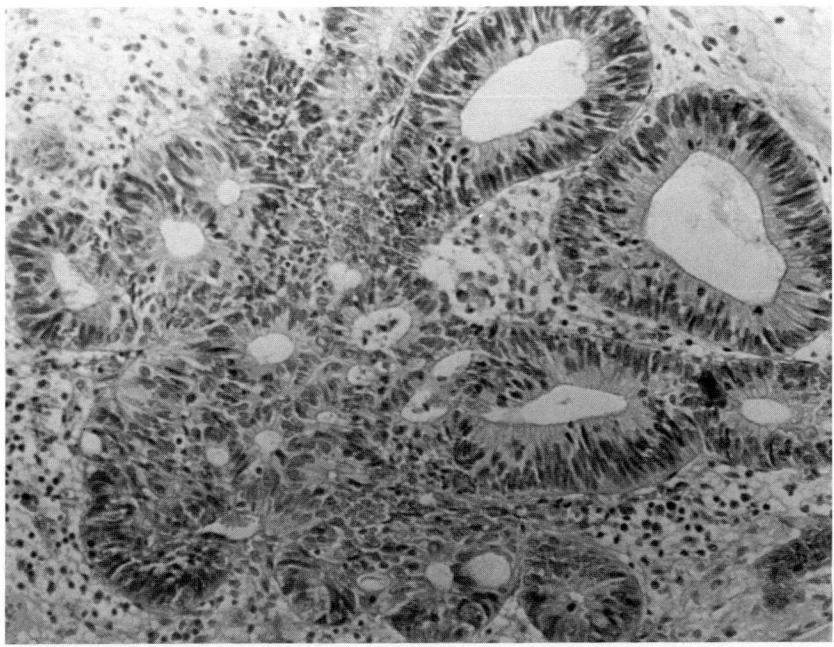

Figure 4-51   *Adenocarcinoma. Well-differentiated glands lined by tumor cells with hyperchromatic nuclei are present. Several glands merge without intervening stroma.*

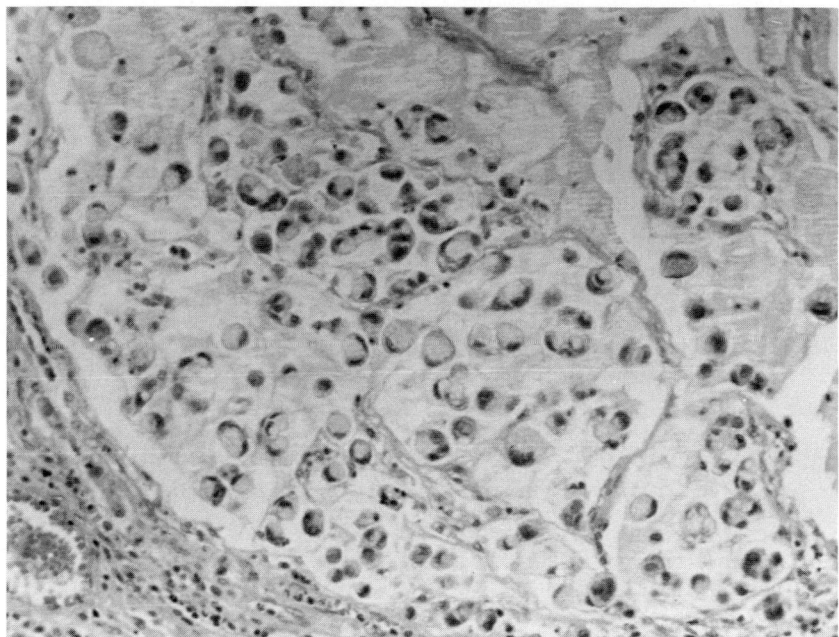

Figure 4-52 *Adenocarcinoma, signet ring cell type. The tumor cells with signet ring appearance are found in pools of extracellular mucin within the wall of the bladder.*

Natural History

The standard treatment for adenocarcinoma of the urinary bladder is radical cystectomy. Radiation therapy appears to give no beneficial effect with this histologic type of bladder carcinoma. The dismal survival rates cited in Table 4-14 reflect primarily the uniformly high stage of vesical adenocarcinomas observed at the time of diagnosis and primary surgical therapy.

Signet-Ring Cell Carcinoma

Signet-ring cell carcinoma is an aggressive, rare histologic variant of adenocarcinoma. It has been reported originating in the urinary bladder in 32 patients (Table 4-15).[545,558,561-576] Eighty-two percent occur in patients older than 50 years, with a reported age range of 38 years to 83 years. Males are affected in 87% of cases. The majority of patients present with dysuria and hematuria, findings that are in no way unique to this form of vesical malignancy. The gross features of the reported cases are variable and nonspecific, with flat, granular, papillary, and ulcerated nodules described. However, these nonspecific features are in the background of diffuse vesical involvement with a rigid and thickened bladder wall, associated with a contracted volume. The combination of all of these features should suggest a bladder malignancy other than the more frequent transitional cell carcinoma, and raise the possibility of a signet-ring carcinoma.

The diagnosis rests on the microscopic identification of the signet-ring cell, for which this adenocarcinoma variant is named. The majority of reported cases of signet-ring carcinoma exhibit a variable pattern of adenocarcinoma, and some contain foci of transitional cell or squamous cell carcinoma. The latter features are limited in extent and the neoplasm is predominantly an adenocarcinoma.

Bladder malignancies of whatever type are to be classified on the basis of the overwhelmingly predominant form of differentiation. This rule holds for signet-ring cell carcinomas that may have focal areas of divergent differentiation. The histologic pattern of the signet-ring cells may be either in mucinous pools separated by fibrous trabeculae, or alternatively, diffusely infiltrating as cords or individual cells typical of the linitis plastica pattern, most commonly encountered in the gastrointestinal tract, especially the stomach. The signet-ring cell is characterized by an intracellular mucin-filled vacuole filling most of the cell and displacing the nucleus to one side, where it appears as slightly curved, hyperchromatic, and compressed against the cell membrane (see Fig. 4-52). The mucin vacuole, appearing clear with routine stains, is PAS- and mucicarmine-positive. Mucin stains similarly is present in extracellular locations of the tumor. Associated Brunn's nests, glandular metaplasia, and squamous metaplastic changes all have been reported in the surface urothelium of involved bladders. Most examples of signet-ring carcinoma exhibit diffuse and deep invasion of the bladder wall, with extension beyond the bladder a frequent observation.

The diagnosis of primary signet-ring cell carcinoma of the urinary bladder is based on the histologic features described previously predominating in a vesical malignancy, and importantly, unequivocal exclusion of alternative primary malignancies (including prostate, stomach, and colon) of identical features metastasizing to the bladder.

At the time of diagnosis and therapy, most signet-ring cell carcinomas of the bladder have achieved high stage (B2, C, or D1). The high stage and apparent poor response to radiation therapy contribute to the poor survival data experienced with the malignancies. I am aware of only one documented patient surviving 5 years, although Fuselier and associates report survival of 8 months to 84 months among 5 cases in their series (Table 4-15). The majority of patients die of tumor-related causes within 2 years of diagnosis.

The histogenesis of this variant of adenocarcinoma has been the subject of much discussion and debate as outlined earlier in this chapter, as have all non-transitional cell carcinomas of the bladder. I regard the histogenetic route of metaplasia and subsequent malignant transformation, both due to unknown underlying causes, as quite adequate to explain the presence of this malignancy within the urinary bladder.

Clear Cell Carcinoma

Clear cell carcinoma is an uncommon histologic variant of adenocarcinoma typically found in the female genital tract. It was originally described by Schiller.[577] The neoplasm is characterized by tubules and papillary histologic patterns in which characteristic malignant clear and hobnail cells are found in varying proportions. Schiller originally called these neoplasms *mesonephromas,* but the consensus reflected in the more recent literature is that it is a malignancy of Müllerian origin.[580] The tumor is most frequent in the endometrium and ovary, but has been observed in the fallopian tube, endocervix, and vagina, in order of decreasing frequency.[580] This neoplasm rarely occurs in the urinary tract, under which circumstances its histogenesis is unsettled. Eight cases in the urethra and six cases in the urinary bladder have been reported in the recent literature (refer to Chap. 5).[558,578-583]

With the exception of the first reported case, which involved a 43-year-old man, all other cases in both the bladder and urethra involved women in the fifth

Table 4-15   *Signet-Ring Cell Carcinoma of the Urinary Bladder*

Author(s)	Year	Age	Sex	Treatment	Follow up
Saphir[561]	1955	60	M	No therapy	D/T, 2 wk
Saphir[561]	1955	50	M	Ureterostomy	D/T, 4 mo
Schroup et al[562]	1955	82	F	None	D/T, "weeks"
Schroup et al[562]	1955	65	F	None	D/T, 1 mo
Schroup et al[562]	1955	59	F	None	D/T, 1 mo
Melicow[563]	1955	*	*	No information (*)	*
Melicow[563]	1955	*	*	No information (*)	*
Winter, Goodwin[539]	1959	69	M	None	D/T, 4 mo
Allen, Henderson[541]	1965	52	F	None	D/T, 10 mo
Payan et al[564]	1966	38	M	Segmental resection	A/NED, "several months"
Rosas-Uribe, Luna[565]	1969	51	M	Segmental cystectomy, radiation	D/T, 7 mo
Rosas-Uribe, Luna[565]	1969	48	F	Biopsy, chemotherapy	D/T, 13 mo
Corwin et al[566]	1971	56	F	Cystectomy, TAHBSO, radiation	A/NED, 10 mo
Johnson et al[545]	1972	†	†	No information (†)	†
Johnson et al[545]	1972	†	†	No information (†)	†
Naeim et al[567]	1972	52	M	Radiation, cystectomy, prostatectomy	No follow up
De Ture et al[568]	1975	62	M	Cystectomy, prostatectomy	D/?T, 30 months
Fuselier et al[570]	1978				D/T,
Fuselier et al[570]	1978	38–69		Surgery—2	D/T,
Fuselier et al[570]	1978	3	F	Surgery, radiation —2	D/T, 8–84 mo
Fuselier et al[570]	1978	2	M	Radiation, chemotherapy—1	D/T,
Fuselier et al[570]	1978				D/Postoperative
Sagalowsky, Donohue[571]	1978	41	M	Left nephrostomy, Cytoxan	A/T, 16 yr
Austin, Safford[569]	1980	54	M	TUR, radiation, cystectomy	D/T, 10 mo
Braun et al[572]	1981	45	M	Cystectomy	A/NED, 3 yr, 9 mo
Poore et al[573]	1981	55	M	Colostomy, nephrostomy	D/T, Postoperative
Yoshida et al[574]	1981	63	M	Cystectomy	A/NED, 19 mo
Gonzalez et al[575]	1982	56	M	None	D/T, 3 mo
Anderstrom et al[558]	1983	‡	‡	No information	‡
Choi et al[576]	1984	61	M	Radical cystectomy	D/T, Postoperative
Choi et al[576]	1984	83	M	Radiation	D/T, 3 mo
Choi et al[576]	1984	50	M	None	D/T, 5 mo

D/T, dead with tumor; A/NED, alive, no evidence of disease; A/T, alive, with tumor; D/?T, dead, tumor status unknown

* Two cases of signet-ring cell carcinoma among 197 cases of bladder adenocarcinoma; no details.

† Two cases among series of 17 cases of adenocarcinoma of bladder; no details.

‡ One case of signet-ring cell carcinoma among 64 vesical adenocarcinoma; no details provided.

to eighth decades.[578] Neither clinical presentation nor radiologic features are specific for this malignancy. This neoplasm shows no site of predilection within the bladder. Four of the reported patients were treated with cystectomy and one was treated with radiation, with apparent favorable response.[581] The latter patient was reported after a 2-year follow up without evidence of recurrence.[581] Among the four patients treated by cystectomy, two died of tumor-related causes within 1 year and two were alive at 10 months and 2 years at the time of reporting.[558,578-583]

The gross features of this histologic type of adenocarcinoma are not unique, and the diagnosis is made on microscopic review. The histologic pattern of tubules, papillary formations, small glands, and occasionally diffuse sheets is characteristic. The diagnostic clear cells and hobnail cells, in variable proportions, constitute the tumor cell population. The clear cells derive their name from the optically clear cytoplasm surrounding the nucleus. The hobnail cells lining the glands and papillary structures and their pleomorphic nuclei oriented toward the luminal side of the cell produce an irregular bumpy outline of the lumen, thus explaining the descriptive name. (Refer to discussion of clear cell carcinoma in Chap. 5.) The tumor cells stain positively with mucicarmine, Alcian blue, PAS without diastase, and oil red O.[582,583]

Carcinomas with Mixed Differentiation

Urothelial neoplasms within the urinary bladder commonly exhibit mixed differentiation. All possible combinations have been observed. The frequency in my experience is greater than generally appreciated, which reflects the limited attention this histologic feature receives in the literature.[537,544,545,550,552,558,560,584] Mention of mixed differentiation is common in reports of large series of bladder carcinoma. The ultimate prognosis, and thus the formal diagnosis rendered on such a case, should reflect the predominant histologic differentiation. When the admixed components are in approximate equal proportions, this should be stated formally in the diagnosis. Transitional cell carcinoma with pseudogland formation is rather common, and is not an example of adenocarcinoma admixed with transitional cell carcinoma.

Carcinoid Tumor

Carcinoid tumors of the urinary bladder have been reported in four patients.[585-588] The same tumor has been observed in the kidney (9 cases), urethra (7 cases), and testis (31 cases), prompting speculation about the histogenesis of this neoplasm in each of these unusual locations. (Refer to corresponding chapters.) Origin from teratomas has been recorded in some of the reported cases occurring in the testis and kidney. This histogenesis has not been recognized underlying any of the four cases originating in the urinary bladder. Two other histogenetic possibilities include migration of chromaffin cells from the neural crest to the bladder during embryologic development, and subsequent neoplastic transformation, or alternatively, *de novo* development of a carcinoid tumor through a two-step process of metaplasia, and subsequent malignant transformation of vesical urothelium. The sequence of events has been elegantly demonstrated in a prostatic carcinoid tumor with the application of immunoperoxidase staining, and electron microscopy (refer to discussion of carcinoid tumor in Chap. 8).

The neoplasms reported in the urinary bladder exhibited a male predominance, with all cases involving middle-aged adults. The tumors, measuring from less than 1 cm to the "size of a hen's egg," produced hematuria in all four patients. The diagnosis of carcinoid tumor was made on either transurethral resection biopsies or only after bladder resection. The diagnostic impression of carcinoid tumor based on routine H and E stained sections was confirmed in all cases with silver stains detecting argyrophil-positive granules, and in three cases, the identification of membrane-bound dense core granules by electron microscopy.[586-588]

The generally indolent behavior of carcinoid tumors was manifested by three of the reported cases occurring in the bladder; however, the reported follow-up periods are relatively short (*i.e.,* 12 months to 22 months).[585-588] One case proved clinically malignant within a brief period, demonstrating local recurrence, distant metastases, and ultimately causing the patient's death within 2 years of cystectomy.[586]

Small Cell Undifferentiated Carcinoma (Oat Cell Carcinoma)

Three cases of small cell undifferentiated carcinoma have appeared in the recent literature.[589-591] These tumors involved two men and one woman, all within the age range of 55 years to 75 years. The patients presented with hematuria. Two of the recorded cases demonstrated systemic manifestations of hypophosphatemia and excess of ACTH hypersecretion related to the tumor.[589,591] The diagnosis in each of the three cases was based on the typical histologic and cytologic features of small cell undifferentiated carcinoma regardless of site of origin. Silver stains for argyrophil granules or ultrastructural demonstration of membrane-bound dense core granules, characteristic of this malignancy, supported the diagnosis in each of the reported cases. Two of the three reported tumors behaved in a manner typical of small cell undifferentiated carcinoma with widespread metastases and death 3 months and 4.5 months after diagnosis.[590,591] The first reported patient was alive without evidence of recurrent tumor 14 months after a partial cystectomy.[589] The true incidence of small cell undifferentiated carcinoma arising in the urinary bladder is undoubtedly not accurately reflected by the limited number of reported cases.

Malignant Melanoma

Primary malignant melanoma of the urinary bladder is distinctly rare, with six cases reported in the literature (Table 4-16). Metastatic malignant melanoma involving the urinary bladder is far more frequent (refer to discussion of metastatic tumors in the bladder).

The most completely documented case of primary melanoma of the urinary bladder is that reported by Wallace Clark and co-workers.[594] The criteria they formulated for the diagnosis of a primary melanoma of the urinary bladder includes the following:

1. Negative history of a cutaneous melanoma
2. Negative physical examination to exclude concurrent cutaneous melanoma
3. Negative appropriate studies to exclude concurrent alternative visceral melanoma
4. No apparent development of alternative primary site found in follow-up examinations
5. Pattern of recurrences consistent with bladder primary neoplasm
6. Neoplasm associated with intramucosal atypical melanocytes at tumor margin

Of the sixteen reported cases of primary malignant melanoma of the urinary bladder, only the case reported by Clark's group and three subsequently reported by Willis and associates and Anichkov and Nikonov can be accepted as proven primary in the urinary bladder.[594-596] The cases reported by Wheelock and by Su and Prince do not satisfy the criteria outlined above, and should be regarded only as possible examples, at best.[592,593] The detection of a malignant melanoma of the scalp 3 weeks after detection of the urinary bladder lesion strongly suggests that the vesical neoplasm reported by Su and Prince represented a metastatic focus.[593]

The diagnosis of malignant melanoma involving the urinary bladder rests on the typical histologic pattern and cytologic features of this malignancy as observed in routinely stained sections. The brown-black pigment present in the tumor cells is identified as melanin by appropriate stains (Fontana–Masson), and further substantiated by ultrastructural studies demonstrating cytoplasmic melanosomes.[594]

The histogenesis of melanocytes and malignant melanomas of the urinary bladder is unsettled.[594,595] Migration of melanocytes from the neural crest, or alternatively, metaplasia of cells arising in the bladder mucosa *de novo,* are two histogenetic possibilities (refer to discussions of blue nevus and melanosis in Chap. 8).

Table 4-16   **Malignant Melanoma**

Author(s)	Year	Age	Sex	Treatment	Follow up
Wheelock[592]	1942	67	F	Partial cystectomy	D/T, 3 yr
Su, Prince[593]	1962	61	F	No treatment	D/T, 8 wk
Ainsworth et al[594]	1976	65	F	Cystectomy	A/T, 1 yr, 5 mo
Willis et al[595]	1980	57	F	Radical cystectomy	D/T, 3 yr
Anichkov, Nikonov[596]	1982	48	M	Partial cystectomy	D/T, 1 yr*
Anichkov, Nikonov[596]	1982	46	M	Cystectomy	LTF, 3 mo

D/T, dead with tumor; A/T, alive with tumor; LTF, lost to follow up
* Autopsy performed.

Benign Mesenchymal Neoplasms

Leiomyoma

Benign smooth muscle neoplasms of the urinary tract are rare to uncommon. The majority originate in the urinary bladder. An accurate number of vesicle leiomyomas is difficult to obtain, because this neoplasm has been reported under different diagnoses including fibroma, fibromyoma, and leiomyoma in the early literature. Early reviews by Kretschmer, Campbell and Gislason, and Zaffagnini recorded 47, 68, and 89 reported cases, respectively.[597-599] An additional 16 cases could be found in the more recent literature of the past 20 years.[600-612]

Vesical leiomyomata have been observed in all age groups from 1.5 years to 75 years, with a peak frequency observed in the fourth to sixth decades. Approximately two thirds of patients are women, consistent with the female predominance observed among leiomyomata of the kidney, ureter, and urethra (refer to corresponding chapters). Patients most commonly present with hematuria and dysuria. Alternatively, the neoplasm may be an asymptomatic mass detected incidentally on intravenous pyelography (IVP). Radiologic examination and cystoscopy reveals a rounded intramural mass, most frequently on the posterior wall. The reported size varies from millimeters to several centimeters. Three forms have been described — endovesical, intramural, and extravesical — dependent on the predominant location of the neoplasm. In reality, this classifi-

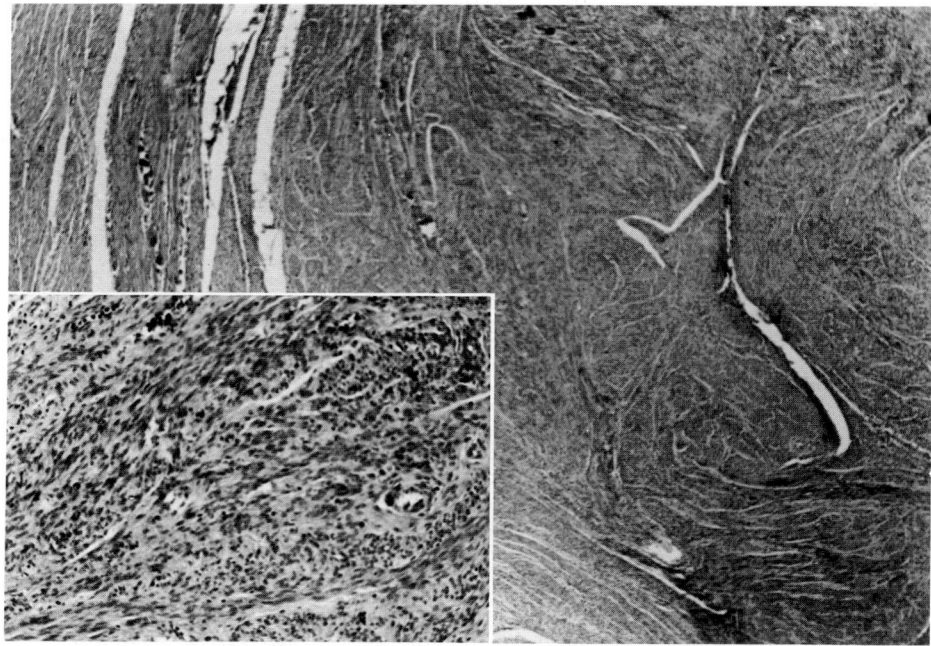

Figure 4-53 *Leiomyoma. The periphery of this benign smooth muscle neoplasm is well demarcated and commonly "cracks" away from the adjacent fibromuscular stroma of the bladder wall. The interlacing bundles of spindle cells typical of benign smooth muscle neoplasms are present* (inset).

cation more closely reflects tumor size, because larger examples, although arising in intramural smooth muscle, tend to protrude into the vesicle lumen.

The vesicle leiomyoma is identical in both gross and microscopic features to examples of this neoplasm observed in more common locations, such as the uterus (Fig. 4-53). Local excision is curative.

Hemangioma

Hemangioma of the urinary bladder with histologic documentation has been reported in 66 patients.[614-629] An additional 20 cases without histologic documentation were found in literature reviews by Segal and Fink.[614] In subsequent review by Hamsher and associates, Fuleihan and Cordonnier, and Hendry and Vinnicombe, the recorded cases came to 52.[615-617] An additional 14 cases have been reported since 1971.[618-629] Association of bladder hemangiomas with similar vascular neoplasms of the skin and gastrointestinal tract, and examples of the

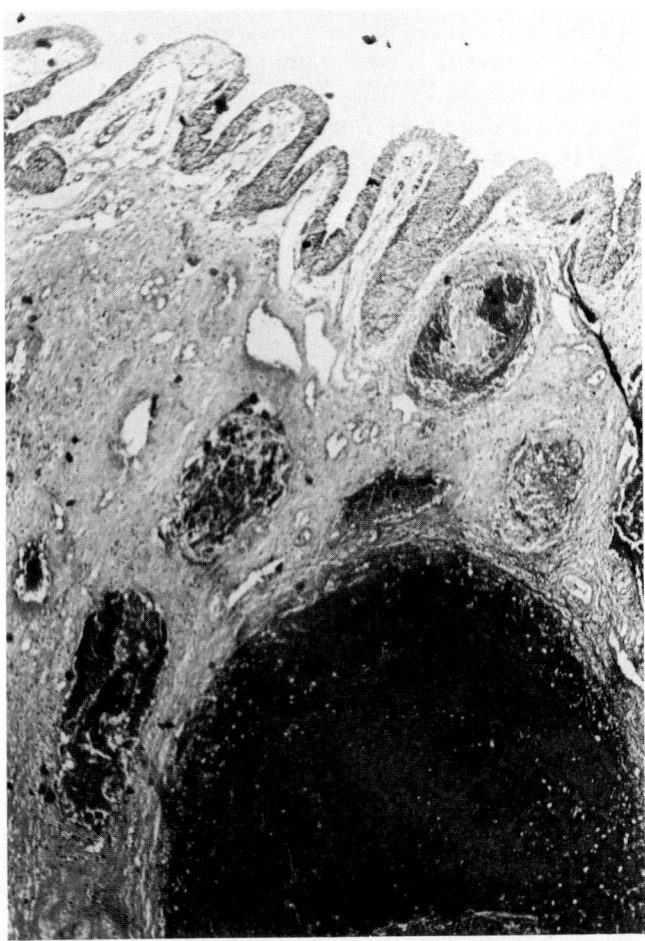

Figure 4-54   *Hemangioma. The numerous vascular channels of this vesical hemangioma are present in the lamina propria of the bladder wall.*

Klippel–Trenaunay syndrome have been documented in more recent reports.[618,622]

Patients range in age from 2 years to 78 years, with 60% younger than 30 years of age. Approximately 60% involve males. Most vesicle hemangiomas present clinically with hematuria and are found to be single nodular lesions on the lateral wall or dome of the bladder. Massive hemorrhage with death by exsanguination rarely has been reported.[613] Biopsy at the time of cystectomy carries with it a significant risk of major hemorrhage.[619,627] Arteriography has been employed as an alternative diagnostic procedure.[620]

The gross and microscopic features of hemangiomas in this unusual location are similar to those observed in more common sites. The majority are cavernous hemangiomas (Fig. 4-54). The most frequent therapy is partial cystectomy, which is curative. Differentiation from angiosarcoma is based on evaluation of the benign cytologic features of the endothelial cells (refer to discussion of angiosarcoma).

Granular Cell Tumor

Seven cases of granular cell tumor originating in the urinary bladder are reported in the literature (Table 4-17).[631-638] A slight female predominance is observed among these patients, who range in age from 23 years to 66 years. Six of the vesical granular cell tumors proved benign as evidenced by the limited follow up. The first reported case by Ravich and associates, involving a 31-year-old man, demonstrated clinical malignant behavior, causing the patient's death within 17 months.[631] Additional cases reported as *granular cell myoblastoma* are most probably examples of vesical rhabdomyosarcomas, in part reflecting the controversial histogenesis of granular cell neoplasms.[630,636,638-640] Evidence based on histochemical and ultrastructural studies has been presented supporting neural, myogenous, and fibroblastic origin of these neoplasms.[636,638-640] The matter remains unresolved, and thus the choice of the descriptively accurate, but histogenetically noncommittal term, *granular cell tumor*.

Morphologically, these neoplasms are generally well-circumscribed, yellowgray, solid tumors composed of the diagnostic polygonal cells with abundant granular, eosinophilic cytoplasm (Fig. 4-55). The central vesicular nuclei show little pleomorphism and no mitotic activity in the typical case. The cells are

Table 4-17   **Granular Cell Tumors**

Author(s)	Year	Age	Sex	Classification	Follow up
Ravich et al[631]	1945	31	M	Malignant	D/T, 17 mo
Andersen, Hoeg[632]	1961	66	M	Benign	A/NED, 3 mo
Seery[634]	1968	31	M	Benign	A/NED, 18 yr
Okuda et al[635]	1969	49	F	Benign	A/NED, 1 yr
Christ, Ozzello[636]	1971	23	F	Benign	No information
Mizutani et al[637]	1973	49	F	Benign	A/NED, 5 yr
Mouradian et al[638]	1974	26	F	Benign	A/NED, 2.2 yr

D/T, dead with tumor; A/NED, alive, no evidence of disease.

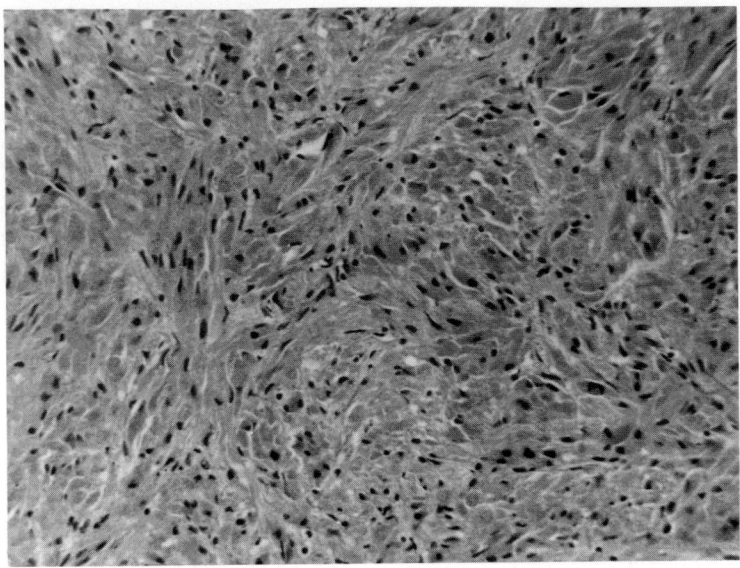

Figure 4-55   *Granular cell tumor. The tumor cells contain relatively small, hyperchromatic nuclei and characteristically abundant eosinophilic granular cytoplasm.*

arranged in irregular nests separated by fibrous or muscular septae. The cytoplasmic granules, deeply eosinophilic on H and E stain, are accentuated by the trichrome and PAS stains.

Conservative surgical therapy has proved adequate for six of the seven reported cases. The one example proving clinically malignant was characterized by greater nuclear pleomorphism, hyperchromaticity, and multinucleation.[631]

Neurofibroma

Bladder neurofibromas are rare, and reported cases are most commonly found in association with other features of neurofibromatosis (von Recklinghausen's disease). Vesicle neurofibromas have been observed in all age groups from infants to the elderly, with a slight male predominance.[641-648] Cameron reviewed 26 previously reported cases in 1964, with occasional cases appearing recorded in the subsequent literature.[645] Clark and co-workers reported an example in a 3-year-old boy and collected previous reports of 14 pediatric patients with vesical neurofibromatosis.[648]

Although some examples are discovered radiologically as incidental findings in asymptomatic patients, the majority present with dysuria, frequency, or hematuria.[645] As noted previously, the majority of bladder neurofibromas are found in patients with von Recklinghausen's disease, and thus neurofibromas and café-au-lait spots accompany the bladder lesion.

The vesical neoplasms present as small intramural nodules or diffuse thickening of the bladder wall. Nodules, measuring millimeters to many centimeters, appear as exophytic smooth nodules, most commonly with an overlying intact urothelial mucosa. The trigone is the site of predilection, but all locations within the bladder have been observed.[645] Associated independent lesions rarely observed within the bladders of patients with neurofibromatosis include diverticula and transitional cell carcinoma.[645]

The microscopic features typical of neurofibromas of the skin are present in the rare cases involving the bladder. Interlacing bundles of delicate spindle cells show focal sites of the characteristic nuclear palisading. Intermingled segments of peripheral nerves arc frequently associated with the neoplastic spindle cells. Microscopic foci with malignant cytologic features have been described in cases reported by de Klerk and Campbell and by Ross, with the latter observing extensive extravesical infiltration and multiple recurrences.[642,643]

In the majority of patients, conservative therapy has proved appropriate, but some patients with concurrent ureteral, prostatic, and urethral involvement require radical cystectomy with urinary diversion.[648]

Miscellaneous Rare Benign Mesenchymal Neoplasms

A single case of ganglioneuroma occurring in the bladder and ureter of a 17-year-old man could be located in the literature.[649] Kracht reported a vesical lipoma removed from a 72-year-old man.[650]

Lymphangioma

Lymphangioma of the urinary bladder has been reported in one patient, a 13-year-old girl who presented with painless hematuria.[651] A partial cystectomy removed a 10 × 5 × 2-cm mass, the bulk of which protruded from the peritoneal aspect of the bladder. The specimen was composed of multiple small cystic cavities filled with proteinaceous fluid. Microscopic features were typical of a cavernous lymphangioma. The patient showed no evidence of recurrence at the time of follow-up examination 1 year after surgery.

Malignant Mesenchymal Neoplasms

Sarcomas of the urinary bladder are uncommon, and are most frequently represented by rhabdomyosarcomas, leiomyosarcomas, or fibrosarcomas, in order of decreasing frequency. Rare examples of other malignant stromal neoplasms are observed, including osteosarcoma, chondrosarcoma, or neoplasms with mixed mesenchymal components (malignant mesenchymomas).

An accurate estimate of the relative frequencies of the histologic forms of sarcoma currently recognized is precluded by the lack of standardization in the nomenclature employed during the 19th and early 20th centuries.[652-654] The descriptive terms applied to mesenchymal neoplasms of all sites at that time suggest a bewildering variety of sarcomas arising in the urinary bladder. The reviews of Wilder, McCrea and Post, and Tripathi and Dick are of historical value, and demonstrate the slow refinement in understanding these malignant neoplasms.[652-654]

Leiomyosarcoma

The first report of a leiomyosarcoma originating in the urinary bladder is attributed to Gusenbauer in 1875.[655] In a comprehensive review of the literature, Silbar and McCrea and Post compiled approximately 40 subsequently recorded cases.[653,657] The cases reported subsequent to, or not included in, the review of McCrea and Post are listed in Table 4-18. A combined total of 83 cases of vesical leiomyosarcoma are reported and serve as a basis for study. A male predominance is observed, with 48 cases (60%) reported in men. No information referable to gender was provided in three patients. The recorded age range is 4 years to 81 years. Fifty-two percent of patients are aged 40 years to 69 years, with 35% of patients younger than 40 years. Most patients present with gross hematuria, with or without dysuria. These neoplasms have been observed in all locations within the bladder, with reported predilection for the trigone or lateral walls.

The pathologic features of bladder leiomyosarcomas are characterized by solid proliferations varying in size from a few to several centimeters. Ulceration of the overlying mucosa is common. The cut surface features as well as the histologic features are typical of leiomyosarcoma in other locations. Nuclear pleomorphism is variable, but generally widespread. Focal areas of hemorrhage and necrosis are not uncommon. All reported cases are of the spindle cell variety, although I have one example of a malignant epithelioid leiomyosarcoma of the urinary bladder in my files. The patient, a woman in the seventh decade, died with widespread intra-abdominal recurrence within 2 years of diagnosis.

Current treatment of leiomyosarcoma of the bladder includes cystectomy with both partial and radical surgical procedures reported in the recent literature.[668,671,672] Adjuvant radiation and chemotherapy appear to have little effect on the outcome of this malignancy. Of the 45 cases reported since the review of McCrea and Post, follow-up information is available on 41 cases. Eleven patients (24%) survived 5 years, and two of these patients subsequently died with tumor recurrence at 6 years and 10 years.[653,658,661,672] Eight patients (18%) died of tumor-related deaths within 5 years of diagnosis and treatment (see Table 4-18). Sixteen patients (36%) were reported alive, with follow-up information fewer than 5 years. Thus, with a total of 45 reported cases, 26 (58%) have no substantive follow-up information.

Rhabdomyosarcoma

Sharing the nomination for major therapeutic advances in pediatric oncology with Wilms' tumor of the kidney, rhabdomyosarcoma of the urinary bladder (and prostate) is currently no longer the invariably rapidly fatal neoplasm it once was.[677,685,686,688,690] The recent progress in combined surgical, radiation, and chemotherapy of genitourinary malignancies of these rare genitourinary malignancies of skeletal muscle has dramatically increased survival of affected patients. The prospective therapy investigations of the Intergroup Rhabdomyosarcoma Study (IRS) deserves much of the credit for these advances.[700]

Rhabdomyosarcoma of the urinary bladder is relatively rare. The majority of the earliest cases were reported as single case studies, which, in combination with occasional small series, have been the subject of comprehensive reviews, by Le-

Table 4-18   *Reported Cases of Leiomyosarcoma not Included in the Literature Review of McRea and Post[653]*

Author(s)	Year	Age	Sex	Follow-up Information
Sadler et al[656]	1954	21	M	A, NED, 2.5 yr
Silbar[657]	1955	20	F	A, NED, 3 yr
Silbar[657]	1955	70	F	A, 1 mo
Silbar[657]	1955	68	M	D, Postoperative
Bohne, et al[659]	1962	37	F	A, NED, 6 mo
Bohne, et al[659]	1962	71	F	D with tumor, 2 mo
Brown[660]	1965	18	F	A, NED, 10 yr
Brown[660]	1965	35	F	A, NED, 4 yr
Reeves[661]	1967	48	F	D with tumor, 6 yr
MacKenzie[662]	1968	59	F	A, NED, 2 mo
MacKenzie[662]	1968	59	F	D with tumor, 4 mo
MacKenzie[662]	1968	68	M	D with tumor, 13 mo
MacKenzie[662]	1968	60	M	A, NED, 7 yr
MacKenzie[662]	1968	69	M	D, Post operative
Tripathi, Dick[663]	1969	NI	NI	NI
Tripathi, Dick[663]	1969	NI	NI	NI
Tripathi, Dick[663]	1969	NI	NI	NI
MacKenzie[664]	1971	7	F	A, NED, 2 yr
MacKenzie[664]	1971	59	M	A, NED, 3 yr
Tara, Mentus[665]	1973	54	F	A, NED, 7 yr
Narayana, et al[706]	1978	57	F	A, 4 yr
Narayana, et al[706]	1978	67	M	D, Postoperative
Narayana, et al[706]	1978	77	M	A, NED, 3 yr
Weitzner[666]	1978	14	F	A, NED, 2 yr
Papacharalambous[667]	1979	63	M	A, NED, 8 mo
Wilson, et al[668]	1979	21	F	A, NED, 2 yr
Savir, Meiraz[669]	1980	62	M	NI
Alabaster, et al[670]	1981	54	M	A, 5 mo
Patterson, Barrett[671]	1983	80	M	D, tumor status ?, 6 mo
Patterson, Barrett[671]	1983	72	M	D with tumor, "shortly thereafter"
Patterson, Barrett[671]	1983	59	F	A, NED, 8 yr
Patterson, Barrett[671]	1983	81	M	D without tumor, 6 mo
Patterson, Barrett[671]	1983	66	M	A, NED, 5 yr
Swartz et al[672]	1985	30	F	A, NED, 9 yr
Swartz et al[672]	1985	19	F	A, NED, 6 yr
Swartz et al[672]	1985	28	F	A, NED, 6 yr
Swartz et al[672]	1985	57	F	A, NED, 5 yr
Swartz et al[672]	1985	55	M	D with tumor, 10 yr
Swartz et al[672]	1985	62	F	D with tumor, 4 yr
Swartz et al[672]	1985	76	M	D with tumor, 2 yr
Swartz et al[672]	1985	59	F	D with tumor, 9 mo
Swartz et al[672]	1985	59	M	D with tumor, 3 mo
Swartz et al[672]	1985	51	M	D, Postoperative, 6 wk
Seo et al[673]	1985	17	M	A, NED, 2 yr*

* Associated with prior cyclophosphamide therapy for Hodgkin's disease.
A, NED — alive, no evidence of disease; A — alive; D — dead.

gier and by MacKenzie and co-workers.[682,688] Tefft and co-workers culled 74 cases of rhabdomyosarcoma of the bladder in children from the literature.[690] An additional 79 cases were found in the more recent literature.[691,693,700,701] Approximately 20 additional examples involving adults have been reported.[685,686,688]

This malignancy is more common in males (approximately 60% of cases). Among children with vesical rhabdomyosarcoma, who as a group constitute 90% of cases, 90% occur before the age of 4 years.[690] These children present with urinary retention and an abdominal mass, with or without hematuria.[690] Cystogram reveals a nonspecific filling defect (Fig. 4-56). At cystoscopy, an edematous polypoid mass is encountered. When a biopsy is done, it will yield the diagnosis.

Historically, this neoplasm has been called myxosarcoma, sarcoma botryoides, rhabdomyosarcoma, and embryonal rhabdomyosarcoma, the last term reflecting the most frequent form of rhabdomyosarcoma encountered in this location. The current classification of skeletal muscle malignancies includes three histologic subtypes: embryonal, alveolar, and pleomorphic rhabdomyosarcomas.[676,702] The typical rhabdomyosarcoma of childhood arising in the urinary bladder appears as an edematous mucosal polypoid mass, likened to a cluster of grapes. When the lesion is small, both the gross features as well as the histologic characteristics superficially resemble polypoid cystitis, and care must be taken not to overlook the features that disclose the true nature of the lesion. When the

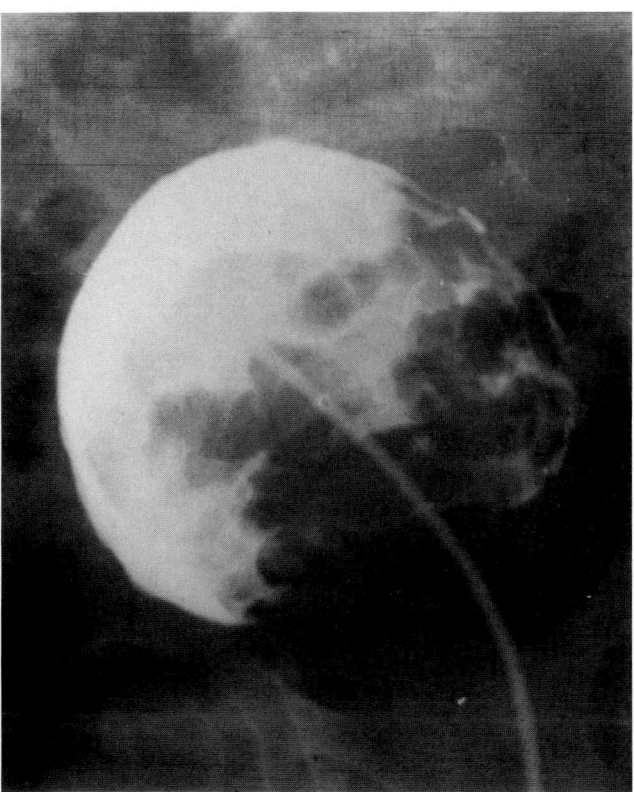

Figure 4-56   *Rhabdomyosarcoma. The cystogram shows a large multilobulated lesion occupying most of the bladder lumen. This appearance is characteristic of rhabdomyosarcoma in children.*

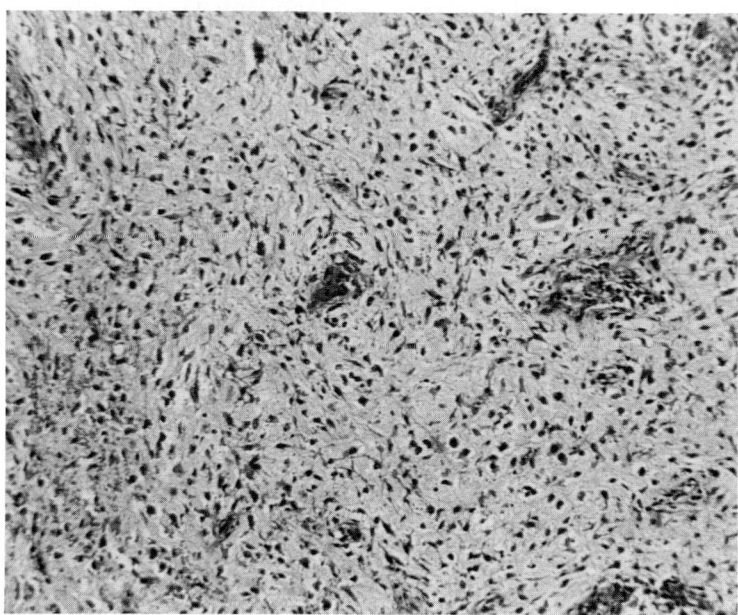

Figure 4-57 *Rhabdomyosarcoma. The stellate, round, and spindle-shaped tumor cells infiltrate an edematous stroma. Nuclei vary in size but are uniformly hyperchromatic.*

tumor is large, the precise origin (bladder or prostate) is difficult to determine. The stroma is edematous and contains the neoplastic rhabdomyoblastic cells in varying density from area to area (Fig. 4-57). A typical feature is a greater concentration of the tumor cells immediately beneath the mucosa, the so-called cambium layer, and also around blood vessels. The nuclei vary in configuration from small and round to large and irregular. The amount of cytoplasm is also variable from virtually none to abundant. Special stains reveal the characteristic cross striations of skeletal muscle-derived cells. In recent years, the increased application of histochemical and immunohistochemical techniques, coupled with electron microscopy, has greatly assisted the surgical pathologist in the reliable

Table 4-19   **Clinical Groups for Rhabdomyosarcoma[694]**

Clinical Group	Extent of Invasion

Group I	Localized disease completely resected
	  No lymph node involvement
	  No 2 organs involved

Group II	A — Grossly resected tumor with microscopic residual tumor
	B — Regional lymph node involvement or contiguous organ involvement no microscopic residual tumor
	C — Regional disease grossly resected, with microscopic residual tumor
Group III	Incompletely resected tumors or biopsy with gross residual disease
Group IV	Metastatic tumor to distant organs

diagnosis of rhabdomyosarcomas in the bladder as well as in more common locations.[695,696,698,702] The demonstration of myoglobin in a tumor apparently devoid of demonstrable cross striations has largely made the debate over such cases moot.

Rhabdomyosarcomas of the urinary bladder and prostate typically show variably extensive bladder wall invasion and local infiltration. The staging of these malignancies has been codified into clinical groups for purposes of investigational studies of therapeutic regimens (Table 4-19). The recent advances in the combined forms of treatment of the sarcomas has resulted in significant increases in survival in both the patient group with localized completely resected, and importantly, the group with incompletely resected tumors.[691,694,700,701]

Fibrosarcoma

The literature records fibrosarcomas originating in the bladder wall, but provides little illustrative histologic documentation and even less clinical information of value. These neoplasms are rare in the bladder. Wilder recorded two previous cases of vesical fibrosarcoma.[703] Because many sarcomas at that time were reported as round cell sarcoma or spindle cell sarcoma, the true number of all types of sarcomas is not known. Fifty years later, McCrea found 19 cases of fibroblastic malignancies arising in the bladder reported under various descriptive names including fibrosarcoma, fibromyxosarcoma, and fibrocellular sarcoma among others.[704] Three additional cases have been found in the literature as reported by Tripathi and Dick, Narayana and associates, and Savir and Meiraz.[705-707]

This sarcoma is most frequent in the first and second decades, with a second group of patients in the sixth to seventh decades.[704] An apparent female predilection is reported.[704] Clinical presentation is not specific for this sarcoma in the bladder. Limited follow-up information is available; however, no patients surviving 5 years could be found in the few reports of bladder fibrosarcoma.

The histologic features of vesical fibrosarcoma are identical to those observed in examples in more typical soft tissue locations.[704-707]

Osteosarcoma and Chondrosarcoma

Bone or cartilage has been observed in a variety of vesical neoplasms, including the following: (1) primary osteosarcomas and chondrosarcomas alone, or in association with an independent carcinoma (collision tumor); (2) sarcomas of mixed differentiation (malignant mesenchymomas); (3) mixed sarcoma mesenchymal and urothelial neoplasms (carcinosarcomas); (4) urothelial carcinomas with malignant mesenchymal differentiation; (5) urothelial carcinomas with osseous metaplasia of the stroma; and (6) in rare examples, extragonadal germ cell tumors (teratomas).[695,709,713,803] (Refer to discussions of malignant mesenchymoma, carcinosarcoma, and germ cell tumors.)

Bone and cartilage within bladder neoplasms, either as a neoplastic or metaplastic component, is distinctly rare. Pang published the most complete review of previously reported cases.[710] Only scattered examples have appeared in the literature in subsequent years.[695] The majority of bone or cartilage-containing neoplasms take the form of carcinosarcomas or collision tumors (refer to the respective sections). The ability of urothelial proliferations to initiate osseous metaplasia of the stroma has been demonstrated in both vesical neoplasms, as reported by Pang, and experimentally as demonstrated by Huggins.[708,710] The pathogenesis of this bone formation is unknown.

The diagnosis of osteosarcoma or chondrosarcoma of the urinary bladder requires the osseous and chrondromatous components to be neoplastic and malignant, and differentiated from metaplastic stromal osteoid, chondroid, bone, or cartilage. This distinction rests on the cytologic characteristics of the osteocytes and chondrocytes that participate in the formation of these heterologous components.

Malignant Mesenchymoma

In 1950, Jones and Ross reported an example of a mixed sarcoma exhibiting areas of leiomyosarcoma, osteosarcoma, and chondrosarcoma in the urinary bladder of a 44-year-old woman.[713] The authors reported the case as an example of an osteogenic leiomyosarcoma. This malignancy satisfies the criteria for neoplasms currently termed malignant mesenchymomas.[712,714] No similar cases were found in the literature.

Miscellaneous Neoplasms

Pheochromocytoma

Extra-adrenal pheochromocytomas originate most commonly in the organ of Zuckerkandl and other sites along the cervical, thoracic, and abdominal paraganglia. In addition, collections of chromaffin cells are found in the abdomen and scrotum and compose the visceral autonomic paraganglia. Pheochromocytomas arising in the urinary bladder originate from chromaffin cells of visceral autonomic paraganglia located within the wall of this organ. A total of 119 reported cases of pheochromocytoma (paraganglioma) of the urinary bladder could be found in the literature.[715-753] Zimmerman and associates reported the first case in 1953.[715] Leestma and Price found 34 previously reported cases, and presented the single largest reported series (24 cases).[727] Ochi and co-workers collected 80 reported cases, and Das and co-workers brought the total to 100 cases.[747,751] An additional 19 cases have been found in the literature, bringing the total to 119 reported cases.[717,740,745,747–749,752,753]

Vesical pheochromocytomas are more common in females (59%) than in males. The age range of the reported cases is 11 years to 78 years with a median patient age in the fourth decade.[747,751] There is a progressive decrease in frequency with increasing age, with only 30% of patients 50 years and older (Table 4-20).

Patients present with symptoms and signs referable both to the vesicle neoplasm and to the excess catecholamines elaborated by the pheochromocytes. Sixty-five percent evidence systemic hypertension.[751] Hypertensive crisis may be experienced during surgical biopsy and resection procedures, and pose an ominous threat for which appropriate precautions must be taken in managing these patients. A history of headaches, palpitations, blurred vision, and sweating temporally related to micturition is common.[751,753] Dysuria and pelvic pain are uncommon, but hematuria is observed in approximately 60% of cases.[751] Less than 20% of vesical pheochromocytomas are hormonally inactive.[751,753] Assay of serum and urine vanillylmandelic acid (VMA) will demonstrate significant elevations in the majority of patients.

At cystoscopy, intramural pheochromocytomas sufficiently large to produce a visible mass appear as a submucosal lesion covered by an intact urothelium. Tumors range in size from a few millimeters to 13 cm, and are most common in the dome and trigone areas.[751] A cauliflower or multinodular mass has been observed in some patients.

Pathologic Features

The cut surface of the resected intramural mass is pink-gray. The neoplasm's color is observed to change characteristically to brown following fixation in formalin.[727] A more reliable test for pheochromocytoma is a brown color developing within 30 minutes following immersion in 10% Zenker's fixative, dichromate solution, or 10% potassium iodate.[727] A white fluorescence is observed following 2 hours of immersion of a frozen section in buffered-formal calcium.[727] Alternatively, formalin-fixed sections may be stained with Fontana–Masson. This procedure is not entirely reliable and may result in false-negative staining results.[727]

Microscopically, the histologic pattern is typified by the characteristic *zellballen* or nests of tumor cells separated by thin fibrovascular septae. Areas of cords or sheets are not uncommon. These neoplasms infiltrate the adjacent muscle and lamina propria of the bladder wall in most examples. Less frequently, some reported cases have been described as sharply circumscribed. The neoplasm is well vascularized and there is a tendency for increased call density to be found in perivascular locations. The tumor cells are polygonal and possess abundant eosinophilic cytoplasm. The oval to round nucleus typically is centrally located, but may be eccentric in location. Nuclear pleomorphism is common, and scattered markedly enlarged, bizarre cells are not uncommon. The nuclei have coarse peripheral chromatin and one or two nucleoli are observed. Focal areas of hemorrhage and necrosis may be observed in pheochromocytomas. Mitosis may be found, but is usually not prominent. None of these features has any reliable

Table 4-20   **Age Distribution of Reported Cases of Pheochromocytoma**

Age (Years)	No. of Cases (%)
10–19	27 (23%)
20–29	23 (20%)
30–39	19 (16%)
40–49	17 (15%)
50–59	18 (15%)
60–69	13 (11%)
70–79	5 (4%)

relationship to clinical behavior. The only reliable criterion of malignancy is the presence of metastates. In some cases even this criterion has proven difficult to apply, as extra vesical pheochromocytoma masses may represent multifocal occurrence of this neoplasm.[751]

Of the 119 reported cases of vesical pheochromocytoma, malignant behavior has been recorded in only 16 patients (13%) (Table 4-21). The age and sex distribution of patients with malignant vesical pheochromocytoma is not significantly different from all other patients with clinically benign tumors. Seventy-five percent of the reported cases of malignant pheochromocytoma were diagnosed in patients younger than 40 years of age. Evidence of malignancy may only become apparent as recurrences diagnosed years after surgical resection of the bladder primary. The true frequency of clinically malignant vesical pheochromocytomas may not be known accurately because the follow-up duration of the majority of reported cases may be too short (51% of all cases have been reported since 1971). In view of the occasional recurrences observed after prolonged symptom-free intervals, protracted follow up of patients with periodic monitoring of blood pressure and serum VMA is appropriate.

Table 4-21   **Reported Cases of Malignant Pheochromocytoma**

Author(s)	Year	Age	Sex	Therapy	Follow-up Information
Lumb, Gresham[716]	1958	48	F	Surgical excision	Recurrent hypertension, 7 yr*
Farley, Smith[718]	1959	16	F	Hemicystectomy	A-NED; NI†
Scott, Eversole[719]	1960	14	M	Radical cystectomy, prostatectomy	Recurrence discovered 14 yr later at dx of renal cell carcinoma‡
Pugh[717]	1958	NI	F	Cystoscopy	Dead post-op; liver, node metastases at autopsy
Pugh[720]	1960	36	F	Cystoscopy	Dead post-op; liver, node metastases at autopsy
Moloncy et al[722]	1966	26	M	Segmented resection	Lung mets, 4 mo; bone mets
Higgins, Tresiddes[723]	1966	14	M	Partial cystectomy	Bladder recurrence, 9 yr later§
Shimbo, Nakano[729]	1974	20	F	Surgery	Metastases at autopsy 4 yr later
Campbell et al[730]	1974	20	F	Partial cystectomy	A-NED 2 yr (bladder, adrenal)
Javaheri, Raafat[732]	1975	44	M	Partial cystectomy and nodes	Dead, 1 yr
Javaheri, Raafat[732]	1975	24	F	Partial cystectomy and nodes	A-NED, 1 yr
Raju et al[737]	1977	18	F	None	Dead preoperatively; pleural metastasis at autopsy
Lang et al[736]	1977	34	M	Multiple surgical resections	Multiple recurrences
Meyer et al[741]	1979	12	F	Segmental cystectomy	A-NED, 2 yr
Flanigan et al[744]	1980	56	M	Radical cystoprostatectomy	Lymph node metastases at surgery; A-NED, 1 yr
Das, Lowe[743]	1980	36	M	Partial cystectomy	Lymph node metastases after 1 yr; A-NED, 2 yr

* Eight-year follow up[724]

† "Metastasis" at bifurcation of hypogastric vessels, or separate pheochromocytoma is unsettled.

‡ Metastatic recurrence[733]

§ Bladder recurrence adherent to posterior symphysis[723]

Plasmacytoma

Extramedullary plasmacytomas originating in the urinary bladder have been reported in five patients (four men and one woman).[754-758] The patients ranged in age from 39 years to 78 years (mean 54 years). There was no evidence of multiple myeloma in any of the patients at the time of diagnosis of the bladder tumor. Local suprapubic recurrence was reported by Gorfain, and Yang and co-workers observed metastatic involvement in regional pelvic lymph nodes.[755,758] Treatment varied, and included subtotal cystectomy, radiation, and chemotherapy. Follow-up information is scanty, but the patient reported by Yang and associates was alive without evidence of recurrence 12 years after diagnosis.[758] As is important for all patients with extramedullary plasmacytomas, regardless of location, close follow up for subsequent systemic involvement is obligatory.

Pathologic Features

Plasmacytoma of the urinary bladder is characterized by a monotonous proliferation of plasma cells of variable differentiation. Immature plasma cells predominate. Occasional mitoses are observed. The plasma cell tumor produces a smooth intramural nodule occupying the lamina propria in biopsies (Fig. 4-58). The characteristic eccentric nucleus, perinuclear halo, and amphophilic cytoplasm identifies the plasma cells (Fig. 4-59). The immaturity of the cells is identified by multinucleation chromatin clumping and nuclear pleomorphism. Assisting in the diagnosis of plasmacytoma are immunoperoxidase stains for immunoglobulins. Plasmacytomas must be distinguished from rare examples of plasma cell

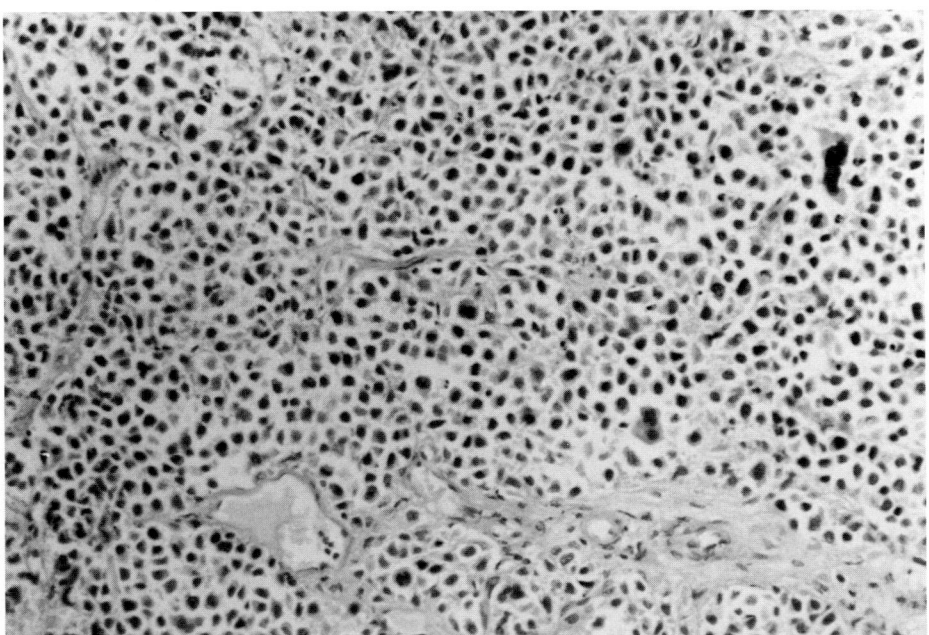

Figure 4-58   *Plasmacytoma. This intramural lesion is composed exclusively of atypical plasma cells invading the stroma. Occasional multinucleated and bizarre cells are present.*

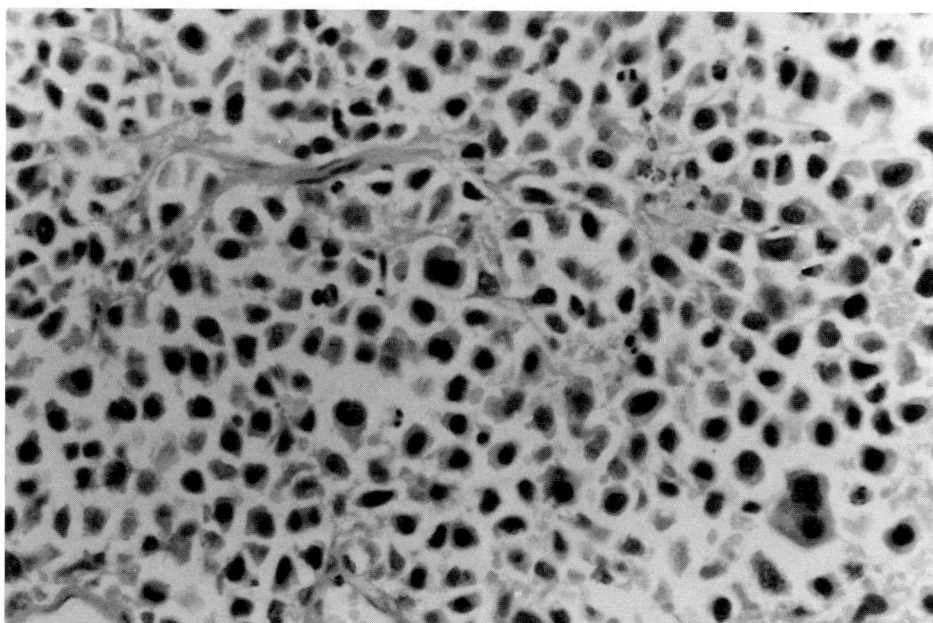

Figure 4-59   *Plasmacytoma. Higher magnification shows the typical cytologic features of plasma cell malignancy. The uniformly hyperchromatic and irregular nuclei are most commonly found eccentrically located within the cell.*

granulomas, an inflammatory lesion that on rare occasions has been reported in the urinary tract, including the urinary bladder (refer to discussion of plasma cell granulomas in this chapter).

The five cases of extramedullary plasmacytomas originating in the urinary bladder contrast with eight cases reported in the kidney and eight arising in the testis, all without evidence of concurrent multiple myeloma (refer to corresponding chapters).

Primary Malignant Lymphoma

Approximately 45 cases of primary malignant lymphoma of the urinary bladder have been reported in the literature.[759-769] Patients most commonly present with hematuria.[760] Cystoscopy typically discloses a single exophytic nodule in the trigone region.[760] Less frequently, multiple nodules are present. Most cases in the past have been treated with segmental resection. Radiation therapy has been employed either as an adjunct or alone.[766]

The diagnosis of primary malignant lymphoma in the urinary bladder requires the obligatory exclusion of systemic lymphoma with bladder involvement. Subsequent to definitive therapy for the bladder lesion, no evidence of systemic involvement for a minimal period of 2 years is required to exclude the possibility of secondary bladder involvement by a malignant lymphoma. The reported cases with sufficient follow up suggest that primary vesical lymphoma is associated with a significantly better prognosis than secondary lymphoma of the bladder.[770] Several cases document 5- and 10-year survival following either surgical or radiation therapy.[760-762,765]

The diagnosis is established by microscopic examination of biopsy fragments of the neoplasm. The frequency of non-Hodgkin's lymphoma exceeds cases of Hodgkin's disease among the examples of primary vesical lymphoma reported in the literature.[759,760,765,766]

Systemic Malignant Lymphoma and Leukemia

Vesical involvement in disseminated extramedullary leukemic infiltration is relatively uncommon, and when present is almost invariably detected only at autopsy.[770] Givler reported that 15.5% of a large series of chronic lymphocytic and chronic myelogenous leukemia patients showed bladder involvement.[770] Patients dying of acute leukemia evidenced bladder involvement slightly more frequently (25.8%).[770] Clinically significant leukemic involvement is distinctly uncommon.[770] Similarly, disseminated malignant lymphoma demonstrates a relatively low frequency of bladder involvement at autopsy, and only rarely is such infiltration detected clinically.[770,771] Non-Hodgkin's lymphoma is consistently observed to involve the bladder more frequently than Hodgkin's disease.[770-772] When clinically apparent, hematuria is the most frequent manifestation.[770-772] Vesical involvement by either malignant lymphoma or leukemia is microscopic in most cases, with only uncommon examples grossly apparent.[770-772] There is no intravesical site of predilection. Multiple foci of infiltration are most common. The uniformity of the cell infiltrate, which is identical to the malignant cell type present in other organs and is established by prior diagnosis, clarifies the nature of the vesical infiltrate.

Mixed Cell Type Neoplasms

Carcinosarcoma

Carcinosarcomas of the urinary bladder are rare malignant neoplasms containing both mesenchymal and epithelial components. These neoplasms must be distinguished from collision tumors and poorly differentiated transitional cell carcinomas showing a spindle cell morphology. Collision tumors actually represent two separate malignancies developing in proximity, with an admixture of their respective epithelial and mesenchymal components in areas of mutual interface. Spindle cell change in an otherwise obvious carcinoma is entirely epithelial in origin, the superficial resemblance of the spindle cell areas to sarcomas notwithstanding.[799]

The classification by Meyers with later modification by Willis has served as the histogenetic explanation of these complex neoplasms.[773,777] Meyers proposed three categories of carcinosarcomas: composition tumors, combination tumors, and collision tumors.[773] Willis objected to the inclusion of collision tumors, and proposed that carcinosarcomas arise as a result of either simultaneous neoplastic transformation of two distinct cell types (in one organ site), or neoplastic transformation of the stroma of a carcinoma.[777] This modification has not been universally accepted, as indicated by the continued reporting of collision tumors as examples of carcinosarcomas (refer to discussion of collision tumors).

The number of reported cases of vesical carcinosarcomas is difficult to quantitate confidently, because many reports lack the requisite details allowing confirmation of their carcinosarcomatous nature.[775,781] Other studies providing adequate details indicate that collision tumors, spindle cell carcinomas as well as examples of vesical teratomatous (germ cell) neoplasms, and extrarenal Wilms' tumors have been incorrectly regarded as carcinosarcomas.[785,811]

Table 4-22   **Carcinosarcoma of the Urinary Bladder**

Author(s)	Year	Age	Sex	Epithelial Component*	Stromal Component
Arnold[776]	1941	43	F	SCC	Undifferentiated, chondrosarcoma
Willis[777]	1950	74	M	TCC	Osteosarcoma
Quilter[778]	1956	21	M	AC	Chondrosarcoma, osteosarcoma
Pang[779]	1958	74	M	TCC	Chondrosarcoma, osteosarcoma
Pang[779]	1958	74	M	TCC	Osteosarcoma
Baranyai, Goracz[780]	1959	59	M	SCC	Rhabdomyosarcoma
Nicolai, Spjut[781]	1959	66	F	SCC	Chondrosarcoma
Fruhling et al[782]	1959	71	M	TCC	Chondrosarcoma
Fruhling et al[782]	1959	65	F	TCC	Fibrosarcoma
Fruhling et al[782]	1959	73	F	TCC	Chondrosarcoma
Fruhling et al[782]	1959	61	M	TCC	Fibrosarcoma
Fruhling et al[782]	1959	47	M	TCC	Fibrosarcoma
Thompson, Coppridge[783]	1959	43	M	SCC	Undifferentiated sarcoma
Thompson, Coppridge[783]	1959	56	M	TCC	Leiomyosarcoma
Thompson, Coppridge[783]	1959	71	F	TCC	Osteosarcoma
Brinton et al[785]	1970	50	M	MC	"Spindle cell sarcoma"
Holtz et al[787]	1972	56	M	MC	Chondrosarcoma, osteosarcoma, rhabdomyosarcoma
Holtz et al[787]	1972	71	M	UC	Chondrosarcoma, osteosarcoma, rhabdomyosarcoma
Holtz et al[787]	1972	79	M	TCC	Undifferentiated sarcoma
Holtz et al[787]	1972	43	M	TCC	Leiomyosarcoma
Delides[788]	1972	82	M	UC	Chondrosarcoma
Delides[788]	1972	56	M	TCC	Chondrosarcoma, osteosarcoma
Shivde, Kherdekar[789]	1973	60	M	SCC	Undifferentiated sarcoma
McCarthy et al[790]	1975	77	F	AC	Chondrosarcoma, osteosarcoma
Patterson, Dale[791]	1976	36	M	TCC	Chondrosarcoma, osteosarcoma
Johansen et al[792]	1979	64	M	AC	Rhabdomyosarcoma
Schoborg et al[793]	1980	71	F	SCC	Rhabdomyosarcoma
Schoborg et al[793]	1980	74	F	UC	Rhabdomyosarcoma
Figueiredo et al[796]	1982	81	M	TCC	Leiomyosarcoma
Figueiredo et al[796]	1982	79	M	TCC	Chondrosarcoma
Smith et al[797]	1983	67	M	SCC	Chondrosarcoma
Smith et al[797]	1983	51	M	SCC	Chondrosarcoma, osteosarcoma
Kusaba et al[798]	1984	34	M	AC	Rhabdomyosarcoma

* TCC, transitional cell carcinoma; SCC, squamous cell carcinoma; AC, adenocarcinoma; MC, mixed carcinoma; UC, undifferentiated carcinoma

A review of the early literature located 33 acceptable examples of vesical carcinosarcomas (Table 4-22). (Refer to following discussions of collision tumors and vesical germ cell tumors.)

The 33 reported examples of carcinosarcoma of the urinary bladder involved patients aged 21 years to 82 years, with a mean age of 60 years, and 75% diagnosed in the sixth to eighth decades. Seventy-five percent of these cases involved men. Patients most commonly present with hematuria. A bulky exophytic neoplasm is detected in cystograms and at cystoscopy. Treatment has most frequently included radical surgery with adjunct radiation and chemotherapy employed in the most recent reports. The provided follow-up information is often of limited duration, but most patients succumb to local recurrence and distant metastases within 3 years of cystectomy. I am aware of only two patients living 3 years, and none living beyond 5 years.[788,793]

Pathologic Features

Carcinosarcomas of the urinary bladder are invariably large bulky masses, with evident surface ulceration, extensive necrosis, and deep invasion of the bladder wall. The most frequent epithelial component is transitional cell carcinoma, with fewer examples of squamous cell carcinoma, adenocarcinoma, mixed carcinoma, or undifferentiated carcinoma (see Table 4-22). The sarcomatous component most commonly evidences chondroid or osteosarcomatous differentiation. Less frequently, rhabdomyosarcomatous, fibrosarcomatous, leiomyosarcomatous, or undifferentiated sarcoma is reported. Holtz and associates reported two cases with osteogenic, chondrosarcoma, and rhabdomyosarcoma components (equivalent to malignant mesenchymoma).[787]

The frequency with which epithelial neoplasms affect a chondroid metaplasia of the tumor stroma, a capability of urothelium observed under experimental circumstances, requires its distinction from true carcinosarcomatous neoplasms with malignant stromal components.[774] As noted previously, carcinosarcomas also must be differentiated from collision tumors and transitional cell carcinomas with spindle cell change. The distinction is difficult in some cases, and is assisted by detailed examination of the gross specimen, adequate histologic sampling of the neoplasm, and ultrastructural study of the stromal components. Future histochemical studies of these tumors employing methods to detect keratin, vimentin, desmin, myosin, and other antigenic substances undoubtedly will prove of value.[795] Such improvements in technology may assist in distinguishing epithelial malignancies with spindle cell change from carcinosarcomas. Fromowitz and co-workers have proposed that these malignancies are indeed of epithelial origin.[799] Methodology to separate vesical carcinosarcoma resulting from dual differentiation of a single undifferentiated transformed cell, and from concomitant malignant transformation of two cell types is a future challenge. (Refer to discussion of collision tumors.)

Collision Tumors

The independent occurrence of two malignant neoplasms in close proximity, one of mesenchymal origin and the other of epithelial derivation, is termed *collision tumor*. Examples of collision tumors have been observed in the gastrointestinal, genital, and urinary tracts. Those within the urinary tract are most commonly observed in the urinary bladder, followed by the kidney and renal pelvis (refer to Chap. 1).

Regardless of their site of origin, they are frequently reported as examples of carcinosarcomas according to the classification of Meyer.[773] Willis correctly excluded collision tumors from carcinosarcomas, the latter representing a single neoplasm with dual mesenchymal and epithelial differentiation.[784] The correct term for these neoplasms is "collision tumors," because they indeed represent the improbable chance occurrence of two independent neoplastic entities that have no recognized common causal factors or other mutual influence or relationship other than close proximity. In some instances, their proximity may result in the contiguous infiltrations and invasion of one neoplasm by the other. The presence and extent of the tumor collision are related to the degree of difficulty of distinguishing a true carcinosarcoma from collision tumors.

The histologic composition of metastases from carcinosarcomas may be either exclusively mesenchymal or epithelial, or alternatively, a mixture of both components. Thus, the duality of the primary neoplasm may not be confirmed by the composition of metastases from carcinosarcomas. This being true of carcinosarcomas, it is obvious that the histologic composition of metastases may not be applied to support or to militate against the diagnosis of collision tumors.

Reported cases of collision tumors arising in the urinary bladder are presented in Table 4-23. The patients range in age from 52 years to 82 years with a median age in the seventh decade. Vesical collision tumors are more common in males (69%). The epithelial neoplasm is transitional cell carcinoma in virtually all cases. Seventy-seven percent of the cases are represented by concomitant leiomyosarcomas, with the remaining represented by fibrosarcomas and one case of osteosarcoma. These 13 cases represent published examples that are supported by sufficient detail to support the diagnosis of collision tumors.[800-807] The earlier

Table 4-23   *Collision Tumors of the Urinary Bladder*

Author(s)	Year	Age	Sex	Epithelial Neoplasm*	Mesenchymal Neoplasm
Balogh[800]	1947	59	F	Carcinoma, NOS	Fibrosarcoma
Mackles et al[801]	1948	52	M	TCC	Leiomyosarcoma
Dent[802]	1955	82	F	TCC	Leiomyosarcoma
Powers et al[803]	1956	79	M	TCC	Osteosarcoma
Fruhling et al[804]	1959	66	M	TCC	Fibrosarcoma
Fruhling et al[804]	1959	53	M	TCC	Leiomyosarcoma
Fruhling et al[804]	1959	64	M	TCC	Leiomyosarcoma
Fruhling et al[804]	1959	66	M	TCC	Leiomyosarcoma
Fruhling et al[804]	1959	63	F	TCC	Leiomyosarcoma
Hejtmancik, Klatt[805]	1960	74	M	TCC	Leiomyosarcoma
Holtz et al[806]	1972	71	F	TCC	Leiomyosarcoma
Holtz et al[806]	1972	67	M	TCC, SCC, AC	Leiomyosarcoma
Kishi et al[807]	1977	61	M	TCC	Leiomyosarcoma

* NOS, not otherwise specified; TCC, transitional cell carcinoma; SCC, squamous cell carcinoma; AC, adenocarcinoma

literature includes a number of published cases, frequently under the title of *carcinosarcoma,* that do not provide sufficient information to determine whether they represent true carcinosarcomas, collision tumors, or poorly differentiated transitional cell carcinomas that evidence a prominent spindle cell component, and are therefore exclusively epithelial neoplasms.[775]

In the background of all this histogenetic hairsplitting, it should be mentioned that the ultimate prognosis of all patients with carcinosarcoma, collision tumors, or transitional cell carcinomas with spindle cell change is uniformly poor. I am unaware of any reported patient with collision tumors of the urinary bladder surviving 5 years.

Germ Cell Neoplasms

Eight acceptable extragonadal germ cell tumors arising in the urinary bladder are reported in the literature.[808-810,812-816] The case reported by Pollack as a teratocarcinoma of the bladder most probably represents an extrarenal Wilms' tumor occurring in an adult (72-year-old man).[811] Of the more convincing cases, four are choriocarcinomas, three are teratomatous, and one represents an extragonadal endodermal sinus tumor (yolk-sac tumor). The rarity of these cases precludes generalizations referable to clinical characteristics. The pathologic features of each of these neoplasms are discussed in Chapter 6. "Mis-migration" of germ cells during embryologic development is the generally accepted histogenetic explanation of extragonadal germ cell tumors (refer to discussion of extragonadal germ cell tumors of the kidney in Chap. 1).

Metastatic Malignancies

The overall frequency of metastases to the urinary bladder as observed at autopsy is less than 5%.[817,819,823,825] The most common primary carcinomas disseminat-

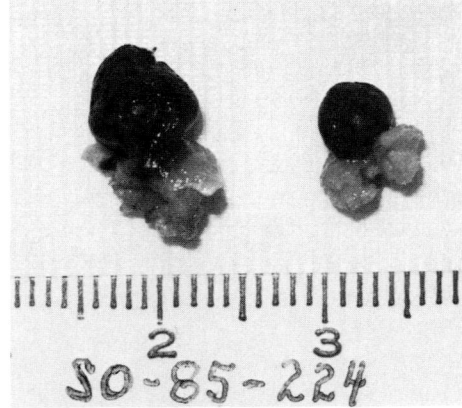

Figure 4-60   *Metastatic malignant melanoma. This black exophytic mucosal nodule has been bisected. On histologic review, it was found to be composed of cytologically malignant melanocytes metastatic from a shoulder lesion.*

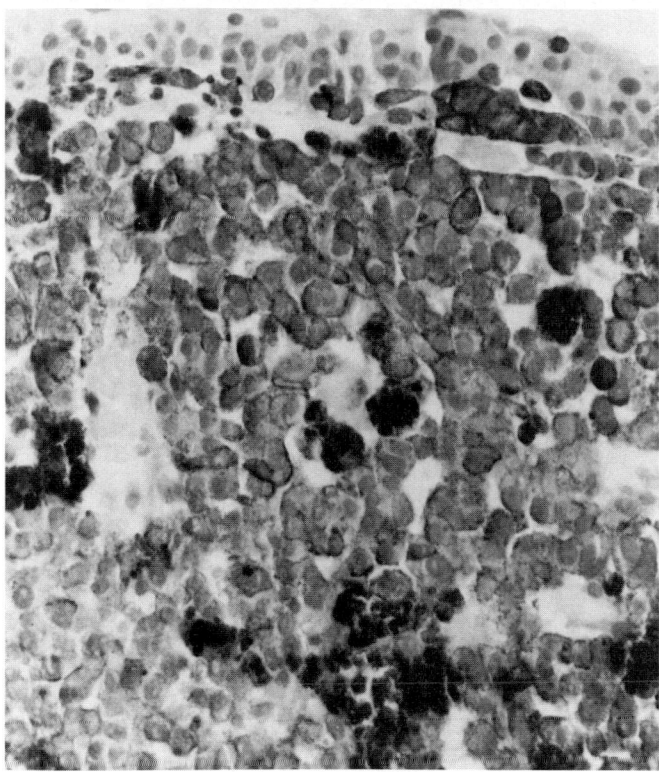

Figure 4-61   *Metastatic malignant melanoma. The heavily pigmented melanocytes found in the gross lesion shown in Figure 4-60 are observed to invade the overlying urothelium focally.*

ing to the bladder are skin (malignant melanoma), stomach, breast, and lung, in order of decreasing frequency.[817,819,820,823,825] Rare examples of distant metastases from renal cell carcinoma, squamous cell carcinoma of the tongue, and carcinoma of the breast and pancreas are reported.[824–826,829] Contiguous spread to the bladder from malignancies of adjacent organs including prostate, cervix, and uterine corpus are far more frequent.

The majority of reported bladder metastases are clinically silent and are discovered only at autopsy. Only rarely does a metastatic lesion in the bladder produce gross hematuria requiring surgical intervention.

In most instances, metastatic involvement of the urinary bladder is a manifestation of more generalized metastases, and thus tends to occur late in the clinical progression of the malignancy.

The metastases of malignant melanoma to the urinary bladder produce characteristic pigmented, brown-black nodules when observed at cystoscopy (Fig. 4-60, 4-61).[818,823,827,830,831] In rare cases, the metastatic tumor burden is of such magnitude that sufficient breakdown products of melanin pigment result in darkening of the urine.[821,822] Such urinary melanin pigment can be identified by chromatography.[821,822]

Urothelial malignancies of the urinary bladder found in association with renal pelvic or ureteral transitional cell carcinomas are regarded as examples of multifocal neoplastic transformation and not as downstream metastases. The latter most probably can occur, especially subsequent to instrumentation, but this is difficult to prove. Downstream implantation metastases of renal cell carcinoma have been reported.[828]

References

Normal Structure

1. Woodburne RT: Anatomy of the bladder and bladder outlet. J Urol 100:474, 1968
2. Gyllensten L: Contribution to the embryology of the human bladder. Part I. The development of the definitive relations between the openings of the Wolffian ducts and the ureters. Acta Anat (Basel) 7:305, 1949
3. Lich R, Howerton LW, Amin M: Anatomy and surgical approach to the urogenital tract in the male. In Harrison JH, Gittes RF, Permutter AD et al (eds): Urology, 4th ed, p 3. Philadelphia, WB Saunders, 1978
4. Muecke EC: The embryology of the urinary tract. In Harrison JH, Gittes RF, Permutter AD et al (eds): Urology, 4th ed, p 1286. Philadelphia, WB Saunders, 1979
5. Moore, KL: The Urogenital System in the Developing Human. Clinically Oriented Embryology, 3rd ed. Philadelphia, WB Saunders, 1982

Congenital Malformations

6. Abrahamson J: Double bladder and related anomalies: Clinical and embryological aspects and a case report. Br J Urol 33:195, 1961
7. Uhlir K: Rare malformations of the bladder. J Urol 99:53, 1968
8. Campbell MF: Embryology and anomalies of the urogenital tract. In Campbell MF, Harrison JH (eds): Urology, 3rd ed. Philadelphia, WB Saunders, 1970
9. Muecke EC: Extrophy, epispadias, and other anomalies of the bladder. IN Harrison JH, Gittes RF, Perlmutter AD et al (eds): Urology, 4th ed, p 1443. Philadelphia, WB Saunders, 1979

Exstrophy

10. Formiggini B: Contributo allo studio della mucosa vesicale extrofica. Riforma Med 36:252, 1920
11. Culp DA: The histology of the exstrophied bladder. J Urol 91:538, 1964
12. Lattimer JK, Smith MJV: Exstrophy closure: A follow-up of 70 cases. J Urol 95:356, 1966
13. Engel RM, Wilkinson HA: Bladder exstrophy. J Urol 104:699, 1970
14. Rudin L, Tannenbaum M, Lattimer JK: Histologic analysis of the exstrophied bladder after anatomical closure. J Urol 108:802, 1972

Malignancy Complicating Exstrophy

15. Montpellier, Goinard P, Karsent, Mele: Extrophie vessicale compliquée de cancer. J Urol (Paris) 39:493, 1935
16. McCown PE: Carcinoma in exstrophy of the bladder. J Urol 43:533, 1940
17. Graham WH: Exstrophy of the bladder complicated by adenocarcinoma, with review of the literature. Br J Surg 30:23, 1942
18. Abeshouse BS: Exstrophy of the bladder complicated by adenocarcinoma of the bladder and renal calculi. A report of a case and review of the literature. J Urol 49:259, 1943
19. Etherington–Wilson W: Primary carcinoma of an ectopic bladder; and primary benign papillomata of the ureter. Br J Urol 8:62, 1945
20. Reid WC, Wescott GW, Summers JE: Carcinoma in exstrophy of the bladder. Am J Surg 75:601, 1948

21. Lange MJ: Un cas de cancer développé sur une vessie exstrophiée et traité par excision et implantation d'aiguilles de radium. J Urol Med Chir 54:183, 1948
22. Comar OB: Extrofia vesicale concerizzata. Gior Ital Chir 6:413, 1950
23. Davidson JA: Report of three cases of carcinoma occurring in exstrophy of the bladder. Urol Cutan Rev 54:206, 1950
24. Goyanna R, Emmett JL, McDonald JR: Exstrophy of the bladder complicated by adenocarcinoma. J Urol 65:391, 1951
25. Bunge RG: Podophyllin in treatment of human adenocarcinoma of bladder. J Urol 68:475, 1952
26. Sanchez RP: Extrofia vesical degenerada. Dos casos personales. J Int Coll Surg 17:528, 1952
27. Wheeler JD, Hill WT: Adenocarcinoma of urinary bladder. Cancer 7:125, 1954
28. Martinez–Peneiro JA: Exstrofia vesical completa. Complicada con adenocarcinoma. Rev Clin Esp 54:353, 1954
29. Mostofi FK, Thompson RV, Dean AL: Mucous adenocarcinoma of urinary bladder. Cancer 8:741, 1955
30. McIntosh JF, Worley G Jr: Adenocarcinoma arising in exstrophy of the bladder: Report of two cases and review of the literature. J Urol 73:820, 1955
31. Scott LS, Sorbie C: The development of carcinoma in an ectopic bladder. Br J Urol 28:264, 1956
32. Staubitz WJ, Oberkircher OJ, Lent MH: Cancer in exstrophy of the bladder. NY J Med 56:386, 1956
33. Wattenberg CA, Beare JB, Tormey AR Jr: Exstrophy of the urinary bladder complicated by adenocarcinoma. J Urol 76:583, 1956
34. Sayeth ES, Ishak KG; Adenocarcinoma associated with schistosomiasis in ectopia vesicae. Br J Surg 44:426, 1957
35. Cordonnier JJ, Spjut HJ: Vesical exstrophy and transitional cell carcinoma and unusual longevity after ureterosignoidostomy. J Urol 78:242, 1957
36. Stuart WT: Carcinoma of the bladder associated with exstrophy. Report of a case and review of the literature. Va Med Mon 89:39, 1962
37. Marshall VF, Muecke EC: Variations in exstrophy of the bladder. J Urol 88:766, 1962
38. Chelloul N, Gubler J–P, Jouannelle A et al: Les tumerus sur exstrophie vesicale. Bull du Cancer 54:447, 1967
39. O'Kane HOJ, Megaw JMcI: Carcinoma in the exstrophic bladder. Br J Surg 55:631, 1968
40. Engel RM, Wilkinson HA: Bladder exstrophy. J Urol 104:699, 1970
41. Semerdjian HS, Texter JH Jr, Yawn DH: Rhabdomyosarcoma occurring in repaired exstrophied bladder: A case report. J Urol 108:354, 1972
42. Kandzari SJ, Majid A, Ortega AM et al: Exstrophy of urinary bladder. Complicated by adenocarcinoma. Urol 3:496, 1974
43. Daroca Jr PJ, Mackenzie F, Reed RJ et al: Primary adenovillous carcinoma of the bladder. J Urol 115:41, 1976
44. Jacobo E, Loening S, Schmidt JD et al: Primary adenocarcinoma of the bladder: A retrospective study of 20 patients. J Urol 117:54, 1977
45. Allen LE: Adult exstrophy of the bladder with adenocarcinoma. J Indiana State Med Assoc 70:639, 1977

Diverticulum

46. Judd ES, Scholl AJ: Diverticulum of the urinary bladder. Surg Gynecol Obstet 38:14, 1926
47. Miller A: The aetiology and treatment of diverticulum of the bladder. Br J Urol 30:87, 1958
48. Fox M, Power RF, Bruce AW: Diverticulum of the bladder — Presentation and evaluation of treatment of 115 cases. Br J Urol 34:286, 1962

49. Kelalis PP, McLean P: The treatment of diverticulum of the bladder. J Urol 98:349, 1967
50. Schiff M, Lytton B: Congenital diverticulum of the bladder. J Urol 104:111, 1970
51. Peterson LJ, Paulson DF, Glenn JF: The histopathology of vesical diverticula. J Urol 110:62, 1973
52. Barrett DM, Malek RS, Kelalis PP: Observations on vesical diverticulum in childhood. J Urol 116:284, 1976

Malignancy Complicating Diverticulum

53. Abeshouse BS, Goldstein AE: Primary carcinoma in a diverticulum of the bladder; A report of four cases and a review of the literature. J Urol 49:534, 1943
54. Pearlman CK, Bobbitt RM: Carcinoma within a diverticulum of the bladder. J Urol 59:1127, 1948
55. Boylan RN, Greene LF, McDonald JR: Epithelial neoplasms arising in diverticula of the urinary bladder. J Urol 65:1041, 1951
56. Thomas EM, Abernathy EL: Leiomyosarcoma in diverticulum of the bladder. J Urol 68:470, 1952
57. Mayer RF, Moore TD: Carcinoma complicating vesical diverticulum. J Urol 71:307, 1954
58. Ward MP: Sarcoma of vesical diverticula. Br J Urol 30:87, 1958
59. Knappenberger ST, Uson AC, Melicow MM: Primary neoplasms occurring in vesical diverticula: A report of 18 cases. J Urol 83:153, 1960
60. Fox M, Power RF, Bruce AW: Diverticulum of the bladder — Presentation and evaluation of treatment of 115 cases. Br J Urol 34:286, 1962
61. Shawdon HH, Doyle FH, Shackman R: Double contrast cystography applied to the diagnosis of tumours in bladder diverticula. Br J Urol 37:536, 1965
62. Kelalis PP, McLean P: The treatment of diverticulum of the bladder. J Urol 98:349, 1967
63. Ostroff EB, Alperstein JB, Young JD Jr: Neoplasm in vesical diverticula: Report of 4 patients, including a 21-year-old. J Urol 110:65, 1973
64. Siegel WH: Neoplasms in bladder diverticula. Urol 4:411, 1974
65. Montague DK, Boltuch RL: Primary neoplasms in vesical diverticula: Report of 10 cases. J Urol 116:41, 1976
66. Ramthor W: Das harnblasendivertikel-karzinom der frau. Z Urol u Nephrol Bd 73:421, 1980
67. Shirai T, Arai M, Sakata T et al: Primary carcinomas of urinary bladder diverticula. Acta Pathol Jpn 34:417, 1984

Urachus

68. Begg RC: The colloid adenocarcinomata of the bladder vault arising from the epithelium of the urachal canal: With a critical survey of the tumours of the urachus. Br J Surg 18:422, 1930
69. Bourne CW, May ME: Urachal remnants: Benign or malignant? J Urol 118:743, 1977
70. Schubert GE, Pavkovic MB, Bethke – Bedurftig BA: Tubular urachal remnants in adult bladders. J Urol 127:40, 1982

Urachal Malignancies

71. Hue L, Jacquin M: Cancer colloide de la lombille et de paroi abdominale antérieure ayant envahi la vessie. Union Med de la Siene-Inf Rouen 6:418, 1863
72. Rankin FW, Parker B: Tumors of the urachus. With report of seven cases. Surg Gynecol Oncol 42:19, 1926
73. Brady L: Solid tumors of the ruachus. Arch Surg 14:46, 1927
74. Greig DM: A case of sarcoma of the uterus. Report of a case of sarcoma of the urachus. Edinburgh Med J 34:425, 1927

75. Voncken, Cambresier: Tumeurs solides de l'ouraque. Arch Med Belges 80:420, 1927

76. Ransom HK: Sarcoma of the urachus. Review of the literature with report of an additional case. Am J Surg 22:187, 1933

77. Hayes JJ, Segal AD: Mucinous carcinoma of the urachus invading the bladder. J Urol 53:659, 1945

78. Higgins CC: Carcinoma of the urachus. Report of two cases. Urol Cutan Rev 50:4, 1946

79. Prentiss RJ: Urachal cysts with malignant invasion of the bladder. Three case reports. Calif Med 67:103, 1947

80. Shaw RE: Sarcoma of the urachus. Report of a case and brief review of the subject. Br J Surg 37:95, 1949

81. Begg RC: Haematuria from an undetected urachal tumour. Lancet 2:18, 1952

82. Carreau EP, Higgins GA: Diseases of the urachus. With three illustrative case reports. Am J Surg 84:205, 1952

83. Sterling JA, Goldsmith R: Lesions of urachus which appear in the adult. Ann Surg 137:120, 1953

84. Slater GS, Torassa GL: Mucinous adenocarcinoma of urachus connected to urinary bladder. Stanford Med Bull 11:19, 1953

85. Wheeler JD, Hill WT: Adenocarcinoma involving the urinary bladder. Cancer 7:119, 1954

86. Garvey FK, Nunnery WE: Mucinous adenocarcinoma of the urachus: Review of the literature and report of a case. J Urol 72:860, 1954

87. Wright HB, McFarlane DJ: Carcinoma of the urachus. Am J Surg 90:693, 1955

88. Schourup K: Rare malignant tumours of the urinary bladder. Acta Path Microbiol Scand (suppl) 105:145, 1955

89. Prentiss RJ, Mullenix RB, Whisenand JM, Feeney MJ: Tumors of the urachus. Report of five cases. Calif Med 84:24, 1956

90. Fisher ER: Transitional-cell carcinoma of the urachal apex. Cancer 11:245, 1958

91. Shaw RE: Squamous-cell carcinoma in a cyst of the urachus. Case report. Br J Urol 30:87, 1958

92. Baglio CM, Crowson CN: Hemangiopericytoma of urachus: Report of a case. J Urol 91:660, 1964

93. Lopez – Engelking R, De La Cruz JV, De Maldonado MEF: Mucinous adenocarcinoma of the urinary tract. Trans Am Assoc Genito-Urinary Surg 58:144, 1966

94. Cornil C, Reynolds CT, Kickham CJE: Carcinoma of the urachus. J Urol 98:93, 1967

95. Raatzsch H, Wehnert J: Zur klinik des urachuskarzinoms. Zeit Urol 60:327, 1967

96. Nadjmi B, Whitehead ED, McKiel CF Jr et al: Carcinoma of the urachus: Report of two cases and review of the literature. J Urol 100:738, 1968

97. Grogono JL, Shepheard BGF: Carcinoma of the urachus. Br J Urol 41:222, 1969

98. Gillenwater JY, Sandusky WR: Mucinous adenocarcinoma of the urachus. Am Surg 35:267, 1969

99. Beck AD, Gaudin HJ, Bonham DG: Carcinoma of the urachus. Br J Urol 42:555, 1970

100. Ohman U, von Garrelts B, Moberg A: Carcinoma of the urachus. Review of the literature and report of two cases. Scand J Urol Nephrol 5:91, 1971

101. Whitehead ED, Tessler AN: Carcinoma of the urachus. Br J Urol 43:468, 1971

102. Rubell D, Porges RF: Carcinoma of the urachus. A case report and review. Obstet Gynecol 39:753, 1972

103. Yu HHY, Leong CH: Carcinoma of the urachus: Report of one case and a review of the literature. Surg 77:726, 1975

104. Lane V: Prognosis in carcinoma of the urachus. Eur Urol 2:282, 1976

105. Lin R – Y, Rappoport AE, Deppisch LM et al: Squamous cell carcinoma of the urachus. J Urol 118:1066, 1977

106. Loening SA, Jacobo E, Hawtrey CE et al: Adenocarcinoma of the urachus. J Urol 119:68, 1978

107. Jakse G, Schneider H–M, Jacob GH: Urachal signet-ring cell carcinoma, a rare variant of vesical adenocarcinoma: Incidence and pathological criteria. J Urol 120:764, 1978

108. Ganguli SK: Urachal carcinoma. J Urol 13:306, 1979

109. Mekras GD, Block NL, Carrion HM, Ishikoff M: Urachal carcinoma: Diagnosis by computerized axial tomography. J Urol 123:275, 1980

110. Noyes D, Vinson RK: Urachal leiomyosarcoma. J Urol 17:279, 1981

111. Kakizoe T et al: Adenocarcinoma of urachus. Report of 7 cases and review of literature. J Urol 21:360, 1983

112. Sheldon CA, Clayman RV, Gonzalez R et al: Malignant urachal lesions. J Urol 131:1, 1984

113. Johnson DE, Hodge GB, Abdul–Karim FW et al: Urachal carcinoma. J Urol 26:218, 1985

Proliferative and Metaplastic Variants of Urothelium

Brunn's Nests, Cystitis Cystica, Cystitis Glandularis

114. von Brunn A: Uber drusenahnliche bildungen in der schleimhaut des nierenbeckens des ureters und der harnblase beim menschen. Arch f Mikro Anat 41:294, 1893

115. Stoerk O, Zuckerkandel O: Ueber cystitis glandularis und den drusenkrebs der harnblase. Z Urol 1:1, 1907

116. Scholl AJ: The potential malignancy in exstrophy of the bladder. Ann Surg 75:365, 1922

117. Morse HD: The etiology and pathology of pyelitis cystica, ureteritis cystica and cystitis cystica. Am J Pathol 4:33, 1928

118. Patch FS, Rhea LJ: The genesis and development of Brunn's nests and their relation to cystitis cystica, cystitis glandularis, and primary adeno-carcinoma of the bladder. Can Med Assoc J 33:597, 1935

119. Stirling C, Ash JE: Chronic proliferative lesions of the urinary tract. J Urol 45:342, 1941

120. Emmett JL, McDonald JR: Proliferation of glands of the urinary bladder simulating malignant neoplasm. J Urol 48:257, 1942

121. Foot NC: Glandular metaplasia of the epithelium of the urinary tract. South Med J 37:137, 1944

122. Lowry MC, Hamm FC, Beard DE: Extensive glandular proliferation of the urinary bladder resembling malignant neoplasm. J Urol 52:133, 1944

123. Sauer, HR, Blick MS: Cystitis glandularis: A consideration of symptom diagnosis and clinical course of the disease. J Urol 61:446, 1948

124. Fagerstrom DP: Proliferative tumors of the ureter and renal pelvis, with further observations on the significance of "epithelial cell nests:" Six case reports. J Urol 59:333, 1948

125. Mostofi FK: Potentialities of bladder epithelium. J Urol 71:705, 1954

126. Mende TJ, Chambers EL: Distribution of mucopolysaccharide and alkaline phosphatase in transitional epithelia. J Histochem Cytochem 5:99, 1957

127. Shaw JL, Gislason GJ, Imbriglia JE: Transition of cystitis glandularis to primary adenocarcinoma of the bladder. J Urol 79:815, 1958

128. Kittredge WE, Brannan W: Cystitis glandularis. J Urol 81:419, 1959

129. Gordon A: Intestinal metaplasia of the urinary tract epithelium. J Pathol Bacteriol 85:441, 1963

130. Bell TE, Wendel RG: Cystitis glandularis: Benign or malignant? J Urol 100:462, 1968

131. Salm R: Combined intestinal and squamous metaplasia of the renal pelvis. J Clin Pathol 22:187, 1969

132. Parker C: Cystitis cystica and glandularis: A study of 40 cases. Proc Roy Soc Med 63:239, 1970

133. Ward AM: Glandular neoplasia within the urinary tract. The aetiology of adenocarcinoma of the urothelium with a review of the literature. I. Introduction: The origin of glandular epithelium in the renal pelvis, ureter and bladder. Virchows Arch [A] 352:296, 1971

134. Susmano D, Rubenstein AB, Dakin AR et al: Cystitis glandularis and adenocarcinoma of the bladder. J Urol 105:671, 1971

135. Edwards PD, Hurm RA, Jaeschke WH: Conversion of cystitis glandularis to adenocarcinoma. J Urol 108:568, 1972

136. Plumpton K, Morales A: Experimental induction of urothelial metaplasia. Urol 3:651, 1974

137. Davis EL, Goldstein AMB, Morrow JW; Unusual bladder mucosal metaplasia in a case of chronic prostatitis and cystitis. J Urol 111:767, 1974

138. Koss LG: Tumors of the urinary bladder. In Atlas of Tumor Pathology, 2nd Series, Fascicle 11, p 2. Washington, DC, AFIP, 1975

139. Goldstein AMB, Fauer RB, Chinn M et al: New concepts on formation of Brunn's nests and cysts in urinary tract mucosa. J Urol 11:513, 1978

140. Weiner DP, Koss LG, Sablay B et al: The prevalence and significance of Brunn's nests, cystitis cystica and squamous metaplasia in normal bladders. J Urol 122:317, 1979

141. Koss LG; Mapping of the urinary bladder: Its impact on the concepts of bladder cancer. Hum Pathol 5:533, 1979

142. Lin JI, Tseng CH, Choy C et al: Diffuse cystitis glandularis. Associated with adenocarcinomatous change. Urol 15:411, 1980

Squamous Metaplasia (Leukoplakia)

143. Connery DB: Leukoplakia of the urinary bladder and its association with carcinoma. J Urol 69:121, 1953

144. Holley PS, Mellinger GT: Leukoplakia of the bladder and carcinoma. J Urol 86:235, 1961

145. O'Flynn JD, Mullaney J: Leukoplakia of the bladder. A report on 20 cases, including 2 cases progressing to squamous cell carcinoma. Br J Urol 39:461, 1967

146. Mostofi FK, Leestma JE: Lower urinary tract, prostate, and male genitalia. In Anderson WAD (ed): Pathology, pp 836–838. St Louis, CV Mosby, 1971

147. Widran J, Sanchez R, Gruhn J: Squamous metaplasia of the bladder: A study of 450 patients. J Urol 112:479, 1974

148. Witherington R: Leukoplakia of the bladder: An 8-year followup. J Urol 112:600, 1974

149. Reece RW, Koontz WW Jr: Leukoplakia of the urinary tract: A review. J Urol 114:165, 1975

150. Koss LG: Tumors of the urinary bladder. In Atlas of Tumor Pathology, 2nd Series, Fascicle 11, p 103. Washington, DC, AFIP, 1975

151. Morgan RJ, Cameron KM: Vesical leukoplakia. Br J Urol 52:96, 1980

152. Benson RC Jr, Squanson SK, Farrow GM: Relationship of leukoplakia to urothelial malignancy. J Urol 131:507, 1984

Nephrogenic Metaplasia (Adenoma)

153. Davis TA: Hamartoma of the urinary bladder. Northwest Med 48:182, 1949

154. Freidman NB, Kuhlenbeck H: Adenomatoid tumors of the bladder reproducing renal structures (nephrogenic adenomas). J Urol 64:657, 1950

155. Hasen HB: Nephrogenic adenoma of the bladder. J Urol 88:629, 1962

156. Goldman RL: Nephrogenic metaplasia (nephrogenic adenoma, adenomatoid tumor) of the bladder. J Urol 108:565, 1972

157. Christoffersen J, Moller JE: Adenomatoid tumours of the urinary bladder. Scand J Urol Nephrol 6:295, 1972
158. Kalloor GJ, Shaw RE: Nephrogenic adenoma of the bladder. Br J Urol 46:91, 1973
159. Sussman EB, Brice M II, Gray GF: Nephrogenic metaplasia of the bladder. J Urol 111:34, 1974
160. Kaany E, Werner SL: Nephrogenic adenoma of bladder. Urol 4:343, 1974
161. Donhuijsen K, Leistenschneider W: Nephrogenic adenoma. A rare epithelial tumor of the urinary bladder in a child. Beitr Path Bd 155:208, 1975
162. Taneja OP, Aurora AL, Grover NK et al: Nephrogenic adenoma of the urinary bladder. Br J Urol 46:97, 1974
163. Allan E: Nephrogenic adenoma of the bladder. J Urol 113:35, 1975
164. Kaswick JA, Waisman J, Goodwin WE: Nephrogenic metaplasia (adenomatoid tumors) of bladder. Urol 8:283, 1976
165. Molland LA, Trott PA, Paris AMI et al: Nephrogenic adenoma: A form of adenomatous metaplasia of the bladder. A clinical and electron microscopical study. Br J Urol 48:453, 1976
166. Leonard SA, Silverman AJ, Langston JW: Postoperative nephrogenic adenoma of bladder. Urol 7:327, 1976
167. Cremer H, Adolphs H–D: The natural history of nephrogenic adenoma of the urinary bladder. Z Krebsforsch 91:49, 1978
168. Peterson LJ, Matsumoto LM: Nephrogenic adenoma in urethral diverticulum. Urol 11:193, 1978
169. Imahori SC, Magoss IV: Nephrogenic adenoma of bladder. Clinical and ultrastructural study. Urol 16:310, 1980
170. Tannenbaum SI, Kramer SA, Gibson WH, Carson CC: Nephrogenic adenoma of bladder. Urol 15:518, 1980
171. Raghavaiah NV, Noe HN, Parham DM, Murphy WM: Nephrogenic adenoma of urinary bladder associated with malakoplakia. Urol 15:190, 1980
172. Berger BW, Belur S, Bhagavan S et al: Nephrogenic adenoma: Clinical features and therapeutic considerations. J Urol 126:824, 1981
173. O'Shea PA, Callaghan JF, Lawlor JB, Reddy VC: Nephrogenic adenoma: An unusual metaplastic change of urothelium. J Urol 125:247, 1981
174. Bhagavan BS, Tiamson EM, Wenk RE et al: Nephrogenic adenoma of the urinary bladder and urethra. Hum Pathol 12:907, 1981
175. Behesti M, Morales A: Nephrogenic adenoma of bladder developing after renal transplantation. Urol 20:298, 1982
176. Navarre RJ, Loening SA, Platz C et al: Nephrogenic adenoma: A report of 9 cases and review of the literature. J Urol 127:775, 1982
177. Lugo M, Petersen RO, Elfenbein IB et al: Nephrogenic metaplasia of the ureter. Am J Clin Pathol 80:92, 1983
178. Ritchey ML, Novicki DE, Schultenover SJ: Nephrogenic adenoma of bladder: A report of 8 cases. J Urol 131:537, 1984
179. Kay R, Lattanzi C: Nephrogenic adenoma in children. J Urol 133:99, 1985

Inflammatory Disorders

Polypoid Cystitis

180. Mostofi FK: Potentialities of bladder epithelium. J Urol 71:705, 1954
181. Milles G: Catheter-induced hemorrhagic pseudopolyps of the urinary bladder. JAMA 193:196, 1965
182. Koss LG: Tumors of the urinary bladder. In Atlas of Tumor Pathology, 2nd Series, Fascicle 11, p 106. Washington, DC, AFIP, 1975
183. Ekelund P, Johansson S: Polypoid cystitis. A catheter associated lesion of the human bladder. Acta Pathol Microbiol Immunol Scand [A] 87:179, 1979
184. Ekelund P, Anderstrom C, Johansson SL et al: The reversibility of catheter-associated polypoid cystitis. J Urol 130:456, 1983

185. Buck EG: Polypoid cystitis mimicking transitional cell carcinoma. J Urol 131:963, 1984

Eosinophilic Cystitis

186. Brown EW: Eosinophilic granuloma of the bladder. J Urol 83:665, 1960
187. Palubinskas AJ: Eosinophilic cystitis. Case report of eosinophilic infiltration of the urinary bladder. Radiology 75:589, 1960
188. Champion RH, Ackles RC: Eosinophilic cystitis. J Urol 96:729, 1966
189. Frensilli FJ, Sacher EC, Keegan GT: Eosinophilic cystitis: Observations on etiology. J Urol 107:595, 1972
190. Gregg JA, Utz DC: Eosinophilic cystitis associated with eosinophilic gastroenteritis. Mayo Clin Proc 49:185, 1974
191. Marshall FF, Middleton AW Jr: Eosinophilic cystitis. J Urol 112:335, 1974
192. Rubin L, Pincus MB: Eosinophilic cystitis: The relationship of allergy in the urinary tract to eosinophilic cystitis and the pathophysiology of eosinophilia. J Urol 112:457, 1974
193. Kessler WO, Clark PL, Kaplan GW: Eosinophilic cystitis. Urol 6:499, 1975
194. Hellstrom HR, Davis BK, Shonnard JW: Eosinophilic cystitis. A study of 16 cases. Am J Clin Pathol 72:777, 1979
195. Littleton RH, Farah RN, Cerny JC: Eosinophilic cystitis: An uncommon form of cystitis. J Urol 127:132, 1982

Chronic Interstitial Cystitis (Hunner's Ulcer)

196. Hunner GL: A rare type of bladder ulcer in women: Report of cases. Trans South Surg Gynecol Assoc 27:247, 1914
197. Smith BH, Dehner LP: Chronic ulcerating interstitial cystitis (Hunner's ulcer). Arch Pathol 93:76, 1972
198. Farkas A, Waisman J, Goodwin WE: Intertitial cystitis in adolescent girls. J Urol 118:837, 1977
199. Messing EM, Stamey TA: Interstitial cystitis. Early diagnosis, pathology, and treatment. Urol 2:381, 1978

Gangrenous Cystitis

200. Stirling WC, Hopkins GA: Gangrene of the bladder. Review of two hundred seven cases; Report of two personal cases. J Urol 31:517, 1934
201. Cristol DS, Greene LF: Gangrenous cystitis. Etiologic classification and treatment. Surg 18:343, 1945
202. Evans AT: Infections of the kidney and bladder in the adult. In Kendall AR, Kerafin LK (eds): Practice of Surgery: Urology, Vol I, Chapter 14, p 80. Philadelphia, Harper and Row, 1984

Follicular Cystitis

203. Hinman F, Cordonnier J: Cystitis follicularis. J Urol 34:302, 1935
204. Schlomovitz BH: Cystitis follicularis. J Urol 47:168, 1942
205. Kretschmer HL: On the occurrence of lymphoid tissue in the urinary organs. J Urol 68:252, 1952
206. Sarma KP: On the nature of cystitis follicularis. J Urol 104:709, 1970

Emphysematous Cystitis

207. Lund HG, Zingale FG, O'Dowd JA: Cystitis emphysematosa. J Urol 42:684, 1939
208. Bailey H: Cystitis emphysematosa. 19 cases with intraluminal and interstitial collections of gas. Am J Roentgenol 86:850, 1961
209. Hawtrey CE, Williams JJ, Schmidt JD: Cystitis emphysematosa. Urol 3:612, 1974
210. Maliwan N: Emphysematous cystitis associated with clostridium perfringens bacteremia. J Urol 121:819, 1979

Eosinophilic Granuloma

211. Auld D: Pathology of eosinophilic granuloma of the lung. Arch Pathol 62:113, 1957
212. Newton WA Jr, Hamondi AB: Histiocytosis: A histologic classification with clinical correlation. Perspect Pediatr Pathol 1:25, 1973
213. Koss LG: Tumors of the urinary bladder. In Atlas of Tumor Pathology, 2nd Series, Fascicle 11 p 107. Washington, DC, AFIP, 1975
214. Kutzenstein A–L, Askin FB: Pulmonary eosinophilic granuloma. In Surgical Pathology of Non-neoplastic Lung Disease, Vol 13, Major Problems in Pathology, p 356. Philadelphia, WB Saunders, 1982

Plasma Cell Granuloma

215. Tchertkoff V, Lee BY, Wagner BM: Plasma cell granuloma of the lung. Case report and review of the literature. Chest 44:440, 1963
216. Bahafori M, Liebow AA: Plasma cell granulomas of the lung. Cancer 31:191, 1973
217. Jufe R, Molinolo AA, Fefer SA et al: Plasma cell granuloma of the bladder: A case report. J Urol 131:1175, 1984

Malakoplakia

218. Michaelis L, Gutmann C: Ueber einschlusse in blasentumoren. Ztschr Klin Med 47:208, 1902
219. Melicow MM: Malacoplakia: Report of case, review of literature. J Urol 78:33, 1957
220. Goldman RL: A case of malacoplakia with involvement of the prostate gland. J Urol 93:407, 1965
221. Smith BH: Malacoplakia of the urinary tract. A study of twenty-four cases. J Urol 43:409, 1965
222. Yunis EJ, Estevez JM, Pinzon GJ et al: Malacoplakia. Discussion of pathogenesis and report of three cases including one of fatal gastric and colonic involvement. Arch Pathol 83:180, 1967
223. Thorning D, Vracko R: Malakoplakia: Defect in digestion of phagocytized material due to impaired vacuolar acidification. Arch Pathol 99:456, 1975
224. Lewin KJ, Fair WR, Steigbigel RT et al: Clinical and laboratory studies into the pathogenesis of malacoplakia. J Clin Pathol 29:354, 1976
225. Abdou NI, Pombejara CN, Sagawa A et al: Malakoplakia: Evidence for monocyte lysosomal abnormality correctable by cholonergic agonist in vitro and in vivo. N Engl J Med 297:1413, 1977
226. McKay EH: Malakoplakia in ulcerative colitis. Arch Pathol Lab Med 102:140, 1978
227. Schreiber AG, Maderazo EG: Leukocyte function in malakoplakia. Arch Pathol Lab Med 102:534, 1978
228. Griggs WP, Hemstreet GP III: Pathologic and immunologic considerations in malakoplakia. Urol 16:638, 1980
229. Lou TY, Teplitz C: Malakoplakia: Pathogenesis and ultrastructural morphogenesis. A problem of altered macrophage (phagolososomal) response. Hum Pathol 5:191, 1974
230. Damjanov I, Katz SM: Malakoplakia. Pathol Annu 16:103, 1981
231. Stanton MJ, Maxted W: Malacoplakia: A study of the literature and current concepts of pathogenesis, diagnosis and treatment. J Urol 125:139, 1981
232. Streem SB: Genitourinary malacoplakia in renal transplant recipients: Pathogenic, prognostic and therapeutic considerations. J Urol 132:10, 1984

Radiation Cystitis

233. Warren S: VII. Effects of radiation on the urinary system. The kidneys and ureters. Arch Pathol 34:1079, 1942
234. Hueper WC, Fisher CV, de Carvajal–Forero J et al: The pathology of experimental roentgen-cystitis in dogs. J Urol 47:156, 1942

235. Gowing NFC: III. Pathological changes in the bladder following irradiation. A contribution to a symposium on "Treatment of carcinoma of the bladder" at the British Institute of Radiology on January 14, 1960. Br J Radiol 33:484, 1960
236. Koss LG: Tumors of the urinary bladder. In Atlas of Tumor Pathology, 2nd Series, Fascicle 11, p 99. Washington, DC, AFIP, 1975
237. Fajardo LF, Berthrong M: Radiation injury in surgical pathology. Part I. Am J Surg Pathol 2:159, 1978

Chemotherapy-Induced Hemorrhagic Cystitis

238. Philips FS, Sternberg SS, Cronin AP et al: Cyclophosphamide and urinary bladder toxicity. Cancer Res 21:1577, 1961
239. George P: Haemorrhagic cystitis and cyclophosphamide. Lancet 2:942, 1963
240. Forni AM, Koss LG, Geller W: Cytological study of the effect of cyclophosphamide on the epithelium of the urinary bladder in man. Cancer 17:1348, 1964
241. Rubin JS, Rubin RT: Cyclophosphamide hemorrhagic cystitis. J Urol 96:313, 1966
242. Lawrence HJ, Simone J, Aur RJA: Cyclophosphamide-induced hemorrhagic cystitis in children with leukemia. Cancer 36:1572, 1975
243. Millard RJ: Busulphan haemorrhagic cystitis. Case report. Br J Urol 50:210, 1978
244. Beyer–Boon ME, De Voogt HJ, Schaberg A: The effects of cyclophosphamide treatment on the epithelium and stroma of the urinary bladder. Eur J Cancer 14:1029, 1978
245. Koss LG: Diagnostic Cytology and its Histopathologic Basis, Vol II, 3rd ed, p 738. Philadelphia, JB Lippincott, 1979
246. Pode D, Perlberg S, Steiner D: Busulfan-induced hemorrhagic cystitis. J Urol 130:347, 1983

Schistosomal Cystitis

247. Edington GM, von Lichtenberg F, Nwabuebo I et al: Pathologic effects of schistosomiasis in Ibadan, Western State of Nigeria. I. Incidence and intensity of infection; Distribution and severity of lesions. Am J Trop Med Hyg 19:982, 1970
248. von Lichtenberg F, Edington GM, Nwabuebo I et al: Pathologic effects of schistosomiasis in Ibadan, Western State of Nigeria. II. Pathogenesis of lesions of the bladder and ureters. Am J Trop Med Hyg 20:244, 1971
249. Khafagy MM, El Bolkainy MN, Mansour MA: Carcinoma of the bilharzial urinary bladder. A study of the associated mucosal lesions in 86 cases. Cancer 30:150, 1972
250. El Bolkainy MN, Ghoneim MA, Mansour MA: Carcinoma of the bilharzial bladder in Egypt. Clinical and pathological features. Br J Urol 44:561, 1972
251. Warren KS: The relevance of schistosomiasis. N Engl J Med 303:203, 1980
252. Nash TE, Cheever AW, Ottesen EA et al: Schistosome infections in humans: Perspectives and recent findings. Ann Intern Med 97:740, 1982

Condyloma Acuminata

253. Kleiman H, Lancaster Y: Condyloma acuminata of the bladder. J Urol 88:52, 1962
254. Lewis HY, Wolf PL, Pierce JM: Condyloma acuminatum of the bladder. J Urol 88:248, 1962
255. Hotchkiss RS, Rouse AJ: Papillomatosis of the bladder and ureters preceded by condyloma acuminata of the vulva: A case report. J Urol 100:723, 1968
256. Bissada NK, Cole AT, Fried FA: Extensive condylomas acuminata of the entire male urethra and the bladder. J Urol 112:201, 1974
257. Pettersson S, Hansson G, Blohme I: Condyloma acuminatum of the bladder. J Urol 115:535, 1976
258. Masse S, Tosi–Kruse A, Carmel M et al: Condyloma acuminatum of bladder. Urol 17:381, 1981
259. Keating MA, Young RH, Carr CP et al: Condyloma acuminatum of the bladder and ureter: Case report and review of the literature. J Urol 133:465, 1985

Amyloidosis

260. Houtappel HCEM, Lauwers GTH: Primary amyloidosis of the bladder. Report of a case and a review of the literature. Arch Chirurgicum Neerlandicum 12:308, 1960
261. Werner H: Ein primares tumorformiges amyloid der harnblase. Z Urol 54:61, 1961
262. Nagel R: "Amyloidtumor" der blase. Z Urol 54:731, 1961
263. Kinzel RC, Harrison EG Jr, Utz DC: Primary localized amyloidosis of the bladder. J Urol 85:785, 1961
264. Nagel R: Localized amyloidosis of the bladder. J Urol 88:56, 1962
265. Grace DA, Walton KN: Primary localized amyloidosis of the bladder. J Urol 92:655, 1964
266. Krzeski T: Pierwotny amyloidowy guz pecherza moczowego. Nowotwory 14:293, 1964
267. Hudson HC, Tingley JO: Primary amyloidosis of the bladder. J Med Assoc Ala 35:353, 1965
268. Narwani KP, Lingard WF: Primary localized amyloidosis of the urinary bladder. Can Med Assoc J 95:76, 1966
269. Sinkevichis CA, Lyutkus LY: Pervichniy amiloidos machevova puzirya. Urol Nefrol (Mosk) 31:52, 1966
270. Lerut R, Lerut H: Amylose primitive et localisée de la vessie. Acta Urol Belg 35:611, 1967
271. Bender LI, Kelly CE: Secondary amyloidosis of the bladder: A case report. J Urol 102:60, 1969
272. Tripathi VNP, Desautels RE: Primary amyloidosis of the urogenital system: A study of 16 cases and brief review. J Urol 102:96, 1969
273. Missen GAK, Tribe CR: Catastrophic haemorrhage from the bladder due to unrecognised secondary amyloidosis. Br J Urol 42:43, 1970
274. Gerami S, Easley GW, Payan H: Primary localized amyloidosis of the urethra and bladder (Amyloidoma). Am Surg 36:375, 1970
275. Malek RS, Greene LF, Farrow GM: Amyloidosis of the urinary bladder. Br J Urol 43:189, 1971
276. Bergqvist D, Westermark P: Primary isolated amyloidosis of the urinary bladder. Report of a case. Acta Chir Scand 137:287, 1971
277. Montie JE, Stewart BH: Massive bladder hemorrhage after cystoscopy in a patient with secondary systemic amyloidosis. J Urol 109:49, 1973
278. Strong GH, Kelsey D, Hoch W: Primary amyloid disease of the bladder. J Urol 112:463, 1974
279. Hofer P–A, Winblad B, Andersson L et al: Primary localized amyloidosis of the bladder. Scand J Urol Nephrol 8:193, 1974
280. Au KK, Gilbaugh JH Jr: Primary amyloidosis of the bladder. J Urol 114:786, 1975
281. Robertson WH, Crowe AD, Crow JB: Case report. Localized amyloid tumor of the bladder presenting as an anterior pelvic mass. Ala J Med Sci 12:10, 1975
282. Blath RA, Bucy JG: Localised primary amyloidosis of the bladder. Br J Urol 48:219, 1976
283. Carris CK, McLaughlin AP, Gittes RF: Amyloidosis of the lower genitourinary tract. J Urol 115:423, 1976
284. Abramovici I, Chwatt S, Nussenson M: Massive hematuria and perforation in a case of amyloidosis of the bladder: Case report and review of the literature. J Urol 118:964, 1977
285. Thomas SD, Sanders PW III, Pollack H: Primary amyloidosis of urinary bladder and ureter. Urol 9:586, 1977
286. Akhtar M, Valencia M, Thomas AM: Solitary primary amyloidosis of urinary bladder. Light and electron microscopic study. Urol 12:721, 1978
287. Kampehl H–J, Gunther M, Putzke HP: Ein Beitrag zur Harnblasenamyloidose. Z Urol Nephrol 72:441, 1979

288. Glenner GG: Amyloid deposits and amyloidosis, the B – fibrilloses. N Engl J Med 302:1283, 1333, 1980
289. Caldamone AA, Elbadawi A, Moshtagi A et al: Primary localized amyloidosis of urinary bladder. Urol 15:174, 1980
290. Nakajima K, Hisazumi H, Okasyo A et al: Primary localized amyloidosis of bladder. Urol 15:302, 1980
291. Mead MG, Hickinbotham P, Walls J: Amyloidosis localised to the bladder. Br J Urol 54:428, 1982

Endometriosis

292. Judd ES: Adenomyoma presenting as a tumor of the bladder. Surg Clin North Am 1:1271, 1921
293. Sampson JA: Development of the implantation theory for the origin of peritoneal endometriosis. Am J Obstet Gynecol 40:549, 1940
294. Nixon WCW: Endometriosis of the bladder. Lancet 1:405, 1940
295. Kahle PJ, Vickery GW, Maltry E: Endometriosis of the urinary bladder. Report of two additional cases. J Urol 46:52, 1941
296. Moore TD, Herring AL, McCannel DA: Some urologic aspects of endometriosis. J Urol 49:171, 1943
297. Goodall JR: Urinary complications of pelvic endometriosis. Ann Surg 120:891, 1944
298. Kretschmer HL: Endometriosis of the bladder. J Urol 53:459, 1945
299. Fitzgerald WL, Kuhn MAR: Endometriosis of the bladder. J Urol 62:467, 1949
300. Brosset A: Endometriosis in the vaginal scar following vaginal hysterotomy for therapeutic abortion. Acta Obstet Gynecol Scand 33:445, 1954
301. Abeshouse BS, Abeshouse G: Endometriosis of the urinary tract: A review of the literature and a report of four cases of vesical endometriosis. J Int Coll Surg 34:43, 1960
302. Lichtenheld FR, McCauley RT, Staples PP: Endometriosis involving the urinary tract. A collective review. Obstet Gynecol 17:762, 1961
303. Ball TL, Platt MA: Urologic complications of endometriosis. Am J Obstet Gynecol 84:1516, 1962
304. Radman HM: Endometriosis of the bladder. Am J Obstet Gynecol 83:171, 1962
305. Stanley KE Jr, Utz DC, Dockerty MB: Clinically significant endometriosis of the urinary tract. Surg Gynecol Obstet 120:491, 1965
306. Fein RL, Horton BF: Vesical endometriosis: A case report and review of the literature. J Urol 95:45, 1966
307. Iwano JH, Ewing GE: Endometriosis of the bladder. J Urol 100:614, 1968
308. Oliker AJ, Harris AE: Endometriosis of the bladder in a male patient. J Urol 106:858, 1971
309. Stewart WW, Ireland GW: Vesical endometriosis in a postmenopausal woman: A case report. J Urol 118:480, 1977
310. Skor AB, Warren MM, Mueller EO Jr: Endometriosis of bladder. Urol 9:689, 1977
311. Makinen J, Lehtonen T: Endometriosis of the urinary bladder. An unusual cause of haematuria. Report of a case. Ann Chir Gynaecol 66:292, 1977
312. Paniel BJ: L'endometriose urinaire. Gynecologie 29:11, 1978
313. Weinberg RW: Vesical endometriosis. Urol 11:72, 1978
314. Pinkert TC, Catlow CE, Straus R: Endometriosis of the urinary bladder in a man with prostatic carcinoma. Cancer 43:1562, 1979
315. Schrott GR, Alcorn MO, Ibanez J: Endometriosis of the male urinary system: A case report. J Urol 124:722, 1980
316. Fianu S, Ingelman – Sundberg A, Nasiell K et al: Surgical treatment of post abortum endometriosis of the bladder and postoperative bladder function. Scand J Urol Nephrol 14:151, 1980
317. Neto WA, Lopes RN, Cury M et al: Vesical endometriosis. Urol 24:271, 1984

Neoplastic Disorders

Inverted Papilloma

318. Paschkis R: Uber Adenome der Harnblase. Z Urol Chir 21:315, 1927
319. Potts IF, Hirst E: Inverted papilloma of the bladder. J Urol 90:175, 1963
320. Oberman HA: Papillomas of the nose and paranasal sinuses. Am J Clin Pathol 42:245, 1964
321. Salm R: Neoplasia of the bladder and cystitis cystica. Br J Urol 39:67, 1967
322. Trites AEW: Inverted urothelial papilloma: Report of two cases. J Urol 101:216, 1969
323. Borski AA: Hamartoma of the bladder. J Urol 104:718, 1970
324. Assor D, Taylor JN: Inverted papilloma of the bladder. J Urol 104:715, 1970
325. Inada T, Ochiai K: Inverted papilloma of the bladder. Jpn J Cancer Clin 17:776, 1971
326. Sullivan JJ, Watson JG, Kingston CW, Yaxley RP: Inverted papilloma of the urinary bladder. A report of two cases. Aust NZ J Surg 41:60, 1971
327. Pienkos EJ, Iglesias F, Joblokow VR: Inverted papilloma of bladder. Urol 2:178, 1973
328. Cummings R: Inverted papilloma of the bladder. J Pathol 112:225, 1974
329. Matz LR, Wishart VA, Goodman MA: Inverted urothelial papilloma. Pathol 6:37, 1974
330. Klein HL: Inverted papilloma and transitional cell carcinoma of the bladder. Kimbrough Urol Semin 8:45, 1974
331. DeMeester LJ, Farrow GM, Utz DC: Inverted papillomas of the urinary bladder. Cancer 36:505, 1975
332. Hefter LG, Young IS: Inverted papilloma of bladder. Urol 5:688, 1975
333. Hasselstrom AK: Inverteret blaerepapillom. Ugeskr Laeger 137:2834, 1975
334. Henderson DW, Allen PW, Bourne AJ: Inverted urinary papilloma. Report of five cases and review of the literature. Virchows Arch [A] 366:177, 1975
335. Simard CL, Tayot J, Francois H et al: Le papillome "inverse" urothelial de Potts et Hirst. Arch Anat Pathol 23:139, 1975
336. Cameron KM, Lupton CH: Inverted papilloma of the lower urinary tract. Br J Urol 48:567, 1976
337. Tannenbaum M: Inverted papilloma: Urothelial tumor of benign biologic potential. Urol 7:76, 1976
338. Jacques J: Inverted papilloma of the urinary bladder. Arch Pathol Lab Med 100:559, 1976
339. Muretto P, De Maurizi M, Mattioli A: Papilloma invertito della vescica. (Ipotesi istogenetica e presentazione di un caso). Pathologica 68:435, 1976
340. Soret J–Y, Simard CL, Meyer PH et al: Papillome "inverse" urothelial. A propos de 3 cas vésicaux. J Urol Nephrol 82:484, 1976
341. Martinez–Penuela Virseda J, Ipiens Aznar A: Papilloma invertido del tracto urinario. Presentacion de un caso de localizacion vesical. Rev Clin Esp 142:175, 1976
342. Dirschmid K, Breitfellner G, Kiesler J: Das invertierte papillom des urothels. Urologe [Ausg A] 15:180, 1976
343. Virseda JMP, Axnar AI: Papilloma invertido del tracto uranario: Presentation de un caso de localizacion vesical. Rev Clin Esp 142:175, 1976
344. Roberts H, Bergman DG, Hoffberger R: Inverted papilloma of the bladder. J Am Osteopath Assoc 76:514, 1977
345. Gamallo C, Lopez–Rubio F, Tallada M et al: Inverted papilloma of the bladder. Report of a case in a 26-year-old female. Eur Urol 3:188, 1977
346. Kim YH, Reiner L: Brunnian adenoma (inverted papilloma) of the urinary bladder: Report of a case. Hum Pathol 9:229, 1978
347. Lazarevic B, Garret R: Inverted papilloma and papillary transitional cell carcinoma

of urinary bladder. Report of four cases of inverted papilloma, one showing papillary malignant transformation and review of the literature. Cancer 42:1904, 1978

348. Caro DJ, Tessler A: Inverted papilloma of the bladder. A distinct urological lesion. Cancer 42:708, 1978
349. Francis RR: Inverted papilloma in a 14-year-old male. Br J Urol 51:327, 1979
350. Alroy J, Miller AW III, Coon JS IV et al: Inverted papilloma of the urinary bladder. Ultrastructural and Immunologic studies. Cancer 46:64, 1980
351. Uyama T, Nakamura S, Moriwaki S: Inverted papilloma of bladder. Two cases with questionable malignancy and squamous metaplasia. Urol 16:152, 1980
352. Theoret G, Paqin F, Schick E, Martel A: Inverted papilloma of urinary tract. Urol 16:149, 1980
353. Bernheim J, Aronheim M, Griffel B: Papillomes vesicaux à cellules urotheliales de type inverse. J Urol (Paris) 86:57, 1980
354. Ponthieu A, Varette I, Pizzi M et al: Papillome à structure inversée de la vessie: Deux observations. J Urol (Paris) 86:150, 1980
355. Altaffer LF III, Wilkerson SY, Jordan GH, Lynch DF: Malignant inverted papilloma and carcinoma in situ of the bladder. J Urol 128:816, 1982
356. Anderstrom C, Johansson S, Petersson S: Inverted papilloma of the urinary tract. J Urol 127:1132, 1982
357. Iwata H, Yokoyama M, Morita M et al: Inverted papilloma of urinary bladder. Scanning and transmission electron microscopic observation. Urol 19:322, 1982
358. Whitesel JA: Inverted papilloma of the urinary tract: Malignant potential. J Urol 127:539, 1982
359. Kunze E, Schauer A, Schmitt M: Histology and histogenesis of two different types of inverted urothelial papillomas. Cancer 51:348, 1983
360. Stein BS, Rosen S, Kendall AR: The association of inverted papilloma and transitional cell carcinoma of the urothelium. J Urol 131:751, 1984

Transitional Cell Papilloma

361. Ash JE: Epithelial tumors of the bladder. J Urol 44:135, 1940
362. Kretschmer HL, Stika EA: Papilloma of the bladder. JAMA 141:1039, 1949
363. Deming CL: The biological behavior of transitional cell papilloma of the bladder. J Urol 63:815, 1950
364. Ewert EE, Summons HJ: Papillomas of the bladder. Surg Clin North Am 31:653, 1951
365. Dean AL, Mostofi FK, Thomson RV et al: A restudy of the first fourteen hundred tumors in the bladder tumor registry, Armed Forces Institute of Pathology. J Urol 71:571, 1954
366. Melicow MM: Tumors of the urinary bladder. A clinico-pathological analysis of over 2500 specimens and biopsies. J Urol 74:498, 1955
367. Mostofi FK: Pathological aspects and spread of carcinoma of the bladder. JAMA 206:1764, 1968
368. Mostofi FK, Sobin LH, Torloni H: Histological Typing of Urinary Bladder Tumours. International Histological Classification of Tumours, No 10. Geneva, World Health Organization, 1973
369. Koss LG: Papillary tumors without significant cytologic abnormalities. In Tumors of the Urinary Bladder, pp 19–28. In Atlas of Tumor Pathology, 2nd Series, Fascicle 11. Washington, DC, AFIP, 1975
370. Friedell GH, Parija GC, Nagy GK et al: The pathology of human bladder cancer. Cancer 45:1823, 1980

Transitional Cell Carcinoma in Situ

371. Melicow MM: Histological study of vesical urothelium intervening between gross neoplasms in total cystectomy. J Urol 68:261, 1952

372. Franks LM, Chesterman FC: Intra-epithelial carcinoma of prostatic urethra, peri-urethral glands and prostatic ducts. ("Bowen's disease of urinary epithelium"). Br J Cancer 10:223, 1956

373. Eisenberg RB, Roth RB, Schweinsberg MH: Bladder tumors and associated proliferative mucosal lesions. J Urol 84:544, 1960

374. Gowing NFC: Urethral carcinoma associated with cancer of the bladder. Br J Urol 32:428, 1960

375. Cordonnier JJ, Spjut HJ: Urethral occurrence of bladder carcinoma following cystectomy. J Urol 87:398, 1962

376. Melamed MR, Vousta NG, Grabstald, H: Natural history and clinical behavior of in situ carcinoma of the human urinary bladder. Cancer 17:1533, 1964

377. Culp OS, Utz DC, Harrison EG Jr: Experiences with ureteral carcinoma in situ detected during operations for vesical neoplasm. J Urol 97:679, 1967

378. Utz DC, Hanash KA, Farrow GM: The plight of the patient with carcinoma in situ of the bladder. J Urol 103:160, 1970

379. Sharma TC, Melamed MR, Whitmore WF Jr: Carcinoma in-situ of the ureter in patients with bladder carcinoma treated by cystectomy. Cancer 26:583, 1970

380. Shade ROK, Tubingen MD, Durh MD et al: Morphological changes in the ureter in cases of bladder carcinoma. Cancer 27:1267, 1971

381. Yates–Bell AJ: Carcinoma in situ of the bladder. Br J Surg 58:359, 1971

382. Barlebo H, Sorensen BL, Ohlsen S: Carcinoma in situ of the urinary bladder. Scand J Urol Nephrol 6:213, 1972

383. Mostofi FK, Sobin LH, Torloni H: Histological Typing Of Urinary Bladder Tumours. International Histological Classification of Tumours, No 10. Geneva, World Health Organization, 1973

384. Cooper PH, Waisman J, Johnston WH et al: Severe atypia of transitional epithelium and carcinoma of the urinary bladder. Cancer 32:1055, 1973

385. Moloney PJ, Elliott GB, McLaughlin M et al: In situ transitional carcinoma and the non-specifically inflamed contracting bladder. J Urol 111:162, 1974

386. Thelmo WL, Seemayer TA, Madarnas P et al: Carcinoma in situ of the bladder with associated prostatic involvement. J Urol 111:491, 1974

387. Skinner DG, Richie JP, Cooper PH et al: The clinical significance of carcinoma in situ of the bladder and its association with overt carcinoma. J Urol 112:68, 1974

388. Seemayer TA, Knaack J, Thelmo WL et al: Further observations on carcinoma in situ of the urinary bladder: Silent but extensive intraprostatic involvement. Cancer 36:514, 1975

389. Koss LG: Precancerous lesions of the urothelium. In Tumors of the Urinary Bladder, pp 62–69. In Atlas of Tumor Pathology, 2nd Series, Fascicle 11. Washington, DC, AFIP, 1975

390. Althausen AF, Prout GR Jr, Daly JJ: Non-invasive papillary carcinoma of the bladder associated with carcinoma in situ. J Urol 116:575, 1976

391. Schellhammer PF, Whitmore WF Jr: Transitional cell carcinoma of the urethra in men having cystectomy for bladder cancer. J Urol 115:56, 1976

392. Farrow GM, Utz DC, Rife CC: Morphological and clinical observations of patients with early bladder cancer treated with total cystectomy. Cancer Res 36:2495, 1976

393. Farrow GM, Utz DC, Rife CC et al: Clinical observations on sixty-nine cases of in situ carcinoma of the urinary bladder. Can Res 37:2794, 1977

394. Richie JP, Skinner DG: Carcinoma in situ of the urethra associated with bladder carcinoma: The role of urethrectomy. J Urol 119:80, 1978

395. Koss, LG: Mapping of the urinary bladder: Its impact on the concepts of bladder cancer. Hum Pathol 5:533, 1979

396. Chasko SB, Gray GF, McCarron JP Jr: Urothelial neoplasia of the upper urinary tract. Pathol Annu, Part II. 16:127, 1981

397. Murphy WM, Soloway MS: Urothelial dysplasia. J Urol 127:849, 1982

398. Wolf H, Hojgaard K: Prognostic factors in local surgical treatment of invasive bladder cancer, with special reference to the presence of urothelial dysplasia. Cancer 51:1710, 1983

399. Grabstald H: Prostatic biopsy in selected patients with carcinoma in situ of the bladder: Preliminary report. J Urol 132:1117, 1984

Transitional Cell Carcinoma

Epidemiology and Etiology

400. Rehn L: Uber Basentumoren bei Fuchsinarbeitern. Arch Klin Chir 50:588, 1895

401. Gehrmann GH: Papilloma and carcinoma of the bladder in dye workers. JAMA 107:1436, 1936

402. Gay DM: Pathology of anilin tumor of the bladder. J Urol 38:221, 1937

403. Davis E: Chemical carcinogenesis, drugs, dyes, remedies and cosmetics with particular reference to bladder tumors. J Urol 49:14, 1943

404. Miller EC, Miller JA: In vivo combinations between carcinogens and tissue constituents and their possible role in carcinogenesis. Cancer Res 12:547, 1952

405. McDonald DF, Lund RR: The role of the urine in vesical neoplasm. 1. Experimental confirmation of the urogenous theory of pathogenesis. J Urol 71:560, 1954

406. Javadpour N, Mostofi FK: Primary epithelial tumors of the bladder in the first two decades of life. J Urol 101:706, 1969

407. Cole P, Monson RR, Haning H et al: Smoking and cancer of the lower urinary tract. N Engl J Med 284:129, 1971

408. Cole P, Hoover R, Friedell GH: Occupation and cancer of the lower urinary tract. Cancer 29:1250, 1972

409. McGuire EJ, Weiss RM, Baskin AM: Neoplasms of transitional cell origin in first twenty years of life. J Urol 1:57, 1973

410. Radomski JL, Rey AA, Brill E: Evidence for a glucuronic acid conjugate of N-hydroxy-4-aminobiphenyl in the urine of dogs given 4-aminobiphenyl. Cancer Res 33:1284, 1973

411. Kadlubar FF, Miller JA, Miller EC: Hepatic microsomal N-glucuronidation and nucleic acid binding of N-hydroxy arylamines in relation to urinary bladder carcinogenesis. Cancer 37:805, 1977

412. Miller AB: The etiology of bladder cancer from the epidemiological viewpoint. Cancer Res 37:2939, 1977

413. Miller AB, Morrison B: Artificial sweeteners and human bladder cancer. Lancet 2:578, 1977

414. Johnson DE, Hillis S: Carcinoma of the bladder in patients less than 40 years old. J Urol 120:172, 1978

415. Kadlubar FF, Miller JA, Miller EC: Guanyl O^6-arylamination and O^6-arylation of DNA by the carcinogen N-hydroxyl-l-naphthylamine. Cancer Res 38:3628, 1978

416. McCarthy, JP, Gavrell GJ, LeBlanc GA: Transitional cell carcinoma of bladder in patients under thirty years of age. Urol 8:487, 1979

417. Hoover R: Saccharin — bitter aftertaste? N Engl J Med 302:573, 1980

418. Morrison AS, Buring JE: Artificial sweetners and cancer of the lower urinary tract. N Engl J Med 302:537, 1980

419. Cherrie RJ, Lindner A, deKernion, JB: Transitional cell carcinoma of bladder in first four decades of life. Urol 20:582, 1982

420. Lower GM Jr: Concepts in causality: Chemically induced human urinary bladder cancer. Cancer 49:1056, 1982

421. Weinberg DM, Ross RK, Mack TM et al: Bladder cancer etiology. A different perspective. Cancer 51:675, 1983

422. Morrison AS, Cole P, Maclure KM: Epidemiology of urologic cancers. In Javadpour N (ed): Principles and Management of Urologic Cancer, 2nd ed, pp 13–32. Baltimore, Williams & Wilkins, 1983

423. Hartge P, Hoover R, Kantor A: Bladder cancer risk and pipes, cigars, and smokeless tobacco. Cancer 55:901, 1985
424. Gonzalez CA, Lopez – Abente G, Errezola M et al: Occupation, tobacco use, coffee, and bladder carcinoma cancer in the country of Mataro (Spain). Cancer 55:2031, 1985

Bladder Carcinoma Associated with Cyclophosphamide Therapy

425. Dale GA, Smith RB: Transitional cell carcinoma of the bladder associated with cyclophosphamide. J Urol 112:603, 1974
426. Wall RL, Clausen KP: Carcinoma of the urinary bladder in patients receiving cyclophosphamide. N Engl J Med 293:271, 1975
427. Fairchild WV, Spence CR, Solomon HD et al: The incidence of bladder cancer after cyclophosphamide therapy. J Urol 122:163, 1979
428. Ershler WB, Gilchrist KW, Citrin DL: Adriamycin enhancement of cyclophosphamide-induced bladder injury. J Urol 123:121, 1980
429. Glucksman MA: Letter: Bladder cancer after cyclophosphamide therapy. Urol 16:553, 1980
430. Hoover R, Fraumeni JF: Drug-induced cancer. Cancer 47:1071, 1981
431. Chodak GW, Straus FW, Schoenberg HW: Simultaneous occurence of transitional, squamous and adenocarcinoma of the bladder after 15 years of cyclophosphamide ingestion. J Urol 125:424, 1981
432. Carney CN, Stevens PS, Fried FA et al: Fibroblastic tumor of the urinary bladder after cyclophosphamide therapy. Arch Pathol Lab Med 106:247, 1982

Transitional Cell Carcinoma: Clinical Pathologic Studies

433. Aschner PW: The pathology of vesical neoplasms. Its evaluation in diagnosis and prognosis. JAMA 91:1697, 1928
434. Smith GG, Mintz ER: Bladder tumors: Observations on 150 cases. Am J Surg 20:54, 1933
435. Spooner AD: Metastasis in epithelioma of urinary bladder. Trans Am Assoc Genito-Urin Surg 27:81, 1934
436. Colston JAC, Leadbetter WF: Infiltrating carcinoma of the bladder. J Urol 36:669, 1936
437. Parmenter FJ, Leutenegger CJ: Bladder tumors. J Urol 35:316, 1936
438. Ash JE: Epithelial tumors of the bladder. J Urol 44:135, 1940
439. Papanicolaou G, Marshall VF: Urine sediment smears as a diagnostic procedure in cancers of the urinary tract. Science 101:519, 1945
440. Jewett HJ, Strong GH: Infiltrating carcinoma of the bladder: Relation of depth of penetration of the bladder wall to incidence of local extension and metastases. J Urol 55:366, 1946
441. Jewett HJ: Infiltrating carcinoma of the bladder. Application of pathologic observations to clinical diagnosis and prognosis. JAMA 134:496, 1947
442. McDonald JR, Thompson GJ: Carcinoma of the urinary bladder: A pathologic study with special reference to invasiveness and vascular invasion. J Urol 61:435, 1948
443. Royce RK, Ackerman LV: Carcinoma of the bladder; Study of clinical therapeutic and pathological aspects of 135 cases. J Urol 65:66, 1951
444. Jewett HJ: Carcinoma of the bladder: Influence of depth infiltration on the 5-year results following complete extirpation of the primary growth. J Urol 67:672, 1952
445. Marshall VF: The relation of the preoperative estimate to the pathologic demonstration of the extent of vesical neoplasms. J Urol 68:714, 1952
446. McDonald JR: Exfoliative cytology in genitourinary and pulmonary diseases. Am J Clin Pathol 24:684, 1954

447. Bischoff AJ, Fishkin BG: Carcinoma of the urinary bladder with cutaneous metastasis: Report of 4 cases. J Urol 75:701, 1956

448. Foot NC, Papanicolaou GN, Holmquist ND et al: Exfoliative cytology of urinary sediments. Cancer 11:127, 1958

449. Cooling CI: Review of 150 post-mortems of carcinoma of the urinary bladder. In Tumors of the Bladder, p 171. Wallace DM (ed): In Neoplastic Diseases at Various Sites, Vol II. Edinburgh, E and S Livingston, 1959

450. Fetter TR, Bogaev JH, McCuskey B et al: Carcinoma of the bladder: Sites of metastases. J Urol 81:746, 1959

451. Royce RK, Spjut HJ: Transitional cell carcinoma of the bladder, grade 1. (So-called papilloma). J Urol 82:486, 1959

452. Melamed MR, Koss LG, Ricci A et al: Cytohistological observations on developing carcinoma of the urinary bladder in man. Cancer 13:67, 1960

453. Francis RR: Carcinoma of the bladder. J Urol 85:552, 1961

453A. Whitmore WF Jr, Marshall VF: Radical total cystectomy for cancer of the bladder: 230 consecutive cases five years later. J Urol 87:853, 1962

454. Umiker W: Accuracy of cytologic diagnosis of cancer of the urinary tract. Acta Cytol 8:186, 1964

455. Jewett HJ, King LR, Shelley WM: A study of 365 cases of infiltrating bladder cancer: Relation of certain pathological characteristics to prognosis after extirpation. J Urol 92:668, 1964

456. Koss LG, Melamed MR, Ricci A et al: Carcinogenesis in the human urinary bladder. Observations after exposure to pra-aminodiphenyl. N Engl J Med 272:767, 1965

457. Bergkvist A, Ljungqvist A, Moberger G: Classification of bladder tumours based on the cellular pattern. Acta Chir Scand 130:378, 1965

458. Stone JH, Hodges CV: Radical cystectomy for invasive bladder cancer. J Urol 96:207, 1966

459. Maltry E Jr: Carcinoma of the bladder. J Urol 99:165, 1968

459A. Dunham LJ, Rabson AS, Stewart HL et al: Rates, interview, and pathology study of cancer of the urinary bladder in New Orleans, Louisiana. J Natl Can Inst 41:683, 1968

459B. Cordonnier JJ: Cystectomy for carcinoma of the bladder. J Urol 99:172, 1968

460. Esposti PL, Moberger G, Zajicen J: The cytologic diagnosis of transitional cell tumors of the urinary bladder and its histologic basis. A study of 567 cases of urinary-tract disorder including 170 untreated and 182 irradiated bladder tumors. Acta Cytol (Baltimore) 14:145, 1970

461. Sarnecki CT, McCormack LJ, Kiser WS et al: Urinary cytology and the clinical diagnosis of urinary tract malignancy: A clinicopathologic study of 1400 patients. J Urol 106:761, 1971

462. Bell JT, Burney SW, Friedell GH: Blood vessel invasion in human bladder cancer. J Urol 105:675, 1971

463. Long RTL, Grummon RA, Spratt JS Jr et al: Carcinoma of the urinary bladder (Comparison with radical, simple, and partial cystectomy and intravesical formalin). Cancer 29:98, 1972

464. Greene LF, Hanash KA, Farrow GM: Benign papilloma or papillary carcinoma of the bladder? J Urol 110:205, 1973

465. Mostofi FK, Sobin LH, Torloni H: Histological typing of urinary bladder tumours. International Histological Classification of Tumours, No 10. Geneva, World Health Organization, 1973

465A. Utz DC, Schmitz SE, Fugelso PD et al: A clinicopathologic evaluation of partial cystectomy for carcinoma of the urinary bladder. Cancer 32:1075, 1973

465B. Scott R Jr, Koff WJ, Hudgins PT et al: Preoperative irradiation in the surgical treatment of transitional cell cancer of the bladder: Preliminary report based on 12 years of experience. J Urol 109:405, 1973

466. Melicow MM: Tumors of the bladder: A multifaceted problem. J Urol 112:467, 1974

467. Varkarakis MJ, Gaeta J, Moore RH et al: Superficial bladder tumor. Aspects of clinical progression. J Urol 4:414, 1974

468. Richie JP, Skinner DG, Kaufman JJ: Radical cystectomy for carcinoma of the bladder: 16 years of experience. J Urol 113:186, 1975

469. Wajsman Z, Merrin C, Moore R et al: Current results from treatment of bladder tumors with total cystectomy at Roswell Park Memorial Institute. J Urol 113:806, 1975

470. Zincke H, Aguilo JJ, Farrow GM et al: Significance of urinary cytology in the early detection of transitional cell cancer of the upper urinary tract. J Urol 116:781, 1976

471. Althausen AF, Prout GR Jr, Daly JJ: Non-invasive papillary carcinoma of the bladder associated with carcinoma in situ. J Urol 116:575, 1976

472. Frable WJ, Paxson L, Barksdale JA et al: Current practice of urinary bladder cytology. Cancer Res 37:2800, 1977

473. Whitmore WF Jr, Batata MA, Ghoneim MA et al: Radical cystectomy with or without prior irradiation in the treatment of bladder cancer. J Urol 118:184, 1977

474. National Bladder Cancer Collaborative Group A: Cytology and histopathology of bladder cancer cases in a prospective longitudinal study. Cancer Res 37:2911, 1977

475. Williams JL, Hammonds JC, Saunders N: Tl bladder tumours. Br J Urol 49:663, 1977

476. Pearse HD, Reed RR, Hodges CV: Radical cystectomy for bladder cancer. J Urol 119:216, 1978

477. Gilbert HA, Logan JL, Kagan AR et al: The natural history of papillary transitional cell carcinoma of the bladder and its treatment in an unselected population on the basis of histologic grading. J Urol 119:488, 1978

477A. Brannan W, Ochsner MG, Fuselier HA Jr et al: Partial cystectomy in the treatment of transitional cell carcinoma of the bladder. J Urol 119:213, 1978

478. Emmott RC, Javadpour N, Bergman SM et al: Correlation of the cell surface antigens with stage and grade in cancer of the bladder. J Urol 121:37, 1979

479. Koss LG: Mapping of the urinary bladder: Its impact on the concepts of bladder cancer. Hum Pathol 5:533, 1979

480. Young AK, Hammond E, Middleton AW Jr: The prognostic value of cell surface antigens in low grade non-invasive, transitional cell carcinoma of the bladder. J Urol 122:462, 1979

481. Domagala W, Kahan AV, Koss LG: The ultrastructure of surfaces of positively identified cells in the human urinary sediment. A correlative light and scanning electron microscopic study. Acta Cytol (Baltimore) 23:147, 1979

482. Truesdale BH, Johnson RD, Evins SC: Carcinoma of bladder metastatic to breast. Urol 8:430, 1979

483. Rife CC, Farrow GM, Utz DC: Urine cytology of transitional cell neoplasms. Urol Clin North Am 6:599, 1979

484. Holmquist ND: Detection of urinary cancer with urinalysis sediment. J Urol 123:188, 1980

485. El–Bolkainy MN: Cytology of bladder carcinoma. J Urol 124:20, 1980

486. Cummings KB: Carcinoma of the bladder: Predictors. Cancer 45:1849, 1980

487. Nakamura S, Nijima T: Staging of bladder cancer by ultrasonography: A new technique by transurethral intravesical scanning. J Urol 124:341, 1980

488. Babaian RJ, Johnson DE, Llamas L et al: Metastases from transitional cell carcinoma of urinary bladder. Urol 16:142, 1980

489. Friedel GH, Parija GC, Nagy GK et al: The pathology of human bladder cancer. Cancer 45:1823, 1980

490. Slack NH, Prout GR Jr: The heterogeneity of invasive bladder carcinoma and different responses to treatment. J Urol 123:644, 1980

491. Anderstrom C, Johansson S, Nilsson S: The significance of lamina propria invasion of the prognosis of patients with bladder tumors. J Urol 124:23, 1980

492. Loening S, Narayana A, Yoder L et al: Factors influencing the recurrence rate of bladder cancer. J Urol 123:29, 1980

493. Kutscher HA, Leadbetter GW Jr, Vinson RK: Survival after radical cystectomy for invasive transitional cell carcinoma of bladder. Urol 17:231, 1981

494. Chasko SB, Gray GF, McCarron JP Jr: Urothelial neoplasia of the upper urinary tract. Pathol Annu, Part II 16:127, 1981

495. Colleen S, Ekelund L, Henrikson H et al: Staging of bladder carcinoma with computed tomography. Scand J Urol Nephrol 15:109, 1981

496. Coon JS, Weinstein RS: Detection of ABH tissue isoantigens by immunoperoxidase methods in normal and neoplastic urothelium. Comparison with the erythrocyte adherence method. Am J Clin Pathol 76:163, 1981

497. Catalona WJ: Practical utility of specific red cell adherence test in bladder cancer. Urol 18:113, 1981

498. Jacobs JB, Cohen SM, Farrow GM et al: Scanning electron microscopic features of human urinary bladder cancer. Cancer 48:1399, 1981

499. Alroy J, Pauli BU, Weinstein RS: Correlation between numbers of desmosomes and the aggressiveness of transitional cell carcinoma in human urinary bladder. Cancer 47:104, 1981

500. Kishi K, Hirota T, Matsumoto K et al: Carcinoma of the bladder: A clinical and pathological analysis of 87 autopsy cases. J Urol 125:36, 1981

501. Brawn PN: The origin of invasive carcinoma of the bladder. Cancer 50:515, 1982

502. Cieplinski W, Ciesielski TE, Haine C et al: Choroid metastases from transitional cell carcinoma of the bladder. A case report and a review of the literature. Cancer 50:1596, 1982

503. Skinner DG: Management of invasive bladder cancer: A meticulous pelvic node dissection can make a difference. J Urol 128:34, 1982

504. Silverberg E: Cancer statistics, 1982. CA 32:15, 1982

505. Limas C, Lange P: A, B, H antigen detectability in normal and neoplastic urothelium. Cancer 49:2476, 1982

506. Stein BS, Kendall AR: Specific red cell adherence testing and radiotherapy. Cancer 50:2329, 1982

507. Kaye KW, Lange PH: Mode of presentation of invasive bladder cancer: Reassessment of the problem. J Urol 128:31, 1982

508. Nelson RP: New concepts in staging and follow-up of bladder carcinoma. Urol 21:105, 1983

509. Beahrs OH, Myers MH (eds): Bladder. In Manual for Staging of Cancer, 2nd ed, p 171. Philadelphia, JB Lippincott, 1983

510. Heney NM, Ahmed S, Flanagan MJ et al: Superficial bladder cancer: Progression and recurrence. J Urol 130:1083, 1983

511. Hopkins SC, Ford KS, Soloway MS: Invasive bladder cancer: Support for screening. J Urol 130:61, 1983

512. Narayana AS, Loening SA, Slymen DJ et al: Bladder cancer: Factors affecting survival. J Urol 130:56, 1983

513. Matthews PN, Madden M, Bidgood KA et al: The clinicopathological features of metastatic superficial papillary bladder cancer. J Urol 132:904, 1984

514. Wijkstrom H, Gustafson H, Tribukait B: Deoxyribonucleic acid analysis in the evaluation of transitional cell carcinoma before cystectomy. J Urol 132:894, 1984

515. Chin JL, Huben RP, Nava E et al: Flow cytometric analysis of DNA content in human bladder tumors and irrigation fluids. Cancer 56:1677, 1985

Squamous Cell Carcinoma

516. Connery DB: Leukoplakia of the urinary bladder and its association with carcinoma. J Urol 69:121, 1953
517. Sakkas JL: Clinical pattern and treatment of squamous cell carcinoma of the bladder. Int Surg 45:71, 1966
518. Newman DM, Brown JR, Jay AC et al: Squamous cell carcinoma of the bladder. J Urol 100:470, 1968
519. Sarma KP: Squamous cell carcinoma of the bladder. Int Surg 53:313, 1970
520. Bessette PL, Abell, MR, Herwig KR: A clinicopathologic study of squamous cell carcinoma of the bladder. J Urol 112:66, 1974
521. Johnson DE, Schoenwald MB, Ayala AG, Miller LS: Squamous cell carcinoma of the bladder. J Urol 115:542, 1976
522. Richie JP, Waisman J, Skinner DG et al: Squamous carcinoma of the bladder: Treatment by radical cystectomy. J Urol 115:670, 1976
523. Rous SN: Squamous cell carcinoma of the bladder. J Urol 120:561, 1978
524. Morgan RJ, Cameron KM: Vesical leukoplakia. Br J Urol 52:96, 1980
525. Faysal MH: Squamous cell carcinoma of the bladder. J Urol 126:598, 1981
526. Benson RC Jr, Swanson SK, Farrow GM: Relationship of leukoplakia to urothelial malignancy. J Urol 131:507, 1984

Verrucous Carcinoma

527. Loewenstein LW: Carcinoma-like condylomata acuminate of the penis. Med Clin North Am 23:789, 1939
528. Ackerman LV: Verrucous carcinoma of the oral cavity. Surg 23:670, 1948
529. Kraus FT, Perez–Mesa C: Verrucous carcinoma. Clinical and pathologic study of 105 cases involving oral cavity, larynx and genitalia. Cancer 19:26, 1966
530. Profitt SD, Spooner TR, Kosek JC: Origin of undifferentiated neoplasm from verrucous epidermal carcinoma of oral cavity following irradiation. Cancer 30:194, 1972
531. El Sebai I, Sherif M, El Bolkainy MN et al: Verrucose squamous carcinoma of bladder. Urol 4:407, 1974
532. Wyatt JK, Craig I: Verrucous carcinoma of urinary bladder. Urol 16:97, 1980
533. Lowe D, McKee PH: Verrucous carcinoma of the penis. (Buschke–Löwenstein tumour): A clinicopathological study. Br J Urol 55:427, 1983
534. Youngberg GA, Thornthwaite JT, Inoshita T et al: Cytologically malignant squamous-cell carcinoma arising in a verrucous carcinoma of the penis. J Dermatol Surg Oncol 9:474, 1983
535. Johnson DE, Lo RK, Srigley J et al: Verrucous carcinoma of the penis. J Urol 133:216, 1985

Adenocarcinoma

536. Wheeler JD, Hill WT: Adenocarcinoma involving the urinary bladder. Cancer 7:119, 1954
537. Mostofi FK, Thompson RV, Dean AL Jr: Mucous adenocarcinoma of the urinary bladder. Cancer 8:741, 1955
538. Shaw JL, Gislason GJ, Imbriglia JE: Transition of cystitis glandularis to primary adenocarcinoma of the bladder. J Urol 79:815, 1958
539. Winter CC, Goodwin WE: Mucus-secreting adenocarcinoma of the urinary bladder simulating carcinoma of the gastrointestinal tract. Am Surg 25:875, 1959
540. Kittredge WE, Collett AJ, Morgan C Jr: Adenocarcinoma of the bladder associated with cystitis glandularis: A case report. J Urol 91:145, 1964
541. Allen TD, Henderson BW: Adenocarcinoma of the bladder. J Urol 93:50, 1965
542. Lopez–Engelking R, De La Cruz JV, De Maldonado MEF: Mucinous adenocarcinoma of the urinary tract. Trans Am Assoc Genito-Urinary Surg 58:144, 1966

543. Susmano D, Rubenstein AB, Dakin AR, Lloyd FA: Cystitis glandularis and adeno-carcinoma of the bladder. J Urol 105:671, 1971

544. Thomas DG, Ward AM, Williams JL: A study of 52 cases of adenocarcinoma of the bladder. Br J Urol 43:4, 1971

545. Johnson DE, Hogan HM, Ayala AG: Primary adenocarcinoma of the urinary blad-der. South Med J 65:527, 1972

546. Edwards PD, Hurm RA, Jaeschke WH: Conversion of cystitis glandularis to adeno-carcinoma. J Urol 108:568, 1972

547. Kovetz A, Elguezabal A: Primary nonurachal adenocarcinoma of bladder. NY State J Med 72:950, 1972

548. Khafagy MM, El–Bolkainy MN, Mansour MA: Carcinoma of the bilharzial urinary bladder. Cancer 30:150, 1972

549. Daroca PJ Jr, Mackenzie F, Reed RJ et al: Primary adenovillous carcinoma of the bladder. J Urol 115:41, 1976

550. Jacobo E, Loening S, Schmidt JD, Culp DA: Primary adenocarcinoma of the blad-der: A retrospective study of 20 patients. J Urol 117:54, 1977

551. Kramer SA, Bredael J, Croker BP et al: Primary non-urachal adenocarcinoma of the bladder. J Urol 121:278, 1979

552. Jones WA, Gibbons RP, Correa RJ Jr et al: Primary adenocarcinoma of bladder. Urol 15:119, 1980

553. Lin JI, Tseng CH, Choy C et al: Diffuse cystitis glandularis. Urol 15:411, 1980

554. Pallesen G: Neoplastic paneth cells in adenocarcinoma of the urinary bladder: A first case report. Cancer 47:1834, 1981

555. El–Bolkainy MN, Mokhtar NM, Ghoneim MA et al: The impact of schistosomiasis on the pathology of bladder carcinoma. Cancer 48:2643, 1981

556. Kishi K, Hirota T, Matsumoto K et al: Carcinoma of the bladder: A clinical and pathological analysis of 87 autopsy cases. J Urol 125:36, 1981

557. Zuppo V, Ikari O, D'Ancona CAL et al: Adenocarcinoma mucoso de vejiga. Arch Esp Urol 35 (6):385, 1982

558. Anderstrom C, Johansson SL, von Schultz L: Primary adenocarcinoma of the uri-nary bladder. Cancer 52:1273, 1983

559. Aygun C, Patanaphan V, Whitley NO et al: Mucin-producing adenocarcinoma of bladder. Urol 21:135, 1983

560. Nocks BN, Heney NM, Daly JJ: Primary adenocarcinoma of urinary bladder. Urol 21:26, 1983

Signet-Ring Cell Type

561. Saphir O: Signet-ring cell carcinoma of the urinary bladder. Am J Pathol 31:223, 1955

562. Schourup K: Rare malignant tumours of the urinary bladder. Acta Pathol Microbiol Scand (suppl) 105:145, 1955

563. Melicow MM: Tumors of the urinary bladder: A clinico-pathological analysis of over 2500 specimens and biopsies. J Urol 74:498, 1955

564. Payan HM, Mendoza C Jr, Cabinum D et al: Primary signet ring cell carcinoma of the urinary bladder. Arch Surg 92:958, 1966

565. Rosas–Uribe A, Luna MA: Primary signet ring cell Report of two cases. Arch Pathol 88:294, 1969

566. Corwin SH, Tassy F, Malament M et al: Rare signet ring cell variant of mucinous adenocarcinoma of the bladder. J Urol 106:697, 1971

567. Naeim F, Schlezinger RM, de la Maza, L: Primary signet ring cell carcinoma of the bladder: Report of a case and review of the literature. J Urol 108:274, 1972

568. de Ture FA, Dein R, Hackett RL, Drylie DM: Primary signet ring cell carcinoma of bladder exemplifying vesical epithelial multipotentiality. Urol 6:240, 1975

569. Austin GE, Safford J: Signet ring cell carcinoma of bladder. Urol 12:458, 1978

570. Fuselier HA Jr, Brannan W, Ochsner MG et al: Adenocarcinoma of the bladder as the bladder as seen at Ochsner Medical Institutions. South Med J 71:804, 1978
571. Sagalowsky A, Donohue, JP: Sixteen-year survival with metastatic signet ring cell bladder carcinoma. Urol 15:501, 1980
572. Braun EV, Ali M, Fayemi AO et al: Primary signet-ring cell carcinoma of the urinary bladder: Review of the literature and report of a case. Cancer 47:1430, 1981
573. Poore E, Egbert B, Jahnke R et al: Signet ring cell adenocarcinoma of the bladder. Linitis plastica variant. Arch Pathol Lab Med 105:203, 1981
574. Yoshida H, Iwata H, Ochi K et al: Primary signet-ring cell carcinoma of urinary bladder. Urol 17:481, 1981
575. Gonzalez E, Fowler MR, Venable DD: Primary signet ring cell adenocarcinoma of the bladder. (Linitis plastica of the bladder): Report of a case and review of the literature. J Urol 128:1027, 1982
576. Choi H, Lamb S, Pintar K et al: Primary signet-ring cell carcinoma of the urinary bladder. Cancer 53:1985, 1984

Clear Cell Carcinoma

577. Schiller W: Mesonephroma ovarii. Am J Cancer 35:1, 1939
578. Dow JA, Young JD Jr: Mesonephric adenocarcinoma of the bladder. J Urol 100:466, 1968
579. Skor AB, Warren MM: Mesonephric adenocarcinoma of bladder. Urol 10:64, 1977
580. Scully RE: Tumors of the ovary and maldeveloped gonads. In Atlas of Tumor Pathology, 2nd series, Fascicle 16, p 117. Washington, DC, AFIP, 1979
581. Pegoraro V, Cosciani–Cunico S, Granziotti PP et al: L'adenocarcinome mesonephrique de la vessie. J Urol (Paris) 88:531, 1982
582. Kanokogi M, Uematsu K, Kakudo K et al: Mesonephric adenocarcinoma of the urinary bladder: An autopsy case. J Surg Oncol 22:118, 1983
583. Schultz RE, Bloch MJ, Tomaszewski JE et al: Mesonephric adenocarcinoma of the bladder. J Urol 132:263, 1984

Carcinoma with Mixed Differentiation

584. Grace DA, Winter CC: Mixed differentiation of primary carcinoma of the urinary bladder. Cancer 21:1239, 1968

Carcinoid Tumor

585. Feyrter F: Zur Pathologie des urogenitalen Helle-Zellen-Systems. Virchows Arch 320:564, 1951
586. Aoyama H, Yoshida K, Kondo T et al: Primary carcinoid tumor of the urinary bladder. (Report of a case). Jpn J Urol 69:124, 1978
587. Aozasa K, Yokoyama M, Uda H et al: Primary carcinoid tumor in the urinary bladder. A case report. Med J Osaka Univ 30:1, 1979
588. Colby TV: Carcinoid tumor of the bladder. A case report. Arch Pathol Lab Med 104:199, 1980

Small Cell Undifferentiated Carcinoma (Oat Cell Carcinoma)

589. Cramer SF, Aikawa M, Cebelin M: Neurosecretory granules in small cell invasive carcinoma of the urinary bladder. Cancer 47:724, 1981
590. Ibrahim NBN, Briggs JC, Corbishley CM: Extrapulmonary oat cell carcinoma. Cancer 54:1645, 1984
591. Partanen S, Asikainen U: Oat cell carcinoma of the urinary bladder with ectopic adrenocorticotropic hormone production. Hum Pathol 16:313, 1985

Malignant Melanoma

592. Wheelock MC: Sarcoma of the urinary bladder. J Urol 48:628, 1942
593. Su C–T, Prince CL: Melanoma of the bladder. J Urol 87:365, 1962

594. Ainsworth AM, Clark WH Jr, Mastrangelo M et al: Primary malignant melanoma of the urinary bladder. Cancer 37:1928, 1976

595. Willis AJ, Huang AH, Carrol P: Primary melanoma of the bladder: A case report and review. J Urol 123:278, 1980

596. Anichkov NM, Nikonov AA: Primary malignant melanomas of the bladder. J Urol 128:813, 1982

Benign Mesenchymal Neoplasms

Leiomyoma

597. Kretschmer HL: Leiomyoma of the bladder. With a report of a case and a review of the literature. J Urol 26:575, 1931

598. Campbell EW, Gislason GJ: Benign mesothelial tumors of the urinary bladder: Review of literature and a report of a case of leiomyoma. J Urol 70:733, 1953

599. Zaffagnini V: Il liomioma della vescica. Arch Ital Urol 27:184, 1954

600. Williams DI, Schistad G: Lower urinary tract tumours in children. Br J Urol 36:51, 1964

601. De Felice G, Vecchione A: Il leiomioma della vescica. Riv Anat Pat Oncol 33:251, 1968

602. Cukier J, Benhamou G: Leiomyome de la vessie (A propos de deux observations). J Urol Nephrol 76:61, 1970

603. Mutchler RW, Gorder JL: Leiomyoma of the bladder in a child. Br J Radiol 45:538, 1972

604. Thompson IM, Balfour J: Leiomyomatous vesical outlet obstruction. Urol 3:92, 1974

605. O'Connell K, Edson M: Leiomyoma of bladder. Urol 6:114, 1975

606. Katz RB, Waldbaum RS: Benign mesothelial tumor of bladder. Urol 5:236, 1975

607. Bittard M, Carbillet J–P, Paoletti G et al: Les leiomyomes du bas appareil urinaire chéz la femme. A propos de deux observations. J Urol Nephrol 83:226, 1977

608. Bellis JA, Post GJ, Rochman SC, Milam DF: Genitourinary leiomyomas. Urol 13:424, 1979

609. Albert NE: Leiomyoma of bladder. Preoperative diagnosis by ultrasound. Urol 17:486, 1981

610. Lake MH, Kossow AS, Bokinsky G: Leiomyoma of the bladder and urethra. J Urol 125:742, 1981

611. Vargas A, Mendez R: Leiomyoma of bladder. Urol 21:308, 1983

612. Frantz BB, Finkelstein LH, Arsht DB et al: Leiomyoma of the urinary bladder associated with in situ transitional cell carcinoma: Report of a case and review of the literature. J Am Osteopath Assoc 82:574, 1983

Hemangioma

613. Katz A: Cavernous hemangioma of the bladder. J Urol 15:201, 1926

614. Segal AD, Fink H: Cavaernous hemangioma of the bladder. J Urol 47:453, 1942

615. Hamsher JB, Farrar T, Moore TD: Congenital vascular tumors and malformations involving urinary tract: Diagnosis and surgical management. J Urol 80:299, 1958.

616. Fuleihan FM, Cordonnier JJ: Hemangioma of the bladder: Report of a case and review of the literature. J Urol 102:581, 1969

617. Hendry WF, Vinnicombe J: Hemangioma of bladder in children and young adults. Br J Urol 43:309, 1971

618. Hall BD: Bladder hemangiomas in Klippel–Trenaunay–Weber syndrome. N Engl J Med 285:1032, 1971

619. Morales A: Haemangioma of the bladder. Postgrad Med J 48:117, 1972

620. Esguerra A, Carvajal A, Mouton H: Pelvic arteriography in the diagnosis of hemangioma of the bladder. J Urol 109:609, 1973

621. Bocker R, Kollias G: Hamangiom der Harnblase. Urologe [Ausg A] 13:90, 1974

622. Klein TW, Kaplan GW: Klippel – Trenaunay syndrome associated with urinary tract hemangiomas. J Urol 114:596, 1975

623. Anderson RU, Andonian RW, Jamison RL: Multiple hemangiomas involving genitourinary system. Conservative management with streptokinase. Urol 10:246, 1977

624. Proca E: Haemangioma of the bladder. Short case report. Br J Urol 49:60, 1977

625. Bouday E, Dimitrov D, Charles G et al: A propos d'un cas rare d'hemangiome caverneux de la vessie. J Urol Nephrol 3:203, 1977

626. Van Dessel J, Michielsen JP: The haemangioma of the bladder. Case report and review of the literature. Acta Urol Belg 46:369, 1978

627. Gottesman JE, Seale RH: Cavernous haemangioma of the bladder. Br J Urol 55:450, 1983

628. Stenos J, Pavlakis A, Rebelakos A: L'hemangiome caverneux de la vessie. A propos de deux cas. J Urol 89:83, 1983

629. Amr SS, Putong PB, Petersen RO: Hemangioma of the urinary bladder — An unusual clinical presentation. Jordan Med J 17:205, 1983

Granular Cell Tumor

630. Hirsch EF, Brown BM: Myoblastic sarcoma of the urinary bladder. Arch Surg 37:562, 1938

631. Ravich A, Stout AP, Ravich RA: Malignant granular cell myoblastoma involving the urinary bladder. Ann Surg 121:361, 1945

632. Andersen R, Hoeg K: Myoblastoma of the bladder neck: Report of a case. Br J Urol 33:76, 1961

633. Marsh RJ, Ceccarelli FE: Ten-year analysis of primary bladder tumors at Brooke General Hospital. J Urol 91:530, 1964

634. Seery WH: Granular cell myoblastoma of the bladder: Report of a case. J Urol 100:735, 1968

635. Okuda N, Ohkawa T, Nakamura T et al: Granular cell myoblastoma. Acta Urol Jpn 15:505, 1969

636. Christ ML, Ozzello L: Myogenous origin of a granular cell tumor of the urinary bladder. Am J Clin Pathol 56:736, 1971

637. Mizutani S, Okuda N, Sonoda T: Granular cell myoblastoma of the bladder: Report of an additional case. J Urol 110:403, 1973

638. Mouradian JA, Coleman JW, McGovern JH, Gray GF: Granular cell tumor (myoblastoma) of the bladder. J Urol 112:343, 1974

639. Stefansson K, Wollmann RL: S – 100 protein in granular cell tumors (granular cell myoblastoma). Cancer 49:1834, 1982

640. Enzinger FM, Weiss SW: Benign tumors and tumorlike lesions of uncertain histogenesis. In Soft Tissue Tumors, p 745. St Louis, CV Mosby, 1983

Neurofibroma and Neurofibromatosis

641. Mintz ER: Pedunculated neurofibroma of the bladder. J Urol 43:268, 1940

642. de Klerk JN, Campbell WA: Neurofibromatosis of the bladder. J Urol 72:1167, 1954

643. Ross JA: A case of sarcoma of the urinary bladder in Von Recklinghausen's disease. Br J Urol 29:121, 1957

644. Gonzalez – Angulo A, Reyes HA: Neurofibromatosis involving the lower urinary tract. J Urol 89:804, 1963

645. Cameron KM: Neurofibromatosis of the bladder. Br J Urol 56:77, 1964

646. Pesin JI, Bodian M: Neurofibromatosis of the pelvic autonomic plexuses. Br J Urol 36:510, 1964

647. Torres H, Bennett MJ: Neurofibromatosis of the bladder: Case report and review of the literature. J Urol 96:910, 1966

648. Clark SS, Marlett MM, Prudencio RF, Dasgupta TK: Neurofibromatosis of the bladder in children: Case report and literature review. J Urol 118:654, 1977

Ganglioneuroma

649. Wyman HE, Chappell BS, Jones WR Jr: Ganglioneuroma of bladder: Report of a case. J Urol 63:526, 1950

Lipoma

650. Kracht H: Lipom der Harnblasenschleimhaut. Z Urol 59:269, 1966

Lymphangioma

651. Bolkier M, Ginesin Y, Lichtig C et al: Lymphangioma of bladder. J Urol 129:1049, 1983

Malignant Mesenchymal Neoplasms

652. Wilder JA: Primary sarcoma of the bladder. With a report of three cases and review of the literature. Am J Med Sci 129:63, 1905
653. McCrea LE, Post EA: Sarcoma of the bladder. Urol Survey 5:307, 1955
654. Tripathi VNP, Dick VS: Primary sarcoma of the urogenital system in adults. J Urol 101:898, 1969

Leiomyosarcoma

655. Bergman RT, Kugel AI: Leiomyosarcoma of the urinary bladder. Urol Cutan Rev 54:65, 1950
656. Sadler RN, Shelley HS, McCarty JE: Leiomyosarcoma of the urinary bladder: Report of a case. J Urol 72:211, 1954
657. Silbar JD, Silbar SJ: Leiomyosarcoma of bladder: Three case reports and a review of literature. J Urol 73:103, 1955
658. Lash AF: Leiomyosarcoma of the bladder. Follow-up report of a case with thirteen years' survival. Obstet Gynecol 8:213, 1956
659. Bohne AW, Urwiller RD, Pantos TG: Leiomyosarcoma of the urinary bladder with review of the literature. Henry Ford Hosp Med Bull 10:445, 1962
660. Brown HE: Leiomyosarcoma of the blader: Followup report of two cases with 4 and 10 years' survival. J Urol 94:247, 1965
661. Reeves JF Jr, Powell EB, Powell NB: Leiomyosarcoma of the bladder: Case report with autopsy. J Urol 97:486, 1967
662. Mackenzie AR, Whitmore WF Jr, Melamed MR: Myosarcomas of the bladder and prostate. Cancer 22:833, 1968
663. Tripathi VNP, Dick VS: Primary sarcoma of the urogenital system in adults. J Urol 101:898, 1969
664. Mackenzie AR, Sharma TC, Whitmore WF Jr et al: Non-extirpative treatment of myosarcomas of the bladder and prostate. Cancer 28:329, 1971
665. Tara HH, Mentus NL: Leiomyosarcoma of urinary bladder. Urol 2:460, 1973
666. Weitzner S: Leiomyosarcoma of urinary bladder in children. Urol 12:450, 1978
667. Papacharalambous AN, Pavlakis AJ: Leiomyosarcoma of the bladder. Br J Urol 51:321, 1979
668. Wilson TM, Fauver HE, Weigel JW: Leiomyosarcoma of urinary bladder. J Urol 13:565, 1979
669. Savir A, Meiraz D: Malignant mesodermal (mesenchymal) tumors of bladder. J Urol 16:307, 1980
670. Alabaster AM, Jordan WP Jr, Soloway MS et al: Leiomyosarcoma of the bladder and subsequent urethral recurrence. J Urol 125:583, 1981
671. Patterson DE, Barrett DM: Leiomyosarcoma of urinary bladder. Urol 21:367, 1983

672. Swartz DA, Johnson DE, Ayala AG et al: Bladder leiomyosarcoma: A review of 10 cases with 5-year followup. J Urol 133:200, 1985

673. Seo IS, CLark SA, McGovern FD et al: Leiomyosarcoma of the urinary bladder. 13 years after cyclophosphamide therapy for Hodgkin's disease. Cancer 55:1597, 1985

Rhabdomyosarcoma

674. Hirsch EF, Brown BM: Myoblastic sarcoma of the urinary bladder. Arch Surg 37:562, 1938

675. Mostofi FK, Morse WH: Polypoid rhabdomyosarcoma (Sarcoma Botryoides) of bladder in children. J Urol 67:681, 1952

676. Horn RC, Enterline HT: Rhabdomyosarcoma: A clinicopathological study of 39 cases. Cancer 11:181, 1958

677. Thompson IM, Coppridge AJ: The management of bladder tumors in children: A study of sarcoma botryoides. J Urol 82:590, 1959

678. Kohler FP, Murphy JJ: Rhabdomyosarcoma of the male genital tract. J Urol 82:500, 1959

679. Maletta T, Horton B: Botryoidal sarcoma of the bladder in children: A case report. J Urol 82:490, 1959

680. Parker P, Smith PL, Rathmell TK: Sarcoma botryoides of the bladder: Successful therapy by cystectomy. J Urol 82:494, 1959

681. Hellstrom HR, Fisher ER: Embryonal rhabdomyosarcoma of the bladder in the aged. J Urol 86:336, 1961

682. Legier JF: Botryoid sarcoma and rhabdomyosarcoma of the bladder: Review of the literature and report of 3 cases. J Urol 86:583, 1961

683. Bhansali SK: Sarcma botryoides of the bladder in infancy and childhood. J Urol 87:871, 1962

684. Williams DI, Schistad G: Lower urinary tract tumours in children. Br J Urol 36:51, 1964

685. Evans AT, Bell TE: Rhabdomyosarcoma of the bladder in adult patients: Report of three cases. J Urol 94:573, 1965

686. Joshi DP, Wessely Z, Seery WH et al: Rhabdomyosarcoma of the bladder in an adult: Case report and review of the literature. J Urol 96:214, 1966

687. Kafka V, Krolupper M, Palecek L: Rhabdomyosarcoma of the bladder in childhood: Report of a successfully treated case. J Urol 96:210, 1966

688. Mackenzie AR, Whitmore WF Jr, Melamed MR: Myosarcomas of the bladder and prostate. Cancer 22:833, 1968

689. Jarman WD, Kenealy JC: Polypoid rhabdomyosarcoma of the bladder in children. J Urol 103:227, 1970

690. Tefft M, Jaffe N: Sarcoma of the bladder and prostate in children. Rationale for the role of radiation therapy based on a review of the literature and a report of fourteen additional patients. Cancer 32:1161, 1973

691. Heyn RM, Holland R, Newton WA Jr et al: The role of combined chemotherapy in the treatment of rhabdomyosarcoma in children. Cancer 34:2128, 1974

692. Auvert J, Boureau M, Weisgerber G: Embryonal sarcoma of the lower urinary tract in children: 5-year survival in 2 cases after radical treatment. J Urol 112:396, 1974

693. Timmons JW Jr, Burgert EO Jr, Soule EH et al: Embryonal rhabdomyosarcoma of the bladder and prostate in childhood. J Urol 113:694, 1975

694. Maurer HM, Moon T, Donaldson M et al: The intergroup rhabdomyosarcoma study. A preliminary report. Cancer 40:2015, 1977

695. Narayana AS, Loening S, Weimar GW, Culp DA: Sarcoma of the bladder and prostate. J Urol 119:72, 1978

696. Mukai K, Rosai J, Hallaway BE: Localization of myoglobin in normal and neoplastic human skeletal muscle cells using an immunoperoxidase method. Am J Surg Pathol 3:373, 1979

697. Gonzalez–Cruzzi F, Balck–Schaffer S: Rhabdomyosarcoma of infancy and child-hood. Problems of morphologic classification. Am J Surg Pathol 3:157, 1979

698. Sarnat HB, deMello DE, Siddiqui SY: Diagnostic value of histochemistry in em-bryonal rhabdomyosarcoma. Am J Surg Pathol 3:177, 1979

699. McDougal WS, Persky L: Rhabdomyosarcoma of the bladder and prostate in chil-dren. J Urol 124:882, 1980

700. Hays DM, Raney RB Jr, Lawrence W Jr et al: Bladder and prostatic tumors in the intergroup rhabdomyosarcoma study (IRS–I). Results of therapy. Cancer 50:1472, 1982

701. Kaplan WE, Firlit CF, Berger RM: Genitourinary rhabdomyosarcoma. J Urol 130:116, 1983

702. Enzinger FM, Weiss SW: Rhabdomyosarcoma. In Soft Tissue Tumors, p 338. St Louis, CV Mosby, 1983

Fibrosarcoma

703. Wilder JA: Primary sarcoma of the bladder. With a report of three cases and review of the literature. Am J Med Sci 129:63, 1905

704. McCrea LE, Post EA: Sarcoma of the bladder. Urol Survey 5:307, 1955

705. Tripathi VNP, Dick VS: Primary sarcoma of the urogenital system in adults. J Urol 101:898, 1969

706. Narayana AS, Loening S, Weimar GW et al: Sarcoma of the bladder and prostate. J Urol 119:72, 1978

707. Savir A, Meiraz D: Malignant mesodermal (mesenchymal) tumors of bladder. Urol 16:307, 1980

Osteogenic Sarcoma

708. Huggins CB: The formation of bone under the influence of epithelium of the urinary tract. Arch Surg 22:377, 1931

709. Tremblay RG, Crane AR, Harris A: Primary osteogenic sarcoma of bladder. J Urol 51:143, 1944

710. Pang S–C: Bony and cartilaginous tumours of the urinary bladder. J Pathol Bacter-iol 76:357, 1958

711. Nicolai CH, Spjut HJ: Primary osteogenic sarcoma of the bladder. J Urol 82:497, 1959

Malignant Mesenchymoma

712. Stout AP: Mesenchymoma, the mixed tumor of mesenchymal derivates. Ann Surg 127:278, 1948

713. Jones HM, Ross CF: Osteogenic leiomyosarcoma of the bladder. Br J Surg 38:242, 1950

714. Enzinger FM, Weiss SW: Soft Tissue Tumors, p 808. St Louis, CV Mosby, 1983

Miscellaneous Neoplasms

Pheochromocytoma

715. Zimmerman IJ, Biron RE, MacMahon HE: Pheochromocytoma of the urinary bladder. N Engl J Med 249:25, 1953

716. Lumb BRB, Gresham GA: Phaeochromocytoma of the urinary bladder. Lancet 1:81, 1958

717. Pugh RCB: Phaeochromocytoma of the bladder. Br J Urol 30:432, 1958

718. Farley SE, Smith CL: Unusual location of pheochromocytoma in the urinary blad-der. J Urol 81:130, 1959

719. Scott WW, Eversole SL: Pheochromocytoma of the urinary bladder. J Urol 83:656, 1960

720. Pugh RCB, Gresham GA, Mullaney J: Phaeochromocytoma of the urinary bladder. J Pathol Bacteriol 79:89, 1960

721. Barroso–Moguel R, Costero I: Argentaffin cells of the carotid body tumor. Am J Pathol 41:389, 1962

722. Moloney GE, Cowdell RH, Lewis CL: Malignant phaeochromocytoma of the bladder. Br J Urol 38:461, 1966

723. Higgins PMcR, Tresidder GC: Phaeochromocytoma of the urinary bladder. Br Med J 2:274, 1966

724. Yoffa DE, Withycombe JFR: Bladder-phaeochromocytoma metastases. Lancet 2:422, 1967

725. Anton AH, Greer M, Sayre DF et al: Dihydroxyphenylalanine secretion in a malignant pheochromocytoma. Am J Med 42:469, 1967

726. Cummins BH, Hill S, Williams JL: Phaeochromocytoma of the urinary bladder. Br J Urol 41:71, 1969

727. Leestma JE, Price EB Jr: Paraganglioma of the urinary bladder. Cancer 28:1063, 1971

728. Lewis PD: A cytophotometric study of benign and malignant phaeochromocytomas. Virchows Arch [Cell Pathol] 9:371, 1971

729. Shimbo S, Nakano Y: A case of malignant pheochromocytoma producing parathyroid hormone-lide sybstance. Calcif Tissue Res 15:155, 1974

730. Campbell DR, Mason WF, Manchester JS: Angiography in pheochromocytomas. J Can Assoc Radiol 25:214, 1974

731. Fuselier HA Jr: Paraganglioma of the bladder: Report of a case. J Urol 113:42, 1975

732. Javaheri P, Raafat J: Malignant phaeochromocytoma of the urinary bladder—Report of two cases. Br J Urol 47:401, 1975

733. Deklerk DP, Catalona WJ, Nime FA et al: Malignant pheochromocytoma of the bladder: The late development of renal cell carcinoma. J Urol 113:864, 1975

734. Lindsey CM, DeHart HS, Glenn JF: Pheochromocytoma of urinary bladder. Urol 7:210, 1976

735. Leong CH, Wong KK, Saw D: Asymptomatic phaechromocytoma of the bladder co-existing with carcinoma. Br J Urol 48:123, 1976

736. Lang R, Meurer KA, Kaufmann W: Rezidivierendes phaochromozytom. Med Welt 28:157, 1977

737. Raju BS, Vaidyanathan S, Banerjee CK et al: Malignant pheochromocytoma of the urinary bladder associated with dystrophic tumor calcification and a bladder stone. J Assoc Physicians India 25:929, 1977

738. Melicow MM: One hundred cases of pheochromochytoma (107 tumors) at the Columbia-Presbyterian Medical Center, 1926–1976. A clinicopathological analysis. Cancer 40:1987, 1977

739. Mahoney EM, Harrison JH: Malignant pheochromocytoma: Clinical course and treatment. J Urol 118:225, 1977

740. Texter JH Jr, Crane DB, Hietala S–O et al: Paraganglioma of urinary bladder wall. Urol 10:79, 1977

741. Meyer JJ, Sane SM, Drake RM: Malignant paraganglioma (pheochromocytoma) of the urinary bladder: Report of a case and review of the literature. Pediatrics 63:879, 1979

742. Kaufman JJ, Franklin S: Familial pheochromocytoma: Report of 2 cases in a kindred. J Urol 12:801, 1979

743. Das S, Lowe P: Malignant pheochromocytoma of the bladder. J Urol 123:282, 1980

744. Flanigan RC, Wittmann RP, Huhn RG et al: Malignant pheochromocytoma of urinary bladder. Urol 16:386, 1980

745. Higgins PMcR, Tresidder GC: Malignant phaeochromocytoma of the urinary bladder. Br J Urol 52:230, 1980

746. Hurwitz R, Fitzpatrick T, Ackerman I et al: A Neuro-ectodermal tumor in the bladder. J Urol 124:417, 1980

747. Ochi K, Yoshioka S, Morita M et al: Pheochromocytoma of bladder. Urol 17:228, 1981

748. Hamberger B, Arner S, Backman K–A et al: Pheochromocytoma of the bladder. Scand J Urol Nephrol 15:333, 1981

749. Messerli FH, Finn M, MacPhee AA: Pheochromocytoma of the urinary bladder. JAMA 247:1863, 1982

750. Dow DJ, Palmer MK, O'Sullivan JP et al: Malignant pheochromocytoma: Report of a case and a critical review. Br J Surg 69:338, 1982

751. Das S, Bulusu NV, Lowe P: Primary vesical pheochromocytoma. Urol 21:20, 1983

752. Chepurnoi GI, Kobzar ON, Lebedev SA et al: Pheochrocytoma of the urinary bladder. Urol Nefrol (Musk) 5:62, 1984

753. Schutz W, Vogel E: Pheochromocytoma of the urinary bladder — A case report and review of the literature. Urol Int 39:250, 1984

Plasmacytoma

754. Marion G, Leroux: Plasmocytome vesical. J Urol (Paris) 118:121, 1924

755. Gorfain AD: Extramedullary plasmacytoma of the bladder with local metastasis. Calif Med 71:147, 1949

756. Auvigne R, Auvigne J, Kerneis J: Un cas de plasmocytome de la vessie. J Urol (Paris) 62:85, 1956

757. Koss LG: Tumors of the urinary bladder. In Atlas of Tumor Pathology, 2nd Series, Fascicle 11, p 92. Washington, DC, AFIP, 1975

758. Yang C, Motteram R, Sandeman TF: Extramedullary plasmacytoma of the bladder. A case report and review of literature. Cancer 50:146, 1982

Primary Malignant Lymphoma

759. Jacobs A, Symington T: Primary lymphosarcoma of urinary bladder. Br J Urol 25:119, 1953

760. Bhansali SK, Cameron KM: Primary malignant lymphoma of the bladder. Br J Urol 32:440, 1960

761. Borski AA: Lymphosarcoma of the bladder. J Urol 48:551, 1960

762. Parton I: Primary lymphosarcoma of the bladder. Br J Urol 34:221, 1962

763. Pontius EE, Nourse MH, Paz L et al: Primary malignant lymphomas of the bladder. J Urol 90:58, 1963

764. Stitt RB, Colapinto V: Multiple simultaneous bladder malignancies: Primary lymphosarcoma and adenocarcinoma. J Urol 96:733, 1966

765. Wang CC, Scully RE, Leadbetter WF: Primary malignant lymphoma of the urinary bladder. Cancer 24:772, 1969

766. Aquilina JN, Bugeja TJ: Primary malignant lymphoma of the bladder: case report and review of the literature. J Urol 112:64, 1974

767. Makinen J, Alfthan O, Vuori J: Malignant lymphoma of the urinary bladder. Eur Urol 5:45, 1979

768. Mincione GP: Primary malignant lymphoma of the urinary bladder with a positive cytologic report. Acta Cytol (Baltimore) 26:69, 1982

769. Forrest JB, Saypol DC, Mills SE, Gillenwater JY: Immunoblastic sarcoma of the bladder. J Urol 130:350, 1983

Secondary Lymphoma; Leukemia

770. Givler RL: Involvement of the bladder in leukemia and lymphoma. J Urol 105:667, 1971

771. Sufrin G, Keogh B, Moore RH et al: Secondary involvement of the bladder in malignant lymphoma. J Urol 118:251, 1977

772. Winter CC, Puente E, Wall RL: Bladder involvement with lymphoma. J Urol 14:151, 1979

Mixed Cell Type Neoplasms

Carcinosarcoma

773. Meyer R: Beitrag zur Verstandigung uber die Namengebung in der Geschwulstlehre. Z Allg Pathol 30:291, 1920

774. Huggins CB: The formation of bone under the influence of epithelium of the urinary tract. Arch Surg 22:377, 1931

775. Saphir O, Vass A: Carcinosarcoma. Am J Cancer 33:331, 1938

776. Arnold W: Teratoides karzinosarkom der harnblase. Z Allg Path Pathol Anat 77:52, 1941

777. Willis RA: Malignant mixed tumor of bladder. Tex J Med 46:627, 1950

778. Quilter TN: Embryoma of the urinary bladder. J Urol 76:392, 1956

779. Pang LSC: Bony and cartilaginous tumours of the urinary bladder. J Pathol Bacteriol 76:352, 1958

780. Baranyai E, Goracz G: Karzinosarkom der harnblase. Z Allg Path Pathol Anat 99:365, 1959

781. Nicolai CH, Spjut HJ: Primary osteogenic sarcoma of the bladder. J Urol 82:497, 1959

782. Fruhling L, Batzenschlager A, Blum E: Epitheliosarcomes vrais (tumeurs mixtes malignes) et cancers doubles didermiques de la vessie. Ann Anat Pathol 4:5, 1959

783. Thompson IM, Coppridge AJ: Bladder sarcoma. J Urol 82:329, 1959

784. Willis RA: Carcino-sarcoma. In Pathology of Tumors, 4th ed, p 138. New York, Appleton–Century–Crofts, 1967

785. Brinton JA, Ito Y, Olsen BS: Carcinosarcoma of the urinary bladder. Cancer 25:1183, 1970

786. Fujita K, Nakauchi K, Matsumoto K et al: Malignant mixed mesodermal tumor of the urogenital tract: Report of a case developed on the patient of urinary bladder transitional cell carcinoma and discussion on its entity. Jpn J Urol 63:346, 1972

787. Holtz F, Fox JE, Abell MR: Carcinosarcoma of the urinary bladder. Cancer 29:294, 1972

788. Delides GS: Bone and cartilage in malignant tumours of the urinary bladder. Br J Urol 44:571, 1972

789. Shivde AV, Kherdekar MS: Carcinosarcoma of the urinary bladder. A case report and review of literature. Indian J Med Sci 27:932, 1973

790. McCarthy LJ, Wahle WM, Moosey NA: Carcinosarcoma of the urinary bladder — A case report. J Indiana State Med Assoc 68:722, 1975

791. Patterson TH, Dale GA: Carcinosarcoma of the bladder: Case report and review of the literature. J Urol 115:753, 1976

792. Johansen SE, Stenwig AE, Tveter KJ: Carcinosarcoma of the urinary bladder in an adult male. Scand J Urol Nephrol 13:117, 1979

793. Schoborg TW, Saffos RO, Rodriquez AP, Scott C Jr: Carcinosarcoma of the bladder. J Urol 124:724, 1980

794. Uyama T, Moriwaki S: Carcinosarcoma of urinary bladder. Urol 18:191, 1981

795. Brooks JJ: Immunohistochemistry of soft tissue tumours: Progress and prospects. Hum Pathol 13:969, 1982

796. Figueiredo L, Nogueira March JL, Ojea A et al: Carcinosarcoma vesical. A proposito de dos casos. Arch Esp Urol 35:179, 1982

797. Smith JA Jr, Herr HW, Middleton RG: Bladder carcinosarcoma: Histologic variation in metastatic lesions. J Urol 129:829, 1983

798. Kusaba Y, Yushita Y, Suzu H et al: Carcinosarcoma of the bladder. J Urol 131:118, 1984

799. Fromowitz FB, Bard RH, Koss LG: The epithelial origin of a malignant mesodermal mixed tumor of the bladder: Report of a case with long-term survival. J Urol 132:978, 1984

Collision Tumors

800. Balogh F: Hugyholyag carcinosarcoma esete. Orvosok Lapja 3:5, 1947

801. Mackles A, Immergut S, Grayzel DM et al: Carcinoma and sarcoma of bladder: Report of unusual simultaneous occurrence of both tumors. J Urol 59:1121, 1948

802. Dent ED Jr: Carcinosarcoma ("Collision tumor") of the urinary bladder. J Urol 74:104, 1955

803. Powers JH, Hawn CVZ, Carter RD: Osteogenic sarcoma and transitional cell carcinoma occurring simultaneously in the urinary bladder: Report of a case. J Urol 76:263, 1956

804. Fruhling L, Batzenschlager A, Blum E: Epitheliosarcomes vrais (tumeurs mixtes malignes) et cancers doubles didermiques de la vessie. Ann Anat Pathol 4:5, 1959

805. Hejtatmancik JH, Klatt WW: Co-existing carcinoma and sarcoma of the bladder. J Urol 84:320, 1960

806. Holtz F, Fox JE, Abell MR: Carcinosarcoma of the urinary bladder. Cancer 29:294, 1972

807. Kishi H, Komatsu H, Kitagawa R et al: Carcinosarcoma (collision tumor) of the urinary bladder: A case report. Jpn J Urol 68:495, 1977

Germ Cell Neoplasms

808. Djewitzki WST: Uber einen fall von chorionepithelioma der harnblase. Virchows Arch [A] 178:451, 1904

809. Teleky D: Teratoider tumor der weiblichen harnblase. Arch f Klin Chir 97:497, 1912

810. Wright–Smith RJ: Malignant teratoma (teratogenous sarcoma) of the urinary bladder. J Coll Surg (Australia) 2:271, 1929

811. Pollack AD: Malignant teratoma of the urinary bladder. Am J Pathol 12:561, 1936

812. Weinberg T: Primary chorionepithelioma of the urinary bladder in a male. Report of a case. Am J Pathol 15:783, 1939

813. Hyman A, Leiter HE: Extratesticular chorioepithelioma in a male probably primary in the urinary bladder. J Mt Sinai Hosp 10:212, 1943

814. Cauffield EW: Dermoid cysts of the bladder. J Urol 75:801, 1956

815. Ainsworth RW, Gresham GA: Primary chorioncarcinoma of the urinary bladder in a male. J Pathol Bacteriol 79:185, 1960

816. Taylor G, Jordan M, Churchill B et al: Yolk sac tumor of the bladder. J Urol 129:591, 1983

Metastatic Neoplasms

817. Abrams HL, Spiro R, Goldstein N: Metastases in carcinoma. Analysis of 1000 autopsied cases. Cancer 3:74, 1950

818. Corriere JH: Secondary melanoma of the urinary bladder. (Report of a case). West Virginia Med J 51:298, 1955

819. Ganem EJ, Batal JT: Secondary malignant tumors of the urinary bladder metastatic from primary foci in distant organs. J Urol 75:965, 1956

820. Sheehan EE, Greenberg SD, Scott R Jr: Metastatic neoplasms of the bladder. J Urol 90:281, 1963

821. Ghislandi E: Chromotographic analysis of the urinary melanin pigment. Ann NY Acad Sci 100:987, 1963

822. Duchon J, Pechan Z: The biochemical and clinical significance of melanogenuria. Ann NY Acad Sci 100:1048, 1963

823. Bartone FF: Metastatic melanoma of the bladder. J Urol 91:151, 1964

824. Perez–Meza C, Pickren JW, Woodruff MN et al: Metastatic carcinoma of the urinary bladder from primary tumors in the mammary gland of female patients. Surg Gynecol Obstet 121:813, 1965

825. Goldstein AG: Metastatic carcinoma to the bladder. J Urol 98:209, 1967

826. Chalbaud RA, Johnson DE: Adenocarcinoma of tongue metastatic to bladder. Urol 4:454, 1974

827. Meyer JE: Metastatic melanoma of the urinary bladder. Cancer 34:1822, 1974

828. Remigio PA, Ramos CM: Bladder tumor implant from renal adenocarcinoma. Urol 4:334, 1974

829. Haid M, Ignatoff J, Khandekar JD et al: Urinary bladder metastases from breast carcinoma. Cancer 46:229, 1980

830. Chin JL, Sales JL, Silver MM et al: Melanoma metastatic to the bladder and bowel: An unusual case. J Urol 127:541, 1982

831. Stein BS, Kendall AR: Malignant melanoma of the genitourinary tract. J Urol 132:859, 1984

Urethra

5

Normal Histology

The male urethra is anatomically divided into the proximal (posterior) urethra and the distal (anterior) urethra.[1] The posterior urethra begins at the internal urethral orifice of the prostatic urethra, and continues as the membranous urethra. Throughout the length of the prostatic urethra, prostatic duct ostia are present on the posterior-lateral walls. The ostia of the utricle and two ejaculatory ducts are present on the verumontanum, a raised area of the posterior wall of the prostatic urethra. The anterior urethra is anatomically divided into the proximal bulbous urethra and the more distal penile urethra, terminating in the fossa navicularis, immediately internal to the external urethral orifice (meatus).

The proximal male prostatic urethra is lined by transitional cell epithelium in continuity with the bladder urothelium. The transitional epithelium of the prostatic urethra gradually changes to stratified columnar epithelium in the membranous and bulbous portions of the urethra (Figs. 5-1, 5-2). The most distal portion of the urethra, the fossa navicularis, is lined by stratified squamous epithelium continuous with the external urethral orifice.

The bulbourethral, or Cowper's, glands are mucous-secreting glands of tubulo-alveolar type that enter the bulbous portion of the anterior urethra. The bulbourethral glands have a main excretory duct entering the posterior proximal bulbous urethra. The secretory component of the glands is composed of alveoli separated by thin, fibrous septae continuous with the periglandular fibrous capsule. The septation is incomplete in many areas, and adjacent alveoli fuse. The secretory cells are cuboidal to tall columnar with basal nuclei. The lumen of the alveolus is present only when the lining cells are low columnar or cuboidal, and the lumen is obliterated when the lining cells assume greater size. The cytoplasm is clear or granular. Secretions are present in the lumen of both alveoli and ducts. Scattered, shallow depressions of the mucous-secreting glands of Littre are present on the lateral walls of the penile portion of the anterior urethra.

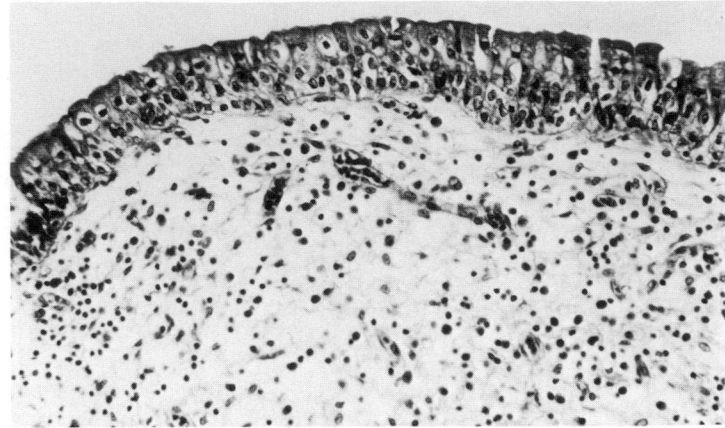

Figure 5-1   *Normal urethra. The stratified columnar epithelium of the urethra overlies the fibrous tissue of the lamina propria. Scattered lymphocytes are present in the lamina propria.*

In the female urethra, as in the male, the transitional epithelium of the bladder is continuous with the proximal urethral lining. The proximal urethral lining gradually makes a transition to stratified columnar epithelium, which in turn makes a transition to stratified squamous epithelium near the external urethral orifice.

Mucosal invaginations with minimal penetration of the periurethral tissue (urethral lacunae) are more common in the proximal urethra. The periurethral glands of Skene, which are histologically similar to the glands of Littre in the male, are more prevalent in the distal urethra.

Congenital Disorders

The congenital disorders of the urethra are as follows:

Hypospadias[3]

Epispadias[4,5]

Duplication[6]

Megalourethra[7]

Posterior urethral valve[8]

Anterior urethral valve[9,10]

Posterior urethral polyp[74,75]

These lesions are of major clinical importance principally in children, but are not commonly encountered by the surgical pathologist.

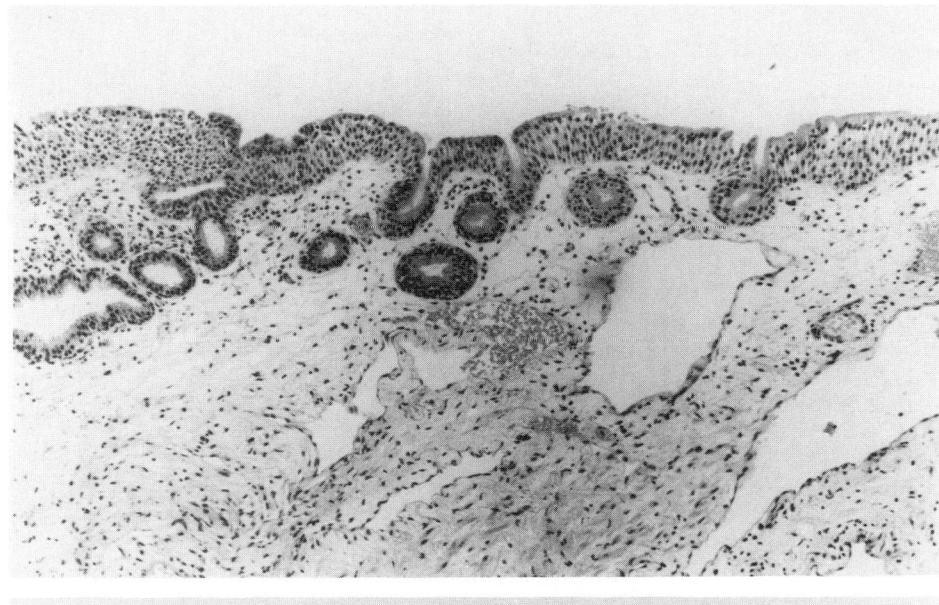

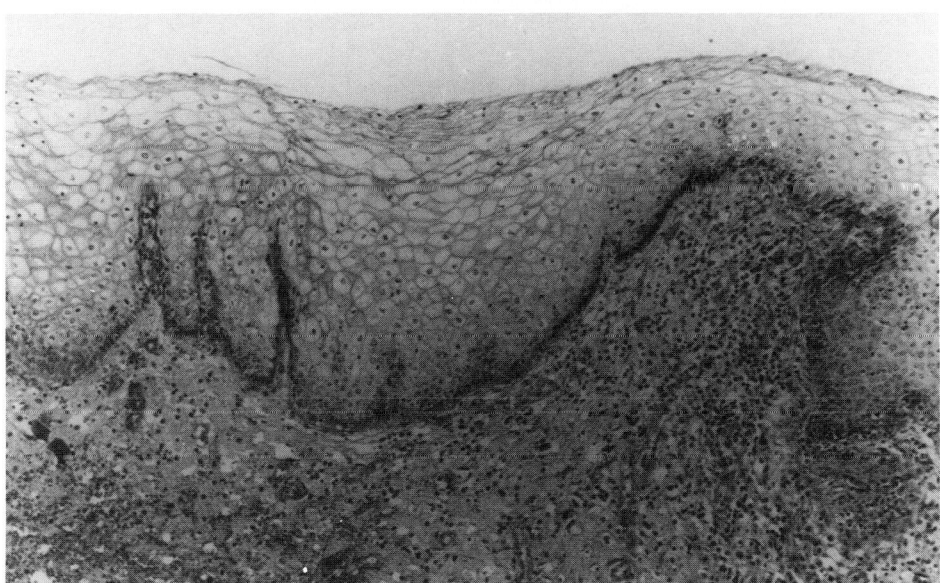

Figure 5-2 *Normal mucosa.* (A) *Transitional cell epithelium, here with urethritis cystica and mucosal invaginations, is characteristic of the proximal urethra.* (B) *The distal urethra is lined by squamous epithelium.*

Inflammatory Disorders

Gonorrhea

Gonorrhea is a venereal disease caused by *Neisseria gonorrhoeae,* a gram-negative intracellular diplococcus. The disease is contracted by direct sexual contact with an infected person. Its incidence in the United States has been increasing during the last two decades.[11] The increase is also recorded among children, who presumably contract gonorrhea from their infected parents.[12]

The urethra is the most common primary site of infection in men. Following a 3 day to 7 day incubation period, there is a viscous yellow discharge associated with urethral irritation. Asymptomatic infections have been reported. The *Neisseria* organisms are strict anaerobes, and the inflammatory discharge is the result of mucosal cell death following release of bacterial endotoxin within the cell cytoplasm. Continued evolution of the untreated local infection commonly results in urethral stricture (Fig. 5-3). In addition, systemic dissemination produces arthritis, meningitis, and uncommonly, pericarditis. The pathogenic strains of *Neisseria* organisms are associated with the presence of IgA protease production by the organisms.[13]

A tentative diagnosis of gonorrhea can be made by the detection of gram-negative intracellular diplococci in smears of the urethral discharge. A definitive diagnosis requires biochemical assay of cultures using Thayer–Martin medium.[14] *Neisseria* organisms ferment glucose, but not sucrose, lactose, or maltose.

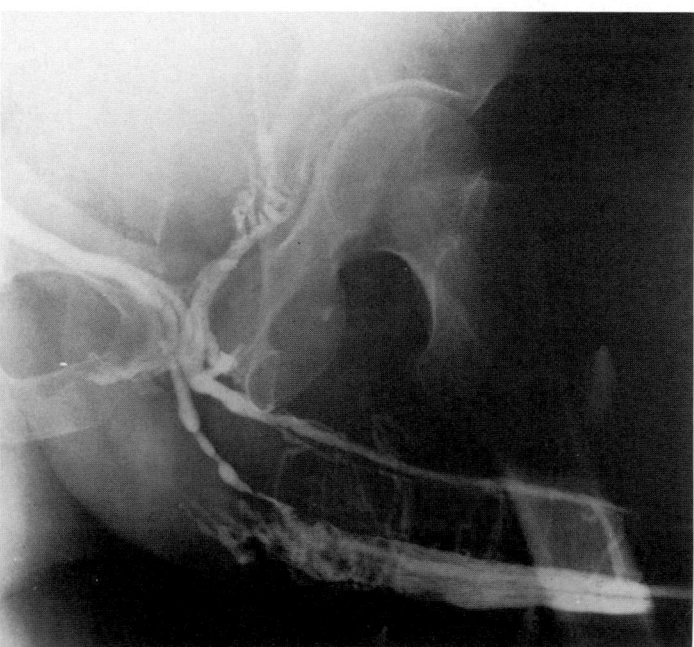

Figure 5-3   *Retrograde urethrography shows a stricture of the proximal membranous urethra. The 52-year-old patient had a long history of multiple dilatation procedures for treatment of gonococcal urethritis.*

Nongonorrheal Urethritis (Nonspecific Urethritis)

The true frequency of staphylococcal, chlamydial, and mycoplasma urethritis is yet to be accurately determined, but there is a general consensus that nonspecific urethritis caused by these organisms is increasing.[15-17] Of the three organisms, chlamydial infections occur most frequently.[15]

Tuberculosis

Tuberculosis of the urethra is rare, with 23 cases reported as of 1979.[23] All reported cases have been associated with tuberculous infection of the upper urinary tract, and the majority have been associated with pulmonary infection.[18-23] Ross reported a frequency of urethral tuberculous infection of 1.9% of cases of renal tuberculosis.[19] Infection of the epididymis and prostate is more common. There is a predilection of the bulbomembranous portion of the urethra.[23] Urethral stricture, dilatation, and less commonly, urethral-cutaneous fistulous tracts are complications of the infection in this site. This urethral infection is reported most commonly in the third to the fifth decades, but it may be observed in older males.[21,22] The diagnosis is made on culturing tuberculous organisms from the urethral discharge, and on detection of the acid-fast organisms in biopsy tissue.

Condyloma Acuminatum

In 1952, Morrow and co-workers reported in an extensive review that urethral condyloma acuminatum constituted only 5% of all infections of the genitourinary systems.[25] In this review, the etiology was reported as "probably a virus."[25] This has now been confirmed, and evidence gathered through the late 1970s up to the present indicates that human papilloma virus (type 6) is the responsible organism.[32-35]

The largest single series (60 cases) of urethral condyloma was reported by Gartman in 1956.[27] The introduction of fluorouracil therapy by Bissada and co-workers and by Dretler and Klein has resulted in cures of both the more typical focal cases and unusual cases of extensive urethral involvement.[29-31] This therapy supersedes the less effective results achieved previously with podophyllin.[24]

Urethral condyloma acuminatum is diagnosed most commonly in men in the second to the fifth decades. The majority of cases are focal exophytic lesions of the distal urethra, near the meatus. Occasionally lesions extend proximal from the fossa navicularis.[25] Rare cases may involve the entire urethra.[26,28,29] Patients experience burning on urination, urinary frequency, and bleeding. Treatment is surgical excision, electrocautery, fluorouracil cream, or the recent introduction of laser therapy. Recurrences are common (Figs. 5-4, 5-5).

The histologic diagnosis of condyloma acuminatum requires excluding another common distal urethral lesion, the squamous papilloma. Squamous papillomas are exophytic lesions with multiple branching papillae. Nonkeratinizing squamous epithelium covers a central fibrovascular core. The characteristic vacuolated epithelial cells, downward projections of the papillae, extensive parakeratosis, and underlying chronic inflammatory cell infiltrate typical of condylomas are absent from squamous papillomas.

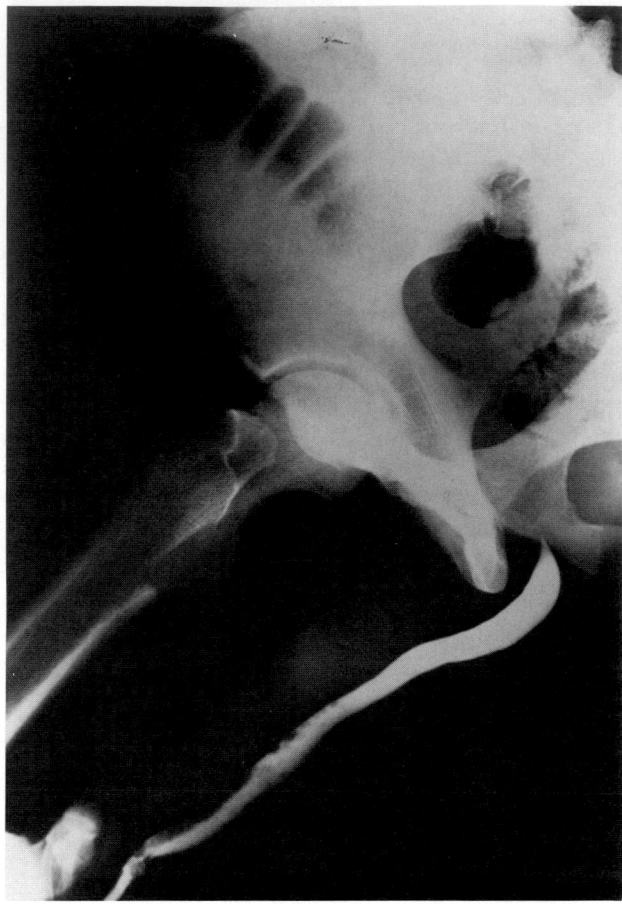

Figure 5-4   *Condyloma. Multiple filling defects in the penile urethra are observed in a retrograde urethrogram of a 27-year-old man with a history of recurrent condylomata.*

Malakoplakia

Three reports of urethral involvement by malakoplakia appear in the literature (Table 5-1).[36-38] All reported patients are in the sixth and seventh decades. Two of the three patients were women.[36,37] In common with this lesion elsewhere in the urinary tract, multifocal sites of involvement are observed. (Refer to discussions of malakoplakia in Chaps. 1 to 4 and 6 to 8.) The histologic picture of urethral malakoplakia is similar to other locations, and the diagnosis requires the

Table 5-1   *Malakoplakia*

Author	Year	Age	Sex	Other Locations
Serra, et al[36]	1974	62	F	None
McClure[37]	1979	59	F	Bladder
Sharma, et al[38]	1981	64	M	None

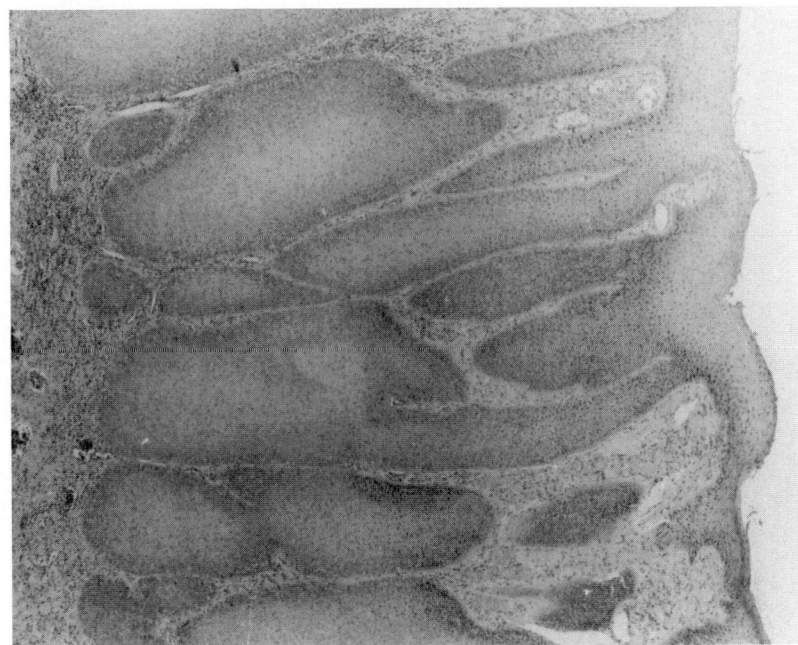

Figure 5-5   *Condyloma acuminatum. The typical bulbous papillae, acanthosis, and focal parakeratosis of the epithelium, associated with chronic inflammatory cells in the lamina propria, identify this 1.3-cm exophytic lesion as a urethral condyloma.*

identification of Michaelis–Gutmann inclusions in the inflammatory cell infiltrate.

Diverticulum

Diverticula of the urethra are virtually limited to women.[39-44] Rare cases associated with infection or prior surgical operations are encountered in men.[21] Anderson found nine urethral diverticula in 300 consecutive female patients for an incidence of 3%.[42] Urethral diverticula are diagnosed most frequently in the third to the sixth decades.[43] The dorsolateral wall of the midurethra is the characteristic location.[42] They have been reported to be more frequent in black women than in white women.[43] Patients present with post-micturition dribbling, urinary frequency, and urgency.[43] As many as 7% of patients are asymptomatic.[41] The diagnosis is made by physical examination, with the detection of a compressible bulge in the anterior vaginal wall. Pressure applied to this location expresses residual urine or pus from the urethral meatus. Urethrography detects many diverticula not apparent on physical examination (Fig. 5-6). Treatment is surgical excision.

Microscopic examination discloses a mucosal surface, frequently inflamed and ulcerated, overlying the attenuated circumferential smooth muscle, and fibrous stroma of the urethral wall.

The pathogenesis of urethral diverticula in the female urethra has been debated for years.[39,41-43] Most studies have concluded that the majority of cases are

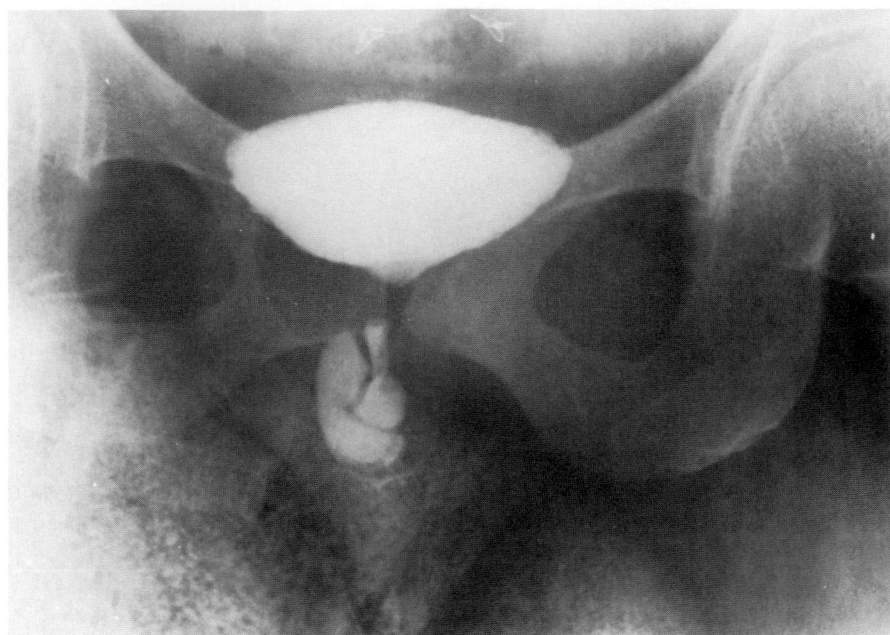

Figure 5-6   *Diverticulum. A septated reflection of contrast measuring 3.5 cm × 2.0 cm is observed on voiding cystourethrography. The patient was a 41-year-old woman with a history of chronic urinary tract infection.*

acquired secondary to trauma or periurethral duct obstruction. One uncontested case of congenital origin involving an infant girl was reported by Rocchi.[40]

On occasion a urethral diverticulum may be the site of stone formation.[43] One case of endometriosis and two cases with nephrogenic metaplasia located within a urethral diverticulum have been reported.[45,46,63]

In 1951, Hamilton and Leach reported the first malignancy complicating a urethral diverticulum.[47] Thirty-five additional cases can be found in the literature subsequent to this report.[48-61] Twenty-two of these reported cases (61%) are adenocarcinoma (Fig. 5-7), 25% are transitional cell carcinomas, and 14% are squamous cell carcinomas (Table 5-2).[47-61] The youngest reported patient was 39 years old; however, two thirds of the reported cases involve women 40 years to 60 years old.[50] The natural history of these neoplasms is not well documented because of inadequate follow-up information provided in the available case reports. Only one reported patient was observed for 5 years.[57]

Table 5-2   **Histologic Distribution of Reported Cases of Carcinoma Complicating Urethral Diverticulum**

Histologic Type	No. of Cases (%)
Adenocarcinoma[47,49,50-61,100]	22 (61%)
Transitional cell carcinoma[48,57]	9 (25%)
Squamous cell carcinoma[93]	5 (14%)

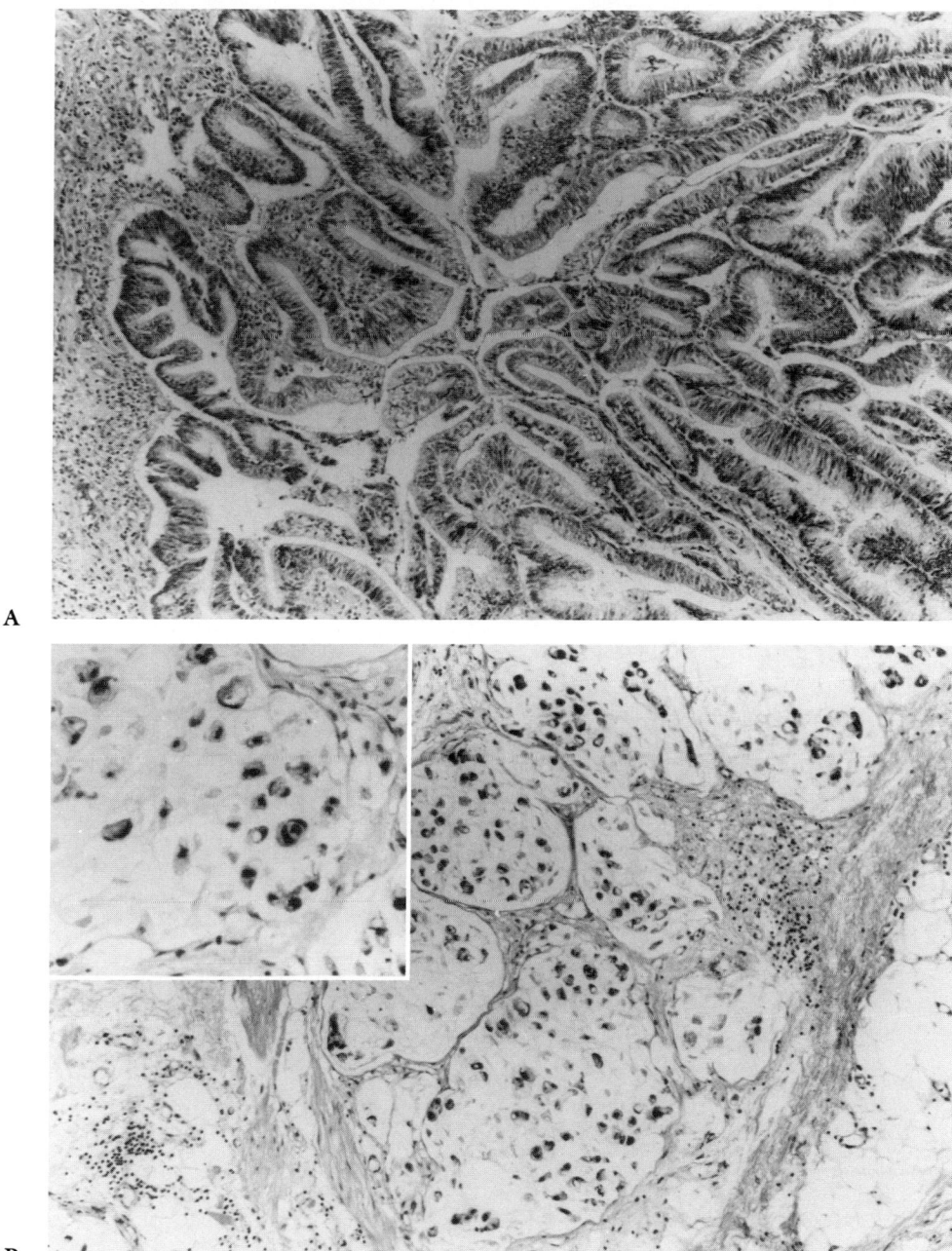

Figure 5-7   ***Adenocarcinoma arising in urethral diverticulum.*** *(A) This well-differentiated adenocarcinoma has a mixed papillary and glandular pattern. (B) A typical mucinous adenocarcinoma with signet-ring cells within expanded pools of mucin* (inset).

Metaplastic Changes

The metaplastic changes described in the renal pelvis, ureter, and urinary bladder also are observed in the urethra. Brunn's nests or buds, urethritis cystica, and glandularis are observed most commonly in the context of TUR fragments. Chronic inflammatory cells subjacent to the urethral urothelium are a frequent associated finding.

Squamous metaplasia occurs in the urethra infrequently. Vijayan and co-workers reported a case and referred to eight previously reported examples in the literature.[63] Extension of vesicle leukoplakia into the posterior urethra may be more common than cases isolated to the anterior urethra.[62] Associated lower urinary tract infection is common among the reported cases of urethral squamous metaplasia.[62,63]

Nephrogenic metaplasia (nephrogenic adenoma), a lesion most commonly observed in the bladder, has been reported in nine patients, seven men and two women.[46,64,65,85] Two of these cases took origin in a urethral diverticulum.[46,63] The histologic features of this lesion are identical to those described elsewhere in the urinary tract. (Refer to discussions of nephrogenic metaplasia in Chaps. 2 to 4.)

Endometriosis

Endometriosis of the female urethra has been reported only once.[66] This lesion is most common in the distal ureter and urinary bladder. (Refer to discussions of endometriosis in Chaps. 3 and 4.)

Amyloidosis

Amyloid deposits of the urethra wall have been reported in two patients.[67,68] The histologic appearance of the amyloid in the urethra is identical to that observed in more frequently encountered locations, such as the urinary bladder. The use of appropriate specific stains and electron microscopy will confirm the deposition in this unusual location to be composed of amyloid fibrils.

Urethral Polyps

Polypoid Urethritis

Polypoid urethritis, also known as inflammatory polyp, and papillary urethritis are the urethral counterparts of polypoid cystitis. Both lesions represent non-neoplastic, proliferative reactive changes to chronic inflammation in their respective sites of origin. Polypoid cystitis is especially common in patients with indwelling catheters. (Refer to discussion of polypoid cystitis in Chap. 4.)

The true frequency of this lesion is unknown and the available literature is sparse.[69,71,88] Within the urethra, as within the bladder, these inflammatory polyps are invariably associated with urinary tract infection. The gross features are described in the name of the lesion. When observed at the time of urethroscopy, the diagnosis is included in the differential of the various types of polypoid and papillary lesions, both neoplastic and non-neoplastic. Polypoid and papillary lesions are as follows:

Nephrogenic metaplasia (adenoma)

Fibroepithelial polyp

Polypoid urethritis

Caruncle (of female urethra)

Condyloma acuminatum

Adenomatous polyps with prostatic epithelium

Squamous papilloma

Transitional cell papilloma

Transitional cell carcinoma

Microscopically, polypoid or papillary exaggerations of the urethral mucosa are observed. The surface epithelium is normal, hyperplastic, or shows squamous metaplasia. Von Brunn's buds and nests are common. The underlying lamina is edematous, with variable numbers of dilated, thin-walled vascular structures. A chronic inflammatory cell infiltrate is present in the stroma.

The histologic diagnosis of polypoid urethritis requires differentiation from other papillary and polypoid urethral lesions, including papillary transitional cell carcinoma, ectopic prostatic tissue, squamous papilloma, and condyloma acuminatum. The relatively abundant stromal stalks and the absence of mucosal features of urothelial malignancy differentiate this lesion from papillary transitional cell papilloma and carcinoma. The paucity of prostatic ducts and acini in the stromal stalk and the urothelial nature of the surface epithelium differentiate polypoid urethritis from ectopic prostatic tissue. The other lesions, squamous papilloma, caruncle, and condyloma acuminatum are distinguished by their greater epithelial proliferation, and in the case of condyloma, the typical perinuclear cytoplasmic clearing. Schinella and co-workers described a papillary lesion in the prostatic urethra of an elderly man with active urinary tract infection.[71] He termed the lesion "proliferative papillary urethritis." This lesion most probably represents a variant of polypoid urethritis. The possibility that urethral fibroepithelial polyps represent another variant of polypoid urethritis is discussed in the following section.

Fibroepithelial Polyps

The term *fibroepithelial polyp of the urethra* is both accurately descriptive and pathogenetically noncommittal. Fibroepithelial polyps are composed of a fibrovascular core covered by transitional or squamous epithelium. Approximately 70% of cases have been reported in boys in the first decade of life.[1] Histologically similar cases have been observed in patients as old as 54 years.[76] Patients have urethral obstruction caused by the polyps, which originate in the proximal (posterior) urethra.[76,77]

The histogenesis of these polyps is unsettled. There is no evidence that they represent true neoplasms. Their similarity with ureteral fibroepithelial polyps is striking, and suggests that they represent the urethral counterpart. (Refer to discussion of fibroepithelial polyps in Chap. 3.) Downs regards all such polyps as congenital disorders.[76] The wide spectrum of ages of the reported patients does not support this pathogenetic explanation in all cases. A congenital (hamartomatous) pathogenesis may underlie some cases observed in children as suggested by the presence of nerve fibers and muscle in one third of reported cases.[76] Alternatively, some examples, composed only of fibrovascular tissue, diagnosed in adults may have their origin in earlier, more typical lesions of polypoid urethritis, a pathogenesis previously suggested by Mostofi and Price.[77]

Caruncle

Urethral caruncles occur exclusively in women, most frequently of postmenopausal age.[72-74] Caruncles are inflammatory lesions that are found near the urethral meatus and are clinically associated with pain and bleeding. The etiology and pathogenesis are unsettled, but prolapse of the urethral mucosa with associated chronic inflammation has been suggested.[72-74]

The constant microscopic features of caruncles are intense acute and chronic inflammation involving the mucosa and lamina propria (Fig. 5-8). The mucosa is either squamous cell or transitional cell epithelium frequently exhibiting ulcer-

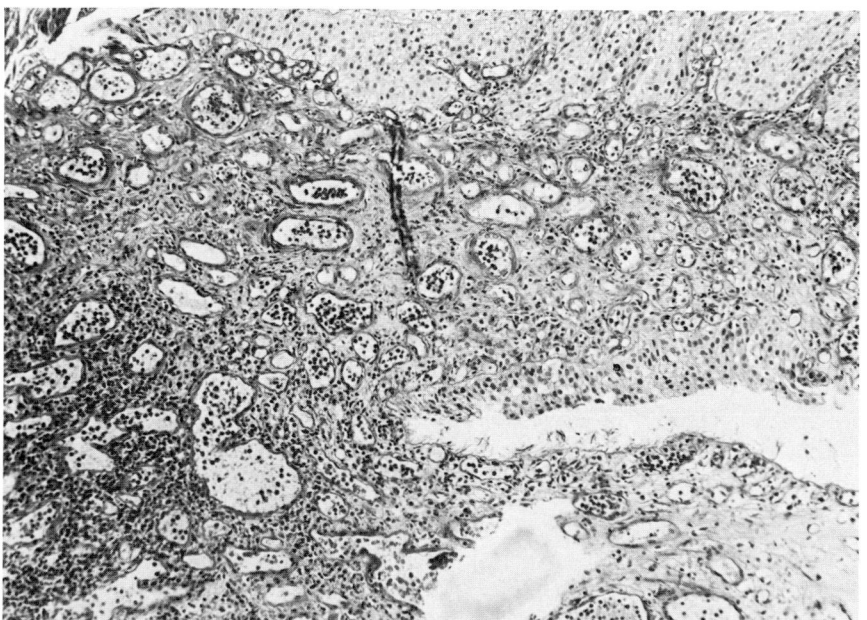

Figure 5-8   *Caruncle. The submucosa of the distal urethral segment contains numerous thin-walled blood vessels. Numerous acute and chronic inflammatory cells are present in the intervening stroma. Focal hyperplasia of the overlying mucosa is seen at the top.*

ation, hyperplasia, and hyperkeratosis. Complex patterns of papillomatosis and occasional dysplastic features of the epithelium bestow a superficial resemblance to this inflammatory lesion and carcinoma. The epithelial proliferation is accompanied by a variably dense infiltration of acute and chronic inflammatory cells, and increased numbers of thin-walled blood vessels. The blood vessels may be so numerous as to suggest a benign vascular neoplasm. The intervening stroma is edematous. These lesions are further described into three types based on the relative dominance of the major histologic components noted previously: (1) papillomatous caruncle, (2) angiomatous caruncle, and (3) granulomatous caruncle. Elbadawi and co-workers have recently described a fourth histologic variant — the mucinous variant, characterized by numerous glands lined by colonic epithelium with variable production of mucin.[75]

Although urethral malignancy has been reported in patients with caruncle, there is no evidence that caruncles increase the risk of urethral malignancy.[72]

Adenomatous Polyps with Prostatic Epithelium

Adenomatous polyps are exophytic, villoglandular proliferations of prostatic tissue observed in the prostatic urethra (Figs. 5-9 to 5-11). The term has numerous synonyms including ectopic prostatic tissue in urethra, benign polyp of prostatic-type epithelium, prostatic caruncle, villous polyp of urethra, adenomatous polyp of prostatic urethra, prostatic urethral polyp, benign prostatic epithelial polyp, and papillary adenoma of prostatic urethra.[79-84,87] There is an equal lack of unanimity about the pathogenesis of the lesion.

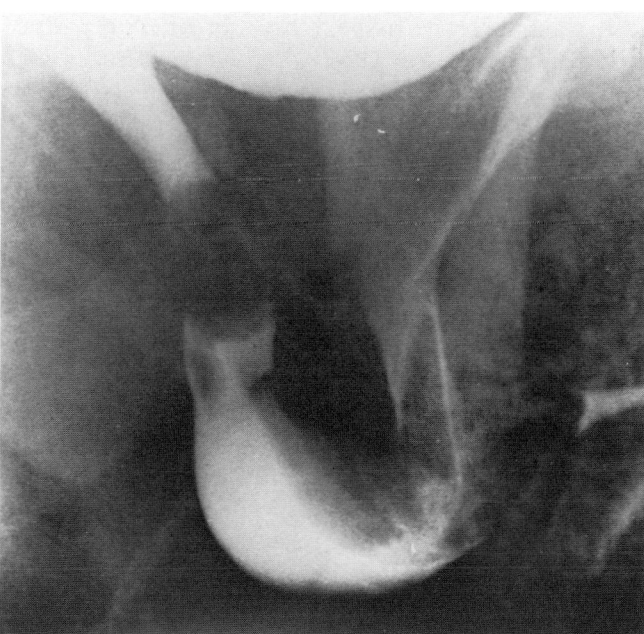

Figure 5-9   *Adenomatous polyps. Voiding cystourethrography demonstrates several polypoid filling defects in this 18-year-old man who had hematuria.*

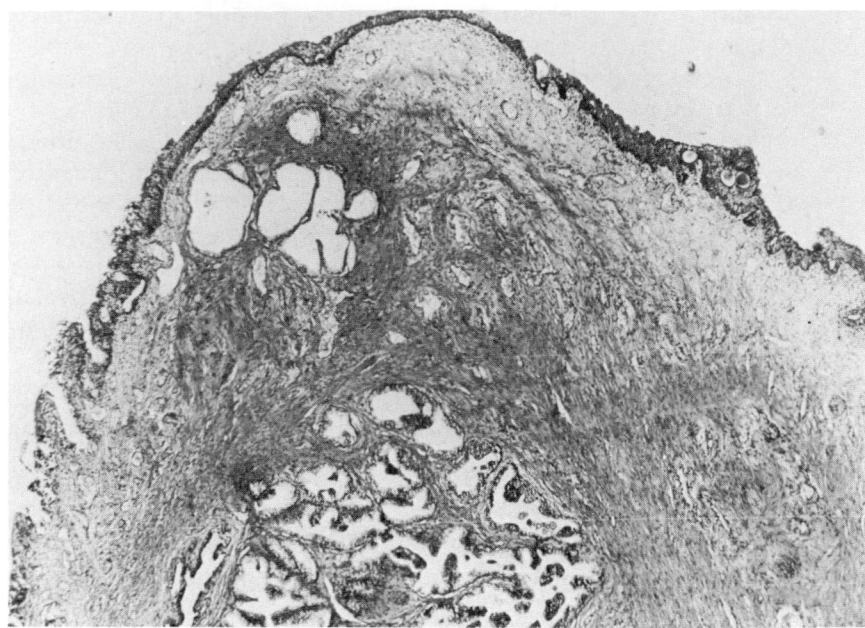

Figure 5-10   *Adenomatous polyp (ectopic prostatic tissue in the urethra). The polypoid structure is covered with transitional cell urothelium. Multiple prostatic acinar structures are scattered throughout the fibromuscular stroma.*

In 1913, Randall described urethral villous polypoid lesions of the prostatic urethra containing prostate tissue.[69] No subsequent reports of such lesions appeared in the literature until 1962 when Nesbit described 12 cases of benign urethral polyps that he interpreted as representing ectopic prostatic tissue.[78] A decade passed before additional studies of this urethral lesion appeared in the literature. In 1971 Butterick and co-workers reported the largest series published to date (68 cases).[79] The male patients ranged in age from 13 years to 63 years with a peak frequency in the second to the fourth decades. Virtually all patients have complaints of hematuria, hemospermia, or both. The prostatic origin of the epithelial component of these villoglandular polyps of the urethra was supported by azo-dye stains demonstrating intracellular acid phosphatase, and by ultrastructural features demonstrated by electron microscopy.[79] Multiple reports appeared in subsequent years, contributing to the recognition of the spectrum of histologic variants of these urethral lesions.[80-88] Positive immunoperoxidase staining for prostatic-specific antigen (PSA) and prostatic acid phosphatase (PAP) confirms the prostatic origin of these lesions.[85-88]

The pathogenesis of these prostatic urethral polyps is unsettled. Nesbit[78] and Butterick and co-workers[79] regarded the polyps as ectopic prostatic tissue. Alternatively, metaplasia of urethral urothelium, prolapse of prostatic ducts, and developmental anomaly of the prostate have all been suggested as the underlying pathogenetic mechanism.[81-87]

As of 1984, approximately 125 cases have been reported.[78-88] All cases, with one exception, have demonstrated a benign clinical course best treated by transurethral resection. In 1982, Walker and co-workers reported an adenocarcinoma

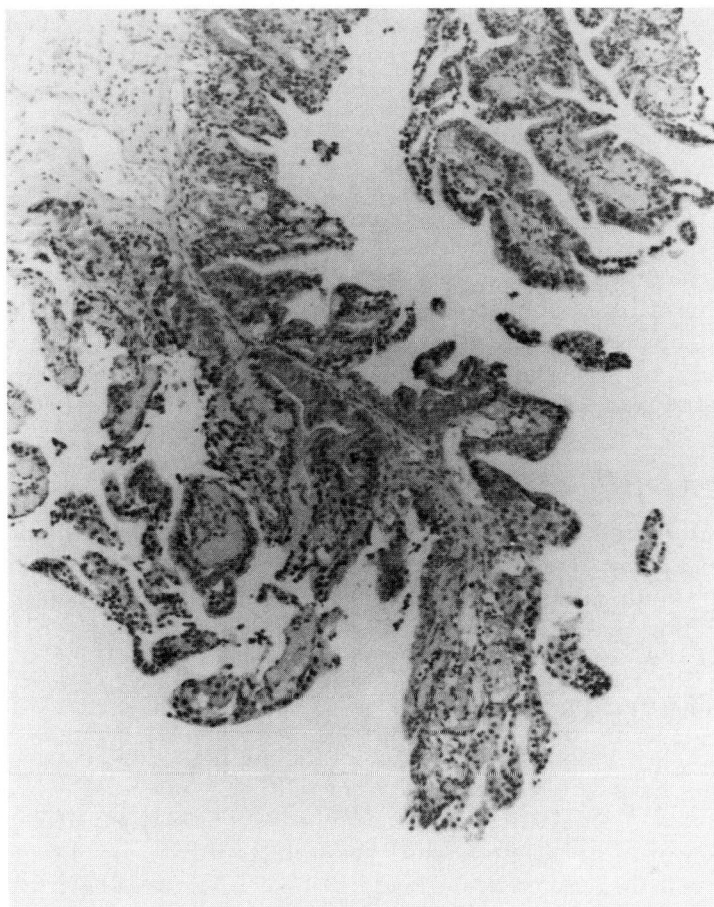

Figure 5-11   *Adenomatous polyp (ectopic prostate tissue). The prostatic origin of this papillary urethral lesion was confirmed by immunoperoxidase staining for prostatic specific antigen (PSA).*

with so-called endometrioid features taking origin in an otherwise typical urethral polyp of prostatic epithelium.[86] The neoplasm stained positively with immunoperoxidase procedures for PSA and PAP, supporting the interpretation of prostatic epithelial origin, and not of Müllerian origin as has been suggested previously.[86] (Refer to discussion of endometrioid carcinoma in Chap. 8.)

Microscopically, these villoglandular polyps are lined by typical prostatic columnar epithelium. Corpora amylacea (acini) have been observed within prostatic glands. Typically, no cytologic atypia or mitotic activity is observed. The surface epithelium can be urothelium, prostatic epithelium, or mixtures of the two types. The villous structures are lined exclusively with prostatic epithelium. As noted earlier, PSA and PAP immunoperoxidase staining confirms the prostatic origin of the epithelium.

The frequency of recurrences following conservative surgery and the frequency of malignant change in these lesions will be known only after greater cumulative experience.

Epithelial Neoplasms

Benign

Squamous Cell Papilloma

Squamous cell papilloma, an uncommon benign epithelial neoplasm, originates in the distal urethra in both sexes.[110,123] Superficially, it resembles condyloma acuminatum, but the central fibrovascular stalks are thin, delicate, and devoid of the inflammatory cell infiltrate present in condylomas. The surface shows no keratinization, which is a constant feature of condylomas. The nuclear and cytoplasmic features characteristic of the cells in a condyloma are not present.

Transitional Cell Papilloma

Transitional cell papilloma is a rare benign neoplasm that originates in the proximal urethra. The diagnosis rests on the same histologic and cytologic criteria outlined in previous chapters. (Refer to discussions of transitional cell papilloma in Chaps. 2 to 4.)

Inverted Papilloma

Five cases of inverted papilloma of the urethra, all in men aged 49 years to 79 years, have been reported.[90,91] None of these five cases was associated with independent urothelial malignancies, nor did the inverted papillomas themselves show malignant change, which has been reported in rare instances when it originates in the renal pelvis and bladder. (Refer to discussion of inverted papilloma in Chaps. 2 and 4.) The histologic appearance of inverted papilloma in the urethra is identical to examples reported elsewhere in the urinary tract.

Malignant

Carcinoma of the urethra is uncommon, with approximately 1400 reported cases. Approximately 72% of all reported cases occur in women. As observed in the upper urinary tract and the bladder, multiple histologic types are encountered, including squamous cell carcinoma (Fig. 5-12), transitional cell carcinoma, adenocarcinoma (Fig. 5-13), and malignant melanoma, in order of decreasing frequency. The four histologic varieties comprise 98% of all urethral carcinomas. Rare reports of clear cell carcinoma, cloacogenic carcinoma, adenoid cystic carcinoma, carcinoid tumors, mixed carcinomas, and carcinomas taking origin in Cowper's gland and Littre's glands appear in the literature. Carcinomas originating in the urethral diverticula are shown in Table 5-2.

The histologic type of urethral carcinoma frequently can be related to its site of origin. In general, the transitional cell carcinomas tend to arise in the proximal urethra, squamous cell carcinomas in the proximal and midurethra, adenocarcinomas in the midurethra, and malignant melanoma in the distal urethra. Exceptions to this site predilection are common. Furthermore, in practice, many ure-

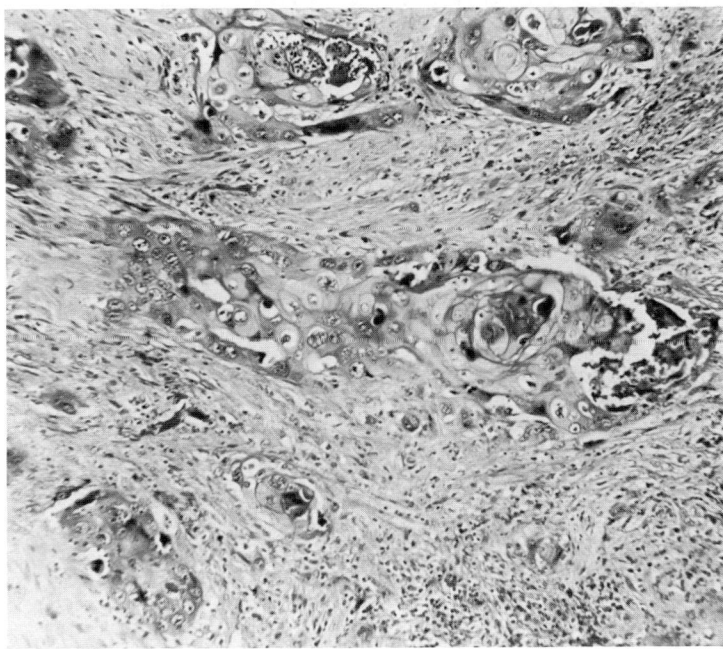

Figure 5-12 ***Squamous cell carcinoma.*** *Sheets and cords of malignant squamous cells invade the adjacent fibrous tissue of the urethral lamina propria.*

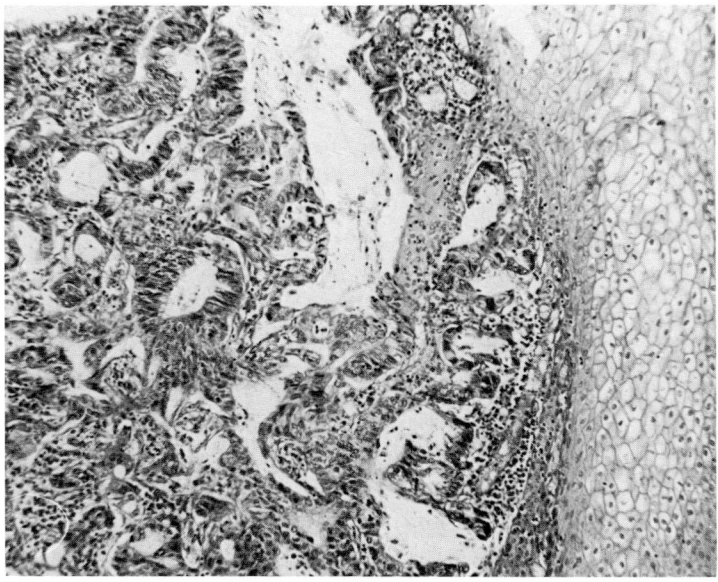

Figure 5-13 ***Adenocarcinoma.*** *Well-differentiated glands of the neoplasm cover the surface to the left of squamous cell epithelium of the distal urethra present on the right. Invasion of the underlying lamina propria by adenocarcinoma is present.*

Table 5-3   ***Staging Protocol for Female Urethral Carcinoma****

O		Noninvasive; limited to mucosa
A		Invasion limited to lamina propria
B		Invasion limited to periurethral muscle
C		Invasion of adjacent tissues
	C1	Invasion beyond muscle of vaginal wall
	C2	Invasion of bladder, vulva, clitoris
D		Metastases
	D1	Inguinal lymph nodes or pelvic lymph nodes
	D2	Distant sites

* Modification of protocol suggested by Grabstald H, Hilaris B, Henschke U et al: Cancer of the urethra. JAMA 197:835, 1966

Table 5-4   ***Staging Protocol for Male Urethral Carcinoma****

O		Noninvasive; limited to mucosa
A		Invasion limited to lamina propria
B		Invasion limited to corpus spongiosum or to prostate
C		Invasion into structures adjacent to corpus spongiosum, or invasion through prostatic capsule
D		Metastases
	D1	Inguinal lymph nodes or pelvic lymph nodes
	D2	Distant sites

* Modification of protocol suggested by Ray B, Canto AR, Whitmore WF: Experience with primary carcinoma of the male urethra. J Urol 117:591, 1977

thral malignancies are sufficiently advanced when diagnosed that the precise site of origin cannot be determined with confidence.

Staging protocols for carcinoma of the female and male urethras are presented in Tables 5-3 and 5-4. The staging protocols are modifications of protocols originally suggested by Grabstald and co-workers for female and Ray and associates for male urethral carcinomas.[100,123] As discussed below, the majority of urethral carcinomas are high stage at the time of presentation. This is particularly true of those neoplasms originating in the proximal urethra.

Etiology and Epidemiology

The cause of urethral carcinoma is unknown. Disorders frequently associated with it include urethral stricture, prior instrumentation, venereal disease, and importantly, prior or concomitant bladder carcinoma.[93,94,115,116,118,119,123,125–130] Urethral caruncles and squamous metaplasia (so-called leukoplakia) were regarded at one time as premalignant, but, as discussed previously, convincing supportive evidence is not available (see Chaps. 2 to 4). However, both mucosal changes are observed in association with urethral carcinomas.

Carcinoma of the Female Urethra

McCrea collected 523 cases of carcinoma primary in the female urethra reported in the literature from 1833 to 1952.[92] Three hundred and forty of these cases (65%) were not histologically classified (Table 5-5). No cases were identified as transitional cell carcinoma. This extensive review is thus limited to its historical value. The histologic distribution of 644 cases of female urethral carcinoma published in the years subsequent to McCrea's review is also presented in Table 5-5.[93-113] Of the more recent cases, 53% are squamous cell carcinoma, whereas transitional cell carcinoma and adenocarcinoma each constitute 14%. Undifferentiated carcinoma constitutes 2.5%, malignant melanoma 2.3%, and mixed carcinomas (squamous cell carcinoma with either adenocarcinoma or transitional cell carcinoma), 2.0%.

Table 5-5 **Histologic Variants of Carcinoma of the Female Urethra[93-113]**

Author	Year	No. of Cases	SCC*	TCC*	AC*	Undifferentiated Carcinoma (Ca-NOS)	Melanoma	TCC + SCC (SCC + AC)	NI
McCrea	1952	533	116		48	(340)	19		
Ritter	1953	26	23		3				
Fagan	1955	8	4	4					
Staubitz et al	1955	32	28	2	2				
Dean	1956	46							16
Flocks	1956	11							11
Monaco et al	1958	22	19		2		1		
Knoblich	1960	3			3				
Grabstald et al	1966	79	59		12	4	4		
Uhle, Kohler	1966	2	2						
Pointon, Poole-Wilson	1968	92	64	19	4		1		4
Rogers, Burns	1969	35	30		5				
Zeigerman, Gordon	1970	6	3	2	1				
Taggert et al	1972	36	20	11	4	1			
Grabstald	1973	15	6		6		1	(2)	
Desai et al	1973	16	9	2	3	2			
Tiltman	1975	3			3				
Bracken et al	1976	95	33	24	19	3	2		14
Roberts, Melicow	1977	33	9	7	5	1		11	
Allen, Nelson	1978	16	5	4	7				
Turner, Hendry	1980	37	13	12	4	3	5		
Bolduan, Farah	1981	14	6	3	4	1			
Benson et al	1982	17	8	3	4	1	1		
Total		644†	341	93	91	16	15	(2) 11	75
Percentage			53%	14%	14%	2.5%	2.3%	(0.3%) 1.7%	12%

* SCC = squamous cell carcinoma; TCC = transitional cell carcinoma; AC = adenocarcinoma
† Cases reported after McCrea's review.

The age distribution of recently reported cases (subsequent to McCrea's review) is 29 years to 88 years, with the peak frequency occurring in the sixth and seventh decades (approximately 80% of cases).[93,95,96,98,100,103,105,107,109] Reported mean ages of various published series range from 57 years to 64 years.[96,98,102,103,105,109] Most patients complain of urethral bleeding and dysuria, whereas one third of patients evidence urethral obstruction.[98,100,103,104,107,109,113] At the time of diagnosis, 2% to 12% of patients are asymptomatic.[104,109]

The site distribution of urethral carcinomas reported in ten recent studies is presented in Table 5-6. The data reflect the variable classifications of the female urethral anatomy employed in the literature, but the salient fact — that the majority of carcinomas originate in the distal (anterior) urethra, or involve the entire urethra — is apparent.[58,93,94,98,100,103,104,107,110,113] Indeed, presentation with a mass apparent at the meatus is common.

In spite of the relatively accessible location and associated symptoms of these neoplasms, the majority are found to have spread to adjacent tissues, or evidence regional node metastases (stages C and D), at the time of initial presentation (Table 5-7). Monaco and co-workers and Ritter observed that the duration of symptoms experienced by the patient before seeking medical attention was frequently several months.[93,98]

Natural History and Survival

The overall 5-year survival rates reported in six studies is 12% to 32%.[58,95,98,107,109,113] The three most important features of a carcinoma of the female urethra that relate to survival are site of origin, size of tumor, and tumor stage. Neither the histologic type nor the tumor grade has been found to affect survival rates significantly.[95,106,109] The reported 5-year survival rates for patients with distal urethral carcinoma range from 14% to 40%, whereas only 0 to 17% of patients with proximal (anterior) carcinomas survive this duration.[98,103,107,113] Bracken and co-workers observed that survival was inversely proportional to tumor size.[109] Rogers and Burns noted a significant reduction in survival among patients with urethral carcinomas larger than 3 cm.[103] Limited information is available relating tumor stage to survival. However, Bracken and co-workers

Table 5-6   ***Site Distribution of Carcinoma of the Female Urethra***

Author	Year	Total Cases	Proximal
Ritter[93]	1953	24	2 (8%)
Fagan, Hertig[94]	1955	8	1 (12%)
Monaco et al[98]	1958	23	0
Grabstald et al[100]	1966	79	
Rogers, Burns[103]	1969	35	4 (12%)
Ziegerman, Gordon[104]	1970	7*	
Desai et al[107]	1973	16	
Roberts, Melicow[110]	1977	38	6 (18%)
Allen, Nelson[58]	1978	18	
Benson et al[113]	1982	17	10 (59%)

* No site information provided for one patient.

reported that 40% to 45% of patients with stages A and B survived 5 years, in contrast to 18% to 25% of patients with stages C and D surviving the same duration.[109]

Carcinoma of the female urethra, as outlined above, is associated with a very poor prognosis. The overall survival rates are significantly affected by the high frequency of high stage tumors encountered clinically. Earlier detection would increase survival rates.

The frequency of distant metastases from urethral carcinoma is not high. Grabstald and co-workers reported that only 14% of patients in their series developed distant metastases during the course of their disease.[100] Regional lymph node metastases (inguinal and iliac lymph nodes) are more common.[100,107]

Carcinoma of the Male Urethra

In a review of the literature from 1862 to 1966, Kaplan and co-workers (1967) collected 221 previously reported cases of carcinoma of the male urethra, to which they added 11 new cases.[116] In subsequent years, approximately 220 additional cases have been reported for a total of about 450 cases.[58,89,106,117,125]

The distribution of histologic types of male urethral carcinoma reported in the review by Kaplan and co-workers and subsequent studies providing this information is as follows: squamous cell carcinoma constitutes approximately 78%, transitional cell carcinoma 15%, and adenocarcinoma 7%.[116-125] Rare cases of malignant melanoma, cloacogenic carcinoma, adenosquamous carcinoma, and carcinoid tumors are reported (see below).

The age range of male patients with urethral carcinoma is most frequently reported as the fourth to ninth decades.[122-124] A 13-year-old patient was cited in the review by Kaplan and co-workers.[116] The peak age frequency is the sixth to seventh decades, represented by 70% to 80% of all patients.[116,122-124] A history of venereal disease, and stricture are each recorded in about one third of cases.[116,122,123] Three cases of carcinoma of the male urethra developing after urethroplasty for stricture were found in the literature.[119,125] The clinical presen-

Midurethra	Distal	Meatus	Entire	Anterior	Posterior
1 (4%)	1 (4%)	13 (54%)	7 (29%)		
0	1 (12%)	5 (63%)	1 (12%)		
2 (9%)	0	21 (91%)	0		
			48 (61%)	31 (39%)	
			12 (34%)	19 (54%)	
		2 (33%)	4 (67%)		
				10 (62%)	6 (38%)
15 (45%)	17 (52%)				
			7 (39%)	8 (44%)	3 (17%)
	7 (41%)				

tation is related to urethral obstruction, bleeding, or discharge.[116,118,122-124] A palpable mass or urethral fistula is present in 20% to 40% of patients.[116,118] Most cases (38% to 73%) originate in the bulbomembranous urethra, and 27% to 50% arise in the distal (posterior urethra).[115,116,118,122-124] The prostatic urethra is the least frequent site of origin (7% to 33%).[115,116,118,122-124] Because the majority of male urethral carcinomas are squamous cell carcinoma and originate in bulbomembranous portion normally lined by columnar epithelium, neoplasia is preceded by squamous metaplasia at this site. Adenocarcinomas not originating from periurethral glands, including Cowper's glands, also arise from metaplastic cell populations in portions of the urethra normally lined by squamous or transitional cell epithelium.[114]

Natural History and Survival

As observed with female urethral carcinoma, neither histologic type nor tumor grade significantly affects survival.[123] The overall 5-year survival rate ranges from 7% to 39%.[116,118,122-124] Site of origin and tumor stage at presentation are the most important factors affecting prognosis. Tumors originating in the bulbomembranous urethra tend to be higher stage than distal tumors at the time of diagnosis.[123] The majority of carcinomas of the distal urethra are low stage (56% stages A and B), and are associated with correspondingly higher survival rates (30% to 67% 5-year survival).[115,116,123] Neoplasms originating in the bulbomembranous urethra tend to be high stage (14% stages A and B).[123] Ray and coworkers have reported an 86% 5-year survival rate for stages A and B tumors, compared to a 19% 5-year survival rate for stages C and D neoplasms.[123] Unfortunately, 60% to 64% of patients present with high stage urethral neoplasms.[123,124]

Metastatic disease is the most probable cause of inguinal lymphadenopathy when associated with primary urethral neoplasms.[123] This is in contrast to the high frequency of reactive lymphadenopathy associated with penile carcinoma. (Refer to discussion of penile carcinoma in Chap. 9.) Death is most frequently secondary to sepsis complicating local ulceration, or fistula formation.[116] Distant metastases are observed infrequently.[116,123]

Although urine cytology studies and brushings are more frequently positive in cases of urethral carcinoma than experienced with lesions in the more proximal urinary tract, definitive diagnosis requires biopsy studies.[123] Examination of surgically resected urethral carcinomas should accomplish accurate pathologic staging, determination of site of origin, and adequacy of all resection margins.

Table 5-7   *Stage Distribution of Carcinoma of the Female Urethra*

Author	Year	No. of Patients	Stage				
			O	A	B	C	D
Bracken et al[109]	1976	74		11 (15%)	19 (25%)	28 (38%)	16 (22%)
Allen, Nelson[58]	1978	17		5 (29%)	1 (6%)	7 (41%)	4 (24%)
Benson et al[113]	1982	17		2 (12%)	2 (12%)	5 (29%)	8 (47%)
				24%–40%		60%–76%	

Urethral Carcinoma Associated with Bladder Carcinoma

Observations reported during the 1940s and 1950s indicate that urethral carcinoma in association with bladder carcinoma was recognized, but the cumulative information had not clarified the frequency, pathogenesis, or clinical significance of this association.[128] Concurrently, descriptive studies of carcinoma-in-situ advanced the concept of intraepithelial malignancy involving the urothelial mucosa, including that of the urethra.[126,127] In 1960, Gowing reported finding carcinoma-in-situ in 18% of retained urethras in 33 patients who died following cystectomy for bladder carcinoma.[128] The presence of intraepithelial neoplasia gave no support to the hypothesis of "drop metastases" from the previously excised bladder carcinoma. Thus, the 18% represents the frequency of independent neoplasia developing in the retained urethra at the end of the natural history of the bladder carcinoma's clinical evolution.

Multiple studies in subsequent years clarified the frequency and clinical significance further. In summary, concomitant carcinoma-in-situ has been observed in 12% to 22% of urethras surgically excised at the time of cystectomy for bladder carcinoma.[129,130] Subsequent urethral neoplasia has been observed in 4% to 12% of patients previously treated with cystectomy, as reviewed by Shellhammer and Whitmore and Richie and Skinner.[129,130] Multifocal bladder tumors are associated with a higher frequency of associated urethral neoplasia.[129,130] Finally, Richie and Skinner reported that 80% of patients with carcinoma-in-situ in the proximal urethra demonstrated at the time of cystectomy, who subsequently do not have a complete urethrectomy, die of tumor-related causes.[130] When urethrectomy is performed in such patients, the frequency of tumor-related deaths is reduced to 14%.[130]

The practical implications of these cumulative observations underscore the necessity of thorough microscopic examination of the urethral segment excised at the time of cystectomy, beyond merely determining the adequacy of the resection margin.

Uncommon Primary Urethral Carcinomas

Malignant Melanoma

Malignant melanoma originating in the urethra is rare. Sixty cases involving the female urethra and 23 cases arising in the male urethra are reported in the literature.[98,100,102,109,113,131-142] The age range for this urethral malignancy is the same in both sexes: the fourth to eighth decades. Approximately 50% of cases are diagnosed in the sixth and seventh decades. The distal urethra (fossa navicularis and meatus) is the site of predilection, but approximately 20% are reported in the proximal urethra.

The recorded patients present most commonly with dysuria and hematuria. Some are aware of a nodule or mass. Delay in seeking medical attention for all or some symptoms is common. The lesion in situ is blue, black, blue-black, or brown.

Microscopically, pigmented atypical melanocytes with numerous mitoses invading the lamina propria in nests, cords, or sheets are characteristic (Fig. 5-14). An organoid pattern to the nests may or may not be apparent. The amount of melanin pigment is highly variable. Amelanotic cases have been reported.[136,138] Occasional cases are so heavily pigmented that evaluation of other

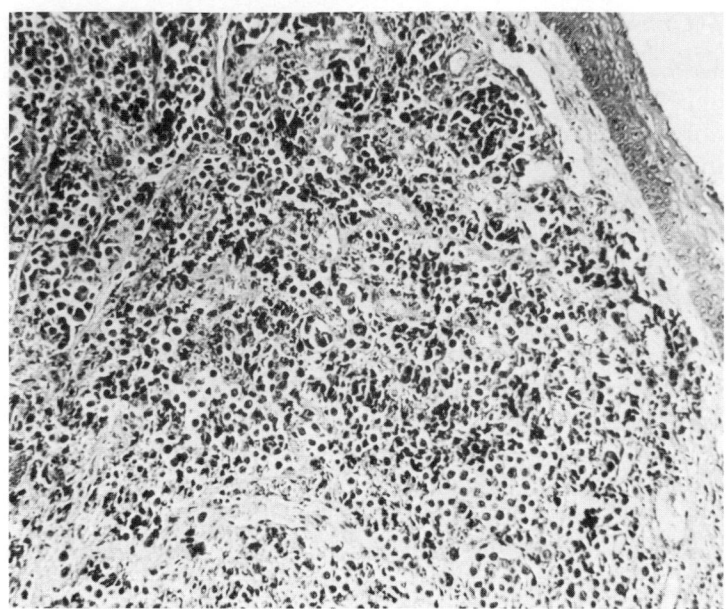

Figure 5-14   *Malignant melanoma. The pigment-containing melanoma cells have infiltrated the lamina propria beneath adjacent normal urothelial lining of the urethra.*

cytologic features is difficult. The Fontana–Masson stain allows differentiating the brown melanin pigment from hemosiderin. The melanocytes may be either epithelioid or spindle shaped, and commonly, both cell types are present. The diagnosis of malignant melanoma is confirmed by the detection of premelanosomes in electron microscopic preparations of the specimen. This can be helpful in small biopsies of poorly differentiated tumors with little or no pigment detected by light microscopy. Origin of the melanoma from the precursor nevus is observed in some of the reported cases.[142] A complete diagnostic evaluation of the resected melanoma specimen includes determining depth of invasion, adequacy of margins, and possible origin from precursor lesion. Identification of such a precursor lesion eliminates the possibility that the urethral melanoma is in fact a metastasis from an undetected primary melanoma elsewhere.

Follow-up information is limited in many reports, but a high percentage of the recorded cases evidence metastases and tumor-related death within 3 years of diagnosis. Three patients surviving 5 years were found in the literature.[131,132,134]

Clear Cell Adenocarcinoma

Eight examples of clear cell adenocarcinoma (so-called mesonephroma) originating in the urethra are found in the literature.[151-156] All reported cases involved women in the fifth to seventh decades with a mean age of 51 years. Three of these cases were reported to originate in urethral diverticula.[60,154] Of the eight cases, no follow-up information was provided in two reports, and in four other cases the follow-up duration was a maximum of 2.5 years. Two patients survived 5 years with tumor, one dying of tumor-related causes 6 years after the diagnosis.[151,153]

Clear cell adenocarcinomas are now regarded to be of Müllerian origin, and not of mesonephric derivation as originally proposed by Schiller in 1939.[143] These neoplasms are most commonly observed in the female ovary, endometrium, cervix, and vagina.[144-150] Three cases have been reported in the urinary bladder. (Refer to discussion of clear cell carcinoma in Chap. 4.)

Histologically, the characteristic features include tubules, and tightly packed small glands lined by hobnail cells or clear cells, focal papillary clusters, or less-differentiated areas showing sheets and cords of tumor cells (Figs. 5-15, 5-16). Glycogen is detected with the PAS stain. Recently the ultrastructural features of urethral clear cell carcinoma were reported by Tanabe and coworkers.[156]

Cloacogenic Carcinoma

Two cases of cloacogenic carcinoma of the urethra have been reported.[159,160] The patients were a 77-year-old man and a 66-year-old woman. Limited follow-up information was provided.

Cloacogenic carcinoma is a term introduced by Grinvalsky and Helwig in reference to carcinomas originating at the anorectal junction.[157] They are thought to arise from persisting transitional epithelium of cloacogenic origin.[157,158] A similar beginning is postulated for tumors originating in the urethra.[159,160]

Three histologic variants are recorded: basaloid type composed of transitional cells; mixed squamous and transitional cells; and small cell type (resembling small cell undifferentiated carcinoma).[158] In the anorectal location, the mixed cell and the small cell variants are the most aggressive.[158]

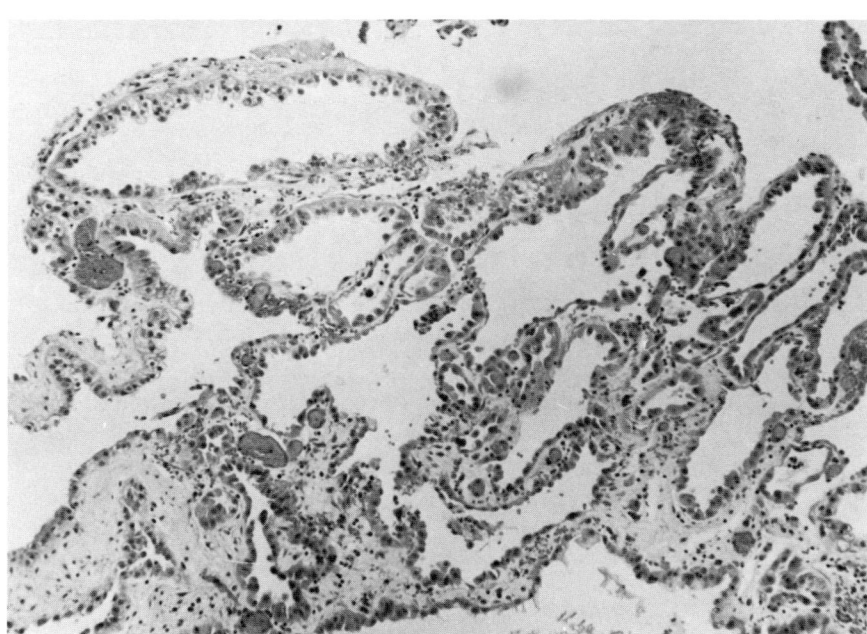

Figure 5-15   *Clear cell carcinoma. Dilated tubulo-glandular structures line tumor cells projecting into the lumen (so-called hobnail cells). Clear cells, for which the tumor is named, were rare in this case, but can be seen lining the largest tubule at the top.*

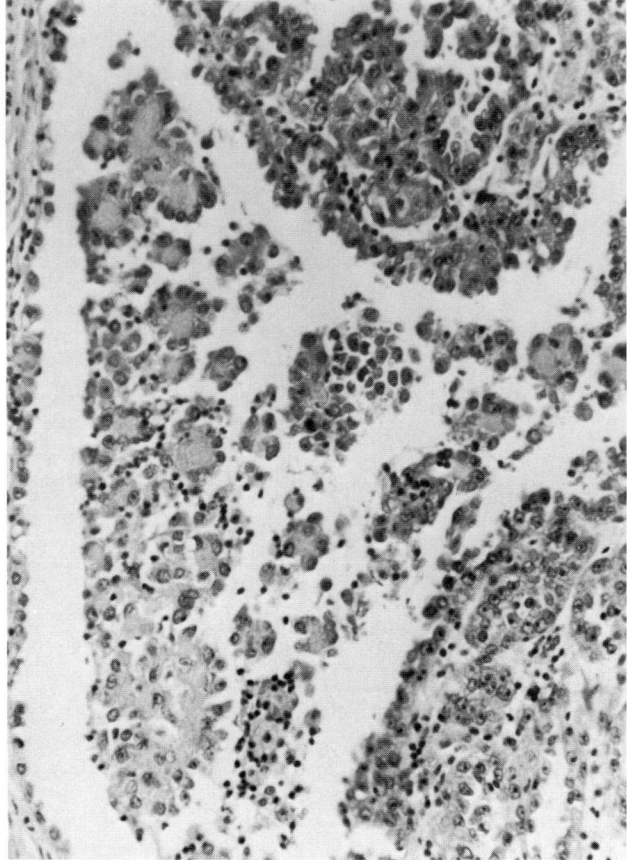

Figure 5-16   *Clear cell carcinoma. Elsewhere in the tumor illustrated in Figure 5-14, clusters of tumor cells surrounding eosinophilic hyalin material appear to float free in a cystic space.*

Mesenchymal Neoplasms

Benign

Mesenchymal neoplasms of all types are rare. A search of the literature indicates that benign mesenchymal neoplasms occur more frequently than their malignant counterparts. The most frequent among the urethral mesenchymal neoplasms are leiomyoma, hemangioma, leiomyosarcoma, and fibrosarcoma in order of decreasing frequency.

Leiomyoma

Shield and Weiss reported a case of leiomyoma of the urethra and cited nine previous cases reported to 1973.[164] An additional 12 cases have been reported to 1983, bringing the total number to 22.[165-173] All reported cases occurred in women in the third to the fifth decades. The largest tumor reported measured

8 cm, but the majority measured 2 cm to 4 cm. Patients present with urinary retention and awareness of a protruding mass in the anterior vaginal wall. Treatment is complete surgical excision. The histologic criteria justifying the diagnosis of leiomyoma have been discussed in Chapters 2 to 4.

Hemangioma

In 1948, McCrea reported a case of urethral hemangioma and reviewed 11 previously reported cases.[174] Nine additional cases have been reported subsequent to McCrea's review for a total of 21 cases.[175-181] Of these 21 cases, 18 were diagnosed in men. The peak age frequency is the second to third decades, but cases have been observed from childhood to the sixth decade. There is no site of predilection within the urethra. Bleeding is the most common presenting clinical picture. Surgical excision is curative if adequate margins are obtained. These neoplasms tend to recur if the surgical excision is inadequate. No examples of angiosarcoma have been reported in the urethra. The histologic features of ure-

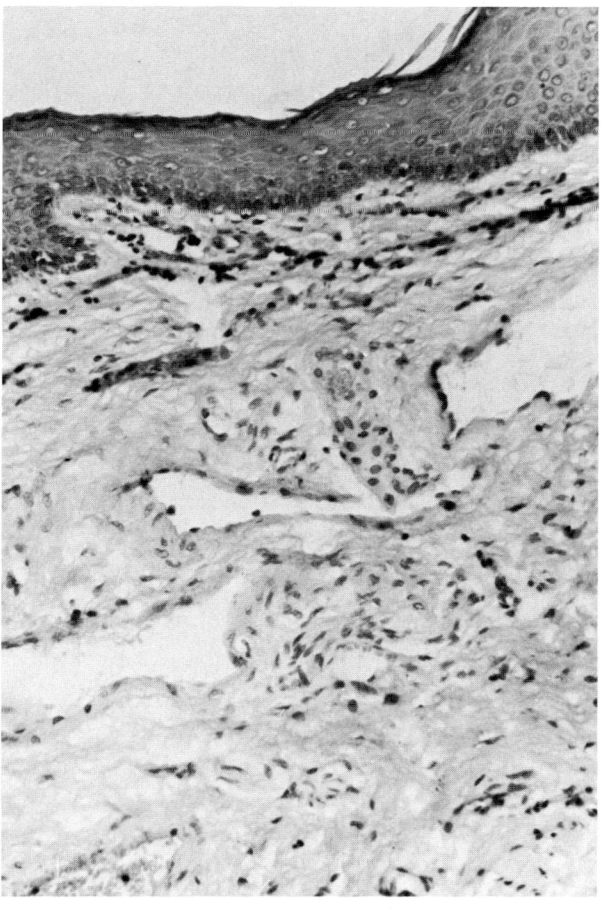

Figure 5-17   *Hemangioma. The distal urethral mucosa overlies multiple vascular channels of a recurrent urethral hemangioma. The lining endothelial cells are flat and devoid of cytologic features suggesting malignancy.*

thral hemangiomas (cavernous or capillary) are identical to their counterparts occurring in more common locations (Fig. 5-17).

Granular Cell Tumor

One reported case of granular cell tumor of the urethra was found in the literature.[110] This neoplasm is more frequently encountered in the urinary bladder. (Refer to discussion of granular cell tumor in Chap. 4.)

Malignant

In 1952, McCrea collected 23 cases of urethral sarcoma reported to that time.[92] Histologic types of primary urethral sarcoma reported since McCrea's review are leiomyosarcoma,[50,110] fibrosarcoma,[93,182] rhabdomyosarcoma,[183] and unclassified sarcoma.[104,105]

Neoplasms Metastatic to the Urethra

Neoplasms metastatic to the urethra are rare, and originate in most instances from the prostate, bladder, and rectum.[184-186] In rare instances, origin from distant sites is observed.[110] Pain, hematuria, and evidence of urethral obstruction in a patient with a known malignancy suggest a diagnosis of metastatic neoplasm. (Refer to discussion of metastatic neoplasms to the penis in Chap. 4.)

References

Normal Histology

1. McCallum RW: The adult male urethra. Normal anatomy, pathology, and method of urethrography. Radiol Clin North Am 17:227, 1979
2. Huffman JW: The detailed anatomy of the paraurethral ducts in the adult human female. Am J Obstet Gynecol 55:86, 1948

Congenital Disorders

3. Sweet RA, Shrott HG, Kirland R et al: Study of incidence of hypospadias. Mayo Clin Proc 49:52, 1974
4. Marshall VF: Variations in exstrophy of bladder. J Urol 88:766, 1962
5. Muecke EC: The role of the cloacal membrane in exstrophy. J Urol 92:659, 1964
6. Olsen JG: Complete urethral duplication. J Urol 95:718, 1966
7. Stephens FD: Congenital Malformations of the Rectum, Anus, and Genito-Urinary Tracts, p 236. Baltimore, Williams & Wilkins, 1963
8. Young HH, Frantz WA, Baldwin JC: Congenital obstruction of the posterior urethra. J Urol 3:289, 1919
9. Kjellberg SR, Ericsson NO, Rhude V: The Lower Urinary Tract in Childhood, p 272. Chicago, Year Book, 1957
10. Williams DI: Discussion on lower urinary obstruction. Arch Dis Child 37:132, 1962

Inflammatory Disorders

Gonorrhea

11. Results of screening for gonorrhea: United States, 6-month period ending June 30, 1978. Morbidity Mortality Weekly Rep 27:448, 1978
12. Meek JM, Askuri A, Belman AB: Prepubertal gonorrhea. J Urol 122:532, 1979
13. Mulks MH, Plaut AG: IgA protease production as a characteristic distinguishing pathogenic from harmless Neisseriaceae. N Engl J Med 299:973, 1978
14. Thayer ID, Martin JE: Improved medium selective for cultivation of N gonorrhoeae and N meningitides. Public Health Rep 82:559, 1966

Nongonorrheal Urethritis (Nonspecific Urethritis)

15. Richmond SJ, Sparking PF: Genital chlamydial infections. Am J Epidemiol 103:428, 1976
16. McDonald MI, Lam MH, Birch DF et al: Ureaplasma urealyticum in patients with acute symptoms of urinary tract infection. J Urol 128:517, 1982
17. Hovelius B, Thelin I, Mardh PA: Staphylococcus saphroticus in the aetiology of nongonococcal urethritis. Brit J Vener Dis 55:368, 1979

Tuberculosis

18. Dourmashkin RL: Urethral stricture: A study of 227 cases J Urol 68:496, 1952
19. Ross JC: Renal tuberculosis. Br J Urol 25:277, 1953
20. Le Brun HI: Tuberculous urethral stricture. Br J Urol 30:82, 1958
21. Chambers RM: Tuberculous urethral fistula. Br J Urol 43:243, 1971
22. Symes JM, Blandy JP: Tuberculosis of the male urethra. Br J Urol 45:432, 1973
23. Raghavaiah NV: Tuberculosis of the male urethra. J Urol 122:417, 1979

Condyloma Acuminatum

24. Culp OS, Kaplan IW: Condyloma acuminata: Two-hundred cases treated with podophyllin. Ann Surg 120:251, 1944
25. Morrow Jr RP, McDonald JR, Emmett JL: Condylomata acuminata of the urethra. J Urol 68:909, 1952
26. Lindner HJ, Pasquier Jr CM: Condylomata acuminata of the urethra. J Urol 72:875, 1954
27. Gartman E: Intraurethral verruca acuminata in men. J Urol 75:717, 1956
28. Bissada NK, Cole AT, Fried FA: Extensive condylomas acuminata of the entire male urethra and the bladder. J Urol 112:201, 1974
29. Bissada NK, Redman JF, Sulieman JS: Condyloma acuminatum of male urethra. Successful management with 5-fluorouracil. Urol 3:499, 1974
30. Dretler SP, Klein LA: The eradication of intraurethral condyloma acuminata with 5 percent 5-fluorouracil cream. J Urol 113:195, 1975
31. Debenedictis TJ, Marmar JL, Praiss DE: Intraurethral condylomas acuminata: Management and review of the literature. J Urol 118:767, 1977
32. zur Hausen H: Human papilloma viruses and their possible role in squamous cell carcinomas. Curr Top Microbiol 78:1, 1977
33. Grissman E, De Villier EM, zur Hausen H: Analysis of human genital warts (condylomata acuminata) and other genital tumors for human papillomavirus type 6 DNA. Int J Cancer 29:143, 1982
34. Dean P, Lancaster W, Chun B et al: Human papillomavirus structural antigens in squamous papillomas of the male urethra. J Urol 129:873, 1983
35. Murphy WM, Fu YS, Lancaster W et al: Papillomavirus structural antigens in condyloma acuminatum of the male urethra. J Urol 130:84, 1983

Malakoplakia

36. Serra CA, Grasso RL, Saade JD: Malacoplakia: A case of unusual localization. J Urol 112:762, 1974
37. McClure J: A case of urethral malacoplakia associated with vesical disease. J Urol 122:705, 1979
38. Sharma TC, Kagan HN, Sheils JP: Malacoplakia of the male urethra. J Urol 125:885, 1981

Diverticulum

39. Couseller VS: Urethral diverticulum in the female: A clinical study. Am J Obstet Gynecol 57:231, 1949
40. Rocchi A: Diverticulo de uretra en una nina recien nacida. Rev Argent Urol 24:723, 1955
41. Wharton Jr LR: Urethral diverticulum. Obstet Gynecol 7:503, 1956
42. Davis HJ, Telinde: Urethral diverticula: An assay of 121 cases. J Urol 80:34, 1958
43. Andersen MJF: The incidence of diverticula in the female urethra. J Urol 98:96, 1967
44. Davis BL, Robinson DG: Diverticula of the female urethra: Assay of 120 cases. J Urol 104:850, 1970

Endometriosis

45. Palagiri A: Urethral diverticulum with endometriosis. Urol 11:271, 1978

Nephrogenic Adenoma

46. Peterson LJ, Matsumoto LM: Nephrogenic adenoma in urethral diverticulum. Urol 11:193, 1978

Malignancy

47. Hamilton JD, Leach WB: Adenocarcinoma arising in a diverticulum of the female urethra. Arch Pathol 51:90, 1951
48. Wishard Jr WN, Nourse MH: Carcinoma in diverticulum of female urethra. J Urol 68:320, 1952
49. Brown EW: Diverticulum of female urethra: Report of 23 cases with adenocarcinoma in one. South Med J 49:982, 1956
50. Hinman Jr F, Cohlan WR: Gartner's duct carcinoma in a urethral diverticulum. J Urol 83:414, 1960
51. DeHaan QC: Paraurethral gland adenocarcinoma. J Fla Med Assoc 52:891, 1965
52. Ney C, Miller HL, Ochs D: Adenocarcinoma in a diverticulum of the female urethra: A case report of mucous adenocarcinoma with a summary of the literature. J Urol 106:874, 1971
53. Torres SA, Quattlebaum RB: Carcinoma in a urethral diverticulum. South Med J 65:1374, 1972
54. Rhamy RK, Boldus RA, Allison RC et al: Therapeutic modalities in adenocarcinoma of the female urethra. J Urol 109:638, 1973
55. Klotz PG: Carcinoma of skene's gland associated with urethral diverticulum: A case report. J Urol 112:487, 1974
56. Cea PC, Ward JN, Lavengood Jr RW et al: Mesonephric adenocarcinomas in urethral diverticula. Urol 10:58, 1977
57. Marshall S, Hirsch K: Carcinoma within urethral diverticula. Urol 10:161, 1977
58. Allen R, Nelson RP: Primary urethral malignancy: Review of 22 cases. South Med J 71:547, 1978
59. Reheis JP, Goldstein IS, Mogil RA: Papillary adenocarcinoma arising in a urethral diverticulum accompanied by adenocarcinoma of the bladder: Case report and review of the literature. J Urol 126:695, 1981

60. Evans KJ, McCarthy MP, Sands JP: Adenocarcinoma of a female urethral diverticulum: A case report and review of the literature. J Urol 126:124, 1981
61. Tesluk H: Primary adenocarcinoma of female urethra associated with diverticula. Urol 17:197, 1981

Metaplastic Changes

Squamous Metaplasia

62. Reece RW, Koontz Jr WW: Leukoplakia of the urinary tract: A review. J Urol 114:165, 1975
63. Vijayan P, Clark PB, Anderson CK: Leukoplakia of the male urethra. Short case report. Br J Urol 48:346, 1976

Adenomatoid Metaplasia

64. Martin SA, Santa Cruz DJ: Adenomatoid metaplasia of prostatic urethra. Am J Clin Pathol 75:185, 1981
65. Bhagavan BS, Tiamson EM, Wenk RE et al: Nephrogenic adenoma of the urinary bladder and urethra. Hum Pathol 12:907, 1982

Endometriosis

66. Goodall JR: Urinary complications of pelvic endometriosis. Ann Surg 20:891, 1944

Amyloidosis

67. Schmid KO: Localized amyloidosis (para-amyloidosis) of the urethra: With a contribution to the knowledge of urethral pseudo tumors. Krebsarzt 11:329, 1956
68. Ullmann AS, Fine G, Johnson AJ: Localized amyloidosis (amyloid tumor) of the urethra. J Urol 92:42, 1964

Urethral Polyps

Polypoid Urethritis

69. Randall A: A study of the benign polyps of the male urethra. Surg Gynecol Obstet 17:548, 1913
70. Carter MF: Polypoid granuloma pyogenicum of the posterior urethra. J Urol 111:616, 1974
71. Schinella R, Thurm J, Feiner H: Papillary pseudotumor of the prostatic urethra: Proliferative papillary urethritis. J Urol 111:38, 1974

Caruncle

72. Walther HWE: Caruncle of the urethra in the female with special reference to the importance of histological examination in the differential diagnosis. J Urol 50:380, 1943
73. Palmer JK, Emmett JL, McDonald JR: Urethral caruncle. Surg Gynecol Obstet 87:611, 1948
74. Marshall FC, Uson AC: Neoplasms and caruncles of the female urethra. Surg Gynecol Obstet 110:923, 1960
75. Elbadawi A, Malhoski WE, Frank IN: Mucinous urethral caruncle. Urol 12:587, 1978

Fibroepithelial Polyps

76. Downs RA: Congenital polyps of the prostatic urethra. A review of the literature and report of two cases. Br J Urol 42:76, 1970
77. Mostofi FK, Price EB: Tumors and tumor-like lesions of the male urethra in tumors of the male genital system, pp 263–276. In Atlas of Tumor Pathology, Second Series, Fascicle 8. Washington, DC, AFIP, 1973

Adenomatous Polyps of Prostatic Epithelium

78. Nesbit RM: The genesis of benign polyps in the prostatic urethra. J Urol 87:416, 1962
79. Butterick JD, Schnitzer B, Abell MR: Ectopic prostatic tissue in urethra: A clinico-pathological entity and a significant cause of hematuria. J Urol 105:97, 1971
80. Craig JR, Hart WR: Benign polyps with prostatic-type epithelium of the urethra. Am J Clin Pathol 63:343, 1975
81. Hara S, Horie A: Prostatic caruncle: A urethral papillary tumor derived from pro-lapse of the prostatic duct. J Urol 117:303, 1977
82. Murad TM, Robinson LH, Bueschen A: Villous polyps of the urethra: A report of two cases. Hum Pathol 10:478, 1979
83. Stein AJ, Prioleau PG, Catalona WJ: Adenomatous polyps of the prostatic urethra: A cause of hematospermia. J Urol 124:298, 1980
84. Goldstein AMB, Bragin SD, Terry R et al: Prostatic urethral polyps in adults: Histo-pathologic variations and clinical manifestations. J Urol 126:129, 1981
85. Walker AN, Mills SE, Fechner RE et al: Epithelial polyps of the prostatic urethra. A light-microscopic and immunohistochemical study. Am J Surg Pathol 7:351, 1983
86. Walker AN, Mills SE, Fechner RE et al: "Endometrial" adenocarcinoma of the prostatic urethra arising in a villous polyp: A light microscopic and immunoperoxi-dase study. Arch Pathol Lab Med 106:624, 1982
87. Eglen DE, Pontius EE: Benign prostatic epithelial polyp of the urethra. J Urol 131:120, 1984
88. Baroudy AC, O'Connell JP: Papillary adenoma of the prostatic urethra. J Urol 132:120, 1984

Benign Epithelial Neoplasms
Papilloma

89. Melicow MM, Roberts TW: Pathology and natural history of urethral tumors in males. Review of 142 cases. Urol 11:83, 1978

Inverted Papilloma

90. Trites AEW: Inverted papilloma: Report of two cases. J Urol 101:216, 1969
91. De Meester LJ, Farrow GM, Utz DC: Inverted papillomas of the urinary bladder. Cancer 36:505, 1975

Malignant Epithelial Neoplasms
Female Urethral Carcinoma

92. McCrea LE: Malignancy of the female urethra. Urol Survey 2:85, 1952
93. Ritter DW: Primary malignancy of the female urethra. A review of the recent litera-ture and report of twenty-five cases. West J Surg 61:420, 1953
94. Fagan GE, Hertig AT: Carcinoma of the female urethra. Review of the literature; report of eight cases. Obstet Gynecol 6:1, 1955
95. Staubitz WJ, Carden LM, Oberkircher OJ et al: J Urol 73:1045, 1955
96. Dean AL: Carcinoma of the male and female urethra: Pathology and diagnosis. J Urol 75:505, 1956
97. Flocks RH: The treatment of urethral tumors. J Urol 75:514, 1956
98. Monaco AP, Murphy GB, Dowling W: Primary cancer of the female urethra. Cancer 11:1215, 1958
99. Knoblich R: Primary adenocarcinoma of the female urethra. Am J Obstet Gynecol 80:353, 1960
100. Grabstald H, Hilaris B, Henschke U et al: Cancer of the urethra. JAMA 197:835, 1966

101. Uhle CAW, Kohler FP: Carcinoma of the female urethra: Report of 2 cases of the urethro-vestibular epidermoid group. J Urol 95:378, 1966

102. Pointon RCS, Poole-Wilson DS: Primary carcinoma of the urethra. Br J Urol 40:682, 1968

103. Rogers RE, Burns B: Carcinoma of the female urethra. Obstet Gynecol 33:54, 1969

104. Zeigerman JH, Gordon SF: Cancer of the female urethra. Obstet Gynecol 36:785, 1970

105. Taggart CG, Castro JR, Rutledge FN: Carcinoma of the female urethra. Am J Roentgenol 114:145, 1972

106. Grabstald H: Tumors of the urethra in men and women. Cancer 32:1236, 1973

107. Desai S, Libertino JA, Zinman L: Primary carcinoma of the female urethra. J Urol 110:693, 1973

108. Tiltman AJ: Primary adenocarcinoma of the female urethra. J Pathol 117:97, 1975

109. Bracken RB, Johnson DE, Miller LS et al: Primary carcinoma of the female urethra. J Urol 116:188, 1976

110. Roberts TW, Melicow MM: Pathology and natural history of urethral tumors in females. Urol 10:583, 1977

111. Turner AG, Hendry WF: Primary carcinoma of the female urethra. Br J Urol 52:549, 1980

112. Bolduan JP, Farah RN: Primary urethral neoplasms: Review of 30 cases. J Urol 125:198, 1981

113. Benson Jr RC, Timca JC, Buchler DA et al: Primary carcinoma of the female urethra. Gynecol Oncol 14:313, 1982

Male Urethral Carcinoma

114. Scott EVZ, Barelare B: Adenocarcinoma of the male urethra. J Urol 68:311, 1952

115. Mandler JI, Pool TL: Primary carcinoma of the male urethra. J Urol 96:67, 1966

116. Kaplan GW, Bulkley GJ, Grayhack JT: Carcinoma of the male urethra. J Urol 98:365, 1967

117. Shuttleworth KED, Lloyd-Davies RW: Radical resection for tumours involving the posterior urethra. Br J Urol 41:739, 1969

118. Guinn GA, Ayala AG: Male urethral cancer: Report of 15 cases including a primary melanoma. J Urol 103:176, 1970

119. Ogreid P: Development of carcinoma urethrae after operation for stricture of the urethra. Case report. Scand J Urol Nephrol 4:178, 1970

120. Milstoc M: New pathologic aspects of primary carcinoma of the prostatic urethra. J Am Geriatr Soc 19:80, 1971

121. Clark MO, Kosanovich M: Primary carcinoma of the male urethra. South Med J 65:1339, 1972

122. Mullin EM, Anderson EE, Paulson DF: Carcinoma of the male urethra. J Urol 112:610, 1974

123. Ray B, Canto AR, Whitmore WF: Experience with primary carcinoma of the male urethra. J Urol 117:591, 1977

124. Bolduan JP, Farah RN: Primary urethral neoplasms: Review of 30 cases. J Urol 125:198, 1981

125. Colapinto V, Evans DH: Primary carcinoma of the male urethra developing after urethroplasty for stricture. J Urol 118:581, 1977

Urethral Carcinoma Associated with Bladder Carcinoma

126. Melicow MM, Hollowell JW: Intra-urothelial cancer: Carcinoma in-situ, Bowen's disease of the urinary system: Discussion of thirty cases. J Urol 68:763, 1952

127. Franks LM, Chesterman FC: Intra-epithelial carcinoma of prostatic urethra, peri-urethral glands and prostatic ducts ("Bowen's disease of urinary epithelium"). Br J Cancer 10:223, 1956

128. Gowing NFC: Urethral carcinoma associated with cancer of the bladder. Br J Urol 32:428, 1960
129. Shellhammer PF, Whitmore WF: Urethral meatal carcinoma following cystoure-threctomy for bladder carcinoma. J Urol 115:61, 1976
130. Richie JP, Skinner DG: Carcinoma in situ of the urethra associated with bladder carcinoma: The role of urethrectomy. J Urol 119:80, 1978

Uncommon Primary Urethral Carcinomas

Malignant Melanoma of the Female Urethra

131. Block NL, Hotchkiss RS: Malignant melanoma of the female urethra: Report of a case with 5-year survival and review of the literature. J Urol 105:251, 1971
132. Katz JI, Grabstald H: Primary malignant melanoma of the female urethra. J Urol 116:454, 1976
133. Turner AG, Hendry WF: Primary carcinoma of the female urethra. Br J Urol 52:549, 1980
134. Sharma SK, Dutta TK, Jain SK et al: Malignant melanoma of female urethra. Indian J Cancer 17:264, 1980
135. Novak P, Strmiska M: Melanoblastome of the female urethra. Int Urol Neprol 12:43, 1980
136. Godec CJ, Cass AS, Hitchcock CR et al: Melanoma of the female urethra. J Urol 126:553, 1981
137. Losappio M, Manneschi L: Melanoma primitivo dell'uretra femminile Osservazione personale e revisione della letteratura. Arch De Vecchi Anat Patol 64:521, 1981
138. Sugaya K, Yazaki T, Ishikawa S et al: A case of amelanotic malignant melanoma of the female urethra. Jpn J Clin Oncol 13:435, 1983
139. Bobin JY, Gaude JM, Gerard JP, Mayer M: Les melanomes malins primitifs de l'urethre. A propos de 4 cas. J Urol (Paris) 89:105, 1983
140. Methfessel HD, Bettzieche H, Methfessel G: Melanom der weiblichen Harnohre. Zentralbl Gynakol 105:796, 1983

Malignant Melanoma of the Male Urethra

141. Kokotas NS, Kallis EG, Fokitis PJ: Primary malignant melanoma of male urethra. Urol 18:392, 1981
142. Weiss J, Elder D, Hamilton R: Melanoma of the male urethra: Surgical approach and pathological analysis. J Urol 128:392, 1982

Clear Cell Carcinoma

143. Schiller W: Mesonephroma ovarii. Am J Cancer 35:1, 1939
144. Teilum G: Histogenesis and classification of mesonephric tumors of the female and male genital system and relationship to benign so-called adenomatoid tumors (mesotheliomas). Acta Pathol Microbiol Scand 34:431, 1954
145. Scully RE, Barlow JF: "Mesonephroma" of ovary. Tumor of Müllerian nature related to endometrioid carcinoma. Cancer 20:1405, 1967
146. Herbst AL, Scully RE: Adenocarcinoma of the vagina in adolescence. A report of 7 cases including 6 clear cell carcinoma (so-called mesonephromas). Cancer 25:745, 1970
147. Norris HJ, Rabinowitz M: Ovarian adenocarcinoma of mesonephric type. Cancer 28:1074, 1971
148. Silverberg SG, De Georgi LS: Clear cell carcinoma of the vagina. A clinical, pathologic, and electron microscopic study. Cancer 29:1680, 1972
149. Hart WR, Norris HJ: Mesonephric adenocarcinomas of the cervix. Cancer 29:106, 1972

150. Silverberg SG, De Georgi LS: Clear cell carcinoma of the endometrium. Cancer 31: 1127, 1973
151. Konnak JW: Mesonephric carcinoma involving the urethra. J Urol 110:76, 1973
152. Altwein JE, Schafer R, Hohenfellner R: Mesonephric carcinoma of the female urethra. Eur Urol 1:248, 1975
153. Tiltman AJ: Primary adenocarcinoma of the female urethra. J Pathol 117:97, 1975
154. Cea PC, Ward JN, Lavengood RW, Gray GF: Mesonephric adenocarcinomas in urethral diverticula. Urol 10:58, 1977
155. Murayama T, Komatsu H, Asano M et al: Mesonephric adenocarcinoma of the urethra in a woman: Report of a case. J Urol 120:500, 1978
156. Tanabe ET, Mazur MT, Schaeffer AJ: Clear cell adenocarcinoma of the female urethra. Cancer 49:372, 1982

Cloacogenic Carcinoma

157. Grinvalsky HT, Helwig EB: Carcinoma of the anorectal junction. Cancer 9:480, 1956
158. Grodsky L: Current concepts on cloacogenic transitional cell anorectal cancers. JAMA 207:2057, 1969
159. Robinson JJ, Jordan WP: Some unusual adult male urogenital tumors with dysontogenetic features. Reports of mesonephroma, mullerian carcinosarcoma, transitional cloacogenic carcinoma and nephroblastoma. J Urol 97:357, 1967
160. Lucman L, Vadas G: Transitional cloacogenic carcinoma of the urethra. Cancer 31:1508, 1973
161. Aronson P, Ronan SG, Briele HA et al: Adenoid cystic carcinoma of female periurethral area. Urol 20:312, 1982
162. Saito R: An adenosquamous carcinoma of the male urethra with hypercalcemia. Hum Pathol 12:383, 1981
163. Sylora HO, Diamond HM, Kaufman M et al: Primary carcinoid tumor of the urethra. J Urol 114:150, 1975

Benign Mesenchymal Neoplasms

Leiomyoma

164. Shield DE, Weiss RM: Leiomyoma of the female urethra. J Urol 109:430, 1973
165. Smith DB, Feder FW, Kelsey JF et al: Leiomyoma of the female urethra. Report of two cases. J Arkansas Med Assoc 72:203, 1975
166. Wani NA, Bhan BL, Guru AA et al: Leiomyoma of the female urethra: A case report. J Urol 116:120, 1976
167. Bittard M, Carbillet J-P, Paoletti G et al: Les leiomyomes du bas appareil urinaire chez la femme. A propos de deux observations. J Urol (Paris) 83:226, 1977
168. Cattolica EV, Klein R, Knigge W: Paraurethral leiomyoma — an imitator. Urol 8:605, 1976
169. Avila del Hierro EG, Saceda JL, Santos J: Leiomioma de uretra femenina. Actas Urol Esp 3:145, 1978
170. Moopan MMU, Kim H, Wax SH: Leiomyoma of the female urethra. J Urol 121:371, 1979
171. Williams JL: Leiomyoma of the urethra. Eur Urol 5:144, 1979
172. Lake MH, Kossow AS, Bokinsky G: Leiomyoma of the bladder and urethra. J Urol 125:742, 1981
173. Ellendt EP-C, Martinez-Pineiro JA, Silva J et al: Leiomyoma of the female urethra and bladder neck. Eur Urol 7:46, 1981

Hemangioma

174. McCrea LE: Angioma of the male urethra. Urol Cutan Rev 52:204, 1948
175. Scholl Jr AJ, Braasch WF: Primary tumors of the urethra. Ann Surg 76:246, 1922

176. Begley BJ: Hemangioma of the male urethra: Treatment by Johanson–Denis Browne technique. J Urol 84:111, 1960
177. Radman HM: Urethral hemangioma. J Urol 94:580, 1965
178. Tilak GH: Multiple hemangiomas of the male urethra: Treatment by Denis Browne–Swinney–Johanson rethroplasty. J Urol 97:96, 1967
179. Manuel ES, Seery WH, Cole AT: Capillary hemangioma of the male urethra: Case report with literature review. J Urol 117:804, 1977
180. Sharma SK, Reddy MJ, Joshi VV et al: Capillary haemangioma of male urethra. Br J Urol 53:277, 1981
181. Roberts JW, Devine Jr CJ: Urethral hemangioma: Treatment by total excision and grafting. J Urol 129:1053, 1983

Malignant Mesenchymal Neoplasms

182. Bailey OT: Fibrosarcoma of the male urethra. J Urol 32:109, 1932
183. Painter MR, O'Shaughnessy EJ, Larson PH et al: Rhabdomyosarcoma of the male urethra. J Urol 99:455, 1968

Metastatic Neoplasms

184. Graf EC, Callahan DH, Sozer I: A study of tumors of the female urethra. J Urol 88:64, 1962
185. Selikowitz SM, Olsson CA: Metastatic ureteral obstruction. Arch Surg 107:906, 1973
186. Kotecha N, Gentile RL: Carcinoma of the prostate with ureteral metastases. Urol 3:85, 1974

Cysts of Cowper's Gland

187. Muschat M: Urethral and perineal cysts of the glands of Cowper. With the report of a case and review of the literature. J Urol 22:239, 1929
188. Cook FE, Shaw JL: Cystic anomalies of the ducts of Cowper's gland. J Urol 85:659, 1961
189. Ansell, JS: Cysts of the ducts of Cowper's glands. J Urol 115:390, 1976

Carcinoma of Cowper's Gland

190. Uhle CAW, Archer GF: Primary carcinoma of Cowper's gland. J Urol 34:128, 1935
191. Gutierrez R: Primary carcinoma of Cowper's gland. Surg Gynecol Obstet 65:238, 1937
192. Griesau WA, Lipphard D: Carcinoma of Cowper's gland. J Urol 65:460, 1951
193. Marshall VF, Pearce JM: Carcinoma of Cowper's gland. J Urol 78:421, 1957
194. le Duc E: Carcinoma of Cowper's gland. Report of the eleventh case. Calif Med 96:44, 1962
195. Arduino LJ, Nuesse WE: Carcinoma of Cowper's gland: Case report. J Urol 102:224, 1969
196. Bourque J-L, Charghi A, Gauthier G-E et al:Primary carcinoma of Cowper's gland. J Urol 103:758, 1970
197. Keen MR, Golden RL, Richardson JF et al: Carcinoma of Cowper's gland treated with chemotherapy. J Urol 104:854, 1970
198. Carpenter AA, Bernardo Jr JR: Adenoid cystic carcinoma of Cowper's gland: Case report. J Urol 106:701, 1971

Adenocarcinoma of Littre's Glands

199. Sacks SA, Waisman J, Apfelbaum HB et al: Urethral adenocarcinoma (possibly originating in the glands of Littre). J Urol 113:50, 1975

Testis

6

Normal Structure

Embryologic Development

The embryologic development of the male genital tract and the urinary tract are related both anatomically and temporally.[8,9] The kidneys and gonads arise from the two urogenital ridges. The mesonephric duct, which initially serves as the excretory duct of the transient mesonephric kidney, ultimately evolves to function as the excretory duct system of the male gonad.

The embryologic development of the internal structure and cytologic components of the testis is incompletely understood. Contrasting with all other components of the gonad, the germ cells arise not from the genital ridge primordia but rather from the yolk sac endoderm. During the third gestational week, the germ cells migrate from their yolk sac origin to the gonadal ridge, where they multiply and take residence in sex cords, the precursors of the seminiferous tubules. The origin of the sex cords, and therefore of the Sertoli cells, remains unsettled. Two possibilities have been debated: origin from the surface epithelium by downgrowth into the gonadal ridge mesenchyme, or by condensation of the gonadal mesenchyme. Proponents of the latter explanation regard the Sertoli cells, within the seminiferous tubules, and the Leydig's cells of the gonadal interstitium as derivative from a common precursor, the gonadal stromal cell. Neoplasms of either cell, Sertoli or Leydig, are regarded as neoplasms of specialized gonadal stroma. The unsettled state of origin of the Sertoli cell is reflected in the World Health Organization classification of these neoplasms as Sex Cord/Stromal Neoplasms (refer to discussion of these neoplasms). The seminiferous tubules containing the germ cells and immature Sertoli cells develop from the cords during the second trimester. Ultimately the seminiferous tubules, straight segments (tubuli recti), and the rete testis tubules emerge from the cords. The production of testosterone in Leydig cells begins in the eighth gestational week.

The testicular excretory ducts, the epididymis, vas deferens, and seminal vesicle are derived from the mesonephric (wolffian) duct. The cephalad mesonephric tubules develop into the efferent ductuli, which connect with the rete testis, completing the excretory duct system. The epididymal appendages are vestigial remnants of mesonephric tubules not making contact with the rete testis tubules. The appendix testis is the cephalad vestigial remnant of the Müllerian duct system.

The normal descent of the testis into the scrotum is described later in the chapter (refer to discussion of cryptorchidism).

Adult Testis

The location, size, and structure of the adult testis are achieved after a prepubertal slow growth phase followed by dramatic growth and maturation achieved at puberty under the influence of the pituitary gonadotropins.[5] The hormonally induced changes at puberty initiate spermatogenesis and the reemergence of the interstitial Leydig cells with an associated marked increase in circulating testosterone. The structure of the adult testis reflects the changes resulting at puberty.[2-7,10]

The normal adult testis measures 4 cm X 3 cm X 3 cm and is located within the lower scrotum. It is invested by the visceral layer of the tunica vaginalis, and is attached to the epididymis along its long axis in the posterolateral aspect of the gonad. The outer capsule of the testis, the tunica albuginea, is a dense fibrous covering with multiple internal septal ramifications that structurally divide the testis into approximately 250 lobules. The coiled seminiferous tubules and minimal interstitial connective tissue fill each lobule. The seminiferous tubular system converges near the mediastinum of the testis.[1] Here multiple seminiferous tubules connect to the rete testis tubules by short straight ducts, called tubuli recti. The rete testis tubules, in turn, connect to the efferent ductuli that constitute the head of the epididymis.

The arterial supply to the testis is through the testicular arteries originating from the abdominal aorta. Venous drainage is a dual system involving the internal pudendal and external iliac vein through the cremasteric vein tributaries, and the internal spermatic vein through the pampiniform plexus that ensheathes the spermatic cord. The right internal spermatic vein drains to the inferior vena cava, and the left to the ipsilateral renal vein, an anatomical difference with implications for metastatic patterns of the left and right kidneys and testes. The lymphatic drainage of the testis is directly to the retroperitoneal para-aortic lymph nodes.

Histology and Age Changes

The testis at birth has the following histologic features: the tubules average 60 μm in diameter, and are filled with undifferentiated cells, including spermatagonia; and Leydig cells are pesent in the interstitium either as single cells or in small clusters (Fig. 6-1).[2,3,10] The Leydig cells thereafter apparently disappear, an absence persisting from age 3 months through 9 years. The seminiferous tubules begin to enlarge during the second year, with increasing numbers of germ cells identifiable within their lumen.[10,30,52]

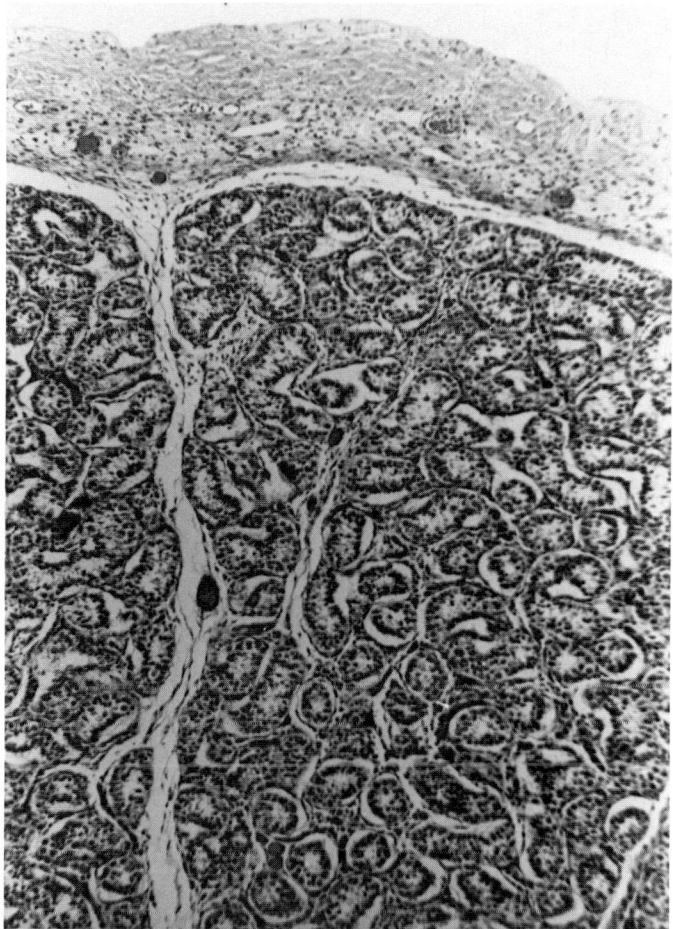

Figure 6-1   ***Normal infant testis.*** *The solid seminiferous tubules are composed of undifferentiated cells in this testis from a 3-month-old infant.*

From age 4 years to 11 years continued tubular enlargement and germ cell maturation are observed.[2,3,10,30,52] Beyond age 12 years the testis evidences uniform active spermatogenesis in all seminiferous tubules, which now contain a lumen (Fig. 6-2). Seminiferous tubular diameter in the adult measures 150 μm to 200 μm in diameter.[3,10,30] The population of germ cells, Sertoli cells, and Leydig cells is thereafter that of the adult testis until the onset of senile atrophy.

Spermatogenesis involves spermatogonia differentiating into primary spermatocytes, which in turn undergo meiotic division to secondary spermatocytes.[5] The secondary spermatocytes undergo the second meiotic division to spermatids, which remain attached to the luminal extension of the Sertoli cells. Upon maturation and release, spermatids become spermatozoa.

Physiologic regression of testicular germ cell production is observed with advancing age. The time of onset and extent of regression are highly variable. With the decrease in germ cells, there is a corresponding increase in Sertoli cells and frequently an increase in Leydig cells. Advanced regressive changes are characterized by tubular sclerosis and interstitial fibrosis (Fig. 6-3).

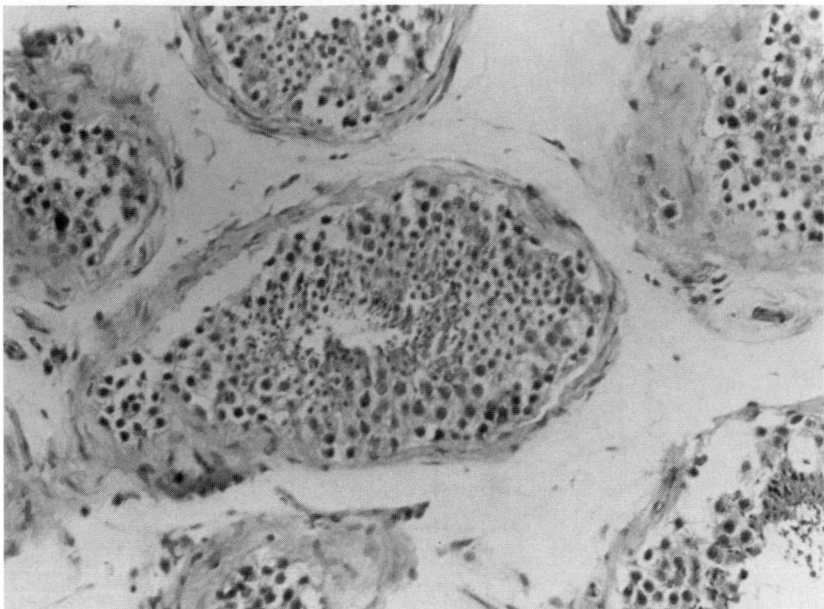

Figure 6-2   *Normal adult testis. Active spermatogenesis is evident in the seminiferous tubules.*

The seminiferous tubules are invested in a thin basement membrane and the tunica propria. The basement membrane is evident only with special stains (PAS or silver stains). The outer tunica propria is composed of layered collagen fibers, myoid cells, and an outer layer of fibroblasts.[4,6] Elastic fibers are evident among the collagen fibers only after puberty.[4,6]

Congenital Disorders

Congenital disorders of the testis include abnormalities of number, location, and formation. Only polyorchidism, cryptorchidism, splenic–gonadal fusion, and disorders of sexual differentiation will be presented here.

Polyorchidism

Polyorchidism is rare, with 55 cases reported in the literature by 1978.[12–14] Four additional cases were found in the subsequent literature, including the first case of bilateral polyorchidism and the first two cases associated with germ cell malignancies.[15–18]

The supernumerary testis may be located anywhere along the route of descent of the normal gonad. In most instances there is complete duplication of the epididymis and testis, which join the vas deferens of the ipsilateral normal testis by a short segment of duplicated vas deferens.[13] The embryologic development of polyorchidism has been discussed by Nocks.[14] The structure and function of the additional testis depends on its location. Intrascrotal examples can be fully functional, the practical importance of which was reported by Hakani and Mo-

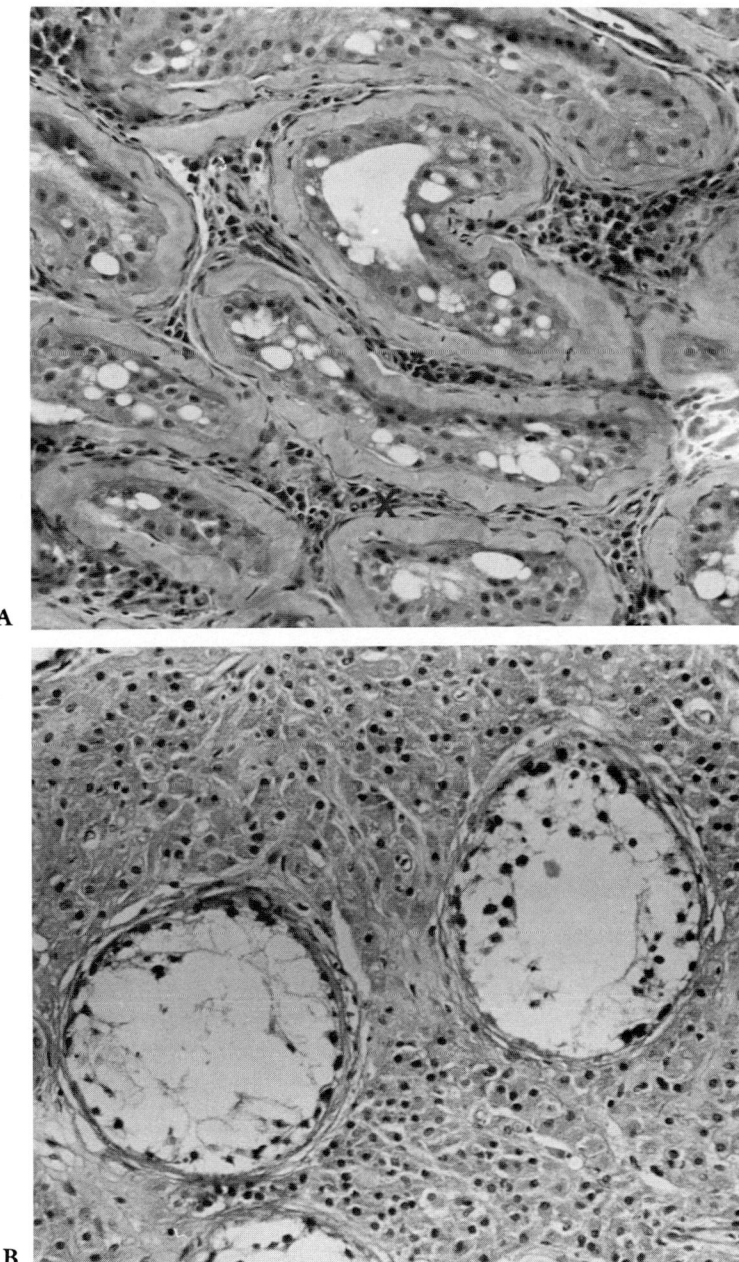

Figure 6-3   ***Physiologic atrophy.*** (A) *There is a marked reduction in tubular diameter, with thickening of the basement membrane and focal tubular sclerosis. Cytoplasmic vacuolization of the Sertoli cells is present.* (B) *Only Sertoli cells remain in the seminiferous tubules. Leydig cell hyperplasia is present in the testicular interstitium.*

zavy, who observed normal sperm counts following a vasectomy in a patient with undiagnosed polyorchidism.[11] Associated congenital anomalies include indirect hernia (30%) and maldescent (15%).[13] Independent of the persistence of fertility under the unique circumstance reported by Hakami and Mozavy, the principal clinical significance of this disorder rests in the differentiation of the extra gonad from other intrascrotal masses, and the rare associated germ cell malignancies noted previously.[11,13,15,16]

Cryptorchidism

Failure of the testis to complete its normal descent into the scrotum is termed *cryptorchidism*. The migration of the male gonad from its intra-abdominal origin commences during the eighth gestational month and is completed by the time of term birth in approximately 96% of male newborns.[24,27] The frequency of cryptorchidism is higher in premature infants (21%) than in normal term infants (4.3%).[24,27] Within 6 weeks of birth the majority of cryptorchid testes have spontaneously descended to the normal scrotal position.[27] Only 0.75% to 0.8% of males have persistent cryptorchidism at age 1 year.[27,44] The prevalence of cryptorchidism among adults is reported to be 0.03% to 0.45%.[25,40] Testicular maldescent is most commonly unilateral, with a slightly greater predilection for the right testis.[23,27]

In the majority of patients with cryptorchidism, the testicular maldescent is an isolated congenital anomaly without apparent cause. Study of large groups of patients allows classification of many into three groups of identifiable causes: (1) anatomical (adhesions, attenuation of inguinal canal); (2) endocrine (disorders involving the hypothalamic–pituitary–testis axis); and (3) dysgenetic (multiple

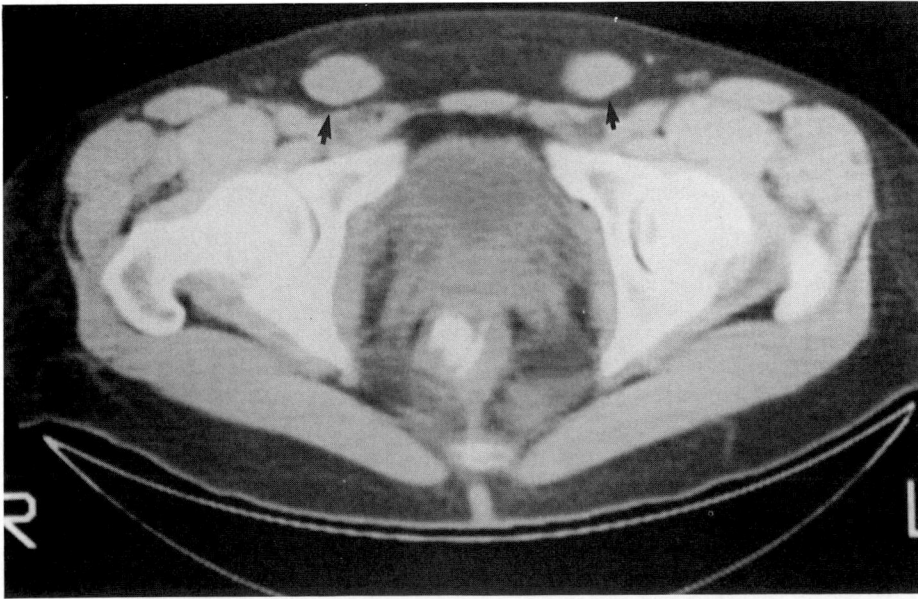

Figure 6-4   *Cryptorchidism, CT scan. Bilateral inguinal canal masses* (arrows) *represent bilateral undescended testicles in a 23-year-old man.*

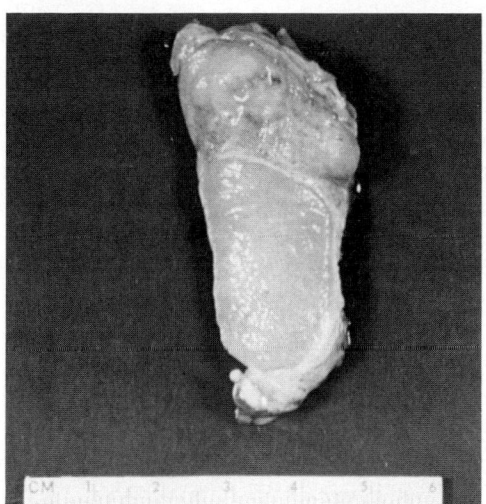

Figure 6-5   ***Cryptorchid testis.*** *This testis from a 19-year-old man is significantly smaller than normal.*

intersex disorders) (Figs. 6-4, 6-5).[45] The most common congenital anomalies accompanying cryptorchidism include hypospadias, atresia of the epididymis, and meningomyelocele.[38,48,49] Although it is congenital, there is no evidence that cryptorchidism is an inherited anomaly, with the apparent exception of rare families with exceptionally high frequencies of this anomaly in the males.[19,29,43,44,51,55] There is no characteristic abnormal karyotype in testicular tissue of cryptorchid patients.[32,36]

The mechanisms operative in the normal descent of the testis are incompletely understood.[47] There is considerable evidence that normal testicular migration into the scrotum requires the action of androgens, which in turn requires a normal hypothalamic–pituitary–testis axis.[47] The mechanism of action of androgen in stimulating testicular descent is unknown.[47] A possible target organ for androgens is the gubernaculum, a fibromuscular band attached to the testis–epididymis and inferiorly to the scrotal wall, which contracts during the last weeks of gestation and draws the testis into its normal scrotal position.[47]

The dominating clinical significance of cryptorchidism relates to the high frequency of compromised fertility and germ cell neoplasms observed in patients with malpositioned gonads. Related to both potential complications is the major clinical decision of the optimal timing of orchiopexy with the intent of minimizing germ cell injury, and thereby increasing the probability of fertility and decreasing the risk of neoplastic transformation. The critical maximum age is currently unknown, as discussed below.

Malignancy Associated with Cryptorchidism

The increased risk of germ cell malignancies complicating cryptorchidism is well established. In a recent review of the literature, Martin reported that an average of 9.8% of testicular germ cell tumors arise in cryptorchid testes.[39,46] The reported frequencies vary from 3.5% to 12%.[46] The calculated increased risk of developing a germ cell malignancy in a malpositioned gonad in an adult male with history of cryptorchidism is approximately 35 times that of the normal adult male population.[20,46] The risk of malignancy in abdominal testes exceeds that of inguinal testes.[40] Martin reviewed 220 previously reported germ cell malignancies arising in patients who had undergone orchiopexy.[39] Ninety-four percent of the patients had surgical correction of the malpositioned gonad at age 10 years or later.[39] Seminomas, embryonal carcinomas, and teratocarcinomas are the most frequent germ cell neoplasms arising in patients with a history of cryptorchidism.[39,40,50]

Importantly, there have been no reported cases of germ cell neoplasms in patients in whom orchiopexy procedure was performed before age 5 years.[39] This must not be equated to an establishment of the critical age for orchiopexy at 5 years. The cumulative data reflect a patient population treated during an era when orchiopexy (for reasons of fertility) was performed after the age of 5 years (refer to following section). The risk of subsequent germ cell malignancy developing in gonads repositioned at ages 1 years to 5 years is currently unknown.

The observation of atypical germ cells in cryptorchid testes has been studied extensively by Muller and Skakkebaek.[53] This has led to the concept of intratubular or in situ germ cell malignancies (refer to discussion of in situ carcinoma in this chapter). The clinical significance and natural history of these lesions awaits further study. A recent report detailed germ cell atypia that progressed to widespread carcinoma in situ and ultimately microinvasive germ cell malignancy in a 21-year-old man who had undergone orchiopexy at age 10 years.[54]

Infertility Associated with Cryptorchidism

With few exceptions, adult males with untreated bilateral cryptorchidism are azoospermic and infertile.[45] Infertility is also observed (although at a lower frequency) in a significant number of adult males with untreated unilateral cryptorchidism.[28,33,35,41] The underlying morphologic changes in the infertile cryptorchid testis included a marked reduction or complete absence of germ cells without evidence of spermatogenesis or tubular, peritubular, and interstitial fibrosis.[21,22,26] Initial surgical attempts to correct infertility in adult cryptorchid males recorded only limited success. There was a preoccupation with debating the relative merits of surgical techniques: *how* the orchiopexy was to be done, rather than the infinitely more important question of *when* the procedure should be done to prevent the clinical infertility and the underlying morphologic changes consistently found in adult cryptorchid testes.

The initial studies indicated that morphologic evidence of injury in the cryptorchid testis was not detected until puberty.[2,3,28] These studies advocated orchiopexy in the late prepubertal years. Subsequent studies detected decreased germ cells and tubular immaturity at progressively younger ages.[26,30,33,34] The most recent investigations report observable changes in the cryptorchid testis as early as 1 year to 2 years of age.[30,33,34,41,52] Correspondingly, the advocated age for orchiopexy has progressively decreased to this same age.[45]

The histologic changes observed in the cryptorchid testis beginning at age 1 year to 2 years and progressing with increasing age include decreased mean tubular diameter (MTD) and germ cell count (GCC) (Figs. 6-6 to 6-8).[30,33,52] Interestingly, the scrotal testis in cases of unilateral cryptorchidism demonstrates similar changes.[28,30,22,41,52]

Accompanying histologic changes in the cryptorchid testis in young children are thickening of the lamina propria, intratubular microlithiasis, focal tubules

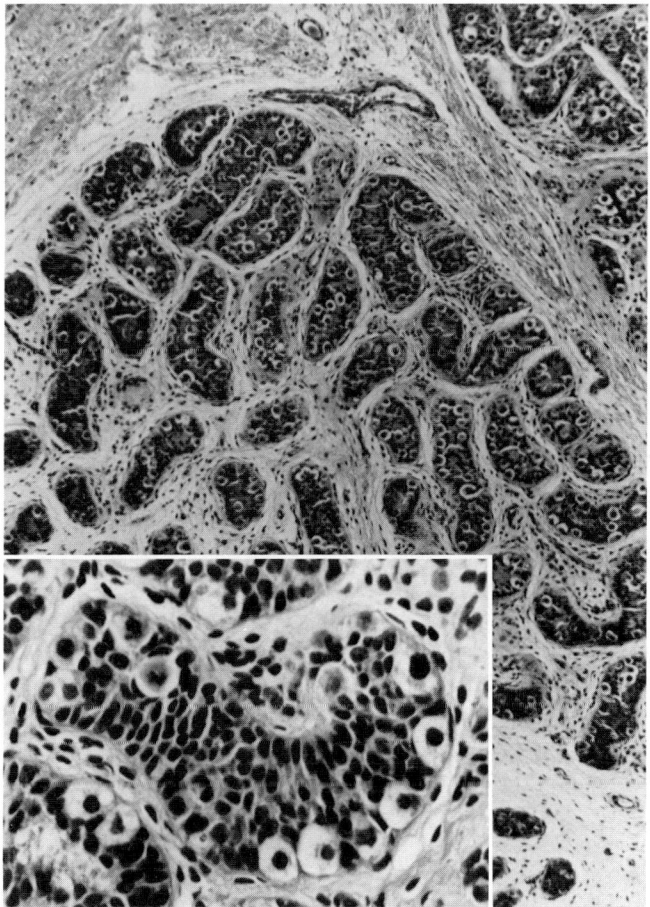

Figure 6-6   ***Cryptorchidism.*** *The mean tubular diameter of these seminiferous tubules is smaller than normal. The germ cells, now readily apparent* (inset), *are reduced in number in this testis from 2-year-old infant. There is slight increase of intratubular fibrosis.*

with Sertoli cell hyperplasia (tubular adenoma of Pick), and abnormalities of germ cell nuclear features.[31,37,41,53,56] The youngest age when cryptorchid testes show a total absence of germ cells is unsettled, but has been reported at 3 years.[33] The point of irreversible damage to the germ cell population, short of germ cell obliteration, beyond which compromised fertility is highly probable, has not been determined. The effect of orchiopexy performed at age 1 year to 2 years on both subsequent fertility and frequency of malignancy is currently unknown.

Splenic – Gonadal Fusion

Splenic–gonadal fusion, a rare congenital anomaly, has been reported in 87 patients.[65] In a comprehensive review, Putschar and Manion detailed the first 30 cases published up to 1956, attributing the first detailed description to Pommer in 1889.[57] Since their review, an additional 57 cases have appeared in the litera-

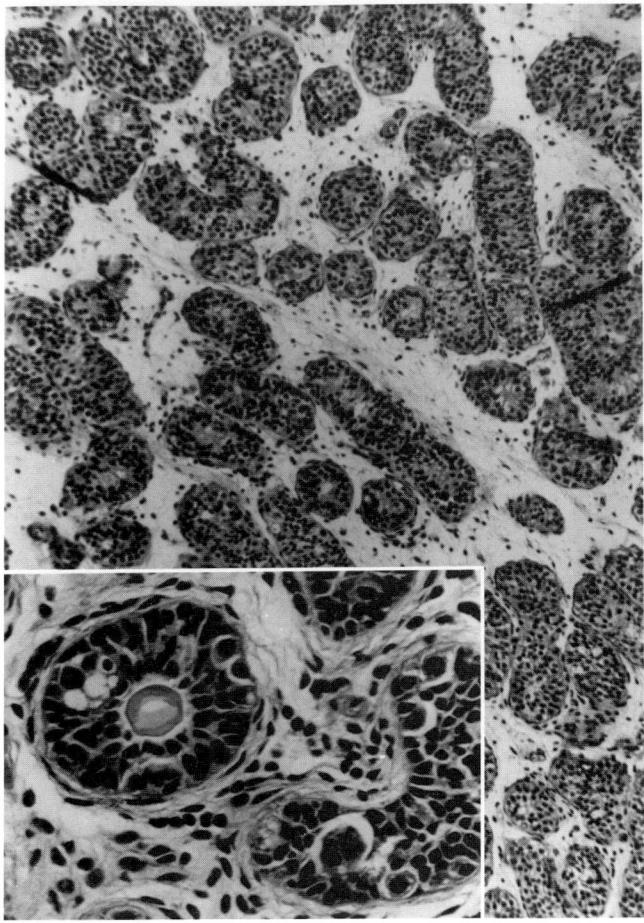

Figure 6-7   **Cryptorchidism.** *The mean tubular diameter is smaller than normal for age (7 years) and the germ cells are markedly reduced. A tubular microlith is present* (inset).

ture, an increase most probably due to an increased awareness and detection of this rare disorder.[58-65] Splenic fusion with the testis is far more common than with the ovary, with only 7 of the 87 cases reported in females.[65] The left gonad is involved almost exclusively, with only a few reported cases involving a right testis.[65]

Putschar and Manion classified examples of splenogonadal fusion into continuous and discontinuous types.[57] Continuous fusion, which is more frequent, evidences a continuous cord of splenic tissue, or a fibrous band from the lower pole of the spleen to the involved gonad. The discontinuous type is characterized by fusion of the accessory or ectopic splenic tissue with the gonad, with loss of all connection to the normally placed spleen.

The cause of splenic–gonadal fusion is unknown. The fusion is tentatively dated to occur during the fifth to eighth gestational weeks, when the splenic and gonadal primordia are differentiating in proximity.[57,63,65] The splenic tissue, fused with the gonad, descends caudally to its ultimate location within the

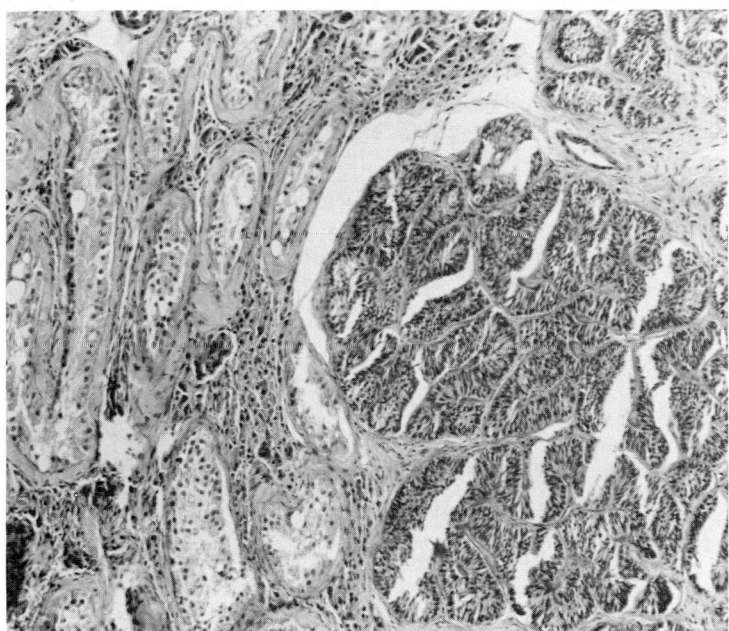

Figure 6-8   *Cryptorchid testis. The tubular basement membrane is markedly thickened with vacuolization of the cytoplasm of the remaining Sertoli cells. A focus of Sertoli cell hyperplasia (tubular adenoma of Pick) is present* (right). *The patient was 28 years old.*

scrotum. Splenogonadal fusion is associated with other congenital anomalies including peromelus, micrognathia, and cardiac malformation.[63,64] These anomalies are associated almost exclusively with splenogonadal fusion of the continuous type, for unknown reasons.[65] Only one case of discontinuous splenic–gonadal fusion associated with other anomalies has been reported.[64]

The disorder has been diagnosed at all ages from newborns to the seventh decade; however, the majority come to clinical attention during the first two decades. The left gonad was involved in 85 of the 87 reported cases.[65] The clinical impression of testicular neoplasm, torsion, or inguinal hernia prompts surgical exploration of the scrotum in most cases. Occasional scattered cases are detected incidentally at autopsy. The correct preoperative diagnosis has been made in only two of the reported cases, utilizing technetium scans of the spleen.[65]

The splenic tissue is fused with the gonad either internal or external to the tunica albuginea, most frequently in the region of the upper pole. Alternatively, the splenic tissue may be associated with the spermatic cord. When found within the testis, it is most commonly encapsulated and separated from the seminiferous tubules.

The clinical significance of splenogonadal fusion is related to the associated congenital anomalies, some of which may not be clinically inapparent (such as cardiac abnormalities), and the necessity of distinguishing the anomaly from testicular neoplasms. There has been a single example of a seminoma arising in an undescended testis showing splenogonadal fusion.[61]

Disorders of Sexual Differentiation

Disorders of sexual differentiation can be broadly classified into three groups: disorders of genetic sex, gonadal sex, or phenotypic sex.[66-68] Each is identified by characteristic karyotype, gonadal structure, and internal and external genitalia, with or without characteristic abnormalities of chromosome karyotype. The clinical significance of the accurate diagnosis relates to the appropriate assignment of gender in all patients, and in some, the increased risk of neoplasms arising in the maldeveloped gonads.[69] The underlying etiology and pathogenesis of most are incompletely understood, but inheritance patterns of some have been delineated.

Disorders of Genetic Sex

Disorders of genetic sex are represented by the following: (1) gonadal dysgenesis (Turner's syndrome) characterized by bilateral gonadal streaks; (2) mixed gonadal dysgenesis, characterized by a testis and contralateral streak gonad; and (3) at the other extreme, true hermaphrodites characterized by bilateral ovaries and testes, or variant combinations with ovotestis. The external genitalia of these disorders of genetic sex are either female (gonadal dysgenesis) or ambiguous (mixed gonadal dysgenesis and true hermaphroditism).

Gonadal dysgenesis (Turner's syndrome) is characterized by 45 XO karyotype, or mosaic patterns.[70-72] The gonadal streaks in young adult patients are composed of fibrous stroma histologically similar to the normal ovary, but lacking germ cells and evidence of differentiation to granulosa cells.[66-68,70,72] Germ cells have been identified in fetal and postnatal ovaries of these patients, but subsequently disappear to give the characteristic histologic features of streak gonads in adults.[72] When neoplasms supervene in streak gonads, they are most frequently gonadoblastomas (refer to discussion of gonadoblastoma in this chapter). The gonadal streaks of mixed gonadal dysgenesis are identical to those observed in Turner's syndrome.[73,76]

The gonads present in true hermaphrodites are represented by structures that have the combined features of an ovary and a testis (an ovotestis).[66,69,77-80] Alternative findings are an ovary and a contralateral testis, or a unilateral ovotestis.[66,68,77-80] The ovotestis, whether unilateral or bilateral, is characterized by unequivocal testicular structures, albeit infantile, in proximity to ovarian primordial follicles.[69,77-80]

Disorders of Gonadal Sex

Examples of disorders of gonadal sex are represented by cases of pure gonadal dysgenesis, characterized by bilateral streak gonads and (usually) female phenotype.[66-68,81,82] These patients have an XX or XY karyotype, and their normal height differs from Turner's patients with XO karyotype and short stature.[68,81,82] The pathogenesis of pure gonadal dysgenesis is currently not established.

Disorders of Phenotypic Sex

The last category, disorders of phenotypic sex, is a large heterogenous group of disorders with ambiguous phenotypic features but with gonads consistent with the genotype of the patients.[83-92] The prototypical examples of phenotypic sex disorders in the male are male pseudohermaphroditism, represented by five distinct metabolic disorders of testosterone synthesis (male adrenogenital syndrome).[84,86-90,92] Alternatively, abnormal peripheral testosterone receptors are identified in testicular feminization.[83,85,91] Phenotypical sexual disorders of the female are represented by female pseudohermaphroditism (adrenogenital syndrome in a genotypic female).[66] In the latter circumstance, enzymatic deficiencies cause congenital hypersecretion of adrenal androgens, producing virilization of the female patient.[66] In male patients the defective testosterone synthesis, or peripheral utilization, results in variable feminization.[18-24] The gonadal morphology of the male reflects the frequent intra-abdominal location.

Infertility

The contribution of testicular biopsy to the clinical evaluation of male infertility was first advocated by Charney and by Engle.[93,94] The procedure was to complement and frequently clarify the clinical and laboratory information in the evaluation of the male's contribution to the dilemma of the childless couple. As the list of recognized clinical disorders underlying male infertility expanded, eight histologic changes evolved in the testicular biopsies of infertile men.[93,94,101,108,112] The initial hope that all clinically recognized forms of male infertility would be associated with a consistent histologic alteration within the testis, and thereby reliably contribute to the diagnosis of and possibly to the therapeutic decisions about male infertility, has proved excessively optimistic. Specifically, it is now recognized that many clinical disorders can produce multiple types of morphologic changes, or alternatively, no apparent histologic change. Furthermore, each of the eight recognized histologic patterns can be produced by infertility disorders of diverse causes.

Several factors underlie the current modest contribution of testicular biopsy interpretation to the study of male infertility. First, virtually nothing is known of the pathogenesis of any of the specific lesions encountered, including maturation arrest, hypospermatogenesis, and tubular and peritubular fibrosis. The investigations into testicular morphology in male infertility have been primarily observational. The rather large body of literature on the subject, detailing an increasing number of hereditary, metabolic, infectious, and traumatic disorders has served not to clarify specific pathogenetic routes of injury, but to confirm the limited patterns of injury demonstrated by the testis, regardless of the nature of the injury agent. Furthermore, insufficient attention has been given to the "time–lesion curve" of testicular injury, with only limited inquiry into the evolution of hypospermatogenesis.[111] Infertility states "characteristically" associated with hypospermatogenesis may progress to the ultimate hypospermatogenic state, germ cell aplasia (Sertoli cell only), with or without associated peritubular fibrosis, and ultimate fibrous obliteration of the seminiferous tubule. The initial insult may also injure the basement membrane or tunica propria. The resultant fibrosis itself may compromise oxygenation of the germ cell population, and thereby independently contribute to the injury of the hypospermatogenic cell population. This pathogenetic interrelationship of tubular and peritubular fibrosis, with maturation arrest and hypospermatogenesis, is currently unknown.

Having detailed the limitations of our knowledge of testicular lesions in infertility, the value of testicular biopsy will be outlined. Under all circumstances the final diagnosis should represent the synthesis of clinical information, including patient age, physical examination, past occupational and medical history, serum follicle-stimulating hormone (FSH), luteinizing hormone (LH), and testosterone, and semen analysis, with the histologic features of the biopsy.

The reported histologic changes observed in testicular biopsies of a wide variety of infertility disorders are as follows:

Normal testicular morphology for age;

Immature testis in postpubertal male;

Maturation arrest;

Intratubular sloughing of germ cells;

Hypospermatogenesis;

Germ cell aplasia (Sertoli cell only);

Peritubular and tubular fibrosis; and

Mixed patterns.

The following features are to be evaluated in testicular biopsies:

1. Adequacy of the biopsy;
2. Number of Leydig cells in interstitium;
3. Presence of interstitial, peritubular, or tubular fibrosis;
4. Presence or absence of elastic fibers in the tunica propria;
5. Mean tubular diameter;
6. Presence of germ cells within the seminiferous tubules;
7. Completeness of maturation of the germ cells;
8. Ratio of germ cells to Sertoli cells;
9. Presence or absence of sloughed immature germ cells;
10. Appropriateness of tubular structure and spermatogenesis referable to age of the patient; and
11. Presence or absence of atypical intertubular germ cells.

Morphologic Classification

Normal Histology

A histologically normal testicular biopsy in the clinical context of infertility is commonly observed in patients with varicocele and tubular obstruction.[113] However, both disorders may produce hypospermatogenesis.[106,107,113,117] In experimental duct obstruction, a transient suppression of spermatogenesis is followed by a return to normal, albeit incomplete.[116]

Immature Testis in Postpubertal Male

The clinical disorder prepubertal hypopituitarism may reflect a panhypopituitary disorder, or may represent a selective deficiency of gonadotropins (hypogonadotrophic eunichoidism).[96,99,100,102,115] In the classic form of each disorder, both FSH and LH secretion are abnormally low, and the testis retains an infantile structure in affected postpubertal males.[96,102,105] Variants of the classic form of hypogonadotrophic eunichoidism show selective deficiency of LH secretion.[99,100] Physical examination, gonadotropin assay, and testicular biopsy will allow distinction of the various forms of prepubertal hypopituitary infertility states.

Maturation Arrest

Maturation arrest is characterized by a cessation of germ cell development beyond the primary spermatocyte stage (Fig. 6-9).[94,108,122] Fewer cases show arrest at the secondary spermatocyte stage.[108,112] Intraluminal sloughing of the arrested spermatocytes is commonly present.[94] This histologic abnormality is among the most commonly encountered in cases of infertility.[108,112] Maturation arrest is encountered in a number of clinical disorders, none of which are uniquely characterized by this histologic finding (Table 6-1).

Intratubular Sloughing of Germ Cells

The sloughing of germ cells is observed occasionally in association with maturation arrest. It is characterized by single cells or clumps of germ cells lying loose in the central lumen of the seminiferous tubule. The pathogenesis of the sloughed

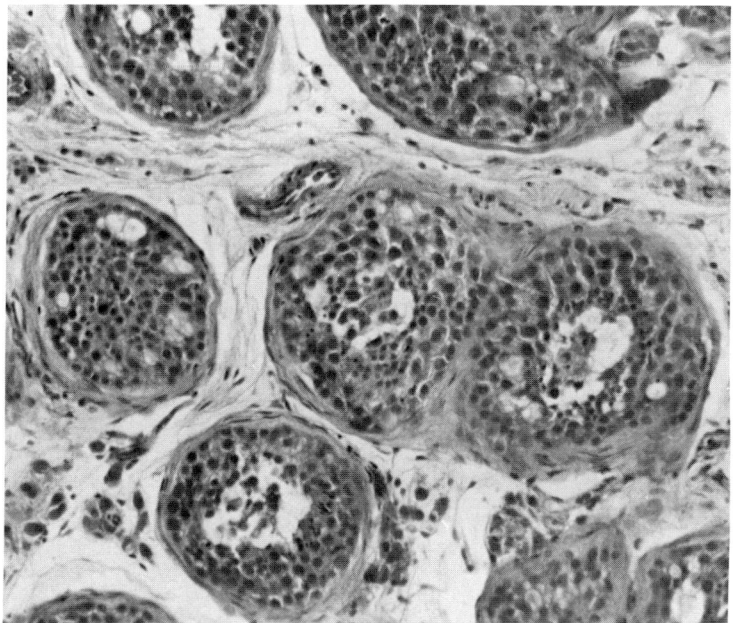

Figure 6-9   *Maturation arrest. The tubules contain germ cells that have uniform cytologic features and a complete absence of spermatid and sperm. Scattered nests of interstitial cells are present.*

germ cells is unknown. It has been reported most commonly in cases of varico-cele and duct obstruction.[107,114]

Hypospermatogenesis

Hypospermatogenesis is characterized by an absolute reduction of germ cells in all stages of maturation (Fig. 6-10).[94,112,124] Importantly, the extant germ cells apparently retain the capacity to undergo complete maturation to sperm.[124] This histologic picture is relatively frequent in infertile males. The underlying causes of hypospermatogenesis are numerous, and include many disorders in which germ cell aplasia and peritubular fibrosis have been reported (see Table 6-1). The severity of the hypospermatogenetic state of the gonad is inversely related to the probability of future restoration of fertility.

Germ Cell Aplasia (Sertoli Cell Only)

The ultimate form of hypospermatogenesis is germ cell aplasia. The seminiferous tubules are populated solely by Sertoli cells (Fig. 6-11). This is regarded as

Table 6-1   Testicular Morphology in Infertility Disorders*

Clinical Disorders	Normal	Hypospermatogenesis	Sertoli Cell Only	Maturation Arrest	Intratubular Sloughing	Immature Testis	Peritubular Fibrosis
Congenital							112
Klinefelter's syndrome		112	112				
Down's syndrome		117					
Reifenstein's syndrome							117
Cystic fibrosis		106					
Cryptorchidism		117	117	117		117	117
Rosewater's syndrome				117			
Diabetes mellitus		104					104
Adrenogenital syndrome			117	117			
Myotonic muscular dystrophy							104
Hypogonadotrophic eunochoidism						96,99,100,102	
DES exposure		†					
Systemic Metabolic							
Malnutrition		117					
Febrile illness		112,117					
Hypothyroidism		115					
Uremia		121					
Cirrhosis	123	123					123
Vascular							
Varicocele	113	106,107,113	120		107,114		

irreversible, and precludes restoration of the germ cell population.[95,108,112] Germ cell aplasia is frequently associated with tubular and peritubular fibrosis. A wide variety of underlying clinical infertility disorders are associated with germ cell aplasia. Most of these same disorders have also been associated with lesser and greater degrees of injury with hypospermatogenesis, and with tubular and peritubular fibrosis (see Table 6-1).

Tubular and Peritubular Fibrosis

As noted previously and as indicated in Table 6-1, tubular and peritubular fibrosis are associated with diverse infertility states. Peritubular fibrosis, in association with Leydig cell hyperplasia, is highly characteristic of Klinefelter's syndrome, a congenital disorder (refer to separate discussion). Appropriate special stains will demonstrate the localization of the fibrosis (*i.e.,* intratubular, basement membrane, or tunica propria). Elastic fibers may be normal, increased, or absent. A decrease or absence of elastic fibers is characteristic of Klinefelter's syndrome.[4,6,112]

Table 6-1 (continued)

Clinical Disorders	Normal	Hypospermatogenesis	Sertoli Cell Only	Maturation Arrest	Intratubular Sloughing	Immature Testis	Peritubular Fibrosis
Infectious Diseases							
Mumps			119		119		
Tuberculosis							144
Physical Injury							
Heat		112					
Radiation injury			121				
Trauma							104
Vasectomy	113	113					
Chemical Injury							
Drugs (antineoplastic agents)			109				109
Exogenous estrogens		103	103	103			
Exogenous androgens		103	103	103			
Exogenous glucocorticoids		105		105			
Neoplastic							
Pituitary neoplasms		115	115	115			115
Sex cord/stromal neoplasms							115

* Numbers refer to references.
† Refer to discussion of DES-Related Abnormalities in Chap. 7.

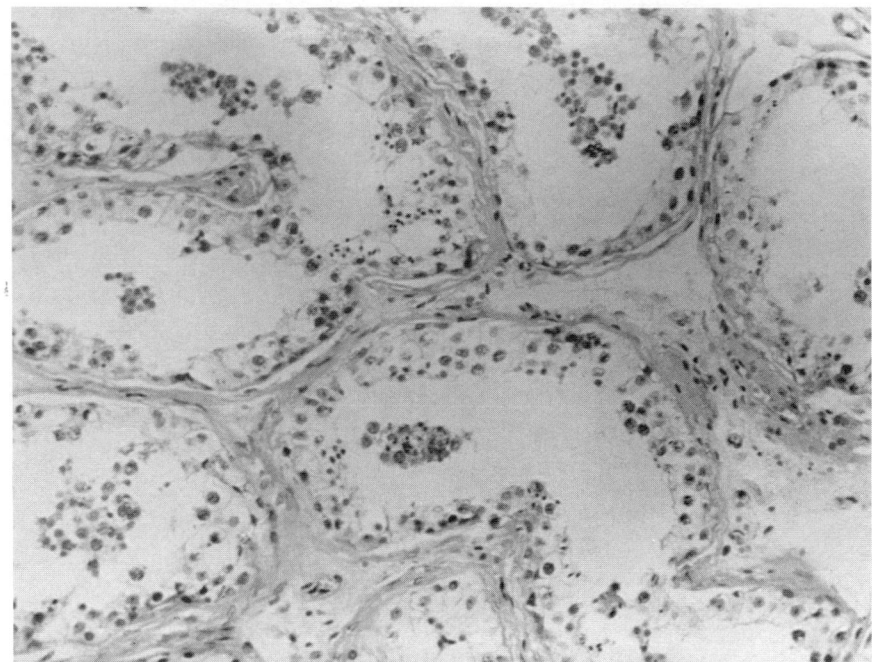

Figure 6-10   *Hypospermia. The numbers of germ cells are markedly reduced in this testis, which did contain some sperm in occasional tubules.*

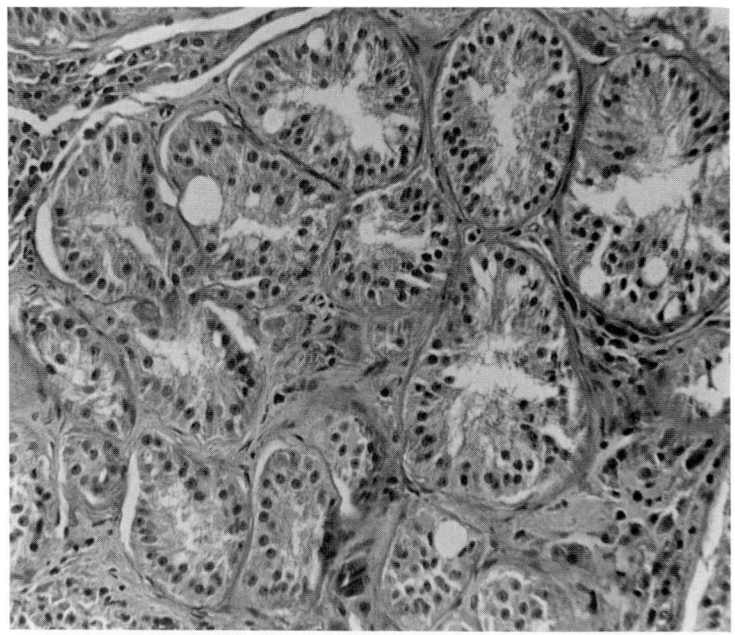

Figure 6-11   *Sertoli cell-only syndrome (germinal cell aplasia). The seminiferous tubules contain only Sertoli cells. The basement membrane of the tubules is not significantly thickened, and there is no interstitial fibrosis.*

Mixed Patterns of Testicular Lesions

Infertility associated with mixtures of the previous features is not uncommon. This reflects the interrelated responses to injury, all of which are poorly understood at present.[108]

Klinefelter's Syndrome

In 1942, Klinefelter and co-workers described a syndrome of male hypogonadism characterized by gynecomastia, spermatogenesis, increased FSH secretion, and apparently normal Leydig cell function among seven patients observed at the Massachusetts General Hospital.[125] Testicular biopsies revealed tubular hyalinization and "normal-appearing interstitial cells."[125] In subsequent decades the association of an abnormal karyotype, most commonly XXY, was detected in these patients.[126,127] Other karyotypes, including XXYY, and mosaic patterns and chromatin-negative patients have been reported.[128,130]

With increasing recognition of Klinefelter's syndrome patients, variability of the clinical features also became apparent. The small testes associated with azoospermia are the most constant findings, with fewer patients showing decreased testosterone, elevated gonadotropins, decreased facial hair, and gynecomastia, in order of decreasing frequency.[131] Most patients are diagnosed in the course of fertility studies. The frequency of Klinefelter's syndrome (0.2% of the male population) makes this disorder the most frequent form of abnormal sexual differentiation.[129]

The histologic features of testicular changes in Klinefelter's syndrome have

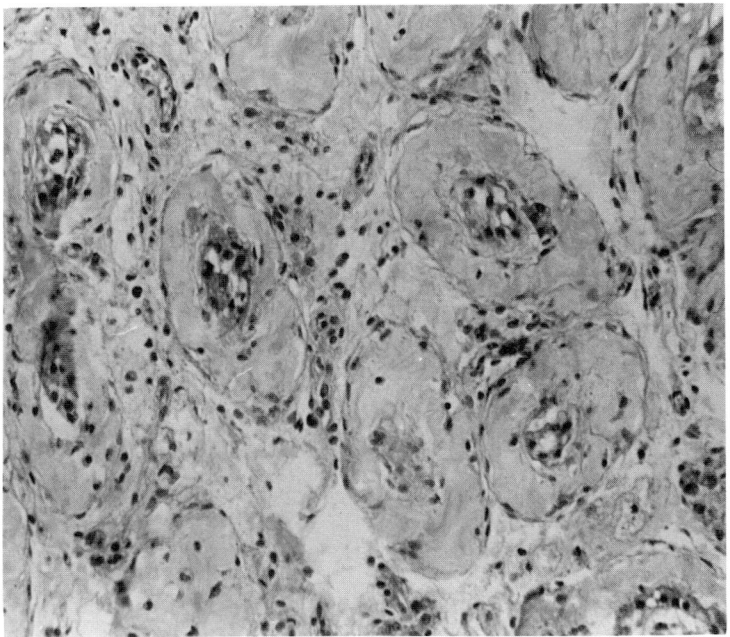

Figure 6-12 **Klinefelter's syndrome.** *There is marked tubular basement membrane thickening, absence of spermatogenesis, rare Sertoli cells, and focal interstitial cell hyperplasia.*

been extensively studied.[108,112,125,132] The earliest abnormality is a reduction in the number of germ cells, with associated atrophy of Sertoli cells. This is progressive, with later total loss of germ cells followed by loss of Sertoli cells, and concomitant tubular atrophy (Fig. 6-12). Initially patchy in distribution, these changes become progressively more uniform throughout the testes. Ultimately the thickening and hyalinization of the tunica propria progresses to complete tubular obliteration. Leydig cells are present in increased numbers. The tubular walls, normally demonstrating elastic fibers after puberty, have been reported to show absent or significantly reduced elastic fibers in Klinefelter's syndrome patients.[108,112]

The histologic diagnosis of Klinefelter's syndrome rests heavily on the combined features of tubular sclerosis with diminished or absent elastic fibers, and increased numbers of Leydig cells within the interstitium. This combination of histologic features, supported by clinical data and karyotype information, will allow differentiation of Klinefelter's syndrome patients from the many other causes of tubular sclerosis including varicocele, alcoholism, physiologic atrophy of aging, diabetes mellitus, trauma, chronic inflammation, and irradiation injury (see Table 6-1).

Inflammatory Disorders

Acute and Chronic Orchitis

Inflammatory disorders of the testis take the clinical forms of acute and chronic, and are frequently associated with involvement of the epididymis. The majority are related to urinary tract infections, which, by means of retrograde spread through the vas deferens, result in epididymo-orchitis. Less frequently, retrograde venous or lymphatic spread accounts for the gonadal inflammation. Only uncommonly do inflamed testes become diagnostic challenges for the surgical pathologist, because most are treated successfully with antibiotics following culture and sensitivity procedures. Gram-negative organisms are most frequently involved, but a wide variety of bacterial species has been identified (Fig. 6-13).[139,145] With significantly lower frequency, viruses, fungi, and rickettsiae have been diagnosed as the underlying cause.[138-146]

Among the viruses, mumps orchitis is the most frequent, reported to complicate 20% of mumps occurring in adults.[133-137] Testicular involvement with marked swelling and pain is most commonly unilateral. The histologic features have been described by Gall and by Charny and Meranze.[133,134] The frequency of compromised sterility subsequent to mumps orchitis is unsettled.[135-137] Testicular swelling and pain of recent onset, with or without evidence of systemic involvement, is the characteristic clinical presentation.

The histologic features of epididymo-orchitis have been reported by Hourihane, who emphasized the frequency of venous thrombosis and testicular infarction.[139] Transition areas with fibrosis and features resembling granulomatous inflammation were observed.

The lack of resolution of the acute inflammatory lesion leads to chronic orchitis, which is histologically classifiable into nongranulomatous and granulomatous types. The latter, granulomatous orchitis, has been associated with ter-

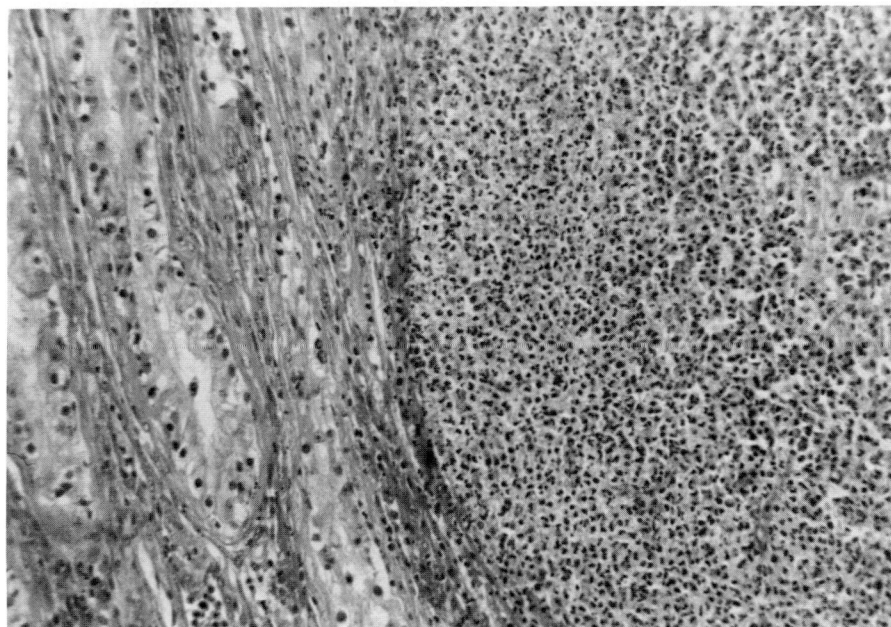

Figure 6-13   *Acute orchitis with abscess. The abscess* (left) *contains innumerable neutrophils in a localized area of parenchymal destruction. Gram-negative organisms were cultured from the abscess.*

tiary syphilis, tuberculosis, sarcoidosis, a variety of fungal agents, and leprosy.[138,140,141,143-145] The specific etiologic agent is identified either by special stains demonstrating organisms in the orchiectomy specimen, or by culturing the lesions. Chronic granulomatous infection of the testis without an identified etiologic agent occurs in two forms, granulomatous orchitis and malakoplakia. Each is discussed briefly below.

Granulomatous Orchitis

In 1926, Grunberg described three patients with orchitis demonstrating granulomatous inflammation.[147] The absence of any demonstrable causal agent characterized these cases and all those subsequently reported in the literature.[148-162] The disorder is uncommon, with approximately 100 cases, virtually all as case studies and small series. The role of trauma, immunologic reaction to sperm, and vascular insufficiency all have been suggested as causally related to this inflammatory disorder.[152,158,159,161,162] Granulomatous orchitis is not analogous to sperm granulomas of the epididymis, as previously proposed.[156] Phagocytosis of sperm fragments, one of the characteristic features of sperm granulomas of the epididymis, is never prominent in granulomatous orchitis, and indeed is not apparent in the majority of cases.[156,162] The proposed immunologic injury underlying granulomatous orchitis, a form of which has been produced experimentally in pigs, does not explain why most cases of granulomatous orchitis observed clinically involve only one testis.[159] The role of prior trauma, recorded in many cases, needs further study. Vascular compromise with testicular ischemia or infarction, followed by immunologic injury perpetuating the lesion, may be the underlying sequence of events, but is currently unsupported by the available studies.[149,161] The granulomatous nature of the inflammatory response may be caused by the reaction to an acid-fast lipid in sperm demonstrated by Berg.[151] Attempts to demonstrate a biologic agent with culture procedures and special stains have proved negative in all reported cases.

Patients present with either acute epididymo-orchitis, or more frequently, a prolonged history of recurrent testicular pain and swelling.[157] Those cases with a more protracted clinical history demonstrated an indurated testis, which clinically suggests either tuberculosis or neoplasm (Fig. 6-14). As noted above, many patients give a history of trauma to the involved testis. Only rarely is the disorder bilateral. Patients range in age from the third to eighth decade, but the majority are in the fifth and sixth decades.[157] The correct diagnosis has not occurred prior to orchiectomy.

Pathologic Features

The testis is commonly moderately enlarged and indurated, with a thickened tunica. The cut surface discloses variably extensive destruction of the tubules with gray-white to tan areas of induration. Microscopically, the characteristics of

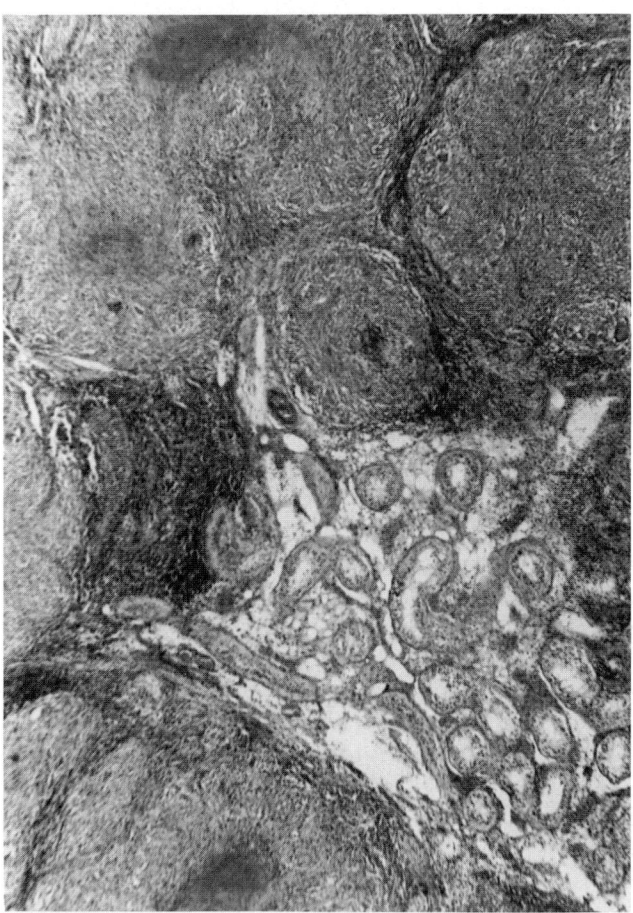

Figure 6-14   *Tuberculosis. Multiple confluent granulomas with central necrosis are present within the testis.*

the lesion depend on the stage of the inflammatory process. Tubular destruction is typically late with extensive fibrosis. Earlier, the tubular structure is retained and the inflammatory process is noted to be predominantly intratubular, with destruction of the germ cells and to a lesser extent the Sertoli cells. Ultimately, all resident cells of the seminiferous tubules are destroyed and replaced by numerous histiocytes with fewer lymphocytes and plasma cells (Fig. 6-15). The interstitium is also infiltrated by the same inflammatory cells. The inflammatory cell infiltrate is usually of such magnitude that the presence of the tubular structures is obscured in routine stained sections. Silver stains will demonstrate the structural remnants of the seminiferous tubules within the inflammatory reactions, outlining the tubular collections of histiocytes, which appear as innumerable noncaseating granulomas.

The diagnosis of idiopathic granulomatous orchitis is based on this clinical and histologic picture, coupled with appropriate special stains and culture procedures that all fail to demonstrate a specific etiologic agent. This inflammatory

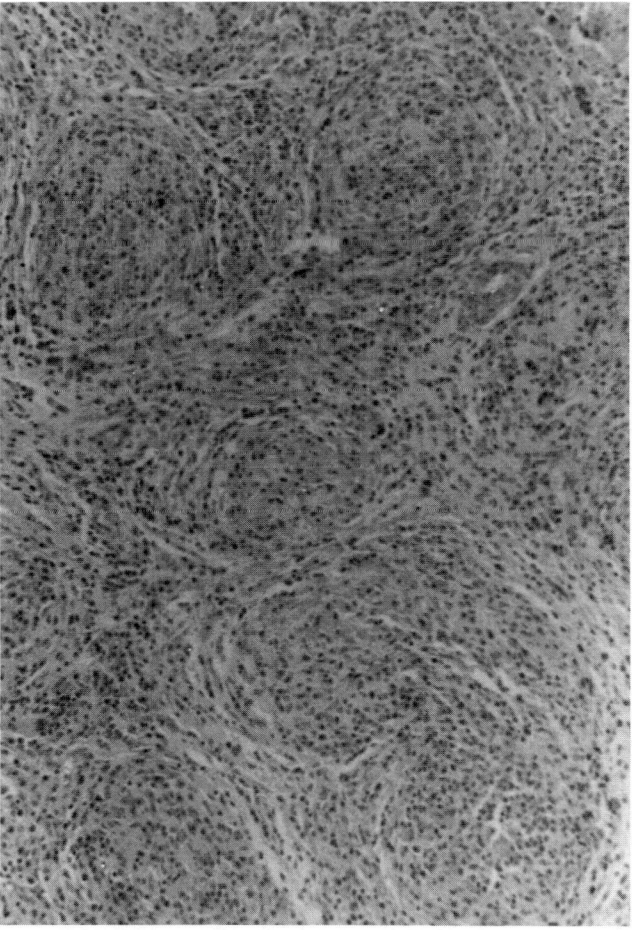

Figure 6-15   ***Granulomatous orchitis.*** *The remnants of destroyed tubules are filled with histiocytes and lymphocytes, creating a nodular pattern. The same inflammatory cells are present in the intertubular interstitium. All cultures and special stains for acid-fast organisms and fungi were negative.*

disorder is to be distinguished from germ cell tumors, especially seminoma and embryonal carcinoma, and lymphomatous involvement of the testis, all of which may bear a superficial resemblance to granulomatous orchitis.

Malakoplakia

Testicular involvement by malakoplakia has been recorded in approximately 30 patients since the first report by Haukohl and Chinchinian.[163-178] Testicular malakoplakia has been observed most frequently between the ages of 40 years to 69 years (75%), but has been observed from the third to eighth decades. Patients commonly present with the clinical symptoms of acute or chronic epididymo-orchitis, but painless testicular enlargement has been observed. The right testis is involved twice as frequently as the left. Urine cultures may disclose bacteria, most commonly *Escherichia coli*.[176] Minimal or no response to antibiotics raises the concern of neoplasm underlying the enlarged testis.

Gonadal malakoplakia is associated with epididymal involvement in about one third of cases.[174] The involved testis is enlarged and discloses tubular destruction of variable extent on the cut surface. Typically the testicular parenchyma is replaced by a yellow-tan, soft to firm, nodular mass. Focal areas of necrosis or cyst formation may be present in the otherwise solid tissue. The tunica albuginea may be thickened. The epididymis is normal in the majority of cases, but may evidence nodular involvement (refer to discussion of malakoplakia of epididymis in Chap. 7).

The destructive inflammatory lesion is characterized by the microscopic features described in all locations: predominance of histiocytes, with both intra- and extracellular Michaelis – Gutmann bodies. The testicular structural framework of the seminiferous tubules can be surprisingly well preserved in early lesions. Either or both intratubular or interstitial inflammatory infiltrates may be observed. More extensive lesions or lesions of longer duration are associated with greater tubular atrophy and destruction.

The differential diagnosis includes all granulomatous inflammatory disorders of the testis of known or unknown etiology. Malakoplakia is identified by the characteristic cell infiltration and the diagnostic inclusions, Michaelis – Gutmann bodies. (Refer to section on malakoplakia in Chaps. 1 and 4 for further discussion of pathogenesis and ultrastructural studies.)

Cysts

Exclusive of cystic neoplasms, two types of cysts are recognized to originate within the testis. These are the epidermoid cyst and the simple cyst. Both types are rare.

Epidermoid Cysts

Epidermoid cysts resemble the common epidermal inclusion cyst of the skin, and are characterized by a squamous cell lining producing the keratin debris filling the lumen (Fig. 6-16).[179,182,187] There are no associated skin appendages in the

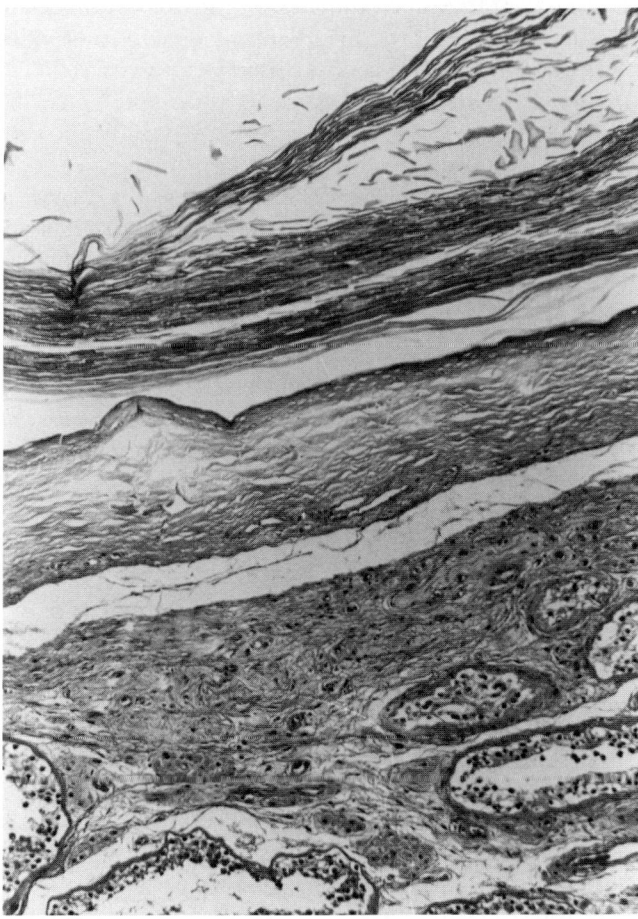

Figure 6-16 *Epidermoid cyst of testis. The squamous cell-lined cyst wall is covered by desquamated keratin debris. Neither skin appendages nor a scar were associated with this intratesticular cyst.*

stroma surrounding the cyst distinguishing it from the mature cystic teratomas ("dermoid" cysts) of germ cell origin. Price further refined the diagnostic criteria by excluding those cysts with an adjacent scar, which could represent a focus of a "burned out" germ cell tumor.[181] This distinction may be artificial, and the difference between epidermoid cyst and cystic teratomas may be only apparent. Some regard the epidermoid cyst as an example of monophasic development of a teratoma.[182,187] However, the histogenesis must be regarded as unsettled with germ cell origin, the current prevailing hypothesis.[180,182]

Epidermoid cysts of the testis were first reported by Dockerty and Priestley.[179] In 1981, Shah and associates reviewed 141 cases reported to 1978, and added three more cases.[187] An additional 10 cases have been reported in the literature.[186,188–190] Patients range in age from the first to the eighth decades, with 85% reported in the second to the fourth decades.[187] Characteristically, cysts produce a painless testicular enlargement, one third of which are detected incidentally during physical examination.[187] These cysts are slightly more common on the right side.[187] Only one case of bilateral epidermoid cysts of the testis has been reported.[183] Recent studies describing ultrasound features of this lesion raise the possibility that future therapy may be more conservative than the standard orchiectomy employed in most cases in the past.[190]

The diagnosis rests on demonstrating a discrete squamous cell-lined cyst within the testis, most commonly apposed to the inside surface of the tunica albuginea. The cut surface has the appearance of a typical epidermal inclusion cyst of the skin, with pasty yellow-white material enclosed within a thin cyst wall. Of those cases reported in the literature, the cyst size varied from 0.5 cm to 10 cm with a mean size of 2 cm.[187] Fibrous stroma surrounds the cyst and separates it from the seminiferous tubules. No skin appendages are present in the stromal tissue, a conclusion that can be made reliably only if the entire cyst is thoroughly examined histologically. Focal calcification has been observed in the cyst wall. The adjacent seminiferous tubules show compression atrophy.

Simple Cyst

A testicular cyst lined by a single layer of flat or low cuboidal epithelium unassociated with other germ cell neoplasm components is termed *simple cyst*.[192] Nine examples could be found in the literature, eight of which are included in the recent review by Takihara and co-workers.[191-194] Affected patients range in age from infants to persons in the ninth decade. The cysts manifest as testicular enlargement with or without pain. Size varies from 1 cm to several centimeters. The cysts have clinically suggested testicular neoplasm, hydrocele, or spermatocele.

On cut surface, a thin-walled unilocular cyst containing clear serous fluid is characteristic within the testis. The smooth cyst lining is covered by flat or cuboidal epithelium. There is no histologic evidence of origin from a teratoma. The adjacent seminiferous tubules are compressed and variably atrophic. Their location within the testis allows distinction of simple cysts from cysts of the tunica albuginea (refer to Chap. 7).

The pathogenesis of these cysts is unknown. The absence of associated inflammation and significant fibrosis suggests they are not the result of prior orchitis. A congenital origin has been suggested.[192] Their clinical significance relates solely to the obligatory clinical distinction of these innocuous cysts from testicular neoplasms.

Finally, cystic dysplasia of the seminiferous tubules has been reported producing a multicystic testis in a 4-year-old boy.[195] This lesion, reported by Leissring and Oppenheimer, represents the only reported example.[195] The pathogenesis of this congenital cystic dilatation of seminiferous tubules is unknown.

Neoplasms

Testicular neoplasms, with important exceptions, are virtually all malignant, and constitute approximately 1% of all cancers in males.[213]

Reflecting the biologic and structural complexity of the male gonad, neoplasms of this organ reflect a diverse spectrum of three major histogenetic categories: germ cell origin; gonadal stromal – sex cord origin; and miscellaneous neoplasms not unique to the gonad (*i.e.,* mesenchymal neoplasms). The current histogenetic views of testicular neoplasms form the basis of the World Health Organization classification presented in Table 6-2.

Neoplasms of germ cell origin constitute more than 90% of all tumors of the male gonad.[212,213,222] The majority of the remaining neoplasms are of stromal – sex cord origin.[212,213,222]

Table 6-2   ***World Health Organization Histologic Classification of Testicular Tumors***

Germ Cell Tumors

Tumors of one histological type

  Seminoma

  Spermatocytic seminoma

  Embryonal carcinoma

  Yolk sac tumor (embryonal carcinoma, infantile type; endodermal sinus tumor)

  Polyembryoma

  Choriocarcinoma

  Teratomas

    Mature

    Immature

    With malignant transformation

Tumors of more than one histological type

  Embryonal carcinoma and teratoma (teratocarcinoma)

  Choriocarcinoma and any other types (specify type)

  Other combinations (specify)

Sex Cord – Stromal Tumors

Well-differentiated forms

  Leydig cell tumor

  Sertoli cell tumor

  Granulosa cell tumor

Mixed forms (specify)

Incompletely differentiated forms

Tumors and Tumor-Like Lesions Containing Both Germ Cell and Sex Cord – Stromal Elements

Gonadoblastoma

Others

Miscellaneous Tumors

Carcinoid

Lymphoid and Hematopoietic Tumors

Secondary Tumors

(Mostofi FK, Sobin LH: Histological typing of testis tumours. In International Histological Classification of Tumours, No. 16. Geneva, World Health Organization, 1977)

Germ Cell Neoplasms

Histogenesis

The germ cell origin of seminomas, questioned only by Masson, has been generally accepted by all others since its original proposal at the beginning of this century.[197] The controversy has centered on the histogenesis of nonseminomatous neoplasms. Competing histogenetic theories included Askanazy's contention that they arose from embryonic totipotential cells that had escaped an organizing influence.[196] Willis accepted this explanation, and the matter remained unsettled until recently.[208] The unsettled state of affairs has been largely clarified as a result of the cumulative experimental work of Stevens, Kleinsmith and Pierce, and Mintz and Illmensee.[200,203,207,219] The occasional observation of extragonadal germ cell tumors, in limited midaxial locations, and the recent studies of intratubular germ cell neoplasms further support the germ cell origin of these neoplasms.[204,205,210,216,247]

As outlined previously, the preponderance of evidence supports the germ cell origin of seminomas, embryonal carcinomas, teratomas, choriocarcinomas, yolk sac tumors, and tumors with combined components. The histogenetic relationship of these neoplasms is currently unsettled. As proposed by Pierce and Abell, neoplastic transformation of a germ cell may give rise either to seminoma (an undifferentiated germ cell neoplasm) or alternatively to embryonal carcinoma (a neoplasm of totipotential cells).[209] Embryonal carcinoma is capable of somatic differentiation (teratoma), or extraembryonic differentiation (yolk sac tumor or choriocarcinoma).[209] Mostofi has recently suggested that all forms of germ cell neoplasms may arise directly from intratubular malignant germ cells.[238] Histologic evidence of direct development of seminoma, yolk sac tumors, and choriocarcinoma within the seminiferous tubules has been recorded.[238]

Metastases of germ cell tumors showing a form of differentiation not present in the primary gonadal tumor is a common observation. The difference may be more apparent than real. The metastases may originate in a small undetected focus of a mixed germ cell tumor that is otherwise uniform in its differentiation. Alternatively, embryonal carcinomas of the testis, capable of differentiating into somatic or extraembryonic structures within the primary site, may retain this capacity in the metastatic site, and thereby result in differentiation divergent from that in the primary tumor. Mostofi suggested that intratubular malignant germ cells serve as a pool of malignant germ cells capable of invading locally, metastasizing, and differentiating along routes completely independent of the manifest differentiation within the clinically apparent testicular primary neoplasm.[238]

Skakkebaek first reported that atypical germ cells within the seminiferous tubules actually represented carcinoma in situ of a testicular germ cell neoplasm.[211] The recognition of in situ malignant changes of germinal epithelium has enormous theoretical and clinical importance. The germ cell origin of nonseminomatous testicular tumors is regarded as established, and does not require additional supportive evidence. The ability of these in situ malignant germ cells to differentiate within the tubule and demonstrate microinvasion has been observed.[239]

The original observation by Skakkebaek involved two infertile men who were reported to develop embryonal carcinomas years after the biopsies that detected the in situ germ cell changes.[211] A similar progression of in situ germ cell changes leading to clinically evident testicular germ cell neoplasms has been recorded in other patients with clinical infertility and previous orchiopexy for cryptorchidism.[215,217,233,239,245,255] Skakkebaek has reported that 50% of 23 patients developed invasive germ cell tumors within 5 years of testicular biopsies that demonstrated carcinoma in situ.[245] Eyben and co-workers reported three patients with germ cell carcinoma in situ associated with microinvasive carcinoma detected prior to clinical evidence of a testicular germ cell neoplasm.[239] In a recent retrospective study by Klein and co-workers, 75% of clinically apparent embryonal carcinomas and 82% of seminomas were accompanied by in situ germ cell changes.[255] The recognition of atypical germ cells with enlarged hyperchromatic nuclei, frequently adjacent to the tubular basement membrane, or alternatively filling the entire tubule, constitute the features of in situ germ cell malignancies.[215,217,233,234,239,245,255] The recognition of in situ malignant changes in testicular biopsies, under the clinical circumstances cited, is obviously of great importance.

Classification

Reflecting the diverse histogenetic views of germ cell neoplasms, various classifications have been proposed. Four are compared in Table 6-3. The classification of Mostofi and Price is based on the classification proposed by Dixon and Moore

Table 6-3   *Histologic Classifications of Testicular Germ Cell Tumors**

Dixon and Moore[199]	Mostofi and Price[213]	British Testicular Tumour Panel[222]	WHO[226]
Seminoma	Seminoma	Seminoma	Seminoma
	Typical	Classic	Typical
	Anaplastic	Spermatocytic	Spermatocytic
	Spermatocytic		
Embryonal	Embryonal carcinoma	Malignant teratoma, undifferentiated (MTU)	Embryonal carcinoma
	Adult		
	Polyembryoma		
Teratoma with embryonal carcinoma ("teratocarcinoma")	Embryonal carcinoma with teratoma ("teratocarcinoma")	Malignant teratoma, intermediate (MTI)	Embryonal carcinoma with teratoma ("teratocarcinoma")
Teratoma, adult	Teratoma	Teratoma, differentiated (MTD)	Teratoma
	Mature		Mature
	Immature		Immature
			With malignant transformation
Choriocarcinoma	Choriocarcinoma	Malignant teratoma, trophoblastic (MTT)	Choriocarcinoma
	Embryonal carcinoma	Yolk sac tumor	Yolk sac tumor
	Infantile		

* This table simplifies the overall comparison of the four classifications. For detailed discussion of comparison of WHO classification and British Testicular Tumor Panel classification, refer to Mostofi.[238]

20 years previously, and in turn influences the WHO classification.[199,213,226] The most significant differences are between these three classifications, and the classification of the British Testicular Tumor Panel, the most recent version of which is presented in Table 6-3.[222] Direct equivalence exists for seminoma, spermatocytic seminoma, mature (or adult) teratoma, differentiated teratoma (MTD), choriocarcinoma (malignant teratoma, trophoblastic), and yolk sac tumor in children (embryonal carcinoma, infantile type; endodermal sinus tumor). Direct comparisons cannot be made between the Mostofi and WHO embryonal carcinomas, teratocarcinomas, and malignant teratomas, and the undifferentiated and intermediate groups of the British classifications.[222] Finally, polyembryoma is not included in the British classification. I urge the adoption of the WHO classification on its merits.

Epidemiology and Etiology

Significant geographic and racial differences in frequency of testicular germ cell tumors are observed. Incidence rates are relatively high in Denmark and the United States, and low in Japan.[251] Incidence rates are 6 to 10 times higher in whites than in blacks, a disparity that is observed in all geographic locations and in all age groups.[227,240] Three peak age groups are observed in infants and children, in young adults in the third and fourth decades, and in men older than 50 years as noted previously.[213,230,252] Genetic influences are suggested in rare cases involving twins or fathers and sons.[220,223,254]

The role of previous trauma and infections (*i.e.,* mumps) is unsettled, but a history of these possible causes is elicited in only 10% of patients.[213]

The role of maldescent of the testis in causing testicular malignancies is unquestioned.[214,235] (Refer to discussion of cryptorchidism.) The risk of developing a germ cell malignancy in an adult with cryptorchid testis has been variously estimated as 20 to 40 times that of the normal male population.[20,214] Javadpour found a 6.5% incidence of cryptorchidism among 1,865 patients with testicular germ cell tumors reported in six previous series.[232] In a similar review Martin found a reported range of 3.5% to 12% with an average of 9.8% incidence of cryptorchidism among 13,089 patients with testicular tumors.[46] The mechanism(s) operative in increasing the risk of neoplastic transformation are unknown. Any future explanation must address the increased frequency of germ cell tumors observed in the normally positioned testis in patients with unilateral cryptorchidism.[214] The effectiveness of orchiopexy performed in young children in reducing the incidence of subsequent germ cell neoplasms is unsettled.[235] Seminomas are the single most frequent germ cell neoplasm arising in cryptorchid testes.[235]

Bilateral testicular germ cell tumors occur with a frequency of 1% to 3%.[218,225] This is equivalent to a 500 times greater risk of developing a second germ cell neoplasm than the risk of developing the first tumor.[225]

The ultimate explanation for this frequency is currently unknown, but undoubtedly is related to the unidentified causal factors producing the first malignancy continuing to influence the contralateral gonad germ cell population. Most commonly the bilateral tumors are asynchronous, with 50% detected within 5 years of diagnosis of the first germ cell neoplasm.[231] Prolonged follow up is required, because 3% of the second asynchronous tumors are detected after an interval of 20 years.[231] All histologic types have been observed in the recorded bilateral tumors; however, the overwhelming number (91%) involve seminomas in one or both of the involved testes.[231]

Clinical Features

Patients with germ cell neoplasms present with testicular swelling, pain, or symptoms of metastases, or any combination of these features. Symptoms of metastases are most common in patients who have testicular choriocarcinomas. At the initial presentation, metastases from seminomas and embryonal carcinomas are present in 10% to 33% of patients.[213] Metastases at initial presentation are uncommon with teratoma, yolk sac tumor, and spermatocytic seminoma.[213]

All testicular germ cell tumors exhibit age predilections (with considerable overlap). Yolk sac tumors and teratomas are most common in the first decade, choriocarcinomas in the second and third decades, embryonal carcinoma in the third decade, seminoma in the fourth decade, and spermatocytic seminoma in the fifth decade.

The relatively recent introduction of tumor marker assays into the clinical management of testicular germ cell neoplasms involves two tumor products detectable in the serum, namely, human chorionic gonadotropin (HCG) and alpha-fetoprotein (AFP).

The elevations of serum HCG typically found in patients with choriocarcinoma are also observed occasionally in patients with embryonal carcinoma or seminoma.[243] Kurman and co-workers reported that 92% of patients with elevated serum HCG demonstrated positive staining for it in sections of their tumors as demonstrated by the immunoperoxidase technique.[228] More recently, a direct correlation was found between tumor tissue concentration of HCG and immunoperoxidase staining for HCG in testicular neoplasms.[253] The HCG is localized exclusively in the syncytiotrophoblasts. The multinucleated giant cells in seminomas and embryonal carcinomas, which stain positively for HCG, are identified unequivocally as syncytiotrophoblasts. This explains why some patients with these nonchoriocarcinomatous neoplasms demonstrate serum elevations of HCG.[228,253]

Alpha-fetoprotein is usually synthesized by the yolk sac and the liver only during embryologic development.[229] During this time AFP is present in the serum. Following birth the synthesis of this glycoprotein ceases, and serum levels fall to virtually undetectable levels during the first year of life.[229] The reemergence of AFP of neoplastic origin was first observed associated with hepatomas, and subsequently elevated serum AFP associated with testicular germ cell tumors was reported by Abelev and co-workers.[206] Later, the association of elevated AFP and yolk sac tumors of the testis (and ovary) was established.[228,236,316,320] Further studies have demonstrated a correlation of AFP concentrations in tumor tissue and serum, and the frequency of positive immunoperoxidase staining for this substance in microscopic sections of tumors.[228,242,253] Although characteristic of yolk sac tumors, AFP was found not to be specific for them, because serum elevations are observed in a low percentage of seminomas and embryonal carcinomas.[228,237] Possible explanations for these findings include undetected foci of yolk sac tumor within the primary testicular neoplasm, or yolk sac differentiation in metastatic sites.[237,248] Elevations of either AFP or HCG or both are found in 86% to 94% of nonseminomatous tumors; therefore, they serve as useful markers of possible tumor recurrence.[243]

Currently, utilizing tumor markers in the management of germ cell malignancies frequently raises as many questions as it answers. Serial determination of these tumor markers is undoubtedly of great assistance in accurate staging and early detection of tumor recurrence. However, determination of the true frequency of false-positive and false-negative assay results is required for the development of reliable markers to monitor seminomas.[241,244]

Natural History

The extent of tumor spread has been described in numerous proposed staging protocols. An example currently used at the National Cancer Institute is outlined in Table 6-4.[249] The more elaborate TNM staging protocol for testicular cancer is reproduced in Table 6-5.[250]

With the exception of choriocarcinoma, testicular germ cell neoplasms disseminate primarily by metastatic spread to regional lymph nodes (iliac and para-aortic) and thence to the lungs by the thoracic duct (Fig. 6-17).[213] Choriocarcinoma disseminates primarily by hematogenous routes to the lung.

The distribution pattern of testicular germ cell tumor metastases, with two exceptions, shows no significant features attributable to specific tumors.[199,213,221,246] In order of decreasing frequency, the retroperitoneal lymph nodes, lungs, liver, and mediastinal lymph nodes are most commonly involved by metastases.[199,213,221,246] The two exceptions relate to the propensity of seminomas to metastasize to bone, and the greater frequency of brain metastases demonstrated by choriocarcinoma observed in some studies.[221,246] Independent of histologic type of germ cell tumor, bone metastases most frequently involve the vertebral column.[221]

The majority of tumor recurrences manifest as distant metastases in the first 2 years following initial surgical therapy.[198] Decreasing numbers of patients recur in each subsequent year, with recurrence after 5 years uncommon. Anecdotal examples of recurrences after 10 years are observed, but are distinctly rare.

Finally, the metastases of germ cell malignancies may demonstrate histologic features divergent from that of the testicular primary tumor. The frequency of this phenomenon is unique to each specific germ cell malignancy. Seminomas manifest nonseminomatous metastases in 26% to 44% of cases.[199,213,221,224,246] Embryonal carcinoma and choriocarcinoma are the most frequent nonseminomatous components observed in metastatic sites.[199,213,221,224,246] Similarly, embryonal carcinomas and choriocarcinomas demonstrate histologically divergent metastases in 17% to 31% of cases.[199,213,221,224,246] Teratocarcinomas (embryonal carcinoma plus teratoma) primary in the testis commonly gives origin to metastases that are exclusively embryonal carcinoma, but other patterns are also observed.[199,213,221,224,246] The emergence of histologically different metastases has obvious significant therapeutic implications.

Seminoma

Testicular seminomas are malignancies of undifferentiated germ cells. Ninety percent of seminomas are of the "typical" or classic variety, with the remaining represented by variants including the spermatocytic seminoma, the anaplastic seminoma, and a recently described seminoma with syncytiotrophoblastic giant

Table 6-4   **_Clinical Staging of Testicular Cancer_**

Stage I	**_Local Spread_**
A	Confined to testis
B	Involves testicular adnexa
C	Involves scrotal wall
Stage II	**_Confined to Retroperitoneal Lymphatics_**
A	Microscopic
B	Gross involvement without capsular invasion
C	Gross involvement with capsular invasion
D	Massive involvement of retroperitoneum
Stage III	
A	Solitary metastasis
B	Multiple metastases

(Javadpour N: Natural history, diagnosis, and staging of nonseminomatous testicular cancer. In Javadpour N (ed): Principles and Management of Urologic Cancer, 2nd ed, p 293. Baltimore, Williams & Wilkins, 1983)

Table 6-5   **_TNM Classification of Testicular Tumors_**

Primary Tumor (T)

TX	Minimum requirements cannot be met (no orchiectomy)
T0	No evidence of primary tumor
T1	Limited to body of testis
T2	Extension beyond tunica albuginea
T3	Involvement of rete testis or epididymis
T4a	Invasion of spermatic cord
T4b	Invasion of scrotal wall

Nodal Involvement (N)

NX	Minimum requirements to assess metastases cannot be met
N0	No evidence of regional lymph node metastases
N1	Involvement of single ipsilateral lymph node
N2	Involvement of contralateral, or bilateral, or multiple regional lymph node
N3	Palpable abdominal mass present or fixed inguinal node

Distant Metastases (M)

MX	Minimum requirements to assess distant metastases cannot be met
M0	No (known) distant metastases
M1	Distant metastases present

Postsurgical Treatment Residual Tumor (R)

R0	No residual tumor
R1	Microscopic residual tumor
R2	Macroscopic residual tumor

(American Joint Committee on Cancer: Manual for Staging of Cancer, 2nd ed, p 166. Philadelphia, JB Lippincott, 1983)

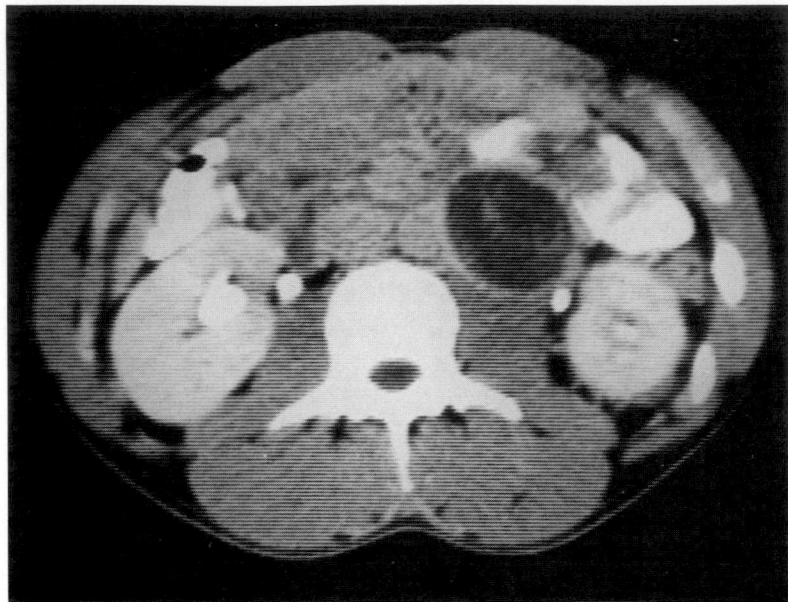

A

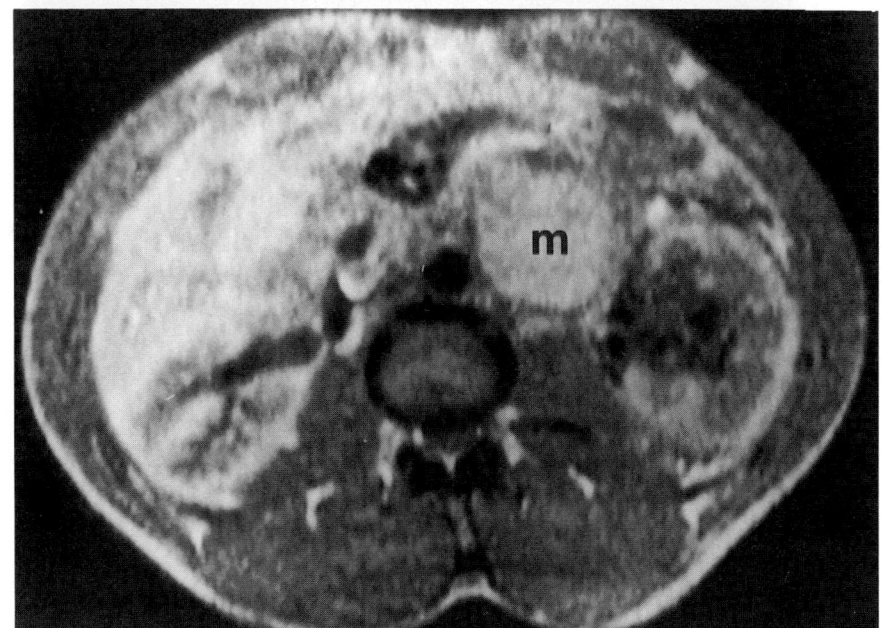

B

Figure 6-17   ***Seminoma metastatic to retroperitoneum.*** *(A) Contrast-enhanced CT scan at the level of the kidneys disclosed a mass in the left para-aortic region. (B) MRI scan using spin echo technique with TE 28/msec and TR 500/msec reveal the mass (m) as a relatively high signal density.*

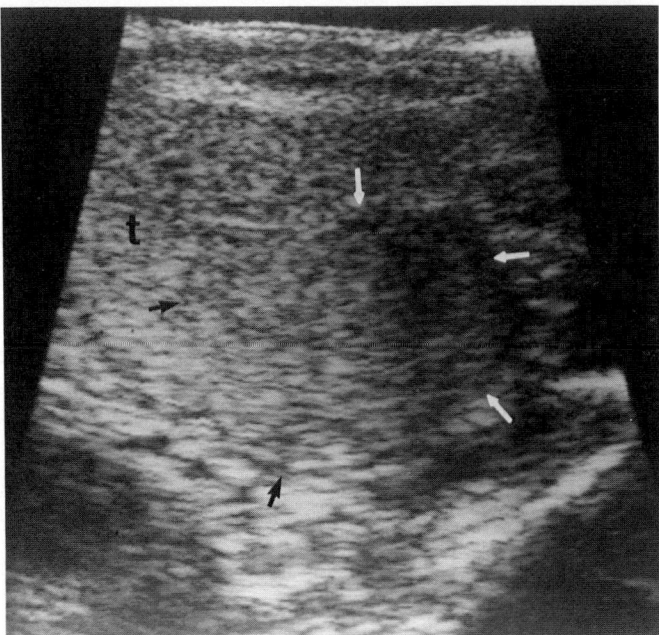

Figure 6-18   *Seminoma. High-resolution realtime ultrasound of superior left testis disclosed a 1.9-cm poorly defined mass (arrows). Much of the mass had an echo texture comparable to the normal testicular parenchyma (t). The neoplasm could not be detected by palpation.*

cells.[260,262] As a group, they comprise approximately 40% to 50% of testicular germ cell tumors.[199,252,256,258] The mean age of patients is reported as 35 years to 42 years, generally older than patients with embryonal carcinoma and choriocarcinoma. Patients present with testicular swelling, or very uncommonly, symptoms of metastases (Fig. 6-18).[213,256,259] Seminomas are the most frequent testicular germ cell neoplasms encountered in patients with bilateral germ cell neoplasms, and germ cell neoplasms complicating cryptorchidism in the adult.[231,235]

Pathologic Features

The testis is enlarged and firm, and the external configuration is usually distorted by the tumor nodule. On cut surface the typical seminoma is homogeneous white-gray, well demarcated, and tends to bulge above the adjacent uninvolved compressed testis (Fig. 6-19). The consistency varies (within the same tumor and from case to case) from soft to firm, attributable to the amount of fibrous stroma within the neoplasm. Areas of necrosis with associated hemorrhage are usually observed only in the larger examples of this neoplasm. The tunica albuginea usually is distorted but structurally intact. Local invasion, if present, is most commonly observed at the testicular mediastinum where it may be contiguous with epididymal invasion. In my experience, this is most commonly detected only at microscopic review of sections of these structures.

The histologic pattern of the typical seminoma is characterized by sheets, nests, or cords of relatively uniform tumor cells proliferating between segregat-

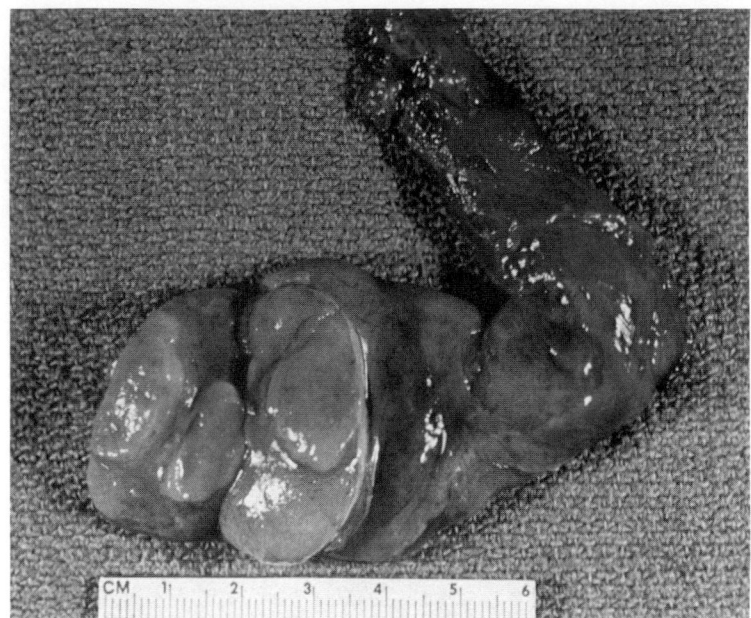

Figure 6-19   ***Classic seminoma.*** *The cut surface shows the solid tumor confined within the testis. Hemorrhage and necrosis of the tumor are not conspicuous.*

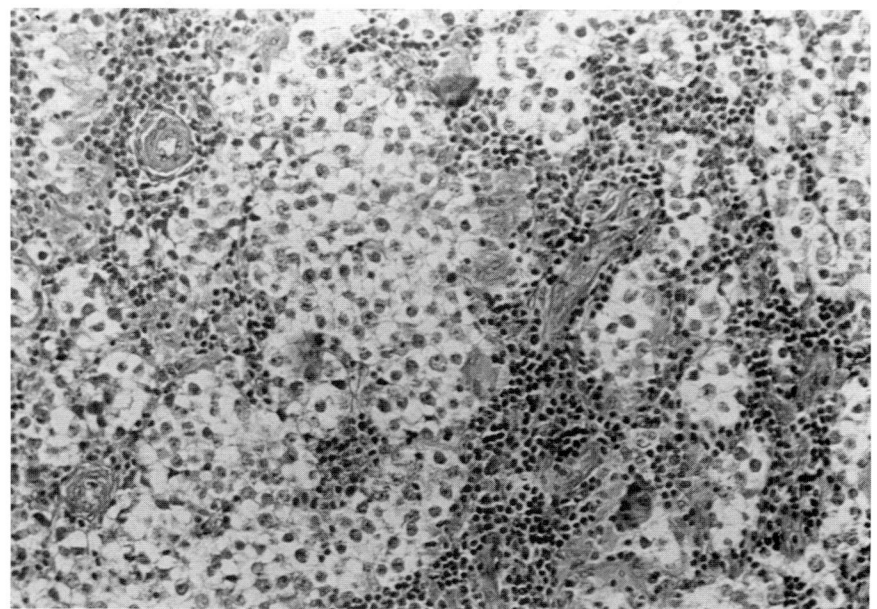

Figure 6-20   ***Classic seminoma.*** *The seminoma cells are present in nests confined by fibrous septae containing numerous lymphocytes.*

ing fibrous trabeculae (Fig. 6-20). Papillary, cystic, tubular, and acinar patterns are not observed in seminomas, and their presence suggests the admixture of other malignant germ cell components. The trabeculae vary in width from area to area, ranging from delicate and thin, to broad irregular fibrous bands containing blood vessels and characteristically a lymphocytic infiltrate. The neoplastic cells infiltrate the interstitium between compressed seminiferous tubules at the advancing margin. Intratubular (in situ) tumor cells may be observed within the intact seminiferous tubules.

The cytologic features of seminomas, indeed, of all testicular germ cell neoplasms, are best demonstrated following fixation in Bouin's fluid, which does not produce the shrinkage artifact resulting from formalin fixation. The typical seminoma is characterized by relatively uniform cells with an enlarged, round to polyhedral nucleus surrounded by clear cytoplasm, and a distinct cell membrane (Fig. 6-21). The hyperchromatic nucleus contains coarse chromatin and one or two prominent nucleoli. Infrequent variations on these typical characteristics include indistinct cell borders, light uniform eosinophilic-staining cytoplasm, and small oval nuclei. These variant features are most frequently focal, and adequate sectioning of the tumor will invariably disclose the areas of more typical morphology, thereby clarifying the true nature of the neoplasm. Mitoses are common, but vary from area to area within the tumor. Seminomas with more than three mitoses per high-power field, which are commonly associated with greater cytologic pleomorphism, have been termed *anaplastic seminomas*.[282-287] (Refer to discussion of anaplastic seminoma.)

The PAS stain demonstrates intracytoplasmic glycogen, a characteristic helpful in identifying metastatic seminoma.[263] Spermatocytic seminomas have little or no cytoplasmic glycogen, and therefore are PAS-negative, a histologic feature aiding in their distinction from classic seminoma (refer to discussion of

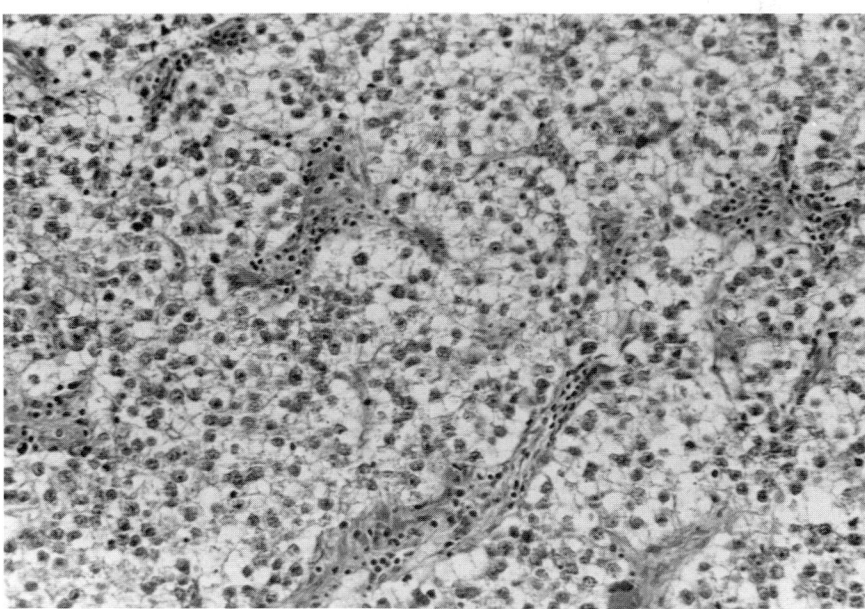

Figure 6-21   *Classic seminoma. The cell borders of the seminoma cells are well defined, and the cytoplasm is clear. The nuclei show minimal variation of size and shape.*

spermatocytic seminoma). Beckstead has recently reported the value of alkaline phosphatase staining in testicular germ cell neoplasms.[264] Additional histologic features in seminomas include focal areas of necrosis (55%), lymphoid aggregates and follicles scattered focally accentuating the lymphocytic infiltrate, and scattered tuberculoid granulomas within the interstitium, on occasion with Langhan's type giant cells (40% of cases).[213,256,259,261] These giant cells are to be differentiated from syncytiotrophoblastic giant cells, which occasionally are observed in seminoma and are associated with a more aggressive clinical behavior.[260,262] The identification of syncytiotrophoblastic giant cells can be readily accomplished by immunoperoxidase staining for HCG.[228,253] With the exception of the syncytiotrophoblastic giant cells noted above, the presence and extent of necrosis, fibrosis, granulomatous reaction, and lymphocytic infiltration have no prognostic significance.[259] Intratesticular venous invasion was reported in 20% to 50% of seminomas, and lymphatic invasion in 60% to 77% of seminomas. However, they were found by Johnson and co-workers to be of no prognostic significance.[256,259]

Ultrastructural characteristics of seminoma cells reflect their primitive nature. The cell membrane is well developed but intercellular connections are rudimentary or absent. Only sparse organelles are found in the cytoplasm, including mitochondria and smooth endoplasmic reticulum. The nucleus is irregular with dispersed chromatin and prominent nucleoli, frequently with irregular contour.[257]

The diagnosis of typical seminoma requires distinguishing it from the anaplastic and spermatocytic variants, lymphomatous involvement of the testis, and examples of granulomatous orchitis. (Refer to corresponding discussions in this chapter.) Distinguishing embryonal carcinoma cells from seminoma cells in poorly fixed specimens can be a diagnostic challenge.

Anaplastic Seminoma

The practice of subclassifying seminomas at the Walter Reed General Hospital was reported in a series of papers published in 1968.[282,283] In addition to the classic seminoma and the spermatocytic variant, a third type, the anaplastic variant, was described. This variant constituted 4.4% of a series of 277 seminomas, but accounted for 6 of the 15, or 40%, of the deaths from all histologic types of seminomas in the study.[282] Although the overall survival rate of this histologic variant was lower than recorded for the classic seminoma cases (74% versus 86% absolute 5-year survival), these differences disappeared when the survival of patients of equivalent stage was compared.[283] A higher percentage of classic seminomas were confined to the testis (stage I) than was observed among the anaplastic seminomas (83% versus 65%), which undoubtedly contributed to the lower overall survival rate of the anaplastic seminomas.[282] Subsequently, two additional studies concluded that the prognosis of classic and anaplastic seminoma was similar when patients of equivalent stages were evaluated.[284,287] Kademian and co-workers, reporting on eight cases of anaplastic seminomas, concluded this variant was more aggressive, even when patients were compared by stage.[285] Others provided only information referable to overall prognosis, which consistently showed a lower survival rate associated with anaplastic seminoma.[256,284] The matter remains unsettled.[238] Anaplastic seminoma is currently

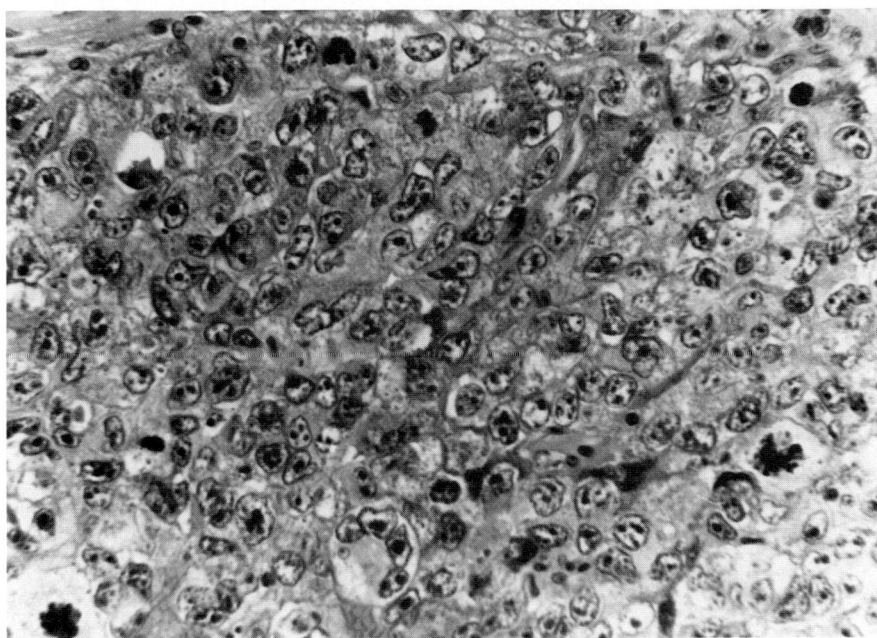

Figure 6-22   *Anaplastic seminoma. Numerous mitoses are associated with anaplastic nuclear features of the tumor cells.*

not a recognized variant in the WHO classification of testicular tumors (see Table 6-3).

The clinical and gross features of anaplastic seminoma are not significantly different from those of classic seminoma.[284] The diagnosis rests on the microscopic findings of pervasive nuclear enlargement and pleomorphism, prominent nucleoli, and three or more mitoses per high power field (Fig. 6-22).[213] The lymphocytic infiltrate is less than observed in classic seminoma, and in some cases, is virtually absent. Granulomas are similarly inconspicuous in anaplastic seminomas. The ultrastructural features of anaplastic seminoma are identical to the classic seminoma tumor cells.[286]

With the exception of an apparent tendency to disseminate earlier in a higher percentage of patients, metastases show temporal and distribution similarities to classic seminoma.[284] Although the histologic criteria noted above allow a diagnosis of anaplastic seminoma, the clinical significance of this entity remains to be clarified.

Spermatocytic Seminoma

Spermatocytic seminomas are germ cell neoplasms unique to the testis. Since the original description of *le seminome spermatocytaire,* or spermatocytic seminoma, by Masson in 1946, a total of 75 cases have been reported, all arising within the testis.[265–281] No examples of this germ cell neoplasm arising in the ovary or in extragonadal sites could be found in the literature. Fewer than 10 spermatocytic seminomas have been reported in men younger than 40 years of age; the majority have been diagnosed in men older than 50 years of age.[267,274] The frequency of bilaterality has been cited as 6%, significantly higher than observed in typical seminomas (2%).[256,271,274,281] Patients most commonly present with painless testicular enlargement. Of great importance is the nonaggressive clinical behavior observed, with only 3 confirmed examples giving origin to distant metastases among the 75 reported cases.[265,280]

Pathologic Features

Compared with typical seminoma, the contrasting clinical features of spermatocytic seminoma are accompanied by equally contrasting pathologic features. Typically, the spermatocytic seminoma is poorly demarcated, soft, yellow-gray, and gelatinous. Microcystic areas are common. Extensive hemorrhage and necrosis are not observed.

Three cell populations, based on size, are observed microscopically, with intermediate cells (10 μm to 20 μm) predominating.[265,267,274,281] Fewer numbers of cells, both larger and smaller, make up the heterogenous neoplasm. Histologic pattern is apparent with cells dispersed in sheets, randomly punctuated by microcysts. The prominent fibrous trabeculae stroma of typical seminomas is not present. In addition, the lymphocytic infiltrate, granulomas, and PAS-positive clear cytoplasm of the tumor cells, which are all characteristic of typical seminomas, are absent in spermatocytic seminomas.[267,274,277,281] Although the nuclei vary in size as noted previously, they exhibit a uniform round configuration (Figs. 6-23, 6-24).[265,267,274] The predominating intermediate-sized cells have eosinophilic cytoplasm. The centrally placed nuclei contain an evenly dispersed

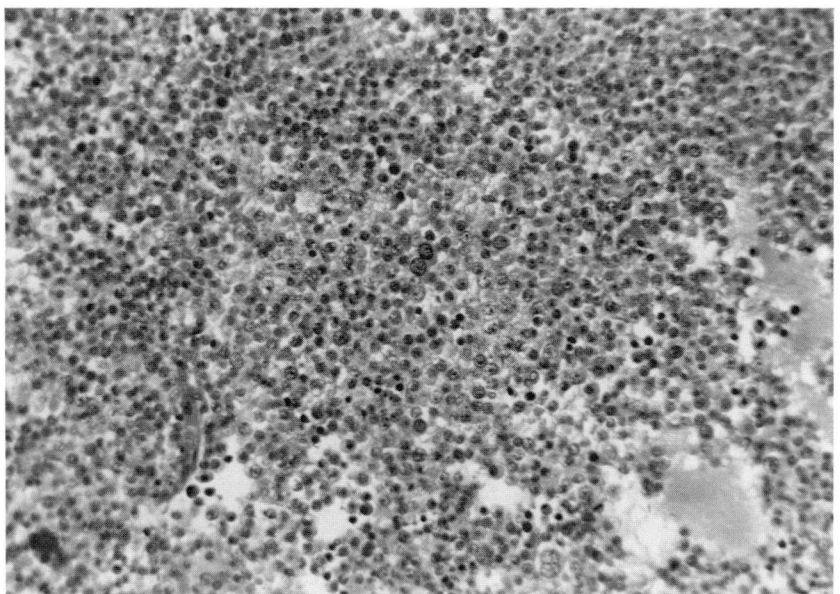

Figure 6-23   *Spermatocytic seminoma. Scattered giant tumor cells are present in this seminoma. The nuclei are uniformly round, but vary in size. The cytoplasm stains lightly eosinophilic. No fibrous septa or lymphocytes are present. Only rare mitoses were present in this tumor.*

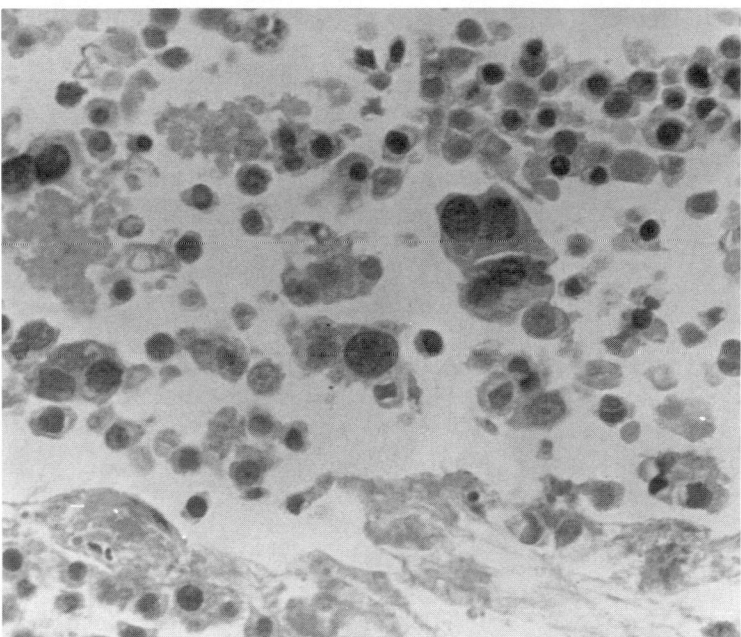

Figure 6-24 **Spermatocytic seminoma.** *Scattered giant tumor cells are present* (center).

granular chromatin, some of which is adjacent to the nuclear membrane, giving this structure an uneven thickness around its circumference. These chromatin features are accentuated in the nuclei of the large cells with the addition of filamentous clumps of chromatin, characterized in the original description by Masson as spirene-like.[265] In contrast, the smallest cells in the tumor have uniformly hyperchromatic nuclei and minimal associated cytoplasm. Finally, in contrast to typical seminomas, the cell borders of the tumor cells of spermatic seminomas are generally poorly delineated. The overall appearance is that of a cohesive syncytium of tumor cells. Mitoses are present, but rarely exceed two per occasional high-power fields.

Ultrastructural features of spermatocytic seminomas have been studied by Rosai and co-workers, who observed prominent nucleoli, well-developed Golgi apparatus, and well-developed intercellular junctions including bridges, the last feature not found in typical seminomas.[275]

The documented histologic features of spermatocytic seminoma allow distinguishing this neoplasm from the more common typical seminoma, and equally uncommon but contrastingly aggressive anaplastic seminoma.

Embryonal Carcinoma

Embryonal carcinoma is a germ cell tumor composed of cytologically primitive epithelial cells, characteristically proliferating in varied acinar, tubular, papillary, or solid histologic patterns. These neoplasms compose the second most frequent type of testicular germ cell tumor, constituting 15% to 35% of this group.[213,253,261]

The term *embryonal carcinoma* as defined by the WHO Classification, refers to the tumor Mostofi and Price called *embryonal carcinoma, adult type,* and some tumors that the British Testicular Tumor Panel classified as *malignant teratoma, undifferentiated type (MTU).*[213,226,296]

Yolk sac tumors, now frequently called embryonal carcinoma (formerly called embryonal carcinoma of infancy), are excluded from the tumors currently called embryonal carcinoma. (Refer to discussion of yolk sac tumor.)

The neoplasms occur most frequently in the third decade, but have been observed from the second to eighth decades.[213,253,289] Mostofi states categorically that they are not found in infants and children.[238] Patients typically present with testicular swelling (Fig. 6-25). Approximately one third of patients present with metastases, indicative of the aggressiveness of this neoplasm.[213] Either AFP or HCG, or both, may be elevated in embryonal carcinoma.[228,243,253] In such cases, foci of yolk sac tumor or syncytiotrophoblasts are present.[228] The frequency of these admixed components is currently a matter of investigation, but preliminary evidence suggests that it is significantly higher than previously appreciated.[318,320,328]

Metastases from embryonal carcinoma show both hematogenous and lymphatic dissemination with periaortic lymph nodes, lung, and liver most frequently involved.[213] The histologic composition of the metastases from testicular embryonal carcinoma show seminomatous, choriocarcinomatous, or teratomatous differentiation in 4% to 8% of cases.[199,213] Prognosis is related most closely to tumor stage at presentation.[288] Recent significant advances in effective chemotherapy have been reported.[290]

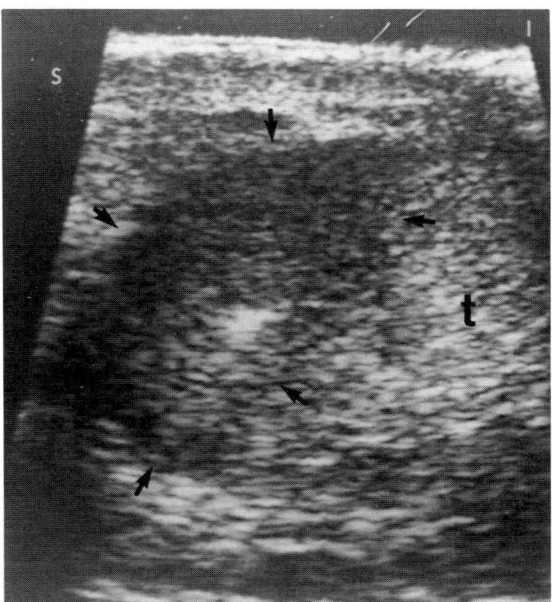

Figure 6-25   *Embryonal carcinoma.* Longitudinal high-resolution realtime ultrasound of the right testicle revealed a hypoechoic mass (arrows) with an area of increased echoes (center). The mass contains fewer echoes than normal parenchyma (t; S, superior; I, inferior).

Pathologic Features

Embryonal carcinomas generally become clinically evident before attaining large size. This is attributable to either metastases or testicular pain. A frequent, if not characteristic, feature of testicular embryonal carcinomas is variably extensive necrosis and hemorrhage, which most probably contribute to the scrotal discomfort. The cut surface discloses a gray-white, bulging, poorly demarcated mass with variably extensive hemorrhage. Extensive invasion of the tunica albuginea and the adjacent epididymis is evident in approximately 20% of cases.[213]

Microscopically, the tumor has a characteristically varied histologic pattern of glands, tubules, microacini, and papillary and solid patterns that assist in differentiating embryonal carcinoma from seminoma. The cells are equally pleomorphic in their features. Ill-defined cell borders, prominent nucleoli, coarse chromatin, and distinct nuclear membranes are most characteristic (Fig. 6-26). Focal or extensive hemorrhage and necrosis and frequent mitoses are likewise characteristic. Variations on these features include occasional multinucleated tumor giant cells, syncytiotrophoblasts (identifiable with immunoperoxidase staining for HCG), and foci demonstrating yolk sac tumor features (Fig. 6-27). The stroma of the tumor is variably edematous or densely fibrous, features that undoubtedly result in part from hemorrhage within the tumor. The ultrastructural features of embryonal carcinoma seen on light microscopy reflect the primitive morphology characteristic of these cells.[213,257] Contrasting with the typically indistinct cell membranes of these tumor cells by light microscopy, electron microscopy reveals well-defined cell membrane.[213,257]

Embryonal carcinoma must be distinguished from seminoma, yolk sac

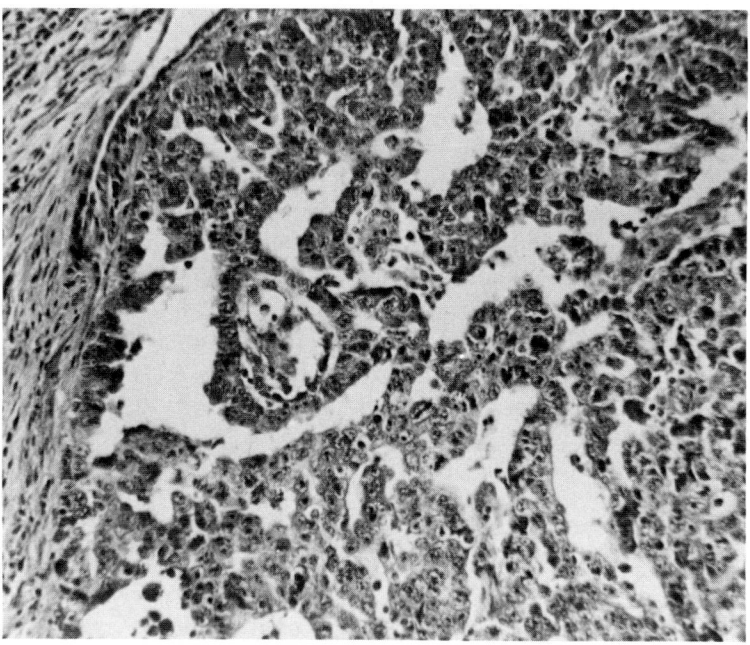

Figure 6-26 *Embryonal carcinoma. A cystic space is lined and almost filled with carcinoma cells without distinct cell membranes. The nuclei are hyperchromatic with prominent nucleoli and lightly eosinophilic cytoplasm.*

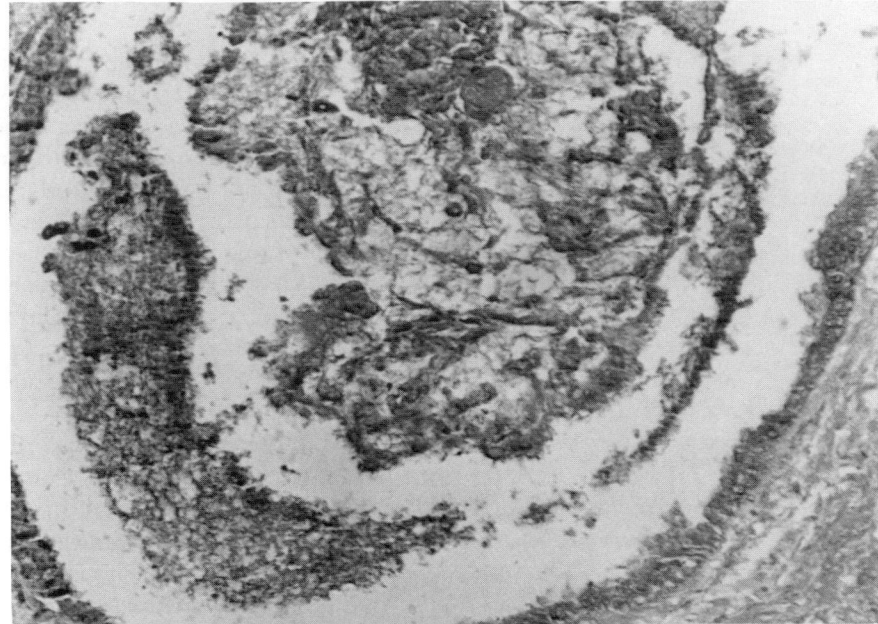

Figure 6-27   *Embryonal carcinoma stained for alpha fetoprotein by immunoperoxidase technique.*

tumor, and lymphomatous involvement of the testis (refer to respective discussions). However, the possible presence of other germ cell components (*i.e.,* seminoma, choriocarcinoma, or yolk sac tumor) in an otherwise predominantly embryonal carcinoma must not be overlooked.

Polyembryoma

The term *polyembryoma* refers to a gonadal neoplasm histologically characterized by innumerable structures called *embryoid bodies*.[213] Such neoplasms are apparently rare.[213] Only one example could be found in the American literature. Simard reported a polyembryonic embryoma arising in an ovary.[292] The significance of this neoplasm in the context of testicular tumors is the occasional finding of an embryoid body, which is the characteristic feature of polyembryomas, in testicular embryonal carcinomas and teratomas. Only when the preponderance of a neoplasm is composed of embryoid bodies is it to be regarded as a polyembryoma.[213]

The embryoid body resembles an embryo of 1 week to 2 weeks gestation with an embryonic disk inserted between a larger cavity lined by flattened cells (recapitulating the amniotic cavity) and a smaller cavity lined by cells suggesting endodermal origin.[213,292] Evans thoroughly studied the histologic variants of these structures.[291] Whether in a polyembryoma, or focally in an embryonal carcinoma or teratoma, the embryoid body's structural features are similar and distinctive.

Teratoma

Testicular teratomas are germ cell neoplasms characterized by tissues from all three germ layers, including ectoderm, endoderm, and mesoderm, assembled in either a disorganized or organoid pattern.[213,238] Three histologic subtypes of testicular teratomas are recognized in the WHO classification: mature, immature, and teratomas with malignant transformation.[226] Immaturity refers to the differentiation of the organoid components in the teratoma, whereas malignant transformation identifies malignant components such as squamous cell carcinoma or sarcoma.[213,226] Their germ cell origin was not universally accepted in the past, with origin from totipotential cells that had escaped the influence of organizers as one suggested alternative.[208] However, the cumulative weight of experimental evidence and clinical observations are overwhelmingly in favor of germ cell origin, which can no longer be doubted. (Refer to discussion of histogenesis.)

The natural history of testicular teratoma relates more closely to the patient's age than to any other factor, including the anticipated clinical behavior implicit in the name (*teratoma* suggests a benign germ cell neoplasm), and the degree or extent of maturity or differentiation of the tissues composing the tumor. Specifically, mature teratomas without any histologic evidence of immaturity or malignant transformation must never be regarded as necessarily benign in adult patients.[238,296] Their clinical behavior is completely unpredictable, with examples metastasizing as teratocarcinoma or choriocarcinoma.[199,213] Two cases of mature teratomas showing only mature teratoma in the metastases in young adult patients have been reported.[295,301] At the other extreme, mature teratomas, including examples with foci of immaturity, arising in infants and children are apparently uniformly benign.[298,300,303] Fraley and Ketcham reviewed the reported testicular teratomas, and were unable to find a single case of testicular teratoma that demonstrated metastases arising in a child.[298] The observation remains without exception to this date.[299,300,302]

Teratomas — mature, immature, and those with malignant transformation — are to be differentiated from teratocarcinoma, a mixed germ cell tumor composed of teratomatous elements admixed with embryonal carcinoma (refer to discussion of mixed germ cell tumors). Teratocarcinomas are uniformly malignant neoplasms that give rise to embryonal carcinoma or teratomatous or teratocarcinomatous metastases.

Rare examples of nonteratomatous germ cell tumors give origin to mature teratomatous metastases with an associated dramatic increase in survival rates.[302] The cause of this apparent maturation of a malignant neoplasm in metastatic sites is unknown.[302] Similar examples have been observed in ovarian germ cell neoplasms and neoplasms arising in the adrenal medulla.

Testicular teratomas compose 4% to 9% of testicular tumors. Most are diagnosed in the first three decades, but some have been observed in older patients. In children, they are exceeded in frequency only by yolk sac tumors (refer to discussion of yolk sac tumors).

Pathologic Features

Testicular teratomas are typically multicystic and solid neoplasms enlarging the testis in a nodular configuration. On cut surface the cysts contain mucinous material. Solid areas may reveal cartilaginous foci, or less frequently, bone formation. Hemorrhage and necrosis may be present focally but are not typical. As in all testicular neoplasms, all areas of hemorrhage are to be examined extensively to exclude underlying choriocarcinoma.

The classification of a testicular teratoma is based on the histologic features of the tumor. Those examples exclusively composed of well-differentiated tissues (representing epidermis, gastrointestinal or respiratory mucosa, thyroid, and

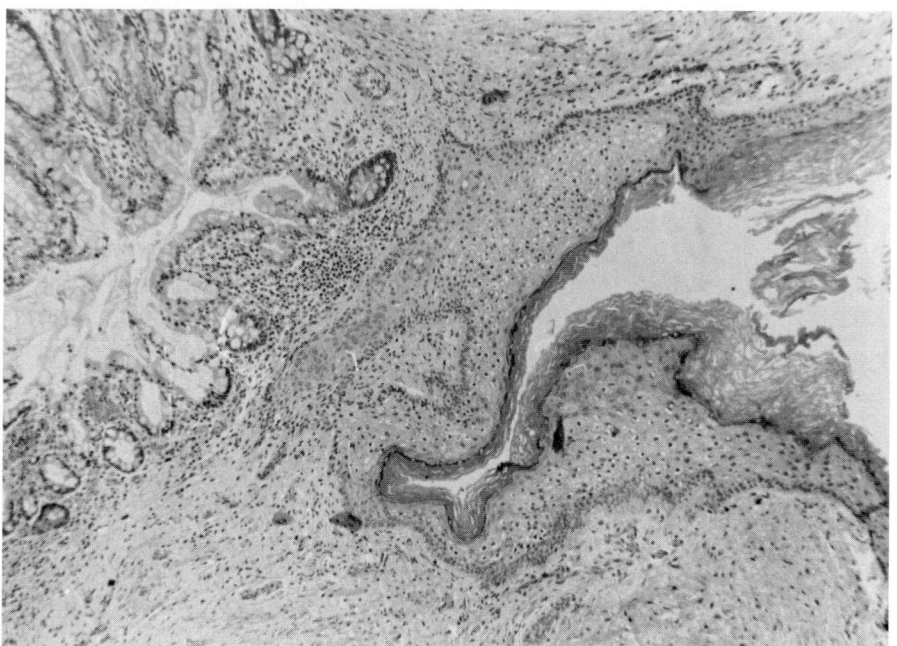

Figure 6-28   *Teratoma. A cyst lined by well-differentiated squamous epithelium is in proximity to a focus of endodermal glands with colonic features.*

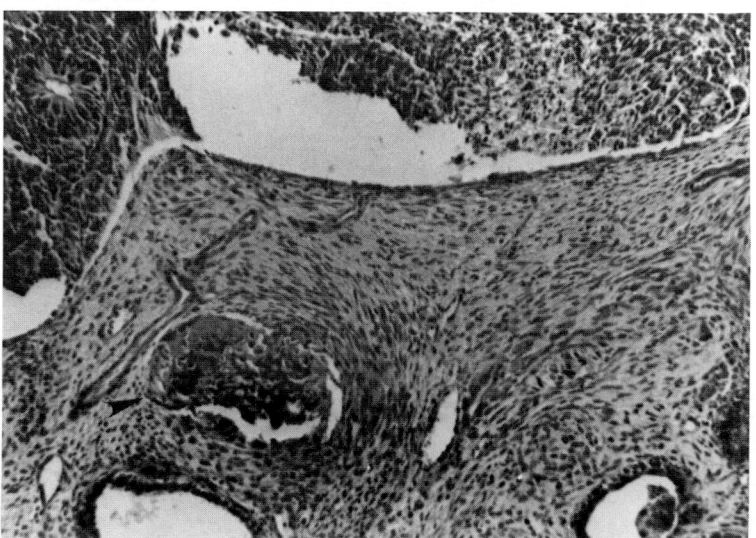

Figure 6-29   *Immature teratoma. Immature neural tissue* (upper left) *and primitive osteoid* (arrow) *are present in the immature stroma of this teratoma.*

pancreatic) or a variety of other organoid structures are termed *mature teratomas* (Figs. 6-28, 6-29). Immature teratomas in pure form are extremely rare, and most commonly are represented by an admixture of mature and immature tissue of neuroectodermal, endodermal, and mesodermal nature. Foci of seminoma, embryonal carcinoma, choriocarcinoma, or yolk sac tumor are not immature forms as such, but represent malignant germ cell components producing a *mixed germ cell tumor* or as classified by the WHO, *tumors of more than one histologic type.*[226] The individual neoplastic components should be stated in the formal diagnosis of such germ cell tumors. The term *teratocarcinoma* is reserved exclusively for those tumors composed of admixed teratomatous and embryonal carcinomatous components (refer to discussion of teratocarcinoma).

Yolk Sac Tumor (Endodermal Sinus Tumor)

Yolk sac tumor is a malignant germ cell neoplasm demonstrating extraembryonic yolk sac differentiation. It has been reported to originate in the ovary, testis, liver, and midline extragonadal retroperitoneal and mediastinal sites.[309,321] Most yolk sac tumors occur in infants and young children, in whom they represent the single most common testicular neoplasm.[213,238] Yolk sac tumors, recapitulating the gene expression of the embryonic mammalian yolk sac, synthesize the α_1-globulin, alpha-fetoprotein.[206,316] AFP is detectable in the serum of patients with yolk sac tumors, providing a tumor marker aiding in the initial diagnosis and postsurgical detection of possible recurrences.[206,316]

Few gonadal neoplasms have traversed such a protracted "gestation" prior to general recognition and acceptance as a nosologic entity. The original description of the yolk sac tumor or endodermal sinus tumor was reported by Teilum.[306] He discovered that the neoplasms reported as *mesonephroma ovarii* by Schiller 20 years previously in reality were a collection of two separate entities.[304,306] Schiller had combined the neoplasm currently known as clear cell carcinoma (or mesonephric carcinoma), and the yolk sac, or endodermal sinus tumor, a germ cell neoplasm that Teilum later described as recapitulating the structure of the rat placenta. Teilum reported examples of this yolk sac tumor in an ovary of a 35-year-old woman and the testis of a 30-year-old man.[306]

For purposes of this historical review, the study of germ cell tumors in the testis of infants can be dated to begin in the 1950s with the publication of a series reported by Magner and co-workers.[305] The pathologic features were sufficiently distinctive that they regarded the neoplasm as unique to infants. Teoh and co-workers confirmed the description of Magner and co-workers and suggested that these neoplasms arose "from the neoplastic counterpart of undifferentiated tubules, analogous to nephroblastomas and other embryonic tumors."[307] Teoh and co-workers suggested the name *orchioblastoma.*

Abell and Holtz reported a series of 29 germ cell tumors in children, and identified a group of embryonal carcinomas that they equated morphologically to embryonal carcinomas in the adult testis.[310] Subsequently, numerous reports of testicular germ cell neoplasms in infants were reported under a variety of names including embryonal carcinoma of childhood, infantile adenocarcinoma, orchioblastoma, or simply embryonal carcinoma.[213,305,307,308,310,314,325]

During the 1960s and 1970s, two growing bodies of literature existed. One recorded cases of embryonal carcinoma in infants, and the other was represented by scattered "minority reports" suggesting that these neoplasms were actually examples of Teilum's yolk sac tumor.[309,314]

The discovery of elevated AFP in patients with testicular "teratocarcinoma" by Abelev and co-workers set the stage for the emergence of Teilum's yolk sac tumor as the actual neoplasm predominating among testicular germ cell neoplasms in infants.[206] Specifically, the elevated levels of AFP characteristically associated with yolk sac tumors served both to identify the neoplasm and to support Teilum's theory of its histogenesis. Yolk sac tumor was formally recognized in both the WHO and the British Testicular Tumor Panel classifications of testicular tumors published.[222,226]

Clinical Features

Our current understanding of the clinical features of yolk sac tumor can be summarized. Germ cell tumors arising in the testes of infants, children, and (rarely) in adults, and previously recorded under a variety of names, including embryonal carcinoma, adenocarcinoma with clear cells, or orchioblastoma, are examples of Teilum's yolk sac tumor. These tumors represent the single most common germ cell neoplasm in the pediatric age group.[213,320] Pure yolk sac tumors of adult testes are uncommon; however, yolk sac tumor foci have been reported by Talerman to be present in 30% to 44% of nonseminomatous germ cell tumors.[318,320,328] Children present with a rapid testicular enlargement.[213] Metastases by both lymphatic and hematogenous routes most commonly involve the lungs, liver, and peritoneum.[325,326]

The collective reviews and individual reported series of yolk sac tumor arising in the infant testis indicate a relatively low rate of retroperitoneal metastases and relatively high survival rates.[315,317,326] The recent reports of Smith and co-workers and Kaplan and Firlit, detailing retroperitoneal lymph node metastases in a significant number of infants with yolk sac tumors, suggests that a reappraisal of the natural history and surgical therapy of this malignancy is appropriate.[327,329]

Pathologic Features

The enlarged testis discloses a poorly defined, lobulated, white-gray or gray-yellow, focally cystic, solid mass of variable consistency. Focal areas of hemorrhage are common. When encountered in the infant testis, yolk sac tumors differ from teratomas, which are generally more prominently cystic and commonly evidence foci of cartilage in the solid areas between the mucin-containing cysts.

The characteristic histologic features of yolk sac tumors include a basic pattern of anastomosing tubules and glands of varying size interspersed with densely cellular areas. Focal microcysts with papillary clusters of cells projecting into the lumen are common. The lining cells within the anastomosing tubules are usually flat, but may be columnar. This variable morphology is highly characteristic. Large areas of some tumors can be devoid of such tubules, and exhibit a reticular pattern created by the prominence of cytoplasmic vacuoles within the tumor cells. The pathognomonic glomeruloid body (Schiller–Duval body) is characterized by a microcystic structure with a glomerulus-like structure, containing a central fibrovascular core surrounded by an outer mantle of tumor cells (Fig. 6-30).[306,319] In addition, both intracellular and extracellular PAS-positive

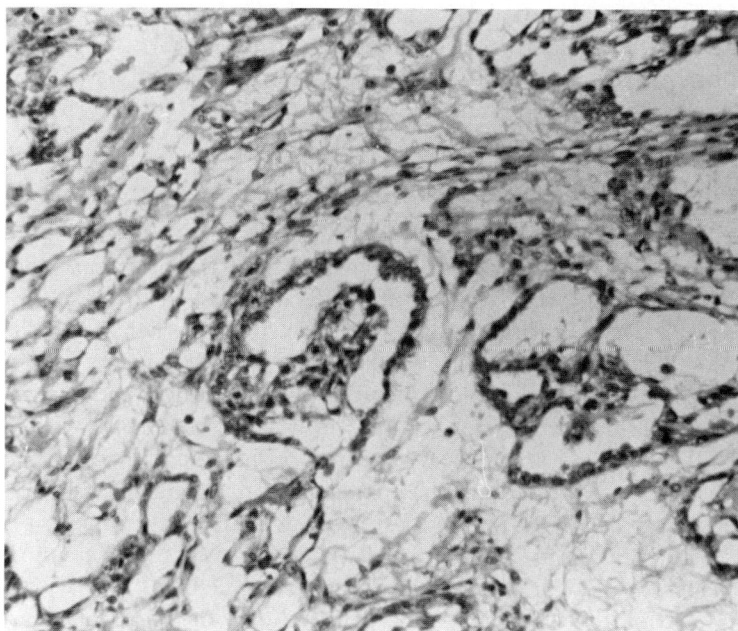

Figure 6-30   *Endodermal sinus tumor (yolk sac tumor). The tumor is composed of multiple dilated tubular spaces lined by flattened cells with an edematous stroma intervening. A glomerulus-like structure is present* (center).

hyaline globules are highly characteristic of this neoplasm.[319,323] Immunofluorescence and immunoperoxidase staining for alpha-fetoprotein identifies this tumor marker within the tumor cells and some of the hyaline globules.[319,324]

The histologic features are distinct from the highly variable patterns of the embryonal carcinoma typical in adult patients.

Choriocarcinoma

Choriocarcinomas are germ cell neoplasms representing differentiation to extraembryonic structures (*i.e.,* placenta), and in pure form are composed exclusively of syncytiotrophoblastic and cytotrophoblastic cells. Choriocarcinomas arising in the testis are uncommon, constituting 0.3% to 3.5% of all germ cell neoplasms.[198,213,335] More frequently, choriocarcinoma is observed as one component in a mixed germ cell tumor in the testis, or in a metastasis.[213,227,261] The identity of some multinucleated giant cells observed in typical seminomas and embryonal cell carcinomas has recently been established as syncytiotrophoblasts by their positive immunoperoxidase staining for HCG.[324] Typically, these syncytiotrophoblasts are not accompanied by cytotrophoblastic cells, as is observed in pure choriocarcinomas or foci of choriocarcinoma in mixed germ cell tumors.

Testicular choriocarcinomas are virtually limited to males in the second and third decades.[213,261] However, Mostofi and Price reported observing this neoplasm in a 50-year-old man.[213] Most patients present with symptoms of metastases, with only minimal testicular enlargement characteristic. Teilum reports that 10% of patients exhibit gynecomastia.[336] Serum levels of HCG are invariably elevated in cases of choriocarcinoma; however, a recent report has documented false-negative assays for serum HCG in the clinical context of residual nonseminomatous germ cell tumor with a choriocarcinomatous component.[244] The true frequency of this finding is currently unknown.

Pathologic Features

Choriocarcinoma is typically an ill-defined mass or nodule, the bulk of which is hemorrhagic and apparently necrotic. Gray-tan soft tissue is admixed within the hemorrhage. Extensive hemorrhage, as observed in pure choriocarcinoma, or focally when choriocarcinoma is admixed with other germ cell components in a mixed germ cell tumor, is the key diagnostic feature.

The requisite histologic features allowing the diagnosis of choriocarcinoma include syncytiotrophoblasts in close association with cytotrophoblastic cells (Fig. 6-31). Masses of these cells in combination with abundant hemorrhage are characteristic of this tumor. Local invasion through the testicular interstitium is common, as is vascular invasion, which may be prominent. The syncytiotrophoblasts take various forms in a manner recapitulating their development in the placenta.[332] Typically, large multinucleated cells with variably dense eosinophilic or vacuolated cytoplasm drop over a cluster of cytotrophoblastic cells. Alternatively, syncytiotrophoblasts may have attenuated cytoplasm, and the nuclei are correspondingly condensed in irregular, bizarre spindle shapes. Regardless of the overall configuration of the syncytiotrophoblast cell, the nuclei are markedly hyperchromatic and atypical, and the close association with the polygonal cytotrophoblasts is maintained. Cytotrophoblasts have well-defined cell borders surrounding pale eosinophilic or clear cytoplasm. The relatively uniform, vesicular nuclei of the cytotrophoblasts contrasts with the hyperchromatic large, irregular, frequently bizarre nuclei of the syncytiotrophoblasts.

The ultrastructural features of choriocarcinomas have been studied by Price and Midgley, who observed a paucity of ER in the cytotrophoblasts in contrast with abundant ER in the syncytiotrophoblasts.[332] In addition, they observed a gradation of cytoplasmic organization supporting the origin of syncytiotrophoblasts from the cytotrophoblasts.[332] They further demonstrated by immunofluorescence that the source of HCG was the syncytiotrophoblast cells, a finding antedating confirmation by immunoperoxidase staining by 14 years (Fig. 6-32).[332,324]

The dramatically poorer prognosis of patients with testicular choriocarcinoma compared to women with uterine examples of this malignancy persists. The neoplasm, by virtue of its tendency to disseminate early, is not amenable to surgery. Further, the tumor is not radiosensitive and no effective chemotherapy regimen has been developed to date.

Finally, diagnostically challenging cases of germ cell malignancies initially manifesting as extragonadal neoplasms (most frequently in the retroperitoneum) have been associated with clinically negative testes.[330,331,333,337] Numerous reports of such cases have described only "burned-out" foci within the extensively examined gonads, characterized by fibrous scars associated with hemosiderin deposition.[337] It is currently thought that such cases represent examples of spontaneous regression of the true primary site, with clinical attention directed to the more apparent metastases.[330,331,333] The majority of such cases are

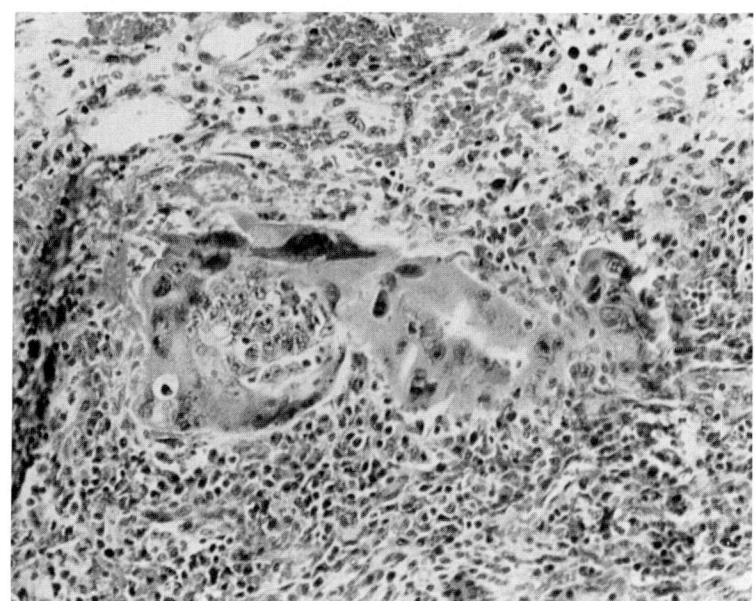

Figure 6-31 *Choriocarcinoma. The syncytiotrophoblast cells surround a cluster of cytotrophoblast cells with evident hemorrhage in the adjacent tissue.*

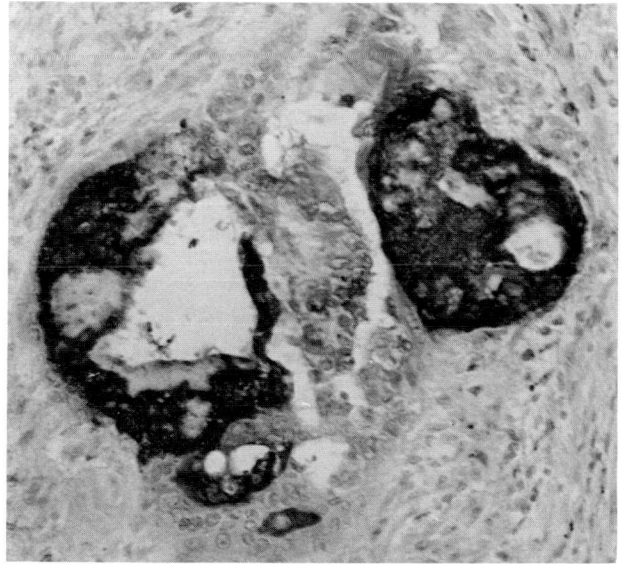

Figure 6-32 *Syncytiotrophoblastic giant cells stained for HCG by immunoperoxidase technique.*

choriocarcinomas, but examples of virtually all histologic forms of testicular germ cell neoplasms have been observed under these circumstances.

Mixed Germ Cell Neoplasms

Teratocarcinoma

Mixed germ cell tumors, that is, tumors composed of more than one histologic type of germ cell neoplasm, constitute 40% to 45% of all primary testicular germ cell neoplasms.[199,213,338] Although the possible combinations exceed a dozen, the three most frequent combinations are teratoma plus embryonal carcinoma (teratocarcinoma), constituting 24% of germ cell tumors; teratoma, embryonal carcinoma, and seminoma, constituting 6.4% of germ cell tumors; and embryonal carcinoma with seminoma, constituting 5% of germ cell neoplasms.[199,213] Talerman recently reported that significant numbers (38% to 44%) of nonseminomatous germ cell neoplasms contain components of yolk sac tumor.[320,328] The demonstration of AFP in nonseminomatous germ cell tumors lends support to the surprisingly high frequencies reported by Talerman.[228,253] The significance of yolk sac components in the clinical behavior of mixed germ cell tumor requires greater elucidation.

Teratocarcinomas, which are tumors containing a teratomatous component in association with embryonal carcinoma, are the most frequently encountered mixed form of germ cell neoplasms, as noted previously. These neoplasms are most frequent during the third decade.[213,338] Mostofi reports that 20% of patients present with metastases that most frequently take the histologic form of embryonal carcinoma.[213] Teratomatous or choriocarcinomatous metastases are observed less frequently.[199,213]

The relative effects of the addition of one histologic form of germ cell neoplasm to another were first reported in the large study by Dixon and Moore.[199] The addition of choriocarcinomatous foci to any other germ cell neoplasm significantly decreases survival, as does the admixture of embryonal carcinoma to either seminoma or teratoma in the adult.[213]

Gonadal Stromal/Sex Cord Tumors

Primary neoplasms of Sertoli, Leydig, granulosa, and theca cell origin constitute approximately 6% of testicular tumors.[213] As a group they are referred to as "tumors of specialized gonadal stroma" by Mostofi, or sex cord/stromal tumors in the WHO classification (see Table 6-2).[213,226] The differences in terminology reflect the unsettled state of histogenesis of these neoplasms. In summary, two views regarding the origin of Sertoli cells and granulosa cells remain unreconciled. One hypothesis, based on the work of Gillman, favors Sertoli and granulosa cell origin from sex cords that develop from the surface germinal epithelium of the gonadal ridge.[368] Alternatively, others favor origin from the gonadal mesenchyme, in common with Leydig cells, and thus neoplasms of these cell types represent "tumors of specialized gonadal stroma."[213,347,367] The WHO terminology is noncommittal about the histogenesis of these tumors. As outlined in the WHO classification, these neoplasms may occur in "pure" form or as mixtures of the cell types in this group.

Leydig Cell Tumors

Leydig cell tumors of the testis, also known as interstitial cell tumors, have been reported in approximately 200 patients.[343-366] This neoplasm occurs at all ages, but with nonuniform frequency.[348,353,360] When it develops in children, it is most common after age 4 years. It is more common in adults, with a peak frequency in the third to sixth decades. Endocrine effects of the tumor are found in all age groups, but are most frequent when the tumor arises in prepubertal children who virtually always evidence precocious physical and sexual development.[344,348,353] When arising in adults, accompanying endocrine effects are less common, with decreased libido, with or without gynecomastia, observed in about 20% of patients.[348] All patients present with testicular enlargement. Rare examples have been reported in cryptorchid testes.[352] Reflecting the clinical evidence of either masculinization, feminization, or absence of endocrine effects, hormone assays show no characteristic pattern, but estrogen and testosterone have been reported elevated.[364] Rare examples of gonadotropin elevation have been reported.[364]

Pathologic Features

Leydig cell neoplasms affect the right and left testis with approximately equal frequency. Bilateral examples are distinctly uncommon, but have been reported.[213,346] These neoplasms are characteristically well defined, some appearing encapsulated, and vary from 1 cm to 10 cm. Their color varies from yellow to mahogany-brown. Fibrous trabeculae are randomly oriented through the neoplasm, and tend to make the cut surface lobulated. The consistency of the tumor is characteristically soft, but larger tumors with significant fibrosis can be firm. The fibrosis is accompanied by focal calcification in some examples. Cyst formation, hemorrhage, and necrosis are not characteristic of these tumors.

Microscopically, the tumor cells are arranged in sheets or broad cords with fibrous trabeculae, often hyalinized, in between. If present, the calcification is located in the fibrous areas, which may also show myxoid stromal change. The tumor cells have no organization within the nests beyond a tendency to show numerous thin-walled blood vessels in a manner characteristic of endocrine neoplasms (Fig. 6-33). The tumor cells are most commonly polygonal, with abundant eosinophilic or vacuolated cytoplasm and a central round or oval nucleus. The cell borders are usually indistinct. Lipofuscin pigment within the cytoplasm is inconstant, but when present it is helpful in identifying the cells as Leydig in nature. Occasional cells may be significantly larger than the bulk of the tumor cells, which characteristically exhibit a limited spectrum of pleomorphism. Occasional multinucleated giant cells may be present. Mitoses are typically rare or absent.

The pathognomonic cytoplasmic inclusion, the Reinke crystal, is inconstant and the diagnosis can be made in its absence. Mostofi and Price report observing this structure in 40% of Leydig cell neoplasms.[213] Typically, it is intensely eosinophilic and rectangular with well-defined borders. The use of the trichrome stain significantly accentuates these structures, making their detection correspondingly easier.

The ultrastructural features of the neoplastic Leydig's cell include abundant smooth endoplasmic reticulum, cytoplasmic lipochrome pigment, mitochondria with tubular cristae, and scattered lysosomes, some with fat vacuoles.[358,359,365,366] Kay and co-workers described cytoplasmic membranous whorls

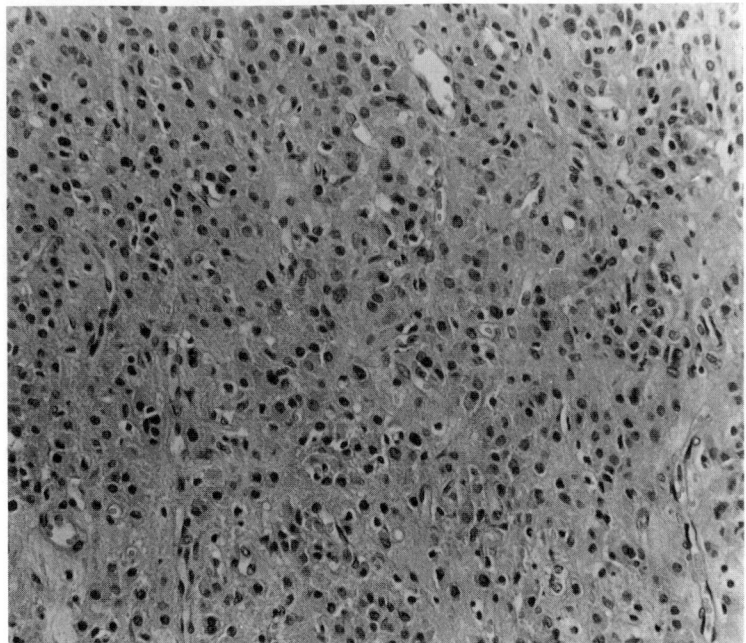

Figure 6-33   *Leydig cell (interstitial cell) tumor. The tumor cells, arranged in sheets, are moderately pleomorphic with abundant eosinophilic cytoplasm. No mitoses are present.*

composed in tightly bound narrow tubules.[359] These features are similar in normal Leydig's cells and in both benign and malignant neoplasms arising from these cells.[358,359,365,366] Kurman and co-workers demonstrated testosterone and estrogen in Leydig cells by the immunoperoxidase technique.[366]

Variants of these histologic features include focal areas of spindle cells, or predominance of vacuolated cells. Typically the advancing border is blunt and there is a fibrous pseudocapsule at the interface between the tumor and the adjacent compressed seminiferous tubules. Occasionally, the tumor extends through this capsule into the adjacent testis interstitium, or into the testicular hilum. Two additional features may be quantitatively different than observed in the typical case. Rare examples may show focal areas of marked vascularity with numerous thin-walled vessels. Also, focal areas in occasional cases may show marked fibrosis imparting a pattern of greater disorganization to a tumor typically showing sheets of tumor cells with minimal fibrosis. Occasional cases show an admixture of Sertoli cells, the features of which are described later under Sertoli cell tumors.

The differential diagnosis of Leydig cell tumors requires their distinction from Leydig cell hyperplasia, metastatic carcinoma (especially poorly differential prostatic carcinoma), lymphomatous involvement of the testis, and adrenal rests.[213] The features allowing the distinction of Leydig cell neoplasia from hyperplasia include the diffuse distribution of the Leydig cells between seminiferous tubules, and the absence of compression atrophy of the seminiferous tubules characteristic of hyperplasia.

The great majority of Leydig cell neoplasms are clinically benign. However, some are malignant and their recognition is possibly the most important differential diagnosis when encountering a Leydig cell tumor. Unfortunately, the surgical pathologist's ability to reliably predict future malignant behavior of Leydig cell tumors is limited, as will be discussed below.

Malignant Leydig Cell Tumors

Twenty-nine documented cases of malignant Leydig cell tumors could be found in the literature. Dalgaard and Hesselberg reviewed previously reported cases and accepted nine examples.[348] Mahon and co-workers reported one case and reviewed the 12 cases previously reported.[357] The number doubled in the subsequent decade with a recent review reported by Chen and co-workers.[365] Four additional cases found in the recent literature brings the total to 29.[363,364,366]

These 29 patients range in age from 29 years to 82 years with 90% older than 40 years.[365] The peak frequency occurs in the seventh decade. Patients present with testicular enlargement as the principal complaint in 80% of cases. In 20% of patients, symptoms relate to established metastases.[365,366] Gynecomastia has been observed in three patients. Elevated estrogens have been recorded in seven patients, with elevated androgens in nine patients.[364,365] Three patients demonstrated elevations of serum gonadotropins.[364,365]

The malignant Leydig cell tumors recorded tend to be larger than those behaving in a benign manner, with the majority of the former 5 cm to 10 cm in diameter. Exclusive of size, and occasional cases with gross evidence of extensive local invasion of the epididymis, no other gross features allow distinction from the clinically benign examples. Microscopically, 75% of the reported malignant Leydig cell tumors show capsular invasion and vascular invasion.[345,365] Importantly, 25% of those proving malignant showed neither. All other morphologic criteria, including number of mitoses, necrosis, fibrosis, and cytologic pleomorphism, are even more unreliable. The prevailing opinion regards the presence of metastases as the only reliable criterion of malignancy among Leydig cell tumors.[213] The role of the surgical pathologist is thus both critical and limited. These neoplasms must be extensively sectioned to detect the possible presence of vascular or local invasion. Their absence, as noted above, does not preclude subsequent metastases. Recurrences (metastases) have been diagnosed as long as 9 years after orchiectomy.[365] Death from such metastases occurs an average of 2.5 years after orchiectomy.[365] Unfortunately, neither radiation nor chemotherapy has proved effective.[365]

Paratesticular Leydig Cell Tumors

The occurrence of Leydig cell tumors in extragonadal sites has been reported in two patients.[367,368] Tedeschi and Burke reported an example arising in a 57-year-old man that proved malignant, with intra-abdominal metastases and death occurring within 45 days of orchiectomy.[367] The tumor arose in the proximal spermatic cord, and the ipsilateral testis was found free of malignancy.[367] The second, and more recently reported, case was described by Maurer and co-workers.[368] The patient was a 40-year-old man in whom a paravesical Sertoli–Leydig gonadal stromal tumor containing Sertoli and Leydig cells was identified. The authors found positive staining for estradiol and testosterone in the Leydig cells as demonstrated by the immunoperoxidase method.[368] The tumor demonstrated vascular invasion, but a retroperitoneal node dissection was found to be free of metastases and the patient was alive without evidence of tumor 2 years after surgical removal of the neoplasm.[368] Incidentally, Reinke crystals were not found in either of these extragonadal sex cord/stromal tumors.[367,368]

Sertoli Cell Tumors

Testicular Sertoli cell tumors (androblastomas) were first described by Teilum.[369,370] He regarded these neoplasms as homologous to the ovarian differentiated arrhenoblastoma. The histogenesis of Sertoli cells and their neoplasms remains unsettled, as does the relationship of Sertoli cell tumors and Leydig cell tumors, as previously discussed.

Approximately 100 cases of testicular Sertoli cell tumors have been reported in the literature since Teilum's first report.[369-393] Gabrilove and co-workers evaluated the first 72 reported cases in a comprehensive review published in 1980.[376] Additional cases were found in the more recent literature.[375,385-388] Of the total number of Sertoli cell tumors reported, 21 have proved clinically malignant (refer to discussion of malignant Sertoli cell tumors).

Sertoli cell tumors have been observed in all age groups from infancy to the ninth decade. Approximately 30% of reported cases involve infants and children in the first decade and an additional 30% of patients are in the third to fourth decades.[376] Thereafter, the frequency declines with increasing age. Patients present with the complaint of a scrotal mass gradually increasing in size. Approximately 20% have associated gynecomastia, a finding more frequently associated with Sertoli cell tumors that prove clinically malignant than with those that are benign.[376] The right and left testes are affected with equal frequency. Two cases of bilateral Sertoli cell tumors are reported.[376,390]

The cut surface of the involved testis reveals a well-delineated, homogenous, yellow-gray or orange-tan nodule devoid of hemorrhage and necrosis. Pure Sertoli cell tumors microscopically demonstrate a tubular arrangement of cuboidal or columnar cells, most commonly in the form of solid cords without lumen (Fig. 6-34). The stroma is composed of delicate supporting fibrous trabeculae serving as basement membranes for the tubular structures. The nuclei, which show minimal pleomorphism, have a distinct nuclear membrane, a single small nucleolus, and fine granular chromatin, most prevalent near the nuclear membrane. In some tumors the tubular arrangement merges with less well organized areas, and transition to polygonal or spindle cells in sheets is observed.[213,347,374] Approximately one third of these neoplasms have admixed Leydig cells, and therefore are examples of mixed gonadal stromal tumors.

Lesions to be distinguished from the clinically benign Sertoli cell tumors include mixed gonadal stromal neoplasms (Sertoli–Leydig cell tumors), undifferentiated gonadal stromal tumors, the so-called tubular adenoma of Pick (observed in cryptorchid testes), and malignant Sertoli cell tumors.[213] (Refer to discussion of cryptorchidism.)

Malignant Sertoli Cell Tumors

A total of 21 malignant Sertoli cell tumors are reported in the literature (Table 6-6).[377-388] The patients range in age from 8 years to 79 years, with no apparent age predilection. These patients typically give a history of a slowly growing scrotal mass. The majority of patients were aware of the swelling for 1 year to 8 years. Of the cases providing information, the majority exhibited gynecomastia.

These malignant neoplasms vary in size from 3 cm to 15 cm, with the major-

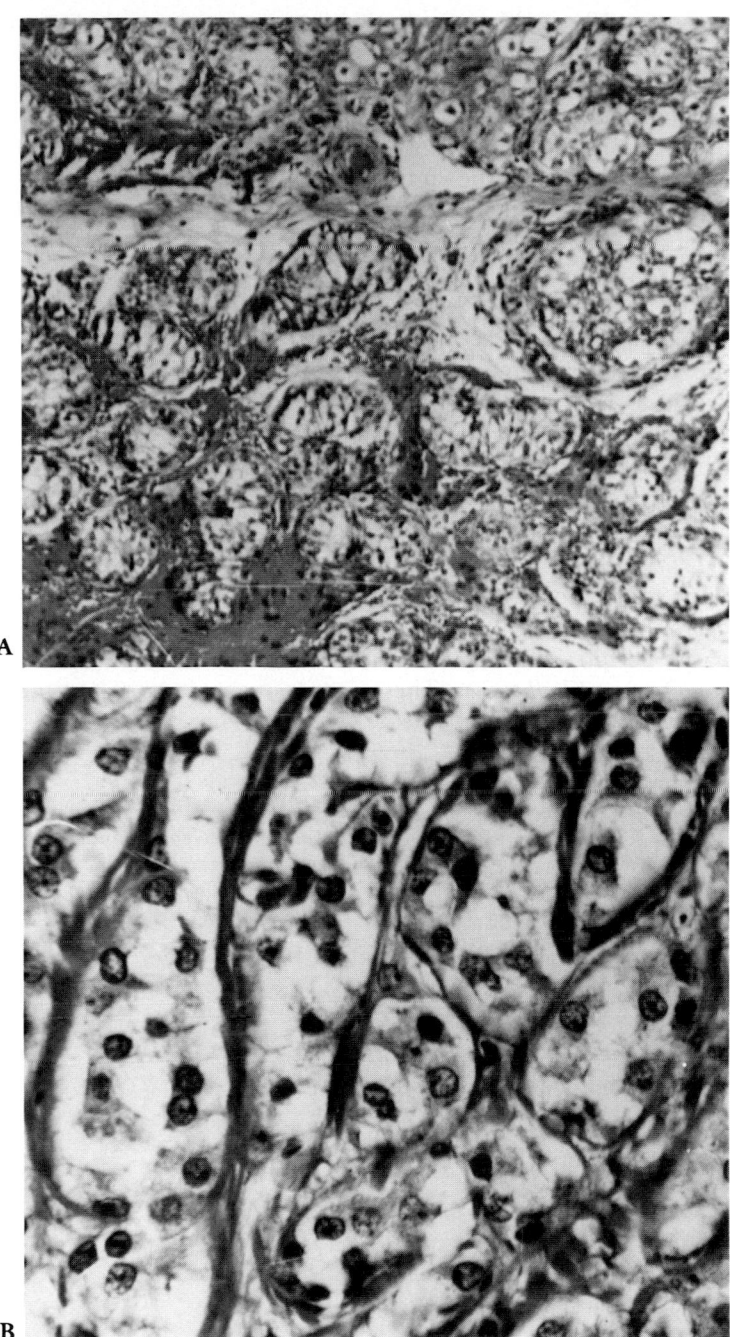

Figure 6-34 *Sertoli cell tumor.* (A) *The neoplastic Sertoli cells are arranged in tubules of variable size.* (B) *Higher magnification shows the vacuolated cytoplasm and round or oval nuclei of the Sertoli cells. The nuclear membrane is characteristically distinct, and a single nucleolus is typical.*

ity 6 cm to 10 cm. Most evidenced local invasion, with some exhibiting focal cystic change within the primary neoplasm. The invasive character of the neoplasm is evident microscopically, with many also demonstrating lymphatic involvement. The basic histologic pattern of Sertoli cell tumors is maintained in those proving malignant. Most patients evidence lymphatic metastases, and the majority succumb to the tumor within 2 years of diagnosis (see Table 6-6). However, two patients demonstrated recurrences 15 years and 18 years after orchiectomy.[374,379,386]

The diagnosis of malignant Sertoli cell tumor rests on macroscopic and microscopic evidence of local invasion of adjacent structures, lymphatics, and blood vessels. Mitotic activity, uncommon in the benign variety, is increased in those proving malignant. The malignant Sertoli cell tumors tend to exhibit necrosis, greater cellular pleomorphism, and a reduced tendency to form tubules.[347,387,388] The presence of metastases, which tend to occur earlier in the clinical evolution than observed in Leydig cell tumors, is unequivocal evidence of malignancy.

Large Cell Calcifying Sertoli Cell Tumors

Proppe and Scully recently described 10 cases of an unusual variant of Sertoli cell tumors characterized by intratubular calcifications and a neoplastic proliferation of large Sertoli cells (Figs. 6-35, 6-36).[391] They called the neoplasm *large cell calcifying Sertoli cell tumor*. These neoplasms were most common in the second

Table 6-6   ***Malignant Sertoli Cell Neoplasms***

Author(s)	Year	Age	Symptom Duration	Gynecomastia*	Follow Up*
Mostofi et al[377]	1959	41	8 yr	+	D, 5 mo
Collins, Symington[371]	1964	27	1 yr	+	D, 3 mo
Nagy et al[378]	1964	35	3 wk	−	D, 1 yr
Nagy et al[378]	1964	62	1 yr	−	D, 10 mo
Rosvoll, Woodard[379]	1968	8	3 yr	−	A/NED, 8 yr†
Hopkins, Perry[380]	1969	63	1 day	+	D, 5 yr
Talerman[381]	1971	79	6 mo	−	D (radiologic), 3 mo
Talerman[381]	1971	19	8 yr	−	A/NED, 8 mo
Morin, Loening[384]	1975	60	1 mo	+	D, 3 yr
Koppikar, Sirsat[382]	1973	33	4 yr	+	A/NED, 2 yr
Hansen[383]	1975	42	3 yr	+	D, 1 yr
Symington, Cameron[374]	1976	‡	NI	NI	1 D, 18 yr
					5 D, <18 mo
Herrera et al[386]	1981	20	NI	NI	A/NED, 17 yr
Campbell, Middleton[385]	1981	16	3 yr	+	A/NED, 6 mo
Eble et al[387]	1984	34	1 yr	−	D, 13 mo
Godec[388]	1985	31	3 days	−	A/NED, 7 mo

* Key—+, present; −, absent; NI, no information; D, dead; A/NED, alive/no evidence of disease
† Original report gives 2-year follow up; Symington and Cameron give 8-year follow up on same patient.[374]
‡ Six cases, no clinical or pathologic details provided

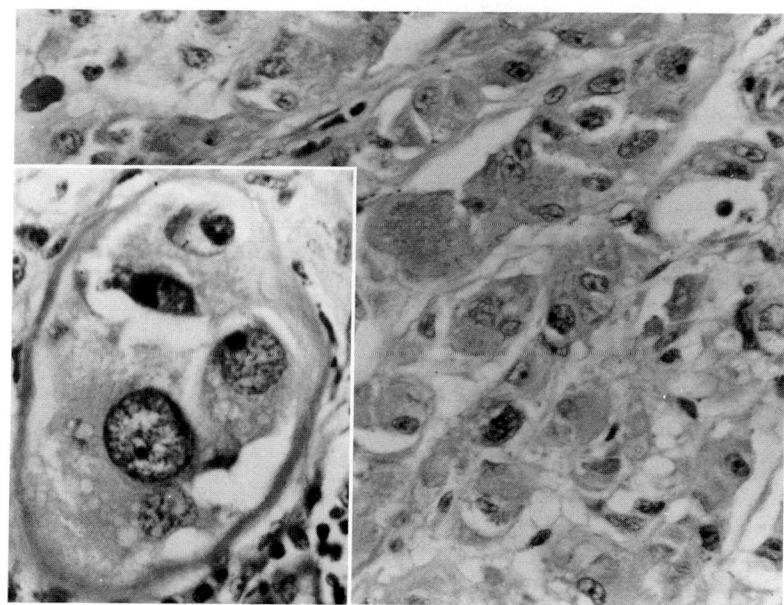

Figure 6-35   *Large cell calcifying Sertoli cell tumor. The large Sertoli cells are arranged in cords or tubules, commonly with distinct basement membrane* (inset). *The cytoplasm of the cells is typically vacuolated.*

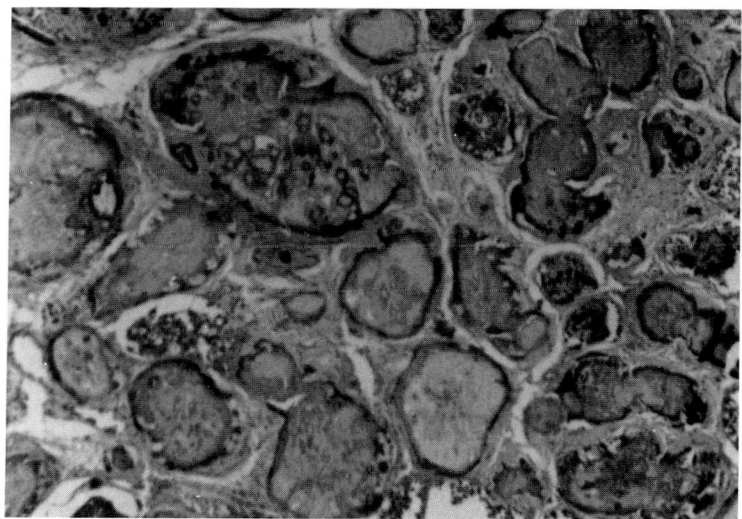

Figure 6-36   *Large cell calcifying Sertoli cell tumor. Characteristic calcification within these neoplasms takes the form of multiple rounded nodular deposits in this example.*

decade, with virtually all occurring before age 20 years. Further characterizing these tumors were the high frequencies of bilaterality (60%) and multifocality (60%). Two patients demonstrated a familial occurrence. Proppe and Scully referred to two previously reported cases as earlier examples of large cell calcifying Sertoli cell tumor.[389,390] Two additional cases have been reported recently by Proppe and Dickerson and by Waxman and co-workers.[392,393] Of the 14 reported cases, only one has proved clinically malignant.[391]

Granulosa Cell Tumors

Granulosa cell tumors of the testis are distinctly rare, with only five cases found in the literature.[394-397] Patients range in age from 20 years to 53 years, and present with a scrotal mass and evidence of hyperestrinism with gynecomastia. The testicular tumor was an incidental finding at autopsy in one patient with gynecomastia.[394]

In addition to the previously mentioned five patients, juvenile granulosa cell tumor, which is a variant of the adult form previously recognized in the ovary, was recently reported arising in the testes of 14 male infants.[398] The neoplasms ranged in size from 0.8 cm to 5.0 cm, and microscopically showed the predominant follicular pattern typical of these neoplasms in the ovary.[398] None evidenced malignant behavior, but follow-up information was available for only 4 of the 14 reported patients.[398]

Gonadoblastoma

Gonadoblastomas are rare neoplasms composed of an intimate admixture of germ cells and immature sex cord/stromal elements, including Sertoli and granulosa cells, and less frequently, Leydig cells.[399,402] These neoplasms arise almost exclusively in dysgenetic gonads.[400-402,406,407] Although gonadoblastomas, per se, have not demonstrated malignant behavior, approximately half of the reported cases are associated with an overgrowth of the germ cell component, and about 10% of germinomas arising in this context have demonstrated metastases.[402] Scully, who originally described gonadoblastomas in 1953, regards these neoplasms as a form of in situ cancer from which clinically malignant germ cell neoplasms may arise.[402]

Since the original description by Scully, approximately 100 cases of gonadoblastomas have been reported.[399-407] Although 80% are diagnosed in phenotypic females, karyotype studies have disclosed a preponderance of 46XY karyotype, and 90% are chromatin negative.[402] About half of the phenotypic females with gonadoblastoma evidence virilization.[402] Among the 20% of cases arising in phenotypic males, only two cases were found in scrotal testes, and the majority of the others arose in males with abdominal testes.[381,405] Bilateral gonadoblastomas are reported in approximately one third of cases.[402] The majority of patients are younger than 20 years old.[399-407]

Pathologic Features

Most gonadoblastomas come to clinical attention as a result of an intra-abdominal mass or the hormonal effects (virilization, defeminization).[402] The neoplasms range in size from microscopic foci in dysgenetic gonads (24% of cases),

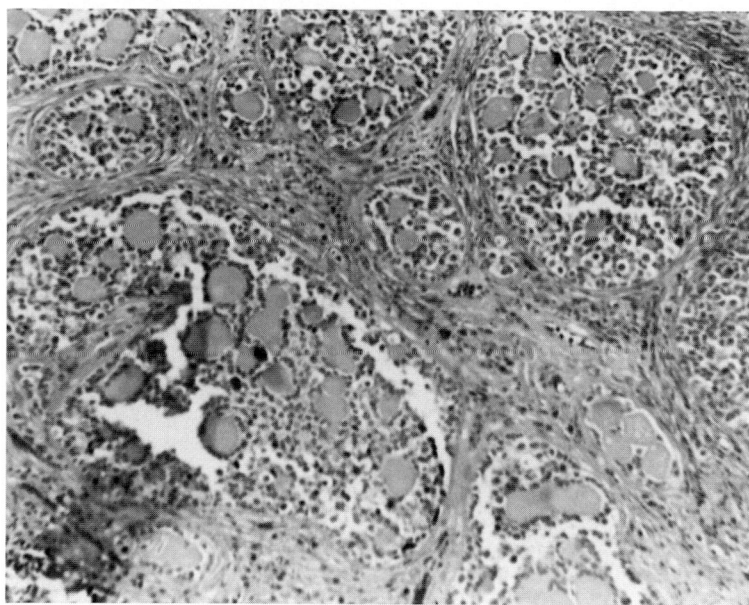

Figure 6-37   *Gonadoblastoma. The neoplasm is composed of mixture of gonadal stromal cells and germ cells arranged in nests arising in dysgenetic gonad.*

to gray yellow masses several centimeters in diameter.[402] The smaller examples commonly exhibit a gritty cut surface reflecting multifocal sites of calcification within the neoplasm. The majority of the larger tumors are associated with superimposed malignant germ cell tumors arising within the gonadoblastoma. In such cases, the features superimposed on the neoplasm reflect the predominant emerging germ cell neoplasm, and not that of the gonadoblastoma from which it originated.

Microscopically, the diagnostic histologic picture is the intimate admixture of gonadal stromal cells and germ cells (Figs. 6-37, 6-38). The gonadal stromal/ sex cord cells are arranged in three patterns. The Sertoli and granulosa-like cells are located around the periphery of nests of germ cells, or individual germ cells. Alternatively, these stromal cells may surround spaces filled with eosinophilic material. Additional features described by Scully include stromal hyalinization, and individual or clustered psammoma bodies, the latter described as mulberry-like calcified masses.[402] Finally, the overgrowth of germ cells, characterized by a unicellular proliferation invading the stroma, may be of such magnitude that neither the original dysgenetic gonad nor the gonadoblastomatous focus of origin may be apparent unless the neoplasm is extensively sectioned (Fig. 6-39). The germ cell neoplasms arising in gonadoblastomas are most frequently germinomas (seminomas, dysgerminomas), but embryonal cell carcinomas, teratomas, and yolk sac tumors also have been observed.[402-406] Under such circumstances metastases have been recorded with the ultimate tumor-related death of the patient. Surgical removal of both gonads has been advocated because approximately one third of gonadoblastomas occur as bilateral neoplasms, commonly in dysgenetic gonads, and some of the clinically aggressive neoplasms have also showed bilaterality.[405]

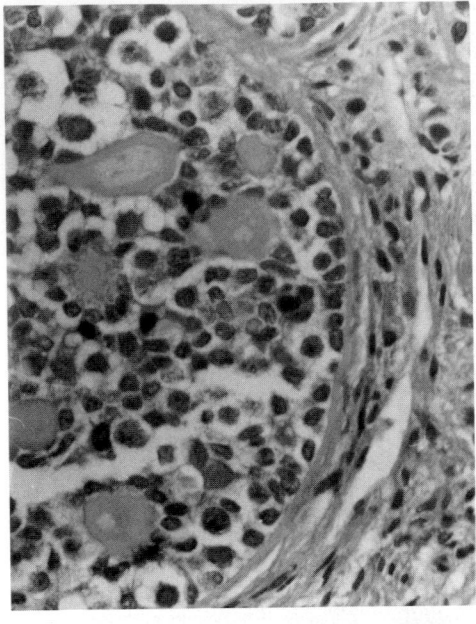

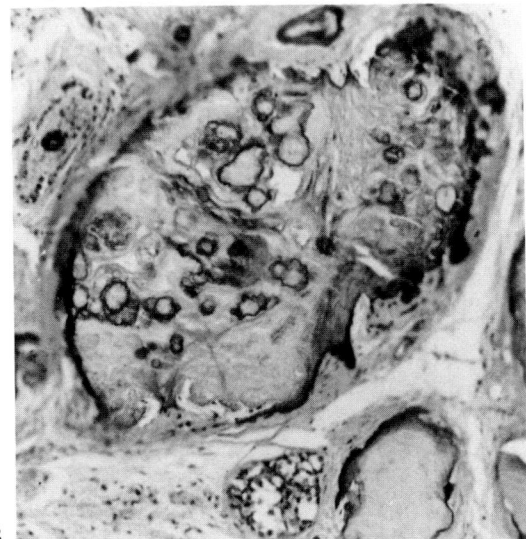

Figure 6-38   *Gonadoblastoma.* (A) *Characteristic nest of
gonadal stromal cells has interspersed germ cells
with clear cytoplasm.* (B) *Calcification is typical of
gonadoblastoma.*

Carcinoid Tumors

Thirty-one testicular carcinoid tumors are reported in the literature (Table 6-7).
Six of these testicular carcinoids were observed originating in teratomas.[408-422]
The case reported by Dockerty and Scheifley was regarded as metastatic in the
testis, but no primary in the intestines was identified at autopsy 12 years later.[409]
Multiple intra-abdominal metastatic foci of carcinoid tumor were found. The

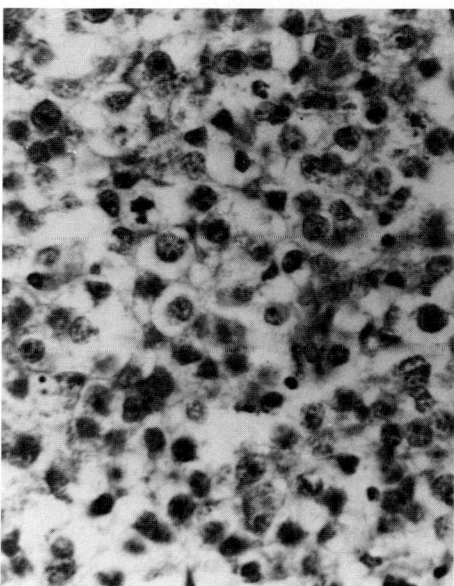

Figure 6-39   *Gonadoblastoma with germinoma. This monocellular proliferation arising in a gonadoblastoma represents a focus of germinoma.*

precise nature of this case is problematic. The patients range in age from 20 years to 76 years, with the peak frequency in the fifth and sixth decades. The neoplasm produces a testicular enlargement that may be either painful or asymptomatic. Only two patients gave symptoms suggesting carcinoid syndrome.[417,418] Of the 30 patients recorded, excluding the problematic case of Dockerty and Scheifley, metastases and tumor-related death were observed in only three patients.[418,421]

Pathologic Features

Tumor size in recorded cases varies from 1 cm to 9 cm in diameter with the majority averaging 3 cm to 5 cm. The cut surface is gray-tan to yellow and lobulated, with focal areas of necrosis commonly superimposed. Fibrous septae separate ill-defined lobules. Focal calcification and minute cysts have been reported in some cases. Testicular carcinoids developing in teratomas are dominated by the typical cystic features of the teratoma. Microscopically, testicular carcinoids are histologically identical to their counterparts in more common locations. Virtually all reported cases have evidenced positive argentaffin staining, and the typical ultrastructural features of carcinoids have been presented in four recent studies.[416,417,420,421]

The histogenesis of testicular carcinoids is unsettled. The most plausible explanation of primary testicular carcinoids is one-sided development of a teratoma.[213,226] Origin from argentaffin cells, which have never been identified within the normal testis, is less probable.

Of greatest importance in making the correct diagnosis of testicular carci-

Table 6-7   *Testicular Carcinoid Tumors*

Author(s)	Year	Age	Presentation	Origin in Teratoma*	Follow Up*
Simon et al[408]	1954	58	Enlarged L testis	+	NI
Dockerty, Scheifley[409]	1955	35	Flushing spells; R testis nodule	Metastatic or primary?	D, tumor metastasis, 12 yr
Berkheiser[410]	1959	54	Painful L testicular enlargement	+	NI
Kemble[411]	1968	53	Enlarged R testis	−	A/NED, 3 yr
Kermarec, Duplay[412]	1968	59	Enlarged L testis	−	NI
Sinnatamby et al[414]	1973	31	Enlarged L testis	+	A/NED, 6 mo
Yalla et al[415]	1974	45	Asymptomatic testicular mass	−	A/NED, 4 yr
Weitzner, Robinson[416]	1976	48	Asymptomatic testicular mass	−	A/NED, 20 mo
Wurster et al[417]	1976	55	Painless testicular mass, diarrhea	−	A/NED, 3 yr
Brown[417a]	1976	†	Painless testicular mass	−	A/NED, 2, 4, 5, 15 yr D, no tumor, 25 yr
Magyar, Talerman[419]	1977	44	Painless L testicular enlargement	−	A/NED, 2 yr
Berdjis, Mostofi[418]	1977	20	Painless L testicular enlargement	−	A/NED, 16 yr
Berdjis, Mostofi[418]	1977	22	Incidental finding	−	NI
Berdjis, Mostofi[418]	1977	45	Testis nodule, flushing	−	A/NED, 6 yr
Berdjis, Mostofi[418]	1977	63	Painless testicular enlargement, 20 yr	−	D, tumor metastasis, 4 yr
Berdjis, Mostofi[418]	1977	50	Painless testicular enlargement, 5 yr	−	D, tumor metastasis, 6 yr
Berdjis, Mostofi[418]	1977	59	Hydrocele, 20 yr	−	D, no tumor, 6 yr
Berdjis, Mostofi[418]	1977	34	L painless testis mass, 4 yr	−	A/NED, 7 yr
Berdjis, Mostofi[418]	1977	53	L painless testis mass, 2 yr	−	A/NED, 3 yr
Berdjis, Mostofi[418]	1977	25	Incidental finding	−	A/NED, 7 mo
Berdjis, Mostofi[418]	1977	51	Small tender mass, R	−	A/NED, 1 yr
Berdjis, Mostofi[418]	1977	40	Incidental L testis mass	+	A/NED, 2.5 yr
Berdjis, Mostofi[418]	1977	22	Hernia; L testis mass	+	A/NED, 4 mo
Talerman et al[420]	1978	71	Painless testicular enlargement	−	A/NED, 10 mo
Sullivan et al[421]	1981	76	Asymptomatic mass; skin nodules	−	D, tumor metastasis, postoperative
Bates et al[422]	1981	53	Tender R testis mass	+	A/NED, 2 yr

* NI, no information; D, dead; A/NED, alive/no evidence of disease; +, present; −, absent

† Six cases: 27 years to 56 years (mean age, 48)

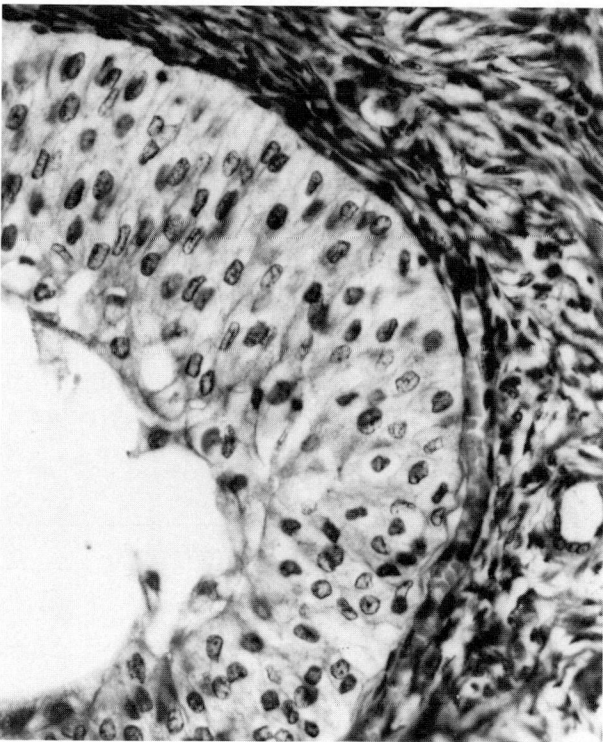

Figure 6-40   *Brenner tumor. The tumor cells are present in nests within a fibrous stroma. The characteristic longitudinal nuclear groove is apparent in the oval nuclei.*

noid is awareness of its occurrence within the testis in the absence of histologic evidence of a teratoma. Exclusion of an extratesticular carcinoid giving origin to testicular metastases, even rarer than primary testicular carcinoid, is obligatory.

Brenner Tumors

Four examples of Brenner tumors of the testis are recorded in the literature, one in association with an adenomatoid tumor.[423-426] The lesions, all relatively small (6 mm to 2.7 cm), were nodules in the tunica albuginea of the testis. The microscopic features are identical to those exhibited by ovarian Brenner tumors, including well-defined nests of polygonal cells containing nuclei with characteristic longitudinal grooves (Fig. 6-40). Most nests are solid, but a central cystic area may be present. Collagenous stroma forms the background of the epithelial nests.

The histogenesis of Brenner tumors is unsettled, but most regard the ovarian counterpart as Müllerian in origin.

Mesenchymal Neoplasms

Intratesticular mesenchymal neoplasms, both benign and malignant, are distinctly rare. Those originating in the tunica albuginea and tunica vaginalis are slightly more common. Reported examples of benign intratesticular hemangiomas, leiomyoma, and myxoid neurofibroma appear in the literature.[428,430] Testicular sarcomas include rhabdomyosarcoma and osteosarcoma.[427,429,431,432] The histologic appearance of each of these neoplasms in this unusual location mimicks that demonstrated by their counterparts in locations where they are more commonly encountered.

Hematopoietic Neoplasms
Plasmacytoma

Twenty-six cases of testicular plasmacytoma appear in the literature (Table 6-8).[433-445] Paladugu and co-workers refer to three additional patients in a reported series of testicular lymphoma.[460] The majority of these reported testicular plasma

Table 6-8   *Plasmacytoma*

Author(s)	Year	Age	Bone	Presentation
Porchownik[433]	1931	39	+ *	
Ulrich[434]	1939	55	− *	Weakness, testicular nodules
Kirshbaum[435]	1947	62	+	Paralysis
Hayes et al[436]	1952	NI	NI	NI†
Melicow, Cahill[437]	1954	54	+	Joint pains in legs
Melicow, Cahill[437]	1954	62	+	Painful epididymal swelling
Melicow, Cahill[437]	1954	63	+	Weakness
Melicow, Cahill[437]	1954	50	+	Scapular pain
Carson et al[438]	1955	72	+	Gingival ulceration, groin and testicular masses
Eckert, Smith[448]	1963	50	NI	Facial swelling, testicular mass
Gowing[449]	1964	50	− *	Painless testicular mass; facial swelling
Gowing[449]	1964	62	+ *	Pneumonia
Gowing[449]	1964	50	NI	Swelling, L side of neck
Osman[439]	1966	53	+	Weight loss, chest nodule
Weitzner[440]	1969	81	+	Weakness, weight loss
Levin, Mostofi[441]	1970	46	− *	Scrotal swelling
Levin, Mostofi[441]	1970	51	+	Lower extremity edema
Levin, Mostofi[441]	1970	66	−	Nosebleed
Levin, Mostofi[441]	1970	26	+ *	Testicular mass
Levin, Mostofi[441]	1970	43	+ *	Shoulder mass
Levin, Mostofi[441]	1970	48	−	Scrotal swelling
Levin, Mostofi[441]	1970	42	−	Scrotal swelling
Oldham, Polmar[442]	1973	44	−	Pneumonia
Steinberg[443]	1975	33	−	Scrotal swelling
Chica et al[444]	1978	64	+ *	Painless scrotal swelling
Chica et al[444]	1978	52	+	Scrotal swelling
Soumerai, Gleason[445]	1980	55	−	Tender scrotal mass

NI, no information; +, present; −, absent

* Bilateral

† One case of testicular involvement among 27 with extramedullary plasmacytomas

cell lesions represent extramedullary manifestations of multiple myeloma, with only eight patients showing no evidence of concurrent medullary plasma cell lesions. This number may actually be excessive by one case, because the patient reported by Eckert and Smith bears a striking resemblance to case 1 in the series of Gowing.[448,449] Among all eight (or seven) patients without evidence of multiple myeloma, the testicular plasmacytomas were associated with other extramedullary plasmacytomas in the CNS, nasopharynx, stomach, lymph nodes or contralateral testis, or retroperitoneal or thigh soft tissues (see Table 6-18). A testicular plasmacytoma, unassociated with either evidence of multiple myeloma or other extramedullary plasmacytomas, is yet to be reported.

The patients range in age from 26 years to 81 years, with 75% in the fifth to seventh decades. Approximately 30% of reported cases show bilateral involvement. Clinical presentations reflect scrotal swelling either alone or in association with systemic manifestations of the more diffuse underlying process, multiple myeloma. Among patients determined to have multiple myeloma with extramedullary testicular involvement, the longest known survival was 21 months, and the majority of patients died within 12 months. The longest survival among those patients with testicular plasmacytomas varies significantly among the reported cases. The tumors are pink to tan, firm, ill-defined or discrete nodules on the cut surface of the testis. There may be a single nodule or clustered smaller nodules, which show no hemorrhage, necrosis, or cyst formation.

Microscopically, the hallmark is an infiltration of immature plasma cells, primarily within the testicular interstitium. The seminiferous tubules are compressed by the infiltration. Invasion of the tubules, vessels, and tunica albuginea is not uncommon. The homogeneity of the cell population — plasma cells — in the absence of associated histiocytes, lymphocytes, and neutrophils allows distinction from inflammatory processes. The invasive features and cytologic immaturity of the plasma cells further identifies the lesion as neoplastic. Soumerai and Gleason suggested using immunoperoxidase staining for immunoglobins to assist in differentiating plasmacytomas from plasma cell granulomas.[445] Evidence of multiple myeloma in bone marrow biopsies, and serum electrophoresis should be evaluated in patients with testicular plasmacytomas. Patients should be closely observed for subsequent development of other extramedullary plasmacytomas.

Lymphoma

Lymphomatous infiltration of the testis was first reported by Malassez in 1877, but few reports appeared in the subsequent literature until the 1950s and 1960s.[446-452] Cohen found six examples reported in the previous decade, and described four additional cases.[447] Ecket and Smith published a series of 34 new cases, and shortly thereafter, Gowing collected 50 previously reported cases.[448,449] Lymphomatous involvement of the testis has been reported with increasing frequency ever since.[451-463]

The question of the existence of a primary lymphoma of the testis emerged in the earliest literature on the subject.[482] The majority of patients initially presenting with lymphomatous involvement of the testis demonstrated systemic dissemination in subsequent months.[454,455,460] This evolution suggested the testicular involvement in these uncommon cases represented only the initial manifestation of an occult systemic lymphoma.[449,453] In the majority of cases of malignant lymphoma, testicular involvement occurs only as a late manifestation of the disseminated disease in approximately 20% of cases, as noted at autopsy.[452] However, patients with malignant lymphoma presenting as a testicular mass who survived 5 years subsequent to an orchiectomy without evidence of recurrence in a nontesticular site continue to be reported. This strongly supports the existence of primary malignant lymphoma of the testis.[454] Such cases are rare and only recently have prognostically important morphologic features been reported.[461-463]

Lymphomatous involvement of the testis has been reported in all age groups; however, 80% occur in men older than 50 years.[449,462,463] Above the age of 60 years, malignant lymphoma is the most common malignant tumor of the testis.[451] The patients present with testicular enlargement, with or without evidence of systemic involvement. Bilateral involvement, either synchronous or asynchronous, is common.[449,461] Staging procedures, including liver and spleen scans, abdominal computed tomography (CT) scans, bone marrow biopsies, and staging laparotomies detect significant numbers of patients who have higher stage lymphoma than is otherwise apparent.[456]

Testicular involvement by malignant lymphoma is virtually limited to non-Hodgkin's lymphoma, with only rare cases of Hodgkin's disease found in the literature.[454] The most frequent histologic variety of non-Hodgkin's lymphoma involving the testis is reticulum cell sarcoma, diffuse histiocytic lymphoma (DHL), or large cell, non-cleaved type, depending on one's taxonomic preference — the Rappaport system, or the Working Formulation of non-Hodgkin's lymphoma.[450,460,462-464] Less frequently, immunoblastic lymphoma, lymphoblastic lymphoma, and large cell, cleaved type lymphomas are observed.[462] Nodular pattern is distinctly rare.[463] The staging protocol for malignant lym-

---

Table 6-9   *Staging Protocol for Malignant Lymphoma*

Stage I

Involvement of single lymph node region (I), or a single extralymphatic organ or site (I_E)

Stage II

Involvement of two or more lymph node regions on same side of diaphragm (II), or an extra lymphatic organ or site of one or more lymph node regions on same side of diaphragm (II_E)

Stage III

Involvement of lymph node regions on both sides of diaphragm (III), which may be accompanied by localized involvement of extralymphatic organ or site (III_E), or by involvement of spleen (III_S), or both (III_{E+S})

Stage IV

Disseminated involvement of one or more extralymphatic organs, with or without associated lymph node involvement. Specific sites are identified as follows: pulmonary, PUL; osseous, OSS; hepatic, HEP; brain, BRA; lymph nodes, LYM; bone marrow, MAR; pleura, PLE; skin, SKI; eye, EYE; other, OTH.

Systemic Symptoms

All cases are further subdivided into "A" and "B" categories depending on absence (A) or presence (B) of systemic symptoms.

(American Joint Committee on Cancer: Manual for Staging of Cancer, 2nd ed, p 227. Philadelphia, JB Lippincott, 1983)

(Carbone PT, Rappaport H, Rosenberg SA et al: Symposium (Ann Arbor): staging in Hodgkin's disease. Cancer Res 31:1707, 1971)

phomas is presented in Table 6-9. The most favorable prognosis is associated with the intermediate grade lymphomas that retain stage IE for 2 years following diagnosis.[462] The survival rate of the majority of patients with lymphomatous involvement of the testis is low, with exceptional cases surviving 5 years without evidence of systemic dissemination.[462] These few patients constitute the group of primary testicular lymphomas. Undoubtedly, other patients, who failed to survive 5 years, may represent dissemination from a testicular primary site.

Pathologic Features

The testis is enlarged, with tumors measuring up to 16 cm reported.[453] Epididymal involvement may be grossly apparent. The cut surface reveals diffuse testicular involvement, or less commonly, multiple nodules within the enlarged testis. Focal hemorrhage and necrosis may alter the otherwise uniform gray or pink-tan lymphomatous tissue. Microscopically, a diffuse infiltration of neoplastic lymphocytes is present in the interstitium with compression, destruction, separation, and infiltration of the seminiferous tubules (Fig. 6-41). Invasion of the tunica albuginea and intratesticular vessels is common. The cytologic features of the malignant infiltrate forms the basis of histologic subclassification in this extranodal site.

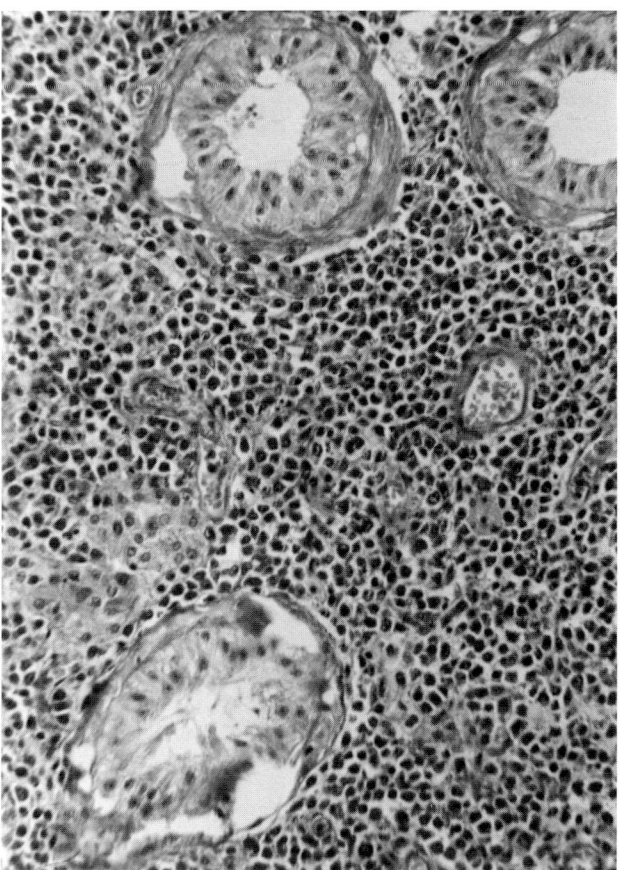

Figure 6-41   *Malignant lymphoma of the testis. The lymphoma cells infiltrate the interstitium. The tubules evidence decreased spermatogenesis.*

The differential diagnosis includes primary testicular germ cell tumor, especially seminomas, which bear a superficial resemblance to poorly differentiated lymphomas involving the testis (refer to discussion of seminoma in this chapter).

Leukemia

Leukemia infiltration of the testis at autopsy is common, with reported frequencies of 64% to 92%.[452,467] Clinically apparent testicular involvement is less frequent, but not uncommon, with reports of 5% to 16% observed.[467,469] Initial presentation of leukemia manifesting as a testicular swelling is distinctly rare, but has been reported.[449,466]

Of greatest clinical concern is the apparent increasing frequency of testicular relapse of leukemias in children following therapy-induced remissions.[465] Testicular relapse has occurred as the first extramedullary relapse at an isolated site, or alternatively, in association with marrow and CNS relapse.[467-469] Leukemic relapses may be unilateral or bilateral, and when occurring in the testis are treated effectively with radiation.[467] Prophylactic radiation has been reported to decrease the testicular relapse rate.[469]

Pathologic Features

The testis is variably enlarged, and the cut surface bulges above the confining tunica albuginea. The infiltrate tends to involve the entire testis uniformly, but ill-defined nodules have been observed in which the seminiferous tubules are apparently absent. The prominent microscopic finding is the diffuse interstitial infiltrate of leukemic cells tending to displace and occasionally invade the seminiferous tubules. The testicular vessel walls and the tunica albuginea typically are infiltrated. The vessels, and less commonly, the seminiferous tubules, show a targeting effect with a concentric layering of leukemic cells around these structures. The compressed seminiferous tubules are atrophic, with reduction of germ cells. Tubules lined exclusively by Sertoli cells are common. Prior radiation therapy consistently produces stromal fibrosis, and undoubtedly, further atrophic changes in the seminiferous tubules.

The diagnosis of leukemic infiltration of the testis generally poses no problem in the clinical context of a known leukemia. In the absence of clinical evidence of an established leukemia, the diagnosis of seminoma has been rendered in the past.[466]

In the clinical evolution of leukemia, testicular relapse is commonly followed within weeks to months by bone marrow relapse.[467-469]

Metastatic Tumors

Metastatic tumors to the testis are uncommon, with a total of 184 reported cases found in the literature (Table 6-10).[470-515] The most common primary sites of metastases to the testis are prostate, lung, malignant melanoma, colon (including rectum), and kidney, in order of decreasing frequency. Malignancies from these sites constitute 80% of testicular metastases. Rare examples of other primary tumors have been observed to disseminate to the testis on occasion, as indicated in the table. Additional examples of systemic disseminated malignancies involving the testis have been discussed previously with plasmacytoma, leukemia, and lymphoma. (Refer also to metastatic tumors of the epididymis and cord, discussed in Chap. 7.)

In the majority of reported cases, metastases to the testis are a late manifestation of a widely disseminated malignancy detected clinically by swelling of the scrotal contents, or diagnosed at autopsy. Bilateral involvement of the testes is observed in about 15% of the reported cases. Rarely, the initial manifestation of an occult malignancy is a metastasis to the testis, 11 examples of which have been found in the literature (Table 6-11). The diagnostic challenge posed by such a presentation is evident from 9 of these 11 cases, 4 of which were initially interpreted as primary testicular malignancies.

Table 6-10   Distribution of Primary Sites of Metastatic Tumors in Testis

Primary Site	Reported Cases		References
	Number	%	
Prostate	59	32	417a, 476, 485, 487–489, 496, 498, 499, 501–503, 507, 509, 513
Lung	33	18	417a, 485, 502, 504, 505, 509
Melanoma	23	12	417a, 471–474, 493, 501, 502, 504, 509
Colon, rectum	17	9	417a, 480, 485, 486, 490, 495, 501, 504, 508, 511
Bladder	7	4	417a, 470, 485, 502, 504, 514
Kidney	14	8	477, 485, 492, 501, 502, 504, 506
Pancreas	6	3	485, 504, 512, 515
Stomach	9	5	478, 479, 485, 491, 494, 500
Others	16	9	475, 478, 481–484, 497, 510

Table 6-11   Testicular Metastases as Initial Presentation of Occult Nongonadal Malignancies

Author(s)	Year	Age	Primary Site	Initial Pathological Diagnosis
Bandler, Roen[477]	1946	47	Kidney	Interstitial cell tumor
London, Grossman[478]	1949	38	Stomach	Embryonal carcinoma
Dockerty, Scheifley[409]	1955	35	Undetermined*	Interstitial cell tumor
Price, Mostofi[485]	1957	54	Prostate	No information
Price, Mostofi[485]	1957	58	Prostate	No information
Kemble[411]	1968	63	Ileum	Primary carcinoid
Talerman, Kniestedt[506]	1974	68	Kidney	Metastatic renal cell carcinoma
Moore et al[511]	1982	61	Colon (cecum)	Metastatic adenocarcinoma
Werth et al[512]	1982	34	Pancreas	Metastatic adenocarcinoma
Haupt et al[515]	1984	34	Pancreas	Metastatic adenocarcinoma
Haupt et al[515]	1984	48	Unknown	Metastatic carcinoma

* Abdominal carcinomatosis at autopsy 14 years after orchiectomy

The ages of the reported patients reflect those most commonly observed with the respective primary malignancies giving origin to testicular metastases, and thus, as a group, tend to be older than the patients with primary germ cell neoplasms. Exceptions include rare cases of primary malignancies of kidney, colon, small intestine, thyroid, and pediatric neoplasms (Wilms' tumor, retinoblastoma, and neuroblastoma), all of which involved patients younger than 3 years.[501,502]

The pathologic features of metastatic malignancy in the testis are highly variable on both the gross and microscopic levels. Many cases, especially those diagnosed at autopsy, demonstrated no grossly observed lesion and are detected only at microscopic review. Clinically diagnosed testicular metastases generally are associated with testicular enlargement, and with intratesticular nodules or masses replacing the testicular parenchyma. The microscopic features vary, and reflect the site of origin of the metastasis. Examples of microscopic foci of metastatic poorly differentiated prostate carcinoma detected in orchiectomy specimens can be diagnostically challenging. Immunoperoxidase staining for PSA and PAP may be of value (refer to Chap. 8). In addition, noting the lipofuscin pigment observed in interstitial cells will assist in the differential diagnosis. Features commonly associated with metastatic lesions of the testis are predominant proliferation in the interstitium and vascular invasion. Appropriate application of stains for epithelial mucin and immunoperoxidase stains for AFP and HCG may be helpful. Knowledge of the complete medical history is required, and frequently will focus diagnostic procedures appropriately. Testicular metastases after prolonged symptom-free intervals have been recorded.

The route of dissemination of metastatic tumors in the testis has been the focus of much discussion in the pertinent literature. There are four possible routes of metastases to the testis: arterial embolism; retrograde venous dissemination; retrograde lymphatic spread; and intraductal spread by means of the vas deferens.[483,501,511–514] Alternatively, transperitoneal spread by means of a congenital hydrocele may produce implantations on the tunica vaginalis with testicular invasion. The demonstration of communicating lymphatics draining the prostate, testis, and epididymis provides the anatomic basis for metastatic prostatic carcinoma within the testis.[513] Cases demonstrating luminal involvement of the vas deferens suggest that retrograde spread by this route underlies testicular metastases. Alternatively, retrograde spread of renal cell carcinomas by means of the left spermatic vein to the ipsilateral testis is possible.

References

Normal Structure

1. Johnson FP: Dissections of human seminiferous tubules. Anat Rec 59:187, 1934
2. Sniffen RC: The testis. I. The normal testis. Arch Pathol 50:259, 1950
3. Charny CW, Conston AS, Meranze DR: Development of the testis. A histologic study from birth to maturity with some notes on abnormal variations. Fertil Steril 3:461, 1952
4. de la Balze FA, Bur GE, Scarpa-Smith F et al: Elastic fibers in the tunical propria of normal and pathologic human testes. J Clin Endocrinol 14:626, 1954
5. Neville AM, Grigor KM: Structure, function and development of the human testis. In Pugh RCB (ed): Pathology of the Testis, pp 1–37. Oxford, Blackwell Scientific Publications, 1975 (Distributed by JB Lippincott)

6. Hermo L, Lalli M, Clermont Y: Arrangement of connective tissue components in the walls of seminiferous tubules of man and monkey. Am J Anat 149:433, 1977
7. Lich R Jr, Howerton LW, Amin A: Anatomy and surgical approach to the urogenital tract in the male. In Harrison JH, Gittes RF, Perlmutter AD et al (eds): Urology, Vol 1, 4th ed, pp 3–33. Philadelphia, WB Saunders, 1978
8. Wilson JD: Embryology of the genital tract. In Harrison JH, Gittes RF, Perlmutter AD et al (eds): Urology, Vol 2, 4th ed, pp 1469–1483. Philadelphia, WB Saunders, 1979
9. Backhouse KM: Embryology of the normal and cryptorchid testis. In Fonkalsrud EW, Mengel W (eds): The Undescended Testis, pp 5–29. Chicago, Year Book Medical Publishers, 1981
10. Mengel W, Wronecki K, Zimmermann FA: Comparison of the morphology of normal and cryptorchid testes. In Fondalsrud EW, Mengel W (eds): The Undescended Testis, pp 57–74. Chicago, Year Book Medical Publishers, 1981

Congenital Disorders

Polyorchidism

11. Hakami M, Mosavy SH: Triorchidism with normal spermatogenesis: An unusual cause for failure of vasectomy. Br J Surg 62:633, 1975
12. Mehan DJ, Chehval MJ, Ullah S: Polyorchidism. J Urol 116:530, 1976
13. Pelander WM, Luna G, Lilly JR: Polyorchidism: Case report and literature review. J Urol 119:705, 1978
14. Nocks BN: Polyorchidism with normal spermatogenesis and equal sized testes: A theory of embryological development. J Urol 120:638, 1978
15. Grechi G, Zampi GC, Selli C et al: Polyorchidism and seminoma in a child. J Urol 123:291, 1980
16. Scott KWM: A case of polyorchidism with testicular teratoma. J Urol 124:930, 1980
17. Feldman S, Drach GW: Polyorchidism discovered as testicular torsion. J Urol 130:976, 1983
18. Snow BW, Tarry WF, Duckett JW: Polyorchidism: An unusual case. J Urol 133:48, 1985

Cryptorchidism

19. Corbus BC, O'Connor VJ: The familial occurrence of undescended testes. Surg Gynecol Obstet 34:237, 1922
20. Campbell HE: Incidence of malignant growth of the undescended testicle. Arch Surg 44:353, 1942
21. Rea C: Histologic character of the undescended testis after puberty. Arch Surg 44:27, 1942
22. Sohval AR: Histopathology of cryptorchidism — A study based upon the comparative histology of retained and scrotal testis from birth to maturity. Am J Med 16:346, 1954
23. Gross RE, Jewett TC Jr: Surgical experiences from 1222 operations for undescended testis. JAMA 160:634, 1956
24. Scorer CG: The incidence of incomplete descent of the testicle at birth. Arch Dis Child 31:198, 1956
25. Campbell HE: The incidence of malignant growth of the undescended testicle: A reply and re-evaluation. J Urol 81:663, 1959
26. Mack WS, Scott LS, Ferguson–Smith MA et al: Ectopic testis and true undescended testis: A histological comparison. J Pathol 82:439, 1961
27. Scorer CG: The descent of the testis. Arch Dis Child 39:605, 1964
28. Hecker WC, Hienz HA: Cryptorchidism and fertility. J Pediatr Surg 2:513, 1967

29. Perrett LJ, O'Rourke O: Hereditary cryptorchidism. Med J Aust 25:1289, 1969
30. Farrington GH: Histologic observations in cryptorchidism: The congenital germinal-cell deficiency of the undescended testis. J Pediatr Surg 4:606, 1969
31. Weinberg AG, Currarino G, Stone IC Jr: Testicular microlithiasis. Arch Pathol 95:312, 1973
32. Mininberg DT, Bingol N: Chromosomal abnormalities in undescended testes. Urol 1:98, 1973
33. Mengel W, Hienz HA, Sippe WG II et al: Studies on cryptorchidism: A comparison of histological findings in the germinative epithelium before and after the second year of life. J Pediatr Surg 9:445, 1974
34. Hadziselimovic F, Herzog B, Seguchi H: Surgical correction of cryptorchism at 2 years: Electron microscopic and morphometric investigations. J Pediatr Surg 10:19, 1975
35. Lipschultz LI: Cryptorchidism in the subfertile male. Fertil Steril 27:609, 1976
36. Klugo R, Van Dyke DL, Weiss L: Cytogenic studies of cryptorchid testes. Urol 11:255, 1978
37. Nistal M, Paniagua R, Diez–Pardo JA: Testicular microlithiasis in 2 children with bilateral cryptorchidism. J Urol 121:535, 1979
38. Marshall FF, Shermeta DW: Epididymal abnormalities associated with undescended testis. J Urol 121:341, 1979
39. Martin DC: Germinal cell tumors of the testis after orchiopexy. J Urol 121:422, 1979
40. Batata MA, Whitmore WF Jr, Chu FCH et al: Cryptorchidism and testicular cancer. J Urol 124:382, 1980
41. Nistal M, Paniagua R, Diez–Pardo JA: Histologic classification of undescended testes. Hum Pathol 11:666, 1980
42. Vegni–Talluri M, Bigliardi E, Vanni MG et al: Testicular microliths: Their origin and structure. J Urol 124:105, 1980
43. Czeizel A, Erodi E, Toth J: Genetics of undescended testis. J Urol 126:528, 1981
44. Czeizel A, Erodi E, Toth J: An epidemiological study on undescended testis. J Urol 126:524, 1981
45. Mengel W, Zimmermann FA, Hecker WCH: Timing of repair for undescended testis. In Fonkalsrud EW, Mengel W (eds): The Undescended Testis, pp 170–183. Chicago, Year Book Medical Publishers, 1981
46. Martin DC: Malignancy and the undescended testis. In Fonkalsrud EW, Mengel W (eds): The Undescended Testis, pp 144–156. Chicago, Year Book Medical Publishers, 1981
47. Elder JS, Isaacs JT, Walsh PC: Androgenic sensitivity of the gubernaculum testis: Evidence for hormonal/mechanical interactions in testicular descent. J Urol 127:170, 1982
48. Fallon B, Welton M, Hawtrey C: Congenital anomalies associated with cryptorchidism. J Urol 127:91, 1982
49. Fram RJ, Garnick MB, Retik A: The spectrum of genitourinary abnormalities in patients with cryptorchidism, with emphasis on testicular carcinoma. Cancer 50:2243, 1982
50. Batata MA, Chu FCH, Hilaris BS et al: Testicular cancer in cryptorchids. Cancer 49:1023, 1982
51. Jones IRG, Young ID: Familial incidence of cryptorchidism. J Urol 127:508, 1982
52. Yunis, NS, Petersen RO, Rathauser F: Bilateral testicular biopsies in the study of cryptorchidism. In Brooks BJ (ed): Controversies in Pediatric Surgery, pp 8–24. Austin, Univ Texas Press, 1983
53. Muller J, Skakkebaek NE: Abnormal germ cells in maldescended testes: A study of cell density, nuclear size and deoxyribonucleic acid content in testicular biopsies from 50 boys. J Urol 13:730, 1984

54. Muller J, Skakkebaek NE, Nielsen OH et al: Cryptorchidism and testis cancer. Cancer 54:629, 1984

55. Savion M, Nissenkorn I, Servadio C et al: Familial occurrence of undescended testes. Urol 23:355, 1984

56. Gaudio E, Paggiarino D, Carpino F: Structural and ultrastructural modifications of cryptorchid human testes. J Urol 131:292, 1984

Splenic – Gonadal Fusion

57. Putschar WGJ, Manion WC: Splenic-gonadal fusion. Am J Pathol 32:15, 1956

58. Mendez R, Morrow JW: Ectopic spleen simulating testicular tumor. J Urol 102:598, 1969

59. Pendse AK, Mathur PN, Sharma MM et al: Splenic-gonadal fusion. Br J Surg 62:624, 1975

60. Halvorsen JF, Stray O: Splenogonadal fusion. Acta Paediatr Scand 67:379, 1978

61. Falkowski WS, Carter MF: Splenogonadal fusion associated with an anaplastic seminoma. J Urol 124:562, 1980

62. Ceccacci L, Tosi S: Splenic-gonadal fusion: Case report and review of the literature. J Urol 126:558, 1981

63. Loomis KF, Moore GW, Hutchins GM: Unusual cardiac malformations in splenogonadal fusion — peromelia syndrome: Relationship to normal development. Teratology 25:1, 1982

64. Mandell GA, Heyman S, Alavi A et al: A cause of microgastria in association with splenic-gonadal fusion. Pediatr Radiol 13:95, 1983

65. Andrews RW, Copeland DD, Fried FA: Splenogonadal fusion. J Urol 133:1052, 1985

Disorders of Sexual Differentiation

66. Federman DD: Abnormal sexual development; a genetic and endocrine approach to differential diagnosis. Philadelphia, WB Saunders, 1967

67. Allen TD: Disorders of sexual differentiation. Urol 7:1, 1976

68. Wilson JD, Walsh PC: Disorders of sexual differentiation. In Harrison JH, Gittes RF, Stamey TA et al (eds): Urology. 4th ed, pp 1484–1532. Philadelphia, WB Saunders, 1979

69. Scully RE: Tumors of the ovary and maldeveloped gonads. In Atlas of Tumor Pathology, 2nd series, Fascicle 16. Washington, DC, AFIP, 1979

Gonadal Dysgenesis

70. Turner HH: A syndrome of infantilism, congenital webbed neck, and cubitus valgus. Endocrinology 23:566, 1938

71. Ferguson – Smith MA: Karyotype-phenotype correlations in gonadal dysgenesis and their bearing on the pathogenesis of malformations. J Med Genet 2:142, 1965

72. Weiss L: Additional evidence of gradual loss of germ cells in the pathogenesis of streak ovaries in Turner's syndrome. J Med Genet 8:540, 1971

Mixed Gonadal Dysgenesis

73. Sohval AR: "Mixed" gonadal dysgenesis: A variety of hermaphroditism. Am J Hum Genet 15:155, 1963

74. Zourlas PA, Jones HW Jr: Clinical, histologic, and cytogenetic findings in male hermaphroditism. III. Male hermaphrodites with asymmetrical gonadal differentiation (mixed gonadal dysgenesis). Obstet Gynecol 26:48, 1965

75. Brosman SA: Mixed gonadal dysgenesis. J Urol 121:344, 1979

76. Robboy SJ, Miller T, Donahoe PK et al: Dysgenesis of testicular and streak gonads in the syndrome of mixed gonadal dysgenesis: Perspective derived from a clinicopathologic analysis of twenty-one cases. Hum Pathol 13:700, 1982

True Hermaphrodite

77. Jones HW, Ferguson–Smith MA, Heller RH: Pathologic and cytogenic findings in true hermaphroditism report of 6 cases and review of 23 cases from the literature. Obstet Gynecol 25:435, 1965
78. Butler LJ, Snodgrass GJAI, France NE et al: True hermaphroditism or gonadal intersexuality. Cytogenetic and gonadal analyses of 5 new examples related to 67 known cases studied cytogenetically. Arch Dis Child 44:666, 1969
79. van Niekerk WA: True hermaphroditism. An analytic review with a report of 3 new cases. Am J Obstet Gynecol 126:890, 1976
80. Roth LM, Cleary RE, Hokum WL: Ultrastructure of an ovotestis in a case of true hermaphroditism. Obstet Gynecol 48:619, 1976

Pure Gonadal Dysgenesis

81. Sohval AR: The syndrome of pure gonadal dysgenesis. Am J Med 38:615, 1965
82. Espiner EA, Veale AMO, Sands VE et al: Familial syndrome of streak gonads and normal male karyotype in five phenotypic females. N Engl J Med 283:6, 1970

Male and Female Pseudohermaphroditism

83. Morris JM: The syndrome of testicular feminization in pseudohermaphrodites. Am J Obstet Gynecol 65:1192, 1953
84. Bongiovanni AM: The adrenogenital syndrome with deficiency of 3B-hydroxysteroid dehydrogenase. J Clin Invest 41:2086, 1962
85. Morris JMcL: Further observations on the syndrome, "testicular feminization." Am J Obstet Gynecol 87:731, 1963
86. Biglieri EG, Herron MA, Brust N: 17-hydroxylation deficiency in man. J Clin Invest 45:1946, 1966
87. Binns JH, Cross RM: Hernia uteri inguinalis in a male. Br J Surg 54:571, 1967
88. Camacho AM, Kowarski A, Migeon CJ et al: Congenital adrenal hyperplasia due to a deficiency of one of the enzymes involved in the biosynthesis of pregnenolone. J Clin Endocrinol 28:153, 1968
89. Zachmann M, Vollmin, JA, Hamilton W et al: Steroid 17, 20-desmolase deficiency: A new cause of male pseudohermaphroditism. Clin Endocrinol (Oxf) 1:369, 1972
90. Brook CGD, Wagner H, Zachmann M et al: Familial occurrence of persistent Mullerian structure in otherwise normal males. Br Med J 1:771, 1973
91. Keenan BS, Meyer WJ III, Hadjian AJ et al: Syndrome of androgen insensitivity in man: Absence of 5-dihydrotestosterone binding protein in skin fibroblasts. Clin Endrocinol Metab 38:1143, 1974
92. Imperato–McGinley J, Peterson RE: Male pseudohermaphroditism: The complexities of male phenotypic development. Am J Med 61:251, 1976

Infertility

93. Charney CW: Testicular biopsy. Its value in male sterility. JAMA 115:1429, 1940
94. Engle ET: The testis biopsy in infertility. J Urol 57:789, 1947
95. del Castillo EB, Trabucco A, de la Balze FA: Syndrome produced by absence of the germinal epithelium without impairment of the Sertoli or Leydig cells. J Clin Endocrinol 7:493, 1947
96. Howard RP, Sniffen RC, Simmons FA et al: Testicular deficiency: A clinical and pathologic study. J Clin Endocrinol 10:121, 1950
97. Heller CG, Nelson WO, Hill IB et al: Improvement in spermatogenesis following depression of the human testis with testosterone. Fertil Steril 1:415, 1950
98. Sniffen RC, Howard RP, Simmons FA: The testis. III. Absence of germ cells; sclerosing tubular degeneration; "male climacteric." Arch Pathol 51:293, 1951

99. Landau RL: Hypogonadism with spermatogenesis: A case report. J Clin Endocrinol Metab 13:510, 1953

100. McCullugh EP, Beck JC, Schaffenburg CA: A syndrome of eunuchoidism with spermatogenesis, normal urinary FSH and low or normal ICSH: ("fertile eunuchs"). J Clin Endocrinol Metab 13:489, 1953

101. Nelson WO: Interpretation of testicular biopsy. JAMA 151:449, 1953

102. Sniffen RC, Howard RP, Simmons FA: The testis. IV. Idiopathic eunochoidism with low FSH; testicular changes secondary to lesions in or near the pituitary and secondary to estrogen therapy. Arch Pathol 57:464, 1954

103. de la Balze FA, Gurtman AI, Janches M et al: Effects of estrogens on the adult human testes, with special reference to the germinal epithelium: A histologic study. J Clin Endocrinol 22:1251, 1962

104. Amelar RD: In Heaton CE (ed): Infertility in Men. Diagnosis and Treatment. Philadelphia, FA Davis, 1966

105. Mancini RE, Lavieri JC, Muller F et al: Effect of prednisolone upon normal and pathologic human spermatogenesis. Fertil Steril 17:500, 1966

106. Kaplan E, Shwachman H, Perlmutter AD et al: Reproductive failure in males with cystic fibrosis. N Engl J Med 279:65, 1968

107. Dubin L, Hotchkiss RS: Testis biopsy in subfertile men with varicocele. Fertil Steril 20:50, 1969

108. Girgis SAM, Etriby A, Ibrahim AA et al: Testicular biopsy in azoospermia. A review of the last ten years' experience of over 800 cases. Fertil Steril 20:467, 1969

109. Richter P, Camalera JC, Morgenfild MC et al: Effect of chlorambucil on spermatogenesis in the human with malignant lymphoma. Cancer 25:1026, 1970

110. Bishop MWH: Ageing and reproduction in the male. J Reprod Fertil (Suppl)12:65, 1970

111. Clark WH Jr: Introduction to the study of disorders of the recently deceased. Philadelphia, Pathology Lecture Series, September, 1973

112. Wong T–W, Strauss FH II, Warner NE: Testicular biopsy in the study of male infertility. I. Testicular causes of infertility. Arch Pathol 95:151, 1973

113. Wong T–W, Strauss FH II, Warner NE: Testicular biopsy in the study of male infertility. II. Posttesticular causes of infertility. Arch Pathol 95:160, 1973

114. Meinhard E, McRae CU, Chisholm GD: Testicular biopsy in evaluation of male infertility. Br Med J 2:578, 1973

115. Wong T–W, Straus FH II, Warner NE: Testicular biopsy in the study of male infertility. III. Pretesticular causes of infertility. Arch Pathol 98:1, 1974

116. Derrick FC Jr, Glover WL, Kanjuparamban Z et al: Histological changes in the seminiferous tubules after vasectomy. Fertil Steril 25:649, 1974

117. Craig JM: The pathology of infertility. Pathobiol Ann 10:299, 1975

118. Sieber SM, Adamson RH: Toxicity of antineoplastic agents in man: Chromosomal aberrations, antifertility effects, congenital malformations, and carcinogenic potential. Adv Cancer Res 22:57, 1975

119. Scott R, Rourke A, Yates A et al: The results of 100 small tissue biopsies of testes in male infertile patients. Postgrad Med J 52:693, 1976

120. Lipschultz LI, Corriere JN Jr: Progressive testicular atrophy in the varicocele patient. J Urol 117:175, 1977

121. Sherin RJ, Howards SS: Male infertility. In Harrison JH, Gittes RF, Perlmutter AD et al: Urology, 4th ed, pp 715–776. Philadelphia, WB Saunders, 1978

122. Levin HS: Testicular biopsy in the study of male infertility. Its current usefulness, histologic techniques, and prospects for the future. Hum Pathol 10:569, 1979

123. Boiesen PT, Lindholm J, Hagen C et al: Histological changes in testicular biopsies from chronic alcoholics with and without liver disease. Acta Pathol Microbiol Immunol Scand A 87:139, 1979

124. Soderstrom K–O, Suominen J: Human hypospermatogenesis. Arch Pathol Lab Med 106:231, 1982

Klinefelter's Disease

125. Klinefelter JF Jr, Reifenstein EC Jr, Albright F: Clinical endocrinology. Syndrome characterized by gynecomastia, aspermatogenesis without A-leydigism and increased excretion of follicle-stimulating hormone. J Clin Endocrinol 2:615, 1942
126. Ferguson–Smith MA: Chromatin-positive Klinefelter's syndrome (primary microorchidism) in a mental-deficiency hospital. Lancet 1:928, 1958
127. Ferguson–Smith MA: The prepubertal testicular lesion in chromatin-positive Klinefelter's syndrome (primary micro-orchidism) as seen in mentally handicapped children. Lancet 1:219, 1959
128. Atkins L, Connelly JP: XXXXY sex-chromosome abnormality. Am J Dis Child 106:514, 1963
129. MacLean N, Harnden DG, Bond J et al: Sex-chromosome abnormalities in newborn babies. Lancet 1:286, 1964
130. Barr ML: The natural history of Klinefelter's syndrome. Fertil Steril 17:429, 1966
131. Paulsen CA, Gorden DL, Carpenter RW et al: Klinefelter's syndrome and its variants: A hormonal and chromosomal study. Recent Prog Horm Res 24:321, 1968
132. Gordon DL, Krmpotic E, Thomas W et al: Pathologic testicular findings in Klinefelter's syndrome. Arch Intern Med 130:726, 1972

Inflammatory Disorders

Mumps

133. Gall EA: The histopathology of acute mumps orchitis. Am J Pathol 23:637, 1947
134. Charny CW, Meranze DR: Pathology of mumps orchitis. J Urol 60:140, 1948
135. Candel S: Epididymitis in mumps, including orchitis: Further clinical studies and comments. An Intern Med 34:20, 1951
136. Ballew JW, Masters WH: Mumps: A cause of infertility. I. Present considerations. Fertil Steril 5:536, 1954
137. Scott LS: Mumps and male fertility. Br J Urol 32:183, 1960

Other Inflammatory Disorders

138. Grobert MJ, Bischoff AJ: Actinomycosis of the testicle: Case report. J Urol 87:567, 1962
139. Hourihane DO'B: Infected infarcts of the testis: A study of 18 cases preceded by pyogenic epididymoorchitis. J Clin Pathol 23:668, 1970
140. Pugh JI, Stringer P: Glove-powder granuloma of the testis after surgery. Br J Surg 60:240, 1973
141. Opal SM, Pittman DL, Hofeldt FD: Testicular sarcoidosis. Am J Med 67:147, 1979
142. Lin JI, Tseng CH, Marsidi PJ et al: Cholesterol granuloma of right testis. Urol 14:522, 1979
143. Akhtar M, Ali MA, Mackey DM: Lepromatous leprosy presenting as orchitis. Am Soc Clin Pathol 73:712, 1980
144. Riehle RA Jr, Jayaraman K: Tuberculosis of testis. Urol 20:43, 1982
145. Mikuz G, Damjanov I: Inflammation of the testis, epididymis, peritesticular membranes, and scrotum. In Sommers SC, Rosen PP (eds): Pathology Annual, Part I, Vol 17, pp 101–128, 1982
146. Weber TR: Hemophilus influenzae epididymo-orchitis. J Urol 133:487, 1985

Granulomatous Orchitis

147. Grunberg H: Uber drei ungewohnliche falle von chronischer orchitis unter dem klinischen bilde eines hodentumors. Frankfurt Z Path 33:217, 1926
148. Friedman NB, Garske GL: Inflammatory reactions involving sperm and the seminiferous tubules: Extravasation, spermatic granulomas and granulomatous orchitis. J Urol 62:363, 1949

149. Lee WR, Nettleship A: A granuloma of the testis of unknown etiology. J Urol 67:342, 1952
150. Dreyfuss W: Acute granulomatous orchiditis. J Urol 71:483, 1954
151. Berg JW: An acid-fast lipid from spermatozoa. Arch Pathol 57:115, 1954
152. Spjut HJ, Thorpe JD: Granulomatous orchitis. Am J Clin Pathol 26:136, 1956
153. Taylor JBL: Spermatic granuloma. Br J Urol 31:196, 1959
154. Hubsmith RJ, Garret R, Photos C: Granulomatous orchitis and epididymitis. J Urol 81:301, 1959
155. Capers TH: Granulomatous orchitis with sperm granuloma of epididymis: A case report. J Urol 87:705, 1962
156. Fajardo LF, Dueker GE, Kosek JC: Light and electron microscopic observations on granulomatous orchitis. Invest Urol 6:158, 1968
157. Lynch VP, Eakins D, Morrison E: Granulomatous orchitis. Br J Urol 40:451, 1968
158. Elicker ER, Evans AT: Granulomatous orchitis. J Urol 113:199, 1975
159. Mazzolli AB, Bustuoabad OD, Barrera C, Mancini RE: A new model for antisperm autoimmunity in guinea pigs. Int J Fertil 21:49, 1976
160. Fauer RB, Goldstein AMB, Green JC, Onofrio R: Clinical aspects of granulomatous orchitis. Urol 12:416, 1978
161. Kahn RI, McAninch JW: Granulomatous disease of the testis. J Urol 123:868, 1980
162. Sporer A, Seebode JJ: Granulomatous orchitis. Urol 19:319, 1982

Malakoplakia

163. Haukohl RS, Chinchinian H: Malakoplakia of the testicle. Report of a case. Am J Clin Pathol 29:473, 1958
164. Blackwell JB, Finley–Jones LR: Malakoplakia of the testis. J Path Bacteriol 78:571, 1959
165. Beskid M, Gawlik Z: Granuloma histiocyticum prostate et testis. Extravesikale lokalisation der malakoplakie. Virchows Arch [A] 339:304, 1965
166. Brown RC, Smith BH: Malacoplakia of the testis. Am J Clin Pathol 47:135, 1967
167. Waisman J, Rampton JB: Malakoplakia of the testis and epididymis. Arch Pathol 86:431, 1968
168. Shaba JK, Black WA: Malacoplakic granuloma of the testis. J Urol 105:687, 1971
169. Tamura H, Iannotti HM: Ultrastructure of Michaelis–Gutmann body. A study of a case of testicular malacoplakia. Arch Pathol 98:409, 1974
170. Csapo Z, Gervain M: A here malakoplakiaja. Orv Hetil 115:87, 1974
171. Dionne GP, Bovill EG, Seemayer TA: New fine structural observations in testicular malakoplakia. Urol 5:828, 1975
172. Rinaudo P, Damjanov I, Stoesser B: Malacoplakia of testis. Int Urol Nephrol 9:249, 1977
173. McClure J, Hadden DR, Mudd DG et al: Adrenocortical hyperactivity with disseminated malacoplakia. J Clin Pathol 30:206, 1977
174. McClure J: Malakoplakia of the testis and its relationship to granulomatous orchitis. J Clin Pathol 33:670, 1980
175. Gonzalez RD, Leiva O, Palacios JJN et al: Testicular malacoplakia. J Urol 127:325, 1982
176. Paquin F, Schick E, Parent C: Malakoplakia of testis. Urol 21:194, 1983
177. Kleinman SZ, Robinson ND, Simon SA: Malakoplakia of testis. Urol 22:194, 1983
178. Saraf P, diSant'Agnese P, Valvo J et al: An unusual case of malacoplakia involving the testis and prostate. J Urol 129:149, 1983

Cysts

Epidermoid Cysts

179. Dockerty MB, Priestley JT: Dermoid cysts of the testis. J Urol 48:392, 1942
180. Halley JBW: Epidermoid cyst of the testicle. J Pathol Bacteriol 82:73, 1961

181. Price EB Jr: Epidermoid cysts of the testis: A clinical and pathologic analysis of 69 cases from the testicular tumor registry. J Urol 102:708, 1969
182. Price EB Jr, Mostofi FK: Epidermoid cysts of the testis in children. A report of four cases. J Pediatr 7:676, 1970
183. Strahlberg M, Brown JS: Concomitant bilateral epidermoid cysts of the testes. J Urol 109:434, 1973
184. Gonzalez BL, Ross LS: Epidermoid cysts of testis. Urol 9:456, 1977
185. Goli VR, Shepherd RR, Hayman WP et al: Epidermoid cyst of the testes. J Urol 123:129, 1980
186. Goldstein AMB, Mendez R, Vargas A et al: Epidermoid cysts of testis. Urol 15:186, 1980
187. Shah KH, Maxted WC, Chun B: Epidermoid cysts of the testis: A report of three cases and an analysis of 141 cases from the world literature. Cancer 47:577, 1981
188. Bates RJ, Perrone TL, Althausen A: Simple epidermoid cysts of testis. Urol 17:560, 1981
189. Rao KG, Lorimer A: Epidermoid cyst of testis: Benign intratesticular tumor. Urol 19:662, 1982
190. Nichols J, Kandzari S, Elyaderani MK et al: Epidermoid cyst of testis: A report of 3 cases. J Urol 133:286, 1985

Simple Cysts

191. Jenkins RH, Deming CL: Cysts of the testicle. N Engl J Med 213:57, 1935
192. Schmidt SS: Congenital simple cyst of the testis: A hitherto undescribed lesion. J Urol 96:236, 1966
193. Tosi SE, Richardson JR Jr: Simple cyst of the testis: Case report and review of the literature. J Urol 114:473, 1975
194. Takihara H, Valvo JR, Tokuhara M et al: Intratesticular cysts. Urol 20:80, 1982
195. Leissring JC, Oppenheimer ROF: Cystic dysplasia of the testis: A unique congenital anomaly studied by microdissection. J Urol 110:362, 1973

Neoplasms

196. Askanazy M: Die teratome nach ihrem bau, ihrem verlauf, ihrer genese und im vergleich zum experimentallen teratoid. Verh Dtsch Pathol Ges 11:39, 1907
197. Masson P: Etude sur le seminome. Rev Ana Biol 5:361, 1946
198. Sauer HR, Watson EM, Burke EM: Tumors of the testicle. Surg Gynecol Obstet 86:591, 1948
199. Dixon FJ, Moore RA: Testicular tumors. A clinicopathological study. Cancer 6:427, 1953
200. Stevens LC, Hummel KPA: A description of spontaneous congenital testicular teratomas in strain 129 mice. J Natl Cancer Inst 18:719, 1957
201. Teoh TB, Steward JK, Willis RA: The distinctive endocarcinoma of the infant's testis: An account of 15 cases. J Pathol Bacteriol 80:147, 1960
202. Pugh RCB, Smith JP: Teratoma. Br J Urol (Suppl)36:28, 1964
203. Kleinsmith LJ, Pierce GB Jr: Multipotentiality of single embryonal carcinoma cells. Cancer Res 24:1544, 1964
204. Phalakornkule S, Woodrudd MW: Extragonadal retroperitoneal seminoma. J Urol 91:579, 1964
205. Abell MR, Fayos JV, Lampe I: Retroperitoneal germinomas (seminomas) without evidence of testicular involvement. Cancer 18:273, 1965
206. Abelev GI, Assecritova IV, Kraevsky NA et al: Embryonal serum-globulin in cancer patients: Diagnostic value. Int J Cancer 2:551, 1967
207. Stevens LC: Origin of testicular teratomas from primordial germ cells in mice. J Natl Cancer Inst 38:549, 1967
208. Willis RA: The teratoma. In Pathology of Tumours, 4th ed, pp 959–1003. New York, Appleton–Century–Crofts, 1967
209. Pierce GB Jr, Abell MA: Embryonal carcinoma of the testis. Pathology Annual,

Sheldon C Sommers, Series ed, pp. 27–60. New York, Appleton–Century–Crofts, 1970

210. Meares EM Jr, Briggs EM: Occult seminoma of the testis masquerading as primary extragonadal germinal neoplasms. Cancer 30:300, 1972

211. Skakkebaek NE: Possible carcinoma-in-situ of the testis. Lancet 2:516, 1972

212. Mostofi FK: Testicular tumors. Epidemiologic, etiologic, and pathologic features. Cancer 32:1186, 1973

213. Mostofi FK, Price EB Jr: Tumors of the male genital system. In Atlas of Tumor Pathology, 2nd Series, Fascicle 8. Washington, DC, AFIP, 1973

214. Gehring GG, Rodriguez FR, Woodhead DM: Malignant degeneration of cryptorchid testes following orchiopexy. J Urol 112:354, 1974

215. Nielsen H, Nielsen M, Skakkebaek NE: The fine structure of a possible carcinoma-in-situ in the seminiferous tubules in the testis of four infertile men. Acta Pathol Microbiol Scand [A] 82:235, 1974

216. Das S, Bovhetto RJ, Alpert LI: Primary retroperitoneal seminoma. Report of a case and review of the literature. Cancer 36:595, 1975

217. Skakkebaek NE: Atypical germ cells in the adjacent "normal" tissue of testicular tumours. Acta Pathol Microbiol Scand [A] 83:127, 1975

218. Lefevre RE, Levin HS, Banowsky LH et al: Bilateral testicular tumors of germ cell origin. J Urol 114:556, 1975

219. Mintz B, Illmensee K: Normal genetically mosaic mice produced from malignant teratorcarcinoma cells. Proc Nat Acad Sci 72:3585, 1975

220. Levey S, Grabstald H: Synchronous testicular tumors in identical twins. Urol 6:754, 1975

221. Johnson DE, Appelt G, Samuels ML, Luna M: Metastases from testicular carcinoma. Study of 78 autopsied cases. Urol 8:234, 1976

222. Pugh RCB, Cameron KM: Teratoma. In Pugh RCB (ed): Pathology of the Testis, pp 199–244. Oxford, Blackwell Scientific Publications, 1976

223. Ghosh P, Jacobs H, Rattner WH: Testicular neoplasm in siblings. Urol 7:212, 1976

224. Bar W, Hedinger C: Comparison of histologic types of primary testicular germ cell tumors with their metastases. Consequences for the WHO and the British nomenclatures? Virchows Arch [A] 370:41, 1976

225. Morris SA, Vaughan ED Jr, Constable WC: Problems in management of primary bilateral germ cell testicular tumors: Report of 3 cases and review of literature. J Urol 115:566, 1976

226. Mostofi FK, Sobin LH: Histological typing of testis tumours. In International Histological Classification of Tumours, No. 16. Geneva, World Health Organization, 1977

227. Mostofi FK: Epidemiology and pathology of tumors of human testis. Recent Results Cancer Res 60:176, 1977

228. Kurman RJ, Scardino PT, McIntire KR et al: Cellular localization of alpha-fetoprotein and human chorionic gonadotropin in germ cell tumors of the testis using an indirect immunoperoxidase technique. A new approach to classification utilizing tumor markers. Cancer 40:2136, 1977

229. Lange PH, Fraley EE: Serum alpha-fetroprotein and human chorionic gonadotropin in the treatment of patients with testicular tumors. Urol Clin North Am 4:393, 1977

230. Braunstein GD, Friedman NB, Sacks SA et al: Germ cell tumors of the testes—Interdepartmental clinical case conference, University of California, Los Angeles (Specialty Conference). West J Med 126:362, 1977

231. Aristizabal S, Davis JR, Miller RC et al: Bilateral primary germ cell testicular tumors. Report of four cases and review of the literature. Cancer 42:591, 1978

232. Javadpour N: The National Cancer Institute experience with testicular cancer. J Urol 120:651, 1978

233. Krabbe S, Berthelsen JG, Volsted P et al: High incidence of undetected neoplasia in maldescended testes. Lancet 1:999, 1979

234. Akhatar M, Sidiki Y: Undifferentiated intratubular germ cell tumor of the testis. Cancer 43:2332, 1979

235. Martin DC: Germinal cell tumors of the testis after orchiopexy. J Urol 121:422, 1979

236. Talerman A, Haije WG, Baggerman L: Serum alphafetoprotein (AFP) in patients with germ cell tumors of the gonads and extragonadal sites: Correlation between endodermal sinus (yolk sac) tumor and raised serum AFP. Cancer 46:380, 1980

237. Javadpour N: Significance of elevated serum alphafetoprotein (AFP) in seminoma. Cancer 45:2166, 1980

238. Mostofi FK: Pathology of germ cell tumors of testis. A progress report. Cancer 45:1735, 1980

239. von Eyben FE, Mikulowski P, Busch C: Microinvasive germ cell tumors of the testis. J Urol 126:842, 1981

240. Daniels JL Jr, Stutzman RE, McLeod DG: A comparison of testicular tumors in black and white patients. J Urol 125:341, 1981

241. Javadpour N, Soares T: False-positive and false-negative alpha-feto protein and human chorionic gonadotropin assays in testicular cancer: A double blind study. Cancer 48:2279, 1981

242. Jacobsen GK, Jacobsen M, Clausen PP: Distribution of tumor-associated antigens in the various histologic components of germ cell tumors of the testis. Am J Surg Pathol 5:257, 1981

243. Bosl GJ, Lange PH, Nochomovitz LE et al: Tumor markers in advanced nonseminomatous testicular cancer. Cancer 47:572, 1981

244. White RDV, Karian S, Hong WK et al: Testis tumor markers: How accurate are they? J Urol 125:661, 1981

245. Skakkebaek NE, Berthelsen JG, Muller J: Carcinoma-in-situ of the undescended testis. Urol Clin North Am 9:377, 1982

246. Bredael JJ, Vugrin D, Whitmore WF Jr: Autopsy findings in 154 patients with germ cell tumors of the testis. Cancer 50:548, 1982

247. Buskirk SJ, Evans RG, Farrow GM et al: Primary retroperitoneal seminoma. Cancer 49:1934, 1982

248. Raghavan D, Sullivan AL, Peckham MJ et al: Elevated serum alphafetoprotein and seminoma. Clinical evidence for a histologic continuum? Cancer 50:982, 1982

249. Javadpour N: Natural history, diagnosis, and staging of nonseminomatous testicular cancer. In Javadpour N (ed): Principles and Management of Urologic Cancer, 2nd ed, pp 293–302. Baltimore, Williams & Wilkins, 1983

250. America Joint Committee on Cancer: Manual for Staging of Cancer, 2nd ed, p 166. Brahrs OH, Myers MH (eds). Philadelphia, JB Lippincott, 1983

251. Morrison AS, Cole P, Maclure KM: Epidemiology of urologic cancers. In Javadpour N (ed): Principles and Management of Urologic Cancer, 2nd ed, pp 12–31. Baltimore, Williams & Wilkins, 1983

252. Brawn PN: The origin of germ cell tumors of the testis. Cancer 51:1610, 1983

253. Morinaga S, Ojima M, Sasano N: Human chorionic gonadotropin and alpha-fetoprotein in testicular germ cell tumors. An immunohistochemical study in comparison with tissue concentrations. Cancer 52:1281, 1983

254. Gedde–Dahl T Jr, Hannisdal E, Klepp OH et al: Testicular neoplasms occurring in four brothers.

255. Klein FA, Melamed MR, Whitmore WF Jr: Intratubular malignant germ cells (carcinoma in situ) accompanying invasive testicular germ cell tumors. J Urol 133:413, 1985

Germ Cell Neoplasms

Seminoma, Classic Type

256. Thackray AC: Seminoma. Br J Urol 36:12, 1964

257. Pierce GB Jr: Ultrastructure of human testicular tumors. Cancer 19:1963, 1966

258. Thackray AC, Crane WAJ: Seminoma. In Pugh RCB (ed): Pathology of the Testis, pp 164–198. Oxford, Blackwell Scientific Publications, 1976

259. Johnson DE, Gomez JJ, Ayala AG: Histologic factors affecting prognosis of pure seminoma of the testis. South Med J 69:1173, 1976

260. Heyderman E, Niville AM: Syncytiotrophoblasts in malgnant testicular tumours. Lancet 2:103, 1976

261. Nochomovitz LE, DeLa Torre FE, Rosai J: Pathology of germ cell tumors of the testis. Urol Clin North Am 4:359, 1977

262. Hedinger C, von Hochstetter AR, Egloff B: Seminoma with syncytiotrophoblastic giant cells. A special form of seminoma. Virchows Arch [A] 383:59, 1979

263. Richter HJ, Leder L–D: Lymph node metastases with PAS-positive tumor cells and massive epithelioid granulomatous reaction as diagnostic clue to occult seminoma. Cancer 44:245, 1979

264. Beckstead JH: Alkaline phosphatase histochemistry in human germ cell neoplasms. Am J Surg Pathol 7:341, 1983

Seminoma, Spermatocytic Type

265. Masson P: Etude sur le seminome. Rev Can Biol 5:361, 1946

266. Martin JF, Feroldi J: Le seminome spermatocytaire. Sem Hop Paris 25:2982, 1949

267. Scully RE: Spermatocytic seminoma of the testis. A report of 3 cases and review of the literature. Cancer 14:288, 1961

268. Martinazzi M: Il seminoma spermatocitario. Arch Ital Path Clin Tumori 5:555, 1962

269. Barr WB Jr, Silberg S: A case report and review of the literature on spermatocytic seminoma of the testis. J Urol 89:464, 1963

270. Jackson JR, Magner D: Spermatocytic seminoma. A variant of seminoma with specific microscopical and clinical characteristics. Cancer 18:751, 1965

271. Giraldo G, Ribacchi R: Il seminoma spermatocitico. Lavori 1st Inst Univ Perugia 26:157, 1966

272. Mikulowski P, Szczudrawa J: Remarks on the pathology and classification of seminoma spermatocyticum. Acta Med Pol 8:129, 1967

273. Fox JE, Abell MR: Spermatocytic seminoma. J Urol 100:757, 1968

274. Rosai J, Silber I, Khodadoust K: Spermatocytic seminoma. I. Clinicopathologic study of six cases and review of the literature. Cancer 24:92, 1969

275. Rosai J, Khodadoust K, Silber I: Spermatocytic seminoma. II. Ultrastructural study. Cancer 24:103, 1969

276. Skudowitz RB, Rippey JJ, Van Blerk PJP: Spermatocytic seminoma of the testis. S Afr Med J 46:9, 1972

277. Talerman A: Spermatocytic seminoma. J Urol 112:212, 1974

278. Dymock RB: Spermatocytic seminoma. Med J Aust 2:18, 1976

279. Weitzner S: Spermatocytic seminoma. Urol 7:646, 1976

280. Schoborg TW, Whittaker J, Lewis CW: Metastatic spermatocytic seminoma. J Urol 124:739, 1980

281. Talerman A: Spermatocytic seminoma. Clinicopathological study of 22 cases. Cancer 45:2169, 1980

Seminoma, Anaplastic Type

282. Maier JG, Sulak MH, Mittemeyer BT: Seminoma of the testis: Analysis of treatment success and failure. Am J Roentgen 102:596, 1968

283. Maier JG, Mittemeyter BT, Sulak MH: Treatment and prognosis in seminoma of the testis. J Urol 99:72, 1968

284. Johnson DE, Gomez JJ, Ayala AG: Anaplastic seminoma. J Urol 114:80, 1975

285. Kademian M, Bosch A, Caldwell WL et al: Anaplastic seminoma. Cancer 40:3082, 1977

286. Janssen M, Johnston WH: Anaplastic seminoma of the testis. Cancer 41:538, 1978

287. Percarpio B, Clements JC, McLeod DG et al: Anaplastic seminoma. An analysis of 77 patients. Cancer 43:2510, 1979

Embryonal Carcinoma (Adult Type)

288. Nefzger MD, Mostofi FK: Survival after surgery for germinal malignancies of the testis. I. Rates of survival in tumor groups. Cancer 30:1225, 1972
289. Tuttle JP Jr, Pratt–Thomas JR, Thomason WB: Embryonal carcinoma of the testis in elderly men. J Urol 118:1070, 1977
290. Einhorn LH, Donohue JP, Peckham MJ et al: Cancer of the testes. In DeVita VT Jr, Hellman S, Rosenberg SA (eds): Cancer. Principles and Practice of Oncology, 2nd ed, pp 979–1011. Philadelphia, JB Lippincott, 1985

Polyembryoma

291. Evans RW: Development stages of embryo-like bodies in teratoma testis. J Clin Path 10:31, 1957
292. Simard L–C: Polyembryonic embryoma of the ovary of parthenogenetic origin. Cancer 10:215, 1957

Teratoma

293. Stevens LC: Studies on transplantable testicular teratomas of strain in 129 mice. J Natl Cancer Inst 20:1257, 1958
294. Pierce GB, Dixon FJ Jr: Testicular teratomas. I. Demonstration of teratogenesis by metamorphosis of multipotential cells. Cancer 12:573, 1959
295. Wogalter H, Scofield GF: Adult teratoma of the testicle metastasizing as adult teratoma. J Urol 87:573, 1962
296. Pugh RCB, Smith JP: Teratoma. Br J Urol (Suppl)36:28, 1964
297. Stevens LC: Origin of testicular teratomas from primordial germ cells in mice. J Nat Cancer Inst 38:549, 1967
298. Fraley EE, Ketcham AS: Teratoma of testis in an infant. J Urol 100:659, 1968
299. Mahour GHJ, Wooley MM, Trivedi SN et al: Teratomas in infancy and childhood: Experience with 81 cases. Surgery 76:309, 1974
300. Riley PA, Sutton PM: Why are ovarian teratomas benign whilst teratomas of the testis are malignant? Lancet 1:1360, 1975
301. Kedia K, Fraley EE: Adult teratoma of the testis metastasizing as adult teratoma: Case report and review of literature. J Urol 114:636, 1975
302. Hong WK, Wittes RE, Hajdu ST et al: The evolution of mature teratoma from malignant testicular tumors. Cancer 40:2987, 1977
303. Dunn D, Hertel B, Kennedy BJ: The management of mature teratoma of the testicle. J Urol 117:259, 1977

Endodermal Sinus Tumor (Yolk Sac Tumor)

304. Schiller W: Mesonephroma ovarri. Am J Cancer 35:1, 1939
305. Magner D, Campbell JS, Wiglesworth FW: Testicular adenocarcinoma with clear cells occurring in infancy. Cancer 9:165, 1956
306. Teilum G: Endodermal sinus tumors of the ovary and testis. Comparative morphogenesis of the so-called mesonephroma ovarri (Schiller) and extraembryonic (yolk sac-allantoic) structures of the rat's placenta. Cancer 12:1092, 1959
307. Teoh TB, Steward JK, Willis RA: The distinctive adenocarcinoma of the infant's testis: An account of 15 cases. J Pathol Bacteriol 80:147, 1960
308. Hodson JM, Perez–Meza C: Infantile adenocarcinoma of the testis. J Urol 89:706, 1963
309. Huntington RW Jr, Morgenstern NL, Sargent JA et al: Germinal tumors exhibiting the endodermal sinus pattern of Teilum in young children. Cancer 16:34, 1963
310. Abell MR, Holtz F: Testicular neoplasms in adolescents. Cancer 17:881, 1964

311. Houser R, Izant RJ Jr, Persky L: Testicular tumors in children. Am J Surg 110:876, 1965

312. Teilum G: Classification of endodermal sinus tumour (mesoblastoma vitellinum) and so-called "embryonal carcinoma" of the ovary. Acta Pathol Microbiol Scand [A] 64:407, 1965

313. Ravich L, Lerman PH, Drabkin JW, Noya J: Embryonal carcinoma of testicle in childhood: Review of literature and presentation of 2 cases. J Urol 96:501, 1966

314. Young PG, Mount BM, Foote FW Jr et al: Embryonal adenocarcinoma in the prepubertal testis. Cancer 26:1065, 1970

315. Pierce GB, Bullock WK, Huntington RW Jr: Yolk sac tumors of the testis. Cancer 25:644, 1970

316. Tsuchida Y, Saito S, Ishida M et al: Yolk sac tumor (endodermal sinus tumor) and alpha-fetoprotein. A report of three cases. Cancer 32:917, 1973

317. Woodtli W, Hedinger C: Endodermal sinus tumor or orchioblastoma in children and adults. Virchows Arch [A] Pathol Anat Histol 364:93, 1974

318. Talerman A: Yolk sac tumor associated with seminoma of the testis in adults. Cancer 33:1468, 1974

319. Teilum G, Albrechtsen R, Norgaard–Pedersen B: The histogenetic-embryologic basis for reappearance of alpha-fetoprotein in endodermal sinus tumors (yolk sac tumors) and teratomas. Acta Pathol Microbiol Scand [A] 83:80, 1975

320. Talerman A: The incidence of yolk sac tumor (endodermal sinus tumor) elements in germ cell tumors of the testis in adults. Cancer 36:211, 1975

321. Hart WR: Primary endodermal sinus (yolk sac) tumor of the liver. Cancer 35:1453, 1975

322. Roth LM, Panganiban WG: Gonadal and extragonadal yolk sac carcinomas. A clinicopathologic study of 14 cases. Cancer 37:812, 1976

323. Nogales–Fernandez F, Silverberg SG, Bloustein PA et al: Yolk sac carcinoma (endodermal sinus tumor). Ultrastructure and histogenesis of gonadal and extragonadal tumors in comparison with normal human yolk sac. Cancer 39:1462, 1977

324. Kurman RJ, Scardino PT, McIntire KR et al: Cellular localization of alpha-fetoprotein and human chorionic gonadotropin in germ cell tumors of the testis using an indirect immunoperoxidase technique. A new approach to classification utilizing tumor markers. Cancer 40:2136, 1977

325. Drago JR, Nelson RP, Palmer JM: Childhood embryonal carcinoma of testes. Urol 12:499, 1978

326. Bracken RB, Johnson DE, Cangir A et al: Regional lymph nodes in infants with embryonal carcinoma of testis. Urol 6:376, 1978

327. Smith AM, Rao RN, Shelor WCN: Clinical dilemma in management of yolk sac tumor of childhood testis. Urol 14:88, 1979

328. Tallerman A: Endodermal sinus (yolk sac) tumor elements in testicular germ-cell tumors in adults: Comparison of prospective and retrospective studies. Cancer 46:1213, 1980

329. Kaplan WE, Firlit CF: Treatment of testicular yolk sac carcinoma in the young child. J Urol 126:663, 1981

Choriocarcinoma

330. Rather LJ, Gardiner WR, Frerichs JB: Regression and maturation of primary testicular tumors with progressive growth of metastases. A report of six new cases and a review of the literature. Stanford Med Bull 12:12, 1954

331. Azzopardi JG, Mostofi FK, Theiss EA: Lesions of testis observed in certain patients with widespread choriocarcinoma and related tumors. Am J Pathol 38:207, 1961

332. Pierce GB Jr, Midgley AR Jr: The origin and function of human syncytiotrophoblastic giant cells. Am J Pathol 43:153, 1963

333. Azzopardi JG, Hoffbrand AV: Retrogression in testicular seminoma with viable metastases. J Clin Pathol 18:135, 1965

334. Greenwood SM, Goodman JR, Schneider G et al: Choriocarcinoma in a man. The relationship of gynecomastia to chorionic somatomammotropin and estrogens. Am J Med 51:416, 1971

335. Bradfield JS, Hagen RO, Ytredal DO: Carcinoma of the testis: An analysis of 104 patients with germinal tumors of the testis other than seminoma. Cancer 31:633, 1973

336. Teilum G: Choriocarcinoma. In Special Tumors of Ovary and Testes. Comparative Pathology and Histological Identification, 2nd ed, pp 404–405. Philadelphia, JB Lippincott, 1976

337. Brendler CB, Dees JE, Older RA et al: Retroperitoneal mass in a 58-year-old man. J Urol 122:535, 1979

Mixed Germ Cell Tumors and Teratocarcinoma

338. Pugh RCB, Thackray AC: Combined tumour. Br J Urol (Suppl)36:45, 1964

339. Friedman M, Pearlman AW: Seminoma with trophocarcinoma. A clinical variant of seminoma. Cancer 26:46, 1970

340. Mostofi FK: Pathology of germ cell tumors of testis. A progress report. Cancer 45:1735, 1980

Gonadal Stromal/Sex Cord Tumors

Interstitial (Leydig) Cell Tumor

341. Fischel A: Uber die entwicklung der keimdrusen des menschen. Z Anat Entwicklungsgeschichte, Abt I, 92:34, 1930

342. Gillman J: Development of gonads in man, with considerations of the role of fetal endocrines and histogenesis of ovarian tumors. Contrib Embryol 32:81, 1948

343. Edmondson HA, Hammack RW: Interstitial cell tumors of the testis. Report of three new cases. Arch Surg 48:415, 1944

344. Scully RE, Parham AR: Testicular tumors. II. Interstitial cell and miscellaneous neoplasms. Arch Pathol 46:229, 1949

345. Gharpure VV: A case of malignant interstitial-cell tumour of the testis in man. J Pathol Bacteriol 62:113, 1950

346. Flynn PT, Severance AO: Bilateral interstitial-cell tumors of the testis. Cancer 4:817, 1951

347. Pomer FA, Stiles RE, Graham JH: Interstitial-cell tumors of the testis in children. Report of a case and review of the literature. N Engl J Med 250:233, 1954

348. Dalgaard JB, Hesselberg F: Interstitial cell tumours of the testis. Acta Pathol Microbiol Immunol Scand 41:219, 1957

349. Mostofi FK, Theiss EA, Ashley DJB: Tumors of specialized gonadal stroma in human male patients. Androblastoma, Sertoli cell tumor, granulosa-theca cell tumor of the testis, and gonadal stromal tumor. Cancer 12:944, 1959

350. Warner NE, Friedman NB, Bomze EJ, Masin F: Comparative pathology of experimental and spontaneous and roblastomas and gynoblastomas of the gonads. Am J Obstet Gynecol 79:971, 1960

351. Arduino LJ, Glucksman MA: Interstitial cell tumor of the testis associated with Klinefelter's syndrome: A case report. J Urol 89:246, 1963

352. Bader LV, Proctor NSF: Interstitial cell tumor in a cryptorchid testis. Arch Pathol 78:260, 1964

353. Collins DH, Cameron KM: Interstitial-cell tumour. Br J Urol (Suppl)36:62, 1964

354. Beals TF, Pierce GB Jr, Schroeder CF: The ultrastructure of human testicular tumors. I. Interstitial cell tumors. J Urol 93:64, 1965

355. Tamoney HJ Jr, Noriega A: Malignant interstitial cell tumor of the testis. Cancer 24:547, 1969

356. Hopkins GB: Interstitial cell tumor of the testis: Case report and review of the literature. J Urol 103:449, 1970

357. Mahon FB Jr, Gosset F, Trinity RG et al: Malignant interstitial cell testicular tumor. Cancer 31:1208, 1973
358. Jones WG, Onofrio R, Goldstein AMB: Interstitial cell tumor of testis in adult. Urol 4:459, 1974
359. Kay S, Fu Y–S, Koontz WW: Interstitial-cell tumor of the testis. Tissue culture and ultrastructural studies. Am J Clin Pathol 63:366, 1975
360. Gabrilove JL, Nicolis GL, Mitty HA et al: Feminizing interstitial cell tumor of the testis: Personal observations and a review of the literature. Cancer 35:1184, 1975
361. Marshall FF, Kerr WS Jr, Kliman B et al: Sex cord-stromal (gonadal stromal) tumors of the testis: A report of 5 cases. J Urol 117:180, 1977
362. Kurman RJ, Andrade D, Goebelsmann U et al: An immunohistological study of steroid localization in Sertoli-Leydig tumors of the ovary and testis. Cancer 42:1772, 1978
363. Sworn MJ, Buchanan R: Malignant interstitial cell tumor of the testis. Human Pathol 12:72, 1981
364. Davis S, Di Martino NA, Schneider G: Malignant interstitial cell carcinoma of the testis: Report of two cases with steroid synthetic profiles, response to therapy, and review of the literature. Cancer 47:425, 1981
365. Chen KTK, Spaulding RW, Flam MS et al: Malignant interstitial cell tumor of the testis. Cancer 49:547, 1982
366. Feldman PS, Kovacs K, Horvath E et al: Malignant Leydig cell tumor: Clinical, histological and electron microscopic features. Cancer 49:714, 1982

Extratesticular Interstitial (Leydig) Cell Tumor

367. Tedeschi CG, Burke FE: Paratesticular interstitial-cell tumor. Cancer 4:312, 1951
368. Maurer R, Taylor CR, Schmucki O et al: Extratesticular gonadal stromal tumor in the pelvis. Cancer 45:985, 1980

Sertoli Cell Tumor

369. Teilum G: Homologous tumors in the ovary and testes. Contribution to classification of the gonadal tumors. Acta Obstet Gynecol Scand 24:480, 1944
370. Teilum G: Arrhenoblastoma-androblastoma, homologous ovarian and testicular tumors; including the so-called "luteomas" and "adrenal tumors" of ovary and interstitial cell tumors of testis. Acta Pathol Microbiol Scand 23:252, 1946
371. Collins DH, Symington T: Sertoli-cell tumour. Br J Urol (Suppl)36:52, 1964
372. Siller JJ, Farah RN: Androblastoma (Sertoli-cell tumor). J Urol 106:565, 1971
373. Weitzner S, Gropp A: Sertoli cell tumor of testis in childhood. Am J Dis Child 128:541, 1974
374. Symington T, Cameron K: Endocrine and genetic lesions. In Pugh RCB (ed): Pathology of the Testis, pp 259–303. Oxford, Blackwell Scientific Publications, 1976
375. Feldman S, Sreckovic I: Gonadal stromal or Sertoli cell tumor. Urol 15:516, 1980
376. Gabrilove JL, Freiberg EK, Leiter E, Nicolis GL: Feminizing and non-feminizing Sertoli cell tumors. J Urol 124:757, 1980

Malignant Sertoli Cell Tumor

377. Mostofi FK, Theiss EZ, Ashley DJB: Tumors of specialized gonadal stroma in human male patients. Androblastoma, Sertoli cell tumor, granulosa-theca cell tumor of the testis, and gonadal stromal tumor. Cancer 12:944, 1959
378. Nagy L, Thurzo R, Pinter J: Zur pathologie der androblastome. Zentralbl Allg Pathol 105:215, 1964
379. Rosvoll RV, Woodard JR: Malignant Sertoli cell tumor of the testis. Cancer 22:8, 1968
380. Hopkins GB, Parry HD: Metastasizing Sertoli-cell tumor (androblastoma). Cancer 23:463, 1969

381. Tallerman A: Malignant Sertoli cell tumor of the testis. Cancer 28:446, 1971

382. Koppikar DD, Sirsat MV: A malignant Sertoli cell tumour of the testis. Br J Urol 45:213, 1973

383. Hansen GVO: Malignant testicular androblastoma with gynecomastia. Dan Med Bull 22:33, 1975

384. Morin LJ, Loening S: Malignant androblastoma (Sertoli cell tumor) of the testis. A case report with a review of the literature. J Urol 114:476, 1975

385. Campbell CM, Middleton AW Jr: Malignant gonadal stromal tumor: Case report and review of the literature. J Urol 125:257, 1981

386. Herrera LO, Wilk H, Wills JS et al: Malignant (androblastoma) Sertoli cell tumor of testes. Urol 18:287, 1981

387. Eble JN, Hull MT, Warfel KA et al: Malignant sex cord-stromal tumor of testis. J Urol 131:546, 1984

388. Godec CJ: Malignant Sertoli cell tumor of testicle. Urol 26:185, 1985

Large Cell Calcifying Sertoli Cell Tumor

389. Lange J, Leger H, Etcheverry M: Androblastome testiculaire. Observation d'un forme bilaterale chez l'enfant. J Urol 66:259, 1960

390. Fligiel Z, Kaneko M, Leiter E: Bilateral Sertoli cell tumor of testes with feminizing and masculinizing activity occurring in a child. Cancer 38:1853, 1976

391. Proppe KH, Scully RE: Large-cell calcifying Sertoli cell tumor of the testis. Am J Clin Pathol 74:607, 1980

392. Proppe KH, Dickersin GR: Large-cell calcifying Sertoli cell tumor of the testis: Light microscopic and ultrastructural study. Hum Pathol 13:1109, 1982

393. Waxman M, Damjanov I, Khapra A et al: Large cell calcifying Sertoli tumor of the testis. Light microscopic and ultrastructural study. Cancer 54:1575, 1984

Granulosa Cell Tumor

394. Cohen J, Diamond I: Leontiasis ossea, slipped epithyses, and granulosa cell tumor of testis with renal disease. Report of a case with autopsy findings. Arch Pathol 56:488, 1953

395. Castleman B, Towne VW: Case records of the Massachusetts General Hospital. Case 41471. Presentation of case. N Engl J Med 253:926, 1955

396. Melicow MM: Classification of tumors of testis: A clinical and pathological study based on 105 primary and 13 secondary cases in adults, and 3 primary and 4 secondary cases in children. J Urol 73:547, 1955

397. Marshall FF, Kerr WS Jr, Kliman B et al: Sex cord-stromal (gonadal stromal) tumors of the testis: A report of 5 cases. J Urol 117:180, 1977

398. Lawrence WD, Young RH, Scully RE: Juvenile granulosa cell tumor of the infantile testis. A report of 14 cases. Am J Surg Pathol 9:87, 1985

Mixed Gonadal Stromal/Sex Cord and Germ Cell Tumors

Gonadoblastoma

399. Scully RE: Gonadoblastoma. A gonadal tumor related to the dysgerminoma (seminoma) and capable of sex-hormone production. Cancer 6:455, 1953

400. Melicow MM, Uson AC: Dysgenetic gonadomas and other gonadal neoplasms in intersexes. Report of 5 cases and review of the literature. Cancer 12:552, 1959

401. Hughesdon PE, Kumarasamy T: Mixed germ cell tumours (gonadoblastomas) in normal and dysgenetic gonads. Case reports and review. Virchows Arch [A] 349:258, 1970

402. Scully RE: Gonadoblastoma. A review of 74 cases. Cancer 25:1340, 1970

403. Gallager HS, Lewis RP: Sequential gonadoblastoma and choriocarcinoma. Obstet Gynecol 41:123, 1973

404. Talerman A: Gonadoblastoma associated with embryonal carcinoma. Obstet Gynecol 43:138, 1974
405. Talerman A, Delemarre FM: Gonadoblastoma associated with embryonal carcinoma in an anatomically normal man. J Urol 113:355, 1975
406. Govan ADT, Woodcock AS, Gowing NFC et al: A clinicopathological study of gonadoblastoma. Br J Obstet Gynecol 84:222, 1977
407. Hung W, Randolph JG, Chandra R et al: Gonadoblastoma in dysgenetic testis causing male pseudohermaphroditism in newborn. Urol 17:584, 1981

Carcinoid Tumors

408. Simon HB, McDonald JR: Argentaffin tumor (carcinoid) occurring in a benign cystic teratoma of the testicle. J Urol 72:892, 1954
409. Dockerty MB, Scheifley CH: Metastasizing carcinoid. Report of an unusual case with episodic cyanosis. Am J Clin Pathol 25:770, 1955
410. Berkheiser SW: Carcinoid tumor of the testis occurring in a cystic teratoma of the testis. J Urol 82:352, 1959
411. Kemble JVH: Argentaffin carcinomata of the testicle. Br J Urol 40:580, 1968
412. Kermarec J, Duplay H: Tumeur carcinoide apparemment primitive du testicule. Arch Anat Pathol 16:56, 1968
413. Enerback L: Specific methods for detection of 5–hydroxytryptamine in carcinoid tumors. Virchows Arch [A] 358:35, 1973
414. Sinnatamby CS, Gordon AB, Griffiths JD: The occurrence of carcinoid tumour in teratoma of the testis. Br J Surg 60:576, 1973
415. Yalla SV, Yalla SS, Morgan JW et al: Primary argentaffinoma of the testis: A case report and survey of the literature. J Urol 111:50, 1974
416. Weitzner S, Robison JR: Primary carcinoid of testis. J Urol 116:821, 1976
417 Wurster K, Brodner O, Rossner JA, Grube D: Case report. A carcinoid occurring in the testis. Virchows Arch [A] 370:185, 1976
417A. Brown NJ: Miscellaneous tumors of epithelial type. In Pugh RCB (ed): Pathology of the Testis, pp 304–316. Oxford, Blackwell Scientific Publications, 1976
418. Berdjis CC, Mostofi FK: Carcinoid tumors of the testis. J Urol 118:777, 1977
419. Magyar E, Talerman A: Primary carcinoid tumor of testis. Urol 10:590, 1977
420. Talerman A, Gratama S, Miranda S et al: Primary carcinoid tumor of the testis. Case report, ultrastructure and review of the literature. Cancer 42:2696, 1978
421. Sullivan JL, Packer JT, Bryant M: Primary malignant carcinoid of the testis. Arch Pathol Lab Med 105:515, 1981
422. Bates RJ, Perrone TL, Parkhurst EC: Insular carcinoid arising in a mature teratoma of the testis. J Urol 126:55, 1981

Brenner Tumor

423. Vechinski TO, Jaeschke WH, Vermund H: Testicular tumors. An analysis of 112 consecutive cases. Am J Roentgen 95:494, 1965
424. Ross L: Paratesticular Brenner-like tumor. Cancer 21:722, 1968
425. Goldman RL: A Brenner tumor of the testis. Cancer 26:853, 1970
426. Nogales Jr F, Matilla A, Ortega I et al: Mixed Brenner and adenomatoid tumor of the testis. An ultrastructural study and histogenetic considerations. Cancer 43:539, 1979

Mesenchymal Neoplasms

427. David AE Jr: Rhabdomyosarcoma of the testicle. J Urol 87:148, 1962
428. Honore LH, Sullivan LD: Intratesticular leiomyoma: A case report with discussion of differential diagnosis and histogenesis. J Urol 114:631, 1975
429. Stein JJ: Hemangioendothelioma of the testis. J Urol 113:201, 1975
430. Livolsi VA, Schiff M: Myxoid neurofibroma of the testis. J Urol 118:341, 1977

431. Cricco CF Jr, Buck AS: Hemangioendothelioma of the testis: Second reported case. J Urol 123:136, 1980
432. Mathew T, Prabhakaran K: Osteosarcoma of the testis. Arch Pathol Lab Med 105:38, 1981

Hematopoietic Neoplasms

Plasmacytoma

433. Porchownik JB: Ein Fall von multiplem Myelom (Plasmocytom). Virchows Arch [A] 280:534, 1931
434. Ulrich H: Multiple myeloma. Arch Intern Med 64:994, 1939
435. Kirshbaum JD: Metastatic plasma cell myeloma of the testicles: With report of a case. Urol Cutan Rev 51:456, 1947
436. Hayes DW, Bennett WA, Heck FJ: Extramedullary lesions in multiple myeloma. Review of literature and pathologic studies. Arch Pathol 53:262, 1952
437. Melicow MM, Cahill GF: Plasmacytoma (multiple myeloma) of testis: A report of four cases and review of the literature. J Urol 71:103, 1954
438. Carson CP, Ackerman LV, Maltby JD: Plasma cell myeloma. A clinical, pathologic and roentgenologic review of 90 cases. Am J Clin Pathol 25:849, 1955
439. Osman R, Morrow JW: Myeloma of the testicle: A case report. J Urol 96:352, 1966
440. Weitzner S: Metastatic plasma cell myeloma in testis. Report of a case and review of the literature. Rocky Mountain Med J 66:48, 1969
441. Levin HS, Mostofi FK: Symptomatic plasmacytoma of the testis. Cancer 25:1193, 1970
442. Oldham RK, Polmar SH: Extramedullary plasmacytomas following successful radiotherapy of Hodgkin's disease. Clinical and immunologic aspects. Am J Med 54:761, 1973
443. Steinberg D: Plasmacytoma of the testis. Report of a case. Cancer 36:1470, 1975
444. Chica G, Johnson DE, Ayala AG: Plasmacytoma of testis presenting as primary testicular tumor. Urol 11:90, 1978
445. Soumerai S, Gleason EA: Asynchronous plasmacytoma of the stomach and testis. Cancer 45:396, 1980

Lymphoma

446. Malassez M: Lymphadenome du testicule. Bull Soc Anat Paris 52:176, 1877
447. Cohen BB, Kaplan G, Liber AF, Roswit B: Reticulum-cell sarcoma with primary manifestation in the testis. Report of four cases. Cancer 8:136, 1955
448. Eckert H, Smith JP: Malignant lymphoma of the testis. Br Med J 2:891, 1963
449. Gowing NFC: Malignant lymphoma of the testis. Br J Urol (Suppl)36:85, 1964
450. Rappaport H: Tumors of the hematopoietic system. In Atlas of Tumor Pathology, Section III, Fascicle 8. Washington, AFIP, 1966
451. Abell MR, Holtz F: Testicular and paratesticular neoplasms in patients 60 years of age and older. Cancer 21:852, 1968
452. Givler RL: Testicular involvement in leukemia and lymphoma. Cancer 23:1290, 1969
453. Kiely JM, Massey BD Jr, Harrison EG Jr et al: Lymphoma of the testis. Cancer 26:847, 1970
454. Hamlin JA, Kagan AR, Friedman NB: Lymphomas of the testicle. Cancer 29:1352, 1972
455. Tanenbaum B, Sanford RS, Elquezabal A et al: Testicular tumor: Presenting sign of lymphoma. Cancer 29:1223, 1972
456. Woolley PV III, Osborne CK, Levi JA et al: Extranodal presentation of non-Hodgkin's lymphomas in the testis. Cancer 38:1026, 1976
457. Silvert MA, Gray CP: Reticulum cell sarcoma of testes. Urol 8:395, 1976

458. Sussman EB, Hajdu SI, Lieberman PH, Whitmore WF: Malignant lymphoma of the testis: A clinicopathologic study of 37 cases. J Urol 118:1004, 1977
459. Tallerman A: Primary malignant lymphoma of the testis. J Urol 118:783, 1977
460. Paladugu RR, Bearman RM, Rappaport H: Malignant lymphoma with primary manifestation in the gonad. A clinicopathologic study of 38 patients. Cancer 45:561, 1980
461. Jackson SM, Montessori GA: Malignant lymphoma of the testis: Review of 17 cases in British Columbia with survival related to pathological subclassification. J Urol 123:881, 1980
462. Turner RR, Colby TV, MacKintosh FR: Testicular lymphomas: A clinicopathologic study of 35 cases. Cancer 48:2095, 1981
463. Tepperman BS, Gospodarowicz MK, Bush RS et al: Non-Hodgkin lymphoma of the testis. Radiology 142:203, 1982
464. The non-Hodgkin's lymphoma pathologic classification project: National Cancer Institute sponsored study of classifications of non-Hodgkin's Lymphomas. Cancer 49:2112, 1982

Leukemia

465. Nies BA, Bodey GP, Thomas LB et al: The persistence of extramedullary leukemic infiltrates during bone marrow remission of acute leukemia. Blood 26:133, 1965
466. Jampol ML, Ohnysty J: Acute leukemia seen as testicular tumor. NY State J Med 67:1903, 1967
467. Stoffel TJ, Nesbit ME, Levitt SH: Extramedullary involvement of the testes in childhood leukemia. Cancer 35:1203, 1975
468. Kuo T–T, Tschang T–P, Chu J–Y: Testicular relapse in childhood acute lymphocytic leukemia during bone marrow remission. Cancer 38:2604, 1976
469. Nesbit ME Jr, Robison LL, Ortega JA et al: Testicular relapse in childhood acute lymphoblastic leukemia: Association with pretreatment patient characteristics and treatment. A report for children's cancer study group. Cancer 45:2009, 1980

Metastatic Neoplasm

470. Brown BH: Primary carcinoma of the urinary bladder. Am J Med Sci 134:849, 1907
471. Coley WB, Hoguet JP: Melanotic cancer. With a report of 91 cases. Ann Surg 64:206, 1916
472. Weller CV: Unusual cardiac and cerebral metastases in melanosarcoma. J Cancer Res 7:313, 1922
473. Gleave HH, Leeds MB: Prognosis in malignant melanoma. A report on forty consecutive cases. Lancet 2:658, 1929
474. Cordes FC, Horner WD: Metastatic melanoma of both eyes. Report of a case. JAMA 95:655, 1930
475. Hirsch EF: Malignant mixed tumor of the thyroid gland with skeletal muscle fibers. Am J Cancer 15:55, 1931
476. Semans JH: Carcinoma of the prostate with metastasis in the testis. J Urol 40:524, 1938
477. Bandler CG, Roen PR: Solitary testicular metastasis simulating primary tumor and antedating clinical hypernephroma of the kidney. Report of a case. J Urol 55:663, 1946
478. London MZ, Grossman SN: Secondary testicular tumor resembling Krukenberg tumor, a case report. J Urol 62:713, 1949
479. Klinger ME: Secondary tumors of the genito-urinary tract. J Urol 65:144, 1951
480. Belsky JB, Konwaler BE: Testicular metastasis from carcinoma of the colon. J Urol 72:712, 1954
481. Kay S, Hennigar GR, Hooper JW Jr: Carcinoma of the testes metastatic from carcinoma of the prostate. Arch Pathol 57:121, 1954

482. Melicow MM: Classification of tumors of testis: A clinical and pathological study based on 105 primary and 13 secondary cases in adults, and 3 primary and 4 secondary cases in children. J Urol 73:547, 1955

483. Howard DE, Hicks WK, Scheldrup EW: Carcinoma of the prostate with simultaneous bilateral testicular metastases: Case report with special study of routes of metastases. J Urol 78:58, 1957

484. Ransom CL, Powell LW Jr, Landes RR: Carcinoma of the prostate with metastases to the testis. Virginia Med Monthly 84:572, 1957

485. Price EB Jr, Mostofi FK: Secondary carcinoma of the testis. Cancer 10:592, 1957

486. Hunter DT Jr, Hutcheson JB: Krukenberg tumor of the testicle, report of a second case. J Urol 81:305, 1959

487. Marble EJ: Testicular metastasis from carcinoma of the prostate: Review of literature and report of a case. J Urol 84:369, 1960

488. Ballanger R: Metastases testiculaires bilaterales d'un cancer prostatique. J Urol Nephrol 67:194, 1961

489. Ichikawa T, Kumamoto Y, Asano M: A case of prostatic carcinoma with metastases to the skin and both testes. J Urol 87:941, 1962

490. Mazzoleni G: Metastasi al testicolo da carcinoma del colon. Riv Anat Pathol Oncol 23:304, 1963

491. Murry LM: Metastasis of gastric carcinoma to the spermatic cord and testis. J Christian Med Assoc 38:511, 1963

492. Tuchschmid D: Quelques cas d'hypernephromes se manifestant cliniquement par des metastases rares. Helv Chir Acta 32:498, 1965

493. Lowell DM, Lewis EL: Melanospermia: A hitherto undescribed entity. J Urol 95:407, 1966

494. Florentin P, Chardot C, Parache RM: Metastase testiculaire d'un epithelioma gastrique mucipare. Ann Anat Pathol 11:315, 1966

495. Bonneau H, Spitalier J–M, Varette I et al: Metastase testiculaire d'un adeno-carcinome du rectum. J Urol Nephrol 73:947, 1967

496. Roque MP, Goldberg HW: Metastatic carcinoma of the prostate — Unusual sites. Chicago Med School Quart 27:42, 1967

497. Bodon GR, Dressler JAW: Metastatic carcinoma of right testicle from primary carcinoma of the appendix. J Urol 97:885, 1967

498. Wolf H, Madsen PO: Metastases to the external genitalia from carcinoma of the prostate: A report of 2 cases. J Urol 99:198, 1968

499. Malek GH, Madsen PO: Carcinoma of the prostate with unusual metastases. Cancer 24:194, 1969

500. Ford ML, Tandan B: Metastatic tumor of the spermatic cord and testis from carcinoma of the stomach: A case report. South Med J 62:352, 1969

501. Hanash KA, Carney JA, Kelalis PP: Metastatic tumors to testicles: Routes of metastasis. J Urol 102:465, 1969

502. Johnson DE, Jackson L, Ayala AG: Secondary carcinoma of the testis. South Med J 64:1128, 1971

503. Jepson PM, Labitzke HG, Bischoff AJ: Solitary testicular metastasis from carcinoma of the prostate. Br J Urol 44:594, 1972

504. Pienkos EJ, Jablokow VR: Secondary testicular tumors. Cancer 30:481, 1972

505. Meares EM Jr, Ho TL: Metastatic carcinomas involving the testis: A review. J Urol 109:653, 1973

506. Talerman A, Kniestedt WF: Testicular tumor as the first manifestation of renal carcinoma. J Urol 111:584, 1974

507. Silverton NP: Testicular metastasis from prostatic carcinoma. Br J Urol 48:498, 1976

508. Cricco RP, Kandzari SJ: Secondary testicular tumors. J Urol 118:489, 1977

509. Tiltman AJ: Metastatic tumours in the testis. Histopathology 3:31, 1979

510. Askari A, Faddoul A, Herrera H: Metastatic carcinoma to testicle. Urol 17:601, 1981

511. Moore JB, Law DK, Moore EE et al: Testicular mass: An initial sign of colon carcinoma. Cancer 49:411, 1982

512. Werth V, Yu G, Marshall FF: Nonlymphomatous metastatic tumor to the testis. J Urol 127:142, 1982

513. Johansson J–E, Lannes P: Metastases to the spermatic cord, epididymis and testicles from carcinoma of the prostate—five cases. Scand J Urol Nephrol 17:249, 1983

514. Binkley WF, Seo IS: Metastatic transitional cell carcinoma of the testis. A case report. Cancer 54:575, 1984

515. Haupt HM, Mann RB, Trump DL, Abeloff MD: Metastatic carcinoma involving the testis. Clinical and pathologic distinction from primary testicular neoplasms. Cancer 54:709, 1984

Testicular Adnexa

7

Testicular Tunics

Hydrocele

The most common cause of scrotal swelling is hydrocele, a collection of serous fluid within the tunica vaginalis sac. When there is an associated patent process vaginalis, it is regarded as congenital in origin. Six percent of newborn male infants have a detectable hydrocele, a frequency that decreases significantly by age 1 year.[1-3] Alternatively, acquired forms are associated with inflammatory disorders of the scrotal contents, especially the epididymis and testis. Hydroceles may mask the presence of neoplasms in these same organs.

Complications of hydrocele include infection (vaginilitis), rupture, and hemorrhage (hematocele). Treatment is surgical removal of the mesothelial cyst. Associated inflammation of the cyst wall may be evident microscopically. Differentiating a spermatocele is important, and occasionally difficult when the lining epithelium is denuded. The finding of sperm in the cyst fluid identifies the cyst as a spermatocele, and therefore of epididymal origin.

Fibrous Pseudotumor

Fibrous pseudotumor previously was regarded as a "fibroma," and was included in reviews of benign neoplasms of the testicular tunics in older literature.[4-6,9] A non-neoplastic pathogenesis was first suggested by Goodwin, who observed associated plasma cells, raising the possibility that some were of an inflammatory nature. He coined the term *proliferative periorchitis*.[7,8] Following a review of cases on file at the Armed Forces Institute of Pathology (AFIP), Mostofi and Price concluded that all cases were reactive, non-neoplastic lesions, prompting them to

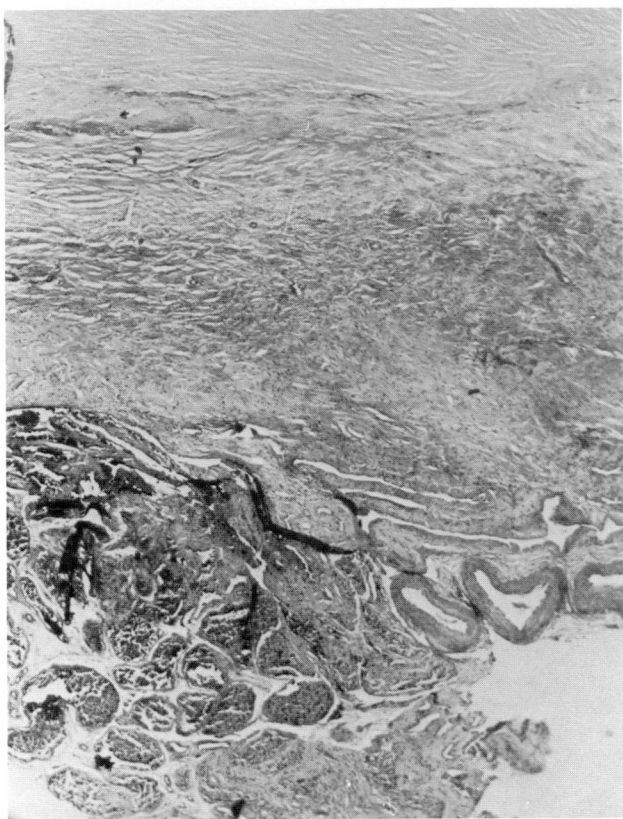

Figure 7-1   *Nodular periorchitis. The tunica albuginea is thickened by dense, acellular collagenous fibrous tissue. Minimal chronic inflammatory cells are scattered in the tunica.*

introduce the term *fibrous pseudotumor*.[10] Patients range in age from 16 years to 80 years, with a peak frequency in the third to the fifth decades.[4-14] Mostofi and Price reported that 45% of cases are associated with a hydrocele, and 30% with a history of trauma or epididymo-orchitis.[10]

The histologic features of these lesions are not constant, but show a spectrum from granulation tissue, with varying amounts of fibrosis, and chronic inflammatory cells, to dense, virtually acellular, hyalinized collagen occasionally with dystrophic calcification (Fig. 7-1). These histologic characteristics are not regarded as variants, but reflect the evolution of a reactive inflammatory process with ultimate fibrosis as the final common pathway.

Because these lesions are not neoplastic, awareness of this entity will allow correct intraoperative diagnosis, and prevent unnecessary radical surgery.

The fibrous nodules may be single or multiple, and take origin from the tunics of the testis, epididymis, or may involve the spermatic cord. One case originating from the parietal tunica vaginalis 4 months after orchiectomy has been reported.[14] They are well circumscribed, firm, with a white-tan, whorled cut surface, and range in size from 4 cm to 8 cm. They show no tendency to invade the underlying structures.

Cysts of the Tunica Albuginea

Frater reported the first tunica albuginea cyst in 1924.[15] Thirteen subsequent reported cases were collected from the literature.[16-20] With the exception of three cases diagnosed in patients 23 years, 31 years, and 38 years old, all other cases occurred in men in the fifth to the eighth decades.[15-20] The cysts measure 0.5 cm to 4.0 cm, contain serous or "chocolate" fluid, and are characteristically located on the anterior-lateral surface of the testis. Origin from the tunica albuginea is suggested from gross examination of the testis, and is confirmed by microscopic review. Unilocular or multilocular cysts lined by flattened or cuboidal epithelium within the dense collagen of the tunica albuginea are typical. Mennemeyer and Mason reported ciliated cells in multilocular cysts suggesting origin from efferent ductules.[18] Alternative histogenetic explanations offered include traumatic or inflammatory cyst development, or mesothelial rests.[15-17] The finding of mesothelial cell clusters in the cyst wall and adjacent tunica albuginea, and acid mucopolysaccharide secretions within one of the reported cysts, lends support to the mesothelial rest pathogenesis.[17] The majority of cases have no history of trauma and no histologic evidence of inflammation. These cysts are to be differentiated from simple cysts originating in the testis. (Refer to Chap. 6.)

One case of an epidermoid cyst of the testicular tunics was reported by Eason and Spaulding.[21] The cyst was lined by squamous epithelium and the cyst contents were composed of abundant keratin debris.[21] Some sections of the cyst wall contained skin appendages. (Refer to discussion of pathogenesis of epidermoid cysts of testis in Chap. 6.)

Walthard's Rests

Rare examples of Walthard's rests have been observed in the paratesticular tissue.[22,23] These structures, more commonly encountered in the ovary, mesovarium, and subserosal surface of the fallopian tube, are of Müllerian origin. When observed in the male genitalia, they reflect remnants of Müllerian tissue. They are of no clinical significance. These well-defined nests of epithelial cells are identical to those observed in the female genital tract. Identification of the longitudinal "groove" or "fold" in the nucleus of the cells in the rest is helpful in making the diagnosis.

Benign Mesothelial Proliferation

Benign mesotheliomas are of two basic histologic types: papillary, and nonpapillary (or adenomatoid tumors). Focal reactive mesothelial cell proliferations histologically resemble the papillary forms of benign mesothelioma; therefore, they are discussed together.

Reactive Mesothelial Cell Hyperplasia and Benign Mesothelioma

The distinction between reactive mesothelial cell hyperplasia and benign mesothelioma is not difficult, but on occasion is arbitrary.[24-28] The most consistently applied criterion is size: reactive mesothelial cell proliferations are most frequently microscopic foci, whereas benign mesotheliomas are grossly apparent lesions. However, occasional mesothelial proliferations are small, grossly apparent nodules, or diffuse, ill-defined fibrous thickenings of hydrocele sacs. Thus, size is a less-than-absolute criterion.

Reactive mesothelial cell proliferations are observed in hydrocele sacs, as noted previously, as incidental findings in orchiectomy specimens removed for a variety of reasons, or as incidental findings in hernia sacs.[27] Surface papillary proliferations, or gland-like structures lined by a single layer of mesothelial cells without atypia, within a fibrous stroma are characteristic. Squamous metaplasia of the mesothelial cells, a rare change reported in mesothelial proliferations elsewhere, has been observed (Fig. 7-2). Focal hyperplastic clusters of the lining cells are common. The overall pattern of glands, papillae, or commonly both, is simple and orderly. The histologic patterns combined with an absence of atypical cytologic features, differentiates this lesion from malignant mesothelioma. At most, only rare mitotic figures are present. Absence of mitotic figures is more characteristic.

Benign mesotheliomas reported in the literature vary in size up to several centimeters. They have cystic and solid components on the cut surface, and frequently have a matted outer surface reflecting the papillary projections observed microscopically. Histologic and cytologic features are similar to those observed in reactive mesothelial cell proliferations. Abundant papillary proliferations are commonly associated with psammoma bodies. Areas of dense hyalinized fibrous tissue are a common component. Mesothelial derivation is determined by noting transitions of normal mesothelial lining cells to the proliferative mesothelial cell lesions, and is supported by the results of special stains (PAS, mucicarmine, and Alcian blue with and without hyaluronidase) and the ultrastructural features. (Refer to discussion later on malignant mesothelioma.)

Nonpapillary Benign Mesotheliomas (Adenomatoid Tumors)

Nonpapillary benign mesotheliomas, the more common of the two histologic types of benign mesotheliomas, are represented by the so-called adenomatoid tumor. It is characterized by a mesothelial cell proliferation in a tubular or syncytial pattern resembling a vascular neoplasm. The mesothelial origin of such neoplasms was first suggested by Evans in 1943.[29] Two years later, Golden and Ash reported 15 cases, the histogenesis of which they were unwilling to accept as mesothelial, prompting them to introduce the descriptive term *adenomatoid tumor*.[30] During the next two decades the histogenesis remained unsettled with suggestions of endothelial, mesonephric, Müllerian, and mesothelial origin suggested.[23,35,40] The weight of evidence supporting mesothelial origin gradually accumulated, and currently there is general acceptance that neoplasms historically regarded as adenomatoid tumors are of mesothelial cell origin. This evidence includes: (1) direct origin from surface mesothelial cells observed in some cases; (2) histochemical staining properties characteristic of normal mesothelial

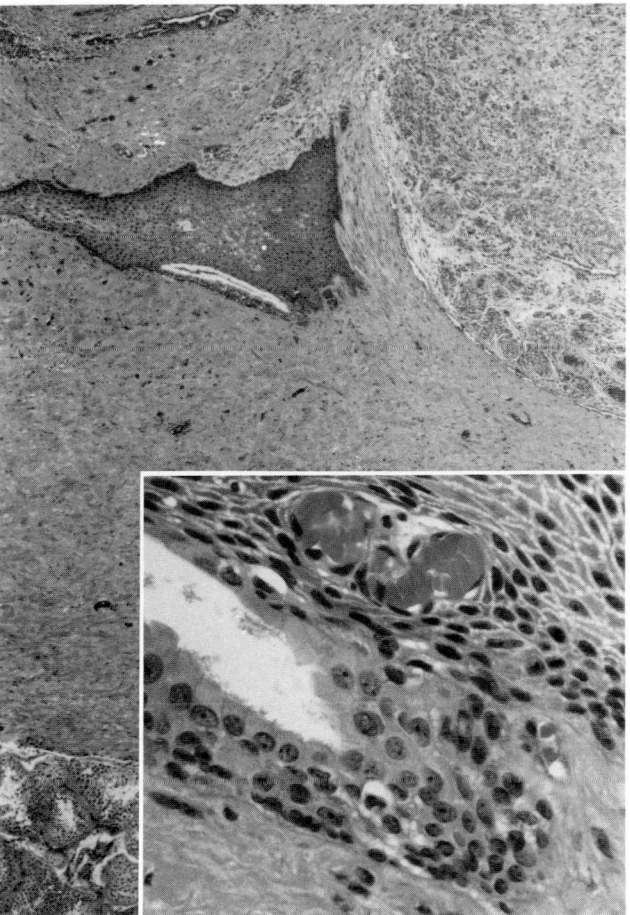

Figure 7-2   *Squamous metaplasia of the tunica vaginalis. Transition of*
the mesothelial cells, which are larger and more prominent than
normal (inset), *to the metaplastic squamous cells is apparent.*
This was an incidental finding in an orchiectomy specimen
removed for therapeutic reasons in a patient with prostatic
carcinoma.

cells and neoplasms of mesothelial cell origin; and (3) ultrastructural features
consistent with mesothelial cell origin (and inconsistent with endothelial cell
origin).[33–36,38,39] With the mesothelial origin established, the term *adenomatoid
tumor* should be discarded for the more appropriated *benign mesothelioma,* a
suggestion previously made by Broth and co-workers.[33]

These neoplasms are located at the lower or upper pole of the epididymis, the
tunica vaginalis of the testis, or the spermatic cord in order of decreasing
frequency.[30–32,37] They are typically a few millimeters to 2 cm in size. Ferenczy
reported one tumor measuring 6 cm in greatest dimensions.[36] Although principally on the surface of these structures, apparent encroachment into the epididymis may suggest malignant behavior. They are well-demarcated white, tan, or
gray nodules with a firm consistency.

Microscopically, the varied histological picture has been classified into three
patterns by Taxy and co-workers: plexiform, tubular, or canalicular, or mixtures

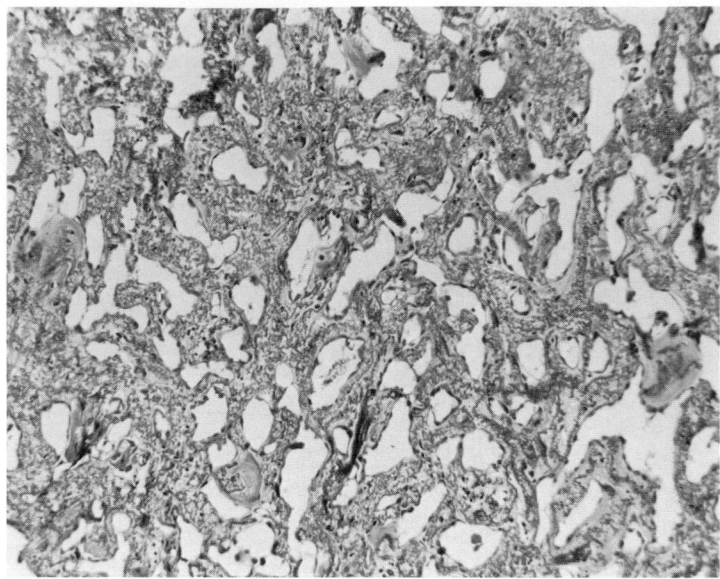

Figure 7-3   *Adenomatoid tumor. The neoplasm contains numerous irregular cysts or tubules lined by flattened epithelium with intervening dense fibrous stroma.*

of these patterns.[38] The lining cells in the tubular and canalicular patterns varied from flat to cuboidal (Fig. 7-3). The intervening tissue is either fibrous or composed of tumor cell nests. Occasional isolated cells (in all patterns) have vacuolated cytoplasm and overall features of signet-ring cells.[26,38] Alcian blue staining of both cells and stroma is diminished by treatment with hyaluronidase. Ultrastructural features consist of epithelial cells resting on basal lamina with numer-

Table 7-1   *Malignant Mesothelioma of the Tunica Vaginalis*

Author	Year	Patient's Age	Histology	Follow Up
Bailey et al	1955	21	Epithelial	A/NED, 15 mon
Abell et al	1968	70	Biphasic	D/TM, 16 mon
Abell et al	1968	78	Biphasic	D/TM, 3.75 yr (45 mon)
Kasdon	1969	56	Biphasic	D/TM, 5 yr
Kasdon	1969	72	Epithelial	A/TM, 5 yr
Johnson et al	1973	23	Epithelial	A/NED, 2 mon
Fishelovitch	1975	60	Epithelial	A/NED, 12 mon
Fliegel	1976	68	Epithelial	D/TM, 20 mon
Eimoto, Inoue	1977	35	Fibrous	A/NED, 1.5 mon
Hamvasi	1977	63	Biphasic	A/NED, 3 mon
Jaffe et al	1978	77	Epithelial	D/TM, 12 mon
Japko et al	1982	30	Epithelial	A/NED, 6 mon
Chen et al	1982	64	Biphasic	D/TM, 2.5 yr
Personal observation	1983	51	Epithelial	A/NED, 2.5 yr

A/NED, alive/no evidence of disease; D/TM, dead/tumor metastases

ous microvilli on the luminal surface, and well-developed desmosomes on the lateral cell surfaces.[34-36,40]

Nonpapillary benign mesotheliomas (adenomatoid tumors) are uniformly benign. If intraoperative diagnosis is established by frozen section, they can be treated by conservative surgical excision.

Malignant Mesothelioma of the Tunica Vaginalis

Thirteen cases of malignant mesothelioma arising in the tunica vaginalis were found in the literature[42-53] (Table 7-1). These patients range in age from 21 years to 78 years with a bimodal distribution of age. Four of the thirteen patients (31%) were in the third and fourth decades and nine patients (69%) were in the sixth to eighth decades.

Microscopically, seven mesotheliomas (54%) were epithelial, five (38%) were biphasic (epithelial and fibrous), and one (8%) was fibrous. The malignant character of these rare mesotheliomas was consistently indicated by the frequency of mitoses, significant nuclear atypia with prominent nucleoli, and invasion of adjacent structures or lymphatics (Figs. 7-4, 7-5). The histologic pattern of the epithelial phase is characterized by numerous papillary projections, either on the surface or into gland spaces. Alternatively, syncytial, microglandular cords or sheets of polygonal cells are seen. Spindle cells in poorly defined fascicles or sheets, with occasional admixed polygonal cells, and variable amounts of collagenous stroma are common in the biphasic and fibrous types of mesothelioma. Special stains (PAS, Alcian blue, and mucicarmine) are helpful in differen-

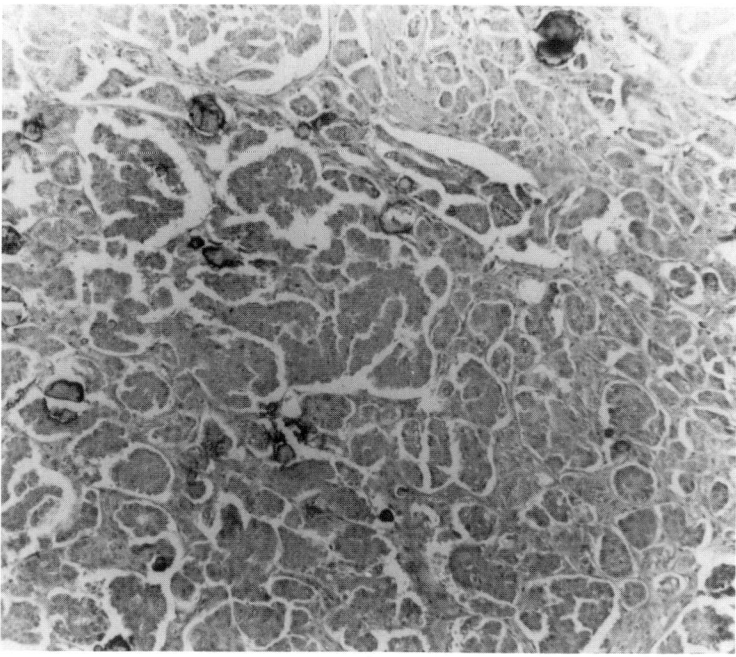

Figure 7-4   *Malignant mesothelioma of the tunica vaginalis. The papillary pattern predominates in this monophasic mesothelioma. Numerous psammoma bodies are present. The cytologic atypia exceeds that observed in reactive mesothelial proliferation.*

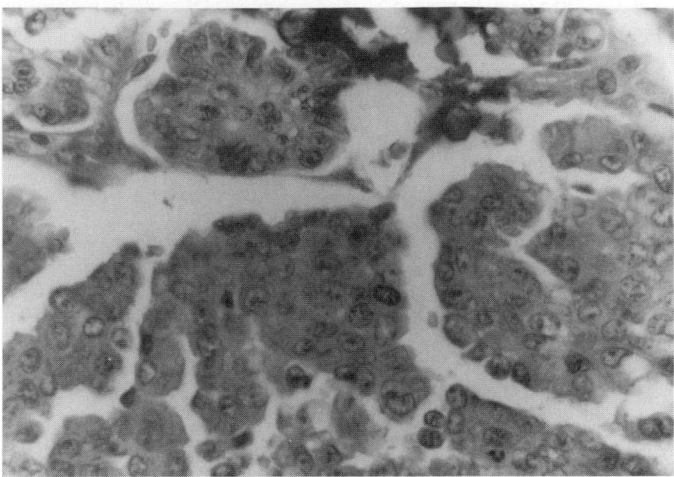

Figure 7-5   *Malignant mesothelioma of the tunica vaginalis (higher magnification of tumor illustrated in Fig. 7-4). The malignant histologic and cytologic features reflected the malignant clinical behavior: two local recurrences with invasion of the scrotal wall within the first 2 years of diagnosis and primary surgical therapy.*

tiating mesotheliomas and metastatic adenocarcinoma. Ultrastructural studies of mesotheliomas identify desmomas and numerous irregular microvilli of variable length, associated with the epithelial component of mesothelioma.[48,50,52] Recently, Japko and co-workers reported the diagnosis of a tunica mesothelioma with specific immunoperoxidase staining for mesotheliomas.[52] Preoperative diagnosis by CT scan and aspiration cytology has been reported.[52]

Among the 13 reported cases of malignant mesothelioma, six died of tumor-related causes with metastases 16 months to 5 years after the diagnosis and surgical therapy (see Table 7-1). One patient was alive at 5 years with evidence of residual tumor. The remaining six cases were reported alive and without clinically apparent residual tumor 1 month to 15 months after the diagnosis. The value of adjunct chemotherapy in treating these neoplasms has not been established at this time.

Miscellaneous Rare Neoplasms

Brenner Tumor

Three cases of Brenner tumors originating in testicular tunics were found in the literature.[54–56] Origin from Müllerian remants in the vicinity of the head of the epididymis is the most probable explanation of this unusual location.

Testicular Appendages

Four small (mm) vestigial structures of Müllerian and mesonephric origin are located on the outer surfaces of the testis, epididymis, and spermatic cord. These structures are inconstant findings. Rolnick and co-workers observed an appendix testis (vestigial cranial portion of Müllerian duct) in 92% of 100 consecutive autopsies.[66] The appendix epididymis (vestigial cranial mesonephric collecting tubules) was present in 34% of the same cases. The paradidymis and vas aberrans (vestigial caudal mesonephric collecting tubules) are rarely present. Other variations referable to these structures include the location, number of each vestige, the frequency of bilaterality, and their structure (pedunculated or sessile).[59-65]

The appendix testis most frequently originates in the groove between the testis and the epididymal head, or on the superior surface of the testis.[61,65] It occurs as a fan-shaped excrescence, or a pedunculated or sessile globular structure.[61] The surface epithelium of this vestigial structure is cuboidal and continuous with the tunica vaginalis near the base. Invaginations of the surface epithelium into the delicate collagenous stroma are common.[61]

The appendix epididymis is most frequently located on the superior surface of the epididymal head. Typically, it is a pedunculated spherical cystic structure. The external surface is lined by flat mesothelial cells. The cyst lining is composed of cuboidal or columnar cells that evidence secretory activity.[61]

The clinical significance of these minute structures is their potential for torsion. The first case of torsion of the testicular appendages was reported by Colt in 1922.[57] Scott collected 85 reported cases up to 1940.[58] By 1958, Fitzpatrick found 151 cases, and by 1970, Skoglund and co-workers collected 321 reported cases, to which they added 43 cases.[63,67] Patients commonly have a history of sudden onset of intrascrotal pain following vigorous physical activity. The peak age frequency is 10 years to 12 years with approximately 90% involving boys 6 years to 14 years.[67] The right and left sides are affected with equal frequency. Of the reported cases, the correct preoperative diagnosis has been made in only 61% of cases.[67] The most frequent incorrect diagnoses were testicular torsion and acute epididymitis. Ninety-two percent of the reported cases involve torsion of the appendix testis, and 7% involve the appendix epididymis.[67] Torsion of the other vestigial remnants is extremely rare.

Treatment involves surgical removal of the twisted appendage, which evidences congestion and ischemic infarction on histologic review.

Epididymis

Normal Structure

The efferent ductules leading from the rete testis converge to form the coiled epididymal duct, which is distally continued as the vas deferens (Fig. 7-6). Throughout most of its length it is highly coiled, and the actual length of the duct is many times that of the superior–inferior length of the in situ epididymis.[68] It is anatomically divided into the head, body, and tail. The mesorchium is a mesenteric attachment to the outer tunica albuginea of the testis. The outer investment, the tunica vaginalis, is continuous with that covering the testis.

The lumen size is smallest in the proximal portion of the head (caput) of the epididymis, increasing progressively toward the body (corpus) and tail (cauda). In contrast to the irregular outline of the lumen of the efferent ductules, the epididymal lumen is relatively round until the terminal portion of the tail, where it again becomes irregular.

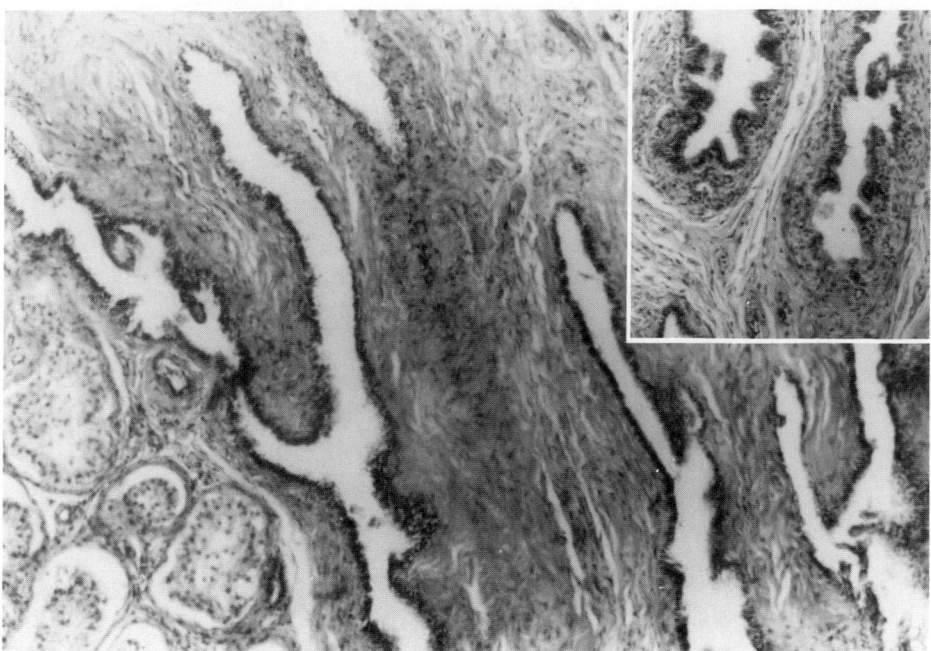

Figure 7-6   *Normal rete testis and epididymis. The seminiferous tubules converge at the mediastinum testis to form the rete testis tubules* (left), *which, in turn, continue as the efferent ductules of the proximal epididymis* (inset).

The epithelial lining of the efferent ducts and the head is pseudostratified, ciliated and nonciliated, columnar cells (Figs. 7-7, 7-8). Distal to the head of the epididymis, the lining epithelium becomes progressively lower and more uniform. The stroma surrounding the basal lamina is composed of vascularized collagen with an external investing sheath of smooth muscle. The smooth muscle sheath constitutes a greater proportion of the total epididymal duct wall as it progresses to the vas deferens. Sperm are normally present within the epididymal lumen throughout its length. Ewing has summarized the evidence of requisite maturational changes occurring in spermatozoa during their transit through the epididymis.[70]

Normal variants of epididymal lining epithelial cells include cytologic atypia, a pseudomalignant change of unknown cause, and intracellular accumulations of brown, lipofuscin-like pigment, producing so-called "brown patches" (Fig. 7-9).[69,71]

Congenital Disorders

Anomalies of the epididymis are rare and include abnormal position, failure of fusion with the testis, and adrenal rests. The epididymis was located anterior to the testis, not at the normal posterior-lateral location, in 14% of a series of patients.[73] This is without clinical significance. Congenital failure of fusion of the mesonephric tubules (ultimately to become the epididymis) and the testis has obvious clinical consequences.[74] This disorder is rare and all of the reported cases have been unilateral.[74] Adrenal rests have been reported in various paratesticular

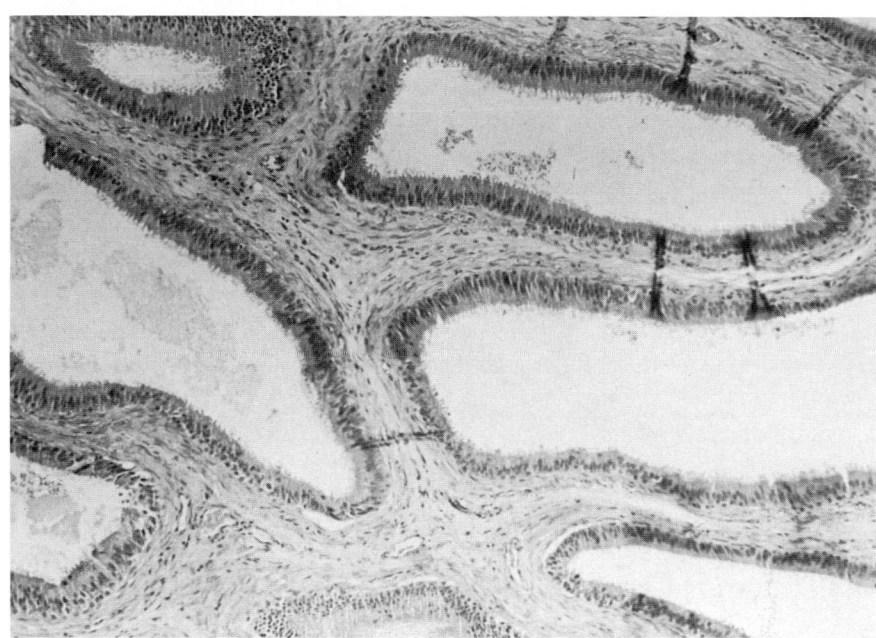

Figure 7-7   ***Normal epididymis.*** *The ducts of the epididymis are lined by uniformly tall columnar epithelium and have a surrounding fibromuscular stroma.*

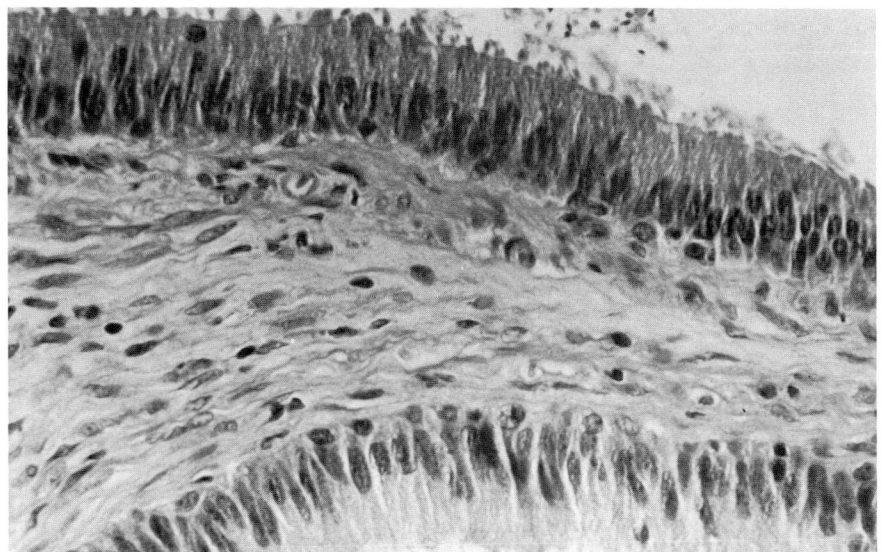

Figure 7-8   ***Normal epididymis.*** *The ciliated pseudostratified columnar epithelium of the epididymis is invested with a layer of smooth muscle.*

locations.[72,75-77] Their frequency in children (7.5%) is higher than that observed in older age groups, suggesting regression with age.[75] Hyperplasia and neoplasia have been rarely reported in such ectopic foci of adrenal tissue.[76,77]

Recently, structural abnormalities of the testis and epididymis have been reported in males exposed to diethylstilbestrol (DES) in utero.[78-81] An increased frequency of both unilateral and bilateral epididymal cysts has been observed.[78,81]

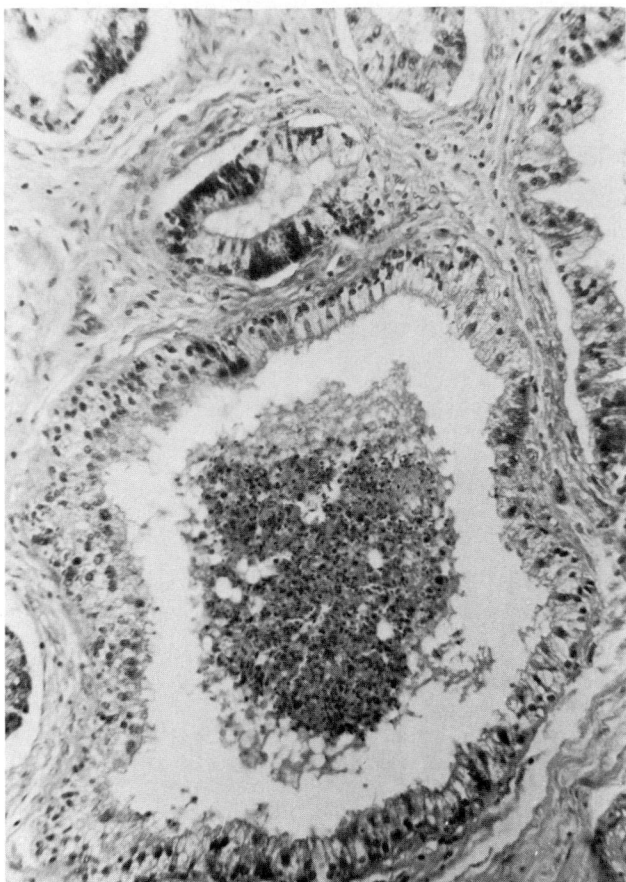

Figure 7-9   **Brown patches of the epididymis.** *The lipofuscin pigment appears as dark granules in the cytoplasm of the epididymal epithelium. Sperm are present in the duct lumen. The brown patches were incidental findings at autopsy.*

Testicular abnormalities include hypoplasia, capsular fibrosis, a high frequency of cryptorchidism, and abnormal semen analyses.[78-81]

Acquired Cysts (Spermatocele)

Cysts of the epididymis, or spermatoceles, originate most commonly from the caput of the epididymis and specifically from the efferent ducts, or the more proximal rete testis.[82,83] They may be unilocular or multilocular, and contain opalescent fluid. They are capable of enlarging to several centimeters. The diagnosis of spermatocele, as opposed to hydrocele (a cyst of the tunica vaginalis) or cyst of the testicular appendages, requires the demonstration of sperm or sperm fragments within the cyst fluid. If needed, a cell block of the cyst fluid will accomplish this evaluation. These are relatively common clinical disorders that have a possible adverse effect on a patient's fertility, a complication not associated with most hydroceles. Distinguishing between the two types of cysts is thus not an academic exercise. Histologically, the cyst wall is composed of fibro-muscular tissue, as are the septae if the specimen is multilocular. The lining epithelium is commonly flattened or denuded. Admixed chronic inflammatory cells are commonly present in the cyst wall.

On rare occasions, microscopic papillary proliferations of the lining cells may be found in spermatocele specimens.[84,85] The papillae are covered by a single layer of columnar epithelium, some cells of which show cytoplasmic vacuolization. No evidence of cytologic atypia or histologic evidence of invasion of the spermatocele wall is present. Mostofi and Price have termed these papillary proliferations *mural papillomas* of spermatoceles.[85] They probably represent variants of cystadenomas of the epididymis, as described originally by Sherrick.[120] (Refer to later discussion of cystadenoma of the epididymis.)

Inflammatory Disorders

Nonspecific Acute and Chronic Epididymitis

With the exception of those cases of epididymitis determined to be of gonococcal, tuberculous, or rarely, fungal origin, most cases in the past were termed *idiopathic* epididymitis.[86] With the decreasing frequency of tuberculosis, an increasing percentage of this inflammatory disorder were therefore of the idiopathic type.[87] In recent years significant advances have been achieved in determining the etiology of acute epididymitis.[88] In summary, the majority of cases involving men younger than 35 years of age are due to *Neisseria gonorrhoeae* and *Chlamydia trachomatis,* whereas *Escherichia coli* is the most common etiologic agent in men older than 35 years.[88] Epididymitis in infants is rare, with 32 cases reported to 1979.[89] There is a significant frequency of associated congenital anomalies of the urogenital tract resulting in urethro-ejaculatory reflex among the reported infants.[89,90] Associated urinary tract infections are common among the older patients with epididymitis of coliform etiology.[68]

The surgical pathologist encounters acutely or chronically inflamed epididymis specimens only uncommonly. In most instances epididymal aspirates or urethral discharge specimens are obtained for smears and culturing.

Histologically, acute inflammation of the epididymis is primarily manifested within the duct lumen with numerous neutrophils admixed with sperm fragments (Fig. 7-10). Focal epithelial ulceration, necrosis, and duct destruction with abscess formation is seen. Squamous metaplasia of the duct epithelium can occur. Persistence of the infection without resolution is associated with increased numbers of plasma cells, histiocytes, and lymphocytes, and a corresponding decrease in neutrophils (Fig. 7-11). Resolution is accompanied by fibrosis, frequently with obliteration and obstruction of the affected duct segments.

Gonorrhea

Epididymal infection following urethral involvement was typical of *N. gonorrhoeae.*[91-94] This association is less typical currently.[91] Histologically the acute inflammatory reaction is nonspecific, but intracellular gram-negative diplococci are diagnostic. Although scrotal (epididymal) pain and tenderness are present in the majority of infected cases, significant numbers of patients are

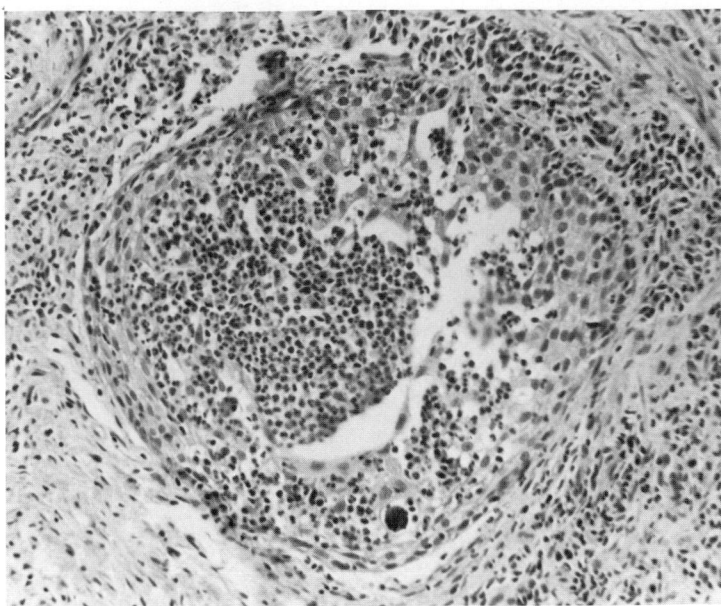

Figure 7-10   *Acute epididymitis. Numerous neutrophils are present in the lumen and the epithelium of the epididymis. The squamous metaplasia of epithelium suggests that the acute inflammation is superimposed on chronic injury to the epididymis.*

asymptomatic and serve as a reservoir for further spread.[93] Epididymal involvement by *N. gonorrhoeae* results in significant destruction with abscess formation, and ultimately fibrosis and sterility. The majority of patients are adults younger than 35 years of age. Systemic dissemination is reported to occur in 1% to 3% of patients.[92-93] (Refer to discussion of gonorrhea in Chap. 5.)

Tuberculosis

Tuberculous involvement of the male genital tract most commonly is associated with previous established renal and pulmonary infection. Epididymal involvement results either from hematogenous dissemination or, more frequently, from infected urine. Concomitant prostatic tuberculosis is common. Patients with genital tuberculosis frequently present because of lower urinary tract symptoms, epididymal pain, or nonspecific constitutional symptoms.[95-98] Epididymal induration, associated with beading of the vas deferens, is typically found on physical examination.

The histologic features of tuberculous infection of the epididymis are identical to the lesions elsewhere. The classic caseating granuloma with Langhans' giant cells, palisading epithelioid histiocytes, and a margin of lymphocytes and plasma cells is observed. Appropriate stains for the acid-fast organisms frequently will demonstrate the tubercle bacilli in the lesion. Ultimate resolution is commonly associated with substantial fibrosis and destruction of the epididymal ducts.

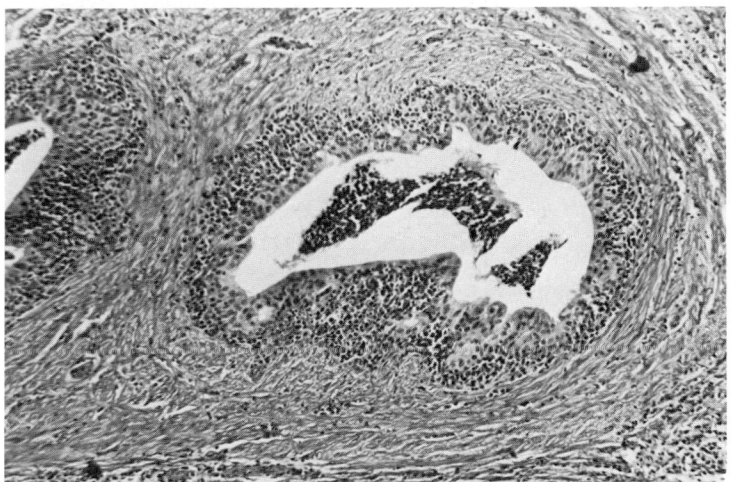

Figure 7-11 *Chronic epididymitis. Numerous lymphocytes surround and infiltrate the wall of the epididymis.*

Fungal Infections

Rare cases of fungal infections of the epididymis have appeared sporadically in the literature. Fungal organisms that infect the epididymis include North American blastomycosis,[99,100,102] South American blastomycosis,[101] histoplasmosis,[103] and coccidiomycosis.[104]

Spermatic Granuloma

The etiology of spermatic granuloma is unsettled.[105,107] The readily apparent effect is the marked inflammatory response to sperm that have gained entrance to the interstitium of the epididymis. Glassy and Mostofi favor ductal epithelial and basement membrane damage secondary to trauma or infection with secondary release of duct contents, including sperm, into the adjacent interstitium.[107] Alternatively, increased intraductal pressure that results in ductal rupture has the same end result.[105]

This lesion is observed in the epididymis and vas deferens, especially in association with prior vasectomy operations. (Refer to discussion of vasitis nodosa of the vas deferens.) In the largest series of such cases published to date, Glassy and Mostofi reported 60 patients ranging in age from 18 years to 74 years.[107] Fifty percent of these patients were in the third decade and about half had a history of epididymitis, vasectomy, or trauma. Bilateral sperm granulomas were present in one infertile male in the series. The majority of patients complained of pain and swelling, in many instances lasting for months to years.[107,108] Some examples were incidental findings, and apparently asymptomatic.

Sperm granulomas of the epididymis are firm to hard nodules averaging less than 1 cm. The largest examples reported by Glassy and Mostofi measured 3 cm.[107] The cut surface is white-cream. The nodules are irregular in outline, but they are well demarcated from the uninvolved epididymis.

Microscopically, the histologic features vary, reflecting the stage of evolution of this inflammatory process. Neutrophils predominate in the earliest le-

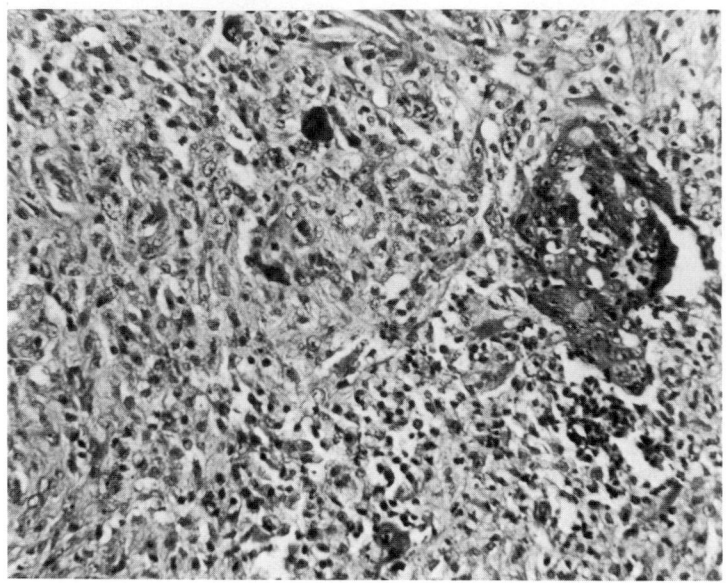

Figure 7-12   ***Sperm granuloma.*** *The inflammatory infiltrate is composed of mixed chronic inflammatory cells including histiocytes with giant cells* (far right). *Numerous sperm fragments are present in the cytoplasm of the giant cells.*

sions and the picture is that of acute epididymitis with extravasated sperm in the interstitium. The evolution of this inflammatory reaction results in the characteristic granuloma formation with predominance of lymphocytes and histiocytes (Fig. 7-12). Multinucleated giant cells are rare. Phagocytosis of sperm by the histiocytes is typical. Interstitial fibrosis in association with the inflammatory lesion is common. The ducts show a variably intense infiltrate of neutrophils and histiocytes, with ulceration, necrosis, and occasionally squamous metaplasia of the ductal epithelium.[105,107] The detection of sperm in the intense inflammatory infiltrate may be assisted by applying the acid-fast stain, which will detect the acid-fast lipid component of sperm originally reported by Berg.[106]

Malakoplakia

Malakoplakia of the epididymis was first reported by Green in 1968.[109] Eleven cases have been subsequently reported.[110–117] The patients range in age from 24 years to 75 years without any apparent intervening age predilection. Six of the reported patients had concurrent involvement of the testis (Table 7-2).

The histologic features supporting the diagnosis are identical to those described in other more common sites of involvement. (Refer to discussion of malakoplakia in Chap. 4.)

Cholesteatoma

Two reported cases of epididymal cholesteatomas occurring in patients with previous scrotal trauma are reported.[118,119] The lesions measured 1 cm to 3 cm and were filled with yellow-brown debris. Microscopically, amorphous eosino-

Table 7-2   ***Malakoplakia of the Epididymis***

Author	Year	Patient's Age	Testicular Involvement
Green	1968	70	No
Waisman, Rampton	1968	40	Yes
Waisman, Rampton	1968	23	Yes
Yang, Murathe	1969	33	Yes
Clay et al	1971	67	No
Shaba, Black	1971	41	Yes
Scheiner et al	1975	61	No
Scheiner et al	1975	24	Yes
Scheiner et al	1975	63	No
Schornagel et al	1976	70	No
Guccion et al	1978	75	Yes
McClure	1980	38	No

philic debris with admixed cholesterol clefts and degenerating cells filled the cyst lumen. Epithelial cells were reported lining one cyst. The cyst wall is composed of fibrous tissue.

The pathogenesis of these cholesteatomas is most probably linked to the prior episodes of trauma in both cases. In one patient this trauma was known to have incised the skin. Possible epidermal fragments were displaced into the scrotum with ultimate development of epidermoid cyst and secondary degeneration and inflammation. Alternatively, squamous metaplasia of the mesothelial cells of the tunica vaginalis could lead to epidermoid cysts. Teratomatous origin is ruled out by the absence of tissue components other than the epithelial lining cells.

Benign Epithelial Neoplasms

Papillary Cystadenoma

Papillary cystadenoma, a rare lesion, was first described by Sherrick in 1956.[120] Approximately 30 cases have been reported in the literature since then. It has been variously regarded as a hyperplastic, hamartomatous, or benign neoplastic proliferation of the lining epithelium.[120,127]

In 1963, Grant and Hoffman reported a case of bilateral epididymal papillary cystadenomas found in association with a cerebellar hemangioblastoma in a 19-year-old patient.[122] In subsequent publications, both unilateral and bilateral cases of this epididymal lesion have been reported in association with von Hippel–Lindau disease, in which cerebellar hemangioblastoma is one component.[123,127] Other components of this syndrome include retinal angioma, hemangiomas of the spinal cord, cysts of the skin, lung, pancreas, or kidneys, and importantly, renal cell carcinoma.[127,130,131] Approximately one third of the cases reported to this time evidence the associated findings of all, or more frequently, only specific components of the von Hippel–Lindau disease.[120-131] The known familial characteristics of this disease have also been demonstrated recently by epididymal papillary cystadenomas, bilateral examples of which were found in three siblings who also manifested the other components of Lindau's disease.[128] Those cases of epididymal papillary cystadenoma without clinical evidence of other components of von Hippel–Lindau disease should be followed closely to detect any other manifestations that subsequently emerge. Price has suggested that unilateral cases of papillary cystadenoma of the epididymis probably represent isolated manifestations of the disease. Such patients will have a lower probability of additional manifestations emerging than those with bilateral epididymal lesions.[127]

The lesion of the epididymis is most frequently reported to arise in the caput. It appears as a 1 cm to 6 cm cystic nodule. The cut surface is variously tan, mucoid, or hemorrhagic. Microscopically, papillary projections emanating from the cyst walls are lined by a single or a double layer of secretory and ciliated columnar cells that are cytologically similar to those normally present in the efferent ductules.[120,122,127] This observation, made by Sherrick in the original description of the lesion, has been confirmed in the ultrastructural studies of Tsuda and co-workers.[128] Many, and in some cases most, of the cells, show cytoplasmic vacuolization.[120,122,127] The papillary projections are generally delicate and vary in their structural complexity. Focal areas show dense hyalinized collagen in the papillary stalks and the cyst wall. Focal areas of the proliferating cells may form solid cords devoid of papillary structure and apear to invade the cyst wall. This is interpreted as encroachment and not true invasion. Secretory substances, both intracellular and within the cyst lumen, are PAS-positive (Figs. 7-13, 7-14).[122,123] Chronic inflammatory cells may be focally present in the cyst wall stroma. The histologic features of cases with and without other associated manifestations of von Hippel–Lindau disease are identical.

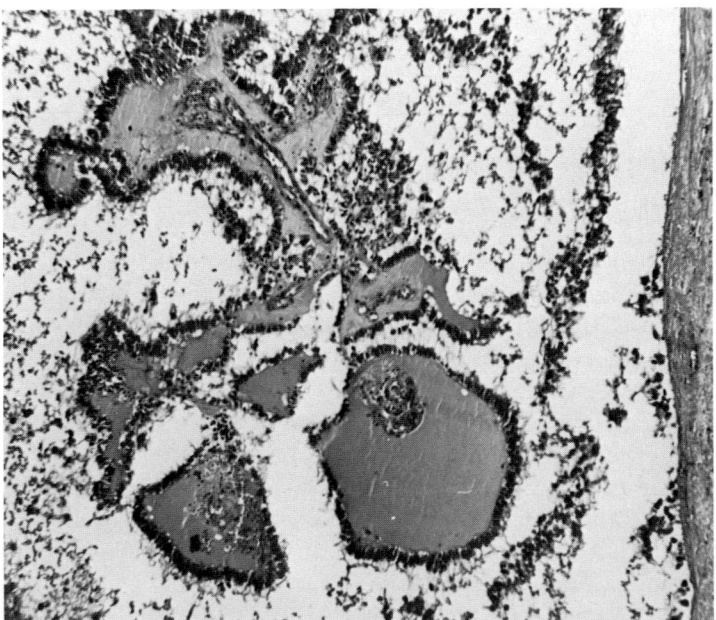

Figure 7-13   *Papillary cystadenoma. The cystic dilatation of the epididymis contains papillary infoldings lined by epithelial cells with cleared cytoplasm and absence of atypical features. PAS-positive secretory material is present in the duct lumen.*

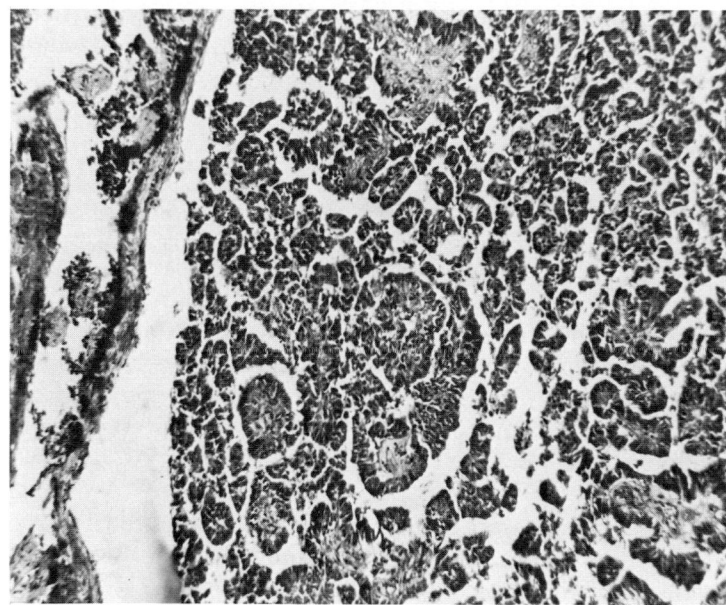

Figure 7-14 *Papillary cystadenoma. The papillary projections are more numerous than those in Figure 7-13. There was no evidence of invasion of adjacent epididymis by the neoplasm.*

Malignant Epithelial Neoplasms

Carcinoma

Carcinoma of the epididymis is rare, with fewer than 20 cases reported to 1969.[136] These neoplasms show histologic heterogeneity with a spectrum of papillary adenocarcinoma, adenocarcinoma, squamous cell carcinoma, and undifferentiated carcinomas, which are all interpreted as primary epididymal carcinoma.[132-136] Included in some earlier reviews are extratesticular germ cell tumors, primarily seminoma, arising in the epididymis.[136]

The reported patients range in age from 22 years to 78 years with 7 (50%) in the third and fourth decades.[136] According to the limited information provided, (1) the tumor size ranges from 3 cm to 6 cm; (2) about half are associated with a hydrocele; and (3) they must be regarded as highly aggressive neoplasms with 8 of 10 patients dying of tumor-related causes within 45 months of diagnosis.[136] Widespread metastases are recorded in many of these cases.

Primary carcinoma of the epididymis, that is, carcinoma originating in the epithelial lining cells of the duct, must be differentiated from benign mesotheliomas (the papillary and the so-called adenomatoid varieties), malignant mesothelioma, extratesticular germ cell neoplasms, and the rare examples of metastatic carcinoma in the epididymis.

Extratesticular Germ Cell Tumors

Ten cases of germ cell tumors originating in the epididymis were collected from the literature by Salm (1969).[136] Six of these cases were seminomas and four were teratomas, teratocarcinomas, or mixed germ cell tumors.[136] These patients range in age from 2 weeks to 13 years, with eight of the ten patients younger than 5 years of age.[136] Because the reported cases span a period beginning in 1914, the recorded survival data is of historical interest only.

Benign Mesenchymal Neoplasms

Leiomyoma

Benign smooth muscle neoplasms of the epididymis are rare. In a collective review published in 1924, Hinman and Gibson found two previously reported cases.[137] Friedman and Grayzel collected 13 cases reported as of 1942.[142] The number reported in English-language literature increased only to 23 cases by 1972, as presented in the review by Spark.[144] Additional cases have been reported in the Japanese literature.[144] Five cases of bilateral epididymal leiomyomas have been reported.[143,144]

The age range of the reported cases is 25 years to 81 years, with 61% of the cases observed in patients in the third and fourth decades.[142,144] Many of the cases have associated hydrocele or inguinal hernia.[144] The reported leiomyomas range in size from less than 1 cm to 8 cm.[144] There is no side predilection. Patient awareness of a slowly growing intratesticular nodule for a prolonged period before seeking medical attention is not uncommon. Some reported cases are incidental findings at autopsy.[144]

Grossly, these lesions are well circumscribed, firm, white, gray, or pink-white nodules showing the typical whorled appearance on the cut surface. Compression of the adjacent epididymal structure is observed. Microscopically, there are typical interlacing fascicles of smooth muscle nuclei. There is no necrosis, significant mitotic activity, or atypia of the cells. Treatment is surgical excision, which in the past has frequently included the testis and involved epididymis. Differential diagnosis includes leiomyosarcoma, of which even fewer cases have been reported arising in the epididymis.

Malignant Mesenchymal Neoplasms

Leiomyosarcoma

Eleven cases of primary leiomyosarcoma of the epididymis were found in the literature.[145-151] The first recorded case was a patient reported from China in 1949 by Kwae.[145] Malignant smooth muscle neoplasms of the epididymis tend to occur more frequently in older patients (64% in the sixth and seventh decades) than do benign mesenchymal neoplasms. However, the age ranges overlap, with leiomyosarcomas reported in patients 6 years to 74 years of age.[145-151] The youngest reported patient (6 years of age) with leiomyosarcoma of the epididymis was recorded by Farrell and Donnelly.[151]

The gross features of the reported cases vary. All of the masses are firm, irregular, or spherical, 2 cm to 8 cm in diameter. Some have been reported as encapsulated and well delineated, whereas others are poorly delineated and fixed to adjacent structures. Thus, the gross features of some do not readily suggest the malignancy discovered on microscopic review. Histologically, variable numbers of mitoses are reported. Unfortunately, mitotic frequency among these neoplasms has not been quantitated uniformly, and thus no well-defined criteria have emerged. Accompanying features suggesting malignancy include foci of necrosis and significant nuclear pleomorphism, neither of which are observed in the benign counterpart at this site. Lymph nodes removed at surgery in two of the reported patients were found free of tumor when reviewed microscopically.[145,146]

To date, none of the 11 reported patients has died of tumor-related causes. One patient was alive with bone metastases after 14 months when reported.[146] Three patients died without evidence of tumor recurrence 1 year to 20 years after surgery.[147] Four patients were reported alive without evidence of tumor recurrence 2 months to 21 years after surgery.[149-151]

Rhabdomyosarcoma

Eleven cases of rhabdomyosarcoma arising in the epididymis were found in the literature.[152-161] Rhabdomyosarcomas more commonly take origin in the spermatic cord and paratesticular tissues. Frequently, the precise site of origin is difficult to determine. The patients ranged in age from 7 years to 36 years, with 64% of cases occurring in patients in their second decade.[152-161]

These neoplasms, ranging in size from a few to several centimeters, are soft or rubbery ill-defined masses that are gray-white or pink on the cut surface. Focal areas of necrosis and hemorrhage are common. The most common histologic variant is embryonal rhabdomyosarcoma, but the pleomorphic and alveolar types also have been observed.[152-161] The rhabdomyoblastic nature of these tumors is determined by the histologic features typical of the four variants, the presence of myosin determined by immunoperoxidase staining, and cross striations detected by PTAH-staining or electron microscopy. (Refer to discussion of rhabdomyosarcoma of the spermatic cord.)

Survival among these 11 patients, all treated by surgery with or without adjunct therapy, is variable: four patients died of tumor-related deaths within 2 years of diagnosis.[157-160] Five patients were alive and without evidence of recurrence 1 year to 14 years after diagnosis.[152-156,160,161]

Primary Lymphoma

One case of a primary histiocytic lymphoma arising in the epididymis of a 26-year-old man is reported in the literature.[162] More frequently, the epididymal involvement by lymphoma reflects extension from testicular lymphoma, or systemic dissemination of lymphoma. (Refer to discussion of malignant lymphoma of the testis in Chap. 6.) In the one case of primary lymphoma of the epididymis, no evidence of tumor recurrence was noted 8 months after orchiectomy and postoperative radiation.[162]

Metastatic Neoplasms

Malignant neoplasms that originate in the testis or spermatic cord and involve the epididymis by direct contiguous spread are not uncommon. Metastatic neoplasms in the epididymis originating from distant sites are distinctly rare. Three examples of prostatic adenocarcinoma metastatic to the epididymis have been reported by Humphrey (1944), Brotherus (1960), and Broth (1968).[165,167,168] Two cases metastatic from the stomach are reported by Katzen (1941) and Brotherus (1960).[164,167] O'Brien reported a case of carcinoid originating in the ileum and metastasizing to the epididymis.[166] Reference is made in the older literature to renal malignancies metastatic from the kidney. Most reported examples of metastatic neoplasms in the epididymis are of little clinical consequence. The ileal carcinoid reported by O'Brien (1951) was discovered when the patient had symptoms referable to the epididymal metastases.[166]

Spermatic Cord

Normal Structures

The spermatic cord (funiculus spermaticus) is composed of the vas deferens (ductus deferens) and accompanying arteries, veins, lymphatics, and nerves, all within a loose fibromuscular and adipose tissue investment.

The vas deferens, the distal continuity of the epididymal duct, ultimately forms the ejaculatory duct with the distal seminal vesicle to terminate in the prostatic urethra at the verumontanum. Three well-developed muscle coats surround the epithelium and the lamina propria. The external and internal longitudinal muscle bundles are separated by an intervening circular muscle bundle. The muscle coats of the wall produce the characteristic irregular, occasionally stellate, lumen in cross sections of the vas. The lining epithelium is composed of pseudostratified columnar cells (Fig. 7-15).

Intranuclear inclusions, the significance of which is not known, are present

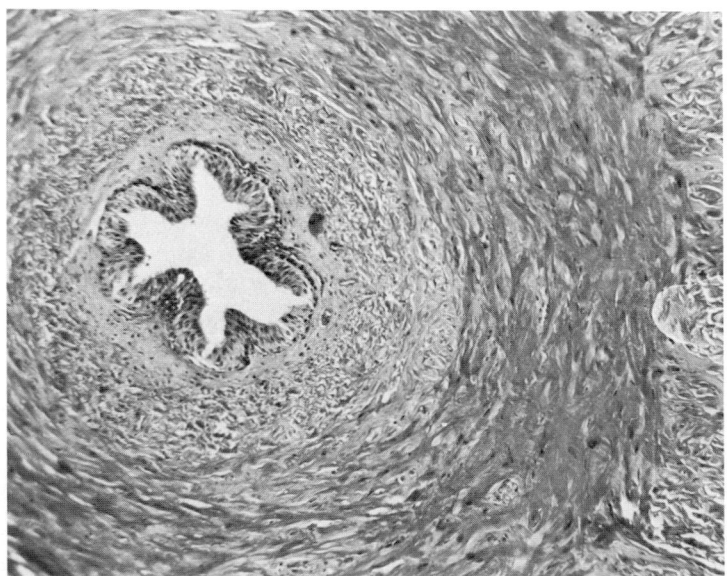

Figure 7-15   *Normal vas deferens. The columnar lining cells of the vas deferens rest on a basement membrane. The surrounding muscle bundles are arranged in longitudinal and circular groups.*

in the epithelial cells lining the vas deferens in adult males.[169] The cytologically atypical cells that are reported to occur normally in both the seminal vesicle and epididymis have not been observed in the vas deferens. In reviewing cross sections of the vas deferens segments removed to achieve desired infertility, the complete wall structure, most importantly including the epithelial lined lumen, must be present to conclude confidently that the operation achieved a segmental interruption of this duct.

Congenital Anomalies

Congenital anomalies of the vas deferens include agenesis, duplication, and ectopia.[170-172]

Inflammatory Disorders

Vasitis Nodosa

The first description of this disorder was reported by Benjamin and co-workers (1943) who introduced the term *vasitis nodosa*.[173] These authors encountered a 27-year-old man who complained of intermittent discomfort in the left spermatic cord for 2 months. Beading of the vas deferens suggestive of tuberculosis was found on physical examination. Microscopic review of a resected segment of the vas deferens disclosed numerous epithelial lined spaces, some containing spermatozoa, within the muscularis and in the peri-vas adventitial tissue. An associated intramural chronic inflammatory cell infiltration accompanied these displaced ductal structures. Possible etiologic factors including infection, diverticula, or developmental defect were considered. Clinically similar and histologically identical lesions were subsequently reported by Graham and O'Connor (1954), who interpreted the lesion as "ductal hyperplasia," and Tamayo and Ruffulo (1967), who interpreted it as "ectopic mesonephric ductules (mesonephric hamartoma)." [174,175]

In 1969, Pugh and Hanley reported normal sperm counts in a patient 13 weeks after segmental resections of the vas deferens.[176] In a second resection of the vas 10 months after the first operation, intramural ductules containing sperm were observed, resulting in a recanalization of the vas deferens. Independent of the medico–legal implications, this observation had pathogenetic ramifications referable to vasitis nodosa. The capacity for regenerative growth was reported in subsequent studies.[177,182,184] It is now recognized that the microscopic evidence of the ductule proliferation and chronic inflammation, including sperm granulomas, are observed in the majority of vas specimens removed at reanastomosis, at variable intervals following previous vasectomy segmental resections.[184] Vasitis nodosa in this context can be asymptomatic, but it is frequently associated with pain.[183] The proliferation of the ductules can superficially resemble invasive adenocarcinoma, especially when this proliferation is found in perineural locations, as has been reported elsewhere.[177,180,181] The etiology of vasitis nodosa occurring in patients without a history of vasectomy is unknown.

The diagnosis is made microscopically upon finding sperm-containing ductules in the muscular coat (Fig. 7-16) or extending into the peri-vas adventitia

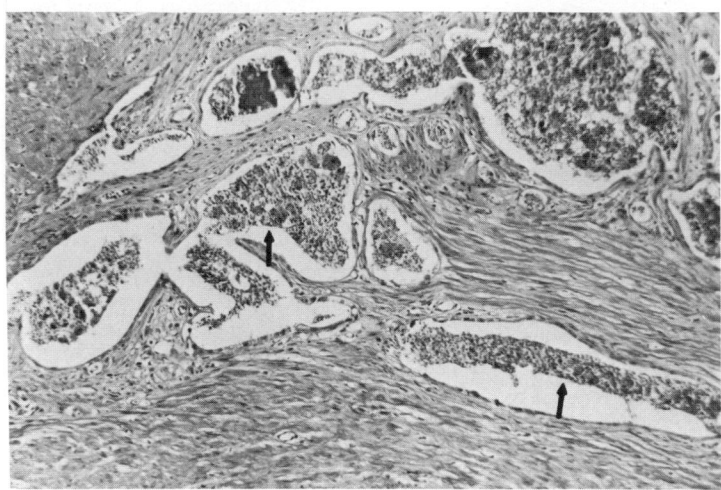

Figure 7-16   ***Vasitis nodosa.*** *The extravasated sperm are present in the outer muscle layers of the vas deferens* (arrows).

in association with chronic inflammation. The latter component may have all the histologic hallmarks of sperm granulomas. (Refer to discussion of sperm granuloma of epididymis.) Serial sections will invariably disclose the intramural ductules originating from the surface epithelium lining the lumen of the vas deferens.

Miscellaneous Inflammatory Disorders

Inflammatory disorders associated with schistosomiasis and foreign bodies have been reported in the vas deferens.[186,187] Tuberculous involvement of the vas deferens is commonly associated with epididymal infection, and both in turn are associated with involvement of the urinary tract.[185]

Benign Mesenchymal Neoplasms

Benign mesenchymal neoplasms of the spermatic cord are relatively common because of the high frequency of lipomas, which constitute more than 90% of all histologic types.[188-191] All other neoplasms, including adenomatoid tumors, lymphangiomas, leiomyomas, neurofibromas, and granular cell tumors, are uncommon to rare in this location.[192-198] The available literature comprises early historical reviews, case reports, and more recent cumulative reviews.[137-140] In many of these reviews, "fibromas" were noted to be the second most common neoplasm.[137-140] As discussed earlier, these lesions are now regarded as non-neoplastic pseudotumors.

Many of intrascrotal benign mesenchymal neoplasms are reported as "paratesticular," and their exact site of origin is not stated. Leyson and co-workers have suggested a classification of intrascrotal lipomas according to site of origin.[190] It should be applied to all intrascrotal neoplasms to achieve a uniformity that is now lacking in the available literature. The histologic features of each of these benign mesenchymal neoplasms are identical to those occurring elsewhere.

Malignant Mesenchymal Neoplasms

With the exception of lipomas of the spermatic cord, sarcomas as a group constitute the second most common type of neoplasm arising in this site.[202] Several specific sarcomas with varying frequency are now recognized to take origin at the site, as shown in the list below (in order of frequency).[199-207]

Rhabdomyosarcoma[208-222]

Leiomyosarcoma[223-235]

Fibrosarcoma[236-241]

Liposarcoma[242-251]

Malignant fibrous histiocytoma[252-256]

Malignant mesenchymoma[258,259]

Angiosarcoma[257]

Undifferentiated sarcoma

Unclassified sarcoma

Rhabdomyosarcomas, the sarcoma arising most frequently in the cord, is most commonly diagnosed in children and adolescents, in contrast to all other types, which typically occur in older adults in the fourth to seventh decades. Rhabdomyosarcomas are also distinguished by their greater tendency to metastasize to regional lymph nodes than that demonstrated by other sarcomas arising in the spermatic cord.[205] All sarcomas show the tendency of dissemination by way of blood vessel invasion.

The older literature contains many reports of histogenetically unclassified spermatic cord sarcomas. Although the vast majority of sarcomas now can be accurately diagnosed with the assistance of histochemical stains, immunoperoxidase stains, and electron microscopy, these neoplasms remain a major diagnostic challenge in many cases. Some cases can be classified only as undifferentiated sarcomas, if their exact histogenesis still is not apparent after thorough study.

No standardized staging protocol for intratesticular sarcomas exists, with the exception of that utilized by the Intergroup Rhabdomyosarcoma Study. A modification of this staging protocol is outlined in Table 7-3.

Table 7-3   ***Staging Protocol for Rhabdomyosarcoma***

Stage I	Tumor confined to organ of origin, completely resected; no microscopic residua, regional lymph nodes negative

Stage II	Regional spread
	   No microscopic residua; regional nodes negative
	   Microscopic residua; regional nodes negative
	   No microscopic residua; regional nodes positive
	   Microscopic residua; regional nodes positive

Stage III	Gross residual disease
Stage IV	Distant metastases

* Modification of Intergroup Rhabdomyosarcoma Study Protocol.[221]

Rhabdomyosarcoma

Sarcomas of skeletal muscle origin are the most common malignant mesenchymal neoplasms of the spermatic cord. Hirsch in 1934 reported the first case in the American literature and reviewed cases of paratesticular rhabdomyosarcomas previously reported in the European literature.[208] Skeel and co-workers in 1975 reported three cases and collected 50 spermatic cord rhabdomyosarcomas from the literature.[209-216,218] Scattered additional cases bring the total to approximately 60.[218-221] This compares with approximately 100 cases of intrascrotal rhabdomyosarcomas originating in paratesticular, testicular, tunica, epididymal, and scrotal wall sites.[221]

The age distribution of reported rhabdomyosarcomas in all intrascrotal sites shows a preponderance of cases in the first two decades.[221] Detection of a mass in the scrotum prompts 97% of patients to seek medical attention. Olney and co-workers noted that the duration of symptoms increased and survival decreased with patient age.[221] When viewed in situ, the neoplasms are commonly large, with extensive local infiltration of epididymis, testis, and the sac of the tunica vaginalis. They are gray-white, firm, and poorly demarcated.

Microscopically, the highly variable histologic pattern of embryonal rhabdomyosarcoma is typical (Figs. 7-17, 7-18). The presence of strap cells, with or without cross striations, bizarre "tadpole" cells, and primitive myoblast-type cells with intense eosinophilic cytoplasm assist in making the diagnosis.[217] Immunoperoxidase staining of myoglobin is confirmatory, as is the detection of the typical ultrastructural features when studied by electron microscopy.

Local recurrence and pelvic lymph node metastases occur frequently with rhabdomyosarcomas.[218-220] Current therapy includes surgery. Adjuvant radia-

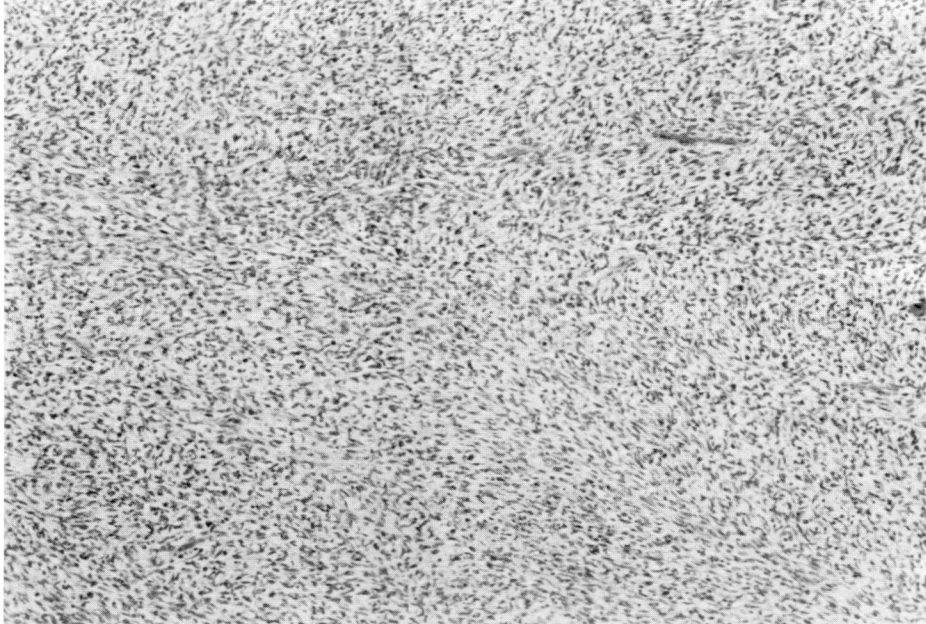

Figure 7-17   *Rhabdomyosarcoma. The highly cellular spindle cell tumor is composed of malignant rhabdomyoblasts, the cytologic features of which are demonstrated in Figure 7-18.*

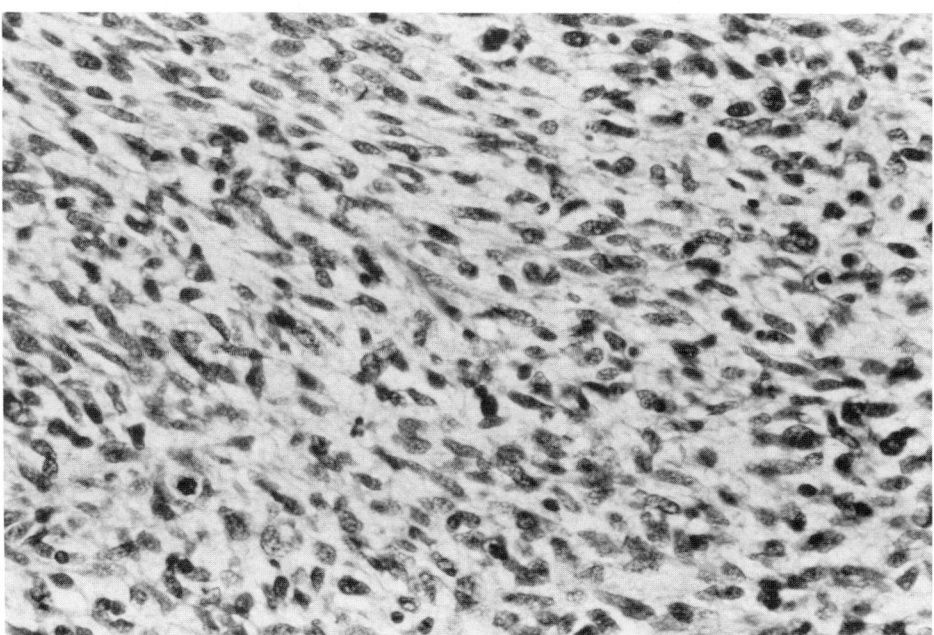

Figure 7-18   *Rhabdomyosarcoma. Higher magnification of the rhabdomyosarcoma of the spermatic cord shows the typical cytologic feature of this neoplasm.*

tion and combination chemotherapy has resulted in significantly improved survival rates, including those patients with documented metastases.[221,222]

Leiomyosarcoma

Nineteen of the collected cases reported by Kyle (1966) are acceptable leiomyosarcomas of the spermatic cord.[229] Two cases incorrectly included in this review took origin from the epididymis (Kwae[145] and Sherwin and Bergman[146]), and are thus excluded.[229] Twenty additional acceptable cases have been reported since Kyle's survey, for a total of 39 cases.[228-235] The reported patients range in age from 15 years to 78 years, with 72% in the sixth to eighth decades. As with fibrosarcomas and liposarcomas of the spermatic cord, there is little demonstrated tendency to metastasize to regional lymph nodes.[226,233] Local recurrence is more typical.[200,205] Origin from a leiomyoma has been reported.[223,224,229] The histologic features of leiomyosarcomas of the cord are similar to those observed in this neoplasm in more common sites of origin (Figs. 7-19, 7-20).

Fibrosarcoma

Fifteen fibrosarcomas of the spermatic cord were collected in a comprehensive literature review by Schulte and co-workers in 1939.[236] Fourteen additional cases were found in the literature, for a total of 29 reported cases.[199-201,204,237-241,243] With the exception of an unusual case involving a 6-year-old boy, reported by Malek, virtually all the other cases of fibrosarcoma involve patients in the sixth to eighth decades.[201] Following surgical excision, prolonged survivals (*e.g.,* 16 years, 18 years, and 24 years) have been reported in some patients.[199,204] Local

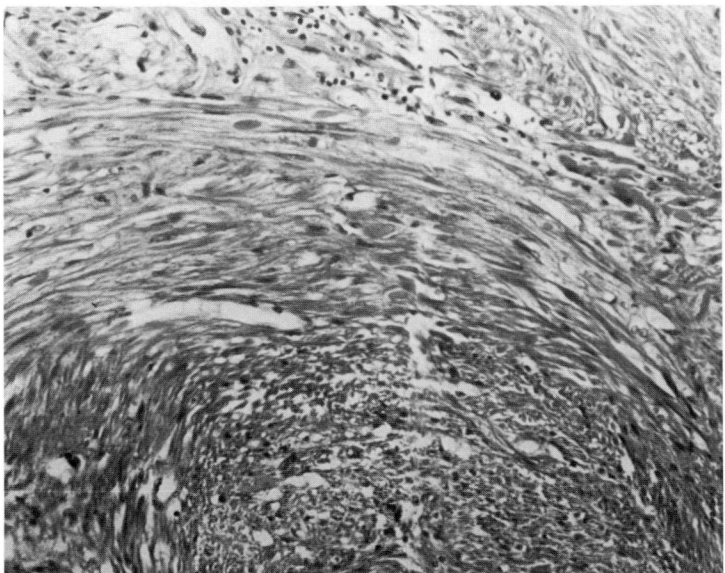

Figure 7-19   *Spermatic cord leiomyoma. Bundles of smooth muscle cells interlace one another. The nuclear features and absence of mitotic figures are typical of the benign smooth muscle tumor.*

recurrences are common. There has been little tendency to metastasize to regional lymph nodes among the few cases reported taking origin in the spermatic cord. Among those reports including sufficient details, the typical feature of interlacing spindle cells in a herringbone pattern, which is characteristic of fibrosarcomas elsewhere, is observed.

Liposarcoma

Twenty-three liposarcomas of the spermatic cord were found in the literature.[201,203,204,242-251] Seventy-five percent of these cases occurred in patients in the sixth to eighth decades. Bissada reported a case in a 29-year-old man, the youngest reported to date.[203] Clinical presentation with a history of a slowly enlarging scrotal mass, known to be present for many weeks to months, and on rare occasions for years, is recorded.[246,250] These neoplasms are capable of attaining large size, as demonstrated by the 13.5 kg (40 cm diameter) neoplasm reported by D'Abrera and Burfitt-Williams.[246] This tumor is treated with radical orchiectomy. Local recurrence has been reported in several cases, with prolonged survival following re-excision.[201,204,250] The majority of liposarcomas of the cord are of the well-differentiated or myxomatous variety. One case reported by Dimacopoulos in 1974 appears to be an example of malignant change in a lipoma.[247]

Miscellaneous Malignant Neoplasms

Rare cases of angiosarcoma, myxosarcoma, and malignant mesenchymoma are found in the literature.[257-260] Malignant fibrous histiocytoma, first described in the spermatic cord in 1972 by Cole and co-workers, has now been reported in a

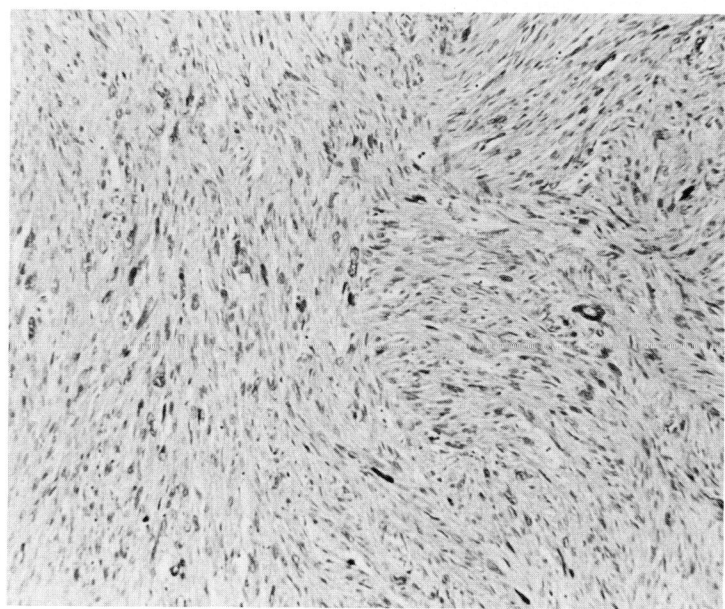

Figure 7-20   *Spermatic cord leiomyosarcoma. The bundles of spindle cells with random orientation constitute the pattern of the neoplasm. Scattered individual cells contain enlarged, hyperchromatic nuclei. Mitoses were common.*

total of nine patients.[252-256] Typical of malignant fibrous histiocytoma in all sites, the majority of the cases reported in the spermatic cord occurred in patients in the sixth to eighth decades.[252-256] The youngest patient with this rare sarcoma in the cord was 32 years old.[256] Unfortunately, the follow-up information supplied in many of these reports is of short duration. Two patients are known to have survived 5 years, with one dying of tumor-related causes 6 years after orchiectomy.[255] Two cases of pheochromocytoma originating in the spermatic cord have been reported in middle-aged men.[261,262] Both neoplasms were hormonally inactive at diagnosis; however, marked elevation of blood pressure was observed during the surgical excision in the case reported by Soejima and coworkers.[262]

Metastatic Neoplasms

Metastatic neoplasms in the spermatic cord are rarely encountered. Thirteen recorded cases were presented in a collective review by Monn and Poticha in 1975.[265] Two additional cases of gastric carcinoma metastatic to the cord and epididymis were found in the literature.[263-264] The clinical significance of these metastases varies among the recorded cases from incidental findings at autopsy, to scrotal masses being the first manifestation of a previously undiagnosed visceral malignancy.[263-265] The stomach was the site of origin for 10 of the 15 cases, with others arising from the colon, appendix, prostate, and kidney.[265] Retrograde lymphatic dissemination is the most probable route of spread to the spermatic cord.

References

Tunica Vaginalis

Hydrocele

1. Campbell MF: Hydrocele of tunica vaginalis. Surg Gynecol Obstet 45:192, 1927
2. Huggins CB, Entz FH: Absorption from normal tunica vaginalis: Hydrocele and spermatocele. J Urol 25:447, 1931
3. Prather GC: Abdominoscrotal hydrocele. N Engl J Med 226:255, 1942

Fibrous Pseudotumor

4. Balloch EA: Fibromata of the tunica vaginalis. Ann Surg 39:396, 1904
5. Hinman F: Tumors of the epididymis, spermatic cord and testicular tunics. A review of the literature and report of three cases. Arch Surg 8:100, 1924
6. Thompson GJ: Tumors of the spermatic cord, epididymis and testicular tunics. Review of the literature and report of forty-one additional cases. Surg Gynecol Obstet 62:712, 1936
7. Goodwin WE, Vermooten V: Multiple fibromata of tunica vaginalis testis or a proliferative type of chronic periorchitis: A report of two cases. J Urol 56:430, 1946
8. Goodwin WE: Multiple, benign, fibrous tumors of tunica vaginalis testis. J Urol 56:438, 1946
9. Lewis HY, Pierce Jr JM: Multiple fibromas of the tunica vaginalis. J Urol 87:142, 1962
10. Mostofi FK, Price Jr EB: Tumors of the male genital system, p 151. In Atlas of Tumor Pathology, 2nd Series, Fascicle 8. Washington, DC, AFIP, 1973
11. Strom GW: Pseudotumor of testicular tunic. J Urol 118:340, 1977
12. Turner Jr WR, Derrick FC, Sanders III P et al: Benign lesions of the tunica albuginea. J Urol 117:602, 1977
13. Gilchrist KW, Benson RC: Multifocal fibrous pseudotumor of testicular tunics. Urol 14:285, 1979
14. Sarlis I, Yakoymakis S, Rebelakos AG: Fibrous pseudotumor of the scrotum. J Urol 124:742, 1980

Cysts of Tunica Albuginea

15. Frater K: Cysts of the tunica albuginea (cysts of the testis). J Urol 21:135, 1929
16. Arcadi JA: Cysts of the tunica albuginea testis. J Urol 68:631, 1952
17. Mancilla-Jimenez R, Matsuda GT: Cysts of the tunica albuginea. Report of 4 cases and review of the literature. J Urol 114:730, 1975
18. Mennemeyer RP, Mason JT: Non-neoplastic cystic lesions of the tunica albuginea: An electron microscopic and clinical study of 2 cases. J Urol 121:373, 1979
19. Sethney HT, Albers DD: Tunica albuginea cyst: Rare testicular mass. Urol 15:285, 1980
20. Warner KE, Noyes DT, Ross JS: Cysts of the tunica albuginea testis: A report of 3 cases with a review of the literature. J Urol 132:131, 1984

Dermoid Cyst

21. Eason AA, Spaulding JT: Dermoid cyst arising in testicular tunics. J Urol 117:539, 1977

Walthard's Rest

22. Hartz PH: Occurrence of Walthard cell rests or Brenner-like epithelium in the serosa of the epididymis. Am J Clin Pathol 17:654, 1947

23. Sundarasivaro D: The Müllerian vestiges and benign epithelial tumors of the epididymis. J Pathol Bact 66:417, 1953

Reactive Mesothelial Cell Proliferations

Papillary Benign Mesothelioma

24. Barbera V, Rubino M: Primary mesothelioma of the tunica vaginalis. Cancer 10:183, 1957
25. Silberblatt JM, Gellman SZ: Mesotheliomas of spermatic cord, epididymis, and tunica vaginalis. Urol 3:235, 1974
26. Mostofi FK, Price EB: Tumors of the male genital system, p 168. In Atlas of Tumor Pathology, Series 2, Fascicle 8. Washington, DC, AFIP, 1973
27. Rosai J, Dehner LP: Nodular mesothelial hyperplasia in hernia sacs: A benign reactive condition simulating a neoplastic process. Cancer 35:165, 1975
28. McDonald RE, Sago AL, Novicki DE et al: Paratesticular mesotheliomas. J Urol 130:360, 1983

Nonpapillary Benign Mesothelioma (Adenomatoid Tumor)

29. Evans N: Mesothelioma of the epididymis and tunica vaginilis. J Urol 50:249, 1943
30. Golden A, Ash JE: Adenomatoid tumors of the genital tract. Am J Pathol 21:63, 1945
31. Longo VJ, McDonald JR: Primary neoplasms of the epididymis. Special reference to adenomatoid tumors. JAMA 147:937, 1951
32. Gray CP, Biorn CL, Drinker HR: Tumors of the epididymis. J Urol 86:620, 1961
33. Broth G, Bullock WK, Morrow J: Epididymal tumors: 1. Report of 15 new cases including review of literature. 2. Histochemical study of the so-called adenomatoid tumor. J Urol 100:530, 1968
34. Marcus JB, Lynn JA: Ultrastructural comparison of an adenomatoid tumor, lymphangioma, hemangioma, and mesothelioma. Cancer 25:171, 1970
35. Maackay B, Benningtonk JL, Skoglund RW: The adenomatoid tumor: fine structural evidence for a mesothelial origin. Cancer 27:109, 1971
36. Ferenczy A, Fenoglio J, Richart RM: Observations on benign mesothelioma of the genital tract (adenomatoid tumor). A comparative ultrastructural study. Cancer 30:244, 1972
37. Glover L, Frensilli FJ, Derrick Jr FC: Simultaneous adenomatoid tumors of epididymis and tunica vaginalis. Urol 2:192, 1973
38. Taxy JB, Battifor H, Oyasu R: Adenomatoid tumors: A light microscopic, histochemical and ultrastructural study. Cancer 34:306, 1974
39. Craig JR, Hart WR: Extragenital adenomatoid tumor. Evidence for the mesothelial theory of origin. Cancer 43:1678, 1979
40. Davy CL, Tang C-K: Are all adenomatoid tumors adenomatoid mesotheliomas? Hum Pathol 12:360, 1981
41. Soderstrom K-O: Origin of adenomatoid tumor. A comparison between the structure of adenomatoid tumor and epididymal duct cells. Cancer 49:2349, 1982

Malignant Mesothelioma

42. Bailey GN, Willis RA, Wilson JV: A case of adenocarcinoma of the appendix testis. J Pathol Bact 69:326, 1955
43. Abell MR, Holtz F: Testicular and paratesticular neoplasms in patients 60 years of age and older. Cancer 21:852, 1968
44. Kasdon EJ: Malignant mesothelioma of the tunica vaginalis propria testis. Report of two cases. Cancer 23:1144, 1969
45. Johnson DE, Fuerst DE, Gallager HS: Mesothelioma of the tunica vaginalis. South Med J 66:1295, 1973

46. Fishelovitch J, Meiraz D, Keinan Z et al: Malignant mesothelioma of the testicular tunica vaginalis. Br J Urol 47:208, 1975

47. Fligiel Z, Kaneko M: Malignant mesothelioma of the tunica vaginalis propria testis in a patient with asbestos exposure. A case report. Cancer 37:1478, 1976

48. Eimoto T, Inoue I: Malignant fibrous mesothelioma of the tunica vaginalis. A histologic and ultrastructural study. Cancer 39:2059, 1977

49. Hamvasi G, Konyar E, Romics I: Uber das mesothelioma der tunica vaginalis. Acta Chir Acad Sci Hung 18:305, 1977

50. Jaffe J, Roth JA, Carter H: Malignant papillary mesothelioma of tunica vaginalis testis. Urol 11:647, 1978

51. Kossow AS, McCann LS: Malignant mesothelioma of the testicular tunic. J Urol 128:272, 1981

52. Japko L, Horta AA, Schreiber K et al: Malignant mesothelioma of the tunica vaginalis testis: Report of first case with preoperative diagnosis. Cancer 49:119, 1982

53. Chen KTK, Arhelger RB, Flam RS et al: Malignant mesothelioma of tunica vaginalis testis. Urol 20:316, 1982

Miscellaneous Rare Neoplasms

Brenner Tumor

54. Vechinski TO, Jaeschke WH, Vermund H: Testicular tumors. An analysis of 112 consecutive cases. Am J Roentgenol 95:494, 1965

55. Ross L: Paratesticular Brenner-like tumor. Cancer 21:722, 1968

56. Goldman RL: A Brenner tumor of the testis. Cancer 26:853, 1970

Testicular Appendages

57. Colt GH: Torsion of the hydatid of Morgagni. Br J Surg 9:464, 1922

58. Scott RT: Torsion of the appendix testis. J Urol 44:755, 1940

59. Seidel RF, Yeaw RC: Torsion of the appendix testis and appendix epididymis: A report of eight cases. J Urol 63:714, 1950

60. Bender RI: Torsion of the appendix of the testis. A review of the literature and presentation of a case. Wis Med J 50:670, 1951

61. Sundarasivarao D: The Müllerian vestiges and benign epithelial tumours of the epididymis. J Pathol Bact 66:417, 1953

62. Ambrose SS, Skandalarkis JE: Torsion of the appendix epididymis and testis: Report of six episodes. J Urol 77:51, 1957

63. Fitzpatrick RJ: Torsion of the appendix testis. J Urol 79:521, 1958

64. Murnaghan GF: The appendages of the testis and epididymis: A short review with case reports. Br J Urol 31:190, 1959

65. Jones P: Torsion of the testis and its appendages during childhood. Arch Dis Child 37:214, 1962

66. Rolnick D, Kawanoue S, Szanto P et al: Anatomical incidence of testicular appendages. J Urol 100:755, 1968

67. Skoglund RW, McRoberts JW, Ragde H: Torsion of testicular appendages: Presentation of 43 new cases and a collective review. J Urol 104:598, 1970

Epididymis

Normal

68. Baumgarten HG, Holstein AF, Rosengren E: Arrangement, ultrastructure and adrenergic innervation of smooth musculature of the ductuli efferentes, ductus epididymis, and ductus deferens of man. Z Zellforsch 120:37, 1971

69. Mitchinson JJ, Sherman KP, Stainer-Smith AM: Brown patches in the epididymis. J Pathol 115:57, 1975

70. Ewing LL: Physiology of male reproduction-5, testis, epididymis. In Harrison JH, Gittes RF, Stanley TA, Welsch PC (eds): Campbell's Urology, 4th ed, p. 134. Philadelphia, WB Saunders, 1978
71. Kuo T-T, Gomez LG: Monstrous epithelial cells in human epididymis and seminal vesicles. A pseudomalignant change. Am J Surg Pathol 5:483, 1981

Congenital Disorders

72. Freeman A: Adrenal cortical adenoma of the epididymis. Arch Pathol 39:336, 1945
73. Waddy SH: The anterior epididymis. Br J Urol 18:24, 1946
74. Lazarus JA, Marks MS: Anomalies associated with undescended testis. J Urol 57:567, 1947
75. Dahl EV, Bahn RC: Aberrant adrenal cortical tissue near the testis in human infants. Am J Pathol 40:587, 1962
76. Morimoto Y, Hiwada K, Nanahoshi M et al: Cushing's syndrome caused by malignant tumor in the scrotum: Clinical, pathologic and biochemical studies. J Clin Endocrinol 32:201, 1971
77. Kirkland RT, Kirkland JL, Keenan BS et al: Bilateral testicular tumors in congenital adrenal hyperplasia. J Clin Endocrinol Metab 44:369, 1977

DES-Related Abnormalities

78. Gill WB, Schumacher GFB, Bibbo M: Structural and functional abnormalities in the sex organs of male offspring of mothers treated with diethylstilbestrol (DES). J Reprod Med 16:147, 1976
79. Bibbo M, Gill WB, Azizi F et al: Follow-up study of male and female offspring of DES-exposed mothers. Obstet Gynecol 49:1, 1977
80. Gill WB, Schumacher GFB, Bibbo M et al: Association of diethylstilbestrol exposure in utero with cryptorchidism, testicular hypoplasia and semen abnormalities. J Urol 122:36, 1979
81. Whitehead ED, Leiter E: Genital abnormalities and abnormal semen analyses in male patients exposed to diethylstilbestrol in utero. J Urol 125:47, 1981

Acquired Cysts (Spermatocele)

82. Huggins C, Noonan WJ: Spermatocele, including x-ray treatment. J Urol 39:784, 1938
83. Wakeley PG: Cysts of the epididymis, the so-called spermatocele. Br J Surg 31:165, 1943
84. Hill Jr RB: Bilateral papillary, hyperplastic nodules of epididymis. J Urol 87:155, 1962
85. Mostofi FK, Price EB: Tumors of the male genital system, p 165. In Atlas of Tumor Pathology, Fascicle 8, 2nd Series. Washington, DC, AFIP, 1973

Inflammatory Disorders

Nonspecific Acute and Chronic Epididymitis

86. Mittemeyer BT, Lennox KW, Borski AA: Epididymitis: A review of 610 cases. J Urol 95:390, 1966
87. Furness G, Kamat MH, Kaminski Z et al: The etiology of idiopathic epididymitis. J Urol 106:387, 1971
88. Berger RE, Alexander ER, Harnisch JP et al: Etiology, manifestations and therapy of acute epididymitis: Prospective study of 50 cases. J Urol 121:750, 1979
89. Williams CB, Litvak AS, McRoberts JW: Epididymitis in infancy. J Urol 121:125, 1979
90. Thomas D, Simpson K, Ostojioc H et al: Bacterimic epididymo-orchitis due to hemophilus influenzae type B. J Urol 126:832, 1981

Gonorrhea

91. Furness G, Kamat MH, Kaminski Z et al: The relationship of epididymitis to gonorrhea. Invest Urol 11:312, 1974
92. Rice PA, Kasper DL: Characterization of gonococcal antigens responsible for induction of bactericidal antibody on disseminated infection: The role of endotoxin. J Clin Invest 60:1149, 1977
93. Fiumara NJ: The sexually transmissable diseases. Dis Month 24:3, 1978
94. Handsfield HH: Gonorrhea and nongonococcal urethritis. Med Clin North Am 62:925, 1978

Tuberculosis

95. Obrent O: Aspects of treatment of urinary tuberculosis. Acta Chir Scand 110:3, 1955
96. Wechsler H, Westfall M, Lattimer JK: The earliest signs and symptoms in 127 male patients with genitourinary tuberculosis. J Urol 83:801, 1960
97. Christensen WI: Genitourinary tuberculosis: A review of 102 cases. Medicine 53:377, 1974
98. Cos LR, Cockett ATK: Genitourinary tuberculosis revisited. Urol 20:111, 1982

Blastomycosis

99. Rolnick D, Baumrucker GO: Genitourinary blastomycosis. J Urol 79:315, 1958
100. Einckemberg HV, Amin M, Lick R: Blastomycosis of the genitourinary tract. J Urol 113:650, 1975
101. Frias FAS, Pasian S, Pires WR et al: South American blastomycosis of epididymis. Urol 14:85, 1979
102. Short KL, Harty JI, Amin M et al: The use of ketoconazole to treat systemic blastomycosis presenting as acute epididymitis. J Urol 129:382, 1983

Histoplasmosis

103. Kauffman CA, Slama TG, Wheat LJ: Histoplasma capsulatum epididymitis. J Urol 125:434, 1981

Coccidioidomycosis

104. Stewart BG: Epididymitis and prostatitis due to coccidioidomycosis: A case report with 5-year follow-up. J Urol 91:280, 1964

Spermatic Granuloma

105. Cronqvist S: Spermatic invasion of the epididymis. Acta Pathol Microbiol Scand 26:786, 1949
106. Berg JW: Differential staining of spermatozoa in sections of testis. Arch Pathol 57:115, 1954
107. Glassy FJ, Mostofi FK: Spermatic granulomas of the epididymis. Am J Clin Pathol 26:1303, 1956
108. Schmidt SS: Spermatic granuloma: An often painful lesion. Fertil Steril 31:178, 1979

Malakoplakia

109. Green Jr WO: Malacoplakia of the epididymis (without testicular involvement). The first reported case. Arch Pathol 86:438, 1968
110. Waisman J, Rampton JB: Malacoplakia of the testis and epididymis. Arch Pathol 86:431, 1968
111. Yang YH, Marathe RL: Malacoplakia of the testis and epididymis (Macrophagie-inclusion epididymo-orchitis). Urol Int 24:364, 1969

112. Clay A, Buffin RP, DuPont A et al: Etude anatomoclinique d'une observation de malacoplasie a localisation epididymaise. Lille Med 16:1089, 1971
113. Shaba JK, Black WA: Malacoplakic granuloma of the testis. J Urol 105:687, 1971
114. Scheiner C, Dor A-M, Basbous D et al: La malacoplasie: formes anatomo-cliniques. Revue de la literature, a propos de 15 observations personnelles. Arch Anat Pathol 23:199, 1975
115. Schornagel JH, Wagenaar SS, de Maat CEM: Malakoplakie. Een zeldzame solitaire lokalisatie in de epididymis. Ned Tijdschr Geneeskd 120:1937, 1976
116. Guccion JG, Thorgiersson UP, Smith BH: Malacoplakia of epididymis. Urol 12:713, 1978
117. McClure J: A case of malacoplakia of the epididymis associated with trauma. J Urol 124:934, 1980

Cholesteatoma

118. Kundert PR: Cholesteatoma of the epididymis. J Urol 56:454, 1946
119. Pingree LJ, Brown DE: Cholesteatoma of the epididymis. J Urol 65:126, 1951

Benign Epithelial Neoplasms

Papillary Cystadenoma

120. Sherrick JC: Papillary cystadenoma of the epididymis. Cancer 9:403, 1956
121. Hill Jr RB: Bilateral papillary, hyperplastic nodules of epididymis. J Urol 87:155, 1962
122. Grant SM, Hoffman EF: Bilateral papillary adenomas of the epididymides. Arch Pathol 76:42, 1963
123. Meyer JS, Roth LM, Silverman JL: Papillary cystadenomas of the epididymis and spermatic cord. Cancer 17:1241, 1964
124. Easton JA, Claridge M: Cystadenoma of the epididymis. Br J Urol 36:416, 1964
125. Chan Y-H, Schinella RA, Draper JW: Papillary clear cell cystadenoma of the epididymis. J Urol 100:661, 1968
126. Broth G, Bullock WK, Morrow J: Epididymal tumors: (1) Report of 15 new cases including review of literature. (2) Histochemical study of the so-called adenomatoid tumor. J Urol 100:530, 1968
127. Price Jr EB: Papillary cystadenoma of the epididymis. A clinicopathologic analysis of 20 cases. Arch Pathol 91:456, 1971
128. Tsuda H, Fukushima S, Takahashi M et al: Familial bilateral papillary cystadenoma of the epididymis. Report of three cases in siblings. Cancer 37:1831, 1976
129. Elsasser E: Tumors of the epididymis. Recent Results Cancer Res 60:163, 1977
130. Fetner CD, Barilla DE, Scott T et al: Bilateral renal cell carcinoma in von Hippel–Lindau syndrome: Treatment with staged bilateral nephrectomy and hemodialysis. J Urol 117:534, 1977
131. Gruber MB, Healey GB, Toguri AG et al: Papillary cystadenoma of epididymis: Component of von Hippel–Lindau syndrome. Urol 16:305, 1980

Malignant Epithelial Neoplasms

Adenocarcinoma

132. Ferrier PA, Foord AG: Primary carcinoma of the epididymis. Urol Cutan Rev 38:646, 1934
133. Whitehead R, Williams AF: Carcinoma of the epididymis. Br J Surg 38:513, 1951
134. Sherwin B, Bergman H: Primary malignant neoplasms of the spermatic cord and epididymis: Two case reports. J Urol 67:208, 1952
135. Fisher ER, Klieger H: Epididymal carcinoma (malignant adenomatoid tumor, mesonephric, mesodermal carcinoma of epididymis). J Urol 95:568, 1966
136. Salm R: Papillary carcinoma of the epididymis. J Pathol 97:253, 1969

Historical Reviews of Mesenchymal Neoplasms

137. Hinman F, Gibson TE: Tumors of the epididymis, spermatic cord and testicular tunics. A review of the literature and report of three new cases. Arch Surg 8:100, 1924
138. Thompson GJ: Tumors of the spermatic cord, epididymis, and testicular tunics. Review of literature and report of forty-one additional cases. Surg Gynecol Obstet 62:712, 1936
139. Strong GH: Lipomyxoma of the spermatic cord: Case report and review of literature. J Urol 48:527, 1942
140. Fitzpatrick RJ, Orr LM, Glanton JB: Tumors of the spermatic cord: Review of literature and report of two cases. JAMA 148:259, 1952

Benign Mesenchymal Neoplasms

Leiomyoma

141. Spivack AH: Leiomyoma of the epididymis: Report of a case and review of the literature. J Urol 34:122, 1935
142. Friedman HH, Grayzel DM: Myomatous tumors of the epididymis. J Urol 47:475, 1942
143. Henderson ID: Bilateral leiomyomas of the epididymis. Br J Surg 44:22, 1956
144. Spark RP: Leiomyoma of epididymis. Arch Pathol 93:18 1972

Malignant Mesenchymal Neoplasms

Leiomyosarcoma

145. Kwae SZ, Liu Y, Chen SC: Leiomyosarcoma of the epididymis: Case report. J Urol 62:349, 1949
146. Sherwin B, Bergman H: Primary malignant neoplasms of the spermatic cord and epididymis: Two case reports. J Urol 67:208, 1952
147. Abell MR: Testicular and paratesticular neoplasms in patients 60 years of age and older. Cancer 21:852, 1968
148. Yadav SB, Patil PN, Karkhanis RB: Primary tumors of the spermatic cord, epididymis and rete testis. J Postgrad Med 15:49, 1969
149. Rushworth GF: Leiomyosarcoma of the epididymis. Proc R Soc Med 64:999, 1971
150. Davides KC, King LM, Paat F: Primary leiomyosarcoma of the epididymis. J Urol 114:642, 1975
151. Farrell MA, Donnelly BJ: Malignant smooth muscle tumors of the epididymis. J Urol 124:151, 1980

Rhabdomyosarcoma

152. Strong GH: Primary malignant tumor of the epididymis (rhabdomyosarcoma). J Urol 48:533, 1942
153. Baurys W, Morton W: Rhabdomyosarcoma of the epididymis. Gutherie Clin Bull 19:201, 1950
154. Horn Jr RC, Enterline HT: Rhabdomyosarcoma: A clinicopathological study and classification of 39 cases. Cancer 11:181, 1958
155. Satter EJ, Heider FC, Wear JB: Primary sarcoma of the spermatic cord and epididymis. J Urol 82:148, 1959
156. Walker WF, Cameron H McD: Rhabdomyosarcoma of the epididymis. Br J Surg 49:319, 1961
157. Ravich L, Lerman PH, Sands A: Intrascrotal extratesticular rhabdomyosarcoma. J Urol 92:144, 1964
158. Arean VM, Kreager JA: Paratesticular rhabdomyosarcoma. Am J Clin Pathol 43:418, 1965

159. Littmann R, Tessler AN, Valensi Q: Paratesticular rhabdomyosarcoma: A case presentation and review of the literature. J Urol 108:290, 1972
160. Olney LE, Norayana A, Loening S et al: Intrascrotal rhabdomyosarcoma. Urol 14:113, 1979
161. Fortune A, Bolton BR: Rhabdomyosarcoma of the paratesticular tissues. J Urol 126:563, 1981

Primary Lymphoma

162. Sched AR, Variakojis D, Straus II FH et al: Primary histiocytic lymphoma of the epididymis. Cancer 43:1156, 1979

Extratesticular Germ Cell Tumors

163. Salm R: Papillary carcinoma of the epididymis. J Pathol 97:253, 1969

Metastatic Neoplasms

164. Katzen P: Metastatic carcinoma of the epididymis: Report of a case. J Urol 46:734, 1941
165. Humphrey MA: Metastasis in the epididymis from cancer of the prostate: Case report. J Urol 51:641, 1944
166. O'Brien JR: Multiple argentaffinomata of ileum revealed by secondary growth in epididymis. Br Med J 2:1315, 1951
167. Brotherus JV: Metastatic tumors of the epididymis and the spermatic cord. J Urol 83:171, 1960
168. Broth G, Bullock WK, Morrow J: Epididymal tumors: (1) Report of 15 new cases including review of literature. (2) Histochemical study of the so-called adenomatoid tumor. J Urol 100:530, 1968

Spermatic Cord

Normal

169. Madara JL, Haggitt RC, Federman M: Intranuclear inclusions of the human vas deferens. Arch Pathol Lab Med 102:648, 1978

Congenital Abnormalities

170. Nelson RE: Congenital absence of the vas deferens: A review of the literature and report of three cases. J Urol 63:176, 1950
171. Beheshti M, Churchill BM, Hardy BE et al: Familial persistent mullerian duct syndrome. J Urol 131:968, 1984
172. van Wingerden JJ, Franz I: The presence of a caput epididymidis in congenital absence of the vas deferens. J Urol 131:764, 1984

Inflammatory Disorders

Vasitis Nodosa

173. Benjamin JA, Robertson TD, Cheetham JG: Vasitis nodosa: A new clinical entity simulating tuberculosis of the vas deferens. J Urol 49:575, 1943
174. Graham JB, O'Connor VJ: Spermatic cord tumors: Review of literature and a case of an unusual vas deferens tumor in an infertility problem. J Urol 72:946, 1954
175. Tamayo JL, Ruffulo EH: Spermatic cord tumor: Mesonephric hamartoma of the vas deferens. Arch Surg 94:430, 1967
176. Pugh RCB, Hanley HG: Spontaneous recanalisation of the divided vas deferens. Br J Urol 41:340, 1969
177. Gruner OPN: Regenerative growth of the vas deferens resembling a low-grade carcinoma: Report of a case. Scand J Urol Nephrol 4:83, 1970
178. Olson AL: Vasitis nodosa. Am J Clin Pathol 55:364, 1971

179. Civantos F, Lubin J, Rywlin AM: Vasitis nodosa. Arch Pathol 94:355, 1972
180. Kovi J, Agbata A: Letter: Benign neural invasion in vasitis nodosa. JAMA 228:1519, 1974
181. Taxy JB: Vasitis nodosa: Two cases. Arch Pathol Lab Med 102:643, 1978
182. Chapman ES, Heidger Jr PM: Spermatic granuloma of vas deferens after vasectomy in rhesus monkeys and men: Light and electron microscopic study. Urol 13:629, 1979
183. Schmidt SS: Spermatic granuloma: An often painful lesion. Fertil Steril 31:178, 1979
184. Taxy JB, Marshall FF, Erlichman RJ: Vasectomy: Subclinical pathologic changes. Am J Surg Pathol 5:767, 1981

Miscellaneous Inflammatory Disorders

185. Garcia JC: Tuberculoma del cordon espermatico. Rev Argent Urol Nefrol 37:10, 1968
186. Bissada NK, Finkbeiner AE, Roundtree GA et al: Foreign bodies in the spermatic cord. J Urol 118:1010, 1977
187. Elbadawi A, Khuri FJ, Cockett ATK: Polypoid granulomatous and sclerosing endophlebitis of spermatic cord: New pathologic type of schistosomal funiculitis. Urol 13: 309, 1979

Benign Mesenchymal Neoplasms

Lipoma

188. Schiller H: Lipoma of the funiculus spermaticus. Ann Surg 68:269, 1918
189. Cecil AB: Intrascrotal lipomata. J Urol 17:557, 1927
190. Leyson JFJ, Doroshow LW, Robbins MA: Extratesticular lipoma: Report of 2 cases and a new classification. J Urol 116:324, 1976
191. Huben RP, Scarff JE, Schellhammer PF: Massive intrascrotal fibrolipoma. J Urol 129:154, 1983

Leiomyoma and Lymphangioma

192. Rubaschow S: Beitrage zur lehre uber die geschwulste der mannlichen geschlechtsorgane. Z Urol Chir 20:290, 1926
193. Rosenfeld A: Zur kasuistik des lymphangioma cysticum nuciculi spermatici. Acta Chir Scand 59:447, 1926
194. Ormond JK, Culp OS: Lymphangioma of spermatic cord: Report of two cases. J Urol 65:906, 1951
195. Chauvin H-F, Farnarier G, Jouve D et al: Lymphangioma kystique du cordon. J Urol Nephrol 68:928, 1962
196. Elbadawi AA, Alghorab MM: Tumors of the spermatic cord: A review of the literature and a report of a case of lymphangioma. J Urol 94:445, 1965

Neurofibroma

197. Schulte TL, McDonald JR, Priestely JT: Tumors of the spermatic cord. Report of a case of neurofibroma. JAMA 112:2405, 1939

Other Rare Neoplasms

198. Chung HD: Granular cell tumor of the spermatic cord: A case report with light and electron microscopic study. J Urol 120:379, 1978

Malignant Mesenchymal Neoplasms

General References

199. Arlen M, Grabstald H, Whitmore Jr WF: Malignant tumors of the spermatic cord. Cancer 23:525, 1969

200. Tripathi VNP, Dick VS: Primary sarcoma of the urogenital system in adults. J Urol 101:898, 1969
201. Malek RS, Utz DC, Farrow GM: Malignant tumors of the spermatic cord. Cancer 29:1108, 1972
202. Beccia DJ, Krane RJ, Olsson CA: Clinical management of non-testicular intrascrotal tumors. J Urol 116:476, 1976
203. Bissada NK, Finkbeiner AE, Redman JF: Paratesticular sarcomas: Review of management. J Urol 116:198, 1976
204. Sogani PC, Grabstald H, Whitmore WF: Spermatic cord sarcoma in adults. J Urol 120:301, 1978
205. Blitzer PH, Dosoretz DE, Proppe KH et al: Treatment of malignant tumors of the spermatic cord: A study of 10 cases and a review of the literature. J Urol 126:611, 1981
206. Gowing NFC: Paratesticular tumours of connective tissue and muscle. In Pugh RCB (ed): Pathology of the Testis. Oxford, Blackwell Scientific Publications, 1976
207. Deluise VP, Draper JW, Gray Jr GF: Smooth muscle tumors of the test. J Urol 121:823, 1979

Rhabdomyosarcoma

208. Hirsch EF: Rhabdomyosarcoma of the spermatic cord (funiculus spermaticus). Am J Cancer 20:398, 1934
209. Shivers CH deT: Rhabdomyosarcoma of the spermatic cord. J Urol 52:266, 1944
210. Gray CP, Biorn CL: Rhabdomyosarcoma of the spermatic cord. J Urol 74:402, 1955
211. Satter EJ, Heidner II FC, Wear JB: Primary sarcoma of the spermatic cord and epididymis. J Urol 82:148, 1959
212. Hoffman WW, Baird SS: A rare tumor of the spermatic cord: Rhabdomyosarcoma. J Urol 84:376, 1960
213. Gray CP, Biorn CL: Myosarcoma of the spermatic cord. J Urol 84:562, 1960
214. Samellas W: Malignant neoplasms of spermatic cord. NY State J Med 64:1213, 1964
215. Lundblad RR, Millinger GT, Gleason DF: Spermatic cord malignancies. J Urol 98:393, 1967
216. Ghazali S: Embryonic rhabdomyosarcoma of the urogenital tract. Br J Surg 60:124, 1973
217. Mostofi FK, Price Jr EB: Tumors of the male genital system, p 154. In Atlas of Tumor Pathology, 2nd Series, Fascicle 8. Washington, DC, AFIP, 1973
218. Skeel DA, Drinker Jr HR, Witherington R: Rhabdomyosarcoma of the spermatic cord: Report of 3 cases with review of the literature. J Urol 113:279, 1975
219. Beall ME, Young IS: Spermatic cord rhabdomyosarcoma: Case report. J Urol 117:807, 1977
220. Cromie WJ, Raney Jr RB, Duckett JW: Paratesticular rhabdomyosarcoma in children. J Urol 122:80, 1979
221. Olney LE, Narayana A, Leoning S et al: Intrascrotal rhabdomyosarcoma. Urol 14:113, 1979
222. Banik S, Guha PK: Paratesticular rhabdomyosarcomas and leiomyosarcomas: A clinicopathological review. J Urol 121:823, 1979

Leiomyosarcoma

223. Wessel HN: Leiomyosarcoma of the spermatic cord. J Urol 69:823, 1953
224. Bevan PG: Malignant leiomyosarcoma of the spermatic cord. Br J Surg 42:101, 1954
225. Cannon EM, Altheide JP, Allen HC: Malignant tumors of the spermatic cord and testicular tunics. South Med J 49:17, 1956
226. Cruze K: Leiomyosarcoma of the spermatic cord. Arch Surg 76:151, 1958

227. Fagundes LA, Hampe O: Leiomyosarcoma of the spermatic cord. J Urol 85:835, 1961
228. Wagner M, Teresi JL: Primary fibroleiomyosarcoma of spermatic cord. Wis Med J 62:342, 1963
229. Kyle VN: Leiomyosarcoma of the spermatic cord: A review of the literature and report of an additional case. J Urol 96:795, 1966
230. Weitzner S: Leiomyosarcoma of spermatic cord. Rocky Mountain Med J 64:73, 1967
231. Sharma CMP: Leiomyosarcoma of the spermatic cord: Case report and review of literature. Br J Urol 40:464, 1968
232. Jenkins DG, Subbuswamy SG: Leiomyosarcoma of the spermatic cord: A case report. Br J Surg 59:408, 1972
233. Weitzner S: Leiomyosarcoma of spermatic cord and retroperitoneal lymph node dissection. Am Surg 39:352, 1973
234. Grinenwald P, Doremieux J, Reziciner S et al: A propos d'un cas de leiomyosarcome du cordon spermatique: Revue de la litterature. J Urol Nephrol 81:440, 1975
235. Deluise VP, Draper JW, Gray Jr GF: Smooth muscle tumors of the testicular adnexa. J Urol 115:685, 1976

Fibrosarcoma

236. Schulte TL, McDonald JR, Priestly JT: Tumors of the spermatic cord. JAMA 112:2406, 1939
237. Laumonier P, Depaulis J: Fibro-sarcomes du cordon a propos d'une observation personnelle. Presse Med 60:1162, 1952
238. Schwartz KG: Fibrosarkom des samenstranges. Zentralbl Chir 79:188, 1954
239. Courbier R: Fibro-sarcome du cordon spermatique. Marseille Chir 8:521, 1956
240. Powell HDW: Fibrosarcoma of the spermatic cord. Br J Urol 28:194, 1956
241. Young TW: Malignant tumours of the spermatic cord. Br J Surg 56:260, 1969

Liposarcoma

242. Angeli A: Su di un caso di lipo-sarcoma del funicolo spermatico. Arch Ital Chir 81:427, 1956
243. Dreyfuss W, Goodsitt E: Tumors of the spermatic cord. J Urol 84:658, 1960
244. Hausfeld KF, Guira AC: Liposarcoma of the spermatic cord. Case report. Ohio State Med J 64:1036, 1968
245. Datta NS, Sigh SM, Bapna BC: Liposarcoma of the spermatic cord: Report of a case and review of the literature. J Urol 106:888, 1971
246. D'Abrera VSTE, Burfitt-Williams W: A giant scrotal liposarcoma. Med J Aust 2:854, 1973
247. Dimacopoulos DG: Paratesticular liposarcoma. Br J Urol 46:347, 1974
248. Mackenzie I, Roberts GH: Liposarcoma of paratesticular origin: A case report. Br J Urol 46:467, 1974
249. Senoh K, Osada Y, Kawachi J: Spermatic cord liposarcoma: Case report. Br J Urol 50:429, 1978
250. Johnson DE, Harris JD, Ayala AG: Liposarcoma of spermatic cord. Urol 11:190, 1978
251. Reyes CV: Spermatic cord liposarcoma. Urol 15:416, 1980

Miscellaneous Malignant Neoplasms

Malignant Fibrous Histiocytoma

252. Cole AT, Straus FH, Gill WB: Malignant fibrous histiocytoma: An unusual tumor. J Urol 107:1005, 1972
253. Farah RN, Bohne AW: Malignant fibrous histiocytoma of spermatic cord. Urol 3:782, 1974

254. Williamson JC, Johnson JD, Lamm DL et al: Malignant fibrous histiocytoma of the spermatic cord. J Urol 123:785, 1980

255. Sclama AO, Berger BW, Cherry JM et al: Malignant fibrous histiocytoma of the spermatic cord: The role of retroperitoneal lymphadenectomy in management. J Urol 130:577, 1983

256. Smailowitz Z, Kaneti J, Sober I et al: Malignant fibrous histiocytoma of the spermatic cord. J Urol 130:150, 1983

Angiosarcoma

257. Prince CL: Malignant tumors of the spermatic cord: A brief review with presentation of a case of angioendothelioma. J Urol 47:793, 1942

Malignant Mesenchymoma

258. Dreyfuss ML, Lubash S: Malignant mixed tumor of the spermatic cord (lipo-osteo-fibrosarcoma). J Urol 44:314, 1940

259. Graves RC, Kickham CJE: Teratoma of the spermatic cord: Case report with a consideration of the prolan test. Am J Surg 47:116, 1940

Myxosarcoma

260. Banowsky LH, Shultz GN: Sarcoma of the spermatic cord and tunics: Review of the literature, case report and discussion of the role of retroperitoneal lymph node dissection. J Urol 103:628, 1970

Malignant Epithelial Neoplasms

Pheochromocytoma

261. Eusebi V, Massarelli G: Pheochromocytoma of the spermatic cord: Report of a case. J Pathol 105:283, 1971

262. Soejima H, Ogawa O, Nomura Y et al: Pheochromocytoma of the spermatic cord: A case report. J Urol 118:495, 1977

Metastatic Neoplasms

263. Lewis LG, Goodwin WE, Randall WS: Carcinoma of the spermatic cord and epididymis extension from primary carcinoma of the stomach. J Urol 51:75, 1944

264. Brotherus JV: Metastatic tumors of the epididymis and the spermatic cord. J Urol 83:171, 1960

265. Monn L, Poticha SM: Metastatic tumors of spermatic cord. Urol 5:821, 1975

Prostate

8

Normal Structure

Embryology

The human prostate develops from epithelial evaginations that initially appear along the prostatic urethra during the third gestational month.[1–3,24] Evaginations in the proximal urethra undergo only minimal further development and give origin to simple periurethral glands (cervical glands of Alberran).[1] Those arising more distally, near the verumontanum, give origin to five independent groups of tubules that grow more extensively to occupy five different regions of the prostate regarded as prostatic "lobes" by Lowsley in 1912.[1] These lobes were reported to maintain their identity throughout fetal development, and in the newborn.[1]

Postnatal Development and Age-Related Changes

There is little subsequent postnatal prostatic development until puberty, when significant prostatic growth occurs (Fig. 8-1; see also Fig. 8-2) achieving an average weight of 20 ± 6 g at age 25 years to 30 years.[2,3,8,13–15,76] Minimal prostatic growth occurs in the two decades thereafter.

Beginning at about 50 years of age, the prostate undergoes progressive atrophy.[3,13–15,20,21,39,47] Alternatively, prostatic enlargement resulting from nodular hyperplasia is observed (see discussion of prostatic hyperplasia; Fig. 8-19).[13,15,20,55] Frequently both changes are present in the prostates of elderly men. Atrophy of the glandular acini, initially nonuniform in distribution, becomes progressively more diffuse with increasing age. By age 80 years, half of the prostatic glandular acini are obliterated.[15]

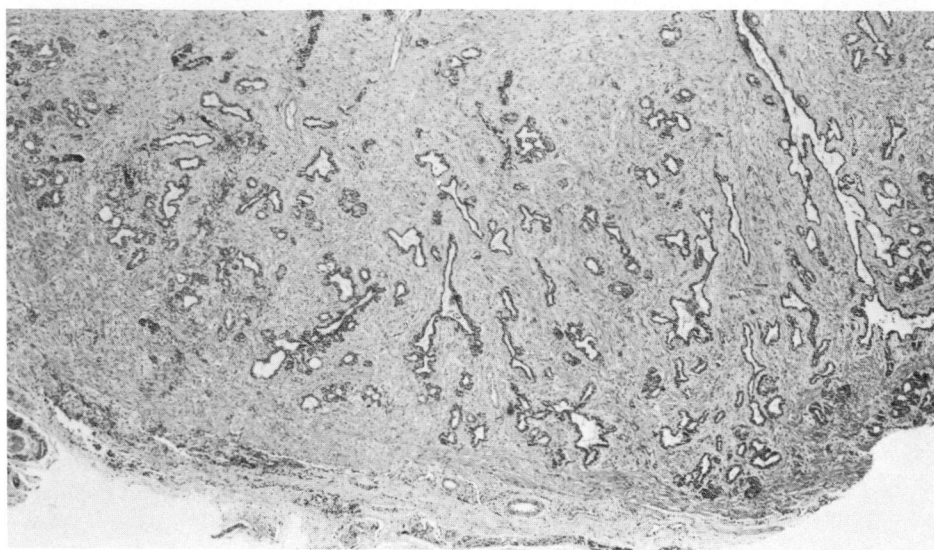

Figure 8-1   *Normal prostate of newborn. Abundant fibromuscular stroma separates the simple ductal system characteristic of the prepubertal prostate. The posterior is at the bottom of the photograph.*

Adult Prostate

Historically there has been considerable interest in relating the origin of major prostatic diseases to specific sites of predilection within the organ. Traditionally, the topography of prostatic disorders is related to prostate lobes (*i.e.*, the posterior lobe, the lateral lobe, and so forth).

Studies of prostate morphology reported in the 19th century concluded that the adult prostate was composed of four lobes: two lateral lobes, a middle lobe, and an inconstant anterior lobe.[11,20] In 1912, Lowsley identified an additional "posterior lobe" in his studies of prostate development in the fetus.[1] In subsequent years, the existence of these five fetal prostate lobes was extrapolated to the clinical study of diseases of the adult prostate. However, the existence of these lobes in the adult prostate has come under increasing criticism.

The basis for the criticism rests on three observations: an inability to identify Lowsley's lobes in the prostates of infants and adults reported in later morphologic studies;[4,8,15,17,20,40,55] the pattern of estrogen-induced changes bearing no relation to lobe boundaries;[10,16] and a similar disregard for lobe boundaries demonstrated by certain prostatic diseases, (*e.g.*, prostatic adenocarcinoma).[34]

These observations strongly suggested that the concept of lobes, as identified in the fetal prostate, has only topographical value in the clinical evaluation of diseases of the adult prostate.

In more recent studies of the adult prostate, Franks described three groups of ducts in the adult prostate distributed in an "inner zone" and a surrounding "outer zone."[20,34] The outer zone of the prostate contains long branching ducts, and the inner zone contains short, simple mucosal and submucosal glands of the urethra. The inner zone was reported to be the exclusive site of nodular hyperplasia, and its location corresponded to the region reported to be responsive to estrogens.[21,23] The outer zone was the site of origin of prostatic adenocarcinoma.

The most recent studies, reported by McNeal, employ serial sections of the adult prostate in a coronal plane, disclosing a different organizational pattern of the adult prostate.[40,48,55,65] Five histologically distinct regions of the prostate have been identified. The anterior zone corresponds to Lowsley's anterior lobe and is composed principally of a fibromuscular stroma with few glands. A peripheral zone, roughly equivalent to Lowsley's lateral and posterior lobes, constitutes approximately 75% of the glandular component of the prostate. This zone is characterized by simple glands and loose stroma, and is the site of origin of the majority of prostatic adenocarcinomas. A central zone is separated from the peripheral zone by fibrous trabeculae. The central zone is located between and surrounds the ejaculatory ducts as they course to the verumontanum. This central zone constitutes about 20% of the prostate, and approximates Lowsley's middle lobe. The periurethral glands are confined within a sleeve of the muscular internal urethral sphincter. This segment of the urethra (proximal to the verumontanum) is called the *preprostatic urethra* and constitutes the fourth zone. A recently described fifth zone, the transitional zone, contains glands that terminate in the distal preprostatic urethra and grow laterally around the distal end of the internal urethral sphincter. This region lies anterior to the central zone, and medial to the peripheral zone. The transitional zone is the site of origin of the majority of hyperplastic nodules. Blacklock has confirmed the essential structural features of the adult prostate as originally reported by McNeal.[66]

The validity of this organizational scheme awaits further study in the continuing effort to relate the regional morphology of the prostate to the pathogenesis of major prostatic diseases.

Microscopic Anatomy

The overall development of the prostatic duct system during the perinatal period is limited. The prostate in the newborn is characterized by simple tubules radiating from the urethra, with abundant intervening primitive fibromuscular stroma.[1,4,17,24] The urethra and distal prostatic ducts show squamous metaplasia induced by maternal estrogen in utero. This histologic feature gradually disappears in the early postnatal months.[1,12,17] Responsiveness to estrogen is retained in the adult prostate, as demonstrated by the squamous metaplasia commonly observed after estrogen therapy for prostatic adenocarcinoma.[18]

During the postpubertal growth period, the microscopic features of the mature adult prostate are achieved (Fig. 8-2). Tubuloalveolar glands are clustered in a fibromuscular stroma that is continuous with the enveloping fibrous capsule. The acinar epithelium is pseudostratified columnar epithelium with a near-constant basal cell layer adjacent to the basal lamina.[2,11,13,15,20,30,40] Similar epithelium lines the excretory ducts throughout most of their length to the urethra, where there is a change to transitional cell epithelium continuous with that of the urethra. Corpora amylacea appear in the first decade and are found in randomly scattered acini in about 25% of men 20 years to 40 years of age. Frequency of corpora amylacea increases with advancing age (Fig. 8-3).[7,15,17,31] Ultrastructural and histochemical studies reveal nucleoproteins and proteins. Their pathogenesis is related to epithelial cell degeneration.[31]

The fibromuscular stroma contains smooth muscle, collagen, and elastic fibers in a circumferential orientation around glands and ducts. Skeletal muscle

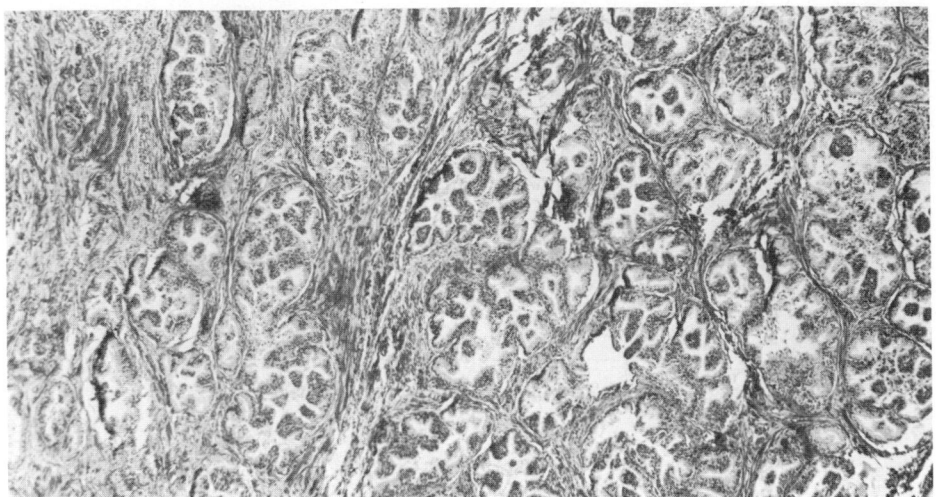

Figure 8-2   *Normal prostate. The prostatic acini are uniformly distributed with intervening fibromuscular stroma.*

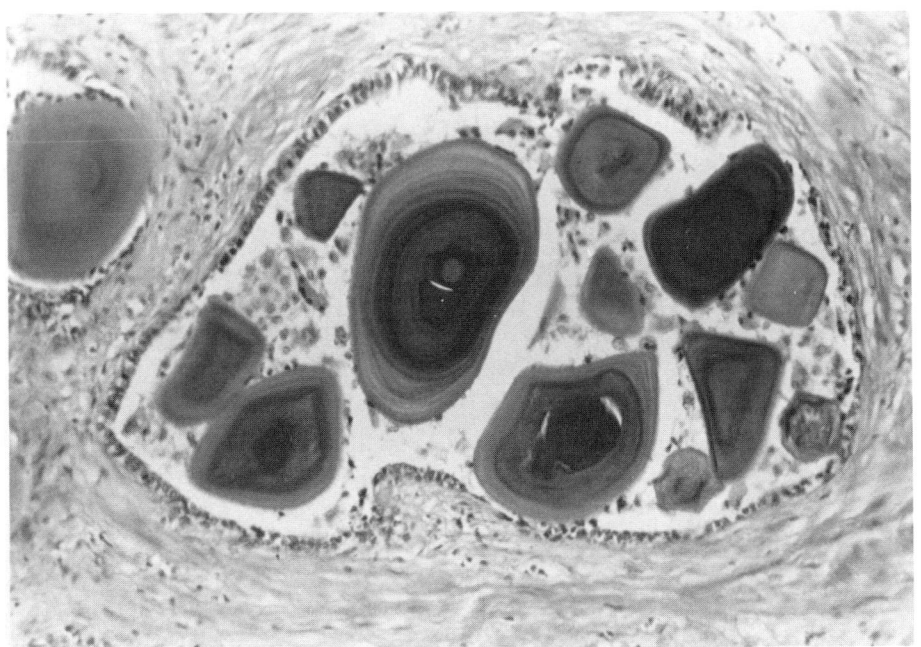

Figure 8-3   *Corpora amylacea. Multiple corpora amylacea with typical concentric laminations are present in the acini of a hyperplastic nodule.*

fibers, most frequent in the anterolateral areas of the prostate, are also commonly observed.[29,32] Intraprostatic vascular tributaries and myelinated nerves are readily apparent in the prostatic stroma. Although their presence was previously denied, injection studies have demonstrated intraprostatic lymphatics.[33,38] These microscopic features are relatively constant until the sixth decade.

During the period of senescent atrophy of the prostate gland, there is progressive acinar obliteration. The remaining acini are smaller, and are lined by

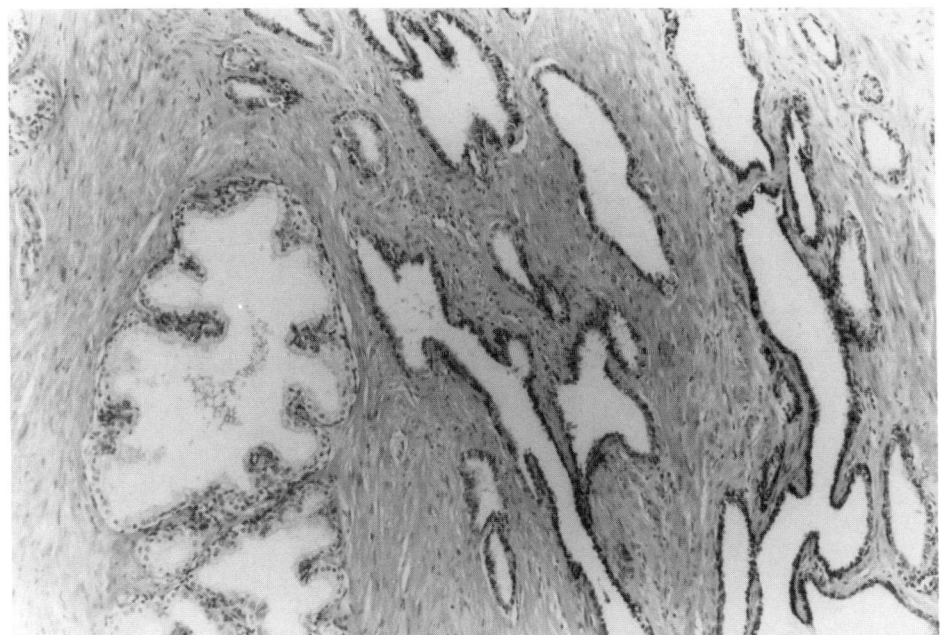

A

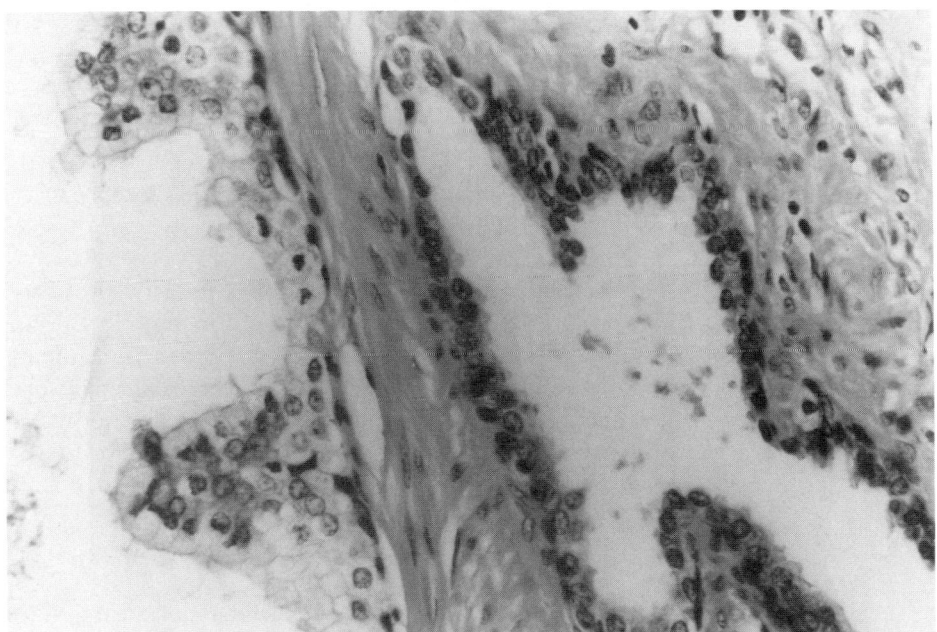

B

Figure 8-4   *Early senescent atrophy.* (A) *The atrophic acinar epithelium contrasts with the acinar epithelium of adjacent hyperplastic glands.* (B) *Higher magnification shows the smaller cells of senescent atrophic acini in comparison to typical epithelium of hyperplastic glands* (left).

cuboidal or flattened epithelium with diminished secretory activity (Figs. 8-4, 8-5).[15,20,21,39,47] The stroma shows collagenous fibrous tissue replacement of smooth muscle. Moore has termed atrophic acini with focal areas of intraglandular papillary hyperplasia *secondary hyperplasia.*[15] Franks (1954) and Liavag (1968) describe solid buds of epithelium growing into the fibrous stroma adjacent to atrophic acini (post-sclerotic hyperplasia).[20,39]

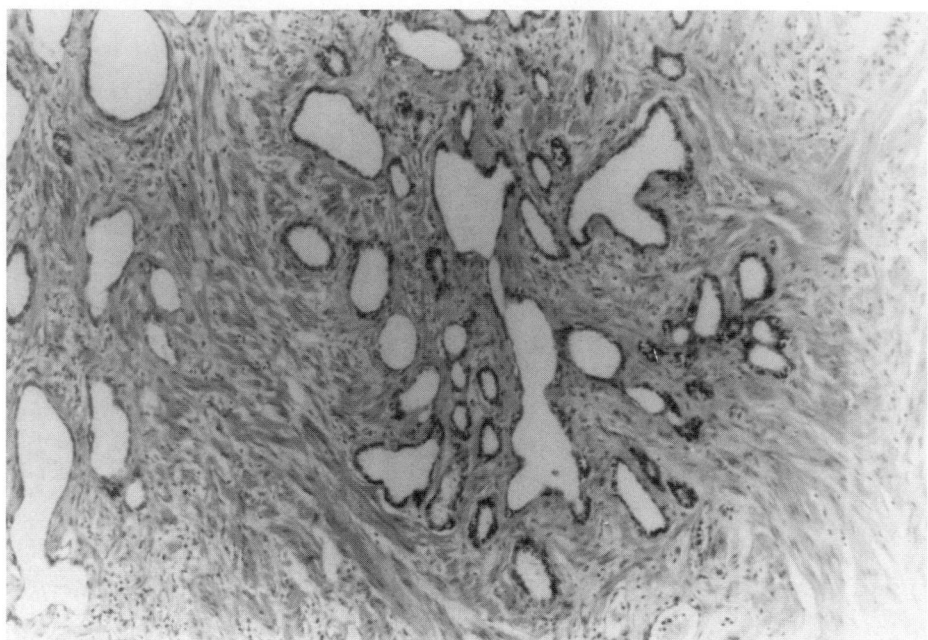

Figure 8-5   *Senescent atrophy. The atrophic acinar and ductal epithelium was typical of the entire prostatic gland in this elderly patient.*

Histochemical and Immunohistochemical Studies

Mucin

Although not prominent in normal or hyperplastic prostate tissue, mucosubstances are detected in prostatic epithelium by appropriate stains. Neutral mucins are demonstrated by the PAS stain both within the epithelial cell cytoplasm and within the lumen of prostatic ducts in normal prostate glands.[28,36] In contrast, neoplastic prostate epithelium of typical adenocarcinomas, characteristically demonstrates only focal acidic mucins detected by Alcian blue (*p*H 2.5) or mucicarmine.[28,36] (Refer to discussion of mucinous adenocarcinoma.)

Melanin

Melanin pigment within the prostate, first reported by Nigogosyan and associates in 1963, remains an enigma.[25] Its true frequency, histogenesis, and biologic significance are not currently understood. Most reported cases are characterized by melanocytes and extracellular melanin deposits within the prostatic stroma, prompting the appellation *blue nevus.*[25,45,46,50,56] Less commonly, melanin is identified within both the cytoplasm of ductal epithelial cells, and the stroma in proximity to the ducts *(prostatic melanosis)* (Fig. 8-6).[43,50,54,68] Rarely, the pigment is limited to the ductal epithelium.[35] Interestingly, two cases of prostatic adenocarcinoma demonstrating focal melanin pigment in the neoplastic epithelial cells have been reported.[54,68]

In the majority of reported cases, the presence of melanin has been suggested

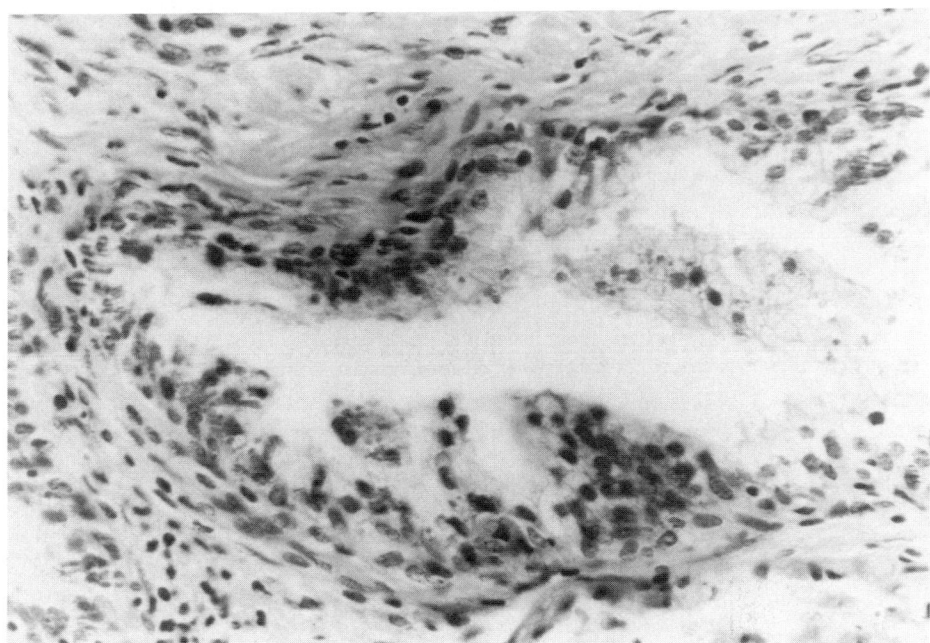

Figure 8-6 *Melanosis. The brown cytoplasmic pigment granules, which were detected in routine stained slides, were iron negative and melanin positive with appropriate stains.*

by dark brown or black coloration apparent on the cut surface of the prostate parenchyma.[25,43,45,54,68] Histologically, the melanin pigment has been differentiated from hemosiderin and lipofuscin with Fontana's stain. Melanocytes within the prostatic stroma have been confirmed by the identification of the characteristic ultrastructural features (premelanosomes and melanosomes) when studied by electron microscopy.[45,56,68] The origin of these stromal melanocytes is unsettled.[68] Similarly, the origin of this pigment within the ductal epithelial cells remains controversial. Goldman (1967) and Tannenbaum (1974) attribute melanogenic properties to these epithelial cells,[35,51] which remains unproven. Alternatively, most authors believe the melanin pigment is synthesized by the stromal melanocytes, and subsequently phagocytized by ductal epithelial cells in proximity to these stromal melanocytes.[25,42,43,50,68]

A total of 32 cases of prostatic melanosis and blue nevus could be found in the literature, but the true frequency is unknown.[25,35,42–46,50,54,56,68] Tannenbaum commented on his observation of melanin in the ductal epithelium of 10% of an unspecified number of prostates studied.[51] This observation remains unconfirmed. It is hoped that future investigations will elucidate the possible melanogenic property of prostatic ductal epithelial cells, and thus clarify the relationship of prostatic melanosis and prostatic blue nevus.

Prostatic Acid Phosphatase

During the 1950s and 1960s numerous histochemical studies demonstrated a variety of enzymes including acid phosphatase in both normal and neoplastic prostate tissue.[19,23,26,27]Gutman and Gutman (1938) had previously established the clinical importance of this enzyme in the context of metastatic prostatic adenocarcinoma.[9] Because parallel histochemical studies had identified acid phosphatase in numerous other normal tissues and nonprostatic malignant neoplasms, the diagnostic value of acid phosphatase histochemical determinations performed on metastatic neoplasms was limited. These histochemical procedures required fresh-frozen tissue, further limiting their practical application in tumor diagnosis.

In 1970, Moncure and Prout demonstrated the antigenicity of an isoenzyme of prostatic acid phosphatase, and thus the organ specificity of this isoenzyme.[41] In 1978, Jobsis and co-workers introduced immunohistochemical identification of an acid phosphatase specific to the prostate with an indirect immunoperoxidase staining technique.[57] Importantly, the technique was applicable to formalin-fixed, paraffin-embedded tissue sections.[60,61] This organ-specific isoenzyme was detected in both normal and neoplastic prostate tissue, and was absent from a multitude of other tissues and nonprostatic neoplasms evaluated.[60,61] Subsequent studies have confirmed the usefulness of this staining technique but have documented some limitations that were not initially apparent. Uniform immunoperoxidase staining of prostatic acid phosphatase (PAP) in epithelium of normal adult prostates and nodules of prostatic hyperplasia have been confirmed (Figs. 8-7, 8-8). This prostate-specific acid phosphatase is inconstant in prepubertal prostates, but is observed regularly at puberty and thereafter.[72] Importantly, it is now known that prostatic neoplasms are not uniformly positive in either the primary tumor or metastatic sites.[70,73] False-negative staining results

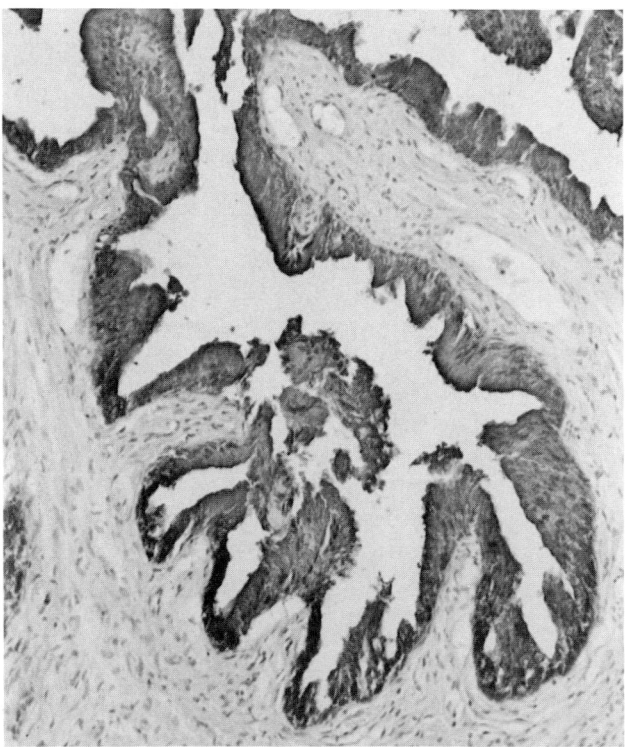

Figure 8-7   *Benign prostatic hyperplasia stained for prostatic acid phosphatase.*

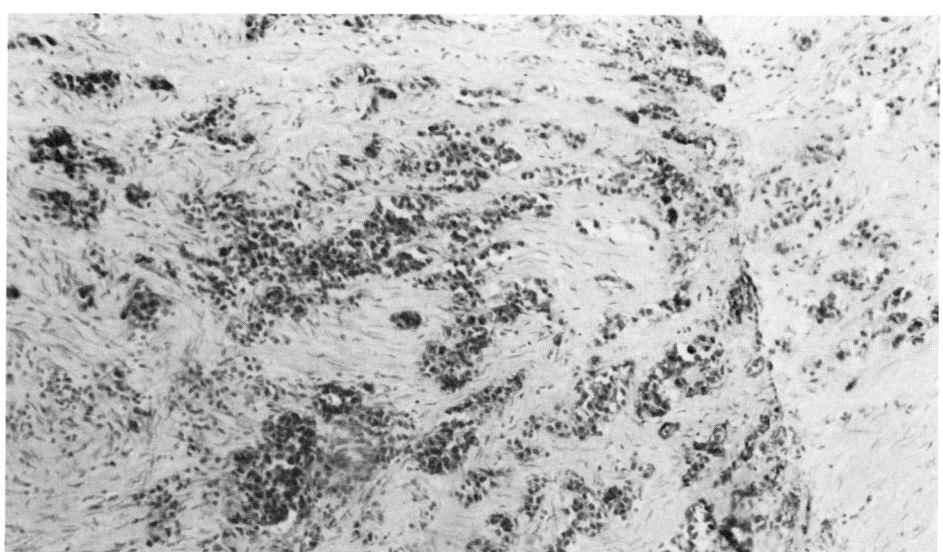

Figure 8-8   *Prostatic adenocarcinoma stained for prostatic acid phosphatase by immunoperoxidase technique.*

are observed most frequently among the most poorly differentiated prostatic adenocarcinomas.[71]

Prostatic-Specific Antigen

In 1979, Wang and associates reported the purification of a second antigen specific to the prostate, which was demonstrated to be independent of prostatic acid phosphatase.[58] This antigen, the prostate-specific antigen (PSA), a glycoprotein of approximately 33,000 molecular weight (mol wt), was found in normal adult prostates, in hyperplastic prostates, and initially, in all prostatic adenocarcinomas studied (Figs. 8-9, 8-10).[62,63] Tissues reported to be devoid of prostatic-specific antigen included seminal vesicle epithelium, urethral and distal prostatic duct urothelium, and squamous metaplastic cells in the vicinity of prostatic infarcts.[62,63,70,71,73] Interestingly, the antigen is absent in prepubertal prostate glands, and appears at the time of pubertal growth of the gland.[72]

According to recent reports, the PSA antigen, like PAP, is not uniformly present in all prostatic carcinomas, as originally reported.[62,63,70,71,73,75] PSA-negative prostatic adenocarcinomas have been observed in both primary and metastatic locations.[70,71,73,75] The observed frequency of false-negative prostatic carcinomas is 20% to 25% among all prostatic neoplasms.[70,71,73] The frequency of false-negative staining results is higher among high grade adenocarcinomas.[71] Finally, demonstrating tumor heterogeneity, examples of PSA-positive primary prostatic adenocarcinomas have been observed to give origin to PSA-negative metastases.[75]

The practical importance of PSA is only slightly diminished by these recent observations of PSA-negative prostatic neoplasms. The application of immunoperoxidase staining for PSA has repeatedly provided definitive evidence of prostatic origin of metastases in cases with dissemination to diverse sites.

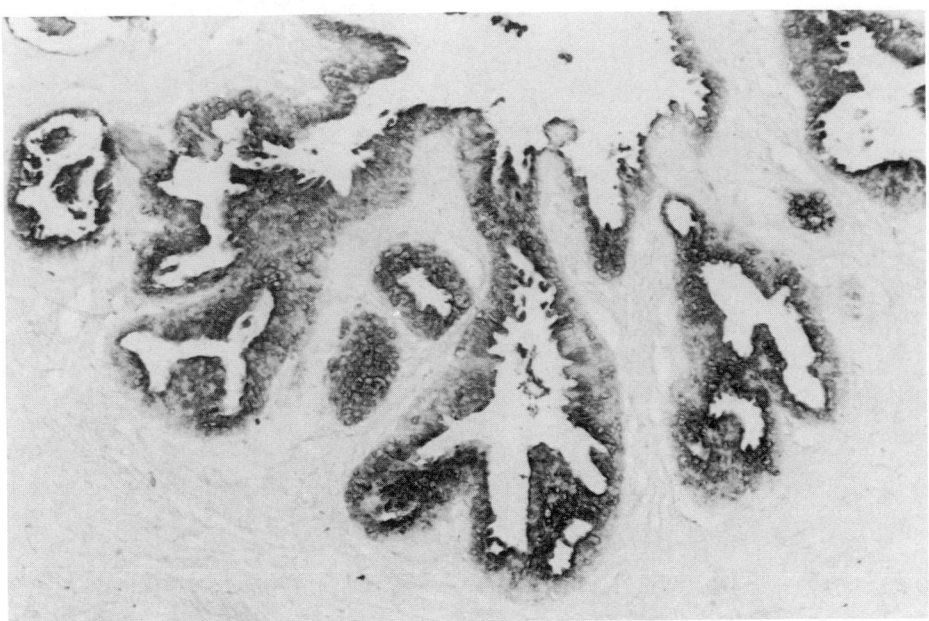

Figure 8-9   *Benign prostatic hyperplasia stained for human prostate-specific antigen.*

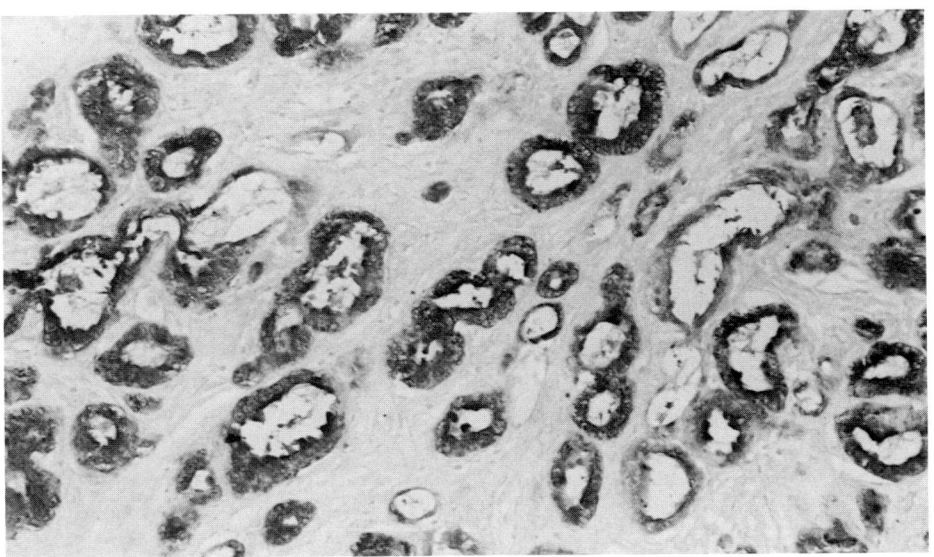

Figure 8-10   *Prostatic adenocarcinoma stained for human prostate-specific antigen by immunoperoxidase technique.*

The significance of the appearance of PSA at testosterone-induced physiologic growth at puberty and its absence in the prepubertal prostate is currently unknown. Interestingly, men castrated before puberty, and presumably lacking PSA-positive prostatic epithelium, apparently do not develop nodular hyperplasia or adenocarcinoma in later life. The application of PSA to studies of prostate growth and structural organization may prove valuable.

Argentaffin and Argyrophil Cells

The presence of argyrophil cells in the normal adult prostate was documented by Grasso (1954), Azzopardi and Evans (1971), and Kazzaz (1974).[22,44,52] Kazzaz reported the cells in a patchy distribution in ducts and acini in all of 50 specimens studied.[52] Detection of these cells by light microscopy requires silver staining: Fontana–Masson for argentaffin cells, and Sevier–Munger for argyrophil cells. Electron microscopy demonstrates neurosecretory granules in the cytoplasm.[77]

The histogenesis and histologic significance of argentaffin and argyrophil cells in the prostate has been clarified in recent years. These cells have been reported both as a minor component in otherwise typical prostatic adenocarcinomas, and in prostatic neoplasms with uniform histologic features of typical carcinoid neoplasms as more commonly observed in the gastrointestinal tract. (Refer to discussion of carcinoid tumors.) Recently, Azumi and associates reported a prostatic carcinoid neoplasm with argyrophil cells demonstrating positive immunoperoxidase staining for both PSA and PAP. (Refer to discussion of carcinoid tumors.) Collectively, these observations indicate that argentaffin and argyrophil cells arise in the prostate by differentiation from prostatic epithelial cells (and are not the result of migration from the neural crest), and that furthermore, they are capable of giving origin to prostatic neoplasms (carcinoid tumors).

Controlling Prostate Growth

In spite of significant progress in our understanding of the controlling influences on prostate growth, much remains to be clarified. Taking origin in clinical observations of previous centuries, experiments examining the influence of sex hormones on prostate growth were initially reported in the 1930s. The results of these studies on experimental animals formed the rational basis for subsequent clinical studies of testosterone in the therapy of abnormal prostatic proliferations (*e.g.*, nodular hyperplasia) and prostatic adenocarcinoma. The discovery of the therapeutic value of estrogen in controlling prostate cancer earned Charles Huggins the Nobel Prize for medicine. (Refer to discussion of adenocarcinoma.)

Current investigations center on the intracellular metabolism of the sex hormones, testosterone and metabolites, and estrogen to understand their role in prostate growth.

Testosterone

The prostatic atrophy resulting from castration of young experimental animals was observed to be reversed following the administration of exogenous testosterone with restoration of normal prostatic growth.[5,6] Clinical correlates of these experiments were observed in prepubertal castrates who failed to show both the normal prostate growth of the second and third decades, and who also were observed to be immune to subsequent nodular hyperplasia or adenocarcinoma. (Refer to discussions of nodular hyperplasia and adenocarcinoma.) Rare cases of testosterone deprivation commencing after puberty, and associated with subsequent development of nodular hyperplasia and adenocarcinoma, were reported. The temporal relationship of prostatic growth with the onset of testosterone synthesis by the testis at puberty reflected these experimental findings. Less clear was the temporal relationship of nodular hyperplasia and prostatic adenocarcinoma when serum levels of testosterone are decreasing, and estrogen increasing.[49,53,67]

More recent studies of testosterone metabolism in the prostate have demonstrated the conversion of this hormone to dihydrotestosterone (DHT) in the presence of the enzyme 5α-reductase.[37] DHT is then coupled to a receptor protein and the complex is transferred to the nucleus, where it combines with chromatin.[59,64,69] As a result of this combination at specific gene sites, DNA, RNA, and thus protein synthesis is affected. Investigative interest thus has centered on the regulation of intracellular metabolism of DHT and possible interrelations with estradiol metabolism.[64,74]

Estrogen

The well-documented influence of estrogens on the progression of prostatic adenocarcinoma has not been matched in studies of estrogen's role in normal prostate proliferation and physiology. The only confirmed morphologic change induced by estrogen is squamous metaplasia of distal prostatic ducts in the periurethral areas of the prostate in the newborn.[17] The same change is commonly observed in prostates of adults receiving estrogen therapy for prostatic carcinoma.[18] Experimental estrogen-induced changes in the prostates of laboratory animals has yielded variable results.[167]

The ultimate elucidation of estrogen's regulatory role of normal and abnormal prostate growth, not apparent from morphologic studies, will be the result of future studies of the intracellular biochemistry of estrogen.

Topographical differences of intracellular biochemistry of the prostate may clarify regional predilections for its major clinical disorders.

Inflammatory Disorders

Acute Prostatitis

Most patients with acute prostatitis characteristically experience intense discomfort on voiding, associated with fever, chills, and perineal pain.[82] Clinically apparent acute prostatitis, which is rarely biopsied, is most commonly diagnosed by examining smears and cultures of prostatic fluid. Most studies have reported gram-negative bacteria, especially *E. coli,* as the most common etiologic agent.[82] However, Drach has reported that gram-positive bacteria are more common.[80] The pathogenesis of most prostatic infections is thought to involve reflux of infected urine into the prostatic ducts.[79,82] Occasionally, infections result from blood-borne bacteria.[80,82]

Prostatic abscesses, most frequently observed in men older than 50 years, are currently uncommon.[78,79] The predisposing circumstances of prostatic abscess formation are unknown.[78]

The histopathology of acute prostatitis is variable numbers of neutrophils and necrotic debris within ducts, acini, and adjacent stroma (Fig. 8-11). Necrosis of the ductal and acinar lining epithelium is present. Microabscesses with destruction of prostatic glands and stroma are frequent.[80,82] These inflamed areas

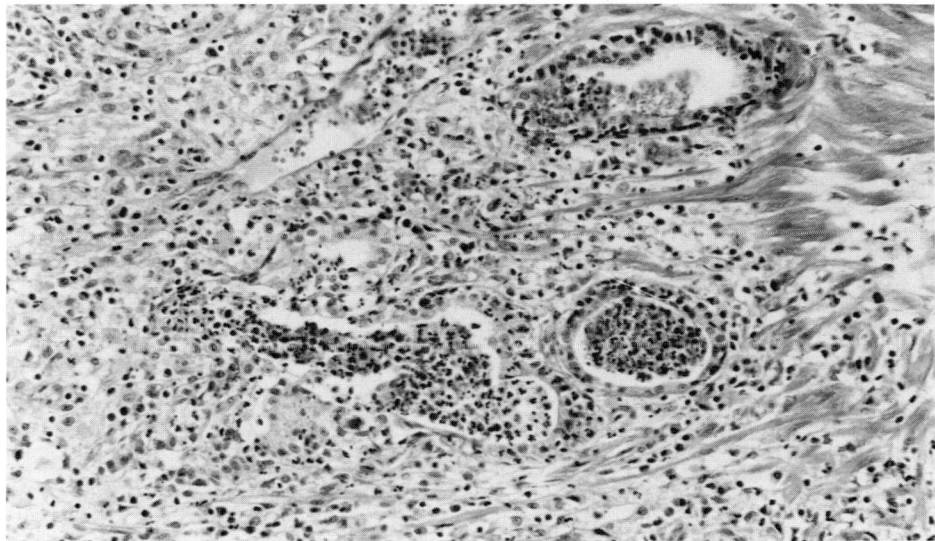

Figure 8-11   *Acute prostatitis. Numerous neutrophils are present within the stroma and acini with focal necrosis of glandular epithelium.*

are most commonly small and localized; less commonly, confluence of microabscesses is observed. Acute inflammation is a common incidental histologic finding in prostatic fragments of nodular hyperplasia obtained by transurethral resection. The etiology and clinical significance of the majority of such cases with incidentally found foci of acute inflammation is unknown and warrants further study.[81]

Chronic Prostatitis

Beyond the impression that chronic prostatitis represents the failure of acute prostatitis to resolve, understanding of this disorder is limited. Chronic prostatitis is most common in men older than 50 years, but has been reported in virtually all age groups.[79] The majority of patients with chronic prostatitis are symptomatic and report suprapubic, perineal, or low back discomfort of gradual onset. A history of acute prostatitis is not uncommon. However, many patients are asymptomatic, and the diagnosis is rendered after examining prostatic fluid or prostate tissue removed for other reasons (*e.g.,* nodular hyperplasia).[81] Schaeffer and associates concluded that 10 or more WBC per high-power field in prostatic fluid supported the diagnosis of prostatitis.[83] Neither the clinical symptoms nor the histologic features are sufficiently specific to suggest a cause, and indeed, no etiologic agent is identified in the majority of cases.[80,82] On occasion, specific causes are identified by examining prostatic fluid cultures and smears. Gram-negative cocci are implicated most frequently; however, this is contested by some investigators.[80,81]

The pathogenesis of chronic prostatitis involves reflux of infected urine into prostatic ducts with associated factors, such as infected prostatic calculi and local prostatic duct obstruction, contributing to the perpetuation of the infection.[82]

In some instances there is evidence of hematogenous spread to the prostate. In those cases where no etiologic agent is identified, the pathogenesis is obscure.

Within the framework of the limited knowledge of this disease, four histologic forms have been described: nonspecific nongranulomatous chronic prostatitis; nonspecific granulomatous prostatitis of unknown etiology, and the eosinophilic variant; granulomatous prostatitis of specific etiology; and malakoplakia.

Nonspecific Nongranulomatous Prostatitis

Nonspecific, nongranulomatous chronic prostatitis is the variety observed most frequently by the surgical pathologist, most commonly in specimens of nodular hyperplasia.[81] The histologic features are entirely nonspecific and the underlying cause is not apparent in routine sections of the lesion (Figs. 8-12, 8-13). Kohnen and Drach observed inflammation in 98% of nodular hyperplasia cases.[81] The histologic features of nonspecific chronic inflammation, with a dense intraglandular and periglandular infiltrate of lymphocytes, plasma cells, and histiocytes, are commonly accompanied by acute inflammatory cells within scattered glands. Focal collections of lymphocytes are not regarded as indicative of active inflammation within the prostate.[95]

Nonspecific Granulomatous Prostatitis of Unknown Etiology

Two forms of chronic nonspecific granulomatous prostatitis are recognized: the eosinophilic type and the noneosinophilic type.[84,86] Patients most commonly have fever and evidence of bladder irritation.[86,87,90-92,97] The age range is the fifth to the ninth decades with a mean age in the seventh decade.[90-92] Cases of the eosinophilic type are characterized clinically with a high frequency of associated systemic or pulmonary allergic diatheses.[86] These associated clinical features are

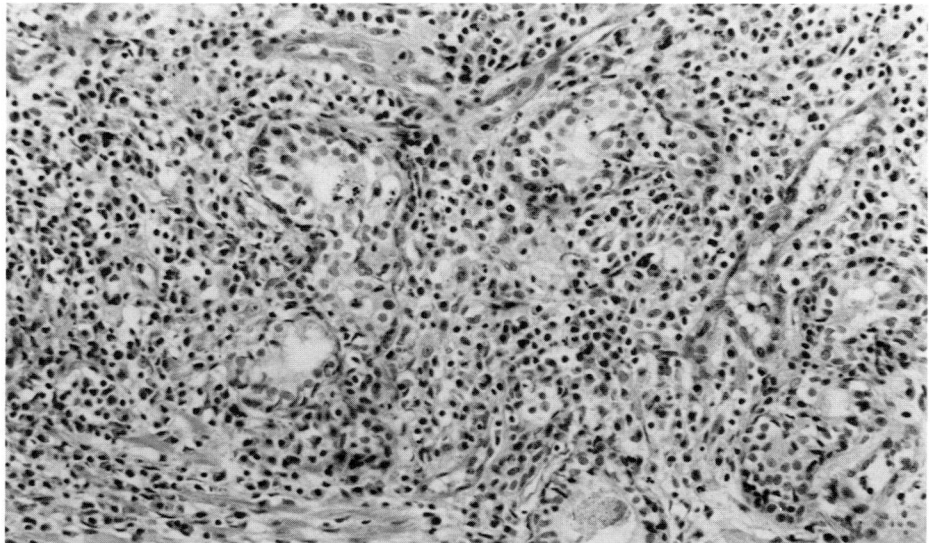

Figure 8-12   *Chronic prostatitis. A dense infiltrate of lymphocytes is present in the stroma and within destroyed prostatic acini.*

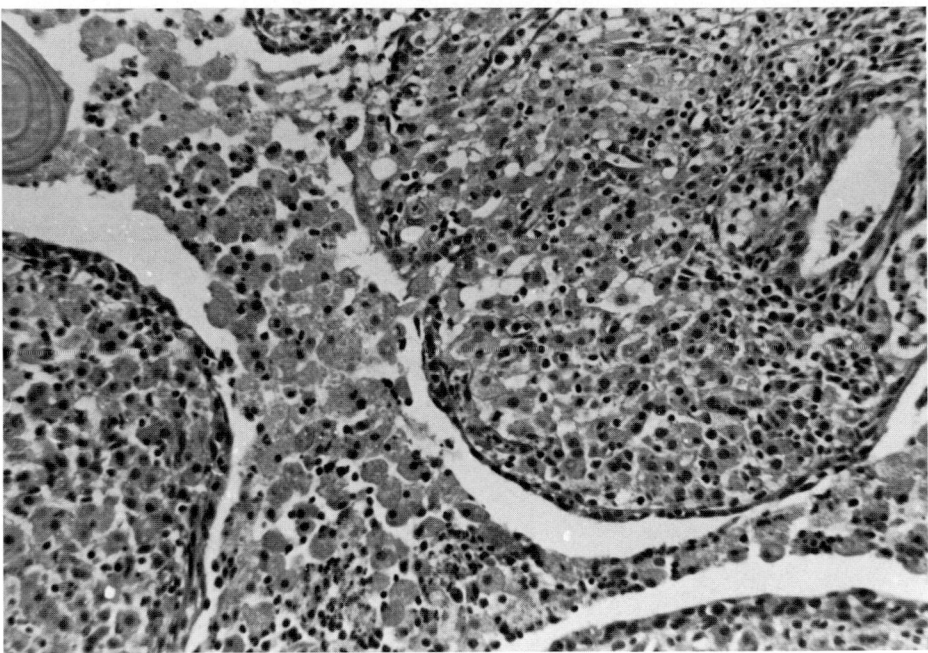

Figure 8-13   **Chronic prostatitis.** *The inflammatory cell infiltrate is composed predominantly of histiocytes with fewer lymphocytes and plasma cells.*

absent in the more common noneosinophilic type, originally described by Tanner and McDonald in 1943.[84] Both types combined constitute no more than 1% to 4% of all specimens of histologically diagnosed prostatitis cases.[84,87,90,93,96]

Clinically, these disorders tend to mimic prostatic carcinoma on physical examination.[85,87,92,97] Microscopically, they must be differentiated from specific infectious granulomas by appropriate histologic strains or culture procedures.[94]

Suggested pathogenetic mechanisms include an inflammatory reaction to inspissated prostatitic secretions or bacterial products resulting from localized prostatic duct obstruction.[84,91,93,94] Recently, lesions resembling rheumatoid granulomas have been described in patients with a history of previous prostate surgery.[98,101] The eosinophilic variety (allergic granuloma of the prostate) may reflect a systemic allergic reaction, as noted previously.[86,88,89,91,94]

Histopathologic features of the noneosinophilic variety include the following (Fig. 8-14): variable numbers of noncaseating granulomas with lymphocytes, plasma cells, and histiocytes, some of which exhibit multinucleation; localized destruction of prostatic ducts and acini; and resultant fibrosis in late stages of the lesion's development.[49,53]

The eosinophilic type has the above features accompanying the following: numerous eosinophils in the inflammatory exudate; granulomas with central fibrinoid necrosis; and rarely, associated necrotizing vasculitis.[94]

In most instances the noneosinophilic form resolves within weeks either spontaneously or with conservative therapy.[92,94,96,97] Some patients with the eosinophilic variety and clinical evidence of asthma have been treated with steroids.[91,94,102]

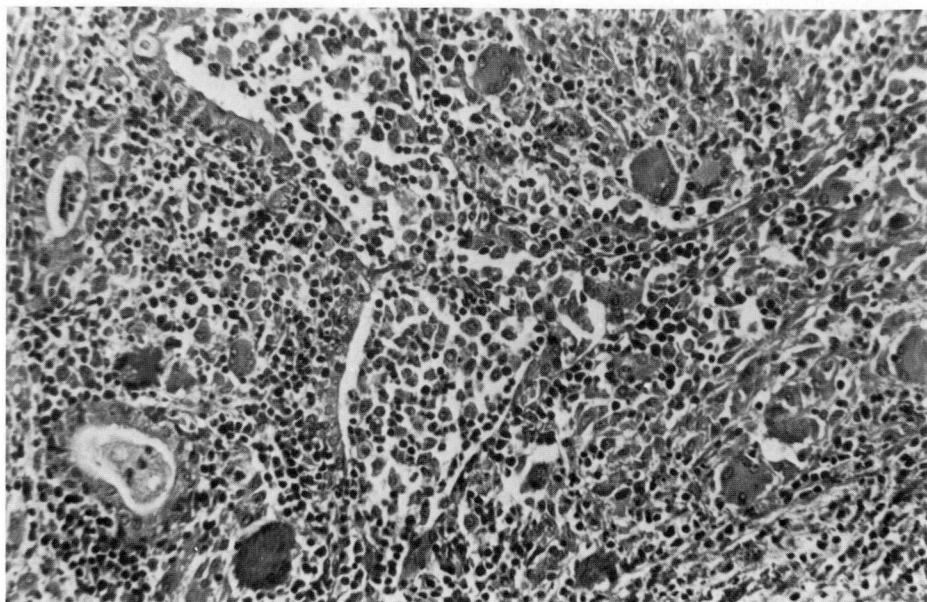

Figure 8-14   *Nonspecific granulomatous prostatitis. Numerous lymphocytes, histiocytes, and giant cells infiltrate the stroma with destruction of the prostatic acini. No organisms were found with the use of special stains.*

Granulomatous Prostatitis of Specific Etiology

Chronic prostatitis with granulomatous inflammatory reactions similar to that observed in more commonly affected sites has been reported associated with prostatic infections by tuberculosis (Fig. 8-15),[103-105] cryptococcosis,[106-109] brucellosis,[110] blastomycosis,[111,112] coccidioidomycosis,[113,116] and echinococcal disease with cyst formation.[117-119] The prostatic infections may be primary, or more commonly, they may reflect one site in a disseminated systemic infection. Appropriate histologic stains and culture of prostatic secretions will assist in identifying the specific etiologic agent.

Malakoplakia

The etiology and pathogenesis of malakoplakia of the prostate are currently unsettled. (See discussion of malakoplakia of the urinary bladder in Chap. 4.) The first case involving the prostate was reported by Carruthers in 1959.[120] About 20 additional cases have been reported.[121-134] It has been reported associated with the same lesion in the bladder.[120,122] The patients, who range in age from the fifth to the ninth decade, most commonly have urinary retention or dysuria.

The histologic and ultrastructural features of malakoplakia in the prostate are similar to the lesion elsewhere.[120-134] The chronic inflammatory cell infiltrate in both prostatic stroma and acini contains a preponderance of histiocytes with fewer plasma cells and lymphocytes. The diagnostic Michaelis–Gutmann bodies are demonstrated in intracellular and extracellular locations with the PAS stain.

As in other locations, malakoplakia of the prostate has been mistaken for

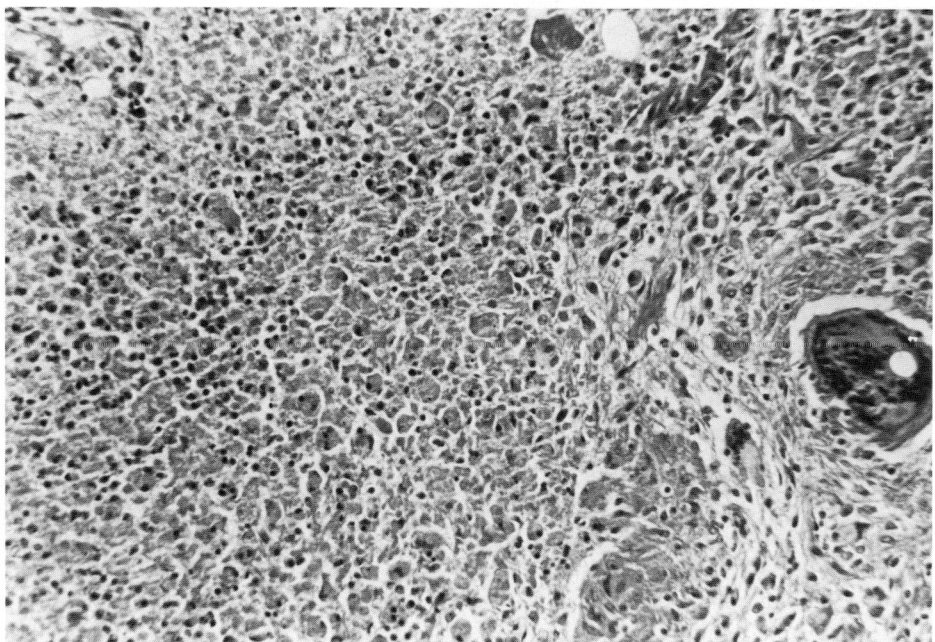

Figure 8-15   *Tuberculosis of the prostate. A Langhans' giant cell on the right is adjacent to an area of necrosis with scattered lymphocytes and histiocytes. Special stain disclosed acid-fast organisms in the lesion.*

carcinoma.[126,127] The rarity of the disorder in any location, especially in the prostate gland, may have contributed to this misdiagnosis in the past.

Prostatic Infarct

Prostatic infarcts were first described by Abeshouse in 1933. He reported three cases associated with prostatic hyperplasia.[135] Subsequent reports brought the number to 30 cases in the next two decades.[136-142] In 1951, Mostofi and Morse reported fifty cases from the Armed Forces Institute of Pathology (AFIP).[143] All studies confirmed the frequent association of prostatic infarcts with prostatic hyperplasia.[135-143] Moore (1943) reported finding infarcts in 25% and Baird (1951) reported infarcts in 18.7% of cases of prostatic hyperplasia.[139,141]

The cause of prostatic infarcts is unsettled. Various authors have speculated that trauma from previous catheterization or extrinsic pressure on regional vascular tributaries by enlarging hyperplastic nodules may result in the observed infarcts.[135,139,140-142] No primary vascular lesions have been identified.[143] Instances of cholesterol emboli in prostatic arteries have been reported,[145] but their rarity precludes a causal relation to most cases of prostatic infarction.

Although prostatic infarcts are often clinically inapparent, Baird has reported an increased frequency of hematuria and acute urinary retention in cases of nodular hyperplasia with associated infarcts compared to cases without infarction.[141]

Histologically, prostatic infarcts vary in size and age. Not uncommonly,

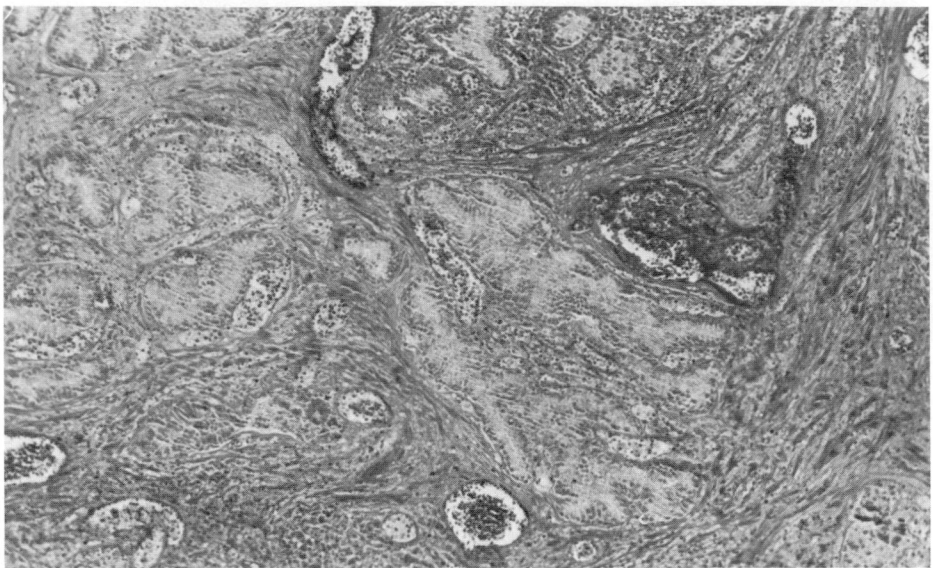

Figure 8-16   *Infarct of the prostate. This recent infarct shows coagulative necrosis and sloughing of the glandular epithelium.*

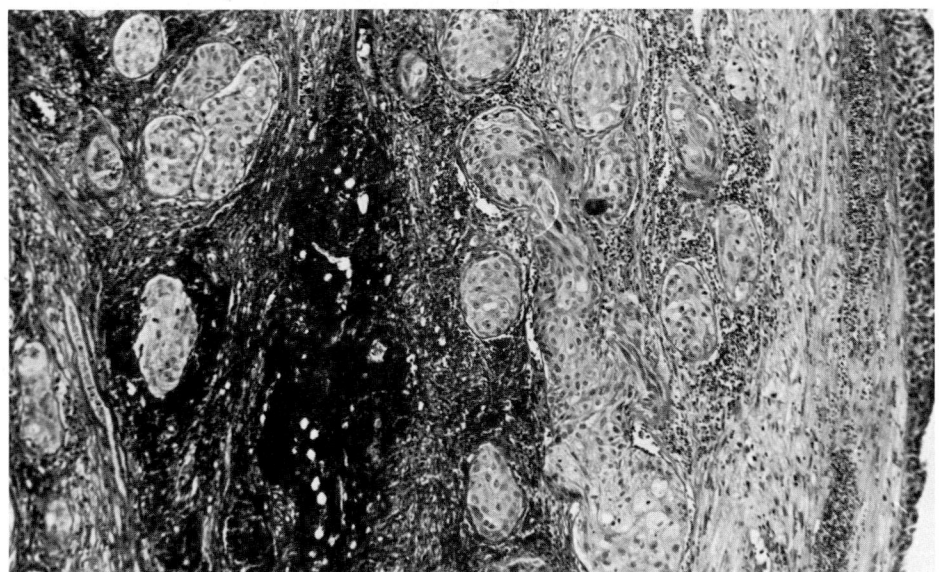

Figure 8-17   *Infarct of the prostate. The hemorrhagic infarct on the left is associated with squamous metaplasia of the adjacent prostatic acini.*

evidence of recent infarction of the ductal and acinar epithelium and surrounding stroma is associated with interstitial hemorrhage and variable numbers of neutrophils at the margin (Figs. 8-16, 8-17). Ducts and acini in the surrounding noninfarcted prostatic tissue show squamous metaplasia, or less frequently, transitional cell or columnar cell metaplasia. These metaplastic changes are apparent within 3 days of experimental prostatic infarction.[139] Indirect evidence suggests the same time frame in clinical prostatic infarction.[140,141] Ultimately, the affected area is identified as a fibrotic scar, frequently with persisting squamous metaplasia of adjacent ducts.

The major importance of infarcts of the prostate is differentiating this lesion clinically and histologically from prostatic carcinoma. Stewart and associates reported the occurrence of elevated serum acid phosphatase in a patient with prostatism and recent infarction.[142] The serum acid phosphatase declined following transurethral resection of the area of infarction. In a series of prostatic hyperplasia, all cases demonstrating elevated serum acid phosphatase (8.3%) were found to have infarcts.[144] Silber and associates reported 30% of prostatic infarcts associated with elevated serum acid phosphatase.[145]

The frequent association of prostatic infarcts with squamous metaplasia of adjacent ducts and acini was first reported by Kasman and Gold,[136] and was confirmed in subsequent studies.[137-143] Culp cautioned against misinterpreting this benign process in a report of eight cases of prostatic infarction, five of which were originally misdiagnosed as squamous cell carcinoma.[138] Mostofi and Morse confirmed the potential danger of misinterpreting these changes as neoplastic.[143]

Nodular Prostatic Hyperplasia

Incidence and Epidemiology

Three factors — geography, race, and age — appear to be related to the incidence of prostatic hyperplasia.[21,153,157,167,172] Marital status, social class, libido, blood type, physiognomy, and concurrent diseases, including cirrhosis, hypertension, and diabetes, apparently have no influence on the risk of developing prostatic hyperplasia as summarized in reviews by Moore (1943) and Rotkin (1976).[157,172]

Geography.   Only sparse information is available about the worldwide variation of the morbidity of prostatic hyperplasia. However, information is available concerning the mortality.[172] Low mortality rates are observed in Central American countries and throughout the Far East. Mortality rates 5 to 50 times greater are reported in most Western European countries. The reported mortality of prostatic hyperplasia in the United States is intermediate between these extremes.[152,172]

Race.   Reflected in the geographical variation, Orientals have a consistently lower mortality attributed to nodular hyperplasia than that reported for whites.[157,172] Evidence suggests an earlier age peak and a slightly greater overall frequency among American blacks than among American whites.[150,153,157,172]

Age.   The peak age of patients with clinical prostatism is the seventh decade.[21,149,153,165] In contrast, autopsy studies show no such peak in the age distribution, but rather a progressive increase in the frequency with age (Table 8-1).[21,47,149,150,153,157,171] The frequency of prostatic hyperplasia in all age groups is far greater at autopsy than is suggested by clinically apparent prostatism. Most reports indicate 75% of men 80 years of age or older have prostatic hyperplasia. Only rare cases have been observed at autopsy in men younger than 40 years of age.[150,157] Predictably, the average weight of prostates with nodular hyperplasia detected at autopsy is less than the weight of prostatectomy specimens from patients with clinical prostatism (33 g versus 52 g) as reported in the recent cumulative review by Berry and associates.[76] The reported frequency of this disorder at autopsy is also related to the thoroughness of the examination (see Table 8-1).

Pathogenesis

Current understanding of nodular hyperplasia can be summarized in its name. Prior to the recognition of its hyperplastic nature, prostatic enlargement in elderly men had been variously interpreted to reflect a neoplastic process (Virchow, 1862–1863), compensatory hypertrophy (Guyon, 1888), a response to inflammation (Ciechanowski, 1901), or arteriosclerosis (Loeschke, 1920), as outlined in the historical reviews by Walker, Moore, and Mostofi.[147,157,167]

Although understanding of the pathogenesis is sufficient to clarify its hyperplastic nature, the earliest histogenetic events leading ultimately to nodular production are not understood. Jores (1894), as cited by LeDuc and Moore, reported hyperplasia of the periurethral glands to be the primary underlying event.[11,157] Pure stromal hyperplasia with nodule production was first reported by Reischauer in 1925.[148] Deming and Newmann, LeDuc, and Moore confirmed this observation.[11,151,155,157] These later investigators regarded the glandular component of prostatic nodules as an event secondary to a stromal stimulus to epithelial proliferation within adjacent ducts, which then infiltrate the hyperplastic stromal nidus.[11,155,157] Evidence of prostatic stromal–epithelial interaction (first suggested by Deming and Newmann in 1939) is supported by the in-vitro experiments of Cunha and associates, who demonstrated an inducing effect of urogenital mesenchyme on epithelial gland formation.[155,168,176] The in-vivo stromal–epithelial interaction in the genesis of human prostatic hyperplasia is yet to be clarified.

Nodule composition, ranging from pure stromal to varying admixtures of stroma and glands, may reflect the extent of epithelial encroachment and intranodular proliferation.[11,21,157,167,173,175] Alternatively, nodular composition may be related to the site of origin. Pure stromal nodules could arise in regions with few prostatic ducts, such as the proximal prostatic urethral submucosa, whereas stromal and ductal epithelial interaction resulting in mixed nodules is more probable in the more lateral areas, which contain more prostatic duct tributaries. McNeal has reported that glandular nodules were more common in the lateral transition zone (see discussion of normal structure), whereas stromal nodules were more common in the submucosa of the proximal prostatic urethra.[55,65,175]

The observation of small nodules composed almost exclusively of prostatic glands suggests that previous stromal nodule formation is not a prerequisite. Thus, there is no evidence that nodules of mixed gland and stromal composition are the result of duct proliferation occurring with any fixed temporal relationship to stromal hyperplasia.[21,167,175]

A possible hormonal stimulus underlying the stromal and glandular hyperplasia of the prostate has long been the subject of investigation.

Testosterone.   The role of testosterone in the hormonal regulation of prostatic growth is well documented (see discussion of normal structure). However, the role of testosterone in the pathogenesis of prostatic hyperplasia is less clearly understood. Although castration before puberty apparently prevents the subsequent development of prostatic hyperplasia,[21,57,156,161,167,169,180] the efficacy of castration in treating established prostatic hyperplasia has produced inconclusive results.[6,156] Huggins and Stevens reported epithelial atrophy but no effect on the stroma of prostatic nodules.[156] Exogenous testosterone has no observable effect on the histology of hyperplastic prostatic nodules, or in areas of the prostate evidencing senile atrophy.[10] Advancing age is associated with a reduction of circulating testosterone in both normal controls and men with prostatic hyperplasia.[49,53,67] However, no reduction in serum dihydrotesterone is observed.[53,177] Siiteri and Wilson have reported increased levels of dihydrotestosterone in specimens of prostatic hyperplasia compared to normal tissue from the same prostate specimen.[166] Recently, Isaacs and associates have reported elevated levels of activity of the enzyme converting testosterone to dihydrotestosterone, offering a partial explanation for the observation of Siiteri and Wilson.[74,166] The experimental production of prostatic hyperplasia in dogs has been reported following administration of dihydrotestosterone or 3α-androstanediol.[174,179]

Estrogen. Serum levels of estrogen are reported to increase with advancing age in men.[53,67] Exogenous estrogens are reported to produce squamous metaplasia of the urethra and distal prostatic ducts, but no significant histologic change in nodules of prostatic hyperplasia.[10,159] The role of estrogens in the production of prostatic hyperplasia is currently not understood.[59,174,179,180]

These observations suggest that testosterone and its more active metabolite, dihydrotestosterone, may have a role in the origin of human prostatic hyperplasia. Further investigation is needed to define more clearly the intracellular metabolism of dihydrotestosterone, its relationship to estrogen metabolism within the prostate, and the exact nature of its role in the production of prostatic hyperplasia.

Pathology

As discussed previously, the origin of early nodular development in nodular hyperplasia has been determined to be in the periurethral submucosa of the proximal urethra, and the recently described *transitional zone.*[65] The precise site of origin is less apparent in typical specimens from patients with clinically significant prostatic nodules when encountered either as prostatic "chips" of a transurethral resection specimen, or on cross section of prostatectomy specimens. Medially, the expanding nodules distort and compress the urethral lumen (Fig. 8-18). Laterally and posteriorly, the nodules eventually compress the normal prostate to an attenuated rim of tissue beneath the prostatic capsule. Each nodule is clearly demarcated from adjacent nodules and normal prostate by an enveloping fibrous pseudocapsule. Secondary changes of focal hemorrhage and infarction may be observed within the nodules. Macrocystic change, on occasion associated with calculi, may be present. Stromal nodules have the gross appearance of uterine leiomyomas.

Histologically, the nodular hyperplasia is the result of proliferation of epithelial cells, smooth muscle cells, and fibroblasts in variable proportions.[21,173] On the basis of the histologic composition, Franks has described five types of nodules: stromal (fibrous); fibromuscular; muscular; fibroadenomatous; and the most common type, fibromyoadenomatous (Figs. 8-19, 8-20).[21,173]

The epithelium lining the ducts and acini within the fibromyoadenomatous

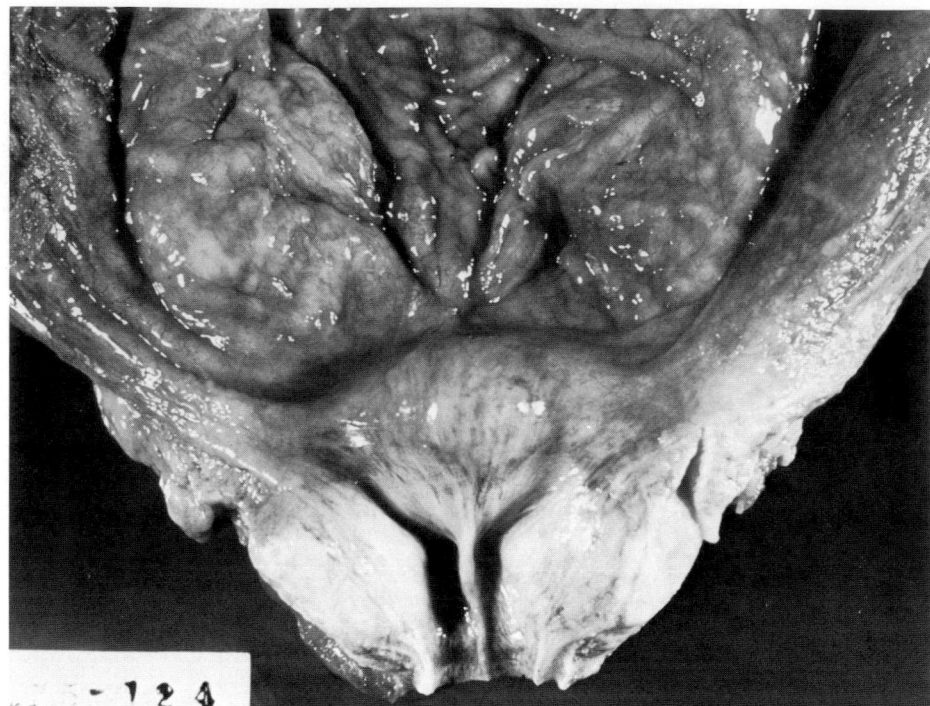

Figure 8-18   ***Prostatic hyperplasia.*** *The enlarged prostate, partially obstructing the vesicle outlet, causes muscular hypertrophy and trabeculation of the bladder wall.*

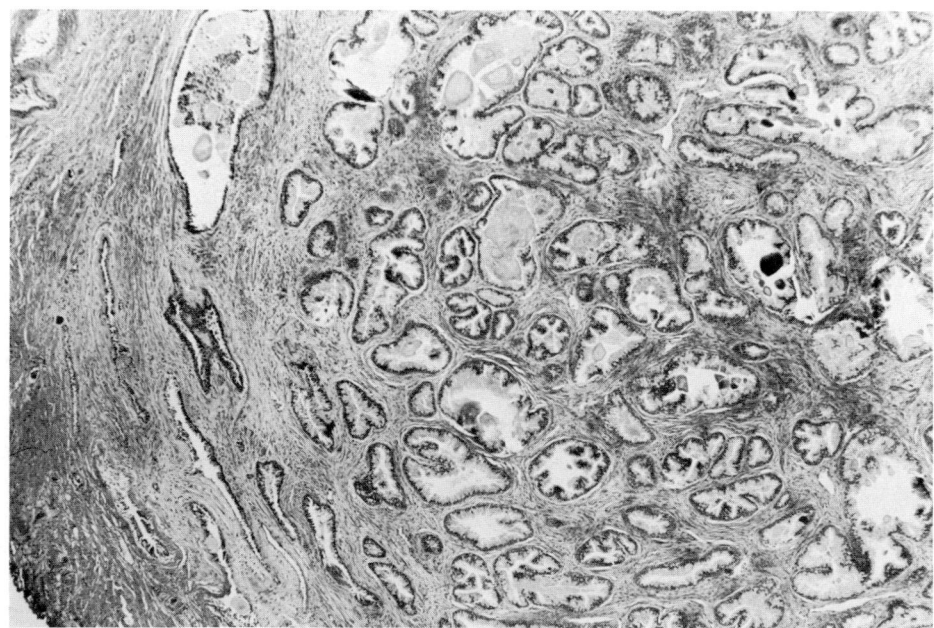

Figure 8-19   ***Prostatic hyperplasia.*** *The columnar acinar-lining epithelium is composed of two layers. Numerous papillary projections are present in the enlarged acini.*

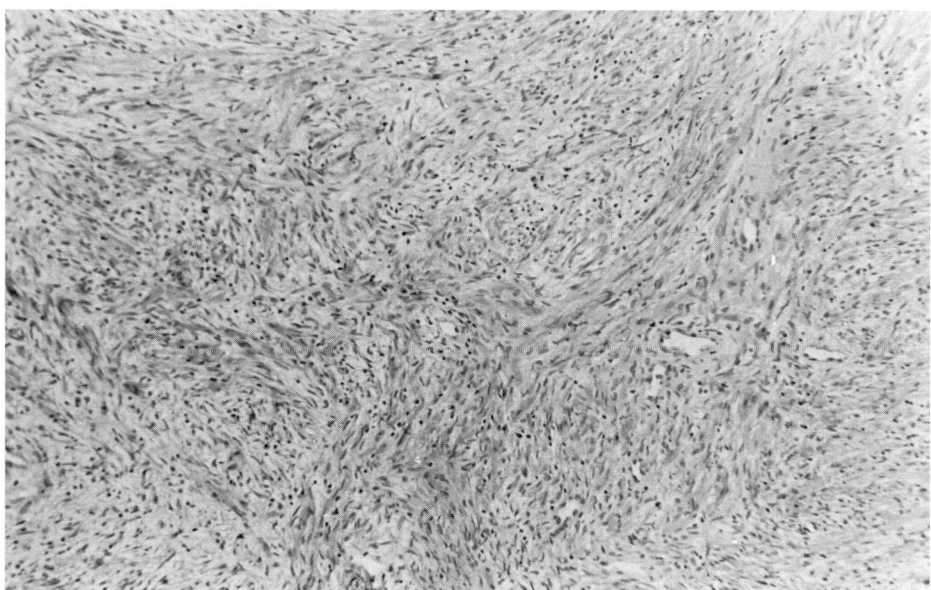

Figure 8-20   *Prostatic hyperplasia. The stromal nodule, devoid of acini, is composed of fibromuscular tissue.*

nodules is generally tall columnar cells overlying a basal cell layer.[163,167,173] This epithelium lines acini of varying sizes, some of microcystic proportions. Intraglandular papillary hyperplasia is characteristic. In contrast, the epithelium of the fibroadenomatous nodules is low cuboidal with frequent foci of transitional cells or squamous metaplasia of the intranodular ducts. The ultrastructural features of the acinar epithelium of hyperplastic nodules and normal prostate are not significantly different.[162–164]

The stroma of each type of nodule differs in composition, as suggested in their descriptive names.[21] Common to all types of nodules is the absence of elastic tissue in the stroma.[11,21,148,154,155,157,172] Franks describes wide stromal septae separating lobules of large hyperplastic nodules in contrast to the more common thin interacinar stromal septae within the lobules.[21,173]

Associated histologic features of hyperplastic nodules commonly observed include the following: cystic dilatation of ducts; chronic inflammatory cell infiltration composed of lymphocytes, plasma cells, and histiocytes within the stroma of the nodule; corpora amylacea within grandular acini; and intranodular infarcts of varying size and vintage (see discussion of prostatic infarct). The glands of the uninvolved (compressed) peripheral regions of the prostate are frequently atrophic.[15,157] Foci of epithelial hyperplasia may be observed in such atrophic glands.[15,20,39,157]

Recent histochemical and electron microscopic studies have detected argentaffin granules and melanin granules in the epithelium of nodular hyperplasia.[42,52,77] Carcinoembryonic antigen (CEA), PSA, and PAP are uniformly present in the epithelium of nodular hyperplasia, as demonstrated by immunoperoxidase staining.[58,62,63,70,71]

Finally, as discussed in the section on prostatic adenocarcinoma, foci of adenocarcinoma will be found in approximately 10% of surgical specimens submitted with the preoperative diagnosis of prostatic hyperplasia.

Table 8-1   *Age Incidence of Prostatic Hyperplasia*

Author	Year	Total Cases	Age Range					
			31–40	*41–50*	*51–60*	*61–70*	*71–80*	*81+*
Autopsy Studies								
Smith, Jaffe[150]	1932	757+*	0%‡	6.4%	13.7%	24.7%	33.8%	50%
Smith, Jaffe[150]	1932	336†	1.8%	4.6%	16.7%	50%	47%	66%
Moore[157]	1943	304	4%	30%	37%	67%	68%	75%
Franks[21]	1954	200	0%	17%	41%	75%	80%	80%
Harbitz, Haugen[47]	1972	165		67%	55%	74%	95%	98%
Pradham, Chandra[171]	1975	161	18%	31%	53%	58%	75%	100%
			<50		*51–60*	*61–70*	*71–80*	*81+*
Clinical Observations								
Hunt[149]	1928	1000	1.6%§		25.8%	56.4%	15.5%	0.7%
Kahle, Beachem[153]	1936	58	10.3%		24.2%	51.7%	15.5%	1.7%
Franks[21]	1954	183	1.5%		15%	48%	26%	9.5%

* Race: white
† Race: black
‡ Expressed as percent of autopsies on males in each decade.
§ Expressed as percent of cases at all ages.

Atypical Forms of Prostatic Hyperplasia

The recent literature contains reports of prostatic hyperplasia with atypical hyperplasia features including proliferations called phyllodes-type hyperplasia, basal cell hyperplasia, and adenosis of the prostate.[182–187]

In the phyllodes-type hyperplasia, the gland and prostatic stromal proliferation is associated with cytologic atypia of both components with a resultant histologic picture resembling cystosarcoma phyllodes of the breast.[182,183]

In basal cell hyperplasia, small acini, or solid nests of cells with high affinity for toluidine blue, are found.[184,185,187] This is characteristic of acini basal cells. There is no cytologic atypia. Basal cell hyperplasia is characteristically associated with "typical" nodular glandular and stromal hyperplasia. The relationship of basal cell hyperplasia to prostatic carcinoma is unknown.

Adenosis of the prostate is a term Brawn has introduced to describe a dysplastic lesion of the prostate characterized by prostatic hyperplasia with gland pattern atypia and mild nuclear pleomorphism.[186] The glands tend to be clustered in well-circumscribed groups, or alternatively, less cohesive groups, suggesting stromal infiltration. The glands are lined by columnar cells, assisting in distinguishing these proliferations from prostatic carcinoma. There is no evidence that any of these forms of hyperplasia, including those with dysplasia, as in adenosis, places the patient at greater risk to develop prostatic carcinoma.[186,187]

Neoplastic Disorders

Prostatic Adenocarcinoma

Epidemiology

Prostatic carcinoma, the second most frequent malignancy in American males, will cause an estimated 26,000 deaths in the United States in 1985, and newly diagnosed cases during the same year will exceed 85,000.[240] The epidemiology of this malignant neoplasm has been the subject of numerous studies and reviews, and the effect of age, geography, race, religion, and social customs on the frequency of prostatic carcinoma has been extensively documented.[206,218,225]

Age

Prostatic adenocarcinoma is a disease of elderly men. Patients younger than 50 years of age constitute less than 1% of cases of prostate carcinoma diagnosed in the United States.[239] At age 50 years, the estimated probability of developing clinically apparent prostatic carcinoma is 9.5% and 11.4% for white and black American men, respectively.[240] Approximately 75% of all patients with clinically diagnosed prostatic carcinoma are 60 years to 79 years old.[218,225,232] Fewer than 20 patients younger than 30 years of age have been recorded in the literature.[235,236]

The true frequency of prostatic carcinoma is significantly higher than is indicated by the clinical frequency, as shown in numerous autopsy studies during the past 50 years (Table 8-2). The term *latent carcinoma* has been applied to clinically undetected prostatic carcinomas diagnosed at the time of autopsy.[198,199,201,203] The true frequency of prostatic carcinomas reflects the combined frequencies of both clinically diagnosed prostatic carcinomas (confirmed at autopsy), and latent carcinomas diagnosed initially at autopsy. As shown in Table 8-2, 67% to 94% of all prostatic carcinomas diagnosed at autopsy are clinically undetected.[188,189,193,199,200,211,214,215]

There is a progressive increase in the frequency of prostatic adenocarcinoma observed at autopsy after age 40 years (Table 8-3). The means of the reported frequencies of prostatic carcinoma at autopsy progressively increase from 4% to 8% among men 40 years to 49 years of age, to 34% to 53% found in men 80 years and older. As is true for prostatic hyperplasia, the frequency of prostatic adenocarcinoma found at autopsy depends on the thoroughness of histologic examination of the organ. The relatively wide range of reported frequencies can be attributed at least partially to variable methods of examination (see Table 8-2). Interestingly, the markedly disparate frequencies of prostatic carcinoma diagnosed clinically in Japan and the United States are not reflected in the similar, higher frequencies of this malignancy observed at autopsy in these two countries, as noted by Oota[203] (see Table 8-2). Guileyardo and associates have made the same observation about white and black men in the United States.[234] There is no completely satisfactory explanation for these observations at present.

Geography

There is considerable geographical variation in the age-adjusted death rates of prostatic carcinoma reported throughout the world.[206,218,225] The highest frequencies are observed in the United States and the Scandinavian countries, whereas the lowest mortality rates are reported in Mexico, Greece, and Japan. Most Western European countries, including England, have intermediate rates. Certain ethnic immigrant groups (*i.e.,* Polish-Americans and Japanese-Americans), demonstrate a higher incidence of prostatic carcinoma than men in their countries of origin.[210,213]

Race

The mortality rate of prostatic carcinoma among black American men is among the highest observed in the world, and significantly exceeds that of white Americans.[218,225,232] The rate among American blacks exceeds that observed among blacks in Africa.[218] American Orientals have the lowest incidence among the three major races in the United States, although it is higher than observed among men in the Orient, as noted previously.[213]

Religion and Social Customs

Newill has reported lower mortality rates among Jewish men compared to Protestant and Catholic men in New York City.[204] Seidman confirmed this and further demonstrated that the lower rates among Jewish men prevailed in all socioeconomic groups.[216] A low frequency of prostatic carcinoma has also been observed among Jewish men in Sweden.[207]

Table 8-2   **Frequency of Prostatic Carcinoma at Autopsy**

Author	Year	Age Range*	Method of Examination†	Total Incidence	Clinical History Positive‡	Clinical History Negative§
Moore[188]	1935	20–90	S	16.8%	3%	13.8%
Rich[189]	1935	>50	R	14%	4.8%	9.2%
Kahler[192]	1939	>50	S	17.3%		
Baron, Angrist[193]	1941	>50	R	14.8%	4.9%	9.9%
Andrews[198]	1949	15–79	S			12%
Edwards et al[199]	1953	>40	S	19.7%	3.4%	16.3%
Franks[201]	1954	20–80	S			38%
Hirst, Bergman[200]	1954	>80	S	53.8%	5%	48.8%
Oota[203]	1961	>45	S			18.1%
Halpert, Schmalhorst[211]	1966	70–80	S	41%	2%	39%
Liavag[39]	1968	>40	R			26.5%
Scott[214]	1969	70–80	S	41%	5%	36%
Scott[214]	1969	>80	S	57%	12%	45%
Lundberg, Berge[215]	1970	>40	R	20.9%	4.8%	16.1%
Lundberg, Berge[215]	1970	>40	S	42.9%	5.3%	37.6%
Harbitz, Haugen[47]	1972	>40	R	34%	2%	32%
Rullis[222]	1975	>80	S			66.7%
Guileyardo et al[234]	1980	25–70+	S			30%

* Age range of population studied at autopsy.

† Method of microscopic examination of prostate gland: R, routine section(s); S, step sections of entire prostate.

‡ Patients with clinically diagnosed prostatic carcinoma confirmed at autopsy, expressed as percent of total autopsies.

§ Patients with clinically undetected prostatic carcinoma diagnosed at autopsy, expressed as percent of total autopsies.

Other Epidemiologic Factors

Socioeconomic status, marital status, fertility, and physiognomy have no apparent influence on the risk of developing prostatic carcinoma.[204,206,218,219,225]

Etiology and Pathogenesis

Viruses

C particles have been detected in specimens of both prostatic hyperplasia and prostatic adenocarcinoma.[228] Sanford and associates have reported evidence of cytomegalovirus in cell cultures of prostatic adenocarcinoma.[229] The significance of the association between viruses and prostatic carcinoma is currently undetermined.

Cadmium Exposure

Industrial exposure to cadmium oxide dust in the electroplating, paint, and plastics industries has been reported to be associated with an increased frequency of lung and prostate carcinoma.[212,226] However, the statistical significance of this increased frequency has been questioned.[227]

Endocrine Influence

Clinical observations suggesting that endocrine factors may play a role in the genesis of prostatic carcinoma include the following: the established testicular (testosterone) control of normal prostate growth (see discussion of normal prostate); the reported absence of both prostatic hyperplasia and carcinoma in men castrated before puberty (in contrast to postpubertal castration);[197,202,223] and the responsiveness of primary and metastatic carcinoma to therapeutic castration and exogenous estrogen, as originally described in the classic observations of Huggins and Hodges.[194]

Table 8-3 **Frequency of Prostatic Carcinoma at Autopsy: Relationship to Age**

Patient Age	Reported Frequency		References
	Range	Mean*	
Consecutive Autopsies with Routine Microscopic Examination			
40–49	0%–8%	4%	39, 47, 189, 214, 215
50–69	10%–32%	16%	39, 47, 189, 193, 205, 214, 215
70–79	17%–40%	27%	39, 47, 189, 193, 205, 214, 215
80+	20%–52%	34%	39, 47, 189, 193, 205, 214, 215
Step-Section Microscopic Examination†			
40–49	4%–17%	8%	188, 191, 198, 199
50–69	10%–40%	22%	188, 191, 193, 198, 201, 203, 215
70–79	21%–67%	37%	148, 188, 193, 199, 201, 203, 214, 215
80+	18%–100%	53%	188, 191, 193, 199, 200, 201, 203, 214, 215, 222

* Represents average of the reported frequencies.

† Many of these step-section studies evaluated the frequency of latent carcinoma, and therefore patients with clinically diagnosed prostatic carcinoma were excluded from the study by design. The true frequency of prostatic carcinoma in each group is the sum of cases observed in a thorough microscopic examination (step-sections) and the clinical frequency of the age group (when these patients are excluded from a study).

Unfortunately, despite considerable research, these empirical observations are not matched by a corresponding increase in an understanding of the role of hormones. Although there is general agreement that serum testosterone levels decrease after 50 years of age, attempts to demonstrate higher levels of this androgen in patients with prostatic carcinoma have not yielded consistent results.[49,53,67,217,233] Elevated urinary estrone/androsterone ratios have been reported in patients with prostatic carcinoma.[208,209] Future studies of tissue dihydrotestosterone (DHT) and androgen receptor concentrations, and 5-reductase enzyme activity levels may clarify the role of testosterone in the control of prostatic cancer progression, if not its role in the genesis of the neoplasm.

Experimental Carcinogenesis

Until recently, experimental production of prostatic carcinoma has had only limited application to the study of the neoplasm as it occurs in humans.[197] The production of squamous cell carcinomas and sarcomas in experimental animals has been reported following the administration of various carcinogens, including 1 : 2 benzpyrene, methylcholanthrene, and nitrosamine.[190,195,196,237] In 1982, Katayama and associates reported the first chemical carcinogen-induced adenocarcinoma in experimental animals following the administration of 3,2'-dimethyl-4-aminobiphenyl (DMAB).[238] Experimental radiation-induced prostatic adenocarcinoma has been reported by Hirose and associates and by Brown and Warren.[224,231] The production of prostatic adenocarcinoma in Nb rats following prolonged administration of testosterone, with or without estrogen, was reported by Noble.[230]

Histogenesis

The cytologic changes preceding adenocarcinoma of the prostate have been the subject of numerous studies. Origin from either hyperplastic nodules (BPH), or peripheral acini with senile atrophy, both frequently observed in prostates harboring adenocarcinoma, has been suggested.[188,192,193,198,241]

The epidemiologic relationship of prostatic hyperplasia and adenocarcinoma has been controversial and remains unsettled. Two large epidemiologic studies published in 1974 arrived at opposite conclusions. After observing 838 patients with prostatic hyperplasia and a similar number of controls for 10 years, Greenwald and associates found no significant difference in the risk of developing prostatic carcinoma.[220] In direct contrast, Armenian and associates reported a 3.7 to 5.1 times higher age-adjusted death rate from prostatic carcinoma among patients with prostatic hyperplasia compared to age-matched controls.[221] Thus, from an epidemiologic perspective, the relative risk of prostate carcinoma attributable to the presence of nodular hyperplasia awaits future clarification.

The possible pathogenetic relationship of nodular hyperplasia and prostatic adenocarcinoma receives little support from morphologic studies. Dossott (1930) and later Andrews (1949) believed prostatic carcinoma arose from nodules of prostatic hyperplasia.[198,241] Later morphologic studies have failed to confirm these findings.[30,188,192,201,242–244] Evidence to the contrary challenging origin from nodular hyperplasia includes the following: the disparate locations of hyperplastic nodules (periurethral or *central*) and adenocarcinoma (subcapsular or *peripheral*); and the absence of observed transitions of nodular hyperplasia to prostatic adenocarcinoma in histologic studies of these diseases.[39,188,192,201,242,244]

Alternatively, origin from foci of epithelial hyperplasia occurring within atrophic peripheral glands has been proposed.[20,39,198] Intraluminal papillary projections or proliferating cell clusters penetrating adjacent stroma have been variously termed *precancerous hyperplasia* (Andrews), *postsclerotic hyperplasia* (Franks), and *small alveolar proliferations* (Liavag).[20,39,198] Supporting the histogenetic role of these focal proliferations is their frequency (reported in 56% of prostates with adenocarcinoma), and the presence of atypical cytologic changes observed in these proliferations.[201,242,244,245] Andrews reported transitions between these hyperplastic foci leading to adenocarcinoma.[198]

McNeal has suggested that adenocarcinoma arises from hyperplastic foci within peripheral glands that have not undergone senile atrophy but have retained active (noninvolutional) morphologic appearance.[242,244] Occasional acini not evidencing the atrophic changes of surrounding glands were reported previously by Moore in his study of the senile involution of the prostate.[15,188] Atypical cytologic features, including those interpreted as carcinoma-in-situ, have been reported within some of these hyperplastic areas of the nonatrophic glands.[246,247] Future studies of these dysplastic changes will elucidate their true biologic significance.

Pathology

Irregular, yellow-white indurations are the most suggestive gross features of prostatic adenocarcinoma. The high frequency of peripheral origin has been reported in several studies.[27,34,191,199,201,271] Multicentricity is common. Any, indeed all, of these features may be absent in individual cases. Localized induration reflecting the desmoplastic reaction to the neoplasm is highly variable, and may be absent, especially in small, well-differentiated adenocarcinomas. Origin in the subcapsular lateral and posterior regions ("lobes") may be obscured by extensive intraprostatic growth to involve more medial areas near the urethra, or by origin from distal prostatic ducts in the periurethral region. Conversely, clinical experience has shown that peripheral nodules represent carcinoma only 50% of the time.[331,341] Benign lesions including granulomatous prostatitis, prostatic infarcts, and nodular prostatic hyperplasia must be distinguished.

Histologically, prostatic carcinomas can be classified with reference to their origin within the gland. I utilize the following classification:

Acinar and proximal duct origin

    Adenocarcinoma with papillary, cribiform, comedo, and acinar patterns

    Mucinous carcinoma (signet-ring cell carcinoma)

    Adenoid cystic carcinoma

    Carcinoid tumor

    Undifferentiated carcinoma, small cell type

Distal ductal origin

    Transitional cell carcinoma

    Squamous cell carcinoma

    Papillary carcinoma

    Ductal carcinoma with endometrial features

Mixed carcinomas

Adenocarcinoma of acinar origin constitutes 98% of all prostatic carcinomas. The pathologic features of the less frequent histologic types are discussed separately.

The microscopic diagnosis of prostatic adenocarcinoma is based primarily on characteristic features of gland formation and pattern, and secondarily on cytologic features (Figs. 8-21 to 8-25). Variability of all features within different areas of the same tumor is so common as to be regarded the rule. Exceptional cases, most commonly small tumors found incidentally, may show little histologic and cytologic variability.

Characteristically the best-differentiated neoplasms show uniform medium-sized or small gland formation throughout the tumor. Most glands are lined by a single layer of neoplastic epithelial cells of uniform height. Progressive loss of differentiation of prostatic adenocarcinomas is characterized by increasing variability of gland size, configuration, and intraglandular patterns of epithelial proliferation. Papillary or cribiform patterns are common in the larger neoplastic gland structures.

Gland fusion is common. Abortive glands composed of infiltrating tumor cells in solid cords or nests with irregular outlines characterize the poorly differentiated tumors. Some of the solid nests exhibit central necrosis of tumor cells, referred to as the "comedo" pattern. Uncommonly, a tumor is composed of small undifferentiated cells growing individually or in sheets without evidence of structural organization. Necrosis of both the tumor and the infiltrated adjacent normal prostate is frequent, in contrast to the infrequency of this finding in better differentiated tumors. Within this spectrum of tumor differentiation, the majority of prostatic adenocarcinomas of acinar origin are observed to be well-differentiated to moderately well-differentiated.[268,273,274,281,282,290,307,357]

The relationship of adenocarcinomas to the intervening and surrounding

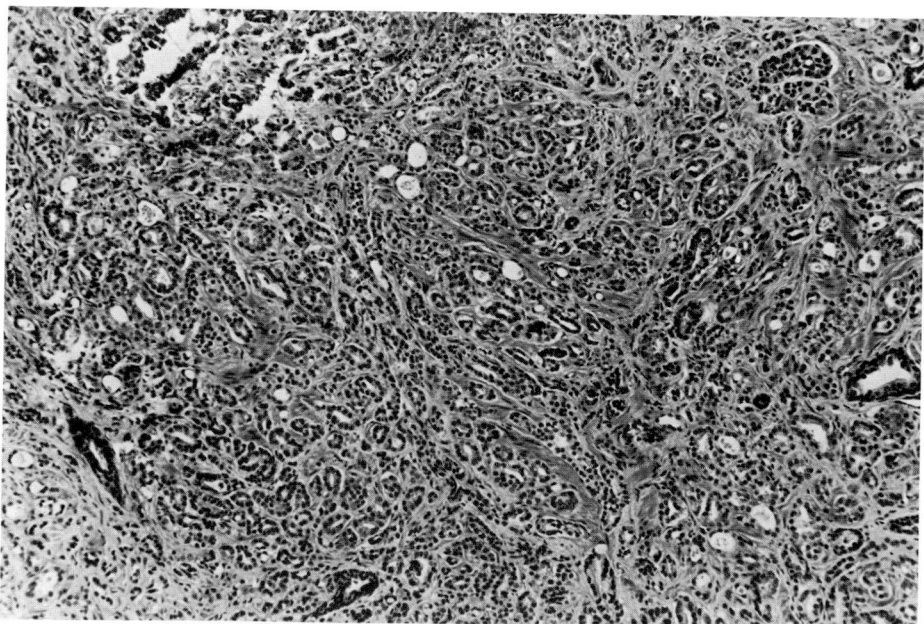

Figure 8-21   *Adenocarcinoma of the prostate, Gleason grade 3. Small single glands and individual tumor cells infiltrate the prostatic stroma.*

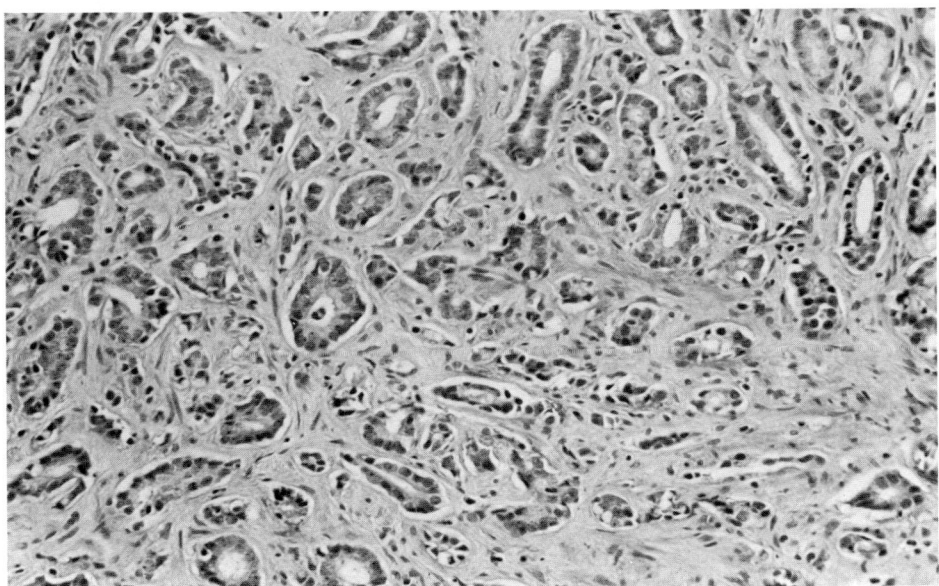

Figure 8-22   *Adenocarcinoma of the prostate, Gleason grade 3. Neoplastic glands lined with a single layer of tumor cells are separated by stroma in which individual tumor cells are infiltrating.*

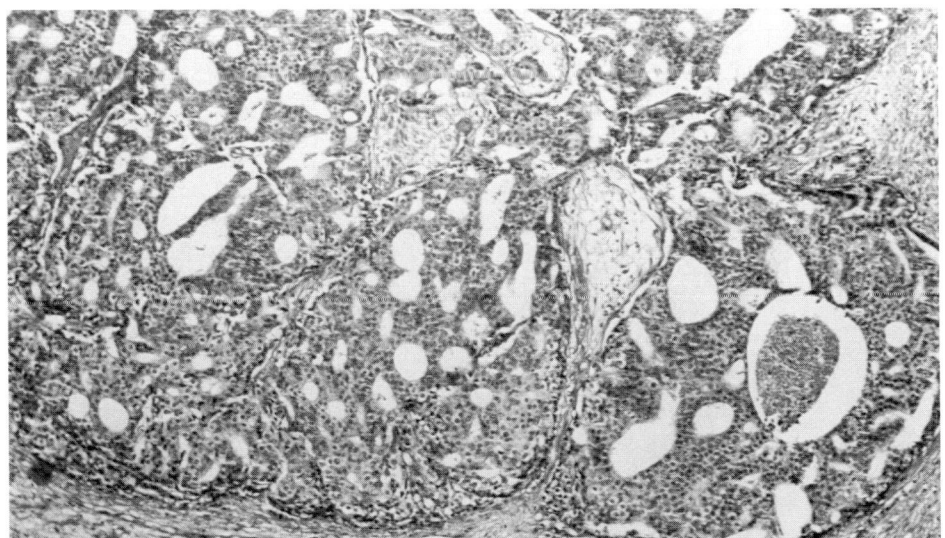

Figure 8-23   *Adenocarcinoma of the prostate, Gleason grade 3. Tumor cells in large nests have a cribriform arrangement. One focus of tumor cell necrosis is present on the right.*

prostatic stroma is diagnostically important. Small foci of well-differentiated tumors tend to have uniformly little stroma between the neoplastic glands and usually a well-demarcated advancing margin abutting against the adjacent normal prostatic tissue. In contrast, poorly differentiated tumors show irregular infiltration of adjacent prostate by clusters of glands or cohesive solid cords of tumor cells. Tumor cells infiltrating and lying immediately adjacent to stromal

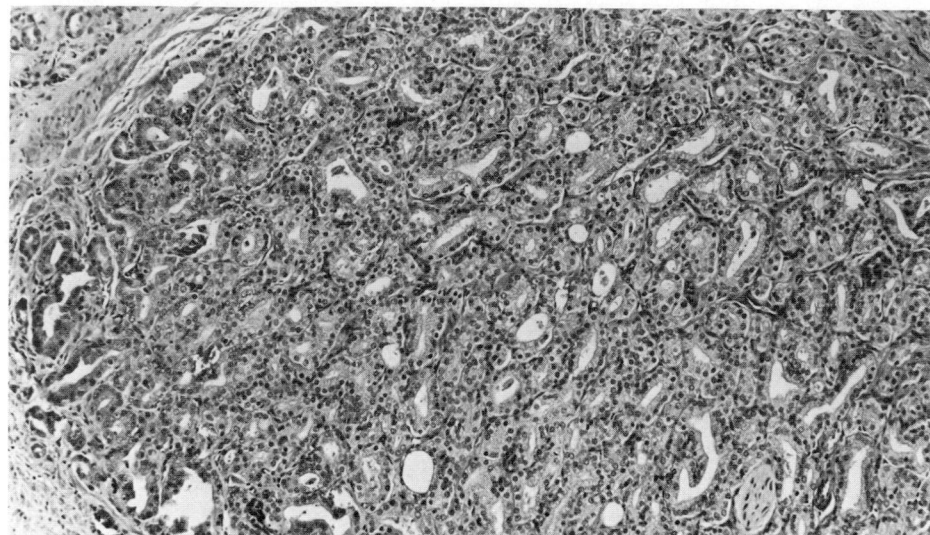

Figure 8-24   *Adenocarcinoma of the prostate, Gleason grade 3. Single neoplastic glands merge into adjacent clusters and cords of tumor cells with no intervening stroma. A nerve (lower right) is surrounded by tumor.*

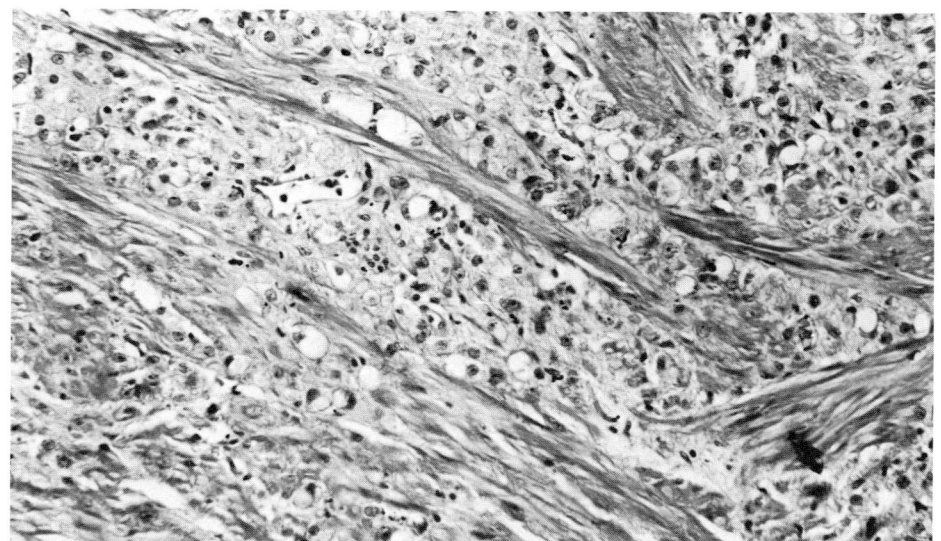

Figure 8-25   *Adenocarcinoma of the prostate, Gleason pattern 5. The tumor cells infiltrate the fibromuscular stroma in cords and single cells with no evidence of gland formation.*

smooth muscle without intervening collagenous investment is characteristic of prostatic adenocarcinoma. The histologic basis for the clinically detected induration associated with adenocarcinoma is attributed to a variably dense desmoplastic response to the infiltrating tumor. Invasion of intraprostatic lymphatics, blood vessels, and perineural space is frequent, and is of diagnostic importance when evaluating prostate biopsies. (Refer to discussion of local spread.)

The cytologic features of prostatic adenocarcinoma exhibit a spectrum from minimal to marked nuclear pleomorphism and hyperchromatism. One or two prominent nucleoli in the background of chromatin clumped near the nuclear membrane are the most frequent nuclear features. The cytoplasm may be vacuolated and appear as the clear cell variety of renal cell carcinoma.[264,284] Alternatively, the cytoplasm stains lightly eosinophilic. The cell borders are usually distinct in the well-differentiated tumors in contrast to indistinct borders more characteristic of poorly differentiated tumors.[280] The single layer of cuboidal cells in neoplastic acini is, from a practical standpoint, the most frequently employed criterion to establish the diagnosis of adenocarcinoma of the prostate.

Prostatic adenocarcinoma must be distinguished from transitional cell metaplasia, adenosis and transitional cell carcinoma of the prostatic ducts, granulomatous prostatitis, malakoplakia, and physiologic senile atrophy of the prostate, all of which have been misinterpreted in the past. The most challenging diagnostic distinction requires separating adenosis of the prostate from well-differentiated adenocarcinoma. (Refer to discussion of atypical forms of prostatic hyperplasia.)

The histologic changes resulting from endocrine and radiation therapy have been the subject of numerous studies.[256,258,305] The classic changes resulting from estrogen therapy include tumor acinar atrophy, with regressive cytologic changes including nuclear pyknosis, loss of nucleoli, cytoplasmic vacuolization, and fragmentation of cell membranes.[256,258] Estrogen-induced squamous metaplasia of non-neoplastic ductal epithelium is typical (Fig. 8-26). Radiation therapy also produces tumor regression characterized by a decrease in the number and size of acini, stromal fibrosis, and radiation-induced vascular injury.[305] Squamous metaplasia of non-neoplastic ductal and acinar epithelium is also observed secondary to radiation therapy.[305]

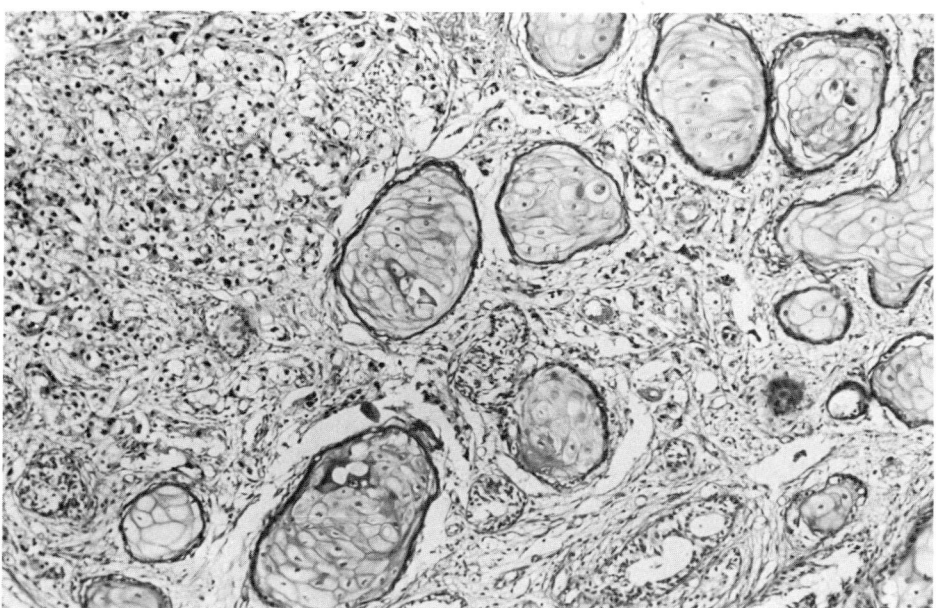

Figure 8-26   *Adenocarcinoma of the prostate with estrogen therapy effect. The poorly differentiated adenocarcinoma (Gleason pattern 5) shows uniform pyknotic nuclei infiltrating the stroma adjacent to glands with squamous metaplasia.*

Tumor Grading

The characteristic histologic variability exhibited by typical prostatic adenocarcinomas apparently has served as a major obstacle to the general acceptance of any one among many proposed tumor grading protocols. Failure to achieve reliability and reproducibility has limited the value and general acceptance of many suggested protocols. The limitations inherent in needle biopsies further compound the difficulty of accurately grading prostatic adenocarcinoma.[299,310,311,313,315]

A common practice in many pathology departments has been the application of a three-grade system: well-differentiated, moderately differentiated, and poorly differentiated adenocarcinoma. The assigned tumor grade reflected either the predominant differentiation, or the poorest differentiation of a given tumor. In practical terms this translates to three categories: the best-differentiated, the worst-differentiated, and the majority in between with little or no objectively applied histologic criteria defining any of the tumor grades. Such informal and subjective grading "systems" are correspondingly of little prognostic value.

The original grading protocol proposed by Broders demonstrated that the percent of a tumor showing differentiation had predictive value prognosticating the ultimate survival of patients with squamous cell carcinoma of the lip, and

Table 8-4   *Tumor Grading Protocols*

Mostofi[277]	*Gleason* *[264,284]	*Brawn et al*[307]
Grade I: tumor composed of well-differentiated glands lined with slight nuclear anaplasia	Pattern 1: closely packed, single, separate, round, uniform glands; well-defined tumor margin	Grade I: 75%–100% of tumor glands (exception—predominantly cribiform-papillary pattern
Grade II: tumor composed of glands lined by cells with moderate nuclear anaplasia	Pattern 2: single, separate, round, less uniform glands separated by stroma up to one gland diameter; tumor margin less well defined	Grade II: 50%–75% of tumor forms glands (includes cribiform-papillary tumors); tumor > 50% of which are cribiform-papillary pattern
Grade III: tumor composed of glands lined by cells with marked nuclear anaplasia or undifferentiated tumors (do not form glands)	Pattern 3: single, separate, irregular glands of variable size; enlarged masses with cribiform or papillary pattern; poorly defined tumor margin	Grade III: 20%–50% of tumor forms glands
	Pattern 4: fused glands in mass with infiltrating cords, small glands, with papillary, cribiform or solid patterns; cells small, dark, or hypernephroid (clear cells)	Grade IV: 0–25% of tumor forms glands
	Pattern 5: few or no glands in background of masses with comedo pattern; cords or sheets of tumor cells infiltrating stroma	

* Gleason tumor grade = dominant pattern + secondary pattern

genitourinary system.[248,249] Broders proposed four grades: grade 1 tumors exhibited features of differentiation in 75% to 100% of neoplasm; 50% to 75% of the tumor was differentiated in grade 2 cases; 25% to 50% of the tumor was differentiated in grade 3 cases; and 0 to 25% of the tumor was differentiated in grade 4 cases. Several modifications of the original Broders system applicable to adenocarcinoma of the prostate have been proposed in the subsequent years.[255,260,262,269,298,307,308] A detailed analysis of these grading systems has been published in a comprehensive review by Mostofi.[278] Three of the most recently proposed grading systems are presented in Table 8-4.

Mostofi classifies tumors into three grades and requires the evaluation of the differentiation (gland structure) and the anaplasia (nuclear features) of the tumor.[277,285] Mostofi has reported that this classification affords good prognostic information.[285] However, recent studies utilizing the Mostofi system have observed limited ability to identify patients at increased risk, and no increased advantage over more simple grading systems, a conclusion supported by Mostofi's own data.[285,307]

In recent years the grading protocol proposed by Gleason has received increasing acceptance, if not uniform support, from numerous published studies evaluating its reproducibility, reliability, and prognostic value.[264,274,284] This grading system recognizes five histologic patterns representing decreasing glandular differentiation (Fig. 8-27, Table 8-4). Variability of histologic pattern within a tumor is recognized and incorporated into the final grade assessment by adding the grade numbers of the predominant and secondary histologic patterns.[284] The value of this grading system, enhanced even further when combined with tumor stage data, has been demonstrated in accurately predicting ultimate survival. Although the Gleason system does recognize the presence of different histologic patterns within a tumor, the histologic grade of the secondary pattern does not consider the proportion of the tumor represented by this component. This is significant, because Mostofi has presented data showing that the prognostic importance of a histologic pattern is achieved only when it exceeds a certain minimum percent of the total tumor.[285]

Numerous studies in recent years have evaluated the reproducibility, reliability, and predictive value of the Gleason grading system. Personal experience confirms the generally reported high marks for reproducibility and reliability of this grading system.[285,307,309,311] Less uniform success has been reported in predicting probability of regional lymph node metastases by Gleason grading. Kramer and associates, Sagalowsky and associates, and Smith and associates reported generally good correlation, whereas Barzell and associates, Olsson and associates, and Zinke and associates reported limited or poor correlation.[286,297,303,304,306,312]

Further studies are required to define more precisely the limits of predictive value of the Gleason system. Finally, several studies utilizing the Gleason grading system have observed significant variation of the grades assigned to the prostatic needle biopsies and the subsequent prostatectomy specimens, a reflection on the representative nature of the biopsy and not the grading system, per se.[299,310,311,313,315]

The M.D. Anderson (MDA) tumor grading system is the most recent presented in the literature.[307] With one modification, it represents the resurrection of the original Broders grading system published 60 years ago.[248,249] The minor

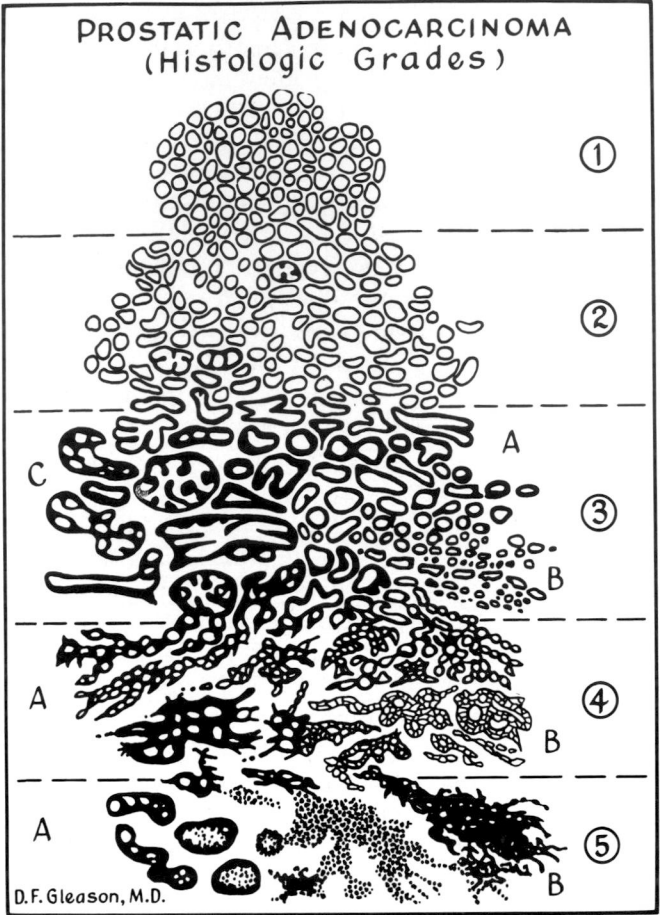

PROSTATIC ADENOCARCINOMA
(Histologic Grades)

Figure 8-27   *Gleason grading system of prostatic adenocarcinoma.*
(Gleason DF, The Veterans Administration Cooperative
Urologic Research Group: Histologic grading and clinical
staging of prostatic carcinoma. In Tannbaum M (ed). Urologic
Pathology: The Prostate. Philadelphia, Lea and Febiger, 1977)

difference concerns the special status of papillary and cribiform patterns, which when present in excess of 50%, places the tumor in grade 2. (Refer to Table 8-4.) In a study of 182 cases of stage C prostatic adenocarcinoma, the MDA grading system exceeded the ability of both the Mostofi and Gleason systems in discriminating patients of low, intermediate, and high risk of tumor-related death.[307] The effectiveness of this grading system to predict lymph node metastases accurately and reliably in clinical stage A and stage B cases is yet to be demonstrated.

Finally, there have been recent findings of increasing tumor grade within the primary neoplasm observed over a period of time.[314] In addition, some studies have reported that 10% to 20% of prostatic adenocarcinomas give rise to metastases demonstrating a grade at variance with that observed in the primary tumor of origin.[75,302] As the frequency of negative immunoperoxidase staining for PSA and PAP increases among high-grade prostatic adenocarcinomas, metastases with such high-grade features may give the erroneous impression that they represent dissemination from nonprostatic sources.

Extraprostatic Spread of Adenocarcinoma
Local Invasion
Perineural Space

The very high frequency of perineural invasion by prostatic adenocarcinoma is documented in numerous studies.[34,188,243,244,250,252,253,262,265,271] Both the prognostic and diagnostic significance traditionally attributed to this histologic feature have been challenged. The studies of Pennington and associates and Byar and Mostofi have shown that perineural invasion per se has no adverse effect on prognosis compared to stage-matched controls.[265,271] The recent observation of benign prostatic glands in perineural locations demands future caution in applying perineural invasion as the sine qua non of malignancy of the prostate.[296,301]

Originally, perineural invasion by prostatic adenocarcinoma was thought to represent invasion of intraprostatic perineural lymphatic channels, a view maintained through the 1960s.[252,265,267] Warren and associates suggested these perineural lymphatics served as a means of local dissemination of the tumor to the pelvic bones and lower vertebral column.[252] In 1967, Rodin and associates challenged the existence of perineural lymphatics within the prostate.[266] By serial sectioning of prostatic carcinomas, he reported that tumor in perineural locations occupied spaces devoid of an endothelial lining. No perineural lymphatics were found when human and canine peripheral nerves were examined by electron microscopy.[266] These findings have been confirmed in subsequent electron microscopic studies of human prostate glands.[263,294,295] The extant perineural vascular structures have the ultrastructural features of blood capillaries, and not lymphatics.[266,294] Based on these results, perineural invasion is currently thought to represent tumor infiltration into a potential tissue space offering a plane of least resistance.[266,294]

Prostatic Capsule

Invasion of the prostatic capsule is frequently observed in surgical and autopsy specimens, and is undoubtedly related to the peripheral location of prostatic adenocarcinoma.[244,271,272] The finding of capsular invasion in 23% of neoplasms smaller than 1 mm³ by McNeal suggests that it is an early event in tumor progression.[244] Increasing size of the tumor is associated with a corresponding increased frequency of capsular invasion and penetration.[244,287] The lower survival observed in cases with capsular penetration is not seen in patients who have capsular invasion without full-thickness penetration.[271]

Seminal Vesicle

Invasion of the seminal vesicles by direct extension occurs in 11% to 31% of clinical stage B prostatic carcinomas, and is observed at autopsy in 14% to 58% of cases.[251,257,259,261,268,287] Seminal vesicle invasion is commonly associated with the finding of prostatic capsular invasion.

Urinary Bladder

Invasion of the urinary bladder by direct extension is less common than capsular penetration and seminal vesicle invasion during the early phases of tumor spread, but is demonstrated in 37% to 50% of cases at autopsy.[251,257,259]

Rectum

Prostatic carcinoma invading the rectum is relatively uncommon, and in published reviews has been reported to occur in an average of 5% of cases with a range of 0.5% to 13%.[251,259,293,336] Rectal obstruction with or without associated bleeding is the most frequent clinical presentation.[270] Invasion of rectal mucosa with ulceration is rare.[257]

Regional and Distant Metastases

At the time of death, the majority of patients with prostatic carcinoma show extraprostatic spread.[251,253,259,272,405] (The pattern of metastases observed at autopsy is presented later in Table 8-14.) This distribution is characteristic of the late stages of the disease and represents cumulative dissemination by both hematogenous and lymphatic routes. Accumulating evidence from surgical staging suggests that the earliest metastases occur in the obturator lymph node, which is often positive when other nodes or bone are negative for metastatic tumor.[275,279,286,339] Subsequent lymphatic dissemination involves the iliac and para-aortic nodes.[275,279,286] Metastases to the lung result both from further lymphatic spread by the thoracic duct, and independently, venous dissemination by the prostatic venous plexus and the inferior vena cava. Metastases to the viscera are the consequence of tumor cells either passing directly through the lung capillaries, or invading pulmonary veins by established pulmonary metastases, and subsequently spreading by the systemic arterial tree.

The high frequency of bone metastases is generally recognized and reflected in the autopsy studies cited later in Table 8-14. Metastases most commonly involve the vertebral column, ribs, and pelvic bones.[251,276,300] Warren and associates postulated that the apparent predilection for these bones was the result of "perineural lymphatic spread" of prostatic carcinoma.[252] Batson demonstrated the valveless venous anastomoses between the periprostatic venous plexus and the vertebral venous plexus, and he suggested that prostatic carcinoma's predilection for these bone sites was by means of these venous anastomoses.[254] Neither Batson's premise (the preferential metastases of prostatic carcinoma to pelvic bones), nor his results were challenged until recently.

Dodds and associates evaluated the technetium bone scans of 73 patients with prostatic carcinoma and a similar number of patients with nonprostatic malignancies of the respiratory, gastrointestinal, and urinary tracts.[300] The distribution of the early skeletal metastases from the prostatic primaries was not significantly different from that of nonprostatic malignancies. Prostatic carcinoma demonstrated no unique predilection for metastases to the pelvic bones and the lumbar vertebrae. Dodds and associates concluded that the venous anastomoses described by Batson served no significant role in the metastatic dissemination of prostatic carcinoma.[300]

Natural History

Tumor Staging

The clinical staging of prostatic carcinoma was introduced by Whitmore.[332] Subsequent modifications, principally by Jewett, have further refined the applicability of Whitmore's staging protocol.[378] More recently, a TNM staging system has been proposed; however, the modified Whitmore–Jewett protocol has received the widest general acceptance in the United States.[390,403] These staging protocols are outlined in Tables 8-5 and 8-6.

Jewett's modification of the Whitmore system is the subdivision of stages A and B cases into A1, A2, and B1, B2 on the basis of extent of tumor, focal or diffuse.[378] In spite of the nonuniform definition of Jewett's terms "focal" and "diffuse," numerous studies have demonstrated the prognostic value of the A1, A2 and B1, B2 stage stratification (refer to following discussion of stages A to D). More recently, stage D has been subdivided into stage D1 cases (metastases limited to regional lymph nodes) and stage D2 cases (metastases to distant sites). Further modifications of this staging system have been suggested in recent years, but have not been formally adopted.[292,387,391,392]

The TNM staging system for prostatic carcinoma is potentially more flexible, and certainly more comprehensive, but its acceptance has been limited. I regard the choice of staging systems to be of lesser importance than the clear communication between pathologist and urologic oncologist achieved when a mutually accepted protocol is consistently applied to tumor staging.

In recent years, technical advances (including more precise serum acid phosphatase determinations, radionuclide bone scans, CT scan, and most recently, NMR of pelvic organs) have greatly increased the accuracy of clinical staging. The distribution of clinical stage of patients with prostatic carcinoma reported in 11 studies is presented in Table 8-7.

Clinical Stage A

The term *incidental carcinoma* is applied to clinically unsuspected prostatic malignancies discovered during microscopic review of specimens surgically removed for nodular hyperplasia, or in prostates obtained at autopsy. The frequency of such carcinomas in clinically benign prostates increases with age and ranges from 1.8% to 24%, with an overall average of 9% among the reported studies (Table 8-8). Incidental carcinomas discovered at autopsy occur in 12% to 46% of all men over the age of 40, rising to 45% to 100% of men over the age of 80 (see Table 8-3). These incidental, or stage A cases, constitute an average of 22% (range, 3% to 53%) of all prostatic carcinomas diagnosed antemortem.[271,272,337,357,361,376,382,388,401] An average of 60% (range, 21% to 83%) of all cases diagnosed at autopsy are clinically unsuspected.[188,189,193,199,215,251,257,259] The thoroughness of examination of prostate specimens influences the frequency of incidental carcinomas, and the nonuniform manner of examination of these specimens by pathologists in different institutions undoubtedly accounts in part for the variation of the reported frequencies.[193,319,348,381,400] The true incidence of prostatic carcinoma in elderly men is more accurately reflected in the data of autopsy studies, which are not affected by the independent frequency of clinically symptomatic nodular hyperplasia, requisite to finding incidental carcinomas in surgical specimens.

The clinical significance of incidental carcinomas has been the subject of considerable interest. The high frequency of incidental prostatic carcinomas found at autopsy prompted speculation that these lesions were biologically different from clinically apparent carcinomas.[199,201,257] This ultimately led to the concept of *latent carcinomas:* lesions morphologically malignant but biologically nonaggressive.[201]

Clinical and pathologic studies of incidental (stage A) carcinomas have clarified our understanding of these neoplasms. Although the vast majority of

Table 8-5   ***Modified Prostate Carcinoma Staging Protocol of Whitmore[332] and Jewett[378]***

Stage	Extent of Invasion
A1	Incidental focal microscopic tumor detected in clinically benign prostate specimen*
A2	Incidental diffuse microscopic tumor detected in clinically benign prostate specimen*
B1	Clinically palpable tumor confined to one lobe of the prostate
B2	Clinically palpable tumor involving more than one lobe of the prostate
C	Locally invasive beyond prostate but without metastases
D1	Metastases to regional pelvic lymph nodes
D2	Distant metastases

* Refer to Golimbu and Morales and Sheldon and co-workers for further discussion of stages A1, A2 and B1, B2.[292,391]

Table 8-6   ***Prostate Carcinoma TNM Staging Protocol[403]***

Stage	Extent of Invasion
Primary Tumor (T)	
TX	Minimum requirements to assess the primary tumor cannot be met
T0	No tumor present
T1a	No palpable tumor; on histologic sections no more than three high-power fields of carcinoma found
T1b	No palpable tumor; histologic sections revealing more than three high-power fields of prostatic carcinoma
T2a	Palpable nodule less than 1.5 cm in diameter with compressible, normal-feeling tissue on at least three sides
T2b	Palpable nodule more than 1.5 cm in diameter or nodule or induration in both lobes
T3	Palpable tumor extending into or beyond the prostatic capsule
T3a	Palpable tumor extending into the periprostatic tissues or involving one seminal vesicle
T3b	Palpable tumor extending into the periprostatic tissues, involving one or both seminal vesicles; tumor size more than 6 cm in diameter
T4	Tumor fixed or involving neighboring structures
Nodal Involvement (N)	
NX	Minimum requirements to assess the regional nodes cannot be met
N0	No involvement of regional lymph nodes
N1	Involvement of a single homolateral regional lymph node
N2	Involvement of contralateral, bilateral, or multiple regional lymph nodes
N3	A fixed mass present on the pelvic wall with a free space between this and the tumor
Distant Metastasis (M)	
MX	Minimum requirements to assess the presence of distant metastasis cannot be met
M0	No (known) distant metastasis
M1	Distant metastasis present. Specify site.*

* Specify sites according to the following notations: distant; lymph nodes, LYM; pulmonary, PUL; osseous, OSS; hepatic, HEP; brain, BRA; pleura, PLE; skin, SKI; eye, EYE; other, OTH.

patients with incidental prostatic carcinomas treated only with transurethral resection suffer no adverse effect on survival relative to age-matched controls, a small percent of these men do evidence clinical progression of disease.[271,340,362,391] Clinically aggressive behavior is associated with diffuse, poorly differentiated tumors.[271,340,362] Small, discrete, and well-differentiated tumors are associated with a good outcome, with rare exceptions.[271,283,340,362]

Table 8-7   *Clinical Stage Distribution of Prostatic Carcinoma*

Author	Year	Clinical Stage			
		A	B	C	D
Anderson[337]	1959	17%	33%	38.7%	10.5%
Flocks et al[339]	1959	← 3% →		56%	41%
VACURG[350]	1967	← 14% →		48%	38%
Corriere et al[357]	1970	3.6%	48.4%	18.7%	29.3%
Carlton et al[361]	1972	3%	32%	27%	38%
Schoones et al[272]	1972	9.3%	10.8%	34%	45.9%
Byar et al[271]	1972	25%	54%	17%	3.5%
Varkarakis et al[376]	1975	4.7%	8.2%	84.7%	2.4%
McMillen, Wettlaufer[382]	1976	5.3%	22%	15%	10%
DeVere White et al[388]	1977	15%	16.5%	35.4%	33%
Murphy et al[401]	1982	25.9%	28.9%	14.9%	25.9%

Table 8-8   *Incidental Adenocarcinoma Found in Clinically Benign Prostatic Surgical Specimens*

Author	Year	Age Range	Surgical Procedure	Frequency of Incidental Carcinoma
Wade[316]	1914	NI	P	10%
Swan[317]	1923	NI	TUR, P	14.3%
McHeffey[319]	1940	NI	TUR, P	4%
Treiger et al[324]	1948	NI	P	12.6%
Smith, Woodruff[328]	1950	NI	P	9.6%
Labess[327]	1952	44–95	P	9.2%
Bergman et al[329]	1955	NI	TUR	3.1%
Green, Simon[330]	1955	NI	TUR	4%
Turner, Belt[334]	1957	NI	P	3.1%
Bauer et al[341]	1960	NI	P	6.5%
Denton[348]	1965	50+	TUR	6%
Denton[348]	1965	50+	TUR	21%*
Lilien et al[352]	1968	NI	P	24%
Melchior et al[373]	1974	NI	TUR	6.5%
Delides et al[381]	1976	NI	P	4%
Heaney et al[281]	1977	50–80	TUR, P	10%

NI, no information; TUR, transurethral resection; P, prostatectomy

* complete histologic exam; all other studies reflect routine examinations.

These findings prompted Jewett to subdivide stage A neoplasms into two subtypes, A1 and A2.[378] Stage A1 lesions were defined as well-differentiated, focal lesions, and stage A2 as diffuse, or poorly differentiated carcinomas. The working definitions of Jewett's criteria for A1 and A2 lesions have not been uniform in the reported studies, and the unsettled state of histologic grading of prostatic carcinomas adds additional variation to the application of Jewett's criteria.[391,400]

These limitations notwithstanding, the cumulative clinical and pathologic experience with stage A1 and stage A2 prostatic carcinoma reported since 1975 is summarized in Table 8-9. The neoplasms identified as clinical stage A2 show a significantly greater tendency to invade the prostatic capsule and seminal vesicle, and importantly, metastasize to pelvic lymph nodes. Thus, significant numbers of clinical stage A2 prostatic carcinomas are in fact pathologic stage C and even stage D1. The recognition of the capability of clinically undetected prostatic carcinoma to invade locally and metastasize to regional lymph nodes constitutes one of the recent major advances in our understanding of prostatic carcinoma. The new perspective has a bearing on clinical management of all prostatic carcinomas: the clinical assessment of tumor stage in the absence of pathologic confirmation invites disaster. The burden of responsibility rests with the surgical pathologist to identify and report histologic features of prostatic carcinomas that predict clinical behavior.

The overall survival of cases of clinical stage A carcinomas of the prostate at 5 years is reported to be 54% to 82%, and at 10 years is 28.5% to 63.6%.[288,391,401] Little data on long-term survival of pathologic stages A1 and A2 are currently available.

Table 8-9 **Comparison of Clinical and Pathologic Stages of Clinical Stage A1 and A2 Prostatic Carcinoma**

Author	Year	Frequency
Clinical Stage A1		*Pathologic Stage C*
Wilson et al[287]	1977	0%
Golimbu et al[290]	1978	0%
		Pathologic Stage D1
Bruce et al[387]	1977	0%
Wilson et al[287]	1977	0%
Donohue et al[384]	1977	0%
Golimbu et al[290]	1978	0%
Prout et al[393]	1980	0%
Clinical Stage A2		*Pathologic Stage C*
Wilson et al[287]	1977	0%
		Pathologic Stage D1
Bruce et al[387]	1977	0%
Wilson et al[287]	1977	0%
Donohue et al[384]	1977	22%
Golimbu, Morales[292]	1979	33%
Prout et al[393]	1980	17%

Clinical Stage B

The palpable prostatic nodule detected by digital rectal examination distinguishes clinical stage B from clinical stage A. Jewett reported that 50% of prostatic nodules in men older than 40 years of age represented carcinoma, data similar to that obtained by Emmett and associates for men 50 years of age and older.[331,341] Both studies demonstrated the limited ability to distinguish benign and malignant nodules reliably.

An additional problem exists. The ability to determine clinically the extent of extraprostatic spread by rectal examination is also limited. The resultant clinical understaging reduces the true incidence of carcinomas confined to the prostate (pathologic stage B).[273,338,369] The reported frequency of clinical stage B prostatic carcinomas varies from 8% to 48% (average 36%) (see Table 8-7). However, 7% to 29% show microscopic invasion of the capsule and 11% to 36% have microscopic invasion of the seminal vesicles (pathologic stage C).[261,268,271,287,292]

Attempts to predict which clinical stage B tumors will evidence clinical aggressiveness were initiated by Jewett.[378] He observed that clinical stage B tumors involving more than one prostatic lobe demonstrated a higher frequency of recurrence than those tumors confined to one lobe. Based on these findings, Jewett subclassified these clinical stage B cases into stages B1 and B2 based on the size and extent of intraprostatic tumor as clinically determined by rectal examination.[378] This subclassification has received general support in studies since 1975. Clinical stage B2 tumors more frequently demonstrate local invasion of the prostatic capsule and seminal vesicles, and metastasis to pelvic lymph nodes than is observed with clinical stage B1 cases (Table 8-10). The limited data available show that a higher proportion of B1 tumors are well differentiated (78% to 96%) than is observed in B2 tumors (40% to 80%).[262,282,292,378] Tumor grading has limited value in predicting clinical aggressiveness of stage B tumors reliably.[292,310,393]

Table 8-10   **Reported Frequency of Metastases to Pelvic Lymph Nodes in Clinical Stage B of Prostatic Adenocarcinoma**

Author(s)	Year	Frequency of Positive Pelvic Lymph Nodes		
		Clinical Stage B	Clinical Stage B1	Clinical Stage B2
Flocks et al[339]	1959	7%		
Arduino, Gluckman[261]	1962	32%		
Castellino et al[365]	1973	44%		
Hilaris et al[275]	1974	21%		
McCullough et al[273]	1974	25%		
Whitmore et al[369]	1974	21%		
Varkarakis et al[376]	1975	14%		
McLaughlin et al[279]	1976		21%	30%
Ray et al[383]	1976		14%	27%
Saltzstein, McLaughlin[385]	1977		16%	29%
Bruce et al[387]	1977		0%	38%
Wilson[287]	1977		14%	45%
Golimbu, Morales[292]	1979		14%	48%

Blanks indicate information not provided.

There is some evidence that clinical stage B1 tumors are less aggressive than stage A2 lesions.[279,287,292,383,384,387] Several studies have demonstrated that clinical stage A2 tumors more frequently exhibit high grade and pelvic lymph node metastases than do clinical stage B1 tumors.[279,287,292,383,384,387] Golimbu and Morales have suggested that clinical stage A2 tumors be reclassified to clinical stage B2, to reflect these observations more accurately.[292]

The 10-year survival rate for clinical stage B tumors ranges from 50% to 79%.[268,283,356,360,383] Only limited data on long-term survival of pathologic stages B1 and B2 are currently available.

Clinical Stage C

In a recent national survey conducted by the American College of Surgeons, 29.8% of 34,245 patients with prostatic carcinoma were clinical stage C.[401] This compares with a 15% to 85% (average 35%) incidence of clinical stage C cases from individual reporting institutions (see Table 8-8). The actual frequency of pathologic stage C prostatic carcinomas is affected by the high frequency of clinical understaging: a significant percent of clinical stage A and B cases show microscopic invasion beyond the prostatic capsule and are thus pathologic stage C tumors; and an average of 55% of prostatic carcinomas clinically judged to be stage C show pelvic lymph node metastases (pathologic stage D1) (Table 8-11).

Elevated serum acid phosphatase is observed in only 20% to 31% of stage C cases, and thus cannot accurately predict local extraprostatic spread.[326,328,333] As previously discussed, the ability of the rectal examination to detect extraprostatic spread is limited and has not been exceeded by any currently available diagnostic test short of histologic examination of radical prostatectomy specimens.

The reported distribution of well-differentiated, moderately differentiated,

Table 8-11   *Frequency of Pelvic Lymph Node Metastases of Clinical Stage C Prostatic Carcinoma*

Author(s)	Year	Frequency of Lymph Node Metastases
Whitmore, Mackenzie[338]	1959	56%
Flocks[339]	1959	38%
Arduino, Glucksman[261]	1962	82.4%
Carlton et al[361]	1972	30%
Flocks[364]	1973	32%
Castellino et al[365]	1973	56%
Dahl et al[370]	1974	69%
Whitmore et al[369]	1974	64.5%
McCullough et al[273]	1974	58.7%
Bagshaw et al[377]	1975	52.2%
Varkarakis et al[376]	1975	47.2%
McLaughlin et al[279]	1975	50%
Ray et al[383]	1976	52%
Barzell et al[286]	1977	63.4%
Nicholson et al[282]	1977	33%
Bruce et al[387]	1977	75%
Wilson et al[287]	1977	53%

and poorly differentiated clinical stage C neoplasms is 0% to 57%, 22% to 50%, and 13% to 60%, respectively.[262,273,282,307,383,401] Ranges of such magnitude reflect the widely divergent histologic criteria employed to grade tumors in different institutions, and very likely also account for the limited ability of tumor grading to predict pelvic lymph node metastases and ultimate survival of clinical stage C cases. Although lymph node metastases are more frequent with high grade carcinomas than with well-differentiated neoplasms, specific predictive limitations of tumor grading studies are apparent. The most important limitations referable to clinical stage C cases are the following: (1) no extant tumor grading system accurately predicts lymph node metastases from moderately differentiated clinical stage C cases;[297,303,396] (2) the low frequency of nodal metastases from well-differentiated (low grade) tumors was not observed by Smith and associates and Olson and associates;[303,312] and (3) the high frequency of nodal metastases from poorly differentiated tumors (greater than 90%) was not confirmed by Sagalowsky and associates, who reported a frequency of 44% to 60%.[297,304] Thus, tumor grading of a large percentage of clinical stage C cases (*i.e.,* moderately differentiated neoplasms) has no predictive value, and the significant number of low grade and high grade tumors behaving in a manner deviant from the majority of cases in these grades further reduces the predictive value of current grading systems.

The overall survival at 5 years and 10 years of clinical stage C cases is reported to be 36% to 61.5% (average 48.6%) and 16% to 51.5% (average 32%).[286,353,364,374,377,383,388] Recently, Brawn and associates have reported a grading system capable of reliably predicting survival of clinical stage C cases.[307] The 5-year survival rates of well-, moderately, and poorly differentiated prostatic carcinomas were 91%, 60%, and 15%, respectively.[307] The applicability of this grading system to predict survival of clinical stage A and stage B cases is yet to be determined.

Clinical Stage D

Prostatic carcinoma with clinically apparent metastases at the time of diagnosis (clinical stage D) constitutes 2% to 46% (average 26%) of reported series of this neoplasm (see Table 8-7). The introduction of radionuclide bone scans and surgical staging operations has clarified the magnitude of clinical understaging of cases judged to be stage A1 to stage C (see Tables 8-9 to 8-11).

Because the earliest metastases from prostatic carcinoma involve the obturator lymph nodes, which are not visualized by pedal lymphangiography, this radiologic technique is not reliable in the clinical evaluation of prostatic carcinoma.[279,342,365,377,383,387] Subsequent dissemination to the iliac and para-aortic lymph nodes is detected by lymphangiography.

The progression of prostatic carcinoma from stage D1 to stage D2 has been studied recently by Prout and associates.[393] During the follow-up period, clinical progression was observed in 18% of stage D1 patients with metastases limited to one pelvic lymph node, in contrast to 76% of patients with multiple positive lymph nodes.[393] When tumor progression was observed, it was virtually always in the form of increasingly widespread bone involvement.

Metastasis to bone most commonly involves the pelvis, vertebral column, and the ribs.[279,342,365,377,383,387] Early bone metastases are most reliably detected by radionuclide bone scans.[380,386] In four reported studies, abnormal bone x-rays were found in only 26% to 68% of patients with positive bone scans.[276,363,371,401]

Serum acid phosphatase (SAP), utilized in the past to detect bone metastases and their response to endocrine therapy, yields both false-positive and false-negative information.[322,372] Elevation of SAP is presumptive, but is not diagnostic evidence of bone metastases, because benign disorders including prostatic infarcts and nodular hyperplasia have been reported associated with elevated SAP.[372] As discussed previously, 20% to 31% of clinical stage C patients without evidence of bone metastases have elevated serum acid phosphatase values.[326,328,333] Conversely, normal levels of SAP have been observed in 26% to 49% of patients with documented metastases in bone.[297,351,367,379] Mobley and Frank have reported normal SAP levels more commonly among grade 3 (45%) than grade 1 (20%) prostatic carcinomas metastatic to bone.[351] The explanation of these observations awaits further study.

The term *occult carcinoma* refers to undiagnosed prostatic carcinoma whose clinical manifestations are caused by metastases (Table 8-12). This is distinctly uncommon, because the majority of patients have local signs and symptoms referable to the urinary outflow tract. When the first manifestations of prostatic carcinoma relate to lymph nodes, lung, skin, or the central nervous system, a diagnostic challenge has presented itself.

Table 8-12   **Prostatic Carcinoma Presenting in Rare Metastatic Sites**

Author(s)	Year	No. of Cases
Supraclavicular Lymph Node		
Brennas[343]	1961	1
Dick[345]	1962	1
Warren, Furlow[355]	1970	5
Butler et al[358]	1971	19
Yam et al[402]	1983	5
Lung		
Greenberg, Young[335]	1958	2
Lome, John[366]	1973	4
Yam et al[402]	1983	2
Intracranial		
Mahavevia et al[394]	1980	1
Rao[397]	1982	1
Bauman et al[404]	1981	1
Skin		
Ronchese[320]	1940	1
Ichikawa et al[344]	1962	1
Razvi et al[375]	1975	1
Abdomen, Retroperitoneum		
Tolia et al[389]	1978	1
Leung, Casciato[398]	1982	1
Orbit		
Tertzakain et al[399]	1982	1

Approximately 30 patients presenting initially with supraclavicular lymph node metastases from undiagnosed prostatic carcinoma have been reported.[343,345,355,358] The rarity of metastases to lymph nodes in the neck at initial presentation contrasts with their greater frequency (32%) in more advanced cases examined at autopsy.[347] The prostatic origin of a recent case of adenocarcinoma metastatic to a supraclavicular lymph node was disclosed by immunoperoxidase staining of prostatic-specific antigen (PSA). Subsequent transrectal needle biopsy confirmed the presence of the previously undetected prostatic carcinoma.

Clinically apparent pulmonary metastases have been reported in approximately 6% of cases of three reported series.[251,257,349] Microscopic evidence of pulmonary metastases at autopsy is observed in 12% to 38% of cases of prostatic carcinoma.[251,257,259,336,349] When observed clinically, metastasis to the lungs manifests either as asymptomatic nodules detected on chest x-ray, or alternatively, as diffuse intrapulmonary lymphangitic spread with associated respiratory insufficiency.[349,359,366] Objective response as measured by reduction of size of lung nodules, or improved pulmonary function has been reported with estrogen therapy.[349,366]

Other rare sites of metastatic occult prostatic carcinoma include meninges (case of mucinous adenocarcinoma of the prostate) and skin.[368,375,394]

Histologic studies of stage D carcinomas show that the majority are high grade, with well-differentiated tumors constituting only 2% to 25% of this group.[351,357,401] Mobley and Frank have reported that tumor grade had no influence on the survival rate of clinical stage D2 prostatic carcinoma patients.[351] The overall survival rate of clinical stage D patients improved from 6% to 13% 5-year survival rate in the preadjuvant period, to 20% to 34% 5-year survival rate after the introduction of estrogen therapy (Table 8-13).

Prostatic Carcinoma at Autopsy

The reported experience with incidental prostatic carcinoma discovered at autopsy has been discussed in the section on stage A. Prostatic carcinomas diagnosed antemortem have disseminated in the majority of cases examined at autopsy.[251,257,259,336,405] Local invasion of the seminal vesicle and the urinary

Table 8-13   ***Survival Rates for Stage D Prostatic Carcinoma***

Author(s)	Year	5-Year Survival	10-Year Survival	Therapy
Bumpus[318]	1926	13%	NI	Preadjuvant era
Nesbit, Plumb[323]	1946	6%	NI	Preadjuvant era
Emmett et al[341]	1960	20%	6.7%	Orchiectomy + estrogens
VACURG[350]	1967	30%	NI	Orchiectomy + estrogens
Corriere et al[357]	1970	24%	NI	Orchiectomy + estrogens
de Vere White et al[388]	1977	31%	9.0%	Orchiectomy + estrogens
Prout et al[393]	1980	34%	NI	Prostatectomy or radiation

NI, no information

bladder is observed in 14% to 53% and 37% to 45% of cases, respectively.[251,257,259,336,405] The distribution of metastases at autopsy is presented in Table 8-14. Pelvic and para-aortic lymph nodes, bone (pelvis, vertebrae, and ribs), and lungs are the most common sites of metastatic involvement. Abdominal viscera (*i.e.,* liver) and the gastrointestinal tract are involved less frequently. Multiple other sites of metastases are observed with a lesser frequency.

Among the patients with clinically diagnosed prostatic carcinoma, the majority succumb to the direct effects of the widely disseminated neoplasm. Carcinomatosis, frequently with terminal pneumonia, sepsis, or renal failure is the most common cause of death.[251,257,259,336,405]

Transitional Cell Carcinoma

Transitional cell carcinoma originating in distal prostatic ducts was not recognized until 1963 when Ende and associates reported seven cases, four of which were associated with prostatic adenocarcinomas.[408] A decade earlier Ortega and associates had reported in situ carcinoma of the prostatic ducts in association with the same lesion involving the prostatic urethra and the urinary bladder.[407]

Since these original descriptions, transitional cell carcinoma of the prostate with origin in prostatic ducts has been reported in approximately 140 patients, 31 of whom had an associated prostatic adenocarcinoma.[409-419, 421-425] During this same period, greater appreciation for urethral and prostatic duct transitional cell carcinoma in situ accompanying bladder urothelial malignancies has also occurred. (Refer to Chap. 4.)

The age range (45 years to 91 years) and mean age (seventh decade) of the reported patients with this histologic type of prostatic carcinoma is similar to that of patients with prostatic adenocarcinoma.[408-419, 421-425] Patients most commonly have urinary bladder outflow obstruction, with or without hematuria.[414,418,419,422] The prominence of obstructive symptoms may be related to the more central location of these neoplasms. Elevations of serum acid phosphatase have been reported in only three patients with prostatic transitional cell carcinoma unaccompanied by an independent adenocarcinoma.[419,422,425]

Histologically, dilated ducts are filled with cytologically malignant urothe-

Table 8-14   *Distribution of Metastases of Prostatic Carcinoma at Autopsy*

Site	Mintz, Smith[251]	Arhneim[257]	Elkins, Mueller[259]	McCrea, Karafin[336]	Petersen *	Saitoh et al[405]
Lymph nodes	60%	"Common"	>71%	54.5%	60%	68%
Bones	39%	48%	65%	NI	68%	67%
Lung	22%	12.5%	38%	36%	40%	49%
Liver	18%	12.5%	22%	24%	24%	36%
GI tract	9%	3%	NI	NI	12%	14%
Pleura	NI	8.5%	11%	NI	4%	8%
Kidney	3%	3.4%	4%	8%	4%	17%
Adrenal	1%	7.4%	12%	4%	12%	11%

NI, no information

* Personal observations based on autopsies of 52 cases of prostatic carcinoma, 1970–1979.

lial cells, most closely resembling the atypical grade 3 transitional cell carcinoma of the bladder or urethra (Fig. 8-28). Uncommonly, the cytologic atypia will be less than grade 3, but only rarely will the in situ form of this ductal carcinoma be differentiated from transitional cell hyperplasia with any degrees of difficulty. The latter proliferation is a common finding in nodular hyperplasia with evidence of chronic prostatitis. The ducts with in situ transitional cell carcinoma commonly exhibit a comedo or cribiform pattern, the latter resulting from pseudogland formation in the epithelium. These patterns are not observed in transitional cell hyperplasia. Infiltration of the prostate stroma takes the form of cords or nests, and less commonly as individual tumor cells. Perineural invasion is reported less frequently.[43] Retrograde spread within the prostatic ductal system is common, as is spread along the basement membrane to involve the urethra and the bladder.[408,410,414] The single most important decision to be made in evaluating a prostate specimen with either in situ or invasive transitional cell carcinoma is the determination of primary site. A primary prostatic transitional cell carcinoma (stage A or B) obviously will evolve and be treated differently than a stage D1 transitional cell carcinoma of the bladder involving the prostate by contigu-

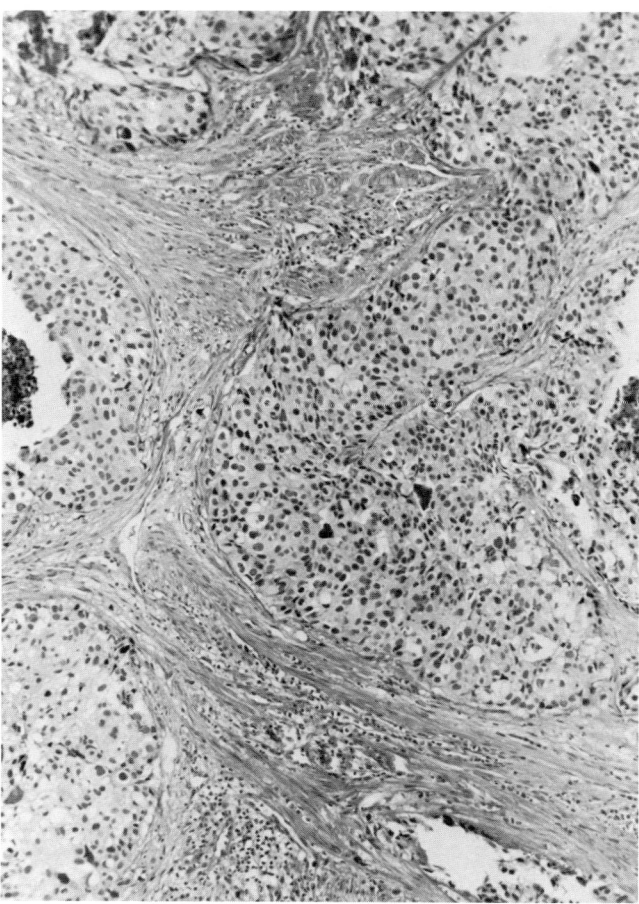

Figure 8-28 *Prostatic transitional cell carcinoma.* The neoplastic *transitional epithelium fills many affected distal prostatic ducts. Necrotic tumor cells are present in the lumen of two ducts.*

ous spread. In some cases that I have personally reviewed, this determination has proved difficult to impossible. The finding of transitional cell hyperplasia with atypia, making a transition to carcinoma in situ within prostatic ducts, establishes this location as primary.[410] Osseous metastases are most frequently osteolytic.[413,416,418,423]

Multiple modes of therapy have been employed including radical surgery, radiation, chemotherapy, and hormone manipulation.[414-418,422,423] These neoplasms are not responsive to hormones, and therefore no benefit is obtained from this therapy. Radical surgery, with or without radiation, currently appears to be most effective.[413-415,419] A clinical response to cisplatin combined with Adriamycin or cyclophosphamide was recently reported.[424,425]

Reported survival data are scant and incomplete. Average survival following surgery with or without postoperative radiation therapy ranges from 17 months to 23 months.[414,419] Rubenstein and Rubnitz reported a 20% 1-year survival.[413] Greene and associates reported survival of 2 months to 6 months in a limited number of untreated patients.[419]

Prostatic Duct Adenocarcinoma

Adenocarcinoma originating in prostatic ducts was first recognized by Belter and Dodson.[426] Including 58 cases from the Mayo Clinic, approximately 80 cases have been reported in the literature.[426-437] To this number should be added 12 cases of the so-called *endometrial carcinoma,* originally thought to arise from the prostatic utricle as described by Melicow and Pachter.[438] As discussed below, evidence accumulating during the past decade supports prostate rather than Müllerian origin of these neoplasms, which are therefore regarded as additional examples of prostatic duct adenocarcinoma.

Clinically, prostatic duct adenocarcinomas exhibit no features that are significantly different from prostatic carcinoma of acinar origin, including patient age and symptoms at presentation.[426-437] Bone metastases are osteoblastic, and in the majority of such cases are associated with elevated serum acid phosphatase.

Dube and associates have classified these neoplasms into two groups: adenocarcinoma of primary prostatic ducts; and adenocarcinoma of secondary prostatic ducts.[428] The histologic characteristics of primary prostatic duct carcinoma are tall and complex papillary formations located in dilated periurethral duct spaces; columnar lining cells with basal nuclei and a moderate amount of pale cytoplasm; and tumor cells showing stainable glycogen and negative stains for mucin (Fig. 8-29).[428] Adenocarcinomas originating in secondary prostatic ducts are characterized by columnar cells with clear to eosinophilic cytoplasm involving small prostatic ducts in low papillary, comedo, or cribiform patterns.[428] Origin from secondary ducts is more common than from primary ducts. Both types may show intraductal extension and invasion of the prostatic stroma. The individual cases reported by Belter and Dodson, Dube and associates, and Catalona and associates appear to have the histologic features of adenocarcinoma of primary prostatic ducts.[426,427,428,431] Examples have been observed showing focal areas of ductal carcinoma admixed with a predominating carcinoma of acinar origin.[428]

The reported survival information for primary and secondary prostatic duct

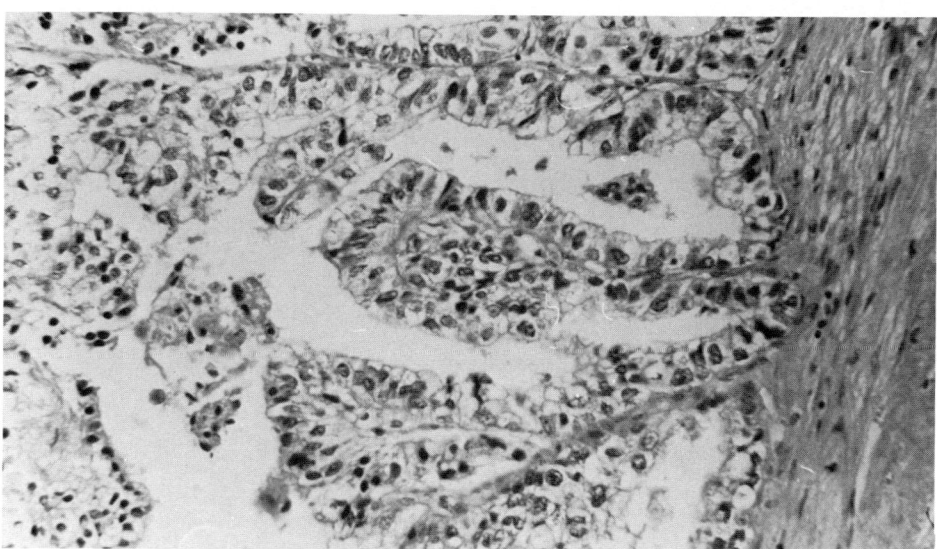

Figure 8-29   *Prostatic duct adenocarcinoma. Dilated prostatic ducts with neoplastic cells in a papillary configuration surround similar cells lying free in the lumen. The cytoplasm of the cells is clear, and there is loss of nuclear polarity.*

adenocarcinomas is 42.8% and 24%, respectively, at 5 years.[428] No apparent benefit was obtained from estrogen therapy.[428]

Endometrial Carcinoma

In 1967, Melicow and Pachter reported a "malignancy, whose pattern was unlike the usual prostatic cancer."[438] They described bands of columnar cells with infoldings and papillary projections in a tumor located near the verumontanum. The overall pattern and cytologic features were interpreted as similar to endometrial carcinoma, and the neoplasm was termed *endometrial carcinoma of the prostatic utricle.*[438] Melicow and Tannenbaum reported six histologically similar cases.[439] In subsequent years, 12 more cases, all histologically similar and located in the periurethral region of the prostate, have been reported.[440-450] Thus, there now exists a small body of literature outlining clinical and pathologic features of what some regard as a unique prostatic carcinoma.

Standard texts of embryology and histology describe the cephalad portion of the verumontanum, the utricle, as the male homologue of the uterus. Thus, neoplasms taking origin from the structure could theoretically have the microscopic features and endocrine responsiveness of endometrium. Castration and estrogen therapy would be inappropriate in such cases.

Of the reported cases, the age range of the patients is 32 years to 87 years, with all but two patients older than 60 years. All neoplasms are in the periurethral region of the prostate, some with involvement of verumontanum.[438-450] The serum acid phosphatase has been normal in all reported cases.

The histologic features of carcinomas interpreted as endometrial carcinomas include masses of neoplastic glands with papillary projections, cribiform pattern,

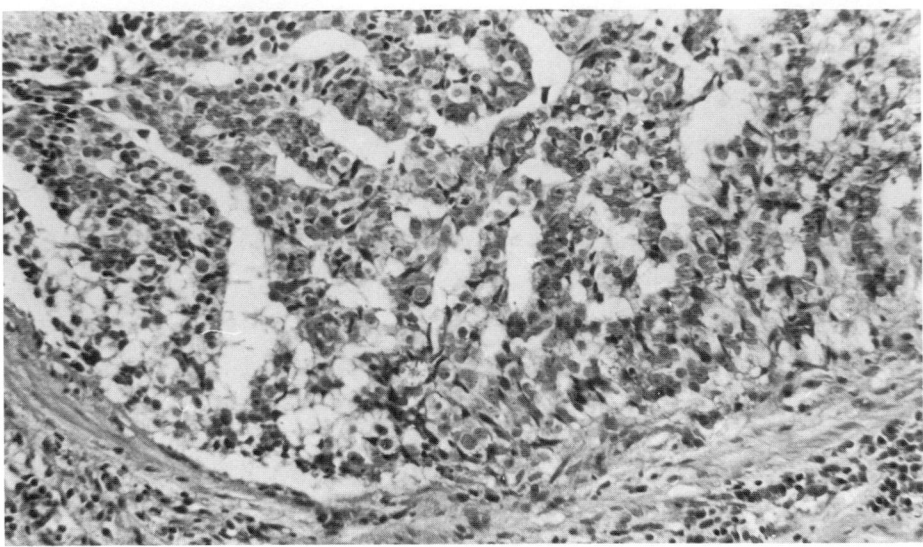

Figure 8-30   ***Endometrial adenocarcinoma of the prostate.*** *The diluted duct is filled with a papillary neoplasm showing bridging and cells with eosinophilic cytoplasm. Elsewhere, the tumor formed glands lined by columnar cells with similar appearance.*

or mixtures of both; glands and papillae lined by tall columnar cells, commonly showing dark eosinophilic cytoplasm and hyperchromatic basal nuclei (Fig. 8-30); and occasional tumors with subnuclear vacuolization or cilia on luminal surface.[439,442,444]

Only two of the reported cases have been observed for 5 years or more, and both were reported without evidence of disease.[439,447] No patient has died of the neoplasm, although two patients had bone metastases at the time of reporting.[439,444]

During this same period, however, further study has raised serious questions about the identity and alleged uniqueness of this neoplasm.[436,437,445,448,450] Electron microscopy and histochemical studies, although limited in number, have not supported the endometrial origin of these neoplasms.[443,445] Tannenbaum reported that the electron microscopic features of a previously publicized case of endometrial carcinoma of the prostatic utricle did not support the original diagnosis.[439,443] The revised diagnosis was metastatic malignancy of prostatic origin.[443] Similarly, Zaloudek and associates reported the following results of electron microscopic and histochemical studies of a neoplasm fulfilling the criteria of endometrial carcinoma by light microscopy: positive histochemical staining for acid phosphatase and lipids and negative staining for alkaline phosphatase; a heterogeneous cell population ("light" and "dark" cells) by electron microscopy with light cells containing multiple secretory granules, lipid droplets, and lysosomes.[445] All of these findings are characteristic of prostatic duct cells and not endometrial gland cells. In addition, one case, interpreted as consistent with endometrial carcinoma of the prostatic utricle by light microscopic criteria, was observed to regress following "inadvertent" orchiectomy.[441] This strongly suggests androgen dependence characteristic of prostatic and not utricular endometrial origin.

Finally, prostatic origin of neoplasms having endometrial features has been demonstrated with positive staining for prostatic-specific antigen (PSA) by the immunoperoxidase technique.[436,437,448,450] Based on this finding, the authors interpreted these adenocarcinomas as prostatic ductal adenocarcinomas and not as neoplasms of the prostatic utricle.

The limited evidence favoring rare tumors originating from the prostatic utricle, and possibly being estrogen-dependent, not androgen-dependent, is not conclusive. Proof of the existence of Müllerian malignancies arising in the utricle (exclusive of neoplasms arising in Müllerian cysts) requires further study.

Squamous Cell Carcinoma

Approximately 50 cases of squamous cell carcinoma of the prostate have been reported in the English literature.[451-460] Detailed clinical information and pathologic features are provided in only scattered reports.[455,457-460]

All reported patients have been older than 50 years with a mean age in the seventh decade. None of the reported patients have evidenced elevated acid phosphatase.[458-460]

Neither the site of origin within the prostate nor the histogenesis of prostatic squamous cell carcinoma is known. Both acinar and ductal epithelium are capable of demonstrating squamous metaplasia under specific circumstances such as hyperestrogen states or in regions of the prostate adjacent to infarction. (Refer to discussion of normal prostate and prostatic infarct.) The reported cases include descriptions of tumors that have an intraductal component, but this does not preclude origin from acini.

Histologically, the neoplasm is characterized by invasive nests or cords of malignant squamous cells evidencing intercellular bridges, and in some instances squamous pearl formation (Fig. 8-31). The cytologic features are that of

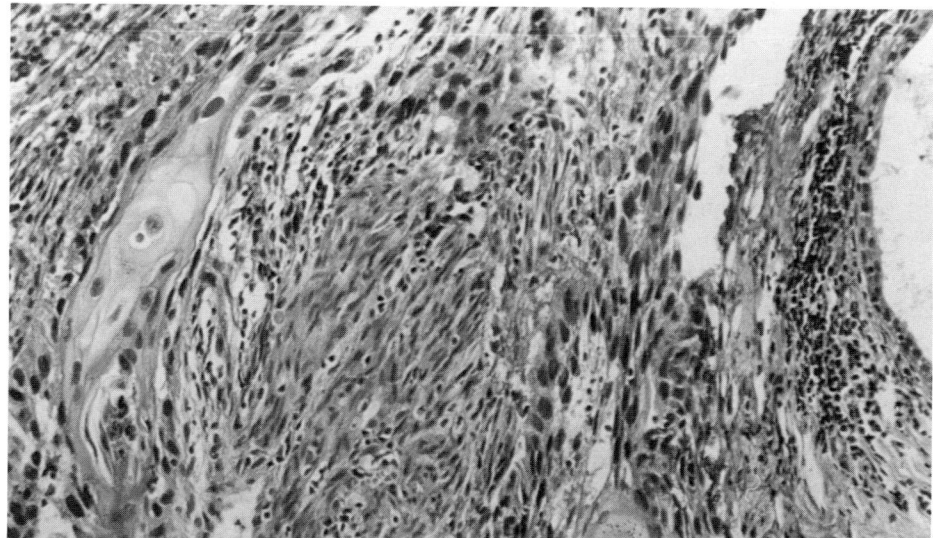

Figure 8-31 *Prostatic squamous cell carcinoma. The neoplasm with uniform and prominent squamous differentiation infiltrates the prostatic stroma. Abundant lymphocytes are intermixed adjacent to the tumor.*

malignant squamous cells with hyperchromatic nuclei, with variable pleomorphism and mitotic activity. These features allow for differentiation from squamous metaplasia in the prostate. Reported bone metastases have been exclusively osteolytic.[459]

Mott noted a mean survival of 14 months with a range of 8 days to 8 years in a review of previously reported cases of prostatic squamous cell carcinoma.[459] None of the reported cases have apparently benefited from estrogen therapy.[455,459]

Mixed Carcinoma

The typical histologic form of prostatic cancer is adenocarcinoma. On occasion, as noted elsewhere in this chapter, the prostate may give origin to transitional cell carcinoma, squamous cell carcinoma, or undifferentiated carcinoma. In rare instances, mixed tumors of adenocarcinoma and transitional cell carcinoma, or squamous cell carcinoma may be observed.[408,413,414,418,419,421,423,452] Approximately 30 cases of adenocarcinoma admixed with tumors, predominantly transitional cell, have been reported.[408,413,414,418,419,421,423] Some of these neoplasms are coincidental with the transitional cell carcinoma and others may represent examples of dual differentiation within a single tumor. Bennett and Edgerton reported an example of prostatic carcinoma with areas of adenocarcinoma, squamous cell carcinoma, and transitional cell carcinoma.[461] Saito and associates recently reported both histologic components of an adenosquamous carcinoma were PAP-positive when stained by immunoperoxidase.[463] Accetta and Gardner reported two cases of prostatic adenocarcinoma, treated with DES, converting to squamous cell carcinoma in multiple metastatic sites.[462] The prostate origin of the metastatic squamous cell carcinoma was determined by positive immunoperoxidase staining for PAP.[462] The authors suggested the conversion of squamous metastases from an adenocarcinoma primary represented a metaplastic process caused by the long-term estrogen therapy.[462]

Mucinous Carcinoma

Mucinous carcinoma, a rare histologic variant of prostatic adenocarcinoma, has been reported in about 25 patients.[464–469,471–481] Because of the limited number of reported cases, definitive clinical description awaits further studies. Of the reported cases, the patients' age and manner of clinical presentation is not significantly different from that reported with other histologic types of prostatic carcinoma. Information related to frequency of elevations of serum acid phosphatase, distant metastases, and overall response to standard surgical, radiation, and hormone therapy is too limited to be meaningful at present.

Histologically, these neoplasms are composed of acini of varying size, filled with extracellular Alcian blue, PAS, and mucicarmine-positive mucin. The tumor cells (columnar, goblet, or typical signet-ring cell types) line the acini or float free in pools of mucin (Fig. 8-32). Intracellular mucin, with the same staining characteristics as observed in the extracellular mucin, is abundant. Merging of this pattern with the more typical pattern of adenocarcinoma of acinar origin has been observed.[477] The rarity of mucinous adenocarcinomas of

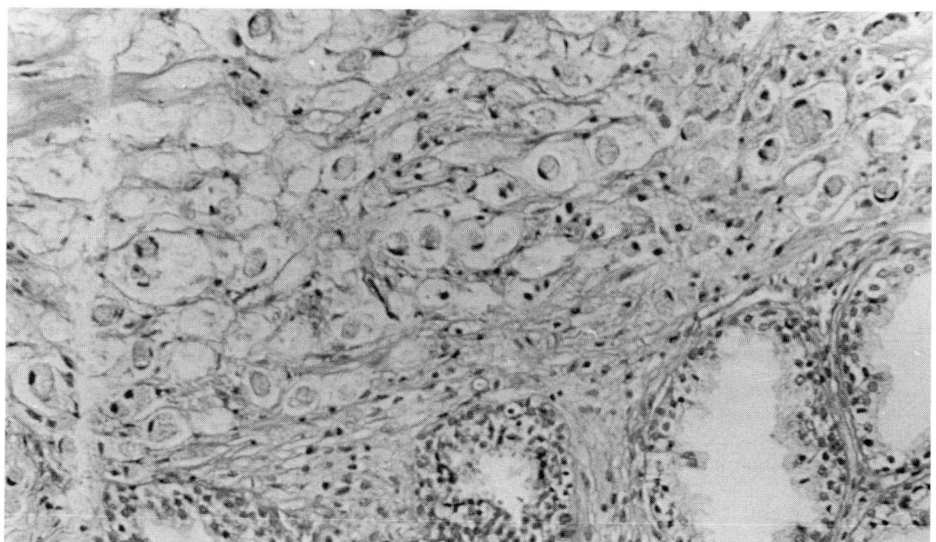

Figure 8-32 *Mucinous adenocarcinoma of the prostate. Signet ring cells, lying in secreted mucin, infiltrate the prostatic stroma.*

the prostate is in contrast to the more typical adenocarcinomas of acinar origin, which are only focally, weakly mucicarmine positive.[470] Proia and associates demonstrated the prostate origin of one case in which they observed positive staining with prostate-specific acid phosphatase.[480] Histologically similar tumors of Cowper's gland origin can be excluded by immunohistochemical means.

Available follow-up information is limited to fewer than half of the reported cases, precluding meaningful evaluation at this time.

Adenoid Cystic Carcinoma

Adenoid cystic carcinoma is common in major and minor salivary glands, and is reported uncommonly in the breast, lung, cervix, and scattered other sites. It is distinctly rare in the prostate, with only four reported cases found in the literature after the illustration of an example without further details by Mostofi and Price.[482,484-486] Dikman and Toker also reported observing ectopic seromucinous glands in the prostate, and correctly predicted the occurrence of adenoid cystic carcinoma in this organ.[483] Manrique and associates reported a malignant mixed tumor of salivary gland type with focal areas containing adenoid cystic carcinoma pattern.[487] In all locations, this neoplasm is characterized by local aggressiveness and a distinct tendency to invade perineural spaces.

The typical microscopic features of adenoid cystic carcinoma are observed in reported examples in the prostate with cylinders, tubules, or nests with prominent microgland (cribiform) pattern. The tumor cells are basaloid in character with minimal cytoplasm. The gland lumina are filled with eosinophilic, PAS-positive, mucinous-appearing material. Perineural invasion by prostatic adenoid cystic carcinoma has been reported.[486] Myoepithelial cells, a component identified in examples of this tumor in salivary glands, have not been identified within the prostate to date.

The clinical behavior of and appropriate therapy for this prostatic neoplasm are currently unknown.

Prostatic Carcinoid

Azzopardi and Evans reported argentaffin- and argyrophil-positive cells in 4 prostatic carcinomas among 50 evaluated.[448] Argentaffin cells demonstrated with the Masson–Fontana stain were found in a high percent of non-neoplastic prostates studied, confirming the findings of Grasso.[22] Seven additional cases of prostatic carcinoid tumors have been reported to this time.[489–492,494–496] The carcinoid nature of these neoplasms has been demonstrated by light microscopy (the presence of argyrophil or argentaffin cells), or by the finding of neurosecretory granules in the cytoplasm by electron microscopy.[489–492,495–496] In approximately half of the reported cases the prostatic carcinoid is either a component of an otherwise typical adenocarcinoma, or is accompanied by an independent adenocarcinoma. Conversely, Ansari and associates reported a prostatic adenocarcinoma with carcinoid features in both the primary and metastatic sites that proved to be argentaffin- and argyrophil-negative.[493] Furthermore, ultrastructural studies failed to demonstrate neurosecretory granules.

Small Cell Undifferentiated Carcinoma

Prostatic epithelial malignancies of high grade (equivalent to Gleason pattern 5) are uncommon, but not rare. Neoplasms of this type may be composed of cells with the cytologic features of small cell undifferentiated carcinoma (oat cell carcinoma). Undifferentiated small cell carcinoma may constitute the entire neoplasm or coexist as a component with a lower grade adenocarcinoma. It is noteworthy that among these heterogenous tumors, the small cell undifferentiated component was prostate-specific antigen (PSA)-negative, whereas the better differentiated adenocarcinoma component was PSA-positive.[500] Among examples of small cell undifferentiated carcinoma of the prostate, four cases associated with ectopic ACTH production have been reported.[497–500] Identification of the small cell carcinoma as the source of the ACTH has been accomplished with immunoperoxidase staining.[499]

In one cited case, Cushing's syndrome developed 3 months after the recurrence of tumor, which was observed to contain a small cell undifferentiated component, not present in the first biopsy at presentation.[499] This tendency of prostatic carcinoma to de-differentiate was previously reported by Stein and associates and Brawn.[75,314] Similar to findings reported in prostatic carcinoid tumors, these tumors show argyrophilia by light microscopy and dense core granules by electron microscopy.[498–500] The prostatic origin of small cell undifferentiated carcinoma arising by de-differentiation of a prostatic adenocarcinoma again demonstrates that cells with neuroendocrine features can originate from the prostate, and are not to be regarded as neural crest in origin.

Mesenchymal Neoplasms

Benign

Leiomyoma

Forty-one cases of prostatic leiomyoma could be found in the literature.[501-503] Thirty-five were published before 1951, as outlined in the literature review by Kaufman and Bernieke.[501] The clinical presentation of the reported patients is indistinguishable from nodular hyperplasia. The diagnosis in each case has been rendered following microscopic examination of the nodular masses. A proliferation of cytologically benign smooth muscle cells in interweaving fascicles has been described. The absence of intermixed glands formed the primary basis for distinguishing these nodular tumors from nodular hyperplasia.

Prostatic leiomyoma has not been universally accepted as a nosologic entity. Some authors, including myself, regard the majority, if not all of the reported cases, as stromal nodules of a hyperplastic nature. Of the 41 reported cases, 5 patients were 24 years to 39 years of age. The remainder were older than 48 years. These five relatively young patients form the only known basis for considering any of the reported cases as neoplastic, rather than hyperplastic. No histologic criteria are available that allow reliable determination of a cytologically benign smooth muscle proliferation as neoplastic. The study of future cases employing methodology other than the microscope may clarify the true nature of these lesions.

Malignant

Leiomyosarcoma

Seventy-six documented cases of malignant smooth muscle neoplasms of prostatic origin could be found in the literature.[505,507,510] The patients range in age from children to the ninth decade. Eight patients younger than 10 years of age are in this group, the majority of whom were 50 years or older.[510,518] The peak frequency is the seventh decade. Most patients have one symptom or a combination of dysuria, urinary retention, and hematuria. Prostatic enlargement is readily detectable by palpation. The correct diagnosis has not been made preoperatively.

Leiomyosarcoma of the prostate is histologically similar to examples in more frequent locations, with interweaving bundles of spindle cells with blunt-ended nuclei, and variable numbers of mitoses. Focal areas of hemorrhage and necrosis may be present. In contrast to leiomyomas and nodular hyperplasia, local invasion of the prostate and surrounding periprostatic tissue is common. Distinguishing cellular leiomyomas (stromal nodules) from low grade leiomyosarcomas in biopsy material remains a challenge when dealing with the prostate and other sites of origin.

Therapy currently includes radical surgery, radiation, and chemotherapy. The longest-surviving patient known lived 13 years following surgery.[510] Few patients (approximately 10%) live beyond 5 years, but the more recent reports indicate that the multimodality therapy is capable of significantly increasing survival durations.[514,517,519,520]

Rhabdomyosarcoma

Sarcomas of skeletal muscle origin occur most commonly in children, with a second age peak after 50 years.[516,517] The variable terminology of sarcomas employed in the past makes precise accounting of reported cases of rhabdomyosarcoma of the prostate impossible.[504] This neoplasm is rare, and in the pediatric age group, it occurs more commonly in the urinary bladder. (Refer to Chap. 4.) In some cases, the location of its origin may not be apparent because of extensive local growth with involvement of both the prostate and contiguous areas of the bladder.

Patients present with urinary retention, hematuria, and pelvic pain. The neoplasm is known for its ability to grow explosively. Prior to 1968, only one patient was reported to have survived 3 years.[508,509] The survival rate has improved in recent years with combined surgery, radiation, and chemotherapy.[509,514] The histologic features of this sarcoma are identical to those occurring in the bladder.[511–513,517] (Refer to discussion of rhabdomyosarcoma in Chap. 4.)

Miscellaneous Other Sarcomas

Examples of osteogenic sarcoma, fibrosarcoma, hemangiopericytoma, and angiosarcomas have been observed.[505,506,515]

Miscellaneous Rare Neoplasms

A single case report of an extragonadal endodermal sinus (yolk sac) tumor arising in the prostate has been reported.[523] Examples of prostatic melanosis or similar lesions reported as prostatic blue nevus appear in the literature (refer to discussion of normal prostate). Finally, four cases of prostatic carcinosarcoma could be found in the literature.[521,522,524,525]

Metastatic Neoplasms

Metastatic neoplasms in the prostate are rare, and when diagnosed are most frequently a manifestation late in the clinical course of the malignancy. Contiguous spread by direct invasion from bladder or urethral carcinomas is much more frequent. Among the recorded malignancies metastatic from distant sites involving the prostate, leukemic infiltration, principally chronic lymphocytic leukemia, metastatic melanoma, and carcinoma of the lung are the most frequently recorded in the literature.[526–528,530–533,535–537] Leukemic infiltration of the prostate produces the clinical picture of acute urinary retention, which has required either surgery or radiation therapy.[530,532,533,535–537] Involvement of the prostate by malignant lymphoma is distinctly rare. Reports of non-Hodgkin's lymphoma involving the prostate exceed reports of involvement by Hodgkin's disease.[526–528,534] Fewer than ten patients with primary lymphoma of the prostate appear in the literature.[529,534] The short follow-up period in some reports of alleged primary lymphoma prompts acceptance of these cases with caution.

References

Normal Structure

1. Lowsley OS: The development of the human prostate gland with reference to the development of other structures at the neck of the urinary bladder. Am J Anat 13:299, 1912
2. Lowsley OS: The human prostate gland in youth. Med Rec 88:383, 1915
3. Lowsley OS: The prostate gland in old age. Ann Surg 62:716, 1915
4. Johnson FP: The later development of the urethra in the male. J Urol 4:447, 1920
5. Moore CR, Price D, Gallagher TF: Rat-prostate cytology as a testis-hormone indicator and the prevention of castration changes by testis-extract injections. Am J Anat 45:71, 1930
6. Deming CL, Jenkins RH, Van Wagenen G: Some endocrinological relationships of prostatic hypertrophy. Clinical and experimental studies; preliminary report. J Urol 33:388, 1935
7. Moore RA, Hanzel RF: Chemical composition of prostatic corpora amylacea and calculi. Arch Pathol 22:41, 1936
8. Moore RA: The histology of the newborn and pre-pubertal prostate gland. Anat Rec 66:1, 1936
9. Gutman AB, Gutman ED: An "acid" phosphatase occurring in the serum of patients with metastasizing carcinoma of the prostate gland. J Clin Invest 17:473, 1938
10. Moore RA, McLellan AM: A histological study of the effect of the sex hormones on the human prostate. J Urol 40:641, 1938
11. LeDuc IE: The anatomy of the prostate and the pathology of early benign hypertrophy. J Urol 42:1217, 1939
12. Brody H, Goldman S: Metaplasia of the epithelium of the prostatic glands, utricle and urethra of the fetus and newborn infant. Arch Pathol 29:494, 1940
13. Swyer GIM: Post-natal growth changes in the human prostate. J Anat 78:130, 1944
14. Tornblom N: Contribution to the discussion on the etiology of prostatic hypertrophy in man. I: The weight of the prostate and seminal vesicles in men of different ages. Acta Med Scand (Suppl) 170:1, 1946
15. Moore RA: The evolution and involution of the prostate gland. J Urol 60:599, 1948
16. Huggins C, Webster WO: Duality of human prostate in response to estrogen. J Urol 59:258, 1948
17. Andrews GS: The histology of the human foetal and prepubertal prostates. J Anat 85:44, 1951
18. Bainborough AR: Squamous metaplasia of prostate following estrogen therapy. J Urol 68:329, 1952
19. Gyorkey F: The appearances of acid phosphatase in human prostate gland. Lab Invest 13:105, 1954
20. Franks LM: Atrophy and hyperplasia in the prostate proper. J Pathol Bact 68:617, 1954
21. Franks LM: Benign nodular hyperplasia of the prostate: A review. Ann Coll Surg Engl 14:92, 1954
22. Grasso R: Sobre las cellulas argentafines de la glandula prostatica. Arch Histol Norm Pathol 5:227, 1954
23. Brandes D, Bourne GH: Histochemistry of the human prostate: Normal and neoplastic. J Pathol Bact 71:33, 1956
24. Glenister TW: The development of the utricle and of the so-called "middle" or "median" lobe of the prostate. J Anat 96:443, 1962
25. Nigogosyan G, De La Pava S, Pickren JW et al: Blue nevus of the prostate gland. Cancer 16:1097, 1963

26. Parkin L, Bylsma G, Torre AV et al: Acid phosphatase in carcinoma of the prostate in man. J Histochem Cytochem 12:288, 1964
27. Kirchheim D, Gyorkey F, Brandes D et al: Histochemistry of the normal, hyperplastic and neoplastic human prostate. Invest Urol 1:403, 1964
28. Franks LM, O'Shea JD, Thomson AER: Mucin in the prostate: A histochemical study in normal glands, latent, clinical, and colloid cancers. Cancer 17:983, 1964
29. Kost LV, Evans GW: Occurrence and significance of striated muscle within the prostate. J Urol 92:703, 1964
30. Brandes D, Kirchheim D, Scott WW: Ultrastructure of the human prostate: Normal and neoplastic. Lab Invest 13:1541, 1964
31. Marx AJ, Gueft B, Moskal JF: Prostatic corpora amylacea. A study with the electron microscope and electron probe. Arch Pathol 80:487, 1965
32. Manley CB: The striated muscle of the prostate. J Urol 95:234, 1966
33. Smith MJV: The lymphatics of the prostate. Invest Urol 3:439, 1966
34. Blennerhassett JB, Vickery Jr AL: Carcinoma of the prostate gland: An anatomical study of tumor location. Cancer 19:980, 1966
35. Goldman RL: Melanogenic epithelium in the prostate gland. Am J Clin Pathol 49:75, 1967
36. Hukill PB, Vidone RA: Histochemistry of mucus and other polysaccharides in tumors. II: Carcinoma of the prostate. Lab Invest 16:395, 1967
37. Bruchovsky N, Wilson JD: The conversion of testosterone to 5a-androstan-17B-ol-3-one by rat prostate in vivo and in vitro. J Biol Chem 243:2012, 1968
38. Connolly JG, Thomson A, Jewett MAS et al: Intraprostatic lymphatics. Invest Urol 5:371, 1968
39. Liavag I: Atrophy and regeneration in the pathogenesis of prostatic carcinoma. Acta Pathol Microbiol Scand 73:338, 1968
40. McNeal JE: Regional morphology and pathology of the prostate. Am J Clin Pathol 49:347, 1968
41. Moncure CW, Prout Jr GR: Antigenicity of human prostatic acid phosphatase. Cancer 25:463, 1970
42. Guillan RA, Zelman S: The incidence and probable origin of melanin in the prostate. J Urol 104:151, 1970
43. Gardner Jr WA, Spitz WU: Melanosis of the prostate gland. Am J Clin Pathol 56:762, 1971
44. Azzopardi JG, Evans DJ: Argentaffin cells in prostatic carcinoma: Differentiation from lipofuscin and melanin in prostatic epithelium. J Pathol 104:247, 1971
45. Jao W, Fretzin DF, Christ ML et al: Blue nevus of the prostate gland. Arch Pathol 91:187, 1971
46. Block NL, Weber D, Schinella R: Blue nevi and other melanotic lesions of the prostate: Report of 3 cases and review of the literature. J Urol 107:85, 1972
47. Harbitz TB, Haugen OA: Histology of the prostate in elderly men. A study in an autopsy series. Acta Pathol Microbiol Scand [Section A] 80:756, 1972
48. McNeal JE: The prostate and prostatic urethra: A morphologic synthesis. J Urol 107:1008, 1972
49. Vermeulen A, Rubens R, Verdonck L: Testosterone secretion and metabolism in male senescence. J Clin Endocrinol 34:730, 1972
50. Langley JW, Weitzner S: Blue nevus and melanosis of prostate. J Urol 112:359, 1974
51. Tannenbaum M: Differential diagnosis in uropathology. III: Melanotic lesions of the prostate: Blue nevus and prostatic epithelial melanosis. Urol 4:617, 1974
52. Kazzaz BA: Argentaffin and argyrophil cells in the prostate. J Pathol 112:189, 1974
53. Pirke KM, Doerr P: Age-related changes in free plasma testosterone, dihydrotestosterone and oestradiol. Acta Endocrinol 80:171, 1975

54. Rios CN, Wright RJ: Melanosis of the prostate gland: Report of a case with neoplastic epithelium involvement. J Urol 115:616, 1976

55. McNeal JE: Development and comparative anatomy of the prostate. In Grayhack JT, Wilson JD, Scherbenske MJ (eds): Benign Prostatic Hyperplasia, p. 1. NIAMDD Workshop Proceedings, DHEW Publication No. (NIH) 76-1113, 1976

56. Kovi J, Jackson AG, Jackson MA: Blue nevus of the prostate: Ultrastructural study. Urol 9:576, 1977

57. Jobsis AC, De Vries GP, Anholt RRH et al: Demonstration of the prostatic origin of metastases. An immunohistochemical method for formalin-fixed embedded tissue. Cancer 41:1788, 1978

58. Wang MC, Valenzuela LA, Murphy GP et al: Purification of a human prostate specific antigen. Invest Urol 17:159, 1979

59. Moore RJ, Gazak JM, Wilson JD: Regulation of cytoplasmic dihydrotestosterone binding in dog prostate by 17B-estradiol. J Clin Invest 63:351, 1979

60. Najdi M, Tabei SZ, Castro A et al: Prostatic origin of tumors. An immunohistochemical study. Am J Clin Pathol 73:735, 1980

61. Li C-Y, Lam WKW, Yam LT: Immunohistochemical diagnosis of prostatic cancer with metastasis. Cancer 46:706, 1980

62. Najdi M, Tabei SZ, Castro A et al: Prostatic-specific antigen: An immunohistologic marker for prostatic neoplasms. Cancer 48:1229, 1981

63. Papsidero LD, Kuriyama M, Wang MC et al: Prostate antigen: A marker for human prostate epithelial cells. JNCI 66:37, 1981

64. Coffey DS, Isaacs JT: Control of prostate growth. Urol 17 (suppl):17, 1981

65. McNeal JE: Normal and pathologic anatomy of prostate. Urol 17 (suppl):11, 1981

66. Blacklock NJ: Morphology in health and disease. Recent Results Cancer Res 78:21, 1981

67. Dai WS, Kuller LH, LaPorte RE et al: The epidemiology of plasma testosterone levels in middle-aged men. Am J Epidemiol 114:804, 1981

68. Aguilar M, Gaffney EF, Finnerty DP: Prostatic melanosis with involvement of benign and malignant epithelium. J Urol 128:825, 1982

69. Trachtenberg J, Bujnovszky P, Walsh PC: Androgen receptor content of normal and hyperplastic human prostate. J Clin Endocrinol Metab 54:17, 1982

70. Stein BS, Petersen RO, Kendall AR: Prostatic carcinoma: Biological markers. 1982

71. Stein BS, Petersen RO, Vangore S et al: Immunoperoxidase localization of prostate-specific antigen. Am J Surg Pathol 6:553, 1982

72. Petersen RO, Stein BS: Unpublished observations, 1982

73. Allhoff EP, Proppe KH, Chapman CM et al: Evaluation of prostate specific acid phosphatase and prostate specific antigen in identification of prostatic cancer. J Urol 129:315, 1983

74. Isaacs JT, Brendler CB, Walsh PC: Changes in the metabolism of dihydrotestosterone in the hyperplastic human prostate. J Clin Endocrinol Metab 56:139, 1983

75. Stein BS, Vangore S, Petersen RO: Immunoperoxidase localization of prostatic antigens. Comparison of primary and metastatic sites. Urol 24:146, 1984

76. Berry ST, Coffrey DS, Walsh PC et al: The development of human benign prostate hyperplasia with age. J Urol 132:474, 1984

77. Di Sant'Agnese PA, De Mesy Jensen KL: Endocrine–paracrine cells of the prostate and prostatic urethra: An ultrastructural study. Hum Pathol 15:1034, 1984

Acute Prostatitis

78. Dajani AM, O'Flynn JD: Prostatic abscess. A report of 25 cases. Br J Urol 40:736, 1968

79. Trapnell J, Roberts M: Prostatic abscess. Br J Surg 57:565, 1970

80. Drach GW, Kohnen PW: Prostatitis. In Tannenbaum M (ed): Urologic Pathology: The Prostate, p 157. Philadelphia, Lea & Febiger, 1977

81. Kohnen PW, Drach GW: Patterns of inflammation in prostatic hyperplasia: A histologic and bacteriologic study. J Urol 121:755, 1979
82. Meares Jr EM: Prostatitis syndromes: New perspectives about old woes. J Urol 123:141, 1980
83. Schaeffer AJ, Wendel EF, Dunn JK et al: Prevalence and significance of prostatic inflammation. J Urol 125:215, 1981

Nonspecific Granulomatous Prostatitis

84. Tanner FH, McDonald JR: Granulomatous prostatitis. Arch Pathol 36:358, 1943
85. Symmers WStC: Non-specific granulomatous prostatitis. Br J Urol 22:6, 1950
86. Melicow MM: Allergic granulomas of the prostate gland. J Urol 65:288, 1951
87. Thompson GJ, Albers DD: Granulomatous prostatitis: A condition which clinically may be confused with carcinoma of prostate. J Urol 69:530, 1953
88. Stewart MJ, Wray S, Hall M: Allergic prostatitis in asthmatics. J Pathol Bact 67:423, 1954
89. Harrison FG, Neander DG: Allergic granuloma of the prostate. J Urol 72:1218, 1954
90. Keuhnelian JG, Guida PM, Pearce JM et al: Experiences with granulomatous prostatitis. J Urol 91:173, 1964
91. Kelalis PP, Harrison Jr EG, Greene LF: Allergic granulomas of the prostate in asthmatics. JAMA 188:963, 1964
92. Kelalis PP, Greene LF, Harrison Jr EG: Granulomatous prostatitis. A mimic of carcinoma of the prostate. JAMA 191:287, 1965
93. Schmidt JD: Nonspecific granulomatous prostatitis: Classification, review and report of cases. J Urol 94:607, 1965
94. Towfighi J, Sadeghee S, Wheeler JE et al: Granulomatous prostatitis with emphasis on the eosinophilic variety. Am J Clin Pathol 58:630, 1972
95. Nielsen ML, Asnaes S, Hattel T: Inflammatory changes in the non-infected prostate gland: A clinical, microbiological and histological investigation. J Urol 110:423, 1973
96. O'Dea MJ, Hunting DB, Greene LF: Non-specific granulomatous prostatitis. J Urol 118:58, 1977
97. Taylor EW, Wheelis RF, Correa Jr RJ et al: Granulomatous prostatitis: Confusion clinically with carcinoma of the prostate. J Urol 117:316, 1977
98. Hedelin H, Johansson S, Nilsson S: Focal prostatic granulomas: A sequel to transurethral resection. Scand J Urol Nephrol 15:193, 1981
99. Lee G, Shepherd N: Necrotising granulomata in prostatic resection specimens: A sequel to previous operation. J Clin Pathol 36:1067, 1983
100. Mies C, Balogh K, Stadecker M: Palisading prostate granulomas following surgery. Am J Surg Pathol 8:217, 1984
101. Schned AR: Prostatic granulomas. Am J Surg Pathol 8:797, 1984
102. Redman JF, Downs RA: Simple eosinophilic granulomatous prostatitis. J Urol 132:358, 1984

Chronic Prostatitis of Specific Etiology

Tuberculosis

103. Moore RA: Tuberculosis of the prostate gland. J Urol 37:372, 1937
104. Sporer A, Auerbach O: Tuberculosis of prostate. Urol 11:362, 1978
105. O'Dea MJ, Moore SB, Greene LF: Tuberculous prostatitis. Urol 11:483, 1978

Cryptococcosis

106. Dreyfuss ML, Simon S, Sommer RI: Granulomatous prostatitis due to *Cryptococcus neoformans (Torula)* with disseminated cryptococcosis and meningitis. NY State J Med 61:1589, 1961

107. Brock DJ, Grieco MH: Cryptococcal prostatitis in a patient with sarcoidosis: Response to 5-fluorocytosine. J Urol 107:1017, 1972
108. Braman RT: Cryptococcosis (Torulosis) of prostate. Urol 17:284, 1981
109. Huynh MT, Reyes CV: Prostatic cryptococcosis. Urol 20:622, 1982

Brucellosis

110. Kelalis PP, Greene LF, Weed LA: Brucellosis of the urogenital tract: A mimic of tuberculosis. J Urol 88:347, 1962

Blastomycosis

111. Bergner DM, Kraus SD, Duck GB et al: Systemic blastomyocosis presenting with acute prostatic abscess. J Urol 126:132, 1981
112. Inoshita T, Youngberg GA, Boelen LJ et al: Blastomycosis presenting with prostatic involvement: Report of 2 cases and review of the literature. J Urol 130:160, 1983

Coccidioidomycosis

113. Gritti EJ, Cook Jr FE, Spencer, HB: Coccidioidomycosis granuloma of the prostate: A rare manifestation of the disseminated disease. J Urol 89:249, 1963
114. Bellin HJ, Bhagavan BS: Coccidioidomycosis of the prostate gland. Report of a case and review of the literature. Arch Pathol 96:114, 1973
115. Sung JP, Sun SS, Crutchlow PF: Coccidioidomycosis of the prostate gland and its therapy. J Urol 121:127, 1979
116. Price MJ, Lewis EL, Carmalt JE: Coccidioidomycosis of prostate gland. Urol 19:653, 1982

Echinococcosis (Hydatid Disease)

117. Kirkland K: Urological aspects of hydatid disease. Br J Urol 38:241, 1966
118. Houston W: Primary hydatid cyst of the prostate gland. J Urol 113:732, 1975
119. Deklotz RJ: Echinococcal cyst involving the prostate and seminal vesicles: A case report. J Urol 115:116, 1976

Malakoplakia

120. Carruthers NC: Malakoplakia: Report of a case. Can J Surg 2:213, 1959
121. Hoffman E, Garrido M: Malakoplakia of the prostate: Report of a case. J Urol 92:311, 1964
122. Goldman RL: A case of malakoplakia with involvement of the prostate gland. J Urol 93:407, 1965
123. Kerr JFR, Gaffney TJ, McGeary HM et al: Malakoplakia: An electron-microscope and chemical study. J Pathol 107:289, 1972
124. Sterrett GF, Heenan PJ, Wyche P et al: Malakoplakia of the prostate: A morphological and biochemical study. Pathology 7:139, 1975
125. Miklos M, Bela R, Denes V: Prostatabol kindulo malakoplakia. Orv Hetil 116:23, 1975
126. Coup AJ: Malakoplakia of the prostate. J Pathol 119:119, 1976
127. Ferreira AA, Alvarenga M: Malakoplakia of the prostate confused with clear cell carcinomas. J Urol 116:828, 1976
128. Konnak JW, Hart WR: Malakoplakia of the prostate in an immunosuppressed patient. J Urol 116:830, 1976
129. Maroti M, Rohonyi B, Vecsey D: Prostata-malakoplakie. Z Urol 69:809, 1976
130. Rhodes RH, Wittmann AL: Malakoplakia of the prostate following chronic urinary tract infection. J Urol 117:808, 1977
131. Doury JC, Berruti A, Garron A et al: Un cas de malacoplasie prostatique. Sem Hop Paris 53:2273, 1977
132. Rubenstein M, Bucy JG: Malacoplakia of the prostate. South Med J 70:351, 1977

133. McClure J: Malakoplakia of the prostate: A report of two cases and a review of the literature. J Clin Pathol 32:629, 1979
134. Kawamura N, Murakami Y, Okada K: Three cases of malakoplakia of prostate. Urol 15:77, 1980

Prostatic Infarct

135. Abeshouse BS: Infarct of the prostate. J Urol 30:97, 1933
136. Kasman LP, Gold J: Metaplastic changes in prostate gland. J Lab Clin Med 19:301, 1933
137. Hubly JW, Thompson GJ: Infarction of the prostate: Its clinical significance. Proc Staff Mayo Clin 13:401, 1938
138. Culp OS: Squamous metaplasia, simulating carcinoma, associated with prostatic infarction. Bull Johns Hopkins Hosp 65:239, 1939
139. Moore RA: Benign hypertrophy of the prostate. A morphological study. J Urol 50:680, 1943
140. Roth RB: Prostatic infarction. J Urol 62:474, 1949
141. Baird HH, McKay HW, Kimmelsteil P: Ischemic infarction of the prostate gland. South Med J 43:234, 1950
142. Stewart CB, Sweetser Jr TH, DeLory GE: A case of benign prostatic hypertrophy with recent infarcts and associated high serum acid phosphatase. J Urol 63:128, 1950
143. Mostofi FK, Morse WH: Epithelial metaplasia in "prostatic infarction." Arch Pathol 51:340, 1951
144. Howard Jr PJ, Fraley EE: Elevation of the acid phosphatase in benign prostatic disease. J Urol 94:687, 1965
145. Silber I, Rosai J, Cordonnier JJ: The incidence of elevated acid phosphatase in prostatic infarction. J Urol 103:765, 1970
146. Knechtges TC, Defever BA: Cholesterol emboli in transurethral curettings: Report of 4 cases. J Urol 114:102, 1975

Nodular Hyperplasia

147. Walker KM: Nature and cause of old-age enlargement of the prostate. Br Med J 1:297, 1922
148. Reischauer F: Die entstehung der sogenannten prostatahypertrophie. Virchows Arch [A] 256:357, 1925
149. Hunt VC: Benign prostatic hypertrophy. A review of one thousand cases. Surg Gynecol Obstet 46:769, 1928
150. Smith KJ, Jaffe RH: The comparative frequency of prostatic hypertrophy in white and colored races. Urol Cutan Rev 36:661, 1932
151. Deming CL, Jenkins RH, van Wagenen G: Further studies in the endocrinological relationships of prostatic hypertrophy: The effect of castration of the sub-urethral glands in the posterior urethra of the rat. J Urol 34:678, 1935
152. Chang HL, Char GY: Benign hypertrophy of the prostate. Chin Med J [Engl] 50:1707, 1936
153. Kahle PJ, Beacham HT: Review of prostatic operations at Charity Hospital, New Orleans, Louisiana. Urol Cutan Rev 40:769, 1936
154. Deming CL, Wolf JS: The anatomical origin of benign prostatic enlargement. J Urol 42:566, 1939
155. Deming CL, Newmann C: Early phases of prostatic hyperplasia. Surg Gynecol Obstet 68:155, 1939
156. Huggins C, Stevens RA: The effect of castration on benign hypertrophy of the prostate in man. J Urol 43:705, 1940
157. Moore RA: Benign hypertrophy of the prostate. J Urol 50:680, 1943

158. Huggins C: The prostatic secretion. Harvey Lect 42:148, 1946–1947
159. Huggins C: The etiology of benign prostatic hypertrophy. Bull NY Acad Med 23:696, 1947
160. Scott WW: What makes the prostate grow? J Urol 70:477, 1953
161. Miller HC, McDonald DF: Klinefelter's syndrome and benign prostatic hypertrophy. JAMA 186:215, 1963
162. Mao P, Nakao K, Bora R et al: Human benign prostatic hyperplasia. Arch Pathol 79:270, 1965
163. Fisher ER, Jeffrey W: Ultrastructure of human normal and neoplastic prostate. Am J Clin Pathol 44:119, 1965
164. Mao P, Nakao K, Angrist A: Acid phosphatase and 5-nucleotidase activities of human nodular prostatic hyperplasia as revealed by electron microscopy. Lab Invest 15:422, 1966
165. Bennett AH, Harrison JH: A comparison of operative approach for prostatectomy, 1948 and 1968. Surg Gynecol Obstet 128:969, 1969
166. Siiteri PK, Wilson JD: Dihydrotestosterone in prostatic hypertrophy. I: The formation and content of dihydrotestosterone in the hypertrophic prostate of man. J Clin Invest 49:1737, 1970
167. Mostofi FK: Benign hyperplasia of the prostate gland. In Campbell's Urology, 3rd ed, p 1065. Philadelphia, WB Saunders, 1971
168. Cunha GR: Tissue interactions between epithelium and mesenchyme of urogenital and integumental origin. Anat Rec 172:529, 1972
169. Tveter KJ: Some aspects of the pathogenesis of prostatic hyperplasia. Acta Pathol Microbiol Scand [Suppl] 248:167, 1974
170. Vermeulen A: Testicular hormonal secretion and aging in males. In Grayhack JT, Wilson JD, Scherbenske M (eds): Benign Prostatic Hyperplasia. NIAMDD Workshop Proceedings, DHEW Publication No. (NIH) 76-1113, 1975
171. Pradhan BK and Chandra K: Morphogenesis of nodular hyperplasia-prostate. J Urol 113:210, 1975
172. Rotkin ID: Epidemiology of benign prostatic hypertrophy: Review and speculations. In Grayhack JT, Wilson JD, Scherbenske MJ (eds): Benign Prostatic Hyperplasia. NIAMDD Workshop Proceedings, DHEW Publication No. (NIH) 76-1113, 1976
173. Franks LM: Benign prostatic hyperplasia: Gross and microscopic anatomy. In Grayhack JT, Wilson JD, Scherbenske MJ (eds): Benign Prostatic Hyperplasia, p 63. NIAMDD Workshop Proceedings, DHEW Publication No. (NIH) 76-1113, 1976
174. Walsh PC, Wilson JD: The induction of prostatic hypertrophy in the dog with androstanediol. J Clin Invest 57:1093, 1976
175. McNeal JE: Origin and evolution of benign prostatic enlargement. Invest Urol 15:340, 1978
176. Cunha GR, Lung B: The importance of stroma in morphogenesis and functional activity of urogenital epithelium. In Vitro 15:50, 1979
177. Bartsch W, Becker H, Pinkenburg F-A et al: Hormone blood levels and their interrelationships in normal men and men with benign prostatic hyperplasia (BPH). Acta Endocrinol 90:727, 1979
178. Marinello MJ, Farnsworth WE, Fisher B et al: Benign prostatic hyperplasia in an XX man. Urol 13:640, 1979
179. Moore RJ, Gazak JM, Quebbeman JF et al: Concentration of dihydrotestosterone and 3-androstanediol in naturally occurring and androgen-induced prostatic hyperplasia in the dog. J Clin Invest 64:1003, 1979
180. Wilson JD: The pathogenesis of benign prostatic hyperplasia. Am J Med 68:745, 1980
181. Frimodt-Moller PC, Jensen KME, Iversen P et al: Analysis of presenting symptoms in prostatism. J Urol 132:272, 1984

Uncommon Benign Proliferations of the Prostate

182. Attah E'B, Nkposong EO: Phyllodes types of atypical prostatic hyperplasia. J Urol 115:762, 1976
183. Attah E'B, Powell ME: Atypical stromal hyperplasia of the prostate gland. Am J Clin Pathol 67:324, 1977
184. Lin JI, Cohen EL, Villacin AB et al: Basal cell adenoma of prostate. Urol 11:409, 1978
185. Dermer GB: Basal cell proliferation in benign prostatic hyperplasia. Cancer 41:1857, 1978
186. Brawn PN: Adenosis of the prostate: A dysplastic lesion that can be confused with prostate adenocarcinoma. Cancer 49:826, 1982
187. Cleary KR, Choi HY, Ayala AG: Basal cell hyperplasia of the prostate. Am J Clin Pathol 80:850, 1983

Prostatic Adenocarcinoma

Epidemiology and Etiology

188. Moore RA: The morphology of small prostatic carcinoma. J Urol 33:224, 1935
189. Rich AR: On the frequency of occurrence of occult carcinoma of the prostate. J Urol 33:215, 1935
190. Moore RA, Melchionna RH: Production of tumors of the prostate of the white rat with 1:2-benzpyrene. Am J Cancer 30:731, 1937
191. Gaynor EP: Zur frage des prostatakrebses. Virchows Arch [A] 301:602, 1938
192. Kahler JE: Carcinoma of the prostate gland: A pathologic study. J Urol 41:557, 1939
193. Baron E, Angrist A: Incidence of occult adenocarcinoma of the prostate after fifty years of age. Arch Pathol 32:787, 1941
194. Huggins C, Hodges CV: Studies on prostatic cancer. I: The effect of castration, of estrogen and of androgen injection on serum phosphatases in metastatic carcinoma of the prostate. Cancer Res 1:293, 1941
195. Dunning WF, Curtis MR, Segaloff A: Methylcholanthrene squamous cell carcinoma of the rat prostate with skeletal metastases, and failure of the rat liver to respond to the same carcinogen. Cancer Res 6:256, 1946
196. Horning ES, Dmochowski L: Induction of prostate tumours in mice. Br J Cancer 1:59, 1947
197. Moore RA: Benign hypertrophy and carcinoma of the prostate: Occurrence and experimental production in animals. In Twambly GH, Pack GT (eds): Endocrinology of Neoplastic Diseases, p 194. New York, Oxford University Press, 1947
198. Andrews GS: Latent carcinoma of the prostate. J Clin Pathol 2:197, 1949
199. Edwards CN, Steinthorsson E, Nicholson D: An autopsy study of latent prostatic cancer. Cancer 6:531, 1953
200. Hirst Jr AE, Bergman RT: Carcinoma of the prostate in men 80 or more years old. Cancer 7:136, 1954
201. Franks LM: Latent carcinoma of the prostate. J Pathol Bact 68:603, 1954
202. Sharkey DA, Fisher ER: Carcinoma of the prostate in the absence of testicular tissue. J Urol 83:468, 1960
203. Oota K: Latent carcinoma of the prostate among the Japanese. Acta Un Int Cancer 17:952, 1961
204. Newill VA: Distribution of cancer mortality among ethnic subgroups of the white population of New York City, 1953–58. JNCI 26:405, 1961
205. Halpert B, Sheehan EE, Schmalhorst RS et al: Carcinoma of the prostate. A survey of 5000 autopsies. Cancer 16:737, 1963
206. King H, Diamond E, Lilienfeld AM: Some epidemiological aspects of cancer of the prostate. J Chronic Dis 16:117, 1963

207. Apt A: Circumcision and prostatic cancer. Acta Med Scand 178:493, 1965

208. Marmorston J, Lombardo Jr LJ, Myers SM et al: Urinary excretion of neutral 17-ketosteroids and pregnanediol by patients with prostatic cancer and benign prostatic hypertrophy. J Urol 93:276, 1965

209. Marmorston J, Lombardo LJ, Myers SM et al: Urinary excretion of estrone, estradiol, and estriol by patients with prostatic cancer and benign prostatic hypertrophy. J Urol 93:287, 1965

210. Staszewski J, Haenszel W: Cancer mortality among the Polish-born in the United States. JNCI 35:291, 1965

211. Halpert B, Schmalhorst WR: Carcinoma of the prostate in patients 70 to 79 years old. Cancer 19:695, 1966

212. Kipling MD, Waterhouse JAH: Cadmium and prostate carcinoma. Lancet 2:566, 1967

213. Haenszel W, Kurihara M: Studies of Japanese migrants. I: Mortality from cancer and other diseases among the Japanese in the United States. JNCI 40:43, 1968

214. Scott Jr R, Mutchnik DL, Laskowski TZ et al: Carcinoma of the prostate in elderly men: Incidence, growth characteristics and clinical significance. J Urol 101:602, 1969

215. Lundberg S, Berge T: Prostatic carcinoma: An autopsy study. Scand J Urol Nephrol 4:93, 1970

216. Seidman H: Cancer death rates by site and sex for religious and socioeconomic groups in New York City. Environ Res 3:234, 1970

217. Moon KH, Flocks RH: Plasma testosterone in patients with prostatic carcinoma and benign prostatic hyperplasia. Urol Dig 9:14, 1970

218. Wynder EL, Mabuchi K, Whitmore Jr WF: Epidemiology of cancer of the prostate. Cancer 28:344, 1971

219. Franks LM: Etiology, epidemiology, and pathology of prostatic cancer. Cancer 32:1092, 1973

220. Greenwald P, Kirmss V, Polan AK et al: Cancer of the prostate among men with benign prostatic hyperplasia. JNCI 53:335, 1974

221. Armenian HK, Lilienfeld AM, Diamond EL et al: Relation between benign prostatic hyperplasia and cancer of the prostate. Lancet 2:115, 1974

222. Rullis I, Shaeffer JA, Lilien OM: Incidence of prostatic carcinoma in the elderly. Urol 6:295, 1975

223. Egle N, Altwein JE: Postpuberal castration and prostatic carcinoma. Urol 6:471, 1975

224. Hirose F, Takizawa S, Watanabe H et al: Development of adenocarcinoma of the prostate in ICR mice locally irradiated with X-rays. Gann 67:407, 1976

225. Owen WL: Cancer of the prostate: A literature review. J Chronic Dis 29:89, 1976

226. Lemen RA, Lee JS, Wagoner JK et al: Cancer mortality among cadmium production workers. Ann NY Acad Sci 271:273, 1976

227. Kolonel L, Winkelstein W: Cadmium and prostate carcinoma. Lancet 2:566, 1977

228. Dmochowski L, Ohtsuki Y, Seman G et al: Search for oncogenic viruses in human prostate cancer. Cancer Treatment Rev 61:119, 1977

229. Sanford EJ, Geder L, Laychock A et al: Evidence for the association of cytomegalovirus with carcinoma of the prostate. J Urol 118:789, 1977

230. Noble RL: The development of prostatic adenocarcinoma in Nb rats following prolonged sex hormone administration. Cancer Res 37:1929, 1977

231. Brown CE, Warren S: Carcinoma of the prostate in irradiated parabiotic rats. Cancer Res 38:159, 1978

232. Levine RL, Wilchinsky M: Adenocarcinoma of the prostate: A comparison of the disease in Blacks versus Whites. J Urol 121:761, 1979

233. Ghanadian R, Puah CM, O'Donoghue EPN: Serum testosterone and dihydrotestosterone in carcinoma of the prostate. Br J Cancer 39:696, 1979

234. Guileyardo JM, Johnson WD, Welsh RA et al: Prevalence of latent prostate carcinoma in two U.S. populations. JNCI 65:311, 1980

235. Shimada H, Misugi K, Sasaki Y et al: Carcinoma of the prostate in childhood and adolescence: Report of a case and review of the literature. Cancer 46:2534, 1980

236. Weitzner S, Sarikaya H, Furness TD: Adenocarcinoma of prostate in a twenty-seven-year-old man. Urol 16:286, 1980

237. Pour PM: A new prostatic model: Systemic induction of prostatic cancer in rats by a nitrosamine. Cancer Lett 13:303, 1981

238. Katayama S, Fiala E, Reddy BS et al: Prostate adenocarcinoma in rats: Induction by 3,2'-Dimethyl-4-aminobiphenyl. JNCI 68:867, 1982

239. Huben R, Nararahan N, Pontes E et al: Carcinoma of prostate in men less than fifty years old. Urol 20:585, 1982

240. Seidman H, Mushinski MH, Gelb SK et al: Probabilities of eventually developing or dying of cancer — United States, 1985. CA 35:36, 1985

Histogenesis

241. Dossot R: Cancer of the prostate: Its origin and extension. J Urol 23:217, 1930

242. McNeal JE: Morphogenesis of prostatic carcinoma. Cancer 18:1659, 1965

243. Kirchheim D, Niles NR, Frankus E et al: Correlative histochemical and histologic studies on thirty radical prostatectomy specimens. Cancer 19:1683, 1966

244. McNeal JE: Origin and development of carcinoma in the prostate. Cancer 23:24, 1969

245. Miller A, Seljelid R: Cellular atypia in the prostate. Scand J Urol Nephrol 5:17, 1971

246. Tannenbaum M: Atypical epithelial hyperplasia or carcinoma of prostate gland. Urol 4:758, 1974

247. Tannenbaum M: Differential diagnosis in uropathology: Carcinoma in situ of prostate gland. Urol 5:143, 1975

Pathology

248. Broders AC: Epithelioma of the genitourinary organs. Ann Surg 75:574, 1922

249. Broders AC: Carcinoma: Grading and practical application. Arch Pathol 2:376, 1926

250. Fergusson RS: Cancer of the prostate. A study of clinical classification and the effects of treatment by irradiation. Am J Cancer 16:783, 1932

251. Mintz ER, Smith GG: Autopsy findings in 100 cases of prostatic cancer. N Engl J Med 211:479, 1935

252. Warren S, Harris PN, Graves RC: Osseous metastasis of carcinoma of the prostate. With special reference to perineural lymphatics. Arch Pathol 22:139, 1936

253. Kahler JE: Carcinoma of the prostate gland: A pathologic study. J Urol 41:557, 1939

254. Batson OV: The function of the vertebral veins and their role in the spread of metastases. Ann Surg 112:138, 1940

255. Evans N, Barnes RW, Brown AF: Carcinoma of the prostate. Correlation between the histologic observations and the clinical course. Arch Pathol 34:473, 1942

256. Schenken JR, Burns EL, Kahle PJ: The effect of diethylstilbesterol and diethylstilbesterol dipropionate on carcinoma of the prostate gland. II. Cytologic changes following treatment. J Urol 48:99, 1942

257. Arnheim FK: Carcinoma of the prostate: A study of the postmortem findings in one hundred and seventy-six cases. J Urol 60:599, 1948

258. Fergusson JD, Franks LM: The response of prostatic carcinoma to oestrogen treatment. Br J Surg 40:422, 1953

259. Elkin M, Mueller HP: Metastases from cancer of the prostate. Autopsy and roentgenological findings. Cancer 7:1246, 1954

260. Shelley HS, Auerbach SH, Classen KL et al: Carcinoma of the prostate. A new system of classification. Arch Surg 77:751, 1958

261. Arduino LJ, Glucksman MA: Lymph node metastases in early carcinoma of the prostate. J Urol 88:91, 1962

262. Vickery Jr AL, Kerr Jr WS: Carcinoma of the prostate treated by radical prostatectomy. A clinicopathological survey of 187 cases followed for 5 years and 148 cases followed for 10 years. Cancer 16:1598, 1963

263. Casley-Smith JR: An electron microscopic study of injured and abnormally permeable lymphatics. Ann NY Acad Sci 116:803, 1964

264. Gleason DF: Classification of prostatic carcinomas. Cancer Chemother Rep 50:125, 1966

265. Pennington JW, Prentiss RJ, Howe G: Radical prostatectomy for cancer: Significance of perineural lymphatic invasion. J Urol 97:1075, 1967

266. Rodin AE, Larson DL, Roberts DK: Nature of the perineural space invaded by prostatic carcinoma. Cancer 20:1772, 1967

267. Case records of the Massachusetts General Hospital (Case 3-1968). N Engl J Med 278:155, 1968

268. Jewett HJ, Bridge RW, Gray Jr GF et al: The palpable nodule of prostatic cancer. JAMA 203:403, 1968

269. Utz DC, Farrow GM: Pathologic differentiation and prognosis of prostatic carcinoma. JAMA 209:1701, 1969

270. Olsen BS, Carlisle RW: Adenocarcinoma of the prostate simulating primary rectal malignancy. Cancer 25:219, 1970

271. Byar DP, Mostofi FK, The Veterans Administration Cooperative Urological Research Group: Carcinoma of the prostate: Prognostic evaluation of certain pathologic features in 208 radical prostatectomies. Cancer 30:5, 1972

272. Schoonees R, Palma LD, Gaeta JF et al: Prostatic carcinoma treated at categorical center. Clinical and pathologic observations. NY State J Med 72:1021, 1972

273. McCullough DL, Prout Jr GR, Daly JJ: Carcinoma of the prostate and lymphatic metastases. J Urol 111:65, 1974

274. Gleason DF, Mellinger GT, The Veterans Administration Cooperative Urological Research Group: Prediction of prognosis for prostatic adenocarcinoma by combined histological grading and clinical staging. J Urol 111:58, 1974

275. Hilaris BS, Whitmore WF, Batata MA et al: Radiation therapy and pelvic node dissection in the management of cancer of the prostate. Am J Roentgenol 121:832, 1974

276. Lentle BC, McGowan DG, Dierich H: Technetium-99M polyphosphate bone scanning in carcinoma of the prostate. Br J Urol 46:543, 1974

277. Mostofi FK: Grading of prostatic carcinoma. Cancer Chemother Rep 59:111, 1975

278. Mostofi FK: Problems of grading carcinoma of prostate. Semin Oncol 3:161, 1976

279. McLaughlin AP, Saltzstein SL, McCullough DL et al: Prostatic carcinoma: Incidence and location of unsuspected lymphatic metastases. J Urol 115:89, 1976

280. Epstein NA: Prostatic carcinoma. Correlation of histologic features of prognostic value with cytomorphology. Cancer 38:2071, 1976

281. Heaney JA, Chang HC, Daly JJ et al: Prognosis of clinically undiagnosed prostatic carcinoma and the influence of endocrine therapy. J Urol 118:283, 1977

282. Nicholson TC, Richie JP: Pelvic lymphadenectomy for stage B1 adenocarcinoma of the prostate: Justified or not? J Urol 117:199, 1977

283. Correa Jr RJ, Gibbons RP, Cummings KB et al: Total prostatectomy for stage B carcinoma of the prostate. J Urol 117:328, 1977

284. Gleason DF: Histologic grading and clinical staging of prostatic carcinoma. In Tannenbaum M (ed): Urologic Pathology: The Prostate, p. 171. Philadelphia, Lea & Febiger, 1977

285. Harada M, Mostofi FK, Corle DK et al: Preliminary studies of histologic prognosis in cancer of the prostate. Cancer Treat Rep 61:223, 1977

286. Barzell W, Bean MA, Hilaris BS et al: Prostatic adenocarcinoma: Relationship of grade and local extent to the pattern of metastases. J Urol 118:278, 1977

287. Wilson CS, Dahl DS, Middleton RG: Pelvic lymphadenectomy for the staging of apparently localized prostatic cancer. J Urol 117:197, 1977

288. Boxer RJ, Kaufman JJ, Goodwin WE: Radical prostatectomy for carcinoma of the prostate: 1951–1976. A review of 329 patients. J Urol 117:208, 1977

289. Veenema RJ, Gursel EO, Lattimer JK: Radical retropubic prostatectomy for cancer: A 20-year experience. J Urol 117:330, 1977

290. Golimbu M, Schinella R, Morales P et al: Differences in pathological characteristics and prognosis of clinical A2 prostatic cancer from A1 and B disease. J Urol 119:618, 1978

291. Murphy GP, Whitmore Jr WF: A report of the workshops on the current status of the histologic grading of prostate cancer. Cancer 44:1490, 1979

292. Golimbu M, Morales P: Stage A2 prostatic carcinoma. Should staging system be reclassified? Urol 13:592, 1979

293. Buck AC, Chisholm GD: Rectovesical fistula secondary to prostatic carcinoma. J Urol 121:831, 1979

294. Hassan MO, Maksem J: The prostatic perineural space and its relation to tumor spread. An ultrastructural study. Am J Surg Pathol 4:143, 1980

295. Paulson DF, Piserchia PV, Gardner W: Predictors of lymphatic spread in prostatic adenocarcinoma: Urooncology research group study. J Urol 123:697, 1980

296. Carstens PHB: Perineural gland in normal and hyperplastic prostates. J Urol 123:686, 1980

297. Kramer SA, Spahr J, Brendler CB et al: Experience with Gleason's histopathologic grading in prostatic cancer. J Urol 124:223, 1980

298. Gaeta JF, Asirwatham JE, Miller G et al: Histologic grading of primary prostatic cancer: A new approach to an old problem. J Urol 123:689, 1980

299. Thomas R, Lewis RW, Sarma DP et al: Accurate clinical staging by histopathologic grading in prostatic cancer (abstr). J Urol (Suppl) 125:168, 1981

300. Dodds PR, Caride VJ, Lytton B: The role of the vertebral veins in the dissemination of prostatic carcinoma. J Urol 126:753, 1981

301. Cramer SF: Benign glandular inclusion in prostatic nerve. Am J Clin Pathol 75:854, 1981

302. Kramer SA, Farnham R, Glenn JF et al: Comparative morphology of primary and secondary deposits of prostatic adenocarcinoma. Cancer 48:271, 1981

303. Olsson CA, Tannenbaum M, Babayan R et al: Prediction of pelvic lymph node metastasis in adenocarcinoma of the prostate (abstr). J Urol (Suppl) 127:137, 1982

304. Sagalowsky AI, Milam H, Reveley LR et al: Prediction of lymphatic metastases by Gleason grading in prostate cancer (abstr). J Urol (Suppl) 127:137, 1982

305. Bostwick DG, Egbert BM, Fajardo LF: Radiation injury of the normal and neoplastic prostate. Am J Surg Pathol 6:541, 1982

306. Zinke H, Farrow GM, Myers RP et al: Relationship between grade and stage of adenocarcinoma of the prostate and regional pelvic lymph node metastases. J Urol 128:498, 1982

307. Brawn PN, Ayala AG, Von Eschenbach AC et al: Histologic grading study of prostate adenocarcinoma: The development of a new system and comparison with other methods — A preliminary study. Cancer 49:525, 1982

308. Bocking A, Kiehn J, Heinzel-Wach M: Combined histologic grading of prostatic carcinoma. Cancer 50:288, 1982

309. Bain GO, Koch M, Hanson J: Feasibility of grading prostatic carcinomas. Arch Pathol Lab Med 106:265, 1982

310. Catalona WJ, Stein AJ, Fair WR: Grading errors in prostatic needle biopsies: Relation to the accuracy of tumor grade in predicting pelvic lymph node metastases. J Urol 127:919, 1982

311. Guileyardo JM, Sarma DP, Johnson WD et al: Incidental prostatic carcinoma: Tumor extent versus histologic grade. Urol 20:40, 1982

312. Smith Jr JA, Seaman JP, Gleidman JB et al: Pelvic lymph node metastasis from prostatic cancer: Influence of tumor grade and stage in 452 consecutive patients. J Urol 130:290, 1983

313. Lange PH, Narayan P: Understaging and undergrading of prostate cancer. Urol 21:113, 1983

314. Brawn PN: The dedifferentiation of prostate carcinoma. Cancer 52:246, 1983

315. Garrett JE, Oyasu R, Grayhack JT: The accuracy of diagnosistic biopsy specimens in predicting tumor grades by Gleason's classification of radical prostatectomy specimens. J Urol 131:690, 1984

Natural History

316. Wade H: Prostatism. Ann Surg 59:321, 1914

317. Swan RHJ: The incidence of malignant disease in the apparently benign enlargement of the prostate. Lancet 2:971, 1923

318. Bumpus Jr HC: Carcinoma of the prostate. A clinical study of one thousand cases. Surg Gynecol Oncol 43:150, 1926

319. McHeffey GJ: Carcinoma of the prostate gland: Efficacy of method of examining prostatic tissue removed by transurethral resection to make a pathologic diagnosis of carcinoma. Proc Staff Mayo Clin 15:458, 1940

320. Ronchese F: Metastases of the scalp simulating turban tumors. Arch Dermatol Syphilology 41:639, 1940

321. Barnes RW: Carcinoma of the prostate. A comparative study of modes of treatment. J Urol 44:169, 1940

322. Huggins C, Stevens Jr RE, Hodges CV: Studies on prostatic cancer. Arch Surg 43:209, 1941

323. Nesbit RM, Plumb RT: Prostatic carcinoma: A follow-up on 795 patients treated prior to endocrine era and comparison of survival rate between these and patients treated with endocrine therapy. Surg 20:263, 1946

324. Treiger P, Welfeld J, Marx J: Suprapubic prostatectomy: A review of 108 cases. Urol Cutaneous Rev 52:8, 1948

325. Smith GG, Woodruff LM: The development of cancer of the prostate after subtotal prostatectomy. J Urol 63:1077, 1950

326. Nesbit RM, Baum WC: Endocrine control of prostatic carcinoma. JAMA 143:1317, 1950

327. Labess M: Occult carcinoma in clinically benign hypertrophy of the prostate: A pathological and clinical study. J Urol 68:893, 1952

328. Woodard HQ: Factors leading to elevation in serum acid glycorophosphatase. Cancer 5:236, 1952

329. Bergman RT, Turner R, Barnes RW et al: Comparative analysis of one thousand consecutive cases of transurethral prostatic resection. J Urol 74:533, 1955

330. Green LF, Simon HB: Occult carcinoma of the prostate: Clinical and therapeutic study of eighty-three cases. JAMA 158:1494, 1955

331. Jewett HJ: Significance of the palpable prostatic nodule. JAMA 160:838, 1956

332. Whitmore Jr WF: Hormone therapy in prostatic cancer. Am J Med 21:697, 1956

333. Ganem EJ: The prognostic significance of an elevated serum acid phosphatase level in advanced prostatic carcinoma. J Urol 76:179, 1956

334. Turner RD, Belt E: A study of 229 consecutive cases of total perineal prostatectomy for cancer of the prostate. J Urol 77:62, 1957

335. Greenberg BE, Young JM: Pulmonary metastasis from occult primary sites resembling cronchogenic carcinoma. Dis Chest 33:496, 1958

336. McCrea LE, Karafin L: Carcinoma of the prostate: Metastases, therapy and survival. A statistical analysis of five hundred cases. J Int Coll Surg 29:723, 1958

337. Anderson R: Carcinoma of the prostate. Clinical observations and treatment. Acta Chir Scand (Suppl) 246, 1959

338. Whitmore Jr WF, Mackenzie AR: Experience with various operative procedures for the total excision of prostatic cancer. Cancer 12:396, 1959

339. Flocks RH, Culp D, Porto R: Lymphatic spread from prostatic cancer. J Urol 81:194, 1959

340. Bauer WC, McGavran MH, Carlin MR: Unsuspected carcinoma of the prostate in suprapubic prostatectomy specimens. Cancer 13:1370, 1960

341. Emmett JL, Greene LF, Papantoniou A: Endocrine therapy in carcinoma of the prostate gland: 10-year survival studies. J Urol 83:471, 1960

342. Fuchs WA, Book-Hederstom G: Inguinal and pelvic lymphography. A preliminary report. Acta Radiol 56:340, 1961

343. Brennaas O: Virchow-Troisiers glandel som forste tegn pa carcinoma prostatae. Nord Med 65:374, 1961

344. Ichikawa T, Kumamoto Y, Asano M: A case of prostatic carcinoma with metastases to the skin and both testes. J Urol 87:941, 1962

345. Dick VS: Carcinoma of the prostate gland with metastases. Surg Clin North Am 42:771, 1962

346. Emmett JL, Barber Jr KW, Jackman RJ: Transrectal biopsy to detect prostatic carcinoma: A review and report of 203 cases. J Urol 87:460, 1962

347. Klingenberg I: Histopathologic findings in the prescalene tissue from 1000 postmortem cases. Acta Chir Scand 127:57, 1964

348. Denton SE, Choy SH, Valk WL: Occult prostatic carcinoma diagnosed by the step-section technique of the surgical specimen. J Urol 93:296, 1965

349. Bolton BH: Pulmonary metastases from carcinoma of the prostate: Incidence and case report of a long remission. J Urol 94:73, 1965

350. Veterans Administration Co-operative Urological Research Group: Treatment and survival of patients with cancer of the prostate. Surg Gynecol Obstet 124:1011, 1967

351. Mobley TL, Frank IN: Influence of tumor grade on survival and on serum acid phosphatase levels in metastatic carcinoma of the prostate. J Urol 99:321, 1968

352. Lilien OM, Schaefer JA, Kilejian V et al: The case for perineal prostatectomy. J Urol 99:79, 1968

353. Scott WW, Boyd HL: Combined hormone control therapy and radical prostatectomy in the treatment of selected cases of advanced carcinoma of the prostate: A retrospective study based on 25 years of experience. J Urol 101:86, 1969

354. Scott Jr R, Mutchnik DL, Laskowski TZ et al: Carcinoma of the prostate in elderly men: Incidence, growth characteristics and clinical significance. J Urol 101:602, 1969

355. Warren MM, Furlow WL: Carcinoma of the prostate presenting as a mass in the neck. JAMA 213:620, 1970

356. Dees JD: Radical perineal prostatectomy for carcinoma. J Urol 104:160, 1970

357. Corriere Jr JN, Cornog JL, Murphy JJ: Prognosis in patients with carcinoma of the prostate. Cancer 25:911, 1970

358. Butler JJ, Howe CD, Johnson DE: Enlargement of the supraclavicular lymph nodes as the initial sign of prostatic carcinoma. Cancer 27:1055, 1971

359. Legge DA, Good CA, Ludwig J: Roentgenologic features of pulmonary carcinomatosis from carcinoma of the prostate. Am J Roentgenol 111:360, 1971

360. Culp OS, Meyer JJ: Radical prostatectomy in the treatment of prostatic cancer. Cancer 32:1113, 1972

361. Carlton Jr CE, Dawoud F, Hudgins P et al: Irradiation treatment of carcinoma of the prostate: A preliminary report based on 8 years of experience. J Urol 108:924, 1972

362. Hanash KA, Utz DC, Cook EN et al: Carcinoma of the prostate: A 15-year followup. J Urol 107:450, 1972

363. Robinson MRG, Constable AR: Strontium-87m and the gamma camera in the study of bone metastases from carcinoma of the prostate. Br J Urol 45:173, 1973

364. Flocks RH: The treatment of stage C prostatic cancer with special reference to combined surgical and radiation therapy. J Urol 109:461, 1973

365. Castellino RA, Ray G, Blank N et al: Lymphangiography in prostatic carcinoma. JAMA 223:877, 1973

366. Lome LG, John T: Pulmonary manifestations of prostatic carcinoma. J Urol 109:680, 1973

367. Nelson CMK, Boatman DL, Flocks RH: Bone marrow examination in carcinoma of the prostate. J Urol 109:667, 1973

368. Schellhammer PF, Milsten R, Bunts RC: Prostatic carcinoma with cutaneous metastases. Br J Urol 45:169, 1973

369. Whitmore Jr WF, Hilaris B, Grabstald H et al: Implantation of 125 I in prostatic cancer. Surg Clin North Am 54:887, 1974

370. Dahl DS, Wilson CS, Middleton RG et al: Pelvic lymphadenectomy for staging localized prostatic cancer. J Urol 112:245, 1974

371. Bisson J, Vickers Jr M, Fagan Jr WT: Bone scan in clinical perspective. J Urol 111:665, 1974

372. Yam LT: Clinical significance of the human acid phosphatases. Am J Med 56:604, 1974

373. Melchior J, Valk WL, Foret JD et al: Transurethral resection of the prostate via perineal urethrostomy: Complete analysis of 7 years of experience. J Urol 111:640, 1974

374. Hill DR, Crews Jr QE, Walsh PC: Prostatic carcinoma: Radiation treatment of the primary and regional lymphatics. Cancer 34:156, 1974

375. Razvi M, Firfer R, Berkson B: Occult transitional cell carcinoma of the prostate presenting as skin metastasis. J Urol 113:734, 1975

376. Varkarakis MJ, Murphy GP, Nelson CMK et al: Lymph node involvement in prostatic carcinoma. Urol Clin North Am 2:197, 1975

377. Bagshaw MA, Ray GR, Pistenma DA et al: External beam radiation therapy of primary carcinoma of the prostate. Cancer 36:723, 1975

378. Jewett HJ: The present status of radical prostatectomy for stages A and B prostatic cancer. Urol Clin N Am 2:105, 1975

379. Johnson DE, Prout GR, Scott WW et al: Clinical significance of serum acid phosphatase levels in advanced prostatic carcinoma. Urol 8:123, 1976

380. Schaffer DL, Pendergrass HP: Comparison of enzyme, clinical, radiographic, and radionuclide methods of detecting bone metastases from carcinoma of the prostate. Radiol 121:431, 1976

381. Delides OS, Baltopoulos G, Papaharalampous NX: Latent carcinoma of the prostate: The probability of identifying small lesions in routine histology. Br J Urol 48:207, 1976

382. McMillen SM, Wettlaufer JN: The role of repeat transurethral biopsy in stage A carcinoma of the prostate. J Urol 116:759, 1976

383. Ray GR, Pistenma DA, Castellino RA et al: Operative staging of apparently localized adenocarcinoma of the prostate: Results in fifty unselected patients. I: Experimental design and preliminary results. Cancer 38:73, 1976

384. Donohue RE, Pfister RR, Weigel JW et al: Pelvic lymphadenectomy in stage A prostatic cancer. Urol 9:273, 1977

385. Saltzstein SL, McLaughlin III AP: Clinicopathologic features of unsuspected regional lymph node metastases in prostatic adenocarcinoma. Cancer 40:1212, 1977

386. Shaffer RB, Reinke DB: Contribution of the bone scan, serum acid and alkaline phosphatase, and the radiographic bone survey to the management of newly-diagnosed carcinoma of the prostate. Clin Nucl Med 2:200, 1977

387. Bruce AW, O'Cleireachain F, Morales A et al: Carcinoma of the prostate: A critical look at staging. J Urol 117:319, 1977

388. de Vere White R, Paulson DF, Glenn JF: The clinical spectrum of prostate cancer. J Urol 117:323, 1977

389. Tolia BM, Nabizadeh I, Bennett B et al: Carcinoma of prostate presenting as retro-peritoneal mass. Urol 12:434, 1978

390. American Joint Committee for Cancer Staging and End Results Reporting: Manual For Staging of Cancer, p 123. New Jersey, Whiting Press, 1978

391. Sheldon CA, Williams RD, Fraley EE: Incidental carcinoma of the prostate: A review of the literature and critical reappraisal of classification. J Urol 124:626, 1980

392. Murphy GP, Gaeta JF, Pickren J et al: Current status of classification and staging of prostate cancer. Cancer 45:1889, 1980

393. Prout Jr GR, Heany JA, Griffin PP et al: Nodal involvement as a prognostic indicator in patients with prostatic carcinoma. J Urol 124:226, 1980

394. Mahadevia PS, Kiely TM: Meningeal carcinomatosis secondary to prostatic carcinoma: Case report. J Urol 124:154, 1980

395. Fowler JE, Whitmore Jr WF: The incidence and extent of pelvic lymph node metastases in apparently localized prostatic cancer. Cancer 47:2941, 1981

396. Smith Jr JA, Middleton RG: Pelvic lymph node metastasis from prostatic cancer: Influence of tumor grade and stage (abstr). J Urol (Suppl) 127:137, 1982

397. Rao KG: Carcinoma of prostate presenting as intracranial tumor with multiple cranial nerve palsies. Urol 19:433, 1982

398. Leung FW, Casciato DA: Carcinoma of prostate presenting as symptomatic abdominal mass. Urol 20:78, 1982

399. Tertzakian GM, Herr HW, Mehta MB: Orbital metastases from prostatic carcinoma. Urol 19:427, 1982

400. Golimbu M, Glasser J, Schinella R et al: Stage A prostate cancer from pathologist's viewpoint. Urol 18:124, 1982

401. Murphy GP, Natarajan N, Pontes JE et al: The national survey of prostate cancer in the United States by the American College of Surgeons. J Urol 127:928, 1982

402. Yam LT, Winkler CF, Janckila AJ et al: Prostatic cancer presenting as metastatic adenocarcinoma of undetermined origin. Cancer 51:283, 1983

403. American Joint Committee on Cancer: Manual for Staging of Cancer, 2nd ed, p 159. Philadelphia, JB Lippincott, 1983

404. Baumann MA, Holoye PY, Choi H: Adenocarcinoma of prostate presenting as brain metastasis. Cancer 54:1723, 1984

405. Saitoh H, Hida M, Shimbo T et al: Metastatic patterns of prostatic cancer: Correlations between sites and number of organs involved. Cancer 54:3078, 1984

Transitional Cell Carcinoma

406. Melicow MM, Hollowell JW: Intraurothelial cancer: Carcinoma in situ, Bowen's disease of the urinary system: Discussion of thirty cases. J Urol 68:763, 1952

407. Ortega LG, Whitmore Jr WF, Murphy AI: In situ carcinoma of the prostate with intraepithelial extension into the urethra and bladder. A Paget's disease of the urethra and bladder. Cancer 6:898, 1953

408. Ende N, Woods LP, Shelley HS: Carcinoma originating in ducts surrounding the prostatic urethra. Am J Clin Pathol 40:183, 1963

409. Bates Jr HR, Thornton JL: Letter to the editor: Carcinoma of prostatic ducts. Am J Clin Pathol 45:96, 1966

410. Ullmann AS, Ross OA: Hyperplasia, atypism, and carcinoma in situ in prostatic periurethral glands. Am J Clin Pathol 47:497, 1967

411. Bates Jr HR: Transitional cell carcinoma of the prostate. J Urol 101:206, 1969

412. Karpas CM, Moumgis B: Primary transitional cell carcinoma of prostate gland: Possible pathogenesis and relationship to reserve cell hyperplasia of prostatic periurethral dusts. J Urol 101:201, 1969

413. Rubenstein AB, Rubnitz ME: Transitional cell carcinoma of the prostate. Cancer 24:543, 1969

414. Johnson DE, Hogan JM, Ayala AG: Transitional cell carcinoma of the prostate. A clinical morphological study. Cancer 29:287, 1972
415. Shenasky II JH, Gillenwater JY: Management of transitional cell carcinoma of the prostate. J Urol 108:462, 1972
416. Greene LF, Mulcahy JJ, Warren MM et al: Primary transitional cell carcinoma of the prostate. J Urol 110:235, 1973
417. Albert PS, Mallouh C, Nagamatsu GR: Transitional-cell carcinoma of prostate: An enigma. Urol 2:128, 1973
418. Rhamy RK, Buchanan RD, Spalding MJ: Intraductal carcinoma of the prostate gland. J Urol 109:457, 1973
419. Greene LF, O'Dea MJ, Dockerty MB: Primary transitional cell carcinoma of the prostate. J Urol 116:761, 1976
420. Schellhammer PF, Bean MA, Whitmore JR WF: Prostatic involvement by transitional cell carcinoma: Pathogenesis, patterns and prognosis. J Urol 118:399, 1977
421. Wendelken JR, Schellhammer PF, Ladaga LE et al: Transitional cell carcinoma: Cause of refractory cancer of prostate. Urol 13:557, 1979
422. Kirk D, Hinton CE, Shaldon C: Transitional cell carcinoma of the prostate. Br J Urol 51:575, 1979
423. Wolfe JHN, Lloyd-Davies RW: The management of transitional cell carcinoma in the prostate. Br J Urol 53:253, 1981
424. Taylor HG, Blom J: Transitional cell carcinoma of the prostate. Response to treatment with adriamycin and cisplatinum. Cancer 51:1800, 1983
425. Alexander SJ, Lee SS, Bekhrad A: Transitional cell carcinoma of the prostate: response to treatment with cisplatinum and cyclophosphamide. J Urol 131:975, 1984

Prostatic Duct Carcinoma

426. Belter LF, Dodson Jr AI: Papillomatosis and papillary adenocarcinoma of prostatic ducts: A case report. J Urol 104:880, 1970
427. Dube VE, Joyce GT, Kennedy E: Papillary primary duct carcinoma of the prostate. J Urol 107:825, 1972
428. Dube VE, Farrow GM, Greene LF: Prostatic adenocarcinoma of ductal origin. Cancer 32:402, 1973
429. Drake WM, Burrows S: Papillary carcinoma of prostatic ducts. Urol 3:621, 1974
430. Rotterdam HZ, Melicow MM: Double primary prostatic adenocarcinoma. Urol 6:245, 1975
431. Catalona WJ, Kadmon D, Martin SA: Surgical consideration in treatment of intraductal carcinoma of the prostate. J Urol 120:259, 1978
432. Kopelson G, Horisiadis L, Romas NA et al: Periurethral prostatic duct carcinoma. Clinical features and treatment results. Cancer 42:2894, 1978
433. Uyama T, Moriwaki S: Papillary and mucus-forming adenocarcinomas of prostate. Urol 13:432, 1979
434. Greene LF, Farrow GM, Ravits JM et al: Prostatic adenocarcinoma of ductal origin. J Urol 121:303, 1979
435. Cantrell BB, Leifer G, DeKlerk DP et al: Papillary adenocarcinoma of the prostatic urethra with clear cell appearance. Cancer 48:2661, 1981
436. Pillarisetti SG, Espinoza CG, Richman AV: Prostatic adenocarcinoma with focal "endometrioid" features: histopathologic and immunocytochemical findings. Lab Invest 48:68A, 1983
437. Kuhajda FP, Gipson T, Mendelsohn G: Papillary adenocarcinomas of the prostate. An immunohistochemical study. Cancer 54:1328, 1984

Endometrial Carcinoma

438. Melicow MM, Pachter MR: Endometrial carcinoma of prostatic utricle (uterus masculinis). Cancer 20:1715, 1967

439. Melicow MM, Tannenbaum M: Endometrial carcinoma of uterus maxulinus (prostatic utricle). Report of 6 cases. J Urol 106:892, 1971
440. Carney JA, Kelalis PP: Endometrial carcinoma of the prostatic utricle. Am J Clin Pathol 60:565, 1973
441. Young BW, Lagios MD: Endometrial (papillary) carcinoma of the prostatic utricle — response to orchiectomy. A case report. Cancer 32:1293, 1973
442. Satter EJ, Blumenfeld CM: Endometrial carcinoma of the prostatic utricle. J Urol 112:505, 1974
443. Tannenbaum M: Endometrial tumors and/or associated carcinomas of prostate. Urol 6:372, 1975
444. Merchant Jr RF, Graham AR, Bucher Jr WC et al: Endometrial carcinoma of prostatic utricle with osseous metastases. Urol 8:169, 1976
445. Zaloudek C, Williams JW, Kempson RL: "Endometrial" adenocarcinoma of the prostate. A distinctive tumor of probable prostatic duct origin. Cancer 37:2255, 1976
446. Buchanan R, Shepherd JH: Endometrial Carcinoma of the prostatic utricle. Br J Urol 49:318, 1977
447. Otnes B, Refsum SB, Husby G et al: Probable endometrial carcinoma of the prostate, crossed renal ectopia and dermatomyositis in a 32-year-old man. J Urol 120:504, 1978
448. Walker AN, Mills SE, Fechner RE et al: "Endometrial" adenocarcinoma of the prostatic urethra arising in a villous polyp. A light microscopic and immunoperoxidase study. Arch Pathol Lab Med 106:624, 1982
449. Nogueira March JL, Figueirdo L, Mata J et al: Coexistent cyst of the utricle and carcinoma of the endometrial type in the prostate. Eur Urol 8:42, 1982
450. Walther MM, Nassar V, Harruff RC et al: Endometrial carcinoma of the prostatic utricle: A tumor of prostatic origin. J Urol 134:769, 1985

Squamous Cell Carcinoma

451. Kahler JE: Carcinoma of the prostate gland. A pathologic study. J Urol 41:557, 1939
452. Thompson GJ: Transurethral resection of malignant lesions of the prostate gland. JAMA 120:1105, 1942
453. Arnheim FK: Carcinoma of the prostate: A study of the postmortem findings in one hundred and seventy-six cases. J Urol 60:599, 1948
454. Thompson GJ, Albess DD, Broders AC: Unusual carcinomas involving the prostate gland. J Urol 69:416, 1953
455. Sieracki JC: Epidermoid carcinoma of the human prostate. Report of three cases. Lab Invest 4:232, 1955
456. Ray GR, Cassady JR, Bagshaw MA: Definitive radiation therapy of carcinoma of the prostate. A report on 15 years of experience. Radiology 106:407, 1973
457. Gray Jr FF, Marshall VF: Squamous carcinoma of the prostate. J Urol 113:736, 1975
458. Corder MP, Cecmil GA: Effective treatment of squamous cell carcinoma of the prostate with adriamycin. J Urol 115:222, 1976
459. Mott LJM: Squamous cell carcinoma of the prostate: Report of 2 cases and review of the literature. J Urol 121:833, 1979
460. Sharma SK, Malik AK, Bapna BC: Squamous cell carcinoma of prostate. Indian J Cancer 17:134, 1980

Mixed Carcinoma

461. Bennett RS, Edgerton EO: Mixed prostatic carcinoma. J Urol 110:561, 1973
462. Accetta PA, Gardner Jr WA: Squamous metastases from prostatic adenocarcinoma. Lab Invest 46:2A, 1982

463. Saito R, Davis BK, Ollapally EP: Adenosquamous carcinoma of the prostate. Hum Pathol 15:87, 1984

Mucinous Carcinoma

464. Klissurow A: Ein fall von carcinoma gelatinosum prostate. Virchow's Arch Pathol Anat 268:515, 1928
465. Ashburn LL: New bone formation in a primary carcinoma of the prostate gland. Arch Pathol 28:145, 1939
466. Bukovics C: Gallertkarzinom der prostata. Krebsarzt 2:167, 1947
467. Thompson GJ, Albers DD, Broaders AC: Unusual carcinomas involving the prostate gland. J Urol 69:416, 1953
468. Edgar WM: Mucin-secreting carcinoma of the prostate. Br J Urol 30:213, 1958
469. Sika JV, Buckley JJ: Mucus-forming adenocarcinoma of prostate. Cancer 17:949, 1964
470. Levine AJ, Foster EA: The relation of mucicarmine-staining properties of carcinomas of the prostate to differentiation, metastasis, and prognosis. Cancer 17:21, 1964
471. Joshi DP, Seery WH, Neier CR: Mucogenic adenocarcinoma of the prostate. J Urol 98:241, 1967
472. Zimmerman G, De Rubertis R: Zur kenntnis schleimbildender prostatacarcinoma. Chirurg 39:559, 1968
473. Lighbourn GA, Abrams M, Seymour L: Primary mucoid adenocarcinoma of the prostate gland with bladder invasion. J Urol 101:78, 1969
474. Alfthan O, Koivuniemi: Mucinous carcinoma of the prostate. Scand J Urol Nephrol 4:78, 1970
475. Mathevet JC, Nedelec M, Auvigne J et al: Tumeur rare de la prostate. A propos d'un cas de cancer muco-secretant. J Urol Nephrol 76:276, 1970
476. Chica G, Johnson DE, Ayala AG: Mucinous adenocarcinoma of the prostate. J Urol 118:124, 1977
477. Uyama T, Moriwaki S: Papillary and mucus-forming adenocarcinomas of prostate. Urol 13:432, 1979
478. Cricco RP, Kassis J: Mucinous adenocarcinoma of prostate. Urol 14:276, 1979
479. Edbadawi A, Craig W, Linke CA et al: Prostatic mucinous carcinoma. Urol 13:658, 1979
480. Proia AD, McCarty Jr KS, Woodard BH: Prostatic mucinous adenocarcinoma. A cowper gland carcinoma mimicker. Am J Surg Pathol 5:701, 1981
481. Giltman LI: Signet ring adenocarcinoma of the prostate. J Urol 126:134, 1981

Adenoid Cystic Carcinoma

482. Mostofi FK, Price Jr EB: Malignant tumors of the prostate, p 244. In Tumors of the Male Genital System, Atlas of Tumor Pathology, 2nd Series, Fascicle 8. Washington, DC, AFIP, 1973
483. Dikman SH, Toker C: Seromucinous gland ectopia within the prostatic stroma. J Urol 109:852, 1973
484. Frankel K, Craig JR: Adenoid cystic carcinoma of the prostate. Report of a case. Am J Clin Pathol 62:639, 1974
485. Tannenbaum M: Adenoid cystic or "salivary gland" carcinomas of prostate. Urol 6:238, 1975
486. Kramer SA, Bredael JJ, Krueger RP: Adenoid cystic carcinoma of the prostate: Report of a case. J Urol 120:388, 1978
487. Manrique JJ, Albores-Saavedra J, Orantes A et al: Malignant mixed tumor of the salivary-gland type, primary in the prostate. Am J Clin Pathol 70:932, 1978

Carcinoid Tumors

488. Azzopardi JG, Evans DJ: Argentaffin cells in prostatic carcinoma: Differentiation from liposuscin and melanin in prostatic epithelium. J Pathol 104:247, 1971
489. Wasserstein PW, Goldman RL: Primary carcinoid of prostate. Urol 13:318, 1979
490. Montasser AY, Ong MG, Mehta VT: Carcinoid tumor of the prostate associated with adenocarcinoma. Cancer 44:307, 1979
491. Miki T, Kuroda M, Kiyohara H et al: Primary carcinoid tumor of the prostate. Report of a case. (Nippon Hinyokika Gakkai Zasshi). Jpn J Urol 71:264, 1980
492. Wasserstein PW, Goldman RL: Diffuse carcinoid of prostate. Urol 18:407, 1981
493. Ansari MA, Pintozzi RL, Choi YS et al: Diagnosis of carcinoid-like metastatic prostatic carcinoma by an immunoperoxidase method. Am Soc Clin Pathol 76:94, 1981
494. Samsanov VA, Kolomiitsev SV: Carcinoid tumor of the prostate. Arkh Patol 44:60, 1982
495. Azumi N, Shibuya H, Ishikura M: Primary prostatic carcinoid tumor with intracytoplasmic prostatic acid phosphatase and prostate-specific antigen. Am J Surg Pathol 8:545, 1984
496. Almagro UA: Argyrophilic prostatic carcinoma. Case report with literature review on prostatic carcinoid and "carcinoid-like" prostatic carcinoma. Cancer 55:608, 1985

Small Cell Undifferentiated (Oat Cell) Carcinoma

497. Newmark SR, Dluhy RG, Bennett AH: Ectopic adrenocorticotropin syndrome with prostatic carcinoma. Urol 2:666, 1973
498. Wenk RE, Bhagavan BW, Levy R et al: Ectopic ACTH, prostatic oat cell carcinoma and marked hypernatremia. Cancer 40:773, 1977
499. Vuitch MF, Mendelsohn G: Relationship of ectopic ACTH production to tumor differentiation: A morphologic and immunohistochemical study of prostatic carcinoma with Cushing's syndrome. Cancer 47:296, 1981
500. Schron DS, Gipson T, Mendelsohn G: The histogenesis of small cell carcinoma of the prostate. An immunohistochemical study. Cancer 53:2478, 1984

Stromal Neoplasms

Leiomyoma

501. Kaufman JJ, Berneike RR: Leiomyoma of the prostate. J Urol 65:297, 1951
502. Michaels MM, Brown HE, Favino CJ: Leiomyoma of prostate. Urol 3:617, 1974
503. Vassilakis GB: Pure leiomyoma of prostate. Urol 11:93, 1978

Sarcoma

504. Lowsley OS, Kimball FN: Sarcoma of the prostate with a review of literature. Br J Urol 6:328, 1934
505. Melicow MM, Pelton TH, Fish GW: Sarcoma of the prostate gland: Review of literature; table of classification; report of four cases. J Urol 49:675, 1943
506. Meeter UL, Richards JN: Osteogenic sarcoma of the prostate. J Urol 84:654, 1960
507. Fitzpatrick TJ, Stump G: Leiomyosarcoma of the prostate: Case report and review of the literature. J Urol 83:80, 1960
508. Mackenzie AR, Whitmore Jr WF, Melamed MR: Myosarcomas of the bladder and prostate. Cancer 22:833, 1968
509. Goodwin WD, Mims MM, Young II HH: Rhabdomyosarcoma of the prostate in a child; first 5-year survival: (combined treatment by preoperative, local irradiation; actinomycin D, intra-arterial nitrogen mustard and hypothermia; radical surgery and ureterosigmoidostomy). J Urol 99:651, 1968
510. Christoffersen J: Leiomyosarcoma of the prostate. 6 new cases and a survey of the literature. Acta Chir Scand (Suppl) 443:75, 1973

511. Sarkar K, Tolnai G, McKay DE: Embryonal rhabdomyosarcoma of the prostate. An ultrastructural study. Cancer 31:442, 1973

512. Mostofi FK, Price Jr EB: Malignant tumors of the prostate, p 253. In Tumors of the Male Genital System, Atlas of Tumor Pathology, 2nd Series, Fascicle 8. Washington, DC, AFIP, 1973

513. Tannenbaum M: Sarcomas of the prostate gland. Urol 5:810, 1975

514. Schmidt JD, Welch Jr MJ: Sarcoma of the prostate. Cancer 37:1908, 1976

515. Reyes JW, Shinozuka H, Garry P et al: A light and electron microscopic study of a hemangiopericytoma of the prostate with local extension. Cancer 40:1122, 1977

516. King DG, Finney RP: Embryonal rhabdomyosarcoma of the prostate. J Urol 117:88, 1977

517. Narayana A, Loening S, Weimar W et al: Sarcoma of the bladder and prostate. J Urol 119:72, 1978

518. Hamann F, Bischoff W: Entartung eines leiomyosarkoms der prostate. Fallbericht. Helv Chir Acta 45:297, 1978

519. Witherow R, Molland E, Oliver T et al: Leiomyosarcoma of prostate and superficial soft tissue. Urol 15:513, 1980

520. Palma PCR, Netto Jr NR, Ikari O et al: Leiomyosarcoma in association with incidental adenocarcinoma of the prostate. J Urol 129:156, 1983

Miscellaneous Rare Neoplasms

521. Hamlin WB, Lund PK: Carcinosarcoma of the prostate: A case report. J Urol 97:518, 1967

522. Haddad JR, Reyes EC: Carcinosarcoma of the prostate with metastasis of both elements: Case report. J Urol 103:80, 1970

523. Benson Jr RC, Segura JW, Carney JA: Primary yolk sac (endodermal sinus) tumor of the prostate. Cancer 41:1395, 1978

524. Martin SA, Fowler M, Catalona WJ et al: Carcinosarcoma of the prostate: Report of a case with ultrastructural observations. J Urol 122:709, 1979

525. Quay SC, Proppe KH: Carcinosarcoma of the prostate: case report and review of the literature. J Urol 125:436, 1981

Metastatic Tumors

526. Watson EM, Sauer HR, Sadugor MG: Manifestations of the lymphoblastomas in genitourinary tract. J Urol 61:626, 1949

527. Waller JI, Shullenberger WA: Lymphosarcoma of the prostate. J Urol 62:480, 1949

528. Lucia SP, Mills H, Lowenhaupt E et al: Visceral involvement in primary neoplastic diseases of the reticuloendothelial system Cancer 5:1193, 1952

529. West WO: Primary lymphosarcoma of prostate gland. Arch Intern Med 109:145, 1962

530. Mitch Jr WE, Serpick AA: Leukemic infiltration of the prostate: A reversible form of urinary obstruction. Cancer 26:1361, 1970

531. Johnson DE, Chalbaud R, Ayala AG: Secondary tumors of the prostate. J Urol 112:507, 1974

532. Melchior J, Valk WL, Foret JD et al: The prostate in leukemia: Evaluation and review of literature. J Urol 111:647, 1974

533. Rader ES: Leukemic infiltration of prostate. Urol 3:779, 1974

534. Cartagena R, Baumgartner G, Wajsman Z et al: Primary reticulum cell sarcoma of prostate gland. Urol 5:815, 1975

535. Mitch WE, Serpick AA: Leukemic infiltration of the prostate. Cancer 38:2442, 1976

536. Dajani YF, Burke M: Leukemic infiltration of the prostate. A case study and clinicopathological review. Cancer 38:2442, 1976

537. Blank B, Hodges CV: Leukemic infiltration of the prostate: a case report. J Urol 123:789, 1980

Penis

9

Normal Structure

The epidermis investing the erectile tissue cylinders and urethra has the microscopic features of true skin covering the shaft and a squamous mucosal surface covering the glans (Fig. 9-1). There is no intervening subcutaneous adipose tissue, but rather two fibrous tunics, an outer dartos tunic and an inner Buck's fascia, which are continuous with fascia of the anterior abdominal muscles. Sebaceous glands, without associated hair follicles and sweat glands, are present in the high dermis. Scattered smooth muscle fibers are continuous with the

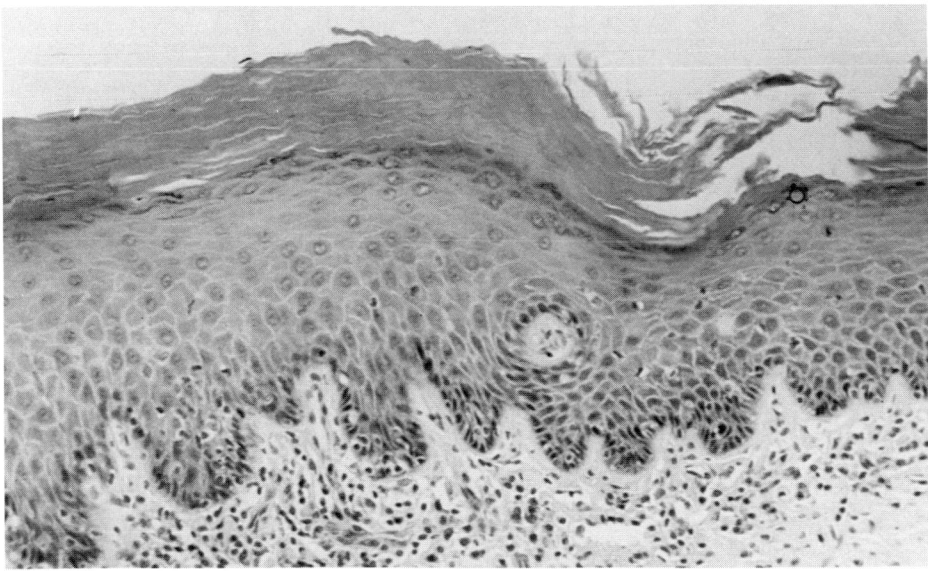

Figure 9-1   **Normal penis.** *The epidermis demonstrates normal maturation to the granular layer with overlying hyperkeratosis.*

smooth muscle in the fibromuscular trabeculae of the centrally located vascular erectile tissue. A fibrous tunic albuginea invests the erectile tissue internal to Buck's fascia. The urethra courses through the corpus cavernosum urethrae. The lymphatic drainage is to the superficial and deep inguinal lymph nodes. Centrally located anastomoses result in bilateral drainage.[1-3]

Congenital Disorders

Congenital disorders of the penis are rare and virtually never come to the attention of the surgical pathologist. The reported congenital disorders are listed here with suggested references for further reading:

Agenesis[4,5]

Canals, cysts of genitoperineal raphe[11-14]

Duplication[9,10]

Hypoplasia[6-8]

Acquired Cysts

Acquired cysts of the penis are rare and are the result of mechanical obstruction in the duct of sebaceous glands. They are basically retention cysts of sebaceous glands.[15] These cysts are observed more commonly in the scrotal skin.

Acquired retention cysts of penile sebaceous glands should be differentiated from congenital cysts of the penis resulting from either ectopic urethral or periurethral gland mucosa, or from ectodermal rests formed during the closure of the genital folds.[11-14] When derived from endoderm, the lining cells are columnar or cuboidal and are capable of mucous production (mucoid cysts).[13] Alternatively, ectodermal-derived cysts are lined by squamous cells and are filled with keratin debris.[14]

Congenital cysts of the type already described are commonly noted to have been present from birth or childhood. Their diagnosis and treatment, however, may not occur until the early adult years.[13] A history of trauma may be associated with acquired cysts.[14]

Disorders of the Prepuce: Balanoposthitis and Phimosis

The surgical removal of the prepuce is virtually always at the time of circumcision of infant males. Less frequently, the prepuce is excised in the clinical circumstances of phimosis or balanoposthitis.

Phimosis, or the inability to retract the prepuce because of an abnormally small preputial orifice, may be of acquired or congenital origin. Chronic inflammation with edema and fibrosis of the prepuce resulting in phimosis is more common than phimosis secondary to a congenitally small preputial orifice. The treatment is circumcision regardless of etiology. Histologic changes present in the preputial specimen include nonspecific chronic inflammation, edema, and fibrosis in the dermis. The epidermis may be ulcerated.

Balanoposthitis is inflammation of the glans and prepuce and is commonly associated with phimosis. Poor personal hygiene and phimosis contribute to the development of this disorder. Alternatively, persistence of the inflammation may contribute in turn to the development of phimosis. Multiple gram-positive and negative organisms have been associated with this inflammatory disorder. The histologic features are entirely nonspecific acute and chronic inflammation.

Inflammatory Disorders

Sclerosing Lipogranuloma of the External Genitalia

Sclerosing lipogranuloma is an inflammatory reactive process to exogenous lipids and waxes gaining access to the dermis (Figs. 9-2 and 9-3). It is reported most frequently in the penis and scrotum in young adults.[16-20] The exogenous nature of the substances prompting the inflammatory response was demonstrated initially by infrared spectrophotometry by Oertel and Johnson and confirmed subsequently by others.[18-20] The circumstances whereby the exogenous lipid substances gain access to the dermis vary and commonly are not clarified by questioning the patient.[18] Recorded instances of topical application of "baby oil" or other similar substances or injection of paraffin clarify the cause in some cases.[20] Several patients relate prior trauma or accidents involving injury to the genital region.[18]

The histologic features of the resulting inflamed fibrous mass excised from the penis are identical to those observed in the scrotum (see Chap. 10).

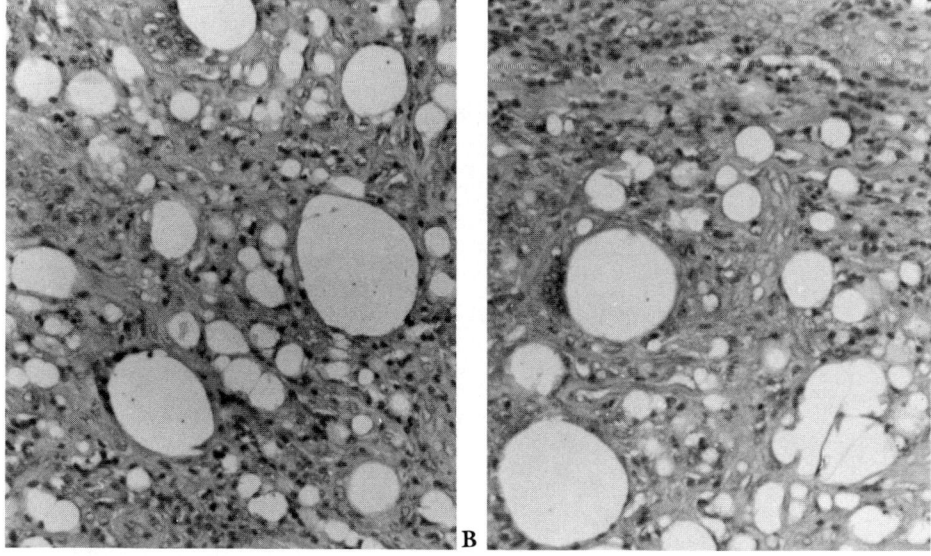

A   **B**

Figure 9-2   *Sclerosing lipogranuloma of penis.* (A, B) *Numerous lacunae, some with evident multinucleated histiocytic giant cells at the periphery, are scattered throughout the fibrous stroma. Chronic inflammatory cells of lymphocytic and histiocytic origin infiltrate the dense fibrosis typical of this reaction to exogenous lipids.*

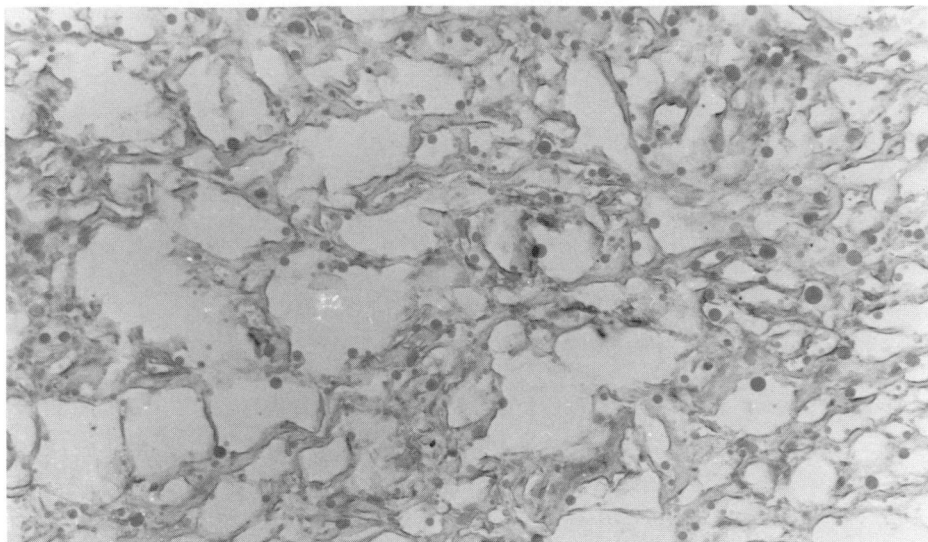

Figure 9-3   *Sclerosing lipogranuloma of penis. The lipid content of the vacuoles (remaining after tissue processing) is identified by the oil-red O stain.*

Syphilis

Syphilis, which is caused by the spirochete *Treponema pallidum* and is transmitted by sexual intercourse, evolves clinically in three stages.

The characteristic lesion of primary syphilis is the chancre at the site of inoculation. The initial small papule ulcerates. Spirochetes are demonstrable in this lesion by use of the Warthin–Starry stain (Fig. 9-4). Histologically, the

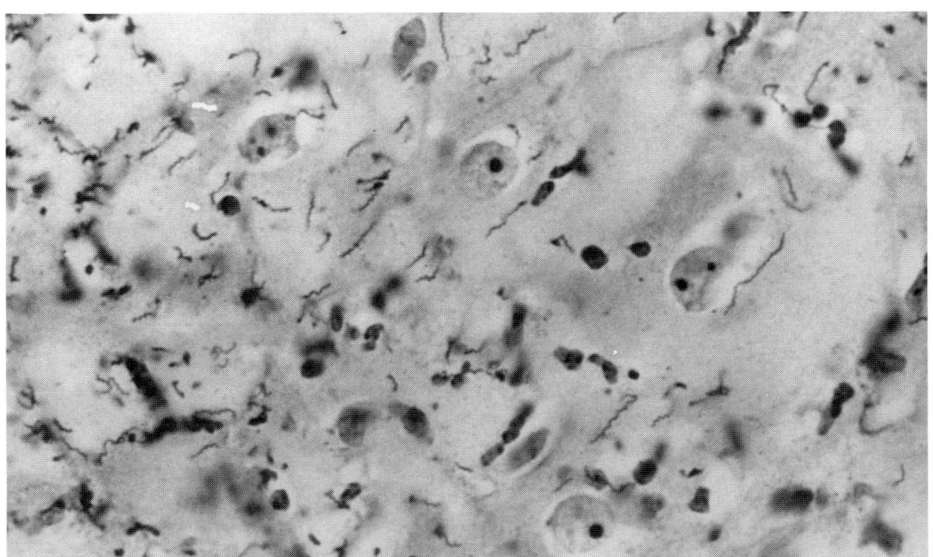

Figure 9-4   *Condyloma lata. Spirochetes are demonstrated in the epidermis by use of the Warthin–Starry stain.*

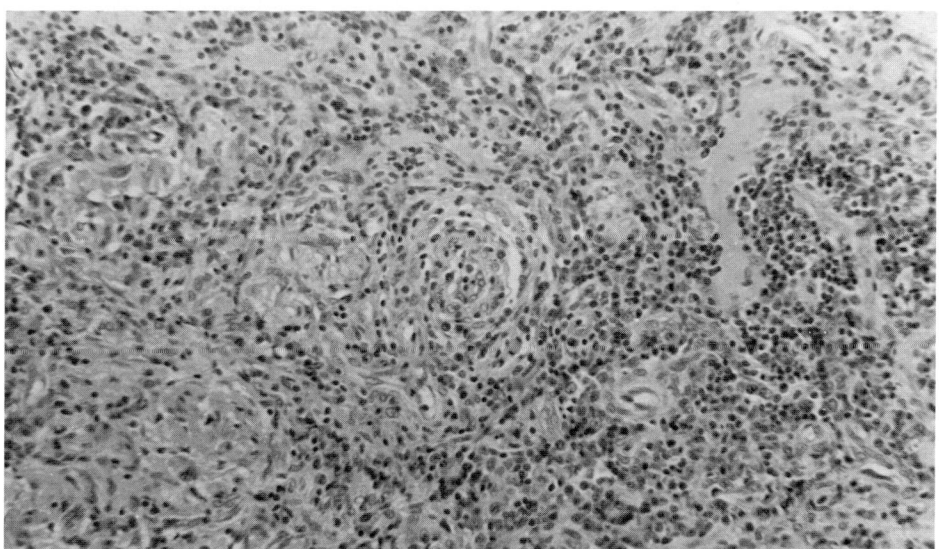

Figure 9-5 *Primary syphilis. A dense infiltrate of plasma cells and lymphocytes surrounds and obliterates the vascular structure in the center.*

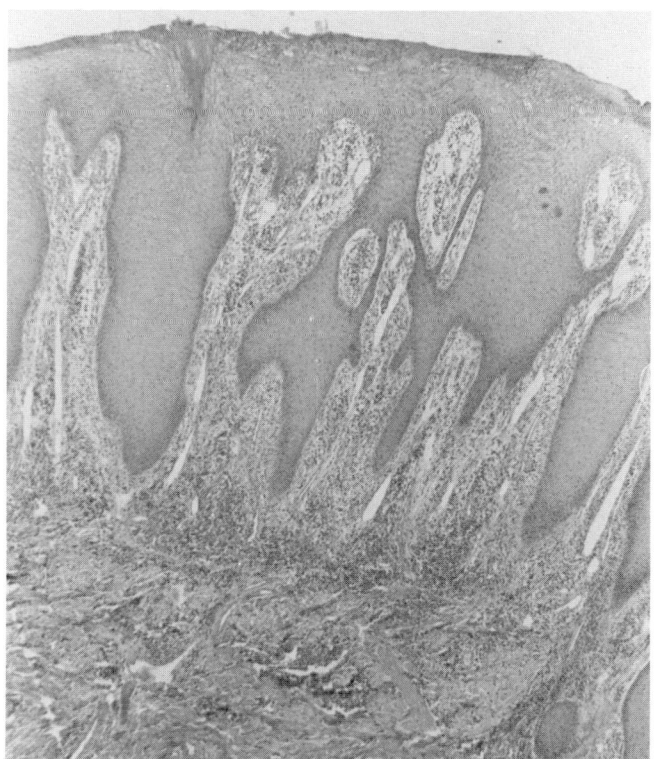

Figure 9-6 *Condyloma lata. The epidermis shows hyperkeratosis and acanthosis. A dense infiltrate of plasma cells and lymphocytes is present in the underlying dermis.*

inflammatory cell infiltrate has a predominance of plasma cells in association with lymphocytes and fewer neutrophils (Fig. 9-5). A prominent feature is the obliterative endarteritis of the vessels in the base of the ulcer. Immunoperoxidase staining allows specific identification of the spirochetes in paraffin-embedded tissue sections.[21]

The characteristic lesion of secondary syphilis is a diffuse maculopapular rash in the area of original inoculation called *condylomata lata* (Fig. 9-6). The histologic features of these lesions are similarly characterized by a predominating perivascular plasma cell infiltrate underlying epidermal hyperplasia with either papillomatosis and acanthosis (psoriaform) or a lichen planus-like pattern.[22]

The gumma, the luetic lesion characteristic of tertiary syphilis, is characterized by an area of central necrosis with surrounding chronic inflammatory cells, occasional giant cells, and abundant collagenous fibrosis within the dermis, or with deeper involvement in the subcutaneous tissue.[21]

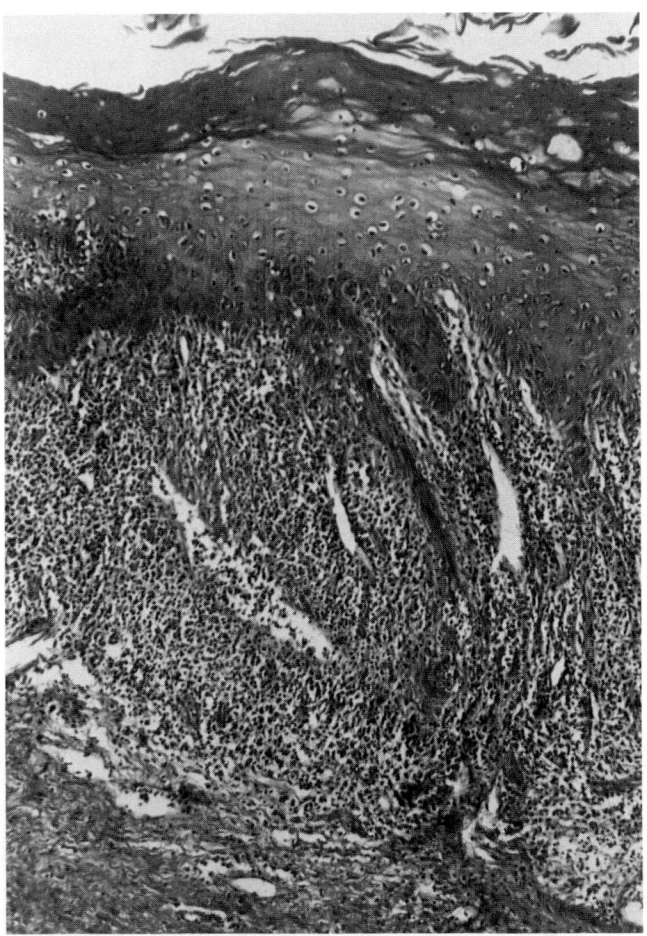

Figure 9-7   *Chancroid. A dense acute and chronic inflammatory cell infiltrate with acute vasculitis is present in the high dermis with papillomatosis of the epidermis adjacent to an ulcer. Gram stain disclosed the gram-negative rods.*

Chancroid (Soft Chancre)

Chancroid is caused by a gram-negative coccobacillus *Hemophilus ducreyi* (Fig. 9-7). Clinically, there is a local ulceration of the epidermis associated with a painful enlargement of the regional lymph nodes.

Histologically, the classic lesion has three "zones."[23,24] The most superficial layer of the ulcer is composed of necrotic tissue overlying a zone composed of an acute inflammatory cell infiltrate with evident acute vasculitis of small vessels. The deepest zone is composed of changes characteristic of resolving acute inflammation, fibroblastic proliferation, and a mixed inflammatory cell infiltrate composed of lymphocytes, plasma cells, histiocytes, and neutrophils. Foci of necrosis with surrounding acute inflammatory cells are also observed in the affected regional lymph nodes in the groin.

Granuloma Inguinale

Granuloma inguinale is caused by the gram-negative coccobacillus *Donovania granulomatis* (Fig. 9-8). Clinically, the initial lesion is a papule that enlarges to an irregular ulcer, frequently with satellite lesions that may ultimately coalesce with the primary ulcer. Satellite ulcers may also occur along the route of lymphatic drainage.

Histologically, the ulcers are composed of necrotic debris on the surface with an underlying exuberant, acute, inflammatory cell infiltration.[25,26] An important histologic feature is the presence of varying numbers of histiocytes containing phagocytized bacteria called Donovan bodies (Fig. 9-9).

The lesion tends to be more destructive and chronic than chancroid. Healing is associated frequently with the production of fibrous scars in the region of the original and satellite ulcers.

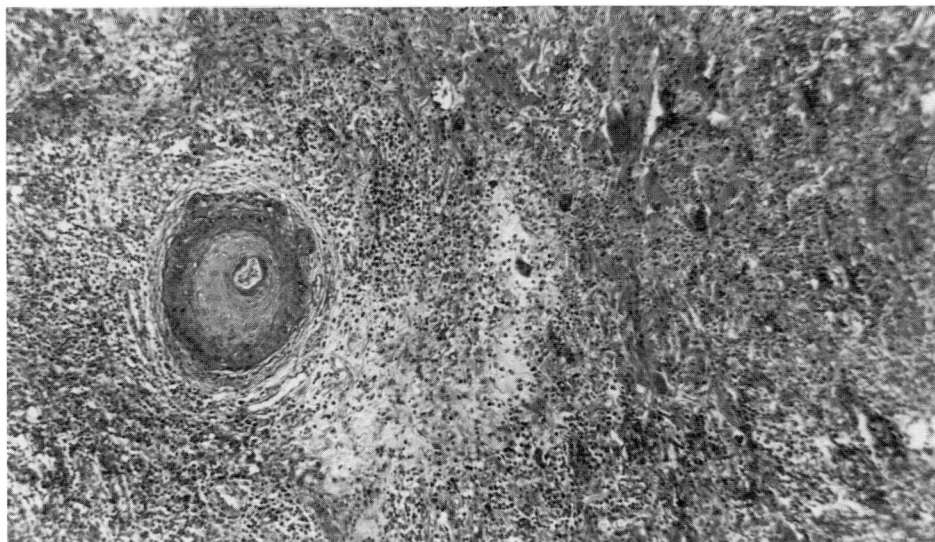

Figure 9-8 *Granuloma inguinale. A dense acute and chronic inflammatory cell infiltrate associated with focal areas of tissue necrosis is present in the dermis.*

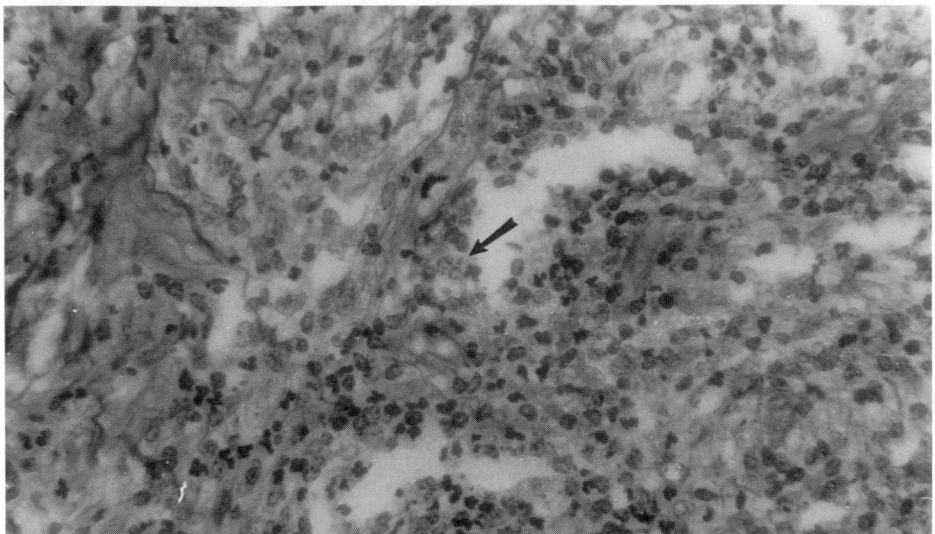

Figure 9-9   *Granuloma inguinale. The inflammatory cells present include neutrophils, lymphocytes, plasma cells, and histiocytes with phagocytized bacteria (Donovan bodies) indicated by the arrow.*

Lymphogranuloma Inguinale (Lymphogranuloma Venereum)

Lymphogranuloma inguinale is the result of venereal inoculation of the L_1, L_2, or L_3 serotypes of *Chlamydia trachomatis* (Fig. 9-10).[28] The infection is characterized by epidermal ulceration on the penis and a prominent enlargement of the regional lymph nodes.

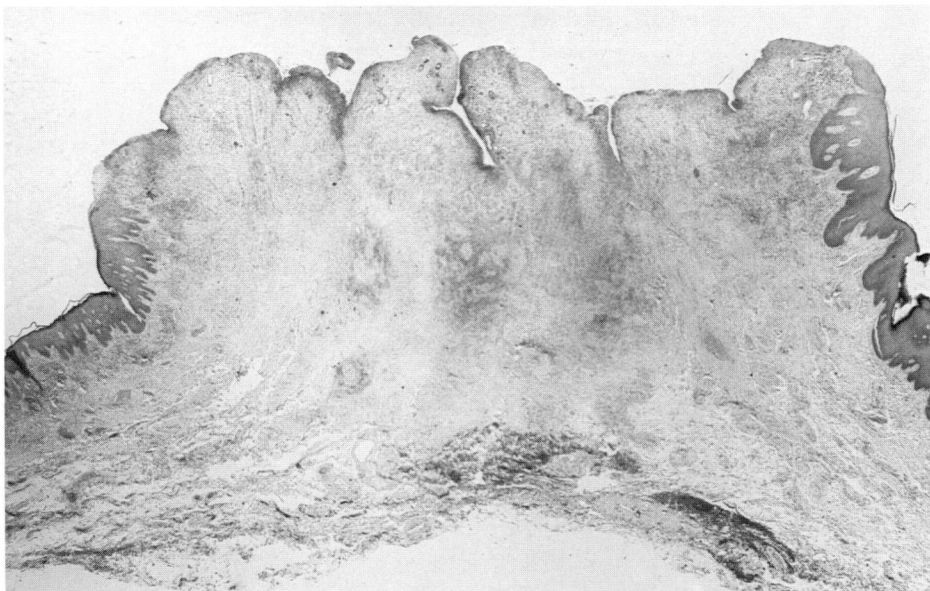

Figure 9-10   *Lymphogranuloma venereum. The dermis and subcutaneous tissue beneath the epidermal ulcer contain all stages of healing with acute inflammation limited to the high dermis. The adjacent epidermis shows papillomatosis and acanthosis.*

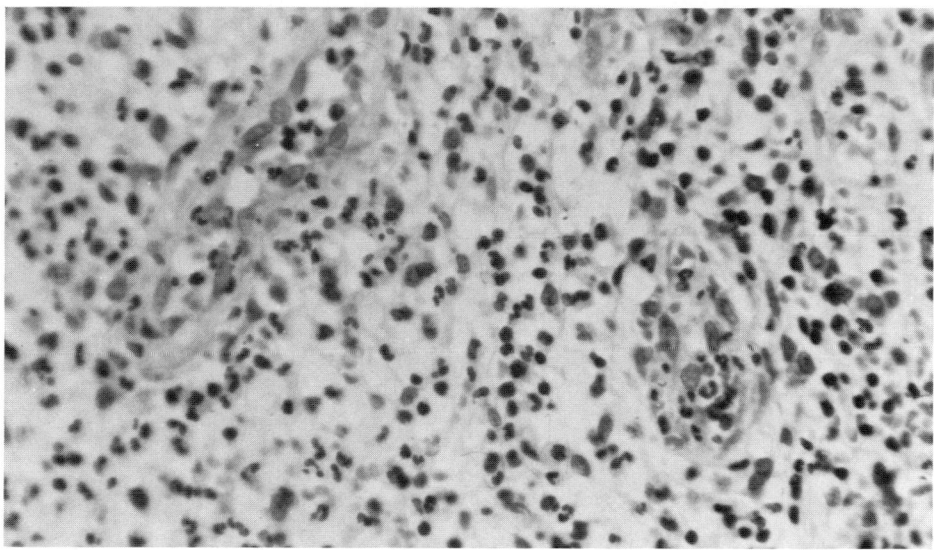

Figure 9-11   *Lymphogranuloma venereum. The inflammatory cell infiltrate of the dermis is nonspecific with neutrophils, lymphocytes, and occasional histiocytes.*

Histologically, the primary lesion is relatively nonspecific with epidermal necrosis, ulceration, and a prominent, acute, inflammatory response (Fig. 9-11).[27,29] The deepest layers of the ulcer have the components of granulation tissue with fibrosis. Ill-defined granulomas with histiocytic giant cells may occasionally be present.

The affected lymph nodes contain a necrotizing acute inflammatory response with prominent necrosis of both the lymphoid tissue and the perinodal tissue that frequently result in the draining of sinus tracts to the overlying skin. The coalescing abscesses in the lymph nodes result in the classic "stellate abscesses" with surrounding acute inflammatory cells and a mantle of histiocytes with occasional giant cells. Resolution results ultimately in a diffuse fibrous scarring and a resultant lymphatic obstruction.

Herpes Genitalis

Herpes genitalis, caused by herpesvirus type II (HVS-2), is subclinical in approximately 90% of cases.[30,31] The clinically apparent cases most commonly affect the prepuce and the glans. The lesions are small (mm) vesicles that rupture resulting in a small ulcer. Regional lymph nodes may be enlarged and tender. The disease is sexually transmitted and the natural history is characterized by multiple recurrences.[30,31]

The characteristic lesion is histologically an intraepidermal vesicle or ulceration. Multinucleated epithelial cells containing intranuclear inclusions in association with epithelial cells with marked ballooning degeneration are diagnostic of herpes infection (Fig. 9-12).[32] The surrounding subcutaneous tissue contains an acute inflammatory cell infiltrate associated with stromal edema.

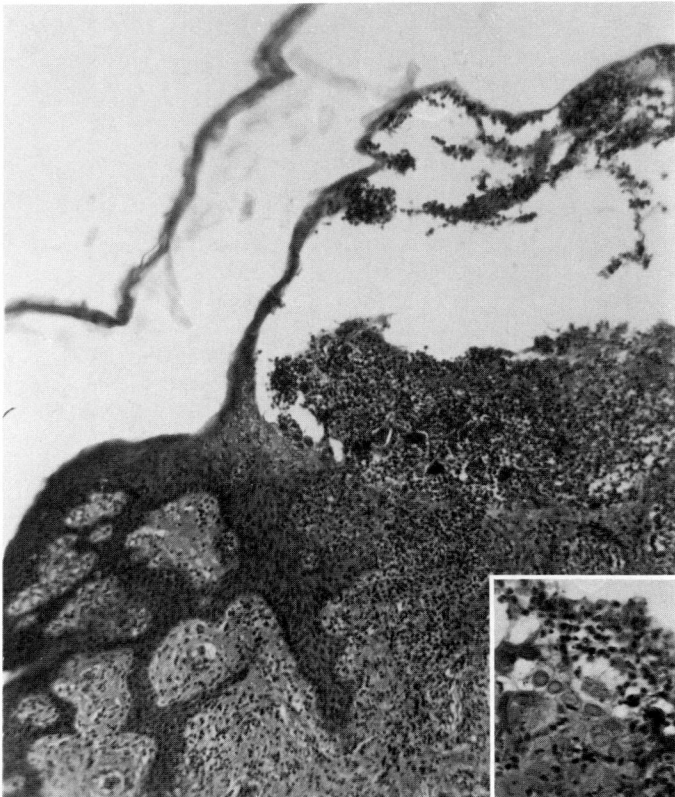

Figure 9-12   *Herpes infection. The shallow epidermal ulcer underlying a ruptured vesicle contains squamous epithelial cells with prominent intranuclear inclusions at the margin* (inset).

Condyloma Acuminatum

Condyloma acuminatum is a wart-like exophytic lesion that is encountered most commonly on the glans and the prepuce in uncircumcised men. The majority of these lesions are millimeters to centimeters in size, but they are capable of extensive superficial growth to ultimately involve the penile shaft.[36] There is evidence of a viral etiology, specifically papillomavirus, HPV_6.[33-35]

The histologic features of condyloma, regardless of size, are epidermal acanthosis, hyperkeratosis, parakeratosis, and papillomatosis (Fig. 9-13).[36] Scattered vacuolated cells in the superficial and deep stratum malpighii are the diagnostic features. Mitoses are variable and may be numerous in the acanthotic epidermis. Typically, the nuclei show no significant atypia. There is a constant accompanying dermal infiltrate of chronic inflammatory cells. The proliferative process is exophytic with little tendency to downward displacement or infiltration of the underlying dermis. Recurrence is not uncommon after surgical therapy.

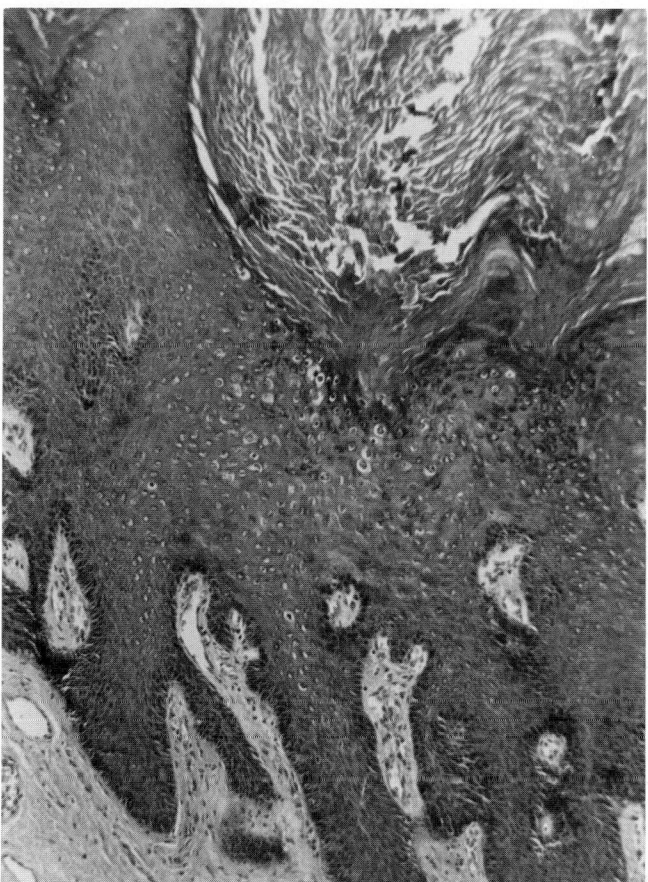

Figure 9-13   ***Condyloma acuminatum.*** *The epidermis shows hyperkeratosis, parakeratosis, acanthosis, and papillomatosis with scattered vacuolated cells.*

Peyronie's Disease

Peyronie's disease, originally described by Francois de la Peyronie in 1743, is characterized by focal, asymmetric fibrosis of the penile shaft (Fig. 9-14). This fibrosis results in pain and curvature of the penis at the time of erection. No consistently reliable therapy has emerged in spite of voluminous literature describing various forms of treatment.[38,39] Furthermore, reports of spontaneous improvement without therapy appear in the literature.[38,39] The causes are unknown.[37,40] An inherited form of Peyronie's disease with autosomal dominant transmission was recently described.[40]

Typically the lesion, 2 cm to 4 cm in dimension, is a penile shaft induration without significant change of the overlying skin.[37,38] Males in the third to seventh decade are most commonly afflicted.[37]

In a review of 26 cases from the Armed Forces Institute of Pathology (AFIP), Smith reported the early lesions were characterized by a chronic inflammatory cell infiltrate in the perivascular tissue deep to Buck's fascia.[37] This inflammatory cell infiltrate diminishes, in time, with a corresponding increase in dense fibrosis involving the corpus cavernosum, Buck's fascia, and the intervening tunica albuginea. Locally, smooth muscle in the septa of the corpus cavernosum is replaced by dense collagen. Focal calcification is not uncommon.[37] The absence of cytologic atypia and lipid vacuoles with histiocytic giant cells differentiates Peyronie's disease from neoplasms of fibroblastic origin and sclerosing lipogranuloma, respectively.

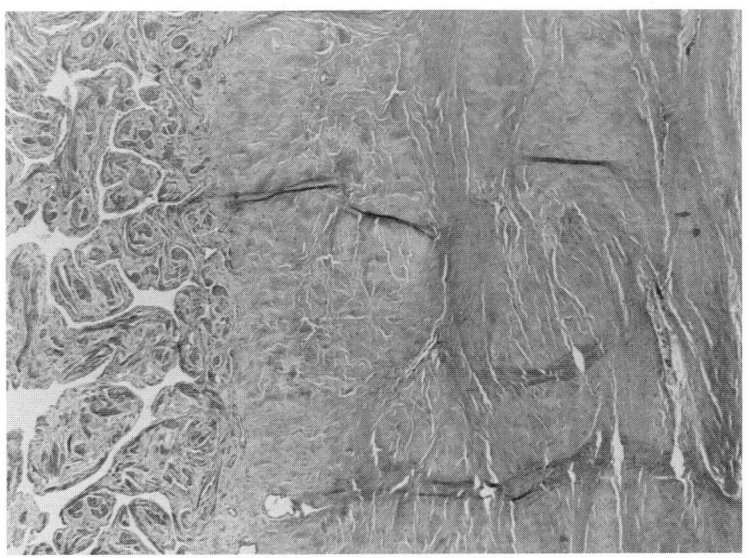

Figure 9-14   *Peyronie's disease. The dermis is markedly thickened by dense collagenous tissue that focally infiltrates into the smooth muscle investing the corpus cavernosum at the left.*

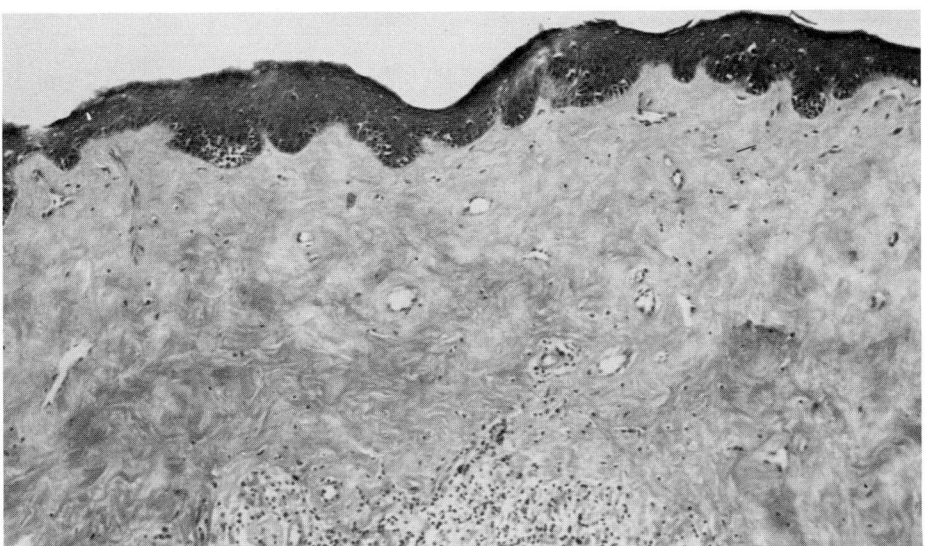

Figure 9-15   *Balanitis xerotica obliterans. The epidermis is thin and shows focal hyperkeratosis. The underlying dermis is composed of amorphous abundant collagen with an associated chronic inflammatory cell infiltrate beneath.*

Balanitis Xerotica Obliterans (Lichen Sclerosis et Atrophicus)

Balanitis xerotica obliterans, most commonly involving the glans penis, prepuce, or both, of elderly men, is characterized clinically by small white macules or larger epidermal plaques.[41-44] Histologically, the epidermis shows a thinned stratum malpighii with associated hyperkeratosis. The underlying papillary dermis is characterized by a homogenization of the collagen in the background of stromal edema (Fig. 9-15). A lymphocytic infiltrate is present typically in the reticular dermis. The cause of this disorder involving dermal collagen and epidermis is unknown. Its association with epithelial malignancy, if any, is unsettled.[43,44]

Neoplastic Disorders

Squamous Cell Carcinoma In Situ

Three clinicopathologic variants of squamous cell carcinoma in situ of the penis appear in the literature: (1) Bowen's disease, (2) erythroplasia of Queyrat, and (3) bowenoid papulosis.[45-49] The uniqueness of bowenoid papulosis, the most recently recognized variant, is generally accepted on the basis of numerous clinical features distinct from the other variants.[49] The same cannot be said for Bowen's disease and erythroplasia of Queyrat. Although some authors maintain that they are separate clinicopathologic entities, others regard them as representing the same pathologic process and believe that erythroplasia of Queyrat represents Bowen's disease of the penis.[48-50] The matter remains controversial and unresolved. All three variants are histologically identical and any differences that exist between them are referable to their respective clinical features and natural history.

The microscopic features of squamous cell carcinoma in situ include: (1) patchy or extensive parakeratosis in association with hyperkeratosis, (2) papillomatosis with broad epidermal papillae, (3) thinning of the granular layer, (4) acanthosis, (5) elongation and broadening of rete ridges, and (6) cytologic atypia of keratinocytes with nuclear hyperchromaticity and pleomorphism involving all layers of the epidermis, (7) mitotic activity at all layers of the epidermis, (8) an intact, sharp epidermal–dermal junction, and (9) chronic inflammatory cell infiltrate in the subjacent dermis.[46,48,49]

Bowen's Disease

Bowen's disease involving the penis typically involves the glans or prepuce of an uncircumcised male older than 50 years.[46] Most lesions are single, discrete, erythematous, scaly plaques.[46,48,51] An increased risk of internal malignancy has been attributed historically to Bowen's disease, an association challenged by Andersen.[46,48,51] Virus-like inclusions have been reported in electron microscopic studies of Bowen's disease.[52] Less than 10% of patients with Bowen's disease develop invasive carcinoma.[48]

Erythroplasia of Queyrat

Penile erythroplasia of Queyrat is reported exclusively on the glans and the prepuce in uncircumcised males (Fig. 9-16).[48] Patients range in age from the third to the ninth decade with a median age of 51 years. The majority of cases are single erythematous plaques. Associated internal malignancy is observed at a lower frequency than with Bowen's disease.[48] These features, outlined in a major study of 100 cases of erythroplasia of Queyrat from the AFIP files, prompted Graham and Helwig to regard it as a clinicopathologic entity separate from Bowen's disease.[48]

Bowenoid Papulosis

The term *bowenoid papulosis* was introduced in 1977 by Kopf and Bart in reference to a clinically distinct form of squamous cell carcinoma in situ regarded originally as unique to penile skin.[53] The lesion has now been recognized to occur on the vulva.[50,54,55] Subsequent reports of this lesion involving the penis all confirm the original observations.[57,58]

Bowenoid papulosis is identical histologically to other forms of squamous cell carcinoma in situ (Bowen's disease and erythroplasia of Queyrat). The im-

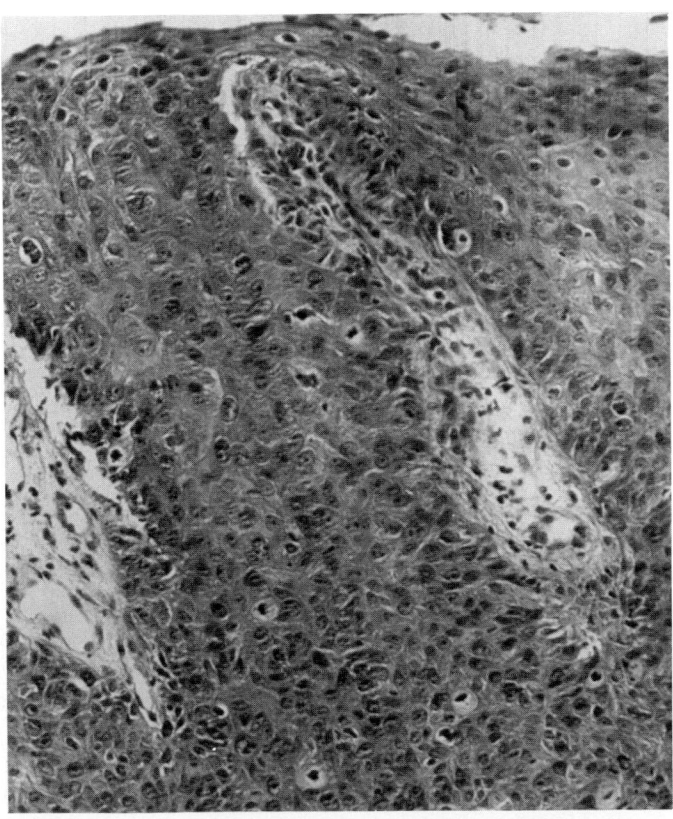

Figure 9-16   *Erythroplasia. The dysplastic cells are found at all levels of the epidermis, which shows acanthosis and papillomatosis.*

portant and distinguishing features of bowenoid papulosis are referable to the clinical features and its natural history. Typically, multiple 2 mm to 10 mm violaceous papules appear over a period of months on the penile shaft in a circumcised male patient 20 to 40 years of age. In contrast, erythroplasia of Queyrat is observed involving the glans and prepuce of uncircumcised older patients. It is more commonly a single larger lesion and 10% of cases are associated with an invasive component (squamous cell carcinoma).[58] In contrast, no case of bowenoid papulosis reported has shown evidence of invasion of the underlying dermis. Spontaneous disappearance of bowenoid papulosis has been reported in rare cases.[54]

The histologic diagnosis of bowenoid papulosis (squamous cell carcinoma in situ) is not predicted prior to biopsy in the reported cases. The clinical diagnoses of the reported lesions include lichen planus, psoriasis, condyloma, and granuloma annulare.[50,54,55]

The microscopic features are identical to Bowen's disease and erythroplasia of Queyrat (Figs. 9-17 and 9-18).[50,54,57,58] Electron microscopic studies failed initially to identify viral particles; however, Zelickson and Prawer reported intranuclear particles.[50,54,56]

The absence of invasion demonstrated by all cases reported should not preclude correctly regarding this lesion as a form of squamous cell carcinoma in situ with the inherent biologic potential of invasion.

The clinical differential diagnosis of penile papules, especially in young adult patients, should include bowenoid papulosis. Following a biopsy diagnosis, treatment and follow-up should be appropriate for this form of squamous cell carcinoma in situ.

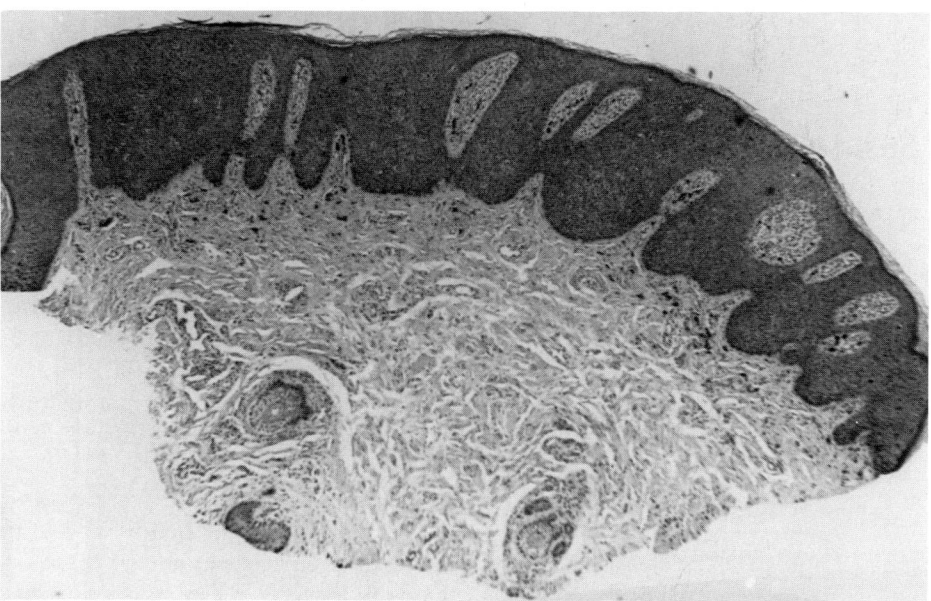

Figure 9-17   *Bowenoid papulosis. The typical features of full-thickness dysplasia in association with blunt papillomatosis were recorded in a 27-year-old man.*

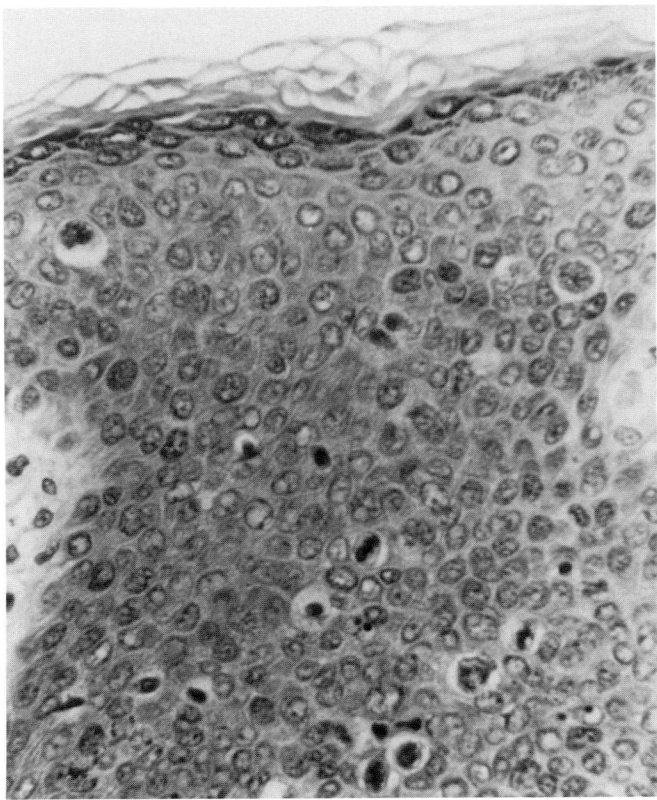

Figure 9-18   *Bowenoid papulosis. Higher magnification of the lesion illustrated in Figure 9-17 shows nuclear atypia and scattered mitoses at all layers of the stratum malpighii.*

Squamous Cell Carcinoma

Epidemiology

The frequency of penile squamous cell carcinoma varies markedly throughout the world with the highest incidence observed in Asian countries (China, Vietnam, Ceylon, Burma, and India), Africa (Uganda), and Central America (Mexico).[59,60] Penile cancer is uncommon in the United States. This variable frequency has been associated with personal, social, and religious practices characteristic of different societies (including personal hygiene and the practice of circumcision).[59,60] Fewer than ten cases of penile cancer have been reported in men circumcised at birth.[61-69]

Related to the lack of circumcision is the possible role of smegma in the causation of squamous cell carcinoma of the penis.[59,60] Thomas identified viral particles similar to those of herpes simplex in two of three cases of penile carcinomas studied with electron microscopy.[70] The role of viruses in the causation of penile carcinoma awaits further study. The role of previous venereal infections (nonviral), race, occupation, and trauma are no longer regarded as being causally significant.

Clinical Features

Squamous cell carcinoma arises most commonly on the glans or the prepuce.[71-73,78] In seven large series of cases in the United States' literature, patients ranged in age from 15 to 91 years with a mean age of approximately 60 years.[74-80] Most cases occur during the sixth to eighth decades.[74-80] Many of the patients have phimosis.[74,81,85] Symptoms that relate to a growing mass on the distal penis, occasionally with ulceration, bleeding, or discharge, are commonly experienced for multiple months prior to seeking medical attention.[74,80] Enlarged inguinal lymph nodes are present in approximately half the patients at the initial presentation.[73,78,82-84]

Pathology

The gross lesion involving the glans may be predominantly infiltrating, or exophytic, frequently with surface ulceration. Typical lesions are 2 cm to 5 cm in greatest dimension but may be larger. The urethral meatus may be destroyed or obscured by the neoplasm. A tumor may partially destroy the prepuce and, on occasion, extend to involve the penile shaft.

Microscopically, moderately well-differentiated tumors are encountered most commonly with uniform or focal keratin production (Fig. 9-19).[73,74,86,87] Poorly differentiated tumors with minimal evidence of their squamous origin are encountered less often. Superimposed acute and chronic inflammatory cells are present commonly within the tumor as well as in the subjacent dermis in association with the infiltrating tumor cells. The epithelium adjacent to the obvious carcinoma may or may not evidence dysplastic changes. The extent of invasion varies, but frequently extensive, deep invasion into the dermis and cavernosa is encountered (Fig. 9-20). Complete examination of the penectomy specimen

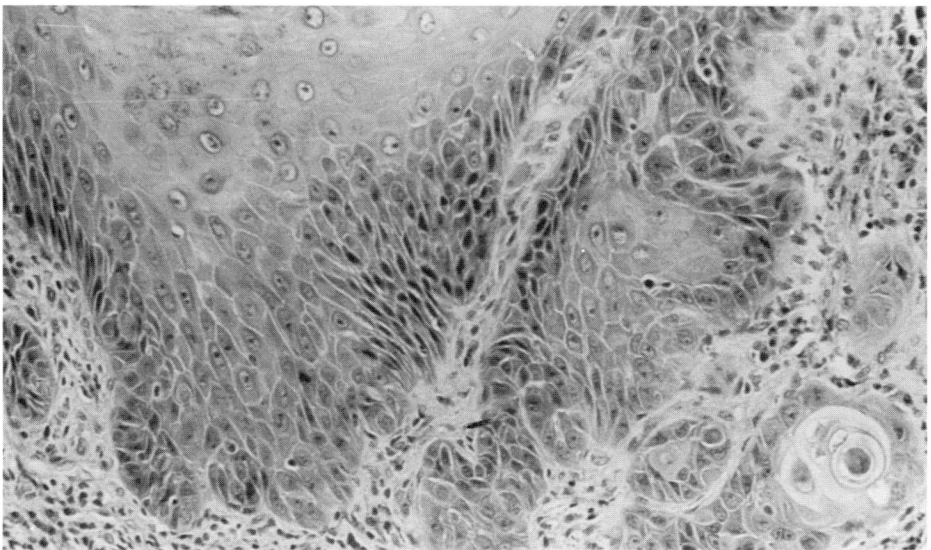

Figure 9-19 *Squamous cell carcinoma. This well-differentiated neoplasm shows clusters of squamous cells infiltrating the underlying dermis at the right. One squamous pearl is present* (lower right).

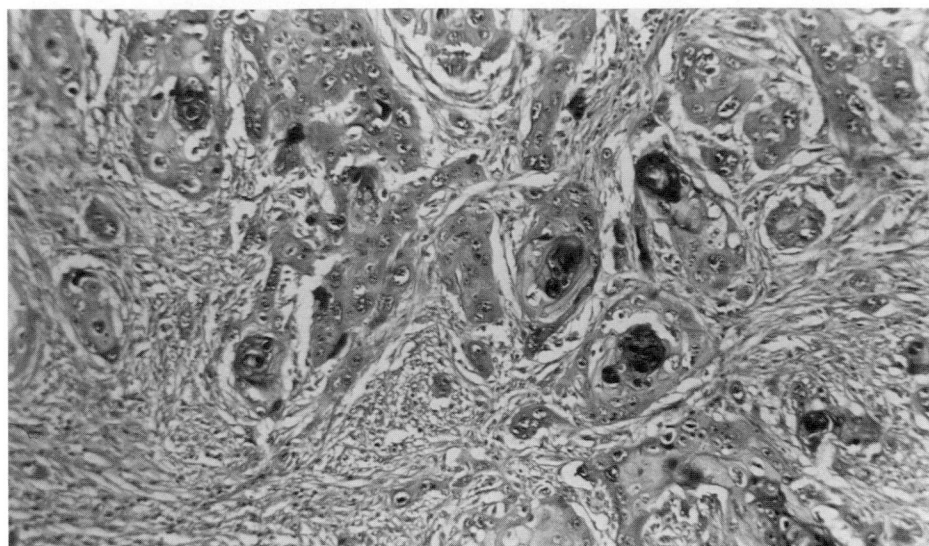

Figure 9-20   *Squamous cell carcinoma. Numerous bizarre squamous cells are present in these nests of invading tumor.*

includes determining the depth of invasion, the presence of lymphatic and vascular invasion, and the adequacy of the surgical resection margin.

The staging of penile carcinoma was introduced originally by Jackson (Table 9-1).[88] Stage I lesions are limited to the glans or prepuce. Stage II lesions show extension to the penile shaft. Metastatic tumors involving groin nodes without distant metastases are classified as stage III. Stage IV cases show distant metastases.

This staging protocol can be utilized for either clinical or pathologic staging. Jackson's original application of this protocol was a retrospective clinical review. Stage III identified cases with groin node metastasis regarded as being operable. Stage IV included cases with inoperable positive groin nodes and cases with distant metastases. Most reported studies of penile carcinoma employ Jackson's protocol, rather than the TNM staging protocol, of the *Union Internationale Contre le Cancer* (UICC) (Table 9-1).[89]

The clinical stage distribution of several published series of penile carcinoma shows stage I, 34% to 60%; stage II, 9% to 47%; stage III, 0 % to 46%; and stage IV, 0% to 14%.[74–78,80,90] These large reported ranges allow only the conclusion that tumors limited to the primary site and distant metastases are the most commonly and most infrequently encountered circumstances, respectively.

The greatest problem referable to penile carcinoma staging is the high frequency of inaccurate clinical staging compared to the pathological stage determined after histologic review of excised groin nodes.[73,74,78,84] In summary, there is a significant frequency of metastases in clinically negative groin nodes and, conversely, a significant frequency of reactive lymphadenopathy found in clinically suspicious lymph nodes. Approximately half of the patients with clinically enlarged lymph nodes actually have no nodal metastases upon histologic review.[73,78,84] This dilemma forms the basis of the historical debate about the therapeutic rationale of inguinal lymph node dissection at the time of definitive surgery for the primary tumor.[80,90–94] Cabanas, employing lymphangiography, identified an inguinal lymph node ("sentinel node") most frequently the initial node to harbor metastases.[3] Biopsy-proven metastases in this node were suggested as the basis for including a groin node dissection in the original definitive therapy.[3] The use of lymphangiography for evaluation of possible groin node metastases, however, is fraught with a high frequency of false-negative and false-positive interpretations and for this reason has little role in the routine clinical evaluation of penile carcinoma.[78,95,96] Subsequent to Cabanas' suggested routine staging procedure of sentinel lymph node biopsy, Perinetti and associates reported a patient with penile carcinoma in whom unresectable iliac lymph node metastases developed within 6 months of bilateral sentinel lymph node biopsies that were interpreted as being free of metastases.[100] This observation suggests that the lymph node identified as a "sentinel lymph node" by Cabanas is not reliable in the staging of this neoplasm.[3,100]

Following dissemination to the inguinal lymph nodes, the neoplasm spreads to the iliac nodes with ultimate distant metastases found most commonly in the lungs.[78]

Treatment of the primary lesion is most frequently partial or complete penectomy with or without inguinal node excision.[78,80,90,91] Radiation therapy of both the primary tumor and the inguinal lymph nodes has been advocated in recent studies.[79,86,97] The role of chemotherapy awaits further investigation, but preliminary studies with methotrexate and cisplatin suggest they may be effective in disseminated disease.[90]

Table 9-1   **Carcinoma of the Penis: Staging Protocols**

Jackson Protocol[88]

Stage I	Tumor confined to glans or prepuce
Stage II	Tumor extension onto penile shaft
Stage III	Metastatic tumor in inguinal lymph nodes (operable)
Stage IV	Metastatic tumor in inguinal lymph nodes (inoperable) or Distant metastases

TNM Protocol[89]

TIS	Carcinoma in situ
T_0	No evidence of primary tumor
T_1	Primary tumor $=$ 2 cm and superficial
T_2	Primary tumor $>$ 2 cm and $<$ 5 cm with minimal invasion
T_3	Primary tumor $>$ 5 cm with deep invasion
T_4	Primary tumor invading adjacent structures
N_0	No palpable nodes
N_1	Movable enlarged unilateral nodes
N_{1A}	Enlarged unilateral nodes clinically benign
N_{1B}	Enlarged unilateral nodes clinically malignant
N_2	Enlarged bilateral nodes
N_{2A}	Enlarged bilateral nodes clinically benign
N_{2B}	Enlarged bilateral nodes clinically malignant
N_3	Fixed lymph nodes
M_0	No distant metastases
M_1	Distant metastases

Survival is related most closely to the stage of the tumor at initial presentation. The predictive value of tumor grade is unsettled.[73,78,87,94,98] Multiple studies have shown that 43% to 61% of deaths among patients treated for penile carcinoma are not related to the neoplasm per se but are attributed to other causes.[74,76,78,80,99] An average of only 42% of deaths are directly related to the penile carcinoma, its metastases, or the therapy.[74,76,78,80,99] No reported cases of Stage IV penile carcinoma surviving 5 years could be found in the literature.[77,78] A range of 27% to 50% of Stage III patients survive 5 years.[75–78,99] Wajsman and associates reported that the mean survival of Stage III patients was 31 months.[78] de Kernion reported a 67% 3-year survival rate, and Williams reported a 50% survival of clinical Stage II patients.[77,84] Stage I patients have a reported survival range of 53% to 70% at 5 years.[76,77,88,92,99] These low survival rates, most pointedly for Stage I disease, illustrate how limited is our ability to predict the natural history of individual patients with this carcinoma. The surgical pathologist currently contributes little of predictive value beyond making the diagnosis.

Verrucous Carcinoma (Carcinoma-like Condyloma [Bushke-Loewenstein Tumor])

In 1939, Loewenstein reported a penile lesion grossly and cytologically similar to condyloma acuminatum, but demonstrating deep, local invasion.[101] He called this lesion carcinoma-like condyloma. Previously, in collaboration with Bushke, Loewenstein had reported three similar cases in the German literature.[102] This penile lesion was subsequently referred to as a Bushke–Loewenstein tumor, a carcinoma-like condyloma, or simply a giant condyloma in the urologic literature.[103-113]

In 1948, without reference to the histologic similarity to the penile lesion described previously by Bushke and Loewenstein, Ackerman reported 31 patients with an exophytic neoplasm of the oral cavity, which he called verrucous carcinoma.[114] During the next decades, additional reports of exophytic tumors of the oral cavity and genital areas appeared in the literature under the names of verrucous carcinoma and Bushke–Loewenstein tumor, respectively.[103-106,115-117] There is no evidence in this literature that the similarities of clinical behavior and histologic features of the two lesions were recognized. In 1963, Goethels and associates, however, mentioned their similarities.[115] Kraus and Perez–Mesa suggested that the two lesions were identical.[116] Smith and associates were the first to equate verrucous carcinoma and Bushke–Loewenstein tumor without equivocation.[117]

Equating a proliferative epithelial lesion, albeit locally aggressive, regarded benign in the original description and subsequent literature (Bushke–Loewenstein tumor) with an accepted malignant squamous neoplasm (verrucous carcinoma) was not universally accepted.[118] Most, but not all, investigators and authors of surgical pathology and dermatology textbooks, regard the two lesions as synonymous.[119-122]

In the original descriptions of both the Bushke–Loewenstein tumor and verrucous carcinoma, the following features were outlined for each lesion:[101,114]

1. A papillary exophytic epithelial proliferation;
2. A marked tendency to infiltrate deeper tissues with local destruction;
3. Broad, club-shaped papillomatosis, acanthosis, hyperkeratosis, intact

basement membrane, and an underlying chronic inflammatory cell infiltrate (Fig. 9-21);

4. Absence of cytologic atypia at all layers of the epithelium (Fig. 9-22);
5. Tendency to recur following inadequate excision.

These features, as abstracted from the original articles describing these two lesions, are superimposable. This similarity and the absence of any clinical features allowing separation of Bushke-Loewenstein tumor and verrucous carcinoma serve as the basis for regarding the two lesions as synonymous.[101,114] The appropriate term, *verrucous carcinoma,* connotes a cytologically benign, exophytic squamous cell malignancy, consistently and characteristically showing locally aggressive behavior and capable of metastases, as observed in a low percentage of patients. Verrucous carcinomas (Bushke–Loewenstein tumors) may be preceded by, or associated with, ordinary condyloma acuminatum lesions at the site of origin.[106,110] Alternatively, focal areas of cytologic dysplasia, in extent equivalent to carcinoma in situ, may be present adjacent to the main neoplasm.[112] Finally, epithelium within or adjacent to the neoplasm may have the morpho-

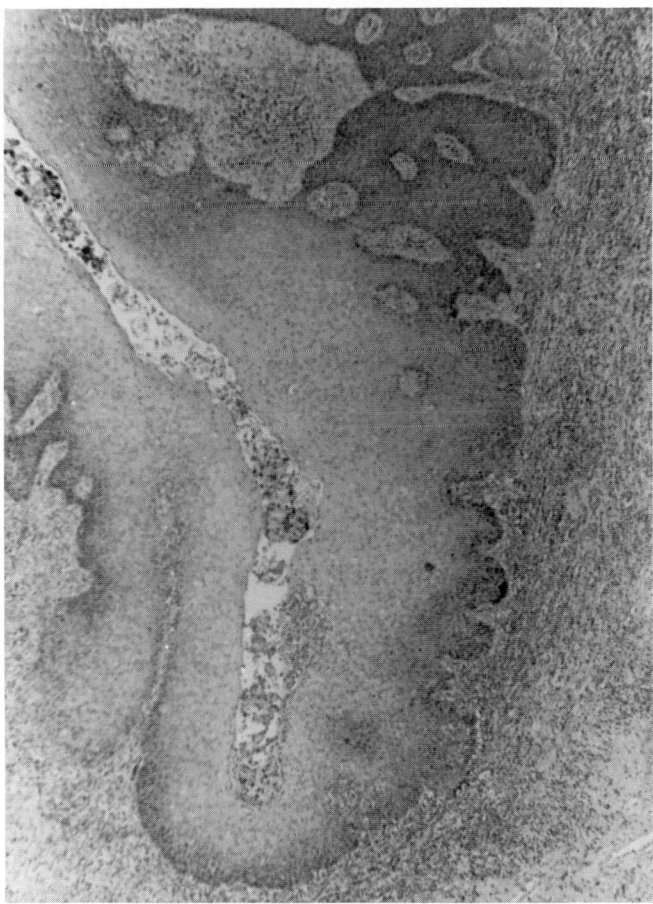

Figure 9-21   *Verrucous carcinoma. The encroaching epithelial neoplasm shows minimal atypia and well-defined interface with the underlying dermis containing numerous chronic inflammatory cells. Minimal cytological atypia is present within the neoplasm.*

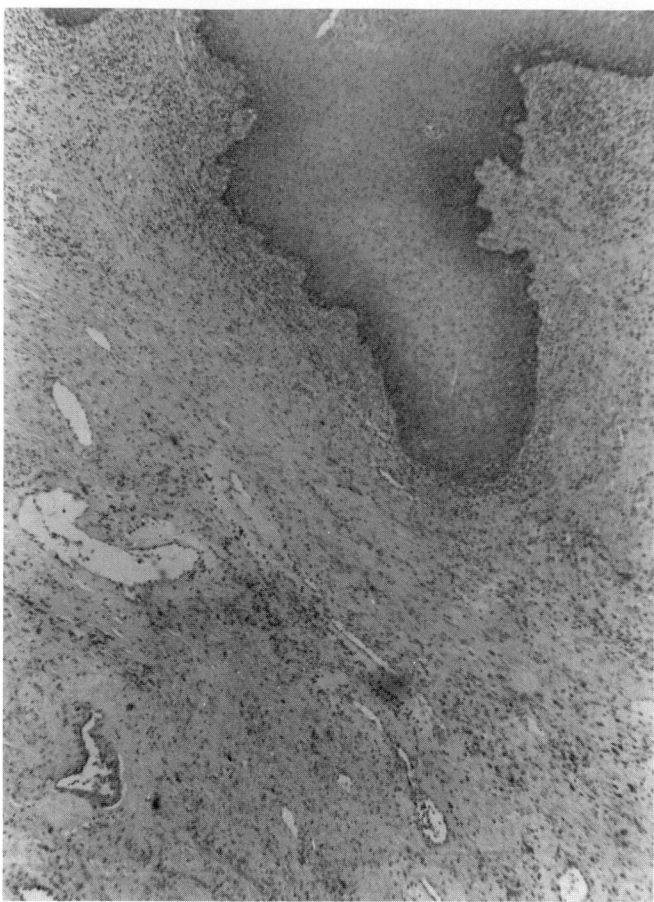

Figure 9-22   *Verrucous carcinoma. The neoplasm encroaches deeply into the penile shaft, compressing vascular channels of the corpus cavernosum.*

logic features of a more typical squamous cell carcinoma with clear evidence of invasion.[103,108,109,111,112,123]

Such foci of more typical (cytologically malignant) squamous cell carcinoma were reported to occur in 20% of a series of otherwise typical verrucous carcinomas of the oral cavity.[124] The emergence of cytologically malignant foci in verrucous carcinoma has been attributed in the past to the effects of radiation therapy.[116,125] The demonstration that this change can occur spontaneously in the absence of prior radiation is prompting a re-evaluation of the role of this form of therapy in the treatment of verrucous carcinoma.[124]

Focal areas of cytologic atypia in association with increased mitosis have also been reported in ordinary condylomas and Bushke – Loewenstein tumors (verrucous carcinomas) following topical treatment with podophyllin.[126] Awareness of this "podophyllin-effect" at the time of microscopic review is important to arrive at an accurate diagnosis and to avoid overinterpretation of such a treated lesion.

As cytologically malignant, "de-differentiated areas" of whatever cause, may be focal, the surgical pathologist's role must include evaluation of all margins for adequacy of excision and extensive sectioning of the neoplasm to identify any possible focal changes divergent from the classically uniformly benign cytologic features typical of verrucous carcinomas.

Finally, in three decades we have only concluded that the Bushke – Loewenstein tumor is synonymous with the low-grade malignant, verrucous carcinoma; the question of etiology remains unanswered.

Spindle Cell Variant

The spindle cell variant of squamous cell carcinoma has been reported to arise on the penis in two patients.[128,129] Manglani and associates demonstrated the epithelial nature of the spindle cells by electron microscopy, confirming previous reports of this histologic variant in the oral cavity.[127,129]

Basal Cell Carcinoma

Basal cell carcinoma, commonly occurring in the head and neck area, rarely originates in the penile and scrotal skin. Eleven cases have been reported on the penis since the original report by Jeck in 1931 (Table 9-2).[130-139] Fourteen cases of scrotal basal cell carcinoma were found in the literature (see Chap. 10). The predilection of this neoplasm for sun-exposed sites has implicated radiation in its causation. Alternative causal factors including prior trauma, dermatitis, and prolonged irritation from a truss have been recorded in some of the patients reported with penile basal cell carcinoma.[133-135,137,138] The age range of the patients is 37 to 78 years. Approximately half of the reported cases were located on the penile shaft and measure 1 cm to 2 cm. The largest lesion, reported by Marsch and Nurnberger, measured 5×2.5 cm.[138] The limited follow-up information reported allows no evidence of recurrence among seven cases from 7 months to 10 years and that no cases have demonstrated metastases from the penile primary site. This is in contrast to metastases occurring in three of the reported 14 cases of scrotal basal cell carcinoma (see Chap. 10).

The histologic picture is typical and characteristic of basal cell carcinomas occurring in the more common locations. Cords and nests of basaloid cells proliferate into the underlying dermis. The neoplastic cells typically have a pe-

Table 9-2   *Basal Cell Carcinoma*

Author	Year	Age	Location
Jeck	1931	67	Meatus
Colon	1952	NI*	NI
Staubitz et al	1955	NI	NI
Kalensky	1960	48	Prepuce
Minami et al	1965	65	Glans
Hartman	1966	48	Shaft
Fox	1966	37	Glans
Hall	1968	43	Shaft
Fegen et al	1970	78	Shaft
Marsch, Nurnberger	1975	79	Shaft
McGregor et al	1982	55	Shaft

* NI — no information

ripheral palisading with lesser degrees of organization in the center of the tumor nests and cords. A desmoplastic response to the invading tumor is typically present in the adjacent dermal stroma. The neoplasm commonly shows central ulceration on the skin surface.

Squamous differentiation of basal cell carcinoma is not uncommon and the differentiation of a basal cell carcinoma with squamous differentiation from a true squamous cell carcinoma can rarely prove to be difficult. Most basal cell carcinomas do not pose a diagnostic challenge.

Malignant Melanoma

In 1924, Joelson reviewed eight patients with penile melanoma reported during the years 1881 to 1924.[140] In the years subsequent, an additional 31 cases have been reported (Table 9-3).[141-165] The age range of all reported patients is 31 to 78 years, although I have seen one primary penile melanoma in an 18-year-old patient. The tumor originates on the glans in patients during the fifth to seventh decades in 80% of the recorded cases. Involvement of the penile shaft has been reported only once.[147] Follow-up information has not been provided for 11 of the 39 reported patients. Fourteen patients died with metastases and only one patient is known to have survived for 5 years.[145]

Unfortunately, only one reported case has been histologically subclassified.[164] Thus, the natural history of each of the histologic variants of melanoma, that is, nodular melanoma, superficial spreading melanoma, and lentigo malignant melanoma when arising in penile skin is unknown. In future cases, histologic subclassification and depth of invasion determination of penile melanomas would be as appropriate in this unusual location as elsewhere.[166]

Paget's Disease

Extramammary Paget's disease involving the penis is rare. In 1937, Weiner's review tabulated only 14 patients reported during the years 1874 to 1937.[167] An additional ten cases, including five cases from an AFIP series have been reported in the more recent literature.[168-172] Most of the reported cases involve men in the seventh and eighth decades. Associated neoplasms with penile Paget's include sweat gland adenocarcinoma and two cases of prostatic carcinoma, one transitional cell and the other adenocarcinoma.[170-172] Penile Paget's disease unaccompanied by other malignancies has been observed.[165] The two patients reported by Fardal and associates survived for 8 and 10 years and ultimately died of metastatic pancreatic carcinoma and recurrent, invasive Paget's disease, respectively.[169] The histogenesis of penile Paget's disease is as controversial as is Paget's disease in all extramammary locations (see Chap. 10).

Mesenchymal Neoplasms

All mesenchymal neoplasms of the penis are rare as reflected in the literature consisting predominantly of case reports and periodic reviews.[173-176] The frequency of malignant neoplasms of mesenchymal origin exceeds benign penile mesenchymal neoplasms. Vascular and smooth muscle and fibrous neoplasms are the most frequent. Most benign mesenchymal neoplasms of the penis occur in the first four decades of life in contrast to their malignant counterparts that are most frequent in the sixth and seventh decades.[176]

Benign Mesenchymal Neoplasms

With the exception of the series of 24 benign penile soft tissue tumors reported from the AFIP by Dehner and Smith, virtually all other available information is obtained from case reports.[176] Vascular neoplasms, both benign and malignant,

Table 9-3   Malignant Melanoma*

Author	Year	Age	Location	Follow-Up
Joelson (8 cases: 1881–1922)	1924	52–75	Glans—6 Prepuce—1 NI—1	4-D/T within 2 yr† 4-NI†
Colby	1929	48	Glans	NI
Wheelock, Clark	1943	49	Glans	NI
Wheelock, Clark	1943	78	Glans	NI
Roberts	1952	62	Glans	A/NED—1 yr†
MacDermott, Kennedy	1955	33	Glans, meatus	D/T—28 mon
Reid	1957	65	Glans, meatus	D/T—12 yr
Buddington et al	1963	65	Coronal sulcus	D/T—2 yr
Sirsat, Shrikande	1965	55	Glans	D/?T—6 mon (no autopsy)
Sirsat, Shrikande	1965	65	Entire penis	NI
Das Gupta, Grabstald	1965	77	Glans	D/?T—14 mon
Das Gupta, Grabstald	1965	59	Prepuce	D/T—8 mon
Schneiderman et al	1965	50	Glans	A/T—23 mon†
Gentil et al	1965	48	Glans	D/T—8 mon
Gentil et al	1965	63	Glans	A/NED—11 mon
Patoria, Junnarkar	1966	35	Glans	Lost to follow-up
Thomas, Fenn	1967	36	Glans	D/T—2 days
Ellis, White	1968	44	Glans	A/NED—21 mon
Fronstin, Hutcheson	1969	70	Glans	D/T—4.5 yr
Fronstin, Hutcheson	1969	66	Glans	A/T—6 mon
Cascinelli	1969	43	Glans	A—8 mon
Troitskii	1971	52	Glans	A/NED—3 yr
Banchieri et al	1971	47	Glans	D/T—4 mon
Gojaseni, Nitiyant	1972	54	Glans	A/NED—2 yr
Bracken, Diokno	1974	45	Glans	A/NED—2 yr
Konigsberg, Gray	1976	59	Glans	D/T—2 yr
Khezri et al	1979	72	Glans	D/T—4 mon
Khezri et al	1979	42	Glans	D/T—13 mon
Crico et al	1980	31	NI	NI
Riveiro, et al	1981	76	Glans	A/?T—3 yr
Jaeger et al	1982	60	Prepuce	A/T—2 yr
Rothenberger et al	1982	61	Glans	D/T—2 yr

* See references 140 to 165.

† NI, no information; D/T, dead with tumors; A/NED, alive, no evidence of disease; A/T, alive with tumor.

develop most frequently in the glans.[176] Both capillary and cavernous heman-giomas have been reported.[176] Neural tumors, both neurofibromas and neuri-lemomas (schwannomas), have been reported in the context of neurofibromato-sis or as solitary lesions.[178-180] Examples of leiomyomas and granular cell tumors have been reported.[172,177] The penile shaft is the most frequent location for the nonvascular neoplasms but all have been observed elsewhere, including the pre-puce.[176] The treatment is complete surgical excision.

Malignant Mesenchymal Neoplasms

Sarcomas of all types taking origin in the penis are rare. In order of decreasing frequency they are angiosarcomas, fibrosarcomas, leiomyosarcomas, Kaposi's sarcoma, followed by all other types. The reported cases in the early literature have been tabulated in extensive reviews by Joelson, Ashley and Edwards, and Abeshouse and associates.[173,174,182] In reviewing the cited reports in these reviews one encounters diagnostic terminology long abandoned and frequently difficult to relate to the current nomenclature of soft-tissue malignancies. Limited micro-scopic descriptions are frequently not supplemented by photomicrographs pre-cluding a critical review of many of the early reports of specific types of sarcomas. A few general observations referable to penile sarcomas can be made from those early reports providing sufficient detail and from the more current literature. They are observed at all ages with a peak frequency in the fifth and sixth decades. With the exception of Kaposi's sarcoma, which is most commonly located in the glans penis, all other sarcomas are most frequently located in the penile shaft. Survival information of long duration is limited, to virtually nonexistent, with only anecdotal reports of patients living beyond 5 years after diagnosis and primary surgical treatment.

Angiosarcoma.   Thirty-two cases of penile angiosarcoma were found in the literature.[176,183-192] The microscopic features are those of angiosarcomas else-where. The application of immunoperoxidase staining for factor VIII, present in normal endothelial cells, is helpful in arriving at the correct diagnosis in the more poorly differentiated cases of angiosarcoma.

Fibrosarcoma.   Twenty-nine cases of fibrosarcoma of the penis were found in the literature.[142,173,175,193-198] Only one patient, cited by Ashley and Edwards, survived 5 years.[169]

Leiomyosarcoma.   Nineteen cases of penile leiomyosarcoma were found in the literature.[173,199-203] These neoplasms arise either deep in the corpus cavern-osum or the smooth muscle of the dermis. As with other penile sarcomas, because of their rarity and the inadequate follow-up information provided in the appro-priate literature, little is known of their natural history. Four patients, known to have died with metastases from their penile leiomyosarcomas, had neoplasms involving the corpus cavernosum at the time of initial diagnosis.[199,202]

Kaposi's Sarcoma.   Ten cases acceptable as Kaposi's sarcoma involving the penis are reported in the literature.[204-211] The case reported by Low and asso-ciates cannot be confirmed upon review of the clinical and pathologic informa-tion provided.[212] The lesions are most commonly red–blue nodules on the glans penis. The correct diagnosis requires microscopic study of a biopsy of the lesion.

Miscellaneous Other Penile Sarcomas. Examples of penile rhabdomyosarcoma, myxosarcoma, neurofibrosarcoma, and malignant schwannoma are noted in the extensive reviews of Ashley and Edwards, Abeshouse and associates, and Dehner and Smith.[173,174,176] Three cases of epithelioid sarcoma, a neoplasm described originally by Enzinger in 1970, have been reported in the penis in recent years.[213-215]

Metastatic Neoplasms

Metastatic neoplasms to the penis are rare.[216-231] Those cases reported in the early literature were tabulated in extensive reviews by McCrea and Tobias and by Abeshouse and Abeshouse.[219,220] The later review found 138 previous reports, with primary neoplasms of the prostate, bladder, and recto-sigmoid constituting approximately 75% of all cases.[220] The scattered case reports published in the more recent literature reflect the distribution of primary sites recorded previously.[221-231] Clinical consequences of such metastases include urinary bladder outlet obstruction, or rarely, priapism.[217,222,225,228,231] In one instance priapism was the initial clinical presentation of a previously occult renal cell carcinoma.[225] Retrograde venous or lymphatic spread has been postulated as the route of most metastatic neoplasms in the penis.[219,220]

References

Normal Structure

1. Morley J, Manch CM: The lymphatics of the scrotum. In relation to the radical operation for scrotal epithelioma. Lancet 2:1545, 1911
2. Daseler EH, Anson BJ, Reiman AF: Radical excision of the inguinal and iliac lymph glands: A study based upon 450 anatomical dissections and upon supportive clinical observations. Surg Gynecol Obstet 87:679, 1948
3. Cabanas RM: An approach for the treatment of penile carcinoma. Cancer 39:456, 1977

Congenital Disorders

4. Richart R, Benirshke, K: Penile agenesis. Arch Pathol 70:752, 1960
5. Johnston WG Jr, Yeatman GW, Weigel JW: Congenital absence of the penis. J Urol 117:508, 1977
6. Schonfeld WA, Beebe GTW: Normal growth and variation in the male genitalia from birth to maturity. J Urol 48:759, 1942
7. Feldman KW, Smith DW: Fetal phallic growth and penile standards for newborn male infants. J Pediatr 86:395, 1975
8. Hinman F: Microphallus: Distinction between anomalous and endocrine types. J Urol 123:412, 1980
9. Seth RE, Peacock AH: Double penis. Urol Cutan Rev 36:590, 1932
10. Nesbit RM, Bromme W: Double penis and double bladder. Am J Roentgenol 30:497, 1933
11. Neff JH: Congenital canals and cysts of the genito-perineal raphe. Am J Surg 31:308, 1936
12. Oshin DR, Bowles WT: Congenital cysts and canals of the scrotal and perineal raphe. J Urol 88:406, 1962

13. Cole LA, Helwig EB: Mucoid cysts of the penile skin. J Urol 115:397, 1976
14. Shah SS, Varea EG, Farsaii A et al: Giant epidermoid cyst of penis. Urol 14:389, 1979

Acquired Cysts

15. Gorro AP, Gamandi AN: Sebaceous cysts of the penis. Urol Cutan Rev 43:195, 1939

Inflammatory Disorders
Sclerosing Lipogranuloma

16. Smetana HF, Bernhard W: Sclerosing lipogranuloma. Arch Pathol 50:296, 1950
17. Marcial–Rojas RA, Colon JE, Figueroa JJ: Sclerosing lipogranulomas in the male genitalia: Report of one case and review of the literature. J Urol 75:334, 1956
18. Oertel YC, Johnson FB: Sclerosing lipogranuloma of male genitalia. Review of 23 cases. Arch Pathol Lab Med 101:321, 1977
19. Holscher AH, Rahlf G, Zimmerman A: Das sklerosierencde lipogranulom des mannlichen genitale. Urolege (Ausg A) 18:106, 1979
20. Winslow PH, Parks S, Whetstone C: Lipogranulomatosis of the genitalia caused by topical application of "baby oil." J Urol 123:127, 1980

Syphilis

21. Lever WF, Schaumburg–Lever G: Histopathology of the Skin, 6th ed., p 320. Philadelphia, JB Lippincott, 1983
22. Jeerapart P, Ackerman AB: Histologic patterns of secondary syphilis. Arch Dermatol 107:373, 1973

Chancroid

23. Sheldon WH, Heyman A: Studies on chancroid. I. Observations on the histology with an evaluation of biopsy as a diagnostic procedure. Am J Pathol 22:415, 1946
24. Lynch PJ: Sexually transmitted diseases: Granuloma inguinale, lymphogranuloma venereum, chancroid, and infectious syphilis. Clin Obstet Gynecol 21:1041, 1978

Granuloma Inguinale

25. Pund ER, Greenblatt RB: Specific histology of granuloma inguinale. Arch Pathol 23:224, 1937
26. Beerman H, Fonk CE: The epithelial changes in granuloma inguinale. Am J Syph 36:501, 1952

Lymphogranuloma Inguinale

27. Smith EB, Custer RP: The histopathology of lymphogranuloma venereum. J Urol 63:546, 1960
28. Schechter J: Chlamydial infection. N Engl J Med 298:428, 1978
29. Johnson WC: Venereal diseases and treponemal infections. In Graham JH, Johnson WC, Helwig EB (eds): Dermal Pathology, p 372. Hagerstown, Harper & Row, 1972

Genital Herpes

30. Young AW: Herpes genitalis. Med Clin North Am 56:1175, 1972
31. Chang TW, Fiumara NJ, Weinstein L: Genital herpes: Some clinical and laboratory observations. JAMA 229:544, 1974
32. Lever WF, Schaumburg–Lever G: Histopathology of the Skin, 6th ed., p 362. Philadelphia, JB Lippincott, 1983

Condyloma Acuminatum

33. zur Hansen H: Human papilloma viruses and their possible role in squamous cell carcinoma. Curr Top Microbiol Immunol 78:1, 1977
34. Gross G, Pfister H, Gagedorn M et al: Correlation between human papillomavirus (HPV) type and histology of warts. J Invest Dermatol 78:160, 1982
35. Almeida JD, Oriel JD, Stannard LM: Characterization of the virus found in human genital warts. Microbios 3:225, 1969
36. Lever WF, Schaumburg – Lever M: Histopathology of the skin, 6th ed., p 373. Philadelphia, JB Lippincott, 1983

Peyronie's Disease

37. Smith BH: Peyronie's disease. Am J Clin Pathol 45:670, 1966
38. Mira JG: Is it worthwhile to treat Peyronie's disease? Urol 16:1, 1980
39. Palomar JM, Halikiopoulos H, Thomas R: Evaluation of the surgical management of Peyronie's disease. J Urol 123:680, 1980
40. Nyberg LM Jr, Bias WB, Hochberg MC, Walsh PC: Identification of an inherited form of Peyronie's disease with autosomal dominant inheritance and association with Dupuytren's contracture and histocompatibility B_7 cross-reacting antigens. J Urol 128:48, 1982

Epithelial Dystrophy: Balanitis Xerotica Obliterans

41. Freeman C, Laymon CW: Balanitis xerotica obliterans. Arch Dermatol Syphil 44:547, 1941
42. Laymon CW, Freeman C: Relationship of balanitis xerotica obliterans to lichen sclerosis et atrophicus. Arch Dermatol Syphil 49:57, 1944
43. Rheinschild GW, Olsen BS: Balanitis xerotica obliterans. J Urol 104:860, 1970
44. Post B, Janner M: Lichen sclerosis et atrophicus of penis. Z Hautkr 50:675, 1975

Malignant Epithelial Neoplasms: Intraepithelial Neoplasia

45. Bowen JT: Precancerous dermatoses: A study of two cases of chronic atypical epithelial proliferation. J Cutan Dis 30:241, 1912
46. Blau S, Hymen AB: Erythroplasia of Queyrat. Acta Derm Venereol (Stockh) 35:341, 1955
47. Queyrat L: Erythroplasie du gland. Bull Soc Fr Dermatol Syphiligr 22:378, 1911
48. Graham JH, Helwig EB: Erythroplasia of Queyrat. Cancer 32:1396, 1973
49. Wade TR, Kopf AW, Ackerman AB: Bowenoid papulosis of the penis. Cancer 42:1890, 1978

Bowen's Disease and Erythroplasia of Queyrat

50. Rosai J: Bowen's disease. In Ackerman's Surgical Pathology, 6th ed, p. 910. St Louis, CV Mosby, 1981
51. Andersen SL, Nielsen A, Reymann F: Relationship between Bowen's disease and internal malignant tumors. Arch Dermatol 108:367, 1973
52. Nordquist RE, Olson RL, Everett MA, Condit PT: Viruslike particles in Bowen's disease. Cancer Res 30:288, 1970

Bowenoid Papulosis

53. Kopf AW, Bart RS: Tumor Conference II: Multiple Bowenoid papules of the penis: A new entity? J Dermatol Surg Oncol 3:265, 1977
54. Berger BW, Hori Y: Multicentric Bowen's disease of the genitalia. Spontaneous regression of lesions. Arch Dermatol 114:1698, 1978
55. Wade TR, Kopf AW, Ackerman B: Bowenoid papulosis of the genitalia. Arch Dermatol 115:306, 1979

56. Zelickson AS, Prawer SE: Bowenoid papulosis of the penis. Demonstration of intranuclear viral-like particles. Am J Dermatopathol 2:305, 1980

57. Kossow AS, Cotelingam JD, MacFarland F: Bowenoid papulosis of the penis. J Urol 125:124, 1981

58. Peters BS, Perry HO: Bowenoid papules of the penis. J Urol 125:482, 1981

Squamous Cell Carcinoma

59. Persky L: Epidemiology of cancer of the penis. Recent results. Cancer Res 60:97, 1977

60. Dodge OG, Lindsell CA: Carcinoma of the penis in Uganda and Kenyan Africans. Cancer 16:1255, 1963

61. Dean AL Jr: Epithelioma of the penis in a Jew who was circumcised in early infancy. Tran Am Ass Genito-Urin Surg 29:493, 1936

62. Marshall VF: Typical carcinoma of the penis in a male circumcised in infancy. Cancer 6:1044, 1953

63. Reitman PH: An unusual case of penile carcinoma. J Urol 69:547, 1953

64. Paquin AJ Jr, Pearce JM: Carcinoma of the penis in a man circumcised in infancy. J Urol 74:626, 1955

65. Amelar RD: Carcinoma of the penis due to trauma occurring in a male patient circumcised at birth. J Urol 75:728, 1956

66. Ledlie RCB, Smithers DW: Carcinoma of the penis in a man circumcised in infancy. J Urol 76:756, 1956

67. Kaufman JJ, Sternberg TH: Carcinoma of the penis in a circumcised man. J Urol 90:449, 1963

68. Melmad EP, Pyne JR: Carcinoma of the penis in a Jew circumcised in infancy. Br J Surg 54:729, 1967

69. Leiter E, Lefkovitis AM: Circumcision and penile carcinoma. NY State J Med 75:1520, 1975

70. Thomas JA: Penile carcinoma and viruses. J Urol 128:307, 1982

71. Kossow JA, Hotchkiss RS, Morales PA: Carcinoma of the penis treated surgically: Analysis of 100 cases. Urol 2:169, 1973

72. Staubitz WJ, Lent MH, Oberkircher OJ: Carcinoma of the penis. Cancer 8:371, 1955

73. Hanash KA, Furlow WL, Utz DC, Harrison EG Jr: Carcinoma of the penis: A clinopathologic study. J Urol 104:291, 1970

74. Hardner GJ, Bhanalaph T, Murphy GP et al: Carcinoma of the penis: Analysis of therapy in 100 consecutive cases. J Urol 108:428, 1972

75. Lenowitz H, Graham A: Carcinoma of the penis. J Urol 56:458, 1946

76. Derrick FC Jr, Lynch KM Jr, Kretkowski RC, Yarbrough WJ: Epidermoid carcinoma of the penis: Computer analysis of 87 cases. J Urol 110:303, 1973

77. Williams JL: Surgical treatment. Proc Roy Soc Med 68:781, 1975

78. Wajsman Z, Moore RH, Merrin CE, Murphy GP: Surgical treatment of penile cancer. A follow-up report. Cancer 40:1697, 1977

79. Orr PS, Habeshaw T, Scott R: Carcinoma of the penis: A review of 42 cases. Br J Urol 49:733, 1977

80. Narayana AS, Olney LE, Loening SA et al: Carcinoma of the penis. Cancer 49:2185, 1982

81. Thomas JA, Small CS: Carcinoma of the penis in Southern India. J Urol 107:273, 1972

82. Beggs JH, Spratt JS: Epidermoid carcinoma of the penis. J Urol 91:166, 1964

83. Harrison CH: Carcinoma of the penis. J Urol 67:326, 1952

84. deKernion JB, Tynberg P, Persky L, Fegen JP: Carcinoma of the penis. Cancer 32:1256, 1973

85. Furlong JH Jr, Uhle CAW: Cancer of penis: A report of eighty-eight cases. J Urol 69:550, 1953
86. Pointon RCS: Discussion. Proc Roy Soc Med 68:779, 1975
87. Frew IDO, Jefferies JD, Swinney J: Carcinoma of penis. Br J Urol 39:398, 1967
88. Jackson SM: The treatment of carcinoma of the penis. Br J. Surg 53:33, 1966
89. Union Internationale Contra le Cancer: TNM classification for malignant tumors. Geneva, International Union Cancer Conference, 1968
90. Merrin CE: Cancer of the penis. Cancer 45:1973, 1980
91. Hoppmann HJ, Fraley EE: Squamous cell carcinoma of the penis. J Urol 120:393, 1978
92. Khezri A, Dunn M, Smith JB, Mitchell A: Carcinoma of the penis. Br J Urol 50:235, 1978
93. Edwards R, Sawyers J: The management of carcinoma of the penis. South Med J 61:843, 1968
94. Baker BH, Spratt JS Jr, Perez–Musa C et al: Carcinoma of the penis. J Urol 116:458, 1976
95. Yu H, Lam P, Lwons CH, Ong GB: Carcinoma of the penis: Report of 52 cases with reference of lymphography and ilioinguinal block dissection. Clin Oncol 4:47, 1978
96. Cosgrove MD, Metzger CK: Lymphangiography in the genitourinary tract. J Urol 113:93, 1975
97. Krieg RM, Luk KH: Carcinoma of the penis. Review of the cases treated by surgery and radiation therapy 1960–1977. Urol 18:149, 1981
98. Bassett JW: Carcinoma of the penis. Cancer 5:530, 1952
99. Skinner DG, Leadbetter WF, Kelley SB: The surgical management of squamous cell carcinoma of the penis. J Urol 107:273, 1972
100. Perinetti E, Crane DB, Catalona WJ: Unreliability of sentinel lymph node biopsy for staging penile carcinoma. J Urol 124:734, 1980

Verrucous Carcinoma

101. Loewenstein LW: Carcinoma-like condylomata acuminate of the penis. Med Clin North Am 23:789, 1939
102. Buschke A, Loewenstein LW: Uber Carcinomahnliche Condylomata Acuminata. Klin Wochenschr 4:1726, 1925
103. Sims DF, Garb J: Giant condylomata acuminata of the penis associated with metastatic carcinoma of the right inguinal lymph node. Arch Dermatol Syphilol 63:103, 1951
104. Gersh I: Giant condylomata acuminata (carcinoma-like condylomata or Buschke–Loewenstein tumors) of the penis. J Urol 69:164, 1953
105. Dreyfuss W, Neville WE: Bushke–Loewenstein tumors (giant condylomata acuminata). Am J Surg 90:146, 1955
106. Lepow H, Leffler N: Giant condylomata acuminata (Bushke–Löwenstein tumor): Report of two cases. J Urol 83:853, 1960
107. Machacek GF, Weakley DR: Giant condylomata acuminata of Buschke and Löwenstein. Arch Dermatol 82:41, 1960
108. Davies SW: Giant condyloma acuminata: Incidence among cases diagnosed as carcinoma of the penis. J Clin Pathol 18:142, 1965
109. Dawson DF, Duckworth JK, Bernhardt H, Young JM: Giant condyloma and verrucous carcinoma of the genital area. Arch Pathol 79: 225, 1965
110. Bulkley G, Wendel R, Grayhack J: Buschke–Loewenstein tumor of the penis. J Urol 97:731, 1967
111. Rhatigan DW, Jimenez S, Chopskie DJ: Condyloma acuminatum and carcinoma of the penis. South Med J 65:423, 1972

112. Schmauz R, Findlay M, Lalwak A et al: Variation in the appearance of giant condyloma in a Ugandan series of cases of carcinoma of the penis. Cancer 40:1686, 1977
113. Hull MT, Eble JN, Priest JB, Mulcahy JJ: Ultrastructure of Buschke–Loewenstein tumor. J Urol 126:485, 1981
114. Ackerman LV: Verrucous carcinoma of the oral cavity. Surgery 23:670, 1948
115. Goethals PL, Harrison EG, Devine KD: Verrucous squamous carcinoma of the oral cavity. Am J Surg 106:845, 1963
116. Kraus FT, Perez–Mesa C: Verrucous carcinoma. Clinical and pathologic study of 105 cases involving oral cavity, larynx and genitalia. Cancer 19:26, 1966
117. Smith RB, Young HH II, Chaffey BT: Verrucous carcinoma of the penis: Report of a case and review. Br J Urol 41:327, 1969
118. Mostofi FK, Price EB: Tumors of the male genital system. In Atlas of Tumor Pathology, Second Series, Fascicle 8, p 273. Washington, D.C., AFIP, 1973
119. Hudson HC, Holcomb FL, Gates W: Giant condyloma acuminatum of the penis: Case reports and review. J Urol 110:301, 1973
120. Tessler AN, Applebaum SM: The Buschke–Loewenstein tumor. Urol 20:36, 1982
121. Rosai J: Verrucous carcinoma. In Ackerman's Surgical Pathology, 6th ed., p. 912. St Louis, CV Mosby, 1981
122. Lever WF, Schaumburg–Lever G: Histopathology of the Skin, 6th ed., p 377. Philadelphia, Lippincott 1983
123. Boxer RJ, Skinner DG: Condylomata acuminata and squamous cell carcinoma. Urol 9:72, 1977
124. Medina JE, Dichtel W, Luna MA: Verrucous-squamous carcinoma of the oral cavity: a clinicopathologic study of 104 cases. Arch Otolaryngol 110:437, 1984
125. Proffitt SD, Spooner TR, Kosek JC: Origin of undifferentiated neoplasm from verrucous epidermal carcinoma of oral cavity following irradiation. Cancer 26:389, 1970
126. Sullivan V, King LS: Effects of resin of podophyllum on normal skin, condylomata acuminata and verrucae vulgares. Arch Dermatol Syphilol 56:30, 1947

Spindle Cell Variant

127. Leifer C, Miller AS, Putong PB, Min BH: Spindle cell carcinoma of the oral mucosa. A light and electron microscopic study of apparent sarcomatous metastasis to cervical lymph nodes. Cancer 34:597, 1974
128. Wood EW, Gardner WA Jr, Brown FM: Spindle cell squamous carcinoma of the penis. J Urol 107:990, 1972
129. Manglani KS, Manaligod RJ, Ray B: Spindle cell carcinoma of the glans penis: A light and electron microscopic study. Cancer 46:2266, 1980

Basal Cell Carcinoma

130. Jeck HS: Unusual tumor of the penis. Trans Am Assoc Genito-Urin Surg 24:315, 1931
131. Colon JE: Carcinoma of the penis. J Urol 67:702, 1952
132. Staubitz WJ, Melbourne HL, Oberkircher OJ: Carcinoma of the penis. Cancer 8:371, 1955
133. Kalensky J: Bazocelularni karcinom predkozky, vznikly po poranemi Cesk Derm 35:115, 1960
134. Minami T, Chino I, Miki M, Kobayashi C: Carcinoma of the penis: Report of two cases and review of the record for the past ten years at the Jikei University Hospital. Acta Urol Jap 11:321, 1965
135. Fox JM: Basal cell epithelioma of the glans penis. Arch Dermatol 94: 807, 1966
136. Hall TC, Britt DB, Woodhead DM: Basal cell carcinoma of the penis. J Urol 99:314, 1968

137. Fegen JP, Beebe D, Persky L: Basal cell carcinoma of the penis. J Urol 104:864, 1970
138. Marsch WC, Nurnberger F: Zur Frage der Haufigkeit des Penisbasalioms. Z Hautkr 50:413, 1975
139. McGregor DH, Tanimura A, Weigel JW: Basal cell carcinoma of penis. Urol 20:320, 1982

Melanoma

140. Joelson JJ: Primary sarcoma of the penis. Report of a case with a review of the literature. Surg Gyn Obstet 38:150, 1924
141. Colby FH: Melanotic sarcoma of the penis. Report of a case. N Engl J Med 201:924, 1929
142. Wheelock MC, Clark PJ: Sarcoma of the penis. J Urol 49:478, 1943
143. Roberts KI: Massive malignant melanoma of the penis occurring in a Malay. Br J Surg 39:561, 1952
144. MacDermott EN, Kennedy JD: A case of melanoblastoma of the penis. Br J Surg 43:213, 1955
145. Reid JD: Melanocarcinoma of the penis. Report of a case. Cancer 10:359, 1957
146. Buddington WT, Kickham CJE, Smith WE: An assessment of malignant disease of the penis. J Urol 89:442, 1963
147. Sirsat MV, Shrikande SS: Malignant melanoma of the penis in Indians. (A report of 2 cases). Indian J Pathol Bacteriol 8:237, 1965
148. Das Gupta T, Grabstald H: Melanoma of the genitourinary tract. J Urol 93:607, 1965
149. Schneiderman C, Simon MS, Levine RM: Malignant melanoma of the penis. J Urol 93:615, 1965
150. Gentil F, Wilson E, Abrao A: Melanoma de penis. Relato de 2 casos. Rev Bras Cir 50:183, 1965
151. Patoria NK, Junnarkar RV: Malignant melanoma of the penis. Report of a case. Indian J Cancer 3:37, 1966
152. Thomas JA, Fenn AS: Malignant melanoma of the penis. (A report of a case and a review of literature.) Indian J Pathol Bacteriol 10:372, 1967
153. Ellis H, White WF: Malignant melanoma of the penis: Endolymphatic therapy with [131]I Lipiodol. Br J Surg 55:238, 1968
154. Cascinelli N: Melanoma maligno del pene. Tumori 55:313, 1969
155. Fronstin MH, Hutcheson JB: Malignant melanoma of the penis: A report of two cases. Br J Urol 41:324, 1969
156. Banchieri FR, Gallizia G, Grandinetti C: Un cas de melanome primitif du penis. J Urol Nephrol 77:138, 1971
157. Troitskii OA: Melanoma of the penis. Urolog Nephrol 36:61, 1971
158. Gojaseni P, Nitiyant P: Malignant melanoma of the penis. Report of a case treated by surgery and chemotherapy. Br J Urol 44:143, 1972
159. Bracken RB, Kiokno AC: Melanoma of the penis and the urethra: 2 case reports and review of the literature. J Urol 11:188, 1974
160. Konisgberg H, Gray GF: Benign melanosis and malignant melanoma of penis and male urethra. Urol 7:323, 1976
161. Khezri AA, Dounis A, Roberts JBM: Primary malignant melanoma of the penis. Two cases and a review of the literature. Br J Urol 51:147, 1979
162. Cricco RP, Lindert DJ, Belis JA: Carcinoma of the penis. South Med J 73:758, 1980
163. Riveiro AP, Sanchez MG, Barreiro JCM et al: Melanoma maligno primitivo de pene. Consederaciones a proposito de un caso. Arch Esp Urol 1:73, 1981
164. Jaeger N, Wirtler H, Tschubel K: Acral lentiginous melanoma of the penis. Eur Urol 8:182, 1982
165. Rothenberger K, Hofstetter A, Pensel J, Keiditsch E: Neodym–YAG–lase–behandlung maligner tumoren des penis. Fortschr Med 100:1806, 1982

166. Clark WH, From L, Bernadino EA, Mihm MC: The histogenesis and biologic behavior of primary human malignant melanomas of the skin. Cancer Res 29:705, 1969

Paget's Disease

167. Weiner HA: Paget's disease of the skin and its relation to carcinoma of the apocrine sweat glands. Am J Cancer 31:373, 1937
168. Helwig EB, Graham JH: Anogenital (extramammary) Paget's disease. A clinico-pathological study. Cancer 16:387, 1963
169. Fardal RW, Kierland RR, Clagett OT, Woolner LB: Prognosis in cutaneous Paget's disease. Postgrad Med 36:584, 1964
170. Ikezawa Z, Ohashi Y, Nakajima H et al: An unusual case of extramammary Paget's disease. Paget's disease of the glans penis probably originating from a prostatic duct carcinoma (transitional cell carcinoma of the prostata). J Dermatol 4:19, 1977
171. Merino MJ, Livolsi VA, Lytton B: Penile Paget's disease and prostatic carcinoma. J Urol 120:121, 1978
172. Mitsudo S, Nakanishi I, Koss LG: Paget's disease of the penis and adjacent skin. Arch Pathol Lab Med 105:518, 1981

Mesenchymal Neoplasms

173. Ashley DJB, Edwards EC: Sarcoma of the penis. Leiomyosarcoma of the penis: Report of a case with a review of the literature on sarcoma of the penis. Br J Surg 45:170, 1957
174. Abeshouse BS, Abeshouse GA, Goldstein AE: Sarcoma of the penis, a review of the literature and a report of a new case; and a brief consideration of melanoma of the penis. Urol Int 13:273, 1962
175. Tripathi VNP, Dick VS: Primary sarcoma of the urogenital system in adults. J Urol 101:898, 1969
176. Dehner LP, Smith BH: Soft tissue tumors of the penis. A clinicopathologic study of 46 cases. Cancer 25:1431, 1970

Benign

177. Haines CE Jr, Garvey FK: Neurosarcoma of penis associated with multiple neurofibromatosis (Von Recklinghausen's Disease). J Urol 63:542, 1950
178. Elliott FG, Eid TC, Lakey WH: Genitourinary neurofibromas: Clinical significance. J Urol 125:725, 1981
179. Das Gupta TK, Brasfield RD, Strong EW, Hajdu SI: Benign solitary schwannomas (neurilemomas). Cancer 24:355, 1969
180. Marsidi PJ, Winter CC: Schwannoma of penis. Urol 16:303, 1980
181. Stone NN, Sun C–C, Brutscher S, Zein T: Granular cell tumor of penis. J Urol 130:575, 1983

Malignant

182. Joelson JJ: Primary sarcoma of the penis. Report of a case with a review of the literature. Surg Gyn Obstet 38:150, 1924

Angiosarcoma

183. Varney DC: Malignant hemangio-endothelioma of the urethra: A case report. J Urol 73:691, 1955
184. Kovacz J, Crouch RD: Sarcoma of the penis. J Urol 80:43, 1958
185. Barnett CP, Low JR: Hemangioendothelioma of the corpus cavernosum penis: Case report. J Urol 83:160, 1960
186. Mecenas HJ, Woodruff MW: Hemangio-endothelioma of the male genitalia. J. Urol 87:560, 1962

187. Garcia AE, Moserrat JM, Martin GG: Hemangioma del pene. Rev Argent de Urol Y Nefrol 37:7, 1968
188. Hodgins TE, Hancock RA: Remangio-endothelial sarcoma of the penis: Report of a case and review of the literature. J Urol 104:867, 1970
189. Deutsch M, Leen RLS, Mercado R Jr: Hemangioendothelioma of the penis with late appearing metastases: Report of a case with review of the literature. J Surg Oncol 5:27, 1973
190. Williams JJ, Mouradian JA, Hagopian M, Gray GF: Hemangioendothelial sarcoma of penis. Cancer 44:1146, 1979
191. Wasmer JM, Block NL, Politano VA, Tejada F: Penile angiosarcoma presenting in bladder. Urol 18:179, 1981
192. Ghandur–Mnaymneh L, Gonzalez MS: Angiosarcoma of the penis with hepatic angiomas in a patient with low vinyl chloride exposure. Cancer 47:1318, 1981

Fibrosarcoma

193. Ju DMC: Fibrosarcoma arising in surgical scars. Plast Reconstr Surg 38:429, 1966
194. Nolazco J, Alonso J, Andrade N: Sarcoma primitivo de pene. Rev Argent Urol 38:66, 1969
195. Das Gupta OP, Chaplot GS, Dube MK: Fibrosarcoma of penis. Indian J Cancer 9:182, 1972
196. Tanimura A, Shigamatsu S, Adachi K, Kobayashi H: Fibrosarcoma of glans penis — case report and review of the literature. Jap J Cancer Clin 21:432, 1975
197. Lue TF, Macchia RJ, Vuletin JC, Rosen Y: Fibrosarcoma of penis. Urol 15:498, 1980
198. Wilson LS, Lockhart JL, Bergman H, Politano VA: Fibrosarcoma of the penis: Case report and review of the literature. J Urol 129:606, 1983

Leiomyosarcoma

199. Greenwood N, Fox H, Edwards EC: Leiomyosarcoma of the penis. Cancer 29:481, 1972
200. Hamal AB: Leiomyosarcoma of the penis — case report and review of the literature. Br J Urol 47:319, 1975
201. Blath RA, Manley CB: Leiomyosarcoma of the prepuce. J Urol 115:220, 1976
202. Elem B, Nieslanik J: Leiomyosarcoma of the penis. Case report. Br J Urol 51:46, 1979
203. Weinberger GI, Wajsman Z, Beckley S, Simpson CL: Primary sarcoma of penis. Urol 19:193, 1982

Kaposi's Sarcoma

204. Barringer BS, Dean AL Jr: Kaposi's disease of the penis. Report of two cases. Trans Am Assoc Genitourin Surg 28:409, 1935
205. Newman BA: Multiple idiopathic hemorrhagic sarcoma (Kaposi) producing urethral stricture. Arch Dermatol Syphil 47:293, 1943
206. McCarthy WD, Pack GT: Malignant blood vessel tumors. A report of 56 cases of angiosarcoma and Kaposi's sarcoma. Surg Gynecol Obstet 91:465, 1950
207. Hopkins JA, Hudson PB: Kaposi's sarcoma: Penile and scrotal lesions. Br J Urol 25:233, 1953
208. Cox JW, Halprin K, Ackerman AB: Kaposi's sarcoma localized to the penis. Arch Dermatol 102:461, 1970
209. Hayes CW, Clark RM, Politano VA: Kaposi's sarcoma of the penis. J Urol 105:525, 1971
210. Summers JL, Wilkerson JE, Wegryn JF: Conservative therapy for Kaposi's sarcoma of the external genitalia. J Urol 108:287, 1972

211. Girgis AS, Bergman H, Rosenthal H, Solomon L: Unusual penile malignancies in circumcised Jewish men. J Urol 110:696, 1973

212. Low HT, Coakley HE, Shontz WC: Kaposi's sarcoma of the penis. J Urol 72:886, 1954

Miscellaneous Other (Rare) Penile Sarcomas

213. Moore SW, Wheeler JE, Hefter LG: Epithelioid sarcoma masquerading as Peyronie's disease. Cancer 35:1706, 1975

214. Enzinger FM: Epithelioid sarcoma: A sarcoma simulating granuloma. Cancer 26:1029, 1970

215. Iossifides I, Ayala AG, Johnson DE: Epithelioid sarcoma of penis. Urol 14:190, 1979

Metastatic Neoplasms

216. Wattenberg CA: Unusual tumors and secondary carcinomas of the penis. Review of the literature and report of a case. J Urol 44:169, 1944

217. Watson EM, Sauer HR, Sodugor MG: Manifestations of lymphoblastomas in the genito-urinary tract. J Urol 61:626, 1949

218. Paquin AJ, Roland SI: Secondary carcinoma of the penis. A review of the literature and a report of nine new cases. Cancer 9:626, 1956

219. McCrea LE, Tobias GL: Metastatic disease of the penis. J Urol 80:489, 1958

220. Abeshouse BS, Abeshouse GA: Metastatic tumors of the penis: A review of the literature and a report of two cases. J Urol 86:99, 1961

221. Sunderland H: Carcinoma of the penis secondary to carcinoma of the bladder. Br J Urol 33:328, 1961

222. Smith MJV, Banacarti AF: Malignant priapism due to clear cell carcinoma: A case report and review of the literature. J Urol 92:297, 1964

223. Hayes WT, Young JM: Metastatic carcinoma of the penis. J Chronic Dis 20:891, 1967

224. Wolf H, Madsen PO: Metastases to the external genitalia from carcinoma of the prostate: A report of 2 cases. J Urol 99:198, 1968

225. Weisman EB, Hardison JE, Burns JB: Priapism as the initial manifestation of renal carcinoma. Arch Intern Med 123:58, 1969

226. Pond HS, Wade JC: Urinary obstruction secondary to metastatic carcinoma of the penis: A case report and review of the literature. J Urol 102:333, 1969

227. Tan HT, Vishniavsky S: Carcinoma of the prostate with metastases to the prepuce. J Urol 106:588, 1971

228. Spreen SA, Keys RH Jr, Evans A: Acute urinary retention secondary to metastatic prostatic carcinoma to the penis: A case report. J Urol 113:59, 1975

229. Patel NP, Ward JN: Carcinoma of prostate metastatic to prepuce and glans penis. Urol 11:269, 1978

230. Smehaug J: Metastases to the penis from carcinoma of the prostate. A case report. Scand J Urol Nephrol 13:205, 1979

231. Knight EL Jr, Post GJ, Morabito RA et al: Leukenic infiltration of penis. Urol 14:83, 1979

Scrotum

10

Normal Structure

The scrotal sac is composed of seven layers investing the testes, adnexa, and distal spermatic cord. Epidermis covers dermis, the deepest layers of which merge with the smooth muscle bundle of the dartos tunic. No intervening subcutaneous adipose tissue layer is present, although scattered adipose cells are commonly present. The dermal adnexa include hair follicles, apocrine and eccrine sweat glands, and sebaceous glands (Fig. 10-1). Three fascial layers (intercrural, cremasteric, and infundibuliform) are deep to the dartos muscle layer. Each layer is continuous with the fascia of the muscles of the anterior abdominal wall. The innermost layer of the scrotal sac is the parietal vaginalis, a monolayer of mesothelial cells.

The scrotal lymphatics drain to the ipsilateral superficial inguinal lymph nodes in three groups according to their location of origin in the scrotal wall: anterior, lateral and posterior.[1] Anastomotic connections to the lymphatics of the contralateral network across the raphe are present.[1]

Congenital Disorders

Congenital disorders of the scrotal sac are uncommon, and are rarely of clinical significance. They include bifid scrotal sacs and hypertrophy (or pendulous scrotum). Underdevelopment of the scrotal sac accompanies persistent cryptorchidism.

Inflammatory Disorders

Inflammatory disorders of the scrotum are of minor clinical significance in the vast majority of cases. Superficial inflammation of the scrotal skin associated with poor hygiene and chafing do not come to the attention of the surgical

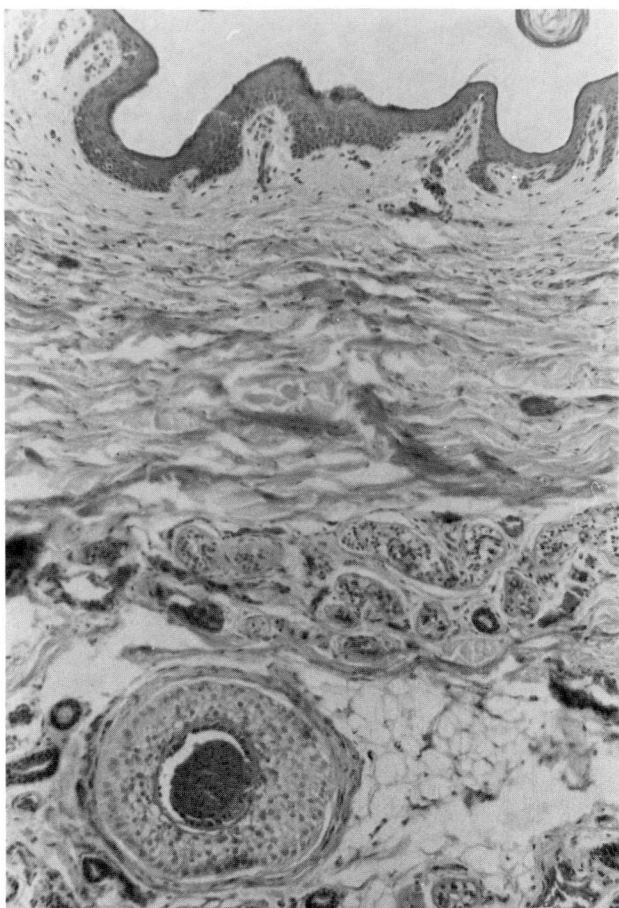

Figure 10-1   *Normal scrotum. The thin scrotal epidermis overlies the dermis that contains the skin appendage structures, including a hair shaft and sweat glands.*

pathologist. Venereal infections primarily involving the penis may show scrotal involvement. These include condyloma acuminatum and herpes genitalis. (See Chap. 9.) Reported cases of hidradenitis suppurativa (due to *Staphylococcus aureus* or *Staphylococcus epidermidis*) and actinomycosis appear in the literature.[2,3]

Sclerosing Lipogranuloma

Petroleum lipids and waxes introduced into the dermis and subcutaneous tissue through the skin elicit a characteristic inflammatory reaction that may be of such magnitude that a localized mass is observed. Most reported patients are younger than 40 years of age. Such lesions, which can attain a size of several centimeters, are firm, frequently tender, and have a greasy cut surface reflecting the lipid component. Histiocytic giant cells in association with lipid vacuoles, with a background of variably dense fibrosis and mixed chronic inflammatory cells, are the characteristic microscopic features. The presence of the lipid is detected by applying oil red-O or other appropriate stains. The lipid vacuoles commonly show a patchy clustering and variability of size. Some vacuoles appear embedded in dense fibrous tissue devoid of significant inflammatory cells, including histiocytes. Smetana and Bernhard introduced the descriptive term *sclerosing lipogranuloma* for such lesions involving either the penis or the scrotum.[4] Previous reports of *paraffinoma* of the genital areas describe an identical histological picture.[5]

The etiology and pathogenesis of this lesion have been the subject of considerable interest.[4,6-8] A definite history of paraffin injection to the local site is obtained from some patients.[5] Oertel and Johnson reported 23 such patients from the Armed Forces Institute of Pathology (AFIP), many of whom had a history of local trauma to the site.[7] Importantly, these authors demonstrated the presence of paraffin hydrocarbons by infrared-absorption spectrophotometry in 21 of the 23 cases, thereby determining conclusively the exogenous nature of the lipid agent inciting the inflammatory reaction. Similar analysis and results were reported more recently by Holscher and associates.[8] The patient reported by these authors had a history of topical application of a paraffin-containing ointment, raising the possibility of percutaneous absorption of paraffin as a possible pathogenetic route in this (and possibly other) cases. (See Chap. 9.)

Treatment is surgical excision of the lesion. Sclerosing lipogranuloma is to be differentiated from traumatic fat necrosis, relapsing nonsuppurative nodular panniculitis, adenomatoid tumors, and lymphangioma.[4,7]

Malignant Epithelial Neoplasms

Squamous Cell Carcinoma

In 1775, Percivall Pott published his observations on "chimney-sweepers cancer," thereby identifying the first occupational group at greater risk of developing carcinoma, in this case, of the scrotal skin.[9] The soot of the chimneys to which the sweeps constantly were exposed was implicated in the cause of scrotal skin cancer. Because no increased frequency of scrotal carcinoma was observed among coal miners, the carcinogenic agents were correctly regarded as products of the combustion of coal.[10] Subsequent studies involving chemical extraction identified numerous specific chemical agents in the chimney soot that demonstrated carcinogenic activity under experimental circumstances.[11-13]

In the latter part of the 19th century and continuing into the 20th, an increasing number of occupations have been identified that apparently increase the risk of developing scrotal carcinoma among workers.[14-23] Men involved in the industrial processing of paraffin, waxes, lubricating oils, metal products (associated with the use of lubricating oils), and cotton and wool spinners (mule spinners) were observed to have an increased frequency of this carcinoma.[14-23] Ray and Whitmore reported an increasing percentage of patients having no prior employment in these high-risk occupations.[24] This contrasts with data from the Connecticut Tumor Registry (1935-1979) showing 77% of 59 patients with prior involvement in an occupation with identified risk.[32] Similar data were reported by Kickham and Dufresne.[25] Among such patients without known occupational exposure, the frequency of scrotal carcinoma was reported higher among workers in low socioeconomic groups than among workers in white-collar and professional occupations.[26] The role of personal hygiene was implicated to explain this observed difference.[26] This neoplasm occurs less frequently in black men than in whites in the United States.[16,19] Although the overall frequency of this skin malignancy appears to be decreasing in both England and the United States, recent data from the Connecticut Tumor Registry indicate no apparent decline in risk for scrotal cancer during the years 1935–1979.[20,21,32]

Clinical Features

Squamous cell carcinoma of the scrotum most frequently is diagnosed in the sixth and seventh decades (Table 10-1). It is rarely observed in patients younger than age 40. The observed age distribution of patients and the tabulated occupational history suggest that the required duration of exposure to carcinogens in the high-risk industries is 10 years to 25 years.[20,28,30] Typically, patients have a scrotal lesion that has enlarged slowly over months, with a more recent onset of discomfort associated with ulceration or bleeding or both. The size varies from millimeters to several centimeters. The lesion is most commonly single and limited to one side of the scrotal sac, with predilection for the anterior inferior surface of the scrotum.[15,17] Southam and Wilson observed that 84% of cases involved the left side; however, others report no side predilection.[15,17,20,24] Approximately half to three quarters of patients will have enlarged inguinal lymph nodes at the time of initial presentation.[24,30,31]

Pathology

Typically, the squamous cell carcinoma is well-differentiated or moderately well-differentiated microscopically (Fig. 10-2). The extent of invasion of the scrotal wall is variable, but most commonly the scrotal contents are not involved. The adjacent epidermis may show hyperkeratosis, acanthosis, and dyskeratosis. Microscopic examination will disclose a reactive lymph node architecture without evidence of metastases in a significant number of patients with clinically enlarged inguinal lymph nodes. Although no currently available formal study relates the size of the primary lesion with the probability of nodal metastases, my experience

Table 10-1   *Squamous Cell Carcinoma*

Author	Year	No. of Patients	Age		Occupational Exposure History	Side Predilection
			Range	*Mean*		
Ray, Whitmore[24]	1977	19	36–76	56	5 (26%)	R = L
Kickham, Dufresne[25]	1967	28*	32–84	NI†	22 (79%)	NI
Tourenc[21]	1964	21	37–81	56	21 (100%)	L > R (65%)
Lione, Denhold[20]	1959	10				R > L (60%)
Dean[30]	1948	27	34–66	56	19 (70%)	NI
Graves, Flo[17]	1940	14	32–76	53	12 (86%)	L = R
Southam, Wilson[15]	1922	141	NI	NI	92 (65%)	L > R (84%)

* Two of 28 patients had basal cell carcinoma.

† NI, no information

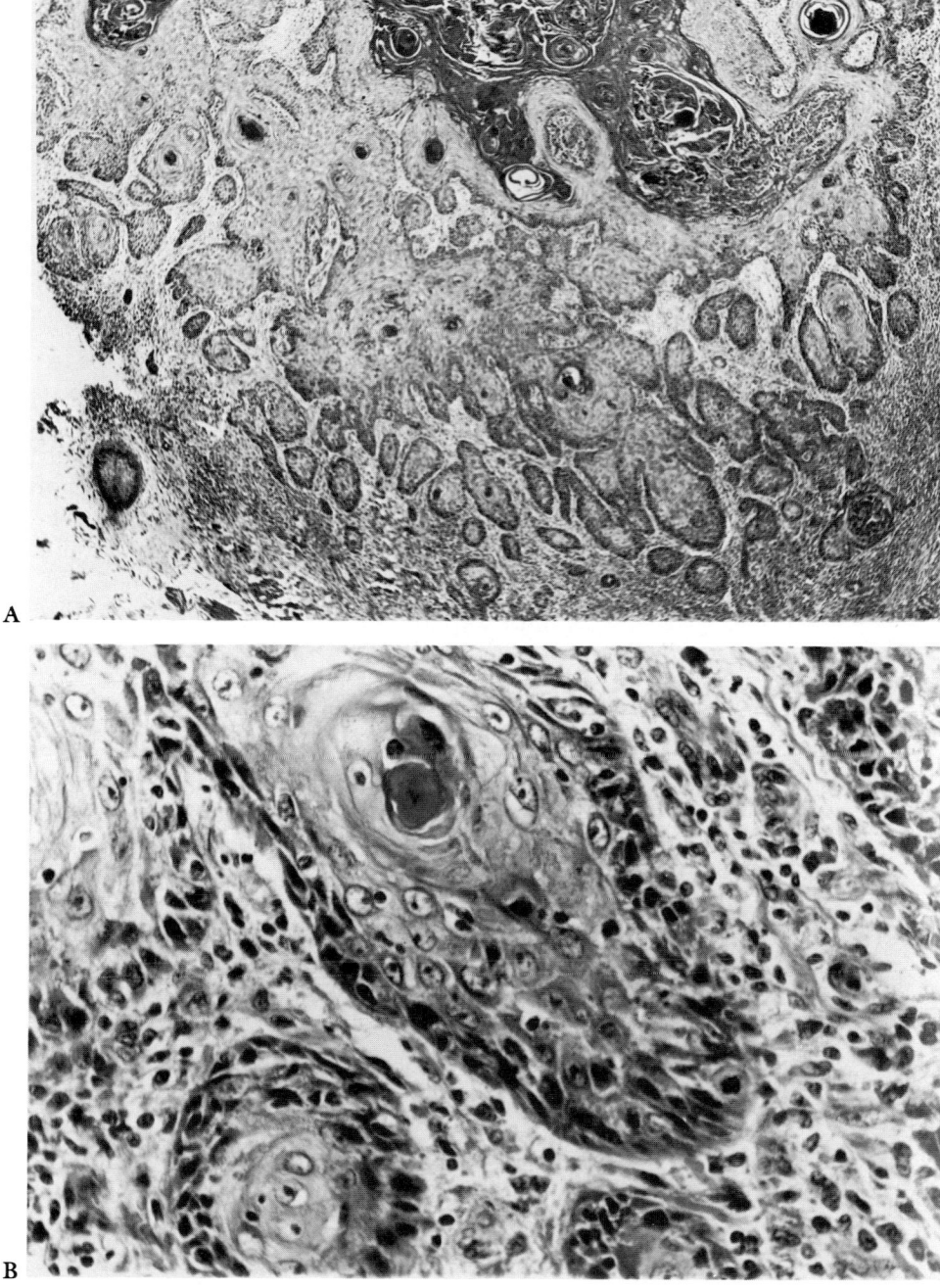

Figure 10-2   **Squamous cell carcinoma.** (A) *The invasive pattern of this well-differentiated squamous cell carcinoma is apparent.* (B) *Higher magnification shows central keratinization of the neoplastic squamous cells.*

and an evaluation of the available literature indicate primary lesions larger than 2 cm have a high risk of associated metastases in the inguinal lymph nodes.

Staging of scrotal carcinomas was not proposed until 1977 by Ray and Whitmore.[24] In 1983, Lowe suggested a modification of the staging protocol, which I have adopted (Table 10-2).[29] The protocol can be used for either clinical or pathologic staging of scrotal carcinoma cases. There is limited information in

Table 10-2 **Staging of Scrotal Carcinoma**

Stage A

    A1   Disease localized to the scrotum

    A2   Locally extensive disease involving adjacent structures (penis, perineum, testis or cord structures, pubic bone) by continuity but without evident metastasis

Stage B

        Regional* metastasis, resectable

Stage C

        Regional metastasis, nonresectable

Stage D

        Distant metastasis (beyond regional nodes)

Ray B, Whitmore Jr WF: Experience with carcinoma of the scrotum. J Urol 117:741, 1977

* Inguinal or ilioinguinal

the available literature referable to stage distribution of scrotal carcinoma; however, clinical stage A1 cases (tumor limited to the scrotal skin) range from 28% to 41% in four reported series.[17,19,24,30] Ray and Whitmore report that 37% of a series of 19 cases were pathologic stage A1.[24]

Treatment and Survival

Surgery remains the principal mode of therapy for scrotal carcinoma. Wide excision of the scrotal skin with split thickness skin grafts for extensive primary lesions is generally employed. Local recurrence (or new primaries) are encountered in 20% to 40% of cases, 5 years to 10 years after the initial surgical therapy.[20,24] Neither radiation nor topical chemotherapy is effective.[31] The appropriateness of inguinal lymph node dissection at the time of primary surgery for scrotal carcinoma remains unsettled.[29] Ray and Whitmore advocate withholding node dissection until there is clinical suspicion of lymph node metastases.[24] As originally described by Morley, the anastomosing pattern of scrotal lymphatics allows for metastases to the contralateral inguinal lymph nodes.[1]

Limited survival data are available. However, two studies report a 65% to 76% 2-year survival rate, and a 22% to 52% 5-year survival rate was reported in three additional studies.[19–21,24,25,30] Lione and Denholme reported an 80% survival rate at 5 years in a series of 10 patients.[20] Ray and Whitmore and McDonald reported lower survival rates associated with increasing clinical stage.[24,31]

Basal Cell Carcinoma

Fourteen basal cell carcinomas involving the scrotal skin have been reported (Table 10-3). Basal cell carcinoma originating in the scrotal skin was first reported by Richter in 1957.[33] Basal cell carcinomas most frequently arise in the head and neck region (80% to 90%).[34] Locally aggressive behavior is not uncommon, but metastases to regional lymph nodes or distant sites have been recorded in fewer than 100 cases.[38] In contrast, 3 patients (21%) among the total of 14 recorded patients with scrotal basal cell carcinoma have demonstrated regional

Table 10-3　　**Basal Cell Carcinoma**

Author	Year	Age	Follow-up
Richter[33]	1957	76	D/T 2 yr, lung metastases
Casal et al[34]	1965	77	A/W 1 yr
Kickham, Dufresne[25]	1967	NI	NI
Kickham, Dufresne[25]	1967	NI	NI
Hughes[35]	1973	47	D/T 2 yr, node metastases
McEleney[37]	1976	60	A/W 3 mon
Ray, Whitmore[24]	1977	NI	NI
Grossman, Sogani[39]	1981	55	A/W 8 mon
Grossman, Sogani[39]	1981	64	A/W 11 yr
McDonald[31]	1982	NI	Lost to follow-up
McDonald[31]	1982	NI	D/no tumor recurrence, 4 yr
McDonald[31]	1982	NI	D/no tumor recurrence, 10 yr
Greider, Vernon[40]	1982	75	A/W 5 mon
Staley et al[41]	1983	58	A/T, node and lung metastases, 2 yr

NI, no information; D/T, dead with tumor; A/W alive and well; A/T, alive with tumor

lymph node or lung metastases (2 patients).[33,36,41] Two of these patients died of their tumor metastases.[33,36] The longest recorded survival without evidence of tumor recurrence following surgical excision is 11 years.[39]

The gross and microscopic features of scrotal basal cell carcinomas show no features unique to the tumor at this site. Nests of basaloid cells taking origin from the epidermis infiltrate the underlying dermis. The nests and cords of tumor cells demonstrate the typical palisading of the peripheral cells with lesser degrees of organization of the more centrally located cells. (Fig. 10-3). The nests and cords may show focal microcyst formation or squamous differentiation. Treatment is surgical excision with wide margins.

Paget's Disease

Since the original description of this neoplasm by Sir James Paget, the histogenesis of the Paget's cells in both mammary and extramammary forms remains unsettled and controversial.[42-49] Histogenetic theories include an unusual form of lymphatic spread of an underlying malignancy to the epidermis; intraepithelial spread of malignant cells from an underlying adnexal carcinoma; or de novo intraepithelial malignant transformation unaccompanied by an underlying or other associated primary malignancy.[42-45] The absence of an associated epithelial malignancy in some cases of Paget's disease can be regarded as more apparent than real, and may simply represent a failure to detect an underlying primary neoplasm. Alternatively, when an associated malignancy is found in a patient with Paget's disease in the skin, it may represent a chance association of two unrelated neoplasms.

Extramammary Paget's disease is uncommon, but is most frequently observed in the anogenital region in women.[43] Scrotal and penile Paget's disease is rare. In a review of the literature in 1937, Weiner accepted only 15 of the

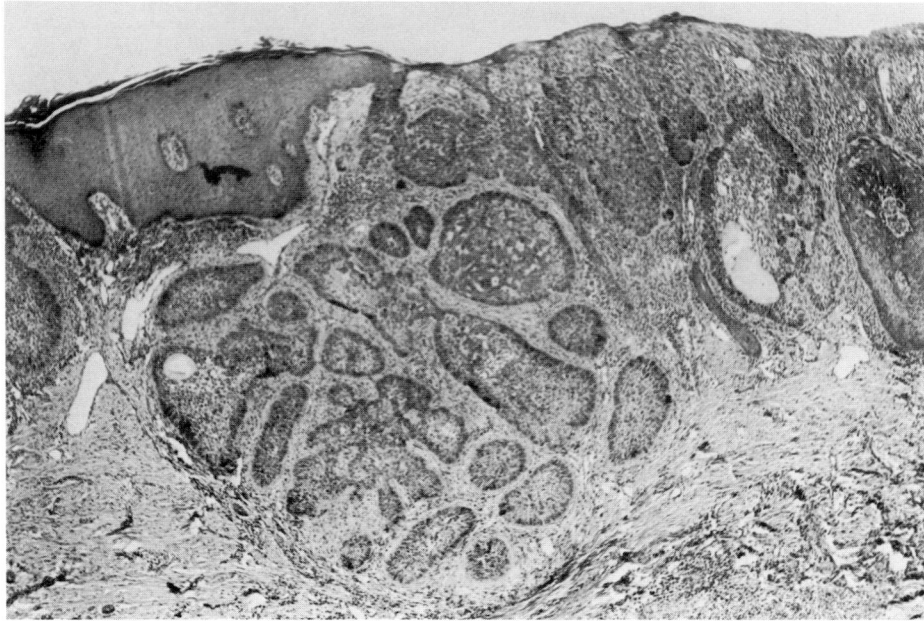

Figure 10-3   **Basal cell carcinoma.** *Basaloid cells proliferate into the underlying dermis with the typical palisading of the tumor cells at the periphery of the nests and cords.*

previously reported 58 cases of extramammary Paget's disease.[43] Only 4 of the 15 cases involved the scrotum. Cases of scrotal Paget's disease reported in the more recent literature are listed in Table 10-4.

Paget's disease of the scrotum is most common in men in the sixth to eighth decades.[43-49] The lesion appears as a slowly enlarging indurated plaque. At the time of initial presentation, it may extend beyond the scrotal skin to involve the penis, anterior abdomen, thigh, and perianal regions.

Microscopically, the Paget's cells appear singly or in clusters within the surface epidermis, typically immediately above the basement membrane at the epidermal–dermal junction (Fig. 10-4). Extension within the epidermis to involve the sheaths of hair shafts may be present. The Paget's cells have abundant cytoplasm showing variable vacuolization. The cytoplasm characteristically

Table 10-4   **Scrotal Paget's Disease**

Author	Year	Patient Age	Survival	Associated Malignancy
Grimes[44]	1959	76	D/T 8 mon*	Prostatic adenocarcinoma
Vermillion, Page[45]	1972	79	A/NED 1 yr	None
Hagan et al[46]	1975	69	D/T 1 mon	None
Feinstein et al[47]	1977	75	A/T	None
Oka et al[48]	1979	65	NI	Prostatic adenocarcinoma
Ueki, Kohda[49]	1979	60	NI	None

* Widespread metastatic prostatic adenocarcinoma present at autopsy

D/T, dead with tumor; A/NED, alive, no evidence of disease; A/T, alive with tumor; NI, no information

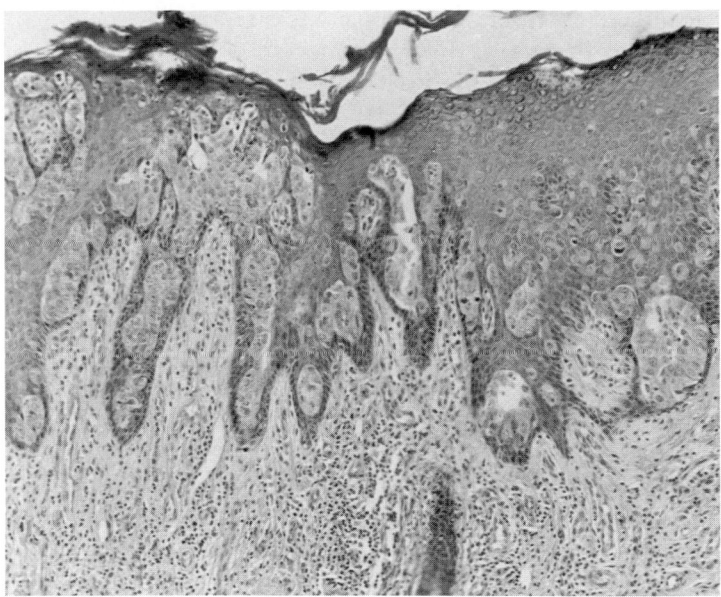

Figure 10-4   *Paget's disease. The enlarged Paget's cells are present in nests adjacent to the basement membrane and single cells scattered throughout the epidermis.*

stains positively with PAS stain (diastase resistant), mucicarmine, and Alcian blue (pH 2.5). Differentiation from melanoma, especially amelanotic melanoma, may pose the greatest diagnostic problem because Paget's cells may contain melanin granules.[50] The mucicarmine stain is especially helpful, because melanoma cells contain no mucin.

Direct invasion of the underlying dermis, when observed, occasionally is associated with regional lymph node metastases.[45]

Treatment is wide surgical excision of the involved scrotal skin. Ultimate survival depends on the extent of the spread of the Paget's disease, and importantly, the clinical evolution of any associated malignancy.[44]

Benign Mesenchymal Neoplasms

Hemangioma

Hemangiomas of the scrotum are rare. The 26 cases reported prior to 1956 are included in reviews by Winslow, Gibson, and Mahoney.[51-53] Eight additional cases have been reported in the more recent literature.[54-62] The peak age frequency of the reported cases is similar to that of lymphangiomas — the third to fifth decades. The age range is newborn to 61 years. Many of the patients report being aware of the lesion years before seeking medical attention. A history of trauma to the scrotum is recorded in some cases.[51] Congenital origin is probable in many cases.

The lesion size varies. Some extend beyond the skin of the scrotum to involve the penis and the thigh. The majority of cases involve the skin of only one side of the scrotum, but extension to the opposite side has been observed.[62] The overlying skin of the smallest lesions has a nonspecific thickened appearance. The larger lesions are typically blue, with evident dilated vascular channels beneath the skin. The arterial supply from the pudendal branches of the femoral artery has been documented.[62]

Most reported cases described the hemangioma to be of the cavernous type. The lesion is located in the high dermis, but extension into the scrotal septum has been reported.[53] Treatment is complete surgical excision.

Lymphangioma

In a review of the world literature, Gueukdjian recorded 15 cases of scrotal lymphangiomas reported from 1829 to 1955.[63] Thirteen additional cases have been reported since then.[64-67] The majority of patients are observed in the third to the fifth decades, although this neoplasm has been reported in the newborn.[63,64] There is evidence that the genesis of these neoplasms is secondary to congenital abnormal development of the local lymphatic communications.[67]

Physical examination suggests an unencapsulated mass, apparently separate from the scrotal contents, involving the dermis of the scrotal skin. The majority are cavernous lymphangiomas with grossly apparent vascular channels present on the cut surface. The endothelial lining cells are flattened, inconspicuous, and without cytologic atypia. The vascular channels are devoid of red blood cells, which assists in differentiating these vascular neoplasms from hemangiomas. The malignant counterpart, lymphangiosarcoma, has not been reported in the scrotum. Treatment is complete surgical excision.

Malignant Mesenchymal Neoplasms

Most so-called scrotal sarcomas are actually intrascrotal in origin, arising from the spermatic cord, epididymis, or the enclosing tunics.[68] Only rare examples of rhabdomyosarcoma, leiomyosarcoma, and liposarcoma originating in the scrotal wall have been reported.[69,70]

References

Normal

1. Morley J, Manch CM: The lymphatics of the scrotum: In relation to the radical operation for scrotal epithelioma. Lancet 2:1545, 1911

Inflammatory Disorders

2. Ray B: Hidradenitis suppurativa of the scrotum. J Urol 118:686, 1977
3. Sarosdy MF, Brock WA, Parsons CL: Scrotal actinomycosis. J Urol 121:256, 1979

Sclerosing Lipogranuloma

4. Smetana HF, Bernhard W: Sclerosing lipogranuloma. Arch Pathol 50:296, 1950
5. Brown AF, Joergenson EJ: Genital mammary paraffin oil granulomas in the male. Ann West Med Surg 1:301, 1947
6. Marcial-Rojas RA, Colon JE, Figueroa JJ: Sclerosing lipogranulomas of the male genitalia: Report of one case and review of the literature. J Urol 75:334, 1956

7. Oertel YC, Johnson FB: Sclerosing lipogranuloma of male genitalia: Review of 23 cases. Arch Pathol Lab Med 101:321, 1977
8. Holscher AH, Rahlf G, Zimmerman A: Das sklerosierencde lipogranulom des mannlichen genitale. Urologe 18:106, 1979

Malignant Epithelial Neoplasms
Squamous Cell Carcinoma

9. Pott P: Cancer scroti. In Humes L, Clarke W, Collins R: Chirurgical Works, Vol 5, p 63. London, Longman, 1775
10. Paget J: Chimney sweep's cancer affecting primarily the inguinal glands: Excision and recovery. M Times and Gaz, NS 5:414, 1952. Surgical Pathology, Philadelphia, p 629, 1865
11. Passey RD: Experimental soot cancer. Br Med J 2:1112, 1922
12. Leitch A: The experimental inquiry into the causes of cancer. Br Med J 2:1, 1923
13. Twort CC, Fulton JD: Experiments on the nature of the carcinogenic agents in mineral oils. J Pathol Bact 32:149, 1929
14. Schamberg JJ: Cancer in tar workers. J Cutan Dis 28:644, 1910
15. Southam AH, Wilson SR: Cancer of the scrotum: The etiology, clinical features and treatment of the disease. Br Med J 2:971, 1922
16. Wilson SR: Cancer in cotton mule-spinners. Br Med J 2:993, 1927
17. Graves RC, Flo S: Carcinoma of the scrotum. J Urol 43:309, 1940
18. Brockbank EM: Mule-spinners' cancer. Br Med J 1:622, 1941
19. Cruickshank CND, Squire JR: Skin cancer in the engineering industry from the use of mineral oil. Br J Ind Med 7:1, 1950
20. Lione JG, Denholm JS: Cancer of the scrotum in wax pressmen: II. Clinical observations. Arch Ind Health 199:530, 1959
21. Tourenc R: Le cancer du scrotum chez les decolleteurs (Apropos de 21 cas). Presse Medic 72:2009, 1964
22. Avellon L, Breine U, Jacobson B et al: Carcinoma of the scrotum induced by mineral oil. Scand J Plast Reconstr Surg 1:135, 1967
23. Roush GC, Kelly JA, Meigs JW et al: Scrotal carcinoma in Connecticut metalworkers. Am J Epidemiol 116:76, 1982
24. Ray B, Whitmore Jr WF: Experience with carcinoma of the scrotum. J Urol 117:741, 1977
25. Kickham CJE, Dufresne M: An assessment of carcinoma of the scrotum. J Urol 98:108, 1967
26. Kennaway EL, Kennaway NM: The social distribution of cancer of the scrotum and cancer of the penis. Cancer Res 6:49, 1946
27. Tucci P, Haralambidis G: Carcinoma of the scrotum: Review of literature and presentation of 2 cases. J Urol 89:585, 1963
28. Henry SA: The study of fatal cases of cancer of the scrotum from 1911 to 1935 in relation to occupation, with special reference to chimney sweeping and cotton mule spinning. Am J Cancer 31:28, 1937
29. Lowe FC: Squamous cell carcinoma of the scrotum. J Urol 130:423, 1983
30. Dean AL: Epithelioma of scrotum. J Urol 61:508, 1948
31. McDonald MW: Carcinoma of scrotum. Urol 19:269, 1982
32. Roush GC, Schymura MJ, Flannery JT: Secular and age distribution of scrotal cancer in Connecticut and a review of United States literature. Cancer 54:596, 1984

Basal Cell Carcinoma

33. Richter G: Subpleurale lungenmetastass bei sog. Basalzellen-carcinoma. Hautarzt 8:215, 1957
34. Lever WF, Schaumberg-Lever G: Histopathology of the skin, 6th ed, pp 562–575. Philadelphia, JB Lippincott, 1983

35. Casal J, Solari JJ, Monserrat JM: Epitelioma del escroto. Rev Argent Urol 34:661, 1965
36. Hughes JM: Metastatic basal cell carcinoma: A report of two cases and a review of literature. Clin Radiol 24:392, 1973
37. McEleney DA: Basal cell carcinoma of the scrotum. Cutis 18:227, 1976
38. Mikhail GR, Nims LP, Kelley Jr AP et al: Metastatic basal cell carcinoma. Review, pathogenesis, and report of two cases. Arch Dermatol 113:1261, 1977
39. Grossman HB, Sogani PC: Basal cell carcinoma of scrotum. Urol 17:241, 1981
40. Greider HD, Vernon SE: Basal cell carcinoma of the scrotum: A case report and literature review. J Urol 127:145, 1982
41. Staley TE, Nieh PT, Ciesielski TE et al: Metastatic basal cell carcinoma of the scrotum. J Urol 130:792, 1983

Paget's Disease

42. Paget J: On disease of the mammary areola preceding cancer of the mammary gland. St. Barth Hosp Rep 10:87, 1874
43. Weiner HA: Paget's disease of the skin and its relation to carcinoma of the apocrine sweat glands. Am J Cancer 31:373, 1937
44. Grimes OF: Extramammary Paget's disease. Surgery 45:569, 1959
45. Vermillion CD, Page DL: Paget's disease of the scrotum: A case report with local lymph node invasion. J Urol 107:281, 1972
46. Hagan KW, Braren V, Viner NA et al: Extramammary Paget's disease in the scrotal and inguinal areas. J Urol 114:154, 1975
47. Feinstein PA, Somberg E, Brodman H: Paget's disease of the scrotum presenting as an inguinal lymph node. J Urol 118:688, 1977
48. Oka M, Saita B: Simultaneous prostatic carcinoma and genital Paget's disease associated with subjacent adenocarcinoma. Br J Urol 51:49, 1979
49. Ueki H, Kohda M: Multilokularer extramarrarer Morbus Paget. Hautarzt 30:267, 1979
50. Taki I, Janovski NA: Paget's disease of the vulva: Presentation and histochemical study of four cases. Obstet Gynecol 18:385, 1961

Benign Mesenchymal Neoplasms

Hemangioma

51. Winslow N: Cavernous hemangioma of the scrotum: Report of a case. Arch Surg 17:829, 1929
52. Gibson TE: Hemangioma of the scrotum. Urol Cutan Rev 41:843, 1937
53. Mahoney MT: Cavernous hemangioma of the scrotum: Report of a case. Urol Cutan Rev 55:744, 1951
54. Gabarro P: The "cheese-board" excision technique: A new technique in the treatment of angioma scrotalis. Br J Plast Surg 10:141, 1957
55. Gotzen FJ: Zur kaswistik intraskrotalar hamangiome. Z Urol 51:107, 1958
56. Gulienetti R: Haemangiomata of the external genitalia. Br J Plast Surg 12:228, 1959
57. Mininberg DT, Harley DP: Scrotal wall hemangioma in an infant. J Urol 106:789, 1971
58. Cooper TP, Anderson RG, Chapman WH: Hemangioma of the scrotum: A case report, review and comparison with varicocele. J Urol 112:623, 1974
59. Ray B, Clark SS: Hemangioma of scrotum. Urol 8:502, 1976
60. Eastridge RR, Carrion HM, Politano VA: Hemangioma of scrotum, perineum, and buttocks. Urol 14:61, 1979
61. Lent V, Stober R, Knecht K: Scrotalhamangiome. Urolege 19:276, 1980
62. Mason JT, Rice JO, Rohrer PA: Massive hemangioma of the scrotum. J Urol 68:367, 1952

Lymphangioma

63. Guenkdjian SA: Lymphangioma of the groin and scrotum. J Int Coll Surg 24:159, 1955
64. Mulcahy JJ, Schileru G, Donmezer MA et al: Lymphangioma of scrotum. Urol 14:64, 1979
65. Thelenbeg G: Prinares spradisches lymphodem mit lymphangioma circumscriptum. Hautarzt 31:491, 1980
66. Koft AW, Bart RS: Tumor conference No. 38. Lymphangioma of the scrotum and penis. J Dermatol Surg Oncol 7:870, 1981
67. Merka, ST, Bhatt KS, Wood FS: Cystic lymphangioma of the scrotum: A case report. J Urol 131:1179, 1984

Malignant Mesenchymal Neoplasms

68. Beccia DJ, Krane RJ, Olsson CA: Clinical management of nontesticular intrascrotal tumors. J Urol 116:476, 1976
69. Waller JI: Liposarcoma of the scrotum. J Urol 87:139, 1962
70. Ray B, Huvos AG, Whitmore Jr WF: Unusual malignant tumors of the scrotum: Review of 5 cases. J Urol 108:760, 1972

Adrenal Gland

11

Normal Structure

The normal adrenal gland is composed of the outer cortex of mesodermal derivation originating in the urogenital ridge and the inner, adrenal medulla derived from the neural crest.[1,2] The weight of the organ is 2 g to 4 g at birth, and increases to 4 g to 6 g in adults.[1] The right and left adrenal glands are of equal

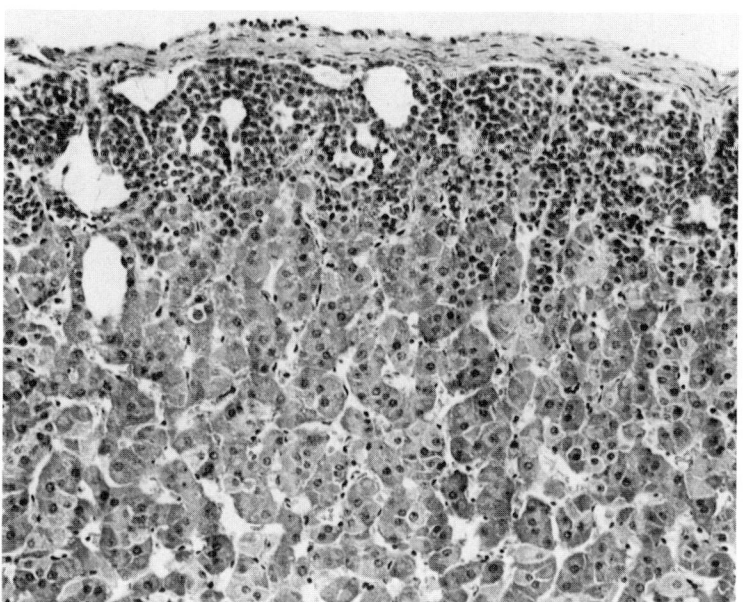

Figure 11-1   ***Normal fetal adrenal gland.*** *The fetal adrenal is composed primarily of a thin rim of small cortical cells that separate the capsule from the provisional or fetal cortex, which is composed of large cells with abundant eosinophilic cytoplasm.*

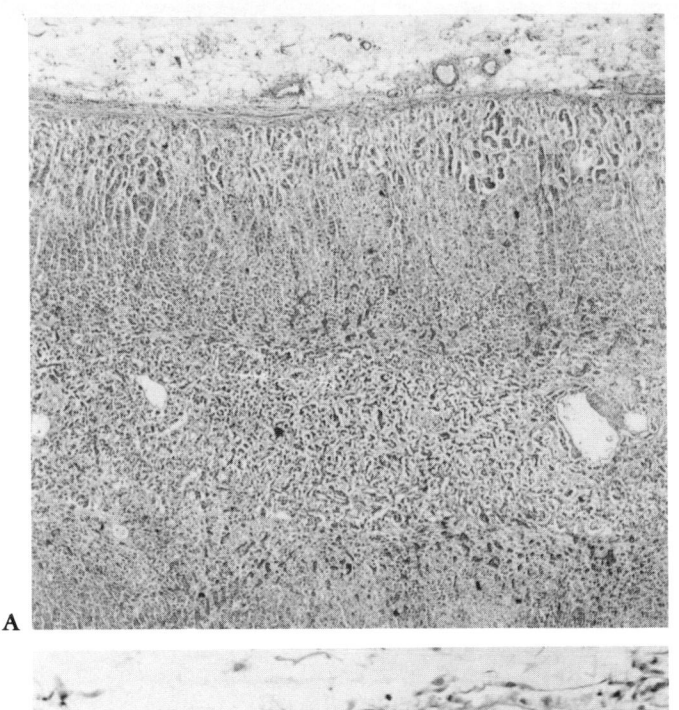

A

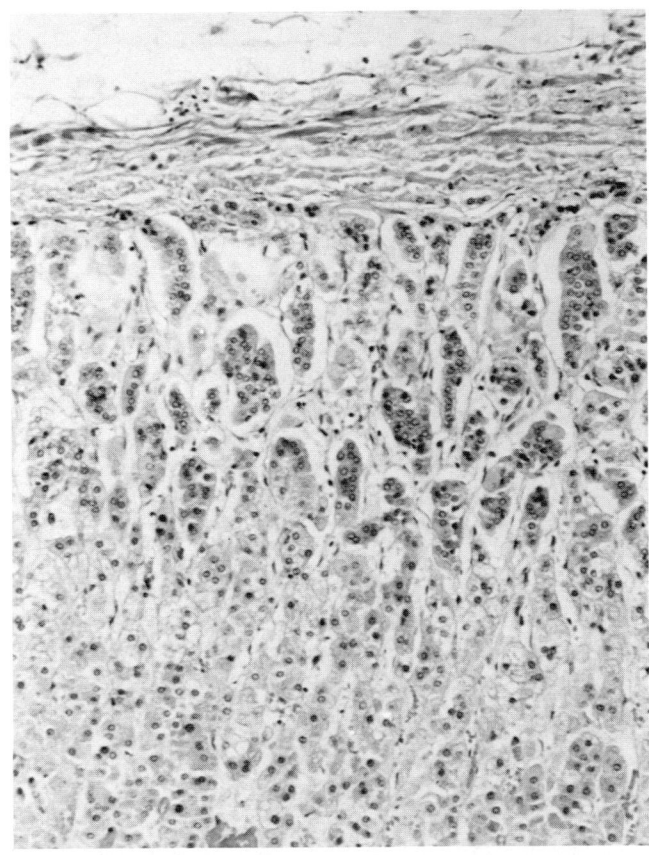

B

Figure 11-2   ***Normal adult adrenal gland.*** *(A) The capsule overlies the three cortical zones—glomerulosa, fasciculata, and reticularis. Adrenal veins and arterial branches are present within the medulla. (B) Normal adult adrenal cortex. The zona glomerulosa cells in nests are smaller than the cells of the zona fasciculata arranged in cords.*

weight. The adrenal glands of adult males are equal in weight to that observed in females.

The structure of the adrenal cortex varies with age. During fetal development the cortex is composed principally of a provisional cortex and a thin rim of subcapsular cells arranged in small nests[2] (Fig. 11-1). Following birth, the provisional or fetal cortex undergoes atrophy and the three cortical zones in the adult adrenal cortex develop. By age 1 year the zona glomerulosa, fasciculata, and reticularis are readily identified (Fig. 11-2).

The zona glomerulosa constitutes approximately 10% of the adult adrenal cortex. The cells are arranged in small nests, in contrast to the cords of cells within the zona fasciculata. The zona glomerulosa is the cytologic source of the mineralocorticoids. The zona fasciculata, which is the source of the glucocorticoids and androgens, comprises approximately 80% of the adrenal cortical cell population. It is composed of well-defined cells that have either a clear or eosinophilic cytoplasm. The clear or light cells of the fasciculata reflect lipid storage, whereas the eosinophilic cytoplasm contains fewer stored steroids. The innermost layer of the adrenal cortex, the zona reticularis, has synthetic functions identical to the zona fasciculata. The zona reticularis is less well organized than the linear cords of the zona fasciculata. The entire zona reticularis constitutes approximately 10% of the adrenal cortex. The cells of the fasciculata and reticularis zones are under the control of ACTH synthesized by the basophil cells of the anterior pituitary gland.

Electron microscopy studies of the normal adrenal cortex reveal differences among the different zones, but all show prominent Golgi apparatus and smooth endoplasmic reticulum.[3,4]

The adrenal medulla contains cells of the chromaffin system of neurectodermal origin. The cells are arranged in groups and nests of varying size throughout the medulla. The use of chromate fixatives produces oxidation of the catecholamines, resulting in readily observed brown cytoplasmic granules. In addition, the adrenal veins with prominent longitudinal muscular coats are present.

Congenital Disorders

Bilateral agenesis of the adrenal gland is quite rare, and is incompatible with survival. Unilateral agenesis is uniformly accompanied by a compensatory enlargement (hyperplasia) of the contralateral adrenal gland. Congenital hypoplasia is bilateral, and frequently familial.[5-11]

The embryologic development of the adrenal cortex from the urogenital ridge accounts for the common findings of heterotopic tissues in proximity to the gonads (testis and ovaries).[13,19-21,23-26,28] In addition, ectopic adrenal tissue is not uncommon in the capsule of the kidney, in the retroperitoneum adjacent to the renal capsule, and in rare reported cases in the mesentery of the appendix, broad ligament, and hernia sacs.[12,14-18,27] Rarely, ectopic renal tissue is observed within the adrenal gland.[22]

Heterotopic hematopoietic elements are a form of metaplasia usually observed as an incidental finding at autopsy. They are commonly found in association with adipose tissue, and on occasion with ectopic bone. When this form of metaplasia is an incidental finding, it is referred to as *myeloid metaplasia*. On

(*Text continues on page 725.*)

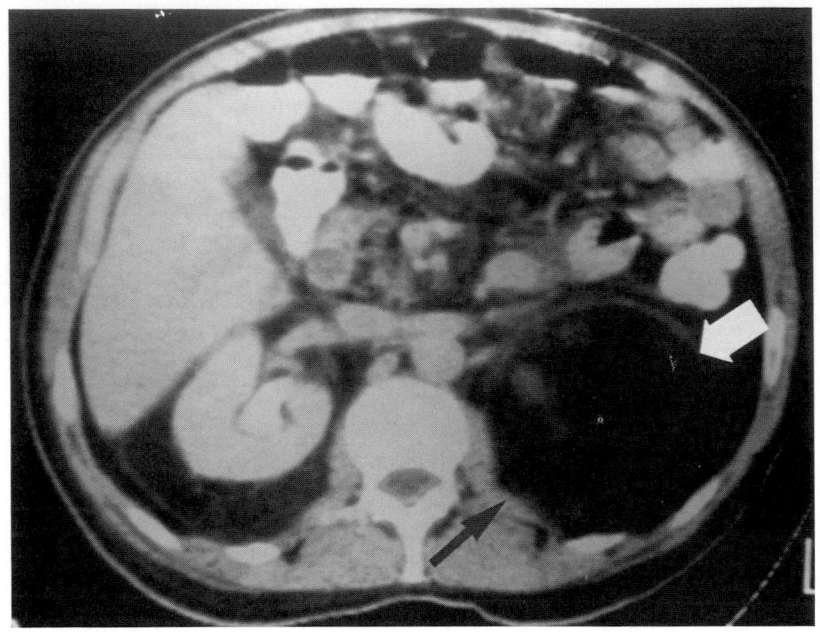

Figure 11-3   *The demonstration of fat in an adrenal mass is helpful in arriving at the radiologic diagnosis of adrenal myelolipoma. Coronal sonogram, with the head of the gland to the left* (L), *shows an echogenic mass* (arrows) *above the rotated, partially hydronephrotic left kidney.*

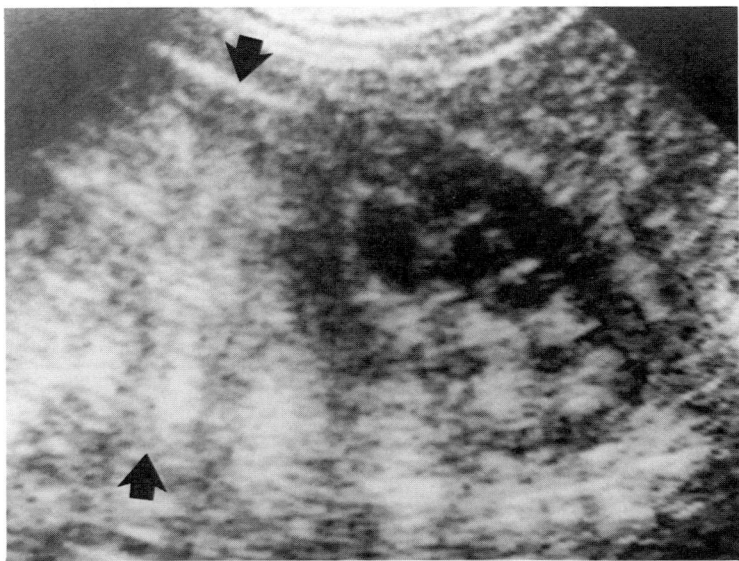

Figure 11-4   ***Adrenal myelolipoma.*** *Sonogram left adrenal mass with apparent fat density* (arrows).

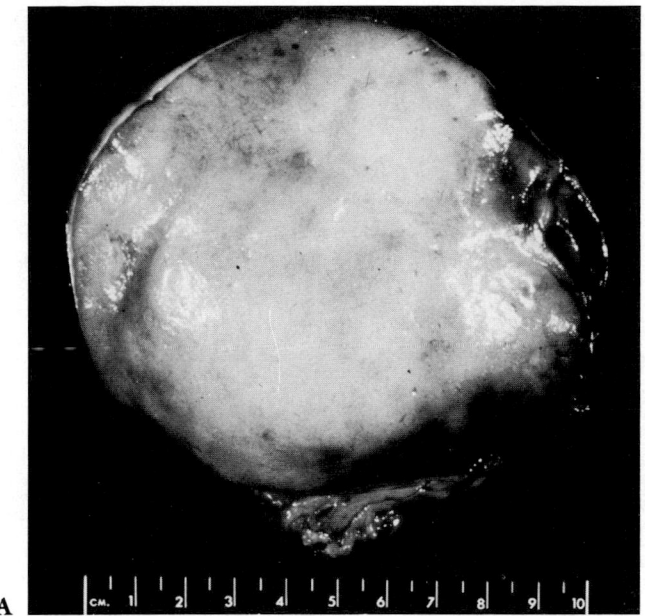

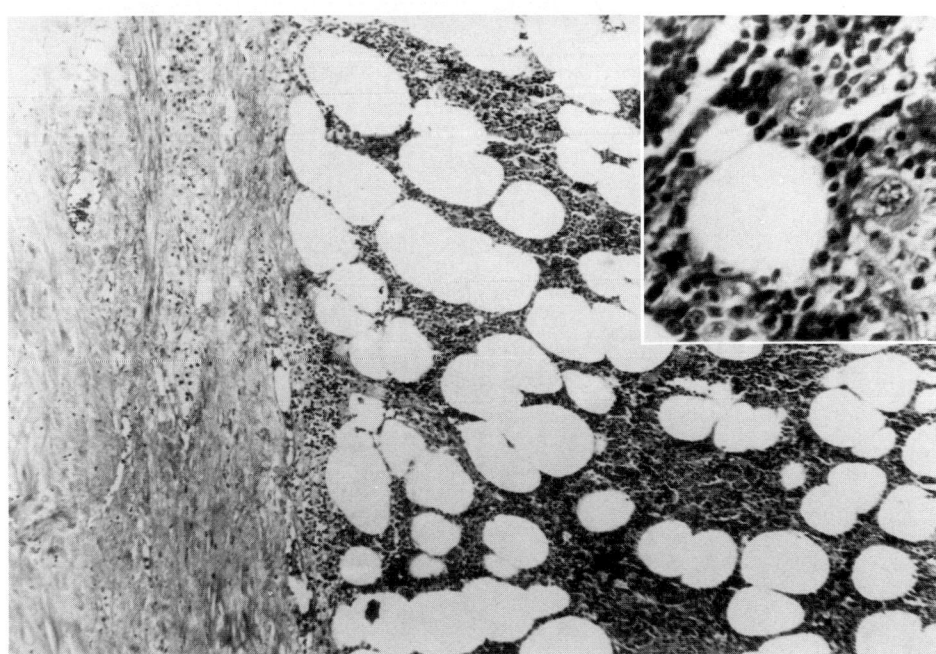

Figure 11-5   *Myelolipoma. (A) The adrenal remnant from which this myelolipoma originated is present at the bottom. (B) A small nest of adrenal cortical cells is adjacent to the fat and hematopoietic tissue (inset) of the myelolipoma. (Courtesy of Harvey Slater, M.D.)*

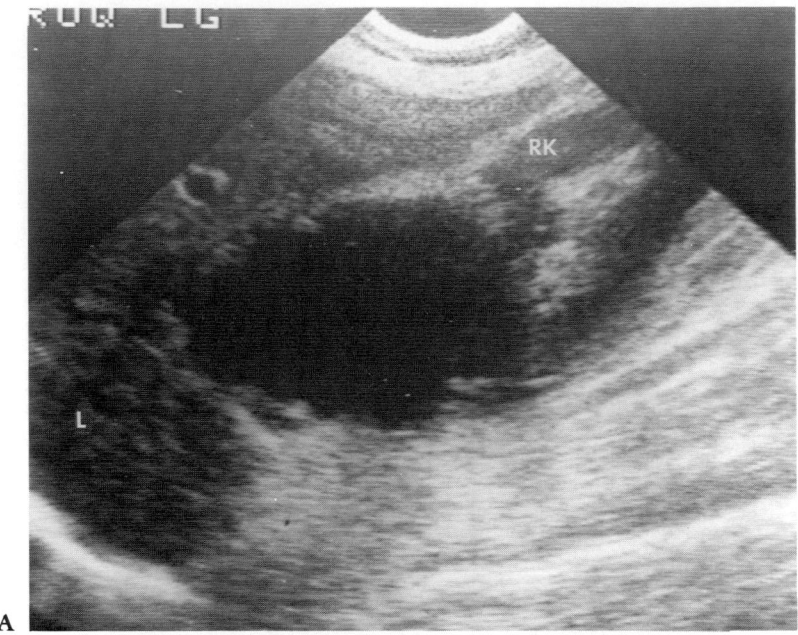

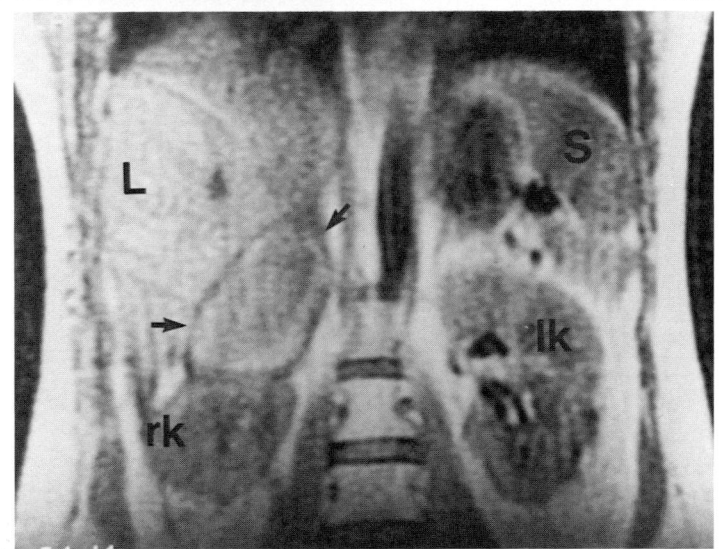

Figure 11-6   ***Adrenal hemorrhage.*** *(A) Longitudinal sonogram of right upper quadrant. The liver (L) and right kidney (RK) are separated by a large hypoechoic mass. (B) Coronal magnetic resonance image (MRI) of the same patient demonstrates the liver (L), spleen (S), left kidney (lk), and right kidney (rk). The suprarenal mass (arrows) has a central medium signal intensity with a low signal rim.*

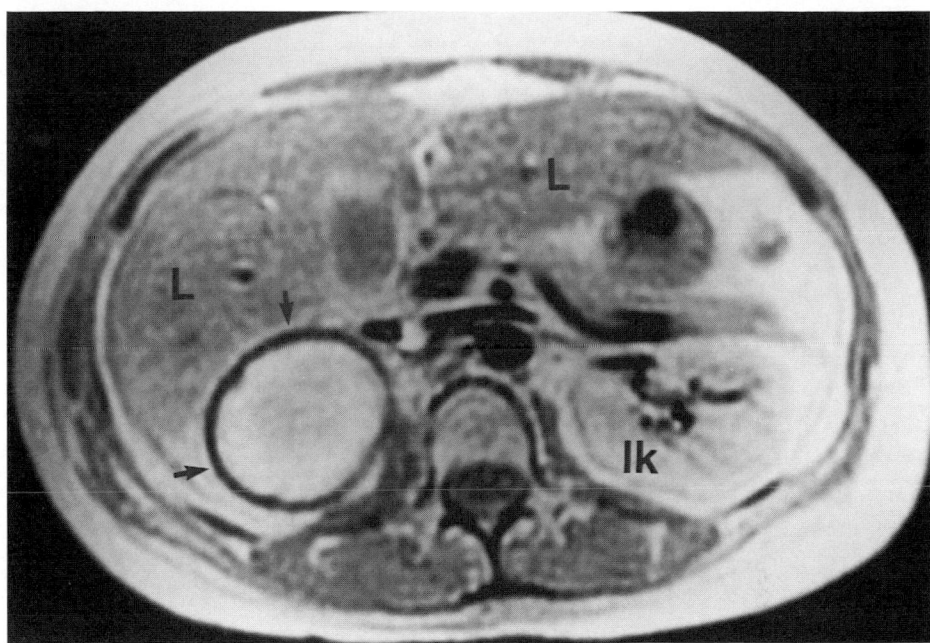

C

Figure 11-6 **Continued** (C) *Transverse axial MRI clearly shows the liver* (L) *and left kidney* (lk). *The right suprarenal mass* (arrows) *is clearly identified.*

occasion these ectopic tissues can attain a size allowing clinical detection.[29-46] Such a tumor is called a *myelolipoma* (Figs. 11-3 to 11-5). One such reported case was associated with Cushing's syndrome.[43]

Adrenal Hemorrhage

The majority of cases of adrenal hemorrhage, a potentially life-threatening lesion, are observed within the first few days of birth.[47-53] Clinical evidence of adrenal insufficiency, with or without an abdominal mass, suggests the presence of adrenal hemorrhage in the newborn. Infants with a history of hypoxia and septicemia are observed to have a higher risk of adrenal hemorrhage. The disorder may involve both adrenals or it may be unilateral. When unilateral, the right is more commonly involved than the left adrenal gland.

The involved adrenal is markedly enlarged, and on cross section the presence of hemorrhage is readily apparent (Figs. 11-6, 11-7). In this age group the affected adrenal gland has gross features similar to that of neuroblastoma, from which it must be differentiated.

Adrenal Cysts

Adrenal cysts are uncommon, with approximately 250 reported cases.[54-56] The majority occur as incidental findings in asymptomatic adults in their third to fifth decades. Rare cases have been reported in infants and children. Traditionally,

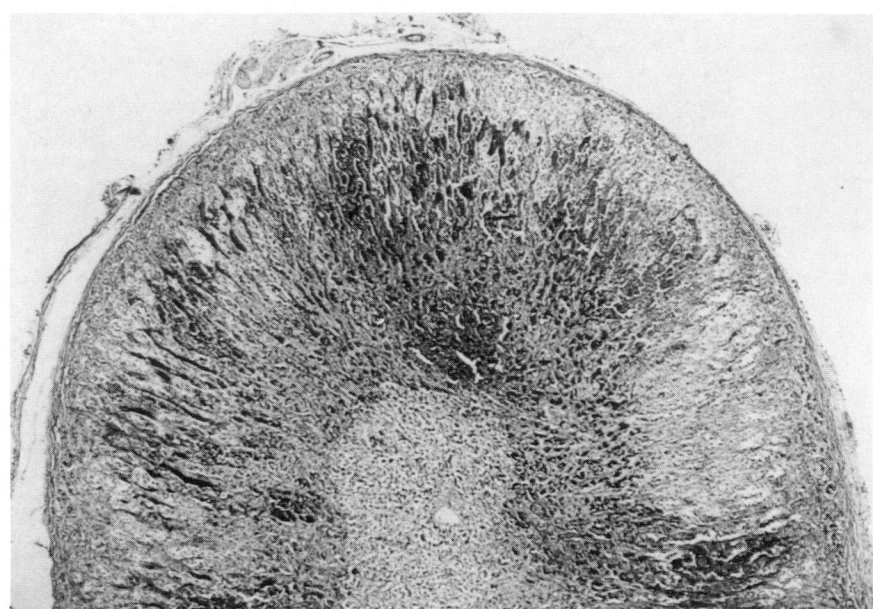

Figure 11-7   ***Adrenal hemorrhage.*** *The intracortical hemorrhage is most prominent in the inner cortex — the zona reticularis and zona fasciculata.*

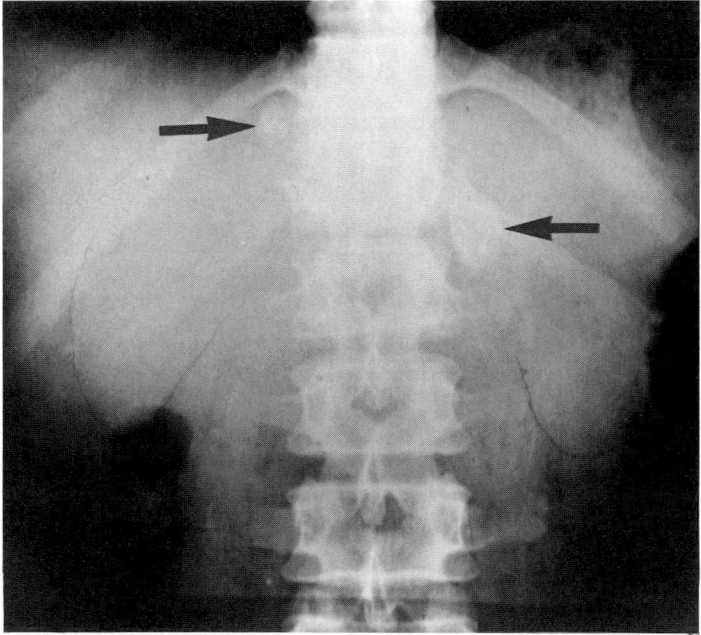

Figure 11-8   *Bilateral densely calcified adrenals (arrows) in an adult with tuberculosis. The differential diagnosis includes old hemorrhage and other granulomatous diseases.*

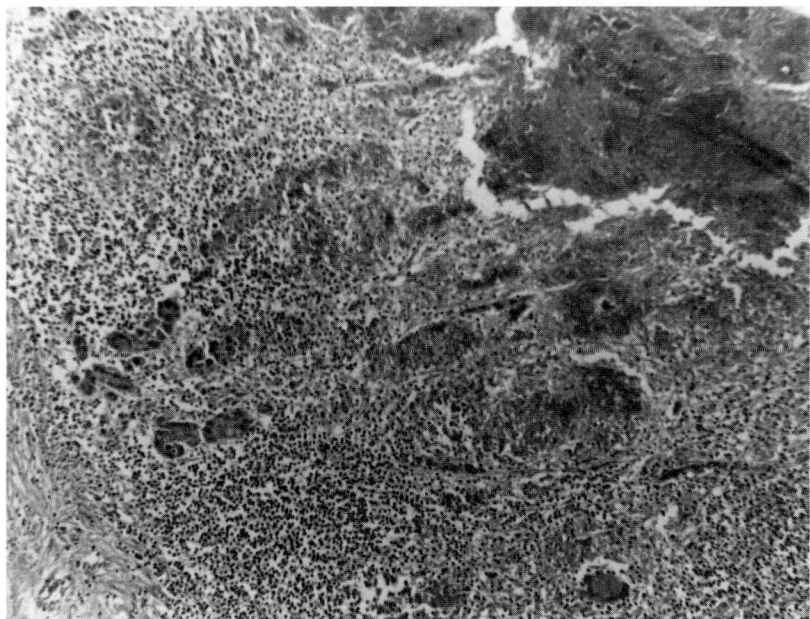

Figure 11-9 *Tuberculosis. The granulomatous inflammation completely destroyed the cortical parenchyma. Central necrosis of the illustrated granuloma is present (upper right).*

four types of adrenal cysts are recognized: endothelial cysts (lymphangiomatous or angiomatous); adrenal pseudocysts resulting from adrenal hemorrhage; epithelial cysts arising from hemorrhage in an adenoma, or as aberrant normal development when observed in premature infants; and parasitic cysts most commonly of ecchinococcal origin.[56] Endothelial cysts and adrenal pseudocysts are the most frequently recorded.

Inflammatory Disorders

Systemic infectious diseases may involve the adrenal glands. This was more common in the past than is observed currently. Tuberculous involvement of the adrenal glands accounted for the majority of cases of adrenal insufficiency prior to the development of antituberculous chemotherapy (Figs. 11-8, 11-9). It is currently uncommon. Autoimmune inflammatory disorders of the adrenal glands are now recognized with increasing frequency. Three cases of extravesical malakoplakia involving the adrenal glands have been reported in the literature.[57-59]

Disorders of the Adrenal Cortex

Nodular and Diffuse Hyperplasia

Hyperplasia of the adrenal cortex may be congenital or acquired. The congenital form is associated with inborn errors of steroid metabolism resulting in one of six identified distinct clinical disorders, the most common being virilizing and salt-losing syndromes (adrenogenital syndromes).[60] In contrast, the majority of cases of acquired hyperplasia observed at autopsy are asymptomatic, without associated hyperfunction of the adrenal cortex.[61] The hyperplasia is always bilateral, although it may be more prominent in one gland than in the contralateral adrenal. The frequency of hyperplastic nodules without associated clinical manifestations increases with age.[61]

When associated with clinical hyperfunction, hyperplasia of the adrenal cortex reflects elevated circulating ACTH, either of pituitary origin or from ectopic sources such as extrapituitary malignant neoplasms. The clinical syndromes most commonly associated with adrenal hyperplasia are Cushing's syndrome and Conn's syndrome.

Microscopically, the hyperplasia of the adrenal cortex may be nodular or diffuse, and affects the zona fasciculata and reticularis in most cases (Fig. 11-10). Conn's syndrome may be associated with a hyperplasia primarily affecting the zona glomerulosa. Evidence of hyperplasia in the contralateral adrenal gland may be minimal or readily apparent. The hyperplastic cortical cells are enlarged, with variable proportions of clear and dark cells intermixed. Variation of nuclear size is common. Hyperplastic nodules do not have surrounding capsules.

Neoplastic Disorders

Adrenal Cortical Adenoma

The vast majority of adenomatous nodules larger than 1 cm in size that are observed at autopsy are nonfunctional.[63] Their frequency in reported autopsy series is approximately 2% of all adults. The nodules are usually discrete and yellow, measuring 1 cm to 5 cm in diameter. Rarely are they larger; however, increased size is associated with areas of necrosis, cystic degeneration, and on occasion, calcification (Figs. 11-11 to 11-13). The adenoma typically, but not invariably, has a surrounding capsule (Fig. 11-14). When present, it is frequently incomplete. The clear cell type is the most commonly encountered histologic form. Variability of nuclear size is common. Mitoses are rare to absent. The ultrastructural features of adrenal cortical adenomas have been extensively studied.[64-66]

Cortical nodules regarded as adenomas vary in size from > 3 mm to > 1 cm. Nodules of smaller dimensions are regarded as examples of nodular hyperplasia, and are frequently multiple and bilateral. The contralateral adrenal is either normal or atrophic depending on the functional status of the adrenal adenoma. When the adenoma is functional, the clinical syndromes reported are adrenogenital syndrome, Cushing's syndrome, or Conn's syndrome. Differentiation of

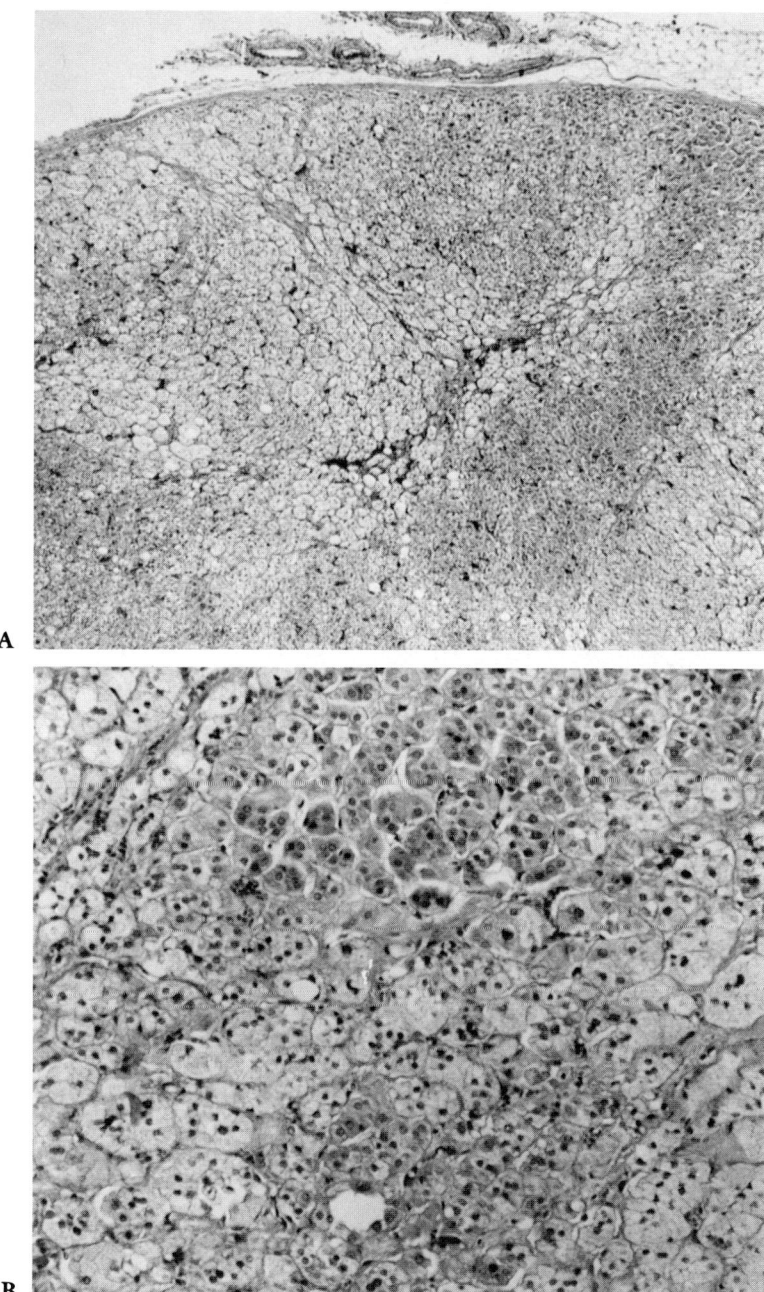

Figure 11-10 *Adrenal cortical hyperplasia.* (A) *The hyperplastic adrenal cortex has a disorganized appearance and is composed of interspersed areas of clear and dark cells.* (B) *Clear cells with abundant vacuolated cytoplasm are interspersed among smaller dark cells with eosinophilic cytoplasm.*

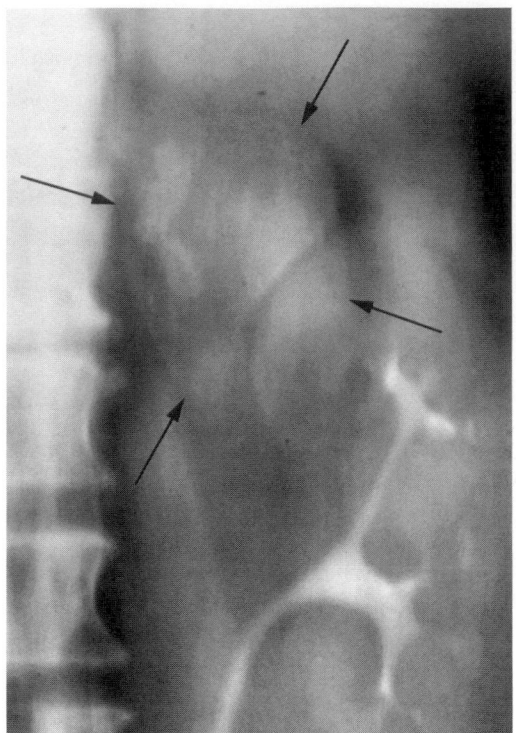

Figure 11-11   ***Adrenal adenoma.*** *Peripheral calcification and lack of necrosis suggest the diagnosis.*

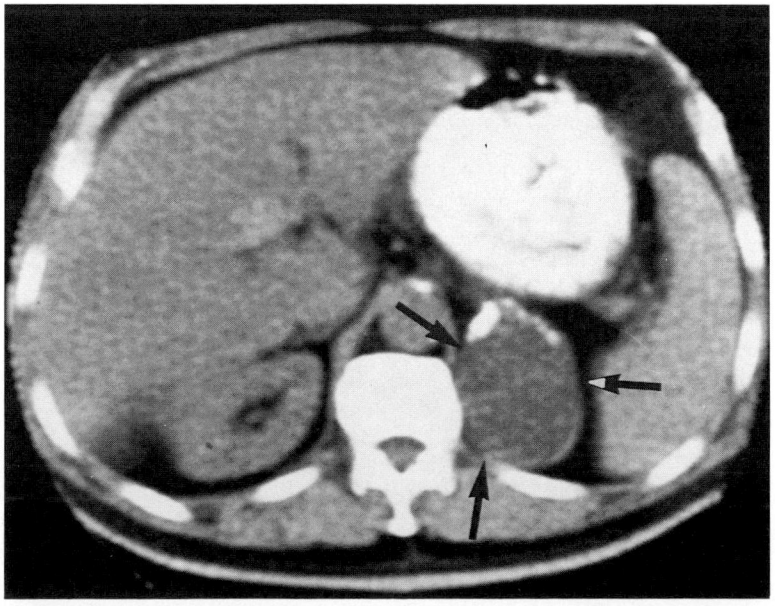

Figure 11-12   ***Adrenal adenoma.*** *Partially calcified left adrenal mass demonstrated on excretory urogram. CT scan shows peripheral calcification and absence of necrosis in left adrenal gland mass* (arrows).

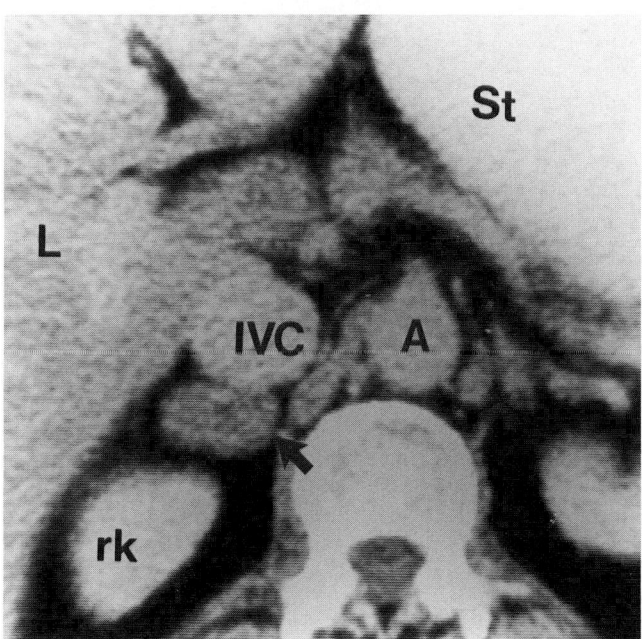

Figure 11-13 *Transverse axial CT scan of adrenal adenoma. A right adrenal mass* (arrow) *is present. The stomach* (St), *aorta* (A), *inferior vena cava* (IVC), *liver* (L), *and right kidney* (rk) *are indicated.*

larger masses (in excess of 5 cm) from those that will behave in a clinically malignant manner must be done with caution. There is general agreement that no criteria short of demonstrating metastasis allows the separation of adrenal cortical adenoma of large size from adrenal carcinoma.

Pigmented Adenoma

A variant of adrenal cortical adenoma termed *pigmented adenoma* has been reported.[67-75] The majority are incidental findings at autopsy and are without apparent function. Rare cases have been reported with virilization, Cushing's syndrome, and Conn's syndrome.[72-75] The black color of the adenoma is attributed to lipofuscin pigment (Fig. 11-15). Histologically, the cells bear greatest resemblance to those of the zona reticularis.

Adrenal Cortical Carcinoma

Adrenal cortical carcinoma is an uncommon adrenal malignancy that may evidence clinical functional activity or may present as a nonfunctional abdominal mass.[76-93] The majority of nonfunctional carcinomas are observed in elderly men; functional carcinomas are more frequent in young women.

Adrenal cortical carcinomas are usually unilateral and solid, and evidence infiltrating margins within the retroperitoneal adipose tissue. The cut surface of the tumor shows multiple areas of necrosis and focal hemorrhage. These neoplasms are characterized histologically by great variation of pattern, cell size, and

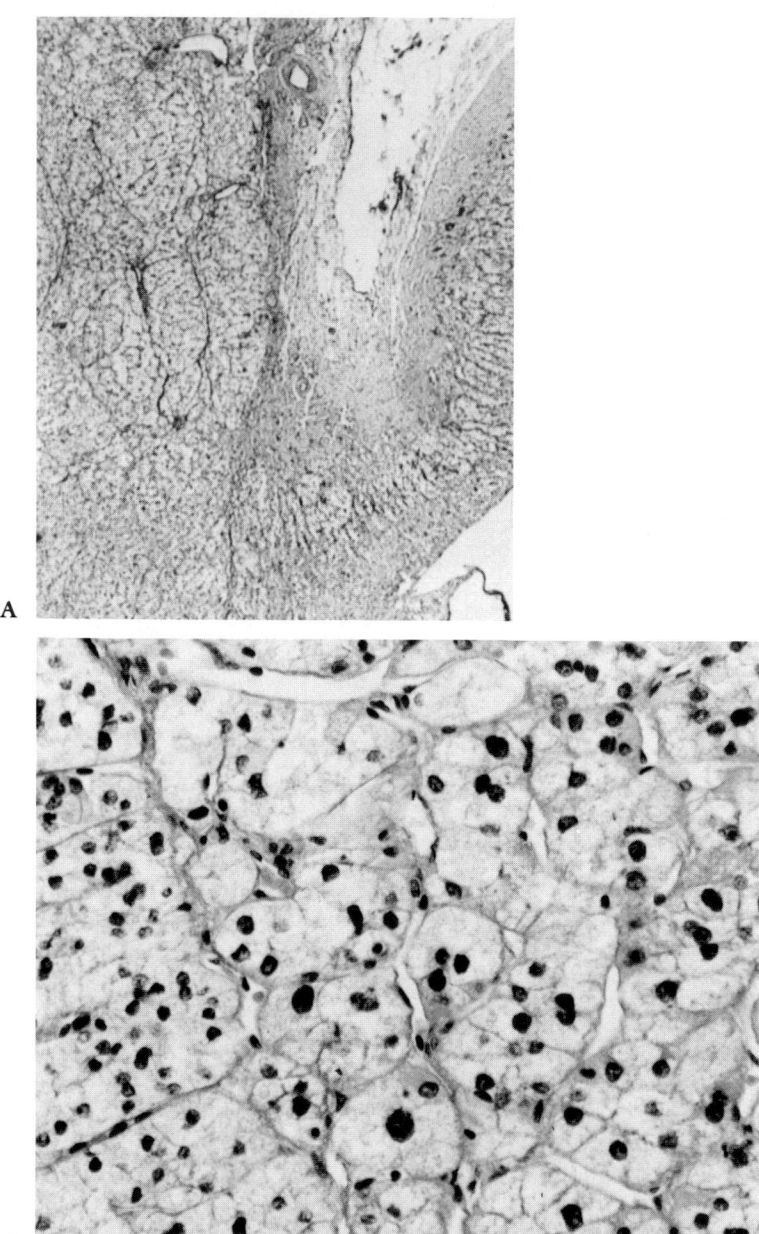

A

B

Figure 11-14   ***Adrenal cortical adenoma.*** (A) *A thin fibrous pseudocapsule separates the adrenal adenoma on the left from the normal adrenal cortex on the right.* (B) *The cells have abundant cytoplasm and are arranged in poorly defined nests with interspersed thin-walled vessels. Variation of nuclear size is readily apparent.*

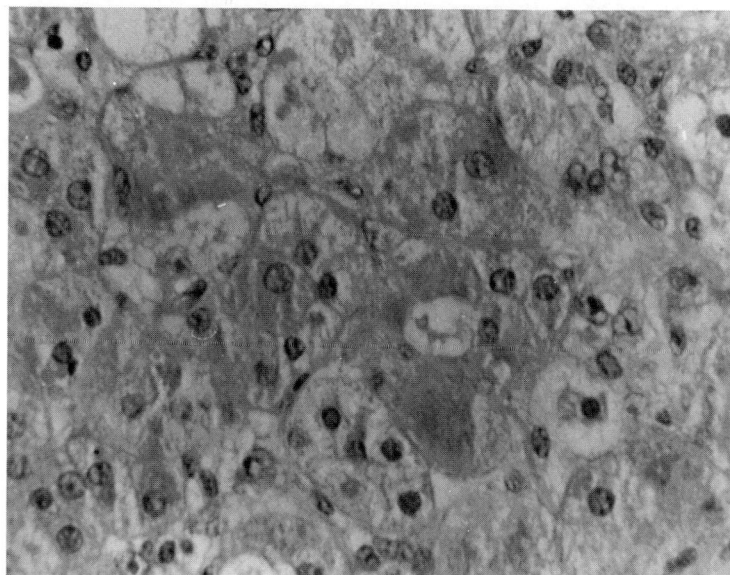

Figure 11-15 *Pigmented adenoma. Abundant brown, granular pigment accumulates in many of the cells of this typical pigmented adenoma of the adrenal gland.*

nuclear staining characteristics (Figs. 11-16, 11-17). Bizarre cells are commonly present, frequently with multiple nuclei. Mitoses are commonly observed. Some cases show incomplete encapsulation, whereas others exhibit no apparent capsule and readily observable invasion of adjacent tissue. Vascular invasion is common. No cytologic or histologic feature serves as an individual reliable criterion for the diagnosis of malignancy. In the past, the only reliable criterion for malignancy has been the presence of distant metastases.[83,84,88] More recent studies suggest that combined histologic parameters may prove helpful in reliably identifying those tumors that will behave in a malignant manner.[89-93] Metastases are most common in the liver, regional lymph nodes, and lungs.[90-93]

Disorders of the Adrenal Medulla

Adrenal Medullary Hyperplasia

In 1977, Rudy and associates proposed diagnostic criteria for medullary hyperplasia of the adrenal gland, including episodic attacks of hypertension associated with increased urinary catecholamines, diffuse expansion of the adrenal medulla, enlarged medullary cells with or without pleomorphism, and an increased medulla/cortex ratio.[100] Prior to this study sporadic reports appeared in the literature describing patients clinically suspected of harboring an adrenal pheochromocytoma, but whose adrenalectomy specimens showed medullary prominence.[94-99] Unfortunately, the morphologic and clinical documentation of the earliest reported cases was incomplete, and the status of medullary hyperplasia was controversial. Later studies, including that of Rudy and associates,

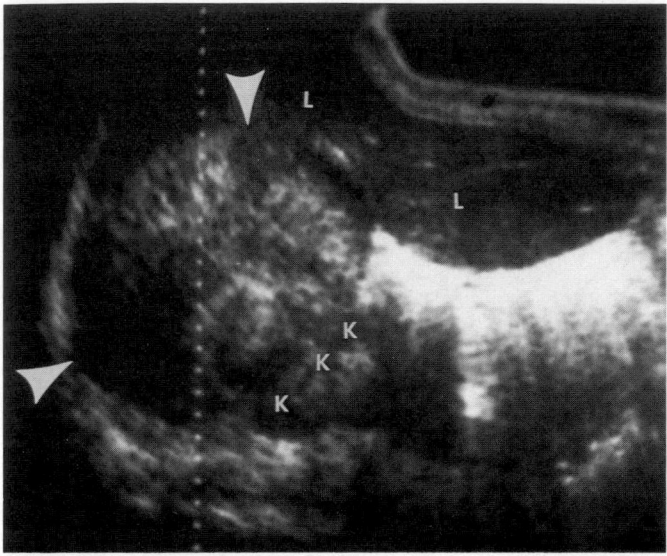

Figure 11-16   ***Adrenal carcinoma.*** *(A) Parasagittal sonogram. A large suprarenal, infrahepatic, partially cystic mass (arrowheads) is present (K, kidney; L, liver). (B) CT scan. Adrenal mass (arrow) displaces the liver (L) and kidney (K). Dark areas in the mass represent necrosis or hemorrhage.*

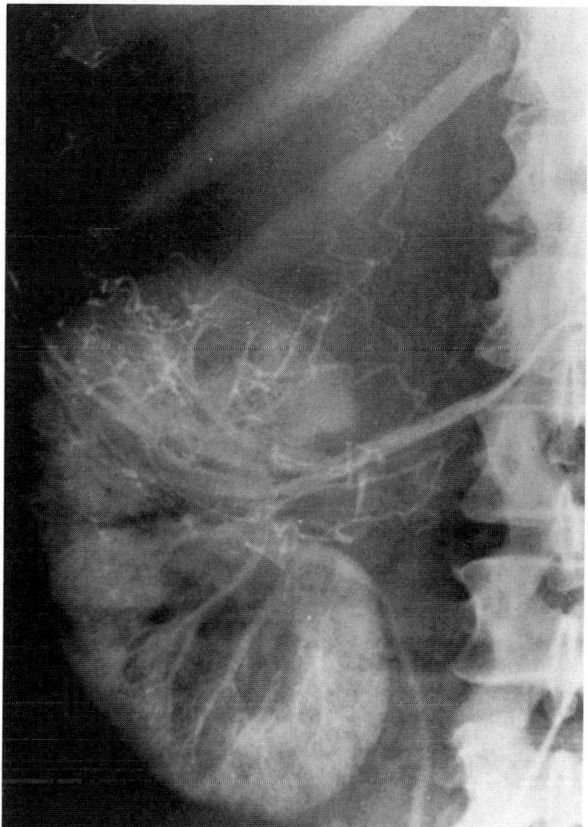

C

Figure 11-16   **Continued** (C) *Right renal arteriogram.*
Hypervascularity of a right adrenal mass.

provided more complete documentation lending support to the entity of medullary hyperplasia.[100] The association of medullary hyperplasia with multiple endocrine neoplasia, type 2 has been reported.[97] Further studies are needed to clarify the true frequency and pathogenesis of this disorder.

Neoplastic Disorders

Pheochromocytoma

Pheochromocytomas are paragangliomas that arise most commonly in the adrenal medulla. Although the majority of pheochromocytomas are not hormonally functional, these tumors may secrete epinephrine, norepinephrine, or both of these catacholamines.[105-107] Although pheochromocytomas are most commonly encountered in the adrenal medulla, they may also be observed in the extra-adrenal retroperitoneum, the mediastinum, and the urinary bladder.[101,109,113,114] Pheochromocytomas constitute a component of the multiple endocrine adenopathies, type 2, in combination with medullary carcinoma of the thyroid and hyperparathyroidism.[104,112,115] These tumors are also reported in

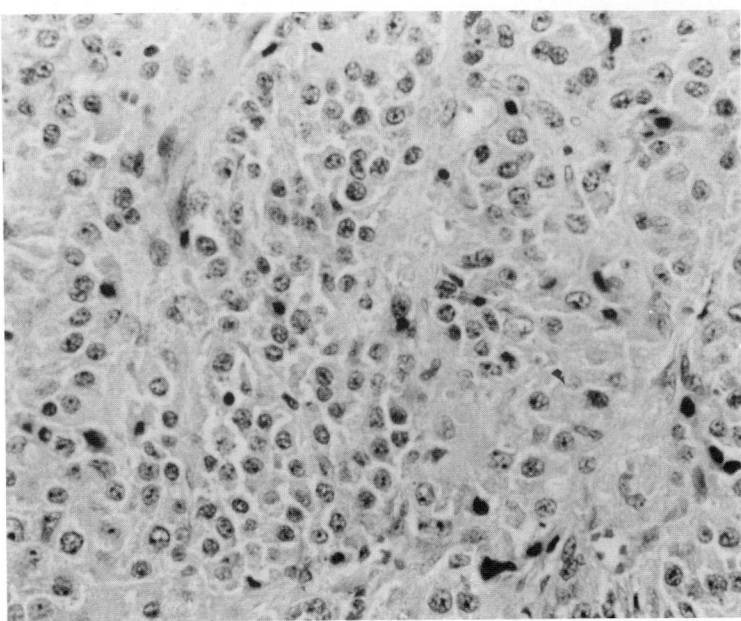

Figure 11-17   *Adrenal cortical carcinoma. The tumor cells grow in sheets without any recognizable organization. Scattered tumor cells contain hyperchromatic irregular, enlarged nuclei. No mitoses are present. The tumor metastasized to the liver and regional lymph nodes.*

association with neural disorders, such as neurofibromatosis and cerebellar hemangioblastomas.

These neoplasms occur most commonly in adults; however, 10% occur in children.[102,103,108,116] The majority of adrenal pheochromocytomas occur unilaterally; the right is involved more frequently than the left. They are highly variable in size, ranging from a few grams to in excess of 2 kg.[110]

Multiple areas of hemorrhage, necrosis, and cyst formation are observed throughout the tumor, which is a soft, red to yellow mass. The most characteristic histologic feature is the pattern of cells in nests called *zellballen* (Fig. 11-18). These nests of cells are separated by thin fibrovascular trabeculae. The cells show moderate variation in size and shape, and have round to oval nuclei with prominent nucleoli. Scattered bizarre cells may be seen, but they have no reliable association with clinical malignancy. The cytoplasm of the tumor cells is finely granular and eosinophilic. As with adrenal cortical carcinoma, experience has demonstrated that there are no reliable histologic features capable of predicting malignant behavior.[116] When metastases are observed, they are most frequently found in bones, especially the ribs and vertebral column. In excess of 80% of these tumors evidence a benign clinical course.[111,116]

Neuroblastoma

Neuroblastomas arise most commonly in the adrenal medulla, and less commonly in the extra-adrenal retroperitoneum. They are virtually confined to the pediatric age group.[117–126] Seventy-five percent of cases are observed in children

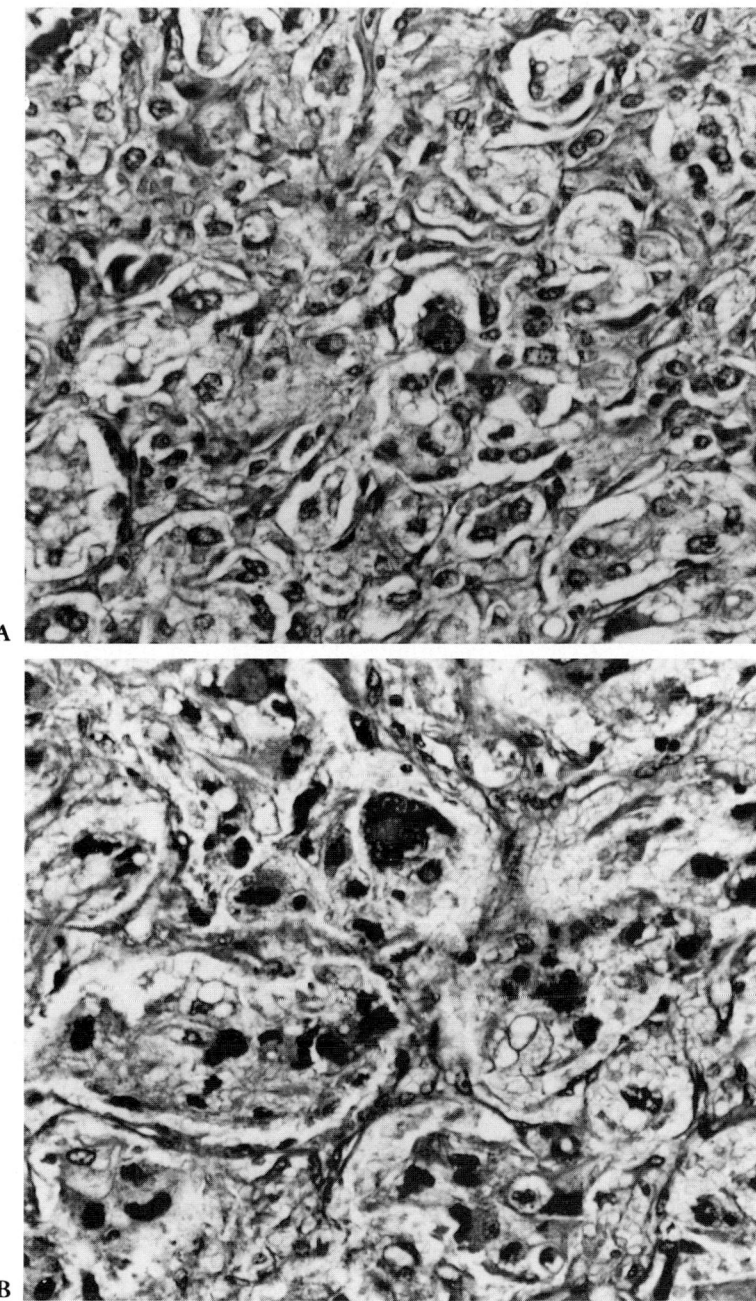

Figure 11-18 **Pheochromocytoma.** (A) *The tumor cells in nests and cords are pleomorphic. Scattered, enlarged, and bizarre nuclei are present.* (B) *The nests of neoplastic cells are separated by thin fibrovascular septa. The variability of the nuclear size and cytoplasm density is apparent.*

younger than 5 years of age. These lesions may be observed as early as birth. The patient's age at diagnosis is correlated with the biological course of these neoplasms.[117,122,124,126] The younger the age at diagnosis, the better the survival rate of the afflicted patient. Tumors diagnosed in patients older than 2 years are consistently aggressive malignancies. Spontaneous regression has been reported in occasional cases. Some neoplasms evidence complete hemorrhagic necrosis with calcification. Alternatively, spontaneously arresting tumors evidence maturation to ganglioneuromas.

These neoplasms are generally very hemorrhagic with multiple areas of necrosis. The necrosis and hemorrhage account for their uniformly soft composition. Infiltration into the adjacent retroperitoneal tissue is common. The tumor is histologically characterized by a densely cellular proliferation of small round cells with minimal cytoplasm and indistinct cell borders. The necrosis and hemorrhage observed grossly is also manifested histologically. The cells proliferate in nests, sheets, or both patterns (Figs. 11-19, 11-20). Occasional true rosettes characterized by tumor cells surrounding a circumscribed area of neurofibrils is a diagnostic feature. These rosettes are highly variable in number, and some cases appear to be devoid of these structures. Some cases contain nests of mature cells with more cytoplasm. In addition, some cases show focal maturation of neuroblasts to ganglion cells.

Clinically, 70% of patients evidence metastases at the initial presentation.[122] The metastases are most common in the liver, lung, and bones.

The entire spectrum of neoplasms involving neuroblasts and cells representing neuroblast maturation is represented by neuroblastomas, which are the most

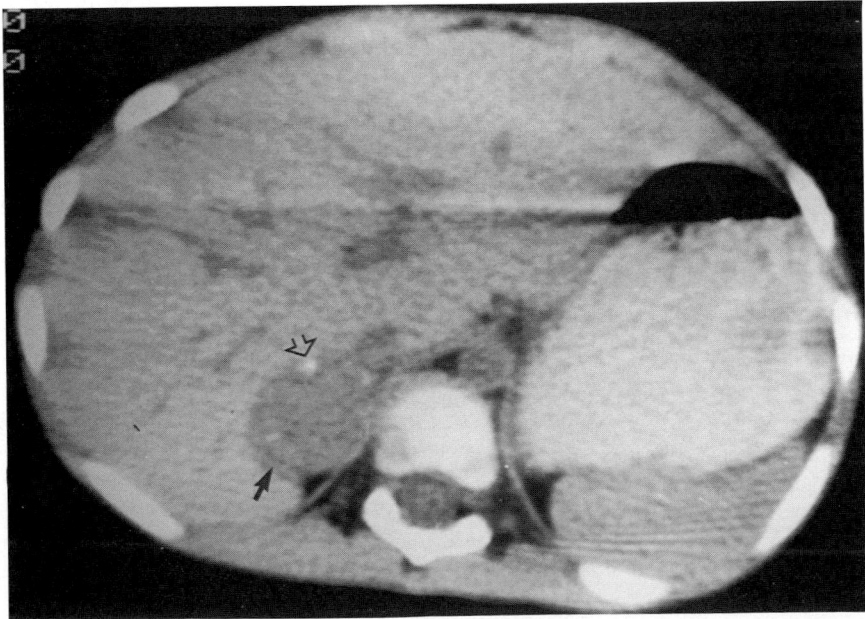

Figure 11-19   *Transverse axial CT scan of neuroblastoma. A right adrenal mass* (arrow) *is present, containing a small focus of calcification* (open arrow). *A radionuclide bone scan showed multiple areas of increased activity. Bone marrow biopsy demonstrated metastatic neuroblastoma.*

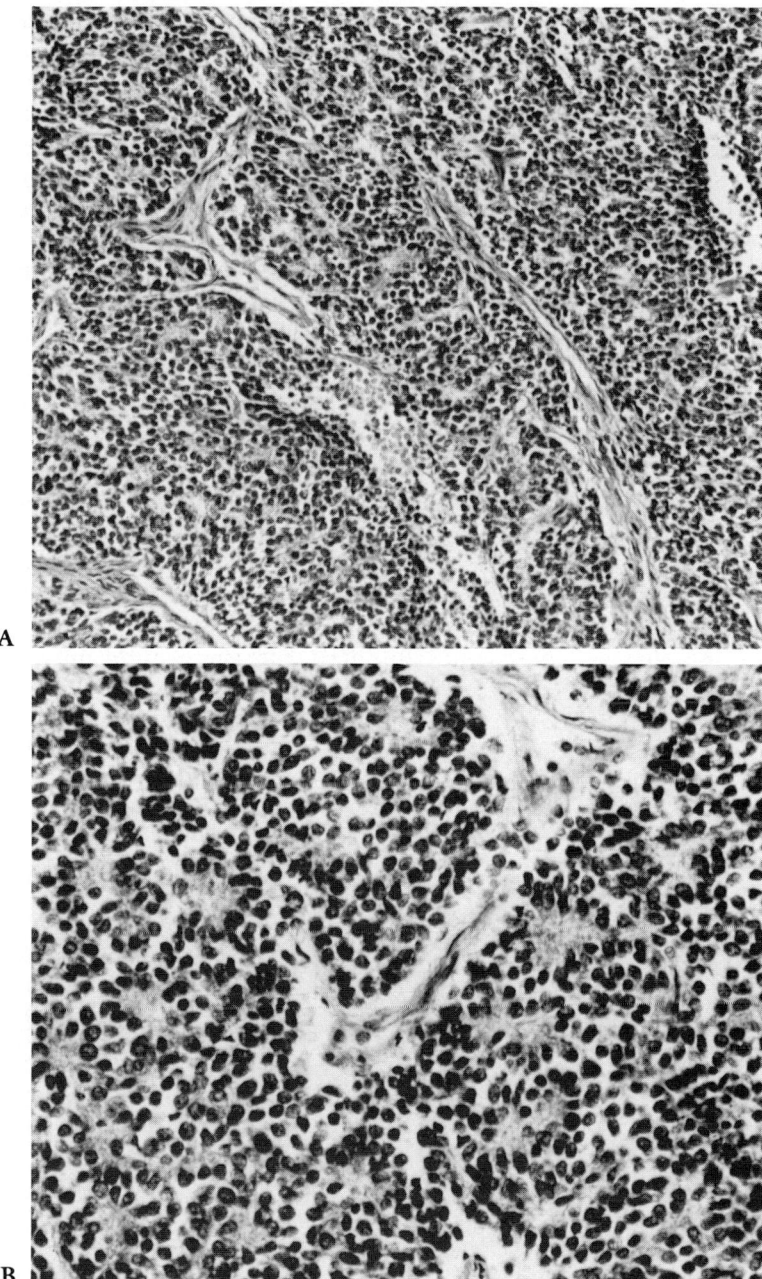

Figure 11-20 ***Neuroblastoma.*** *(A) The tumor is highly cellular and is arranged in large nests and sheets with scattered fibrovascular trabeculae. Occasional clusters of cells suggest rosette formation. (B) Tumor cells arranged around a central acellular fibrillar area constitute the diagnostic rosettes of neuroblastoma. The nuclei are uniform in size and hyperchromaticity, and are virtually devoid of cytoplasm.*

malignant types, and ganglioneuromas, which evidence the greatest extent of maturation and are associated with a clinically benign course. Intermediate between these two neoplasms are ganglioneuroblastomas.

Ganglioneuroma

Ganglioneuromas most commonly arise in the mediastinum and retroperitoneum and only rarely in the adrenal gland. They occur most commonly in adults, in contrast to the predilection for the pediatric age group demonstrated by neuroblastomas. Ganglioneuromas represent the most mature form of neuroblastoma-type tumors.[129–133,138,139]

These neoplasms are entirely encapsulated, solid, gray-white neoplasms. Mature ganglion cells are present in groups or individually, randomly scattered throughout the neoplasm (Fig. 11-21). Hemorrhage and necrosis are distinctly uncommon. There are no cells with the morphology of immature neuroblasts.

Ganglioneuroblastoma

As indicated previously, ganglioneuroblastomas are intermediate in their differentiation between neuroblastomas and ganglioneuromas. As with the latter tumor, they are most commonly found in the mediastinum and retroperitoneum, and only uncommonly within the adrenal.[127,128,134–137] They tend to occur in children, with cases reported only uncommonly in adults.

Ganglioneuroblastomas are characteristically discrete and solid, only occasionally evidencing hemorrhage and necrosis (Fig. 11-22). Histologically, these neoplasms show all stages of neuroblast maturation with variable mixtures of

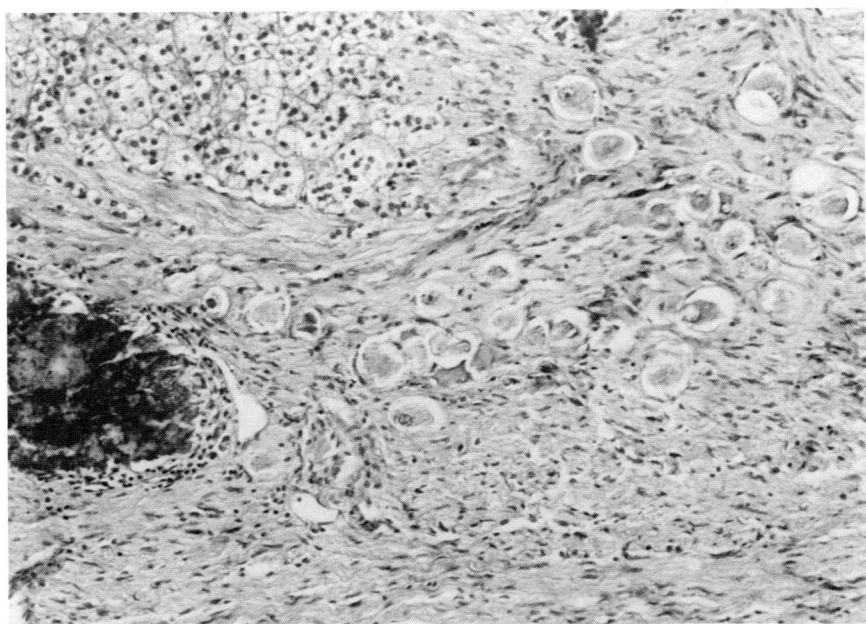

Figure 11-21   *Ganglioneuroma. The neoplastic ganglion cells are scattered in a background of fibrous tissue and occasional nerve fibers. A focus of tumor necrosis with calcification is present on the left.*

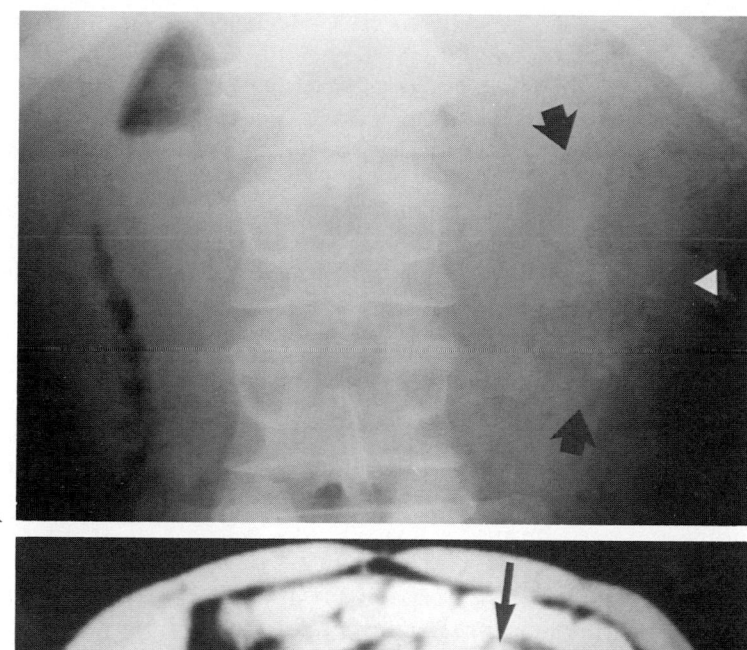

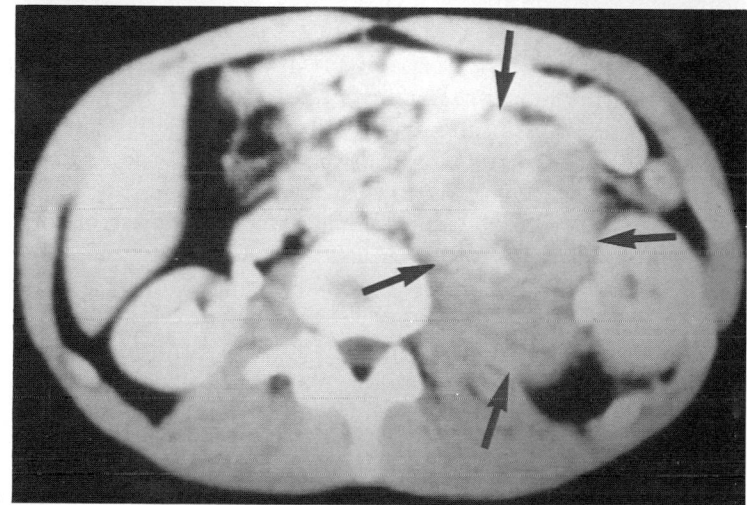

Figure 11-22 *Ganglioneuroblastoma.* (A) *Punctate calcification* (arrows, arrowhead) *is observed in an adrenal mass in an adolescent patient.* (B) *CT scan shows soft tissue component* (arrows) *of adrenal mass.*

immature neuroblasts and variably mature ganglion cells. The immature ganglion cells show variation in nuclear size and number with prominent nuclei.

The biological behavior of these uncommon neoplasms is reported also to be intermediate between neuroblastomas and ganglioneuromas.

Miscellaneous Rare Neoplasms

Malignant Melanoma

Primary malignant melanoma is rare, with 14 recorded cases found in the literature.[149,150] The neural crest origin of the adrenal medulla has provided the explanation for this tumor's histogenesis in the adrenal gland. The authenticity of a primary melanoma requires the exclusion of all other possible sites of origin with metastases to the adrenal gland. In addition, follow-up observation of sufficient duration to allow detection of alternative primary sites (occult at the time of recognition of the adrenal tumor) lends further weight to the diagnosis of primary melanoma of the adrenal. Some of the reported cases of malignant melanoma of the adrenal gland contain neither follow-up information nor autopsy findings, and thus their authenticity is open to question.

The diagnosis in all cases has been made in adults, none of whom evidenced endocrine dysfunction. The tumors are variably large with hemorrhage, necrosis, and local infiltration of periadrenal retroperitoneum. Microscopic features are typical of melanomas with polygonal and elongated cells with abundant cytoplasm and nuclear pleomorphism. Brown pigment granules are present in the cytoplasm. With appropriate stains, they are found to be melanin (Fontana–Masson stain) and not hemosiderin (Prussian blue stain). The cells are arranged in an alveolar nesting pattern.

The diagnosis requires the exclusion of all other possible primary sites, as noted previously, and the demonstration of the histologic and cytologic features typical of melanomas. These neoplasms are to be differentiated from pigmented adenomas and pheochromocytomas. (Refer to discussions of pigmented adenoma and pheochromocytoma.)

Hemangioma

Fourteen examples of adrenal hemangioma appear in the literature.[140-148] Only seven cases were clinically diagnosed. Johnson and Jeppesen reported the first clinically diagnosed and surgically excised adrenal hemangioma.[144] All reported cases have occurred in adults, with a peak frequency in the seventh and eighth decades. Only two of the reported cases were diagnosed in men. The lesions were asymptomatic in all cases discovered at autopsy and in all but one of the seven cases diagnosed clinically.

The reported cases have varied in size from 2 cm to 22 cm. The cut surface reveals numerous vascular channels filled with blood. Stromal calcifications, which are occasionally apparent on abdominal X-ray, have been observed. Microscopic features are typical of hemangiomas in more common sites. Thrombosis within the neoplastic vessels is common.

In addition to the previously noted 14 cases of hemangioma, two cases of "hemangioblastomas" of the adrenal gland have been reported by Menon and Annamalai and by Marten and Meyer.[142,143] The authors regarded these neoplasms as malignant, but no metastases were observed at autopsy. The exact classification of these two cases is indeterminate.

Granulosa-Theca Cell Tumor

Orselli and Bassler reported the first example of an ovarian neoplasm arising in the adrenal.[151] The case had the histologic features characteristic of a granulosa-theca cell tumor. Hormonal changes of the endometrium, commonly found in association with ovarian granulosa-theca cell tumors, were observed in the patient.

Metastatic Neoplasms

The frequency of adrenal metastases from various primary sites found at autopsy is exceeded only by the number observed in the lungs, liver, and bone (Fig. 11-23).[154] Some neoplasms show a predilection for ultimate metastases to the

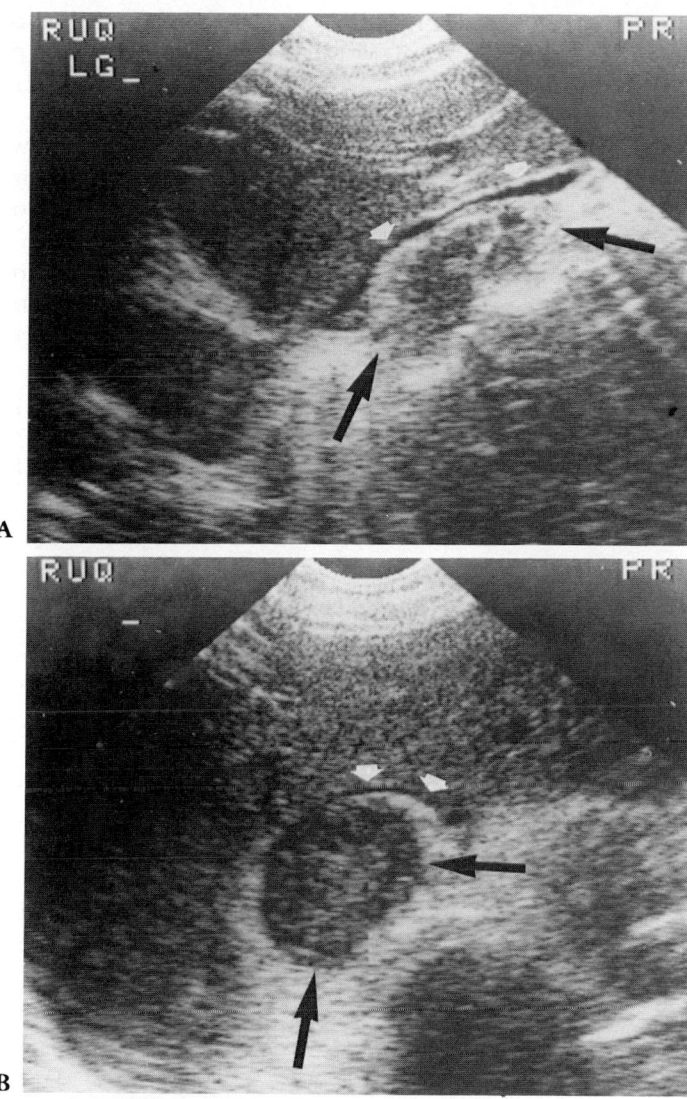

Figure 11-23 **Bilateral adrenal metastases.** (A,B) *Parasagittal and transverse sonograms of a solid right adrenal mass* (black arrows) *elevating and compressing the inferior vena cava* (white arrows).

adrenal glands that is not demonstrated by other malignancies. High frequencies of adrenal metastases are demonstrated by breast and lung carcinomas, followed by renal cell carcinoma.[152,154] The vast majority of such metastases represent hematogenous spread to these organs. Bilateral metastases exceed the frequency of unilateral metastases at autopsy.[154] The majority involve both the cortex and the medulla, with the remaining equally distributed to either the peripheral cortex or the medulla.

Clinical evidence of adrenal insufficiency due to metastatic tumor is uncommon, but has been reported.[155] The same functional failure has also been reported with metastases to, and destruction of, the pituitary gland with secondary effect on the adrenal glands.[155]

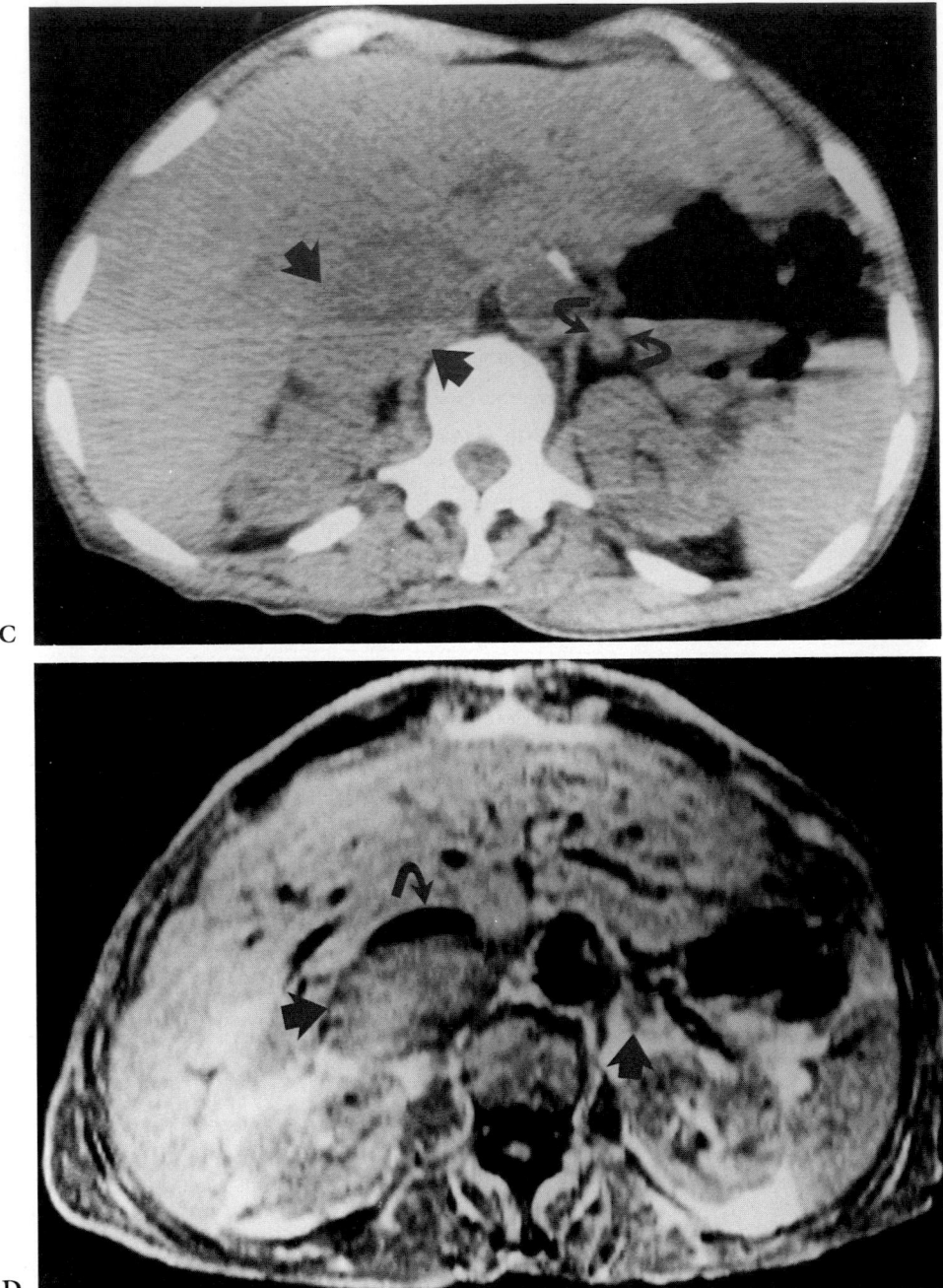

C

D

Figure 11-23   **Continued** (C) *CT scan shows the large solid right adrenal mass* (arrows) *and a similar, but smaller, left adrenal mass* (curved arrows). (D) *MRI shows both masses* (arrows) *and vena cava compression* (curved arrow).

References

Normal Structure

1. Jaffe HL: The suprarenal gland. Arch Pathol 3:414, 1927
2. Gruenwald P: Embryonic and postnatal development of the adrenal cortex, particularly the zona glomerulosa and accessory nodules. Anat Rec 95:391, 1946
3. Long JA, Jones AL: Observations on the fine structure of the adrenal cortex of man. Lab Invest 17:355, 1967
4. McNutt NS, Jones AL: Observations on the ultrastructure of cytodifferentiation in the human fetal adrenal cortex. Lab Invest 22:513, 1970

Congenital Disorders

Aplasia and Hypoplasia

5. Winquist PG: Adrenal hypoplasia. Arch Pathol 71:324, 1961
6. Kerenyi N: Congenital adrenal hypoplasia. Report of a case with extreme adrenal hypoplasia and neurohypophyseal aplasia, drawing attention to certain aspects of etiology and classification. Arch Pathol 71:336, 1961
7. Roselli A, Barbosa LT: Congenital hypoplasia of the adrenal glands. Report of two cases in sisters with necropsy. Pediatrics 35:70, 1965
8. Laverty CRA, Fortune DW, Beischer NA: Congenital idiopathic adrenal hypoplasia. Obstet Gynecol 41:655, 1973
9. Sperling MA, Wolfsen AR, Fisher DA: Congenital adrenal hypoplasia: An isolated defect of organogenesis. J Pediatr 82:444, 1973
10. Pakravan P, Kenny FM, Depp R et al: Familial congenital absence of adrenal glands; evaluation of glucocorticoid, mineralocorticoid, and estrogen metabolism in the perinatal period. J Pediatr 84:74, 1974
11. Mamalle J-C, David M, Riou D et al: Hypoplasie surrenalienne congenitale de type cytomegalique forme recessive liee au sexe. Arch Fr Pediatr 32:139, 1975

Heterotopia (Ectopia)

12. MacLennan A: On the presence of adrenal rests in the walls of hernial sacs. Surg Gynecol Obstet 29:387, 1919
13. Culp OS: Adrenal heterotopia. A survey of the literature and report of a case. J Urol 41:303, 1939
14. Nelson AA: Accessory adrenal cortical tissue. Arch Pathol 27:955, 1939
15. Mitchell N, Angrist A: Adrenal rests in the kidney. Arch Pathol 35:46, 1943
16. Freeman A: Adrenal cortical adenoma of the epididymis. Arch Pathol 39:336, 1945
17. Graham LS: Celiac accessory adrenal glands. Cancer 6:149, 1953
18. Weiner MF, Dallgaard SA: Intracranial adrenal gland: A case report. Arch Pathol 67:228, 1959
19. Dahl EV, Bahn RC: Aberrant adrenal cortical tissue near the testis in human infants. Am J Pathol 40:587, 1962
20. Hamwi GJ, Gwinup G, Mostow JH et al: Activation of testicular adrenal rest tissue by prolonged excessive ACTH production. J Clin Endocrinol Metab 23:861, 1963
21. Schechter DC: Aberrant adrenal tissue. Ann Surg 167:421, 1968
22. Milliser RV, Greenberg SR, Neiman BH: Heterotopic renal tissue in the human adrenal gland. J Urol 102:280, 1969
23. Burke EF, Gilbert E, Uehling DT: Adrenal rest tumors of the testes. J Urol 109:649, 1973
24. Symonds DA, Driscoll SG: An adrenal cortical rest within the fetal ovary: Report of a case. Am J Clin Pathol 60:562, 1973
25. Feldman AE, Rosenthal RS, Shaw JL: Aberrant adrenal tissue: An incidental finding during orchiopexy. J Urol 113:706, 1975

26. Krieger DT, Samojlik E, Bardin CW: Cortisol and androgen secretion in a case of Nelson's syndrome with paratesticular tumors: Response to cyproheptadine therapy. J Clin Endocrinol Metab 47:837, 1978

27. Gutowski III WT, Gray Jr GF: Ectopic adrenal in inguinal hernia sacs. J Urol 121:353, 1979

28. Johnson RE, Scheithauer B: Massive hyperplasia of testicular adrenal rests in a patient with Nelson's syndrome. Am J Clin Pathol 77:501, 1982

Myelolipoma

29. Richardson JC: A tumour of the adrenal gland composed of the elements of bone marrow tissue. Am J Can 25:746, 1935

30. Selye H, Stone H: Hormonally induced transformation of adrenal into myeloid tissue. Am J Pathol 26:211, 1950

31. McDonnell WV: Myelolipoma of adrenal. Arch Pathol 61:416, 1956

32. Plaut A: Myelolipoma in the adrenal cortex. (Myeloadipose structures). Am J Pathol 34:487, 1958

33. Parsons Jr L, Thompson JE: Symptomatic myelolipoma of the adrenal gland. Report of a case and review of the literature. New Engl J Med 260:12, 1959

34. Figueroa G, Tedeschi L: Myelolipoma of the adrenal gland. Boston Med Quart 17:34, 1966

35. Engelking RL, Esparza XI, Velasco DJ et al: Myelolipoma of the adrenal gland and kidney adenocarcinoma: Clinical case. J Urol 98:419, 1967

36. Newman PH, Silen W: Myelolipoma of the adrenal gland. Report of the third case of a symptomatic tumor and review of the literature. Arch Surg 97:637, 1968

37. Whitaker LD: Myelolipoma of the adrenal gland. Surgical removal. Arch Surg 97:628, 1968

38. Tulcinsky DB, Deutsch V, Bubis JJ: Myelolipoma of the adrenal gland. Br J Surg 57:465, 1970

39. Olsson CA, Drane RJ, Klugo RC et al: Adrenal myelolipoma. Surgery 73:665, 1973

40. Rubin HB, Hirose F, Benfield JR: Myelolipoma of the adrenal gland. Angiographic findings and review of the literature. Am J Surg 130:354, 1975

41. Boudreaux D, Waisman J, Skinner DG et al: Giant adrenal myelolipoma and testicular interstitial cell tumor in a man with congenital 21-hydroxylase deficiency. Am J Surg Pathol 3:109, 1979

42. Ayyat F, Fosslin E, Kent R et al: Myelolipoma of adrenal gland. Urol 16:415, 1980

43. Bennett BD, McKenna TJ, Hough AJ et al: Adrenal myelolipoma associated with Cushing's disease. Am J Clin Pathol 73:443, 1980

44. Ishikawa H, Tachibana M, Hata M et al: Myelolipoma of the adrenal gland. J Urol 126:777, 1981

45. Fernandez-Sanz J, Galera H, Garcia-Donas A et al: Adrenal myelolipoma simulating a retroperitoneal malignant neoplasm. J Urol 126:780, 1981

46. Georgiades A, Slater H, Goldfarb IW: Myelolipomas: is surgery indicated? Penn Med 39:32, 1985

Hemorrhage

47. Thrash AM, Iri H: Adrenal infarction. Six case reports. Arch Pathol 75:94, 1963

48. Case records of the Massachussets General Hospital: Case 14-1969. New Engl J Med 280:772, 1969

49. Donohue JP, Garrett RA, Holland TF et al: Obscure abdominal distress and vascular collapse in a man. J Urol 122:83, 1979

50. Smith Jr JA, Middleton RG: Neonatal adrenal hemorrhage. J Urol 122:674, 1979

51. Hensle T, Romas NA, Habif Jr DV: Abdominal mass in the newborn. Urol 14:620, 1979

52. Swift DL, Lingeman JE, Baum WC: Spontaneous retroperitoneal hemorrhage: A diagnostic challenge. J Urol 123:577, 1980
53. Khuri FJ, Alton DJ, Hardy BE et al: Adrenal hemorrhage in neonates: Report of 5 cases and review of the literature. J Urol 124:684, 1980

Cysts

54. Oppenheimer EH: Cyst formation in the outer adrenal cortex. Arch Pathol 87:653, 1969
55. Wilson JM, Woodhead DM, Smith RB: Adrenal cysts. Diagnosis and management. Urol 4:248, 1974
56. Ghandur-Mnaymneh L, Slim M, Muakassa K: Adrenal cysts: Pathogenesis and histological identification with a report of 6 cases. J Urol 122:87, 1979

Malakoplakia

57. Povysil C: Extravesical malakoplakia. Arch Pathol 97:273, 1974
58. Sinclair-Smith C, Kahn LB, Cywes S: Malakoplakia in childhood. Arch Pathol 99:198, 1975
59. Benjamin E, Fox H: Malakoplakia of the adrenal gland. J Clin Pathol 34:606, 1981

Adrenal Cortex

Nodular Hyperplasia

60. Cohen RB, Chapman WB, Castleman B: Hyperadrenocorticism (Cushing's disease): A study of surgically resected adrenal glands. Am J Pathol 35:537, 1959
61. Dobbie JW: Adrenocortical nodular hyperplasia: The ageing adrenal. J Pathol 99:1, 1969
62. Shenoy BV, Carpenter PC, Carney JA: Bilateral primary pigmented nodular adrenocortical disease. Rare cause of the Cushing syndrome. Am J Surg Pathol 8:335, 1984

Cortical Adenoma

63. Spain DM, Weinsaft P: Solitary adrenal cortical adenoma in elderly female. Frequency. Arch Pathol 78:231, 1964
64. Sommers SC, Tezakis JA: Ultrastructural study of aldosterone-secreting cells of the adrenal cortex. Am J Clin Pathol 54:303, 1970
65. Macadam RF: Fine structure of a functional adrenal cortical adenoma. Cancer. 26:1300, 1970
66. Akhtar M, Gosalbez T, Young I: Ultrastructural study of androgen-producing adrenocortical adenoma. Cancer 34:322, 1974

Pigmented Adenoma

67. Baker MR: A pigmented adenoma of the adrenal. Arch Pathol 26:845, 1938
68. Macadam RF: Black adenoma of the human adrenal cortex. Cancer 27:116, 1971
69. Robinson MJ, Rywlin AM: The adrenal black adenoma: Clinical and pathologic correlations. Lab Invest 26:488, 1972
70. Fisher ER, Danowski TS: Ultrastructural study of virilizing adrenocortical adenoma. Am J Clin Pathol 59:480, 1973
71. Garret R, Ames RP: Black-pigmented adenoma of the adrenal gland. Arch Pathol 95:349, 1973
72. Caplan RH, Virata RL: Functional black adenoma of the adrenal cortex. Am J Clin Pathol 62:97, 1974
73. Bahu RM, Battifora H, Shambaugh III G: Functional black adenoma of the adrenal gland. Light and electron microscopical study. Arch Pathol 98:139, 1974
74. Visser JW, Boeijinga JK, Meer CvD: A functioning black adenoma of the adrenal cortex: A clinico-pathological entity. J Clin Pathol 27:955, 1974

75. Givens JR, Andersen RN, Wiser WL et al: A gonadotropin-responsive adrenocortical adenoma. J Clin Endocrinol 38:126, 1974

Cortical Carcinoma

76. Rapaport E, Goldberg MB, Gordan GS et al: Mortality in surgically treated adrenocortical tumors. II. Review of cases reported for the 20 year period 1930–1949, inclusive. Postgrad Med 2:325, 1952
77. Wood KF, Lees F, Rosenthal FD: Carcinoma of the adrenal cortex without endocrine effects. Br J Surg 45:41, 1957
78. Heinbecker P, O'Neal LW, Ackerman LV: Functioning and nonfunctioning adrenal cortical tumors. Surg Gynecol Obstet 105:21, 1957
79. Knight CD, Trichel BE, Mathews WR: Nonfunctioning carcinoma of the adrenal cortex. Ann Surg 151:349, 1960
80. Lipsett MB, Hertz R, Ross GT: Clinical and pathophysiologic aspects of adrenocortical carcinoma. Am J Med 35:374, 1963
81. Constantinou E: Nonfunctioning malignant tumor of the adrenal cortex: A case presentation. Arch Pathol 78:226, 1964
82. Huvos AG, Hajdu SI, Brasfield RD et al: Adrenal cortical carcinoma: Clinicopathologic study of 34 cases. Cancer 25:354, 1970
83. Lewinsky BS, Grigor KM, Symington T et al: The clinical and pathologic features of "non-hormonal" adrenocortical tumors: Report of 20 new cases and review of the literature. Cancer 33:778, 1974
84. Tang CK, Gray GF: Adrenocortical neoplasms: Prognosis and morphology. Urol 5:691, 1975
85. Hajjar RA, Hickey RC, Samaan NA: Adrenal cortical carcinoma: A study of 32 patients. Cancer 35:549, 1975
86. Sullivan M, Boileau M, Hodges CV: Adrenal cortical carcinoma. J Urol 120:660, 1978
87. O'Hare MJ, Monaghan P, Neville AM: The pathology of adrenocortical neoplasia: A correlated structural and functional approach to the diagnosis of malignant disease. Hum Pathol 10:137, 1979
88. Hough AJ, Hollifield JW, Page DL et al: Prognostic factors in adrenal cortical tumors: A mathematical analysis of clinical and morphologic data. Am J Clin Pathol 72:390, 1979
89. Hogan TF, Gilchrist KW, Westring DW et al: A clinical and pathological study of adrenocortical carcinoma: Therapeutic implications. Cancer 45:2880, 1980
90. Didolkar MS, Bescher RA, Elias EG et al: Natural history of adrenal cortical carcinoma: A clinicopathologic study of 42 patients. Cancer 47:2153, 1981
91. Nader S, Hickey RC, Sellin RV et al: Adrenal cortical carcinoma. Cancer 52:707, 1983
92. Weiss LM: Comparative histologic study of 43 metastasizing and nonmetastasizing adrenocortical tumors. Am J Surg Pathol 8:163, 1984
93. Slooten HV, Schaberg A, Smeenk D et al: Morphologic characteristics of benign and malignant adrenocortical tumors. Cancer 55:766, 1985

Adrenal Medulla

Medullary Hyperplasia

94. Drukker W, Formijne P: Hyperplasia of the adrenal medulla. Br Med J 1:186, 1957
95. Montalbano FP, Baronofsky ID, Ball H: Hyperplasia of the adrenal medulla. A clinical entity. JAMA 182:264, 1962
96. Bialestock D: Hyperplasia of the adrenal medulla in hypertension of children. Arch Dis Child 36:465, 1961
97. Carney JA, Sizemore GW, Tyce GM: Bilateral adrenal medullary hyperplasia in

multiple endocrine neoplasia, type 2. The precursor of bilateral pheochromocytoma. Mayo Clin Proc 50:3, 1975

98. Visser JW, Axt R: Bilateral adrenal medullary hyperplasia: A clinicopathological entity. J Clin Pathol 28:298, 1975

99. DeLessis RA, Wolfe HJ, Gagel RF et al: Adrenal medullary hyperplasia: morphometric analysis in patients with familial medullary thyroid carcinoma. Am J Pathol 83:177, 1976

100. Rudy FR, Bates RD, Cimorelli AJ et al: Adrenal medullary hyperplasia: A clinicopathologic study of four cases. Hum Pathol 11:650, 1980

Pheochromocytoma

101. Isaacson C, Rosenzweig D, Seftel HC: Malignant pheochromocytoma of the organs of Zuckerkandl. Arch Pathol 70:725, 1960

102. Cone Jr TE, Pearson HA: Malignant pheochromocytoma: Report of a case in a 12-year-old girl. Pediatr 32:531, 1963

103. Engelman K, Sjoerdsma A: Chronic medical therapy for pheochromocytoma. A report of four cases. Ann Intern Med 61:229, 1964

104. Schimke RN, Hartman WH, Prout TE et al: Syndrome of bilateral pheochromocytoma, medullary thyroid carcinoma and multiple neuromas. A possible regulatory defect in the differentiation of chromaffin tissue. New Engl J Med 279:1, 1968

105. Lauper NT, Tyce GM, Sheps SG et al: Pheochromocytoma. Fine structural, biochemical and clinical observations. Am J Cardiol 30:197, 1972

106. Warren S, Chute RN: Pheochromocytoma. Cancer 29:327, 1972

107. Brown WJ, Barajas L, Waisman J et al: Ultrastructural and biochemical correlates of adrenal and extra-adrenal pheochromocytoma. Cancer 29:744, 1972

108. Buzanowski ZZ, Jorgensen EO, Rahimi A: Pheochromocytoma in obstetric practice. Obstet Gynecol 39:120, 1972

109. Scharf Y, Nahir AM, Better OS et al: Prolonged survival in malignant pheochromocytoma of the organ of Zuckerkandl with pharmacological treatment. Cancer 31:746, 1973

110. Daughtry JD, Susan LP, Straffon RA et al: A case of a giant pheochromocytoma. J Urol 118:840, 1977

111. Mahoney EM, Harrison JH: Malignant pheochromocytoma: Clinical course and treatment. J Urol 118:225, 1977

112. Janson KL, Roberts JA, Varela M: Multiple endocrine adenomatosis: In support of the common origin theories. J Urol 119:161, 1978

113. Simon H, Carlson DH, Hanelin J et al: Intrarenal pheochromocytoma: Report of a case. J Urol 121:805, 1979

114. Lack EE, Cubilla AL, Woodruff JM et al: Extra-adrenal paragangliomas of the retroperitoneum: A clinicopathologic study of 12 tumors. Am J Surg Pathol 4:109, 1980

115. Webb TA, Sheps SG, Carney JA: Differences between sporadic pheochromocytoma and pheochromocytoma in multiple endocrine neoplasia, type 2. Am J Surg Pathol 4:121, 1980

116. Medeiros LJ, Wolf BC, Balogh K et al: Adrenal pheochromocytoma: A clinicopathologic review of 60 cases. Hum Pathol 16:580, 1985

Neuroblastoma

117. Redman JL, Agerty HA, Barthmaier OF, et al: Adrenal neuroblastoma. Am J Dis Children 56:1097, 1938

118. Haber SL, Bennington JL: Maturation of congenital extra-adrenal neuroblastoma. Arch Pathol 76:121, 1963

119. Beckwith JB, Perrin EV: In situ neuroblastomas: A contribution to the natural history of neural crest tumors. Am J Pathol 43:1089, 1963

120. Shanklin DR, Sotelo-Avila C: In situ tumors in fetuses, newborns, and young infants. Biol Neonate 14:286, 1969

121. Turkel SB, Itabashi HH: The natural history of neuroblastic cells in the fetal adrenal gland. Am J Pathol 76:225, 1974

122. Koop CE, Schnaufer L: The management of abdominal neuroblastoma. Cancer 35:905, 1975

123. Yunis EJ, Agostini Jr RM, Walpusk JA et al: Glycogen in neuroblastomas. A light- and electron-microscopic study of 40 cases. Am J Surg Pathol 3:313, 1979

124. Evans AE: Staging and treatment of neuroblastoma. Cancer 45:1799, 1980

125. Kramer SA, Bradford WD, Anderson EE: Bilateral adrenal neuroblastoma. Cancer 45:2208, 1980

126. Triche TJ, Askin FB: Neuroblastoma and the differential diagnosis of small-, round-, blue-cell tumors. Hum Pathol 14:569, 1983

Ganglioneuroma and Ganglioneuroblastoma

127. Cushing H, Wolback SB: The transformation of a malignant paravertebral sympathicoblastoma into a benign ganglioneuroma. Am J Pathol 3:203, 1927

128. Wahl HR, Craig PE: Multiple tumors of the sympathetic nervous system. Report of a case showing a distinct ganglioneuroma, a neuroblastoma and a cystic calcifying ganglioneuroblastoma. Am J Pathol 14:797, 1938

129. Potter EL, Parrish JM: Neuroblastoma, ganglioneuroma and fibroneuroma in a stillborn fetus. Am J Pathol 18:141, 1942

130. Stowens D: Neuroblastome and related tumors. Arch Pathol 63:451, 1957

131. Scully RE, Cohen RB: Ganglioneuroma of adrenal medulla containing cells morphologically identical to hilus cells. (Extraparenchymal Leydig cells). Cancer 14:421, 1961

132. Carpenter WB, Kernohan JW: Retroperitoneal ganglioneuromas and neurofibromas. A clinicopathological study. Cancer 16:788, 1963

133. Hamilton JP, Koop CE: Ganglioneuromas in children. Surg Gynecol Obstet 121:803, 1965

134. Greenfield LJ, Shelley WM: The spectrum of neurogenic tumors of the sympathetic nervous system: Maturation and adrenergic function. J Natl Cancer Inst 35:215, 1965

135. Dyke PC, Mulkey DA: Maturation of ganglioneuroblastoma to ganglioneuroma. Cancer 20:1343, 1967

136. Misugi K, Misugi N, Newton Jr WA: Fine structural study of neuroblastoma, ganglioneuroblastoma, and pheochromocytoma. Arch Pathol 86:160, 1968

137. McLaughlin JE, Urich H: Maturing neuroblastoma and ganglioneuroblastoma: A study of four cases with long survival. J Pathol 121:19, 1977

138. Romansky SG, Crocker DW, Shaw KNF: Ultrastructural studies on neuroblastoma. Evaluation of cytodifferentiation and correlation of morphology and biochemical and survival data. Cancer 42:2392, 1978

139. Tertzakian GM, Herr HW: Ganglioneuroma arising in accessory adrenal gland. Urol 15:401, 1980

Miscellaneous Rare Neoplasms

Hemangioma

140. Scotti G: Contribution a l'etude de l'ossification de la capsule surrenale. Arch Med Exper Anat Pathol 22:762, 1910

141. Muller-Stuler M: Doppelseitiges, kaversonse hamangiom der nebennieren. Virchows Arch [A] 290:177, 1933

142. Menon TB, Annamalai DR: A haemangeiomblastoma of the adrenal gland. J Pathol 39:591, 1934

143. Marten M, Meyer LM: Hemangioblastoma of the adrenal. Am J Cancer 40:485, 1940
144. Johnson CC, Jeppesen FB: Hemangioma of the adrenal. J Urol 74:573, 1955
145. Weiss JM, Schulte JW: Adrenal hemangioma: A case report. J Urol 95:604, 1966
146. Ruebel AAL: Adrenal hemangioma. Urol 2:289, 1973
147. Rothberg M, Bastidas J, Mattey WE et al: Adrenal hemangiomas. Radiology 126:341, 1978
148. Vargas AD: Adrenal hemangioma. Urol 16:389, 1980

Malignant Melanoma

149. Kniseley RM, Baggenstoss AH: Primary melanoma of the adrenal gland. Arch Pathol 42:345, 1946
150. Sasidharan K, Babu AS, Pandey AP et al: Primary melanoma of the adrenal gland: A case report. J Urol 117:663, 1977

Granulosa-Theca Cell Tumor

151. Orselli RC, Bassler TJ: Theca granulosa cell tumor arising in adrenal. Cancer 31:474, 1973

Metastatic Neoplasms

152. Caranasos G, Ruebner BH: Adrenal width and metastasis in bronchogenic carcinoma. Arch Pathol 76:263, 1963
153. Lumb G, Mackenzie DH: The incidence of metastases in adrenal glands and ovaries removed for carcinoma of the breast. Cancer 12:521, 1959
154. Willis RA: Metastasis. In Pathology of Tumors, 4th ed, p 175. New York, Appleton-Century-Crofts, 1967
155. Modhi G, Bauman W, Nicolis G: Adrenal failure associated with hypothalamic and adrenal metastases: A case report and review of the literature. Cancer 47:2098, 1981

Index

Page numbers followed by *f* indicate figures; *t* following a page number indicates tabular material.